KNEE
SURGERY

VOLUME 2

KNEE
SURGERY

VOLUME 2

FREDDIE H. FU, M.D.
Blue Cross of Western Pennsylvania Professor of Orthopaedic Surgery
Executive Vice Chairman
Department of Orthopaedic Surgery
Head Team Physician, Athletic Department
University of Pittsburgh
Pittsburgh, Pennsylvania

CHRISTOPHER D. HARNER, M.D.
Assistant Professor
Chief, Division of Sports Medicine
Department of Orthopaedic Surgery
Associate Medical Director
Center for Sports Medicine and Rehabilitation
University of Pittsburgh
Pittsburgh, Pennsylvania

KELLY G. VINCE, M.D., F.R.C.S. (C)
Assistant Clinical Professor
Department of Orthopaedic Surgery
University of California, Irvine
School of Medicine
Associate Surgeon
The Kerlan-Jobe Orthopaedic Clinic
Inglewood, California

ASSOCIATE EDITOR
MARK D. MILLER, M.D.
Clinical Assistant Professor of Surgery
Uniformed Services University of Health Sciences
F. Edward Herbert School of Medicine
Bethesda, Maryland
Department of Orthopaedic Surgery
United States Air Force Academy Hospital
Associate Team Physician
United States Air Force Academy
United States Air Force Academy, Colorado

Williams & Wilkins

BALTIMORE • PHILADELPHIA • HONG KONG
LONDON • MUNICH • SYDNEY • TOKYO

A WAVERLY COMPANY

Editor: Darlene Cooke, Timothy H. Grayson
Project Manager: Kathleen Courtney Millet
Copy Editor: Harriet Felscher, Kathleen L. Marks, Anne K. Schwartz
Designer: Norman W. Och
Illustration Planner: Wayne Hubbel

Copyright © 1994
Williams & Wilkins
428 East Preston Street
Baltimore, Maryland 21202, USA

Accurate indications, adverse reactions, and dosage schedules for drugs are provided in this book, but it is possible that they may change. The reader is urged to review the package information data of the manufacturers of the medications mentioned.

Printed in the United States of America

Library of Congress Cataloging in Publication Data

Knee surgery / edited by Freddie H. Fu, Christopher D. Harner, Kelly G. Vince.
   p. cm.
   ISBN 0-683-03389-1
   1. Knee—Surgery. 2. Knee—Wounds and injuries. 3. Knee—Diseases.
 .I. Fu, Freddie H. II. Harner, Christopher D. III. Vince, Kelly G.
   [DNLM: 1. Knee—surgery. WE 870 K68 1994]
   RD561.K584 1994
   617.5'82059—dc20
   DNLM/DLC
   for Library of Congress   93-28416
                                     CIP

                    94 95 96 97 98
       1 2 3 4 5 6 7 8 9 10

To my parents, Mr. and Mrs. Ying Foo, my wife, Hilda, my son, Gordon, and my daughter, Joyce.

FHF

To my parents, James and Kathryn Harner, for their inspiration and support. To my wife, Cindy, and our children, Christopher, Andrew, and Nina, for their love, patience, and understanding.

To my teachers, especially George Paulus, for their constant intellectual stimulation and encouragement.

CDH

To our patients with painful knees. May we improve our care by organizing and studying current knowledge.

KGV

FOREWORD

Many textbooks on the knee have been written, but their focus is usually narrow, focused, for example, on total knee replacement or on sports injuries. *Knee Surgery* is decidedly different. This encyclopedic two-volume text covers all aspects of knee surgery, including nonsurgical treatment options as well as current controversies, yet the exhaustive scope does not obscure important details. The authors—authorities in their respective fields—present in-depth reviews of the newest treatment techniques and technologies. The illustrations are also outstanding.

The book begins with a clinically relevant review of basic science, including anatomy, biomechanics, kinematics, and proprioception. Volume 1 continues with evaluation techniques, from the physical examination to the use of rating scales and instrumentation, followed by new imaging techniques. Other segments address special pediatric problems and issues as well as new techniques in rehabilitation and bracing. A large part of Volume 1 is devoted to a thorough review of injuries to the ligaments, tendons, and meniscus, integrating with discussions of the latest treatments and technology. This section includes chapters on the use of lasers, meniscal transplants, and the current status of prosthetic augmentation in revision knee ligament surgery. Volume 2 examines articular cartilage disorders, with review of osteotomies, patellofemoral disorders, and total knee replacement. Controversial issues such as uses of fresh osteochondral allografts, the role of arthroscopy in arthritis, and the management of complications of articular cartilage disorders are explored extensively.

I have had the privilege of being associated with Dr. Freddie Fu and Dr. Christopher Harner at the University of Pittsburgh Medical Center for the past six years. They, with Dr. Vince and their colleagues, have established a world-class sports medicine center with a comprehensive clinical program, outstanding teaching conferences, and clinical and basic research involving soft-tissue injuries and reconstruction about the knee. Their clinical activities as well as their research studies include innovative anterior/posterior cruciate ligament surgery for the treatment of combined injuries, and complex revision surgical procedures. Both expertise and experience make all three editors highly qualified to produce this sweeping review of contemporary knee surgery.

I am very happy to see this book published. I think it is a landmark text that will benefit the practicing orthopaedist as well as senior residents and fellows in sports medicine and adult reconstructive surgery. I know all will find this wonderful textbook to be a valued resource.

James H. Herndon, M.D.

PREFACE

The knee is a frequent site of soft tissue and bony trauma. In addition, its predilection for arthritic changes, especially of the patellofemoral joint, make it one of the most intriguing joints in the human body. Perhaps no other joint has received more attention than the knee. It is a major focus of both basic science and clinical research. Numerous books, both text and clinical, have been written; numerous symposia have been held; innumerable scientific papers and reviews have been written and presented on this single joint. So, when Williams & Wilkins approached us with the task of editing a book on the knee, our goal was clearly one of synthesis—to gather the best multidisciplinary information available and to present it thoroughly and understandably, going beyond the idea of a textbook. We had three specific aims:

1. To present, in a practical and readily comprehensible way, the most current basic science and clinical information on the knee;

2. To present current surgical approaches and techniques, ones that would be readily accessible to the practicing orthopaedist;

3. To provide a single, comprehensive textbook of reliable information to assist the practicing orthopaedic surgeon and the resident-in-training in managing problems of the knee.

Obviously, such an undertaking could not have been achieved without strong contributions from the many knowledgeable colleagues who have worked with us to create the volumes of this textbook. We hope this endeavor will prove its worth in improved understanding, diagnosis, and treatment of injuries and diseases about the knee.

Freddie H. Fu
Christopher D. Harner
Kelly G. Vince

ACKNOWLEDGMENTS

We gratefully acknowledge Nancy Lyscik, Mary Yocum, and Lucille Johnson for their superb secretarial assistance and efforts with preparation of this textbook. We are forever indebted to Brenda Miller and Katey Millet for their guidance and continued support throughout this project.

CONTRIBUTORS

Paul J. Abbott, Jr., M.D.
Staff Orthopaedic Surgeon
Vail-Summit Orthopaedics and Sports Medicine
Vail, Colorado

Abdul M. Ahmed, M.D.
Professor and Chairman
Mechanical Engineering Department
McGill University
Montreal, Canada

Jose A. Alicea, M.D.
Knee Fellow
Insall-Scott-Kelly Institute for Orthopaedics and Sports
Medicine
New York, New York

Louis C. Almekinders, M.D.
Assistant Professor of Orthopaedic Surgery
Department of Surgery
University of North Carolina
Chapel Hill, North Carolina

Allen F. Anderson, M.D.
Director of the Lipscomb Sports Medicine
Fellowship and The Lipscomb Clinic
Foundation for Education and Research
Nashville, Tennessee

Steven Paul Arnoczky, D.V.M., A.C.V.S.
Wade O. Brinker Endowed Professor of Surgery
Director, Laboratory for Comparative Orthopaedic
Research
College of Veterinary Medicine
Professor of Surgery
College of Human Medicine
Michigan State University
East Lansing, Michigan

Gerard A. Ateshian, Ph.D.
Assistant Professor, Mechanical Engineering
Associate, Orthopaedic Research
Columbia University
New York, New York

Bernard R. Bach, Jr., M.D.
Director, Sports Medicine Section
Department of Orthopaedic Surgery
Rush Medical College
Rush-Presbyterian—St. Luke's Medical Center
Chicago, Illinois

Anita M. Bagley, M.S.
Director of Gait and Motion Analysis
Gait and Motion Analysis Laboratory
Orthopedic Biomechanics Institute
Salt Lake City, Utah

Champ L. Baker, Jr., M.D.
Assistant Clinical Professor, Department of Orthopaedics
Tulane University School of Medicine
New Orleans, Louisiana
Chief of Surgery
Director of Sports Medicine Fellowship
Hughston Orthopaedic Sports Medicine Hospital
Columbus, Georgia

Kim C. Bertin, M.D.
LDS Hospital
Assistant Clinical Professor
Division of Orthopaedic Surgery
University of Utah College of Medicine
Salt Lake City, Utah

Michel Bonnin, M.D.
Centre Hospitalier
Clinique Chirurgical Orthopedique et Traumatologique
Pierre-Benite, France

James V. Bono, M.D.
Junior Attending Orthopaedic Surgeon
The Hospital for Special Surgery
Senior Clinical Associate of Surgery
Cornell University Medical College
New York, New York

Robert E. Booth, Jr., M.D.
Department of Orthopaedic Surgery
Thomas Jefferson University
Philadelphia, Pennsylvania

Paul A. Borsa, M.S., A.T.C.
Doctoral Candidate in Exercise Physiology
Clinical Instructor/Athletic Trainer
University of Pittsburgh
Pittsburgh, Pennsylvania

Dale W. Boyd, M.D.
Orthopaedic Surgeon
Southeast Orthopaedic Clinic
Wilmington, North Carolina

James P. Bradley, M.D.
Clinical Assistant Professor
Department of Orthopaedic Surgery
University of Pittsburgh
Team Physician
The Pittsburgh Steelers
Pittsburgh, Pennsylvania

Robert C. Bray, M.D., F.R.C.S.(C), M.Sc.
Associate Professor, Department of Surgery
The University of Calgary
Calgary, Alberta, Canada

Cynthia A. Britton, M.D.
Assistant Professor of Radiology
Department of Radiology
University of Pittsburgh Medical Center
Pittsburgh, Pennsylvania

J. Timothy Bryant, Ph.D.
Professor
Department of Mechanical Engineering
Queen's University
Kingston, Ontario
Canada

David N.M. Caborn, M.D.
Director
University of Kentucky Sports Medicine Center
Lexington, Kentucky

Gary J. Calabrese, M.D.
Director
Mt. Sinai Sports Medicine
Mt. Sinai Medical Center
Cleveland, Ohio

James E. Carpenter, M.D.
Medical Sport Orthopaedic Surgery
Department of Surgery
University of Michigan Medical Center
Ann Arbor, Michigan

Robert W. Chandler, M.D.
Associate
The Kerlan-Jobe Orthopaedic Clinic
Inglewood, California
Associate Clinical Professor
University of Southern California
Los Angeles, California

Edmund Y.S. Chao, Ph.D.
Vice Chairman and Director of Research
Department of Orthopaedics
Consultant and Professor of Bioengineering
Mayo Medical School
Mayo Clinic and Foundation
Rochester, Minnesota

Michael G. Ciccotti, M.D.
Assistant Professor of Orthopaedic Surgery
Rothman Institute, Pennsylvania Hospital, and Thomas
Jefferson University
Philadelphia, Pennsylvania

John P. Collier, D.E.
Professor of Engineering
Thayer School of Engineering
Director, Dartmouth Biomedical Engineering Center
Dartmouth College
Hanover, New Hampshire

William W. Colman, M.D.
Frank E. Stinchfield Fellow
Department of Orthopaedic Surgery
Columbia University
New York, New York

Clifford W. Colwell, Jr., M.D.
Head, Division of Orthopaedic Surgery
Scripps Clinic and Research Foundation
La Jolla, California
Department of Orthopaedics and Rehabilitation
University of California
San Diego School of Medicine
San Diego, California

T. Derek V. Cooke
Professor and Chairman
Department of Orthopaedics and Rehabilitation
Services
King Faisal Specialist Hospital and Research Centre
Riyadh, Saudi Arabia

Daniel E. Cooper, M.D.
W. B. Carrell Memorial Clinic
Associate Attending
Baylor University Medical Center
Clinical Instructor—Orthopaedics
University of Texas Southwestern Medical Center
Dallas, Texas

Paul S. Cooper, M.D.
Assistant Professor
Department of Orthopaedic Surgery
University of Connecticut School of Medicine
Farmington, Connecticut

Christopher V. Cox, M.D.
Attending Physician
Department of Orthopaedic Surgery
California Pacific Medical Center
San Francisco, California

Jay S. Cox, M.D.
Associate Clinical Professor
Uniform Health Sciences
Orthopedic Consultant
Pennsylvania State University
State College, Pennsylvania

Henri DeJour, M.D.
Centre Hospitalier
Clinique Chirurgical Orthopedique et
Traumatologique
Pierre-Benite, France

Jesse C. DeLee, M.D.
Clinical Professor, Orthopaedics
University of Texas Health Science Center
San Antonio, Texas

Nick M. DiGiovine, M.D.
Clinical Instructor
Department of Orthopaedic Surgery
University of Pittsburgh School of Medicine
Assistant Team Physician
The Pittsburgh Steelers
Pittsburgh, Pennsylvania

Michael Dolecki, M.D.
Instructor
Department of Orthopaedic Surgery
University of Pittsburgh School of Medicine
Pittsburgh, Pennsylvania

Kimberly A. Dwyer, M.S.
Anderson Orthopaedic Research Institute
Arlington, Virginia

Scott F. Dye, M.D.
Assistant Clinical Professor of Orthopaedic Surgery
University of California, San Francisco
President, Bay Area Knee Society
San Francisco, California

Robert W. Eberle
Research Coordinator Joint Implant Surgeons, Inc.
Grant Orthopaedic Institute
Grant Medical Center
Columbus, Ohio

Edward Eissmann, M.D.
Fellow
The Kerlan-Jobe Orthopaedic Clinic
Inglewood, California

Neal S. El Attrache, M.D.
Associate, The Kerlan-Jobe Orthopaedic Clinic
Inglewood, California
Team Physician, The Los Angeles Rams
Assistant Clinical Professor
Department of Orthopaedic Surgery
University of Southern California
Los Angeles, California

Roger H. Emerson, Jr., M.D.
Clinical Associate Professor, Orthopaedic
Surgery
Southwestern Medical School
Presbyterian Hospital of Dallas
Dallas, Texas

Gerard A. Engh, M.D.
Assistant Clinical Professor
University of Maryland
Baltimore, Maryland
Assistant Clinical Professor
Georgetown University
Washington, D.C.

Agustín Escalante, M.D.
Assistant Professor of Medicine
Department of Medicine
Section of Rheumatology
The University of Texas Health Science Center at
San Antonio
San Antonio, Texas

Christopher H. Evans, Ph.D.
Associate Professor
Departments of Orthopaedic Surgery, Molecular Genetics,
and Biochemistry
University of Pittsburgh School of Medicine
Pittsburgh, Pennsylvania

Philip M. Faris, M.D.
Center for Hip and Knee Surgery
Mooresville, Indiana

Stephen Fealy, B.A.
Medical Student
College of Physicians & Surgeons
Columbia University
New York, New York

Peter J. Fowler, M.D., F.R.C.S(C)
Professor of Orthopaedic Surgery
Head, Section of Sports Medicine
University of Western Ontario
London, Ontario
Canada

E. Paul France, Ph.D.
Director
Orthopedic Biomechanics Institute
Salt Lake City, Utah

Cyril B. Frank, M.D., F.R.C.S.(C)
Professor, Department of Surgery
Chief, Division of Orthopaedics
The University of Calgary
Calgary, Alberta
Canada

Warren G. Froese, M.D., F.R.C.S.(C)
Clinical Fellow
Sports Medicine Orthopaedic Surgery
University of Western Ontario
London, Ontario
Canada

Freddie H. Fu, M.D.
Blue Cross of Western Pennsylvania Professor of
Orthopaedic Surgery
Executive Vice Chairman, Clinical Department of
Orthopaedic Surgery
Chief, Division of Sports Medicine
Head Team Physician, Athletic Department
University of Pittsburgh
Pittsburgh, Pennsylvania

John P. Fulkerson, M.D.
Professor of Orthopaedics
University of Connecticut School of Medicine
Farmington, Connecticut

Jorge O. Galante, M.D.
Professor and Chairman
Department of Orthopaedic Surgery
Rush Medical College
Rush-Presbyterian—St. Luke's Medical Center
Chicago, Illinois

Ralph A. Gambardella, M.D.
Associate, The Kerlan-Jobe Orthopaedic Clinic
Inglewood, California
Assistant Clinical Professor
Department of Orthopaedics
University of Southern California School of Medicine
Orthopaedic Consultant, The Los Angeles Dodgers
Los Angeles, California

William G. Gardner, M.D.
Chief, Infectious Diseases
Akron General Medical Center
Akron, Ohio
Professor of Medicine
Northeastern Ohio Universities College of Medicine
Rootstown, Ohio

Jonathan P. Garino, M.D.
Adult Reconstructive Fellow
Department of Orthopaedic Surgery
University of Pennsylvania
Philadelphia, Pennsylvania

Victor M. Goldberg, M.D.
Department of Orthopaedic Surgery
University Hospitals of Cleveland
Case Western Reserve University
Cleveland, Ohio

Ronald P. Grelsamer, M.D.
Assistant Professor of Orthopaedic Surgery
Columbia University
Columbia-Presbyterian Medical Center
New York, New York

Allan E. Gross, M.D.
A. J. Latner Professor and Chairman
Division of Orthopaedic Surgery
Mt. Sinai Hospital
University of Toronto
Toronto, Ontario
Canada

W. Doug Gurley, M.D.
Orthopaedic Surgeon in Private Practice
Denver Orthopaedic Specialists, PC
Denver, Colorado

Ramon Gustilo, M.D.
Musculoskeletal Sepsis Unit
Hennepin County Medical Center
Minneapolis, Minnesota

Kenneth Gustke, M.D.
Arthritis Surgery and Joint Reconstruction
Florida Orthopedic Institute
Attending, Tampa Orthopedic Program
Clinical Associate Professor of Orthopedic Surgery
University of South Florida College of Medicine
Tampa, Florida

Steven B. Haas, M.D., M.P.H.
Assistant Attending Orthopaedic Surgeon
The Hospital for Special Surgery
Clinical Instructor in Surgery
Cornell University Medical College
New York, New York

Edgar G. Handal, M.D.
Assistant Clinical Instructor and Fellow in Total Joint and
Reconstructive Surgery of the Hip and Knee
Department of Orthopaedic Surgery
University of California, San Diego
San Diego, California

Arlen D. Hanssen, M.D.
Consultant and Assistant Professor of Orthopaedics
Department of Orthopaedics
Mayo Medical School
Mayo Clinic Foundation
Rochester, Minnesota

Christopher D. Harner, M.D.
Assistant Professor
Chief, Division of Sports Medicine
Department of Orthopedic Surgery
Associate Medical Director
Center for Sports Medicine & Rehabilitation
University of Pittsburgh
Pittsburgh, Pennsylvania

David A. Hart, Ph.D.
Professor, Departments of Microbiology and Infectious
Diseases/Medicine
Chairman, Joint Injury and Arthritis Research Group
The University of Calgary
Calgary, Alberta, Canada

David A. Harwood, M.D.
University Orthopaedic Associates
New Brunswick, New Jersey

Aaron A. Hofmann, M.D.
Professor
Division of Orthopaedic Surgery
University of Utah
Salt Lake City, Utah

William J. Hozack, M.D.
Associate Professor
Department of Orthopaedic Surgery
Jefferson Medical College and The Rothman Institute
Philadelphia, Pennsylvania

Greg L. Hung, M.D.
Research Fellow
Ferguson Laboratory
Musculoskeletal Research Center
Department of Orthopaedic Surgery
University of Pittsburgh
Pittsburgh, Pennsylvania

Robert E. Hunter, M.D.
Clinical Associate Professor
Department of Orthopaedic Surgery
University of Colorado
Denver, Colorado

James J. Irrgang, M.S., P.T., A.T.C.
Director of Outpatient Physical Therapy and Sports
Medicine
University of Pittsburgh Medical Center
Assistant Professor, Department of Physical Therapy
University of Pittsburgh School of Health & Rehabilitation
Sciences
Clinical Instructor, Department of Orthopaedic Surgery
University of Pittsburgh School of Medicine
Pittsburgh, Pennsylvania

Douglas W. Jackson, M.D.
Southern California Center for Sports Medicine
Long Beach, California

Christopher M. Jobe, M.D.
Associate Professor, Orthopaedic Surgery
Loma Linda University, School of Medicine
Loma Linda, California

Darren L. Johnson, M.D.
Assistant Professor
Division of Orthopaedics
Section of Sports Medicine
University of Kentucky
Lexington, Kentucky

Greg A. Johnson, Ph.D.
Musculoskeletal Research Center
Department of Orthopaedic Surgery
University of Pittsburgh
Pittsburgh, Pennsylvania

Michael A. Kelly, M.D.
Director
Insall-Scott-Kelly Institute for Orthopaedics and Sports
Medicine
New York, New York

Nicholas A. King, M.D.
Captain, Medical Corps, United States Army
Orthopaedic Surgery Service
Walter Reed Army Medical Center
Washington, D.C.

Neil E. Klein, M.D.
Private Practice
Downey, California

Mininder S. Kocher, M.D.
Instructor of Orthopaedic Surgery
Department of Orthopaedic Surgery
Harvard Medical School
Boston, Massachusetts

Dieter Kohn, M.D.
Orthopaedische Klinik
Medizinische Hochschule Hannover
Hannover, Germany

Shingi Koshiwaguchi, M.D.
Division of Sports Medicine
Department of Orthopaedic Surgery
University of Tokushima
Tokushima, Japan

Matthew J. Kraay, M.S., M.D.
Assistant Professor of Orthopaedic Surgery
Case Western Reserve University
University Hospitals of Cleveland
Cleveland, Ohio

Christian Krettek, M.D.
Medizinische Hochschule Hannover
Zentrum Chirurgie
Unfallchirurgische Klinik
Hannover, Germany

Peter R. Kurzweil, M.D.
Southern California Center for Sports Medicine
Long Beach, California

Richard S. Laskin, M.D.
Professor of Clinical Orthopaedic Surgery
Cornell University Medical School
Attending Orthopaedic Surgeon
The Hospital for Special Surgery
New York, New York

Scott M. Lephart, Ph.D., A.T.C.
Director, Sports Medicine/Athletic Training
Assistant Professor of Education
Assistant Professor of Orthopaedic Surgery
University of Pittsburgh School of Medicine
Pittsburgh, Pennsylvania

Stephen H. Liu, M.D.
Assistant Professor
Department of Orthopaedic Surgery
Sports Medicine Section
University of California at Los Angeles School of
Medicine
Los Angeles, California

Glen A. Livesay, M.S.
Research Associate
Department of Orthopaedic Surgery
University of Pittsburgh
Pittsburgh, Pennsylvania

Philipp Lobenhoffer, M.D.
Assistant Professor
Medizinische Hochschule Hannover
Zentrum Chirurgie
Unfallchirurgische Klinik
Hannover, Germany

Barbara J. Loitz, Ph.D., P.T.
Postdoctoral Fellow
Department of Surgery
The University of Calgary
Calgary, Alberta
Canada

Adolphe V. Lombardi, Jr., M.D., F.A.C.S.
Associate, Joint Implant Surgeons, Inc.
Clinical Assistant Professor
Division of Orthopaedic Surgery
The Ohio State University
Attending Staff
Grant Medical Center
Columbus, Ohio

Paul A. Lotke, M.D.
Professor of Orthopaedic Surgery
Hospital of the University of Pennsylvania
Philadelphia, Pennsylvania

Michael G. Maday, M.D.
Orthopaedic Surgeon
Midland Orthopaedic Associates
Chicago, Illinois

Thomas H. Mallory, M.D., F.A.C.S.
Senior Associate, Joint Implant Surgeons
Clinical Assistant Professor
Division of Orthopaedic Surgery
The Ohio State University
Director, Joint Implant Surgery Fellowship
Chairman, Section of Joint Implant Surgery
Grant Medical Center
Columbus, Ohio

Paul H. Marks, M.D., F.R.C.S.(C)
Orthopaedic & Arthritic Hospital
Division of Orthopaedics
Department of Surgery
Faculty of Medicine
University of Toronto
Toronto, Ontario
Canada

Leonard Marmor, M.D., F.A.C.S.
Active Staff, St. John's Hospital
President, Knee Society
Santa Monica, California

Scott E. Marwin, M.D.
Chief of Adult Reconstructive Surgery
Department of Orthopaedic Surgery
Long Island Jewish Medical Center
New Hyde Park, New York

John R. Matyas, Ph.D.
Postdoctoral Fellow
Department of Medicine
The University of Calgary
Calgary, Alberta
Canada

Michael B. Mayor, M.D.
Professor of Surgery in Orthopaedics
Department of Orthopaedics
Dartmouth Hitchcock Medical Center
Lebanon, New Hampshire

Kathleen J. McCann, P.T.A.
Department of Physical Medicine and Rehabilitation
Virginia Mason Medical Center
Seattle, Washington

Daniel J. McKernan, M.D.
Teaching Faculty, Orthopaedic Residency Program
Department of Orthopaedics
Hamot Medical Center
Erie, Pennsylvania

James L. McNamara, M.E.
Thayer School of Engineering
Dartmouth College
Hanover, New Hampshire

Lyle J. Micheli, M.D.
Director, Division of Sports Medicine
The Children's Hospital
Associate Clinical Professor of Orthopaedic
Surgery
Harvard Medical School
Boston, Massachusetts

Drew V. Miller, M.D.
Assistant Attending Orthopaedic Surgeon
St. Joseph's Hospital
Northside Hospital
Atlanta, Georgia

Mark D. Miller, M.D.
Clinical Assistant Professor of Surgery
Uniformed Services University of Health Sciences
F. Edward Herbert School of Medicine
Bethesda, Maryland
Department of Orthopaedic Surgery
United States Air Force Academy Hospital
Associate Team Physician
United States Air Force Academy
United States Air Force Academy, Colorado

Anthony Miniaci, M.D.
Head of Orthopaedic Sports Medicine
The Toronto Hospital and the University of Toronto
Department of Surgery
The Toronto Hospital Western Division
Toronto, Ontario, Canada

David R. Morawski, M.D.
Assistant Clinical Instructor and Fellow in Total Joint and
Reconstructive Surgery of the Hip and Knee
Department of Orthopaedic Surgery
University of California, San Diego
San Diego, California

Phillip J. Mosca, M.D.
Research Fellow
Knee Service
The Hospital for Special Surgery
New York, New York

Van C. Mow, Ph.D.
Professor of Mechanical Engineering and Orthopaedic
Bioengineering
Director, Orthopaedic Research Laboratory
Columbia University
Columbia-Presbyterian Medical Center
New York, New York

David C. Neuschwander, M.D.
Clinical Instructor
Department of Orthopaedics
University of Pittsburgh School of Medicine
Pittsburgh, Pennsylvania

Kenneth E. Newhouse, M.D.
Idaho Orthopaedics and Sports Clinic
Pocatello, Idaho

Peter M. Newton, M.D.
Orthopaedic Research Laboratory
Department of Orthopaedic Surgery
Columbia-Presbyterian Medical Center
New York, New York

Philippe Neyret, M.D.
Centre Hospitalier
Clinique Chirurgical Orthopedique et Traumatologique
Pierre-Benite, France

Michael P. Nogalski, M.D.
Attending Orthopaedic
St. John's Mercy Medical Center
St. Louis, Missouri

Stephen J. O'Brien, M.D.
Associate Attending Orthopaedic Surgeon
The Hospital for Special Surgery
Associate Professor (Orthopaedics)
Cornell University Medical College
New York, New York

Eric J. Olson, M.D.
Major, Medical Corps, United States Army
Director, Sports Medicine Clinic
Orthopaedic Surgery Service
Walter Reed Army Medical Center
Washington, D.C.
Assistant Professor of Surgery
Uniformed Services University of Health Sciences
Bethesda, Maryland

Thomas B. Pace, M.D.
Clinical Instructor
Division of Orthopaedic Surgery
University of Utah Medical Center
Salt Lake City, Utah

Richard D. Parker, M.D.
Staff Physician
Section of Sports Medicine
Department of Orthopaedic Surgery
Cleveland Clinic Foundation
Cleveland, Ohio

Lonnie E. Paulos, M.D.
Medical Director
Orthopedic Biomechanics Institute
The Orthopedic Specialty Hospital
Salt Lake City, Utah

William R. Post, M.D.
Assistant Professor of Orthopaedics
Section of Sports Medicine
Department of Orthopaedics
West Virginia University School of Medicine
Morgantown, West Virginia

Bart P. Rask, M.D.
Fellow in Sports Medicine
The Children's Hospital
Boston, Massachusetts

Paul R. Reiman, M.D.
Medical Director, Northeast Ohio Sports Medical Institute
Akron General Medical Center
Akron, Ohio
Assistant Professor of Orthopaedic Surgery
Northeast Ohio Universities College of Medicine
Rootstown, Ohio

Joseph R. Ritchie, M.D.
Major, United States Air Force
Department of Orthopaedic Surgery
Wilford Hall Medical Center
Lackland Air Force Base, Texas

Raymond P. Robinson, M.D.
Director, Adult Hip and Knee Reconstructive Service
Virginia Mason Medical Center
Clinical Associate Professor
Department of Orthopaedics
University of Washington
Seattle, Washington

Aaron G. Rosenberg, M.D.
Associate Professor, Rush Medical College
Director of Orthopaedics Education
Department of Orthopaedic Surgery
Rush Presbyterian—St. Luke's Medical Center
Chicago, Illinois

Thomas D. Rosenberg, M.D.
Co-Director
Orthopedic Biomechanics Institute
The Orthopedic Specialty Hospital
Salt Lake City, Utah

Leif Ryd, M.D., Ph.D.
Associate Professor
Department of Orthopaedics
University Hospital
Lund, Sweden

Stephen C. Saddler, M.D.
The Hospital for Special Surgery
Cornell University Medical School
New York, New York
Clinical Associate
Cincinnati Sports Medicine and Orthopaedic Center
Cincinnati, Ohio

Robert B. Salisbury, M.D.
Chief of Orthopaedics
Kaiser-Permanente Medical Group
Associate Professor of Clinical Orthopaedics
University of Southern California
Bellflower, California

Richard F. Santore, M.D., F.A.C.S.
Senior Surgeon
Department of Orthopaedic Surgery
Sharp Memorial Hospital
Associate Clinical Professor
Orthopaedic Surgery
University of California, San Diego
San Diego, California

R. Allan Scudamore, M.A., Ph.D.
Scientist
Departments of Orthopaedics and Biological Medical
Research
King Faisal Specialist Hospital and Research Centre
Riyadh, Saudi Arabia

Giles R. Scuderi, M.D., F.A.C.S.
Attending Orthopaedic Surgeon
Insall-Scott-Kelly Institute for Orthopaedics and Sports
Medicine
Beth Israel Medical Center—North Division
New York, New York

Dana Seltzer, M.D.
Chief of Sports Medicine and Shoulder Surgery
Phoenix Orthopaedic Residency Program
Maricopa Medical Center
Phoenix, Arizona

Clarence L. Shields, Jr., M.D.
Associate, The Kerlan-Jobe Orthopaedic Clinic
Inglewood, California
Associate Clinical Professor of Orthopaedics
University of Southern California School of Medicine
Orthopaedic Consultant, Los Angeles Rams
Los Angeles, California

Jeffrey Shiffrin, M.D.
Director of Anesthesia
Vail Valley Medical Center
Vail, Colorado

**Nigel G. Shrive, M.A., D.Phil., P.Eng.,
C.Eng.**
Professor and Head
Department of Civil Engineering
The University of Calgary
Calgary, Alberta, Canada

Peter T. Simonian, M.D.
Department of Orthopaedic Surgery
University of Washington Medical Center
Seattle, Washington

Domenick J. Sisto, M.D.
Fellowship Director
Los Angeles Orthopaedic Institute
Sherman Oaks, California

Brian A. Smith, M.D.
Department of Orthopaedic Surgery
University of Pittsburgh
Pittsburgh, Pennsylvania

Kurt P. Spindler, M.D.
Assistant Professor
Department of Orthopaedics and Rehabilitation
Vanderbilt University Medical Center
Nashville, Tennessee

Steven H. Stern, M.D.
Assistant Professor
Department of Orthopaedic Surgery
Northwestern University
Chicago, Illinois

Michael J. Stuart, M.D.
Assistant Professor of Orthopaedic Surgery
Mayo Medical School
Co-Director, Sports Medicine Center
Mayo Clinic Foundation
Rochester, Minnesota

Victor A. Surprenant, B.A.
Thayer School of Engineering
Dartmouth College
Hanover, New Hampshire

Timothy N. Taft, M.D.
Max M. Novich Professor and Director of Sports
Medicine
Department of Surgery
University of North Carolina at Chapel Hill
Chapel Hill, North Carolina

George Thabit III, M.D.
Clinical Instructor
Department of Orthopaedic Surgery
Stanford University Medical Center
Stanford, California
Sports Orthopaedic and Rehabilitation Medicine
Associates
Menlo Park, California

F. Leland Thaete, M.D.
Assistant Professor of Radiology
University of Pittsburgh School of Medicine
Pittsburgh, Pennsylvania

Alfred J. Tria, Jr., M.D.
Associate Clinical Professor
Division of Orthopaedic Surgery
Robert Wood Johnson Medical School
New Brunswick, New Jersey

Harald Tscherne, M.D.
Professor
Medizinische Hochschule Hannover
Zentrum Chirurgie
Unfallchirurgische Klinik
Hannover, Germany

Dean T. Tsukayama, M.D.
Medical Director, Musculoskeletal Sepsis Unit
Hennepin County Medical Center
Minneapolis, Minnesota

Kelly G. Vince, M.D. F.R.C.S.(C)
Assistant Clinical Professor
Department of Orthopaedic Surgery
University of California, Irvine
School of Medicine
Associate Surgeon
The Kerlan-Jobe Orthopaedic Clinic
Inglewood, California

Robert N. Walker, M.D.
Fellow in Sports Medicine
Vanderbilt University Medical Center
Nashville, Tennessee

Larry W. Watson, M.D.
Private Practice
Riverside Sports Medicine
Riverside Methodist Hospital
Columbus, Ohio

Jon J.P. Warner, M.D.
Assistant Professor of Orthopaedic Surgery
University of Pittsburgh
Pittsburgh, Pennsylvania

Jackie E. Wilson, B.A.
Research Assistant
Department of Surgery
The University of Calgary
Calgary, Alberta, Canada

Russell E. Windsor, M.D.
Associate Professor of Surgery (Orthopaedics)
Cornell University Medical College
Associate Attending Orthopaedic Surgeon
Associate Chief of the Knee Service
The Hospital for Special Surgery
New York, New York

Carl J. Wirth, M.D.
Orthopaedische Klinik
Medizinische Hochschule Hannover
Hannover, Germany

Edward M. Wojtys, M.D.
Associate Professor
Department of Surgery
Assistant Medical Director
Sports Medicine Program
University of Michigan Medical Center
Ann Arbor, Michigan

Savio L-Y Woo, Ph.D.
Professor and Vice Chairman for Research
Department of Orthopaedic Surgery
Professor, Department of Mechanical Engineering
Director, Musculoskeletal Research Center
University of Pittsburgh
Pittsburgh, Pennsylvania

Steven T. Woolson, M.D.
Private Practice
Menlo Park, California
Clinical Associate Professor
Division of Orthopaedic Surgery
Stanford University Medical School
Stanford, California

Michael Wright, M.D.
Instructor of Orthopaedic Surgery
Research Fellow in Spine Surgery
Rush Medical College
Rush Presbyterian—St. Luke's Hospital
Chicago, Illinois

Timothy M. Wright, Ph.D.
Director, Department of Biomechanics
The Hospital for Special Surgery
Professor of Applied Biomechanics in Surgery
(Orthopaedics)
Cornell University Medical College
New York, New York

Marguerite Wrona, M.E.
Johnson & Johnson Orthopaedics
Raynham, Massachusetts

Kenneth Yaw, M.D.
Assistant Professor
Department of Orthopaedic Surgery
University of Pittsburgh Medical Center
Pittsburgh, Pennsylvania

CONTENTS

VOLUME 1

VOLUME 2

SECTION

X

General Concepts and Nonsurgical Treatment in Disorders of Articular Cartilage

50

Biomechanical Factors in Alignment and Arthritic Disorders of the Knee

T. Derek V. Cooke, J. Timothy Bryant, and R. Allan Scudamore

Alignment and arthritic disorders of the knee are commonly associated with deformities of the lower limb and are usually manifest as an abnormal alignment of the limb segments, patellar dysfunction, or impaired flexion-extension. The pattern of limb involvement is often one of bilateral symmetry. Thus a common pattern of deformity in osteoarthritis (OA) is bilateral varus knee alignment occurring with a focus of arthritic changes in the medial compartment of the knee (19, 48, 75). Another is valgus limb alignment with the damage primarily in the lateral compartment (11, 13, 21, 37).

Although associations between disease states and deformities are well recognized, the pathogenetic relationships are poorly understood. That deformity can lead to arthritis is often generally assumed so that developmental abnormalities of childhood are viewed as factors likely to contribute to arthritic disease in later life. The reverse also holds true—that deformities occur as a consequence of progression of arthritic disease. A better understanding of the pathogenetic relationships between diseases and deformities holds promise for the development of earlier and more appropriate management strategies for patients diagnosed as having arthritis with dysfunctional malalignments.

This chapter describes some of the more common patterns of disease and deformity that we have encountered. Also described are biomechanical data considered "normal" (from young healthy adult volunteers), which have served as a baseline for the evaluation of data arising from the patients (17, 52).

Biomechanics of the Knee

Measuring Knee Alignment

We used a standardized radiographic approach to describe the alignment and geometry of the knee in stance (Fig. 50.1). Standardization of patient positioning just before the exposures is emphasized in this technique. The system includes a set of markers for correction of parallax errors, images of which are digitized along with key bone landmarks. The data are processed by a custom software program to provide values of key parameters in a standard format (Fig. 50.2). In a clinical setting, angular measurements were found to be reproducible within ±1.3 degrees (18, 72, 74).

Major parameters of alignment are shown in Figure 50.3 (9). The line from the hip to the ankle is the mechanical or load axis, and in the ideal case the knee is centered close to this line. Deviation from this is defined as the angle between the lines from the hip to the knee center and from the knee center to the ankle (i.e., the hip-knee-ankle angle [HKA]). By convention, varus deviation is indicated in degrees negative and valgus deviation in degrees positive. The articulating surfaces of the distal femur and proximal tibia are located in the coronal plane by drawing a tangent to the outline of the femoral condyles and a line connecting the lateral margins of the tibial plateau, respectively. The orientation of these surfaces is measured with respect to hip and ankle centers by the condylar-hip (CH) and plateau-ankle (PA) angles. The deviation from 90 degrees for these angles is expressed as degrees negative for varus and degrees positive for valgus. The angle between the knee joint surfaces is given by the condylar-plateau (CP) angle. Geometrically, the angles are related by the expression:

$$HKA = CH + PA + CP \qquad (1)$$

Axes of Femoral and Tibial Rotation

The femur and tibia link at the knee with the sesamoidal patella-quadriceps apparatus to form a balanced tricompartmental articulation. This linkage promotes sagittal-plane motion (flexion-extension) of 160 degrees or more, axial rotation of 10 to 15 degrees, and an element of varus-valgus motion. There is no general agreement concerning the axes about which knee movement occurs. For the femur, we proposed a mechanical axis arising at

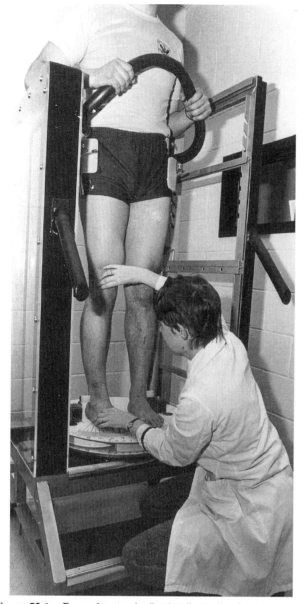

Figure 50.1. Frame for standardized radiography of the lower limb (Questor Precision Radiographs, PARTEQ, Queen's University, Kingston, Ontario, Canada). The patient climbs on to a turntable contained within a frame. Placement of the feet is standardized within ankle blocks, and the degree of foot rotation is noted after the limbs have been rotated to bring the knees into a straight-ahead position (i.e., plane of flexion coinciding as nearly as possible with the sagittal plane). Rotation of the turntable through increments of 90 degrees serves to align the patient for anteroposterior (AP) or lateral radiographic views without change to the initial positioning. Cassette holders are seen on the right of the frame, and a plexiglass panel containing reference markers is attached to the left side. The x-ray source is off the picture to the left.

the center of the femoral head and extending distally through the intercondylar notch between the cruciate ligament attachments (78) (Fig. 50.4). The mechanical long axis for the tibia may be defined as a line from the center of the plateau (interspinus intercruciate midpoint) to the center of the distal articulating surface (79).

The assessment of axial rotation of the femur and tibia is difficult using anteroposterior and lateral radiographic views alone. One method of assessing femoral rotation has been to note the relative position of medial and lateral condylar outlines on lateral radiographic views. In neutral rotation, the medial condyle extends distally and posteriorly beyond the lateral one. Computer scanning methods are preferred for precise definition of the axial rotations (42, 77).

Flexion of the tibia around the femur throughout the entire range involves adduction-abduction and axial rotation of the tibia. This may be explained on the basis of multiple axes of rotation (27, 34, 76) or a biaxial system in which the two axes are not perpendicular to each other (40). For most of the flexion range, the transverse axis may be usefully approximated by a line running parallel to (and very close to) the transepicondylar line (TEL) (77, 78). The TEL also serves as a reference for assessing axial rotation of the femoral condyles and proximal femur (i.e., the angle of anteversion (ϕ degree) (77) (Fig. 50.5, *A*). For the proximal tibia, the transverse axis may be described by a line bisecting the articular surface and running parallel to the anterior margins. The anteroposterior axis of the plateau is then defined as a line running normal to the transverse axis through the knee center. Axial rotation of the tibial plateau is then measured as the angle (ϑ degrees) between the anteroposterior axis and a line projected from the tibial tubercle to the knee center (Fig. 50.5, *B*). The tibial tubercle (attachment site of the patellar tendon), the position of which dictates in part the tracking pattern of the patella, usually has a small lateral deviation from the anteroposterior axis.

The Patellofemoral Joint

The knee is a triarticular composite, the third component of which is the patella-quadriceps mechanism and its articulation with the femur. Patellofemoral alignment may be described by the Q angle, which is the angle between the line connecting the anterior superior iliac spine (ASIS) to the patella center and the line connecting the tibial tubercle to the patella center (44) (Fig. 50.4). This has a mean value of about 11 degrees valgus ± 6 degrees SD (12). The movement of the patella is complex. Despite extensive literature on the subject, patellofemoral joint mechanics are still poorly defined (28–30, 43, 50, 53, 56, 58). As the knee flexes, the patella enters and tracks centrally along the trochlear groove without obvious tilt. In a three-dimensional analysis of patella movement, Ahmed et al. (2) related tracking to the geometry of the femoral sulcus with which it articulates. Tracking also is controlled by orientation of the quadriceps muscle pull proximally and by location of the tibial tubercle distally (2, 44).

A dynamic linkage between the patellofemoral joint and the tibiofemoral compartments serves to distribute loads across the femur and to the tibia during diverse activities of the limb. According to our analysis, the loading of the patella in the femoral sulcus during flexion (e.g., squatting, stair climbing) provides a three-

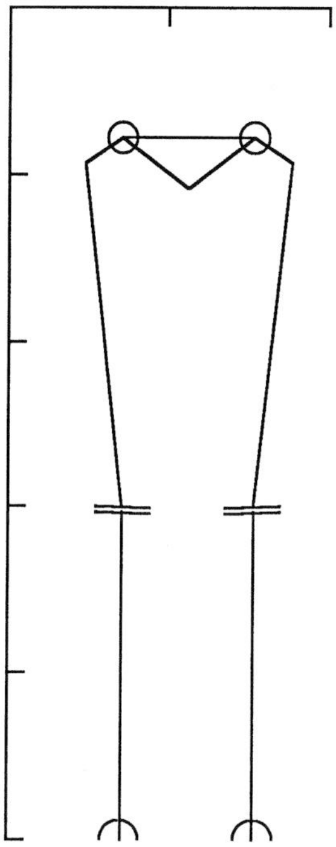

		Don CR:NM29-1 DOB: *: Varus(-), Valgus(+)	QPR:27-02-1986 Dr.Cooke XR:29 OP		Save?	
					RIGHT	LEFT
A N G L E *	CMTS	Hip-Knee-Ankle	0		0	-2
	CMXC	Condylar-Hip (>90)	4		4	6
	TPTS	Plateau-Ankle (>90)	-3		-4	-7
	CMFS	Hip-Knee-Femoral Shaft	5		5	5
	FNFS	Femoral Neck-Femoral Shaft	131		134	133
	FSXC	Condylar-Femoral Shaft (>90)	9		9	10
	FSTS	Femoral Shaft-Tibial Shaft	5		5	3
	CMCM	Knee-Hip-Ankle	0		0	-1
	FLEX	Hip-Knee-Ankle Flexion	0		8	10
	FROT	Foot Rotation (Ext'l [+])	10		12	10
D I S T A N C E		Femoral Length (mm)			473	469
		Tibial Length			385	386
		Standing Leg Length			861	859
		Condylar Width			75	76
		Lateral Condylar Depth			73	70
		Plateau Width			74	79
		Medial Plateau Depth			43	46
		Lateral Joint Space	5		4	8
		Medial Joint Space	5		5	7
		Coronal Subluxation			3	7
		A/P Knee Radiograph Reduction (%)			82	81
		LAT Knee Radiograph Reduction (%)			95	95

Figure 50.2. Standardized radiography output format. Bone landmarks and reference markers on the standardized radiographs are digitized, and their coordinates processed by a software program (Questor) to provide a list of critical angular and linear parameters that describe the static biomechanics of the lower limbs. These parameters are corrected for parallax error. The column of data before the right and left limb entries is included for comparison: These are mean values obtained from a population of healthy young adults.

point load distribution whereby compressive forces are transmitted across the distal condylar surfaces of the femur and supported by the surfaces of tibial plateau (unpublished data). This mechanism appears to be reflected in the bone architecture of the distal femur, which features arrays of trabeculae aligned between the femoral sulcus and the condyles (Fig. 50.6, A). The inference is that the anteroposterior and oblique alignment of the trabeculae represent lines of principal compressive and tensile stress, respectively (64). In the intercondylar notch, the bone is extremely dense, which is appropriate for resisting compressive loads that tend to force the condyles apart (Fig. 50.6, B).

Role of Ligaments in Biomechanics of the Knee

A major contribution to knee stability (resistance to buckling) is made by the soft tissue constraints, of which the collateral ligaments and the cruciate ligaments play a major part (63). Normal motion is contingent on adequate stiffness of these structures. When the ligaments are lax, shear forces may lead to subluxation. A "hysteresis loop" is evident when the knee is tested for varus-valgus motion (moment-rotation pattern) at 0 degrees flexion. This is shown in Figure 50.7, in which tibial displacement around the femur involves a cycle of rapidly increasing tension, then relaxation, in the collateral and cruciate ligaments (7). Similar patterns have been reported for various positions of flexion and for motion in the sagittal plane (55, 59). Hysteresis patterns of joint motion have some diagnostic value: Joints affected with rheumatoid arthritis usually feature broad hysteresis loops indicative of ligamentous laxity, whereas osteoarthritic joints (in which soft tissue contractures are common) tend to feature narrower loops (8).

During stance, the neutrally aligned knee resists mediolateral buckling in proportion to the axial load, indicating that, in this situation, geometry of the congruent bearing surfaces plays a major role in stability (55, 68). When a limb is malaligned, there is an increased tendency for the knee to buckle, which must be resisted by the muscles and ligaments. An example of this malfunction is the tendency for varus knees with ACL deficiency to buckle (65).

The Knee in Action

The functioning knee, like any other joint, may be modeled as a balanced interaction of mechanical and biologic factors. Factors in the mechanical category may be described as either static or dynamic. Static factors include the alignment of the limb segments, the geometry of the joint surfaces, and the degree of joint laxity as determined by the state of the ligamentous tissues that surround it. Dynamic mechanical factors are those that pertain to joints in use, including the variable distribution of loads during such functions as gait and stair climbing, and to proprioceptive and other neuromuscular factors that may regulate stress levels in joints. An imbalance in the interaction of mechanical factors may lead to joint dysfunction (17, 13, 26). Within the category of biologic factors, one may include the effects of connective tissue disease on the proper functioning of

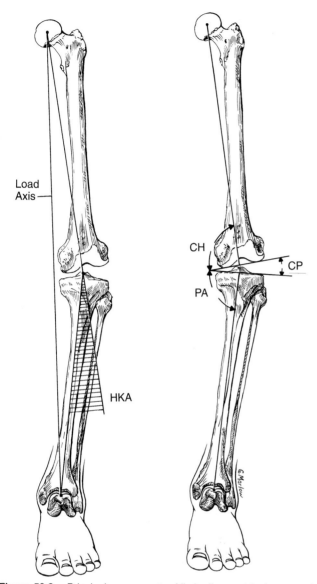

Figure 50.3. Principal components of limb alignment in the coronal plane. The load axis of the limb is defined as the line passing from the hip center to the ankle center. The mechanical axis of the femur is the *line* from the hip center to the knee center, and for the tibia it is from the knee center to the ankle center. In an ideally aligned limb, the knee center falls in line with the load axis (i.e., the hip-knee-ankle angle (*HKA*) is close to 0. (In the example shown, the limb has a marked varus alignment.) The tilt of the femoral condylar surface is measured by the condylar-hip angle (*CH*), whereas that of the tibial plateau is measured by the plateau-ankle (*PA*) angle. CH and PA are recorded as degrees deviation from 90 degrees. The angle between the condylar and tibial articulating surfaces is the condylar-plateau angle (*CP*). All angles have the conventional negative for varus and positive for valgus.

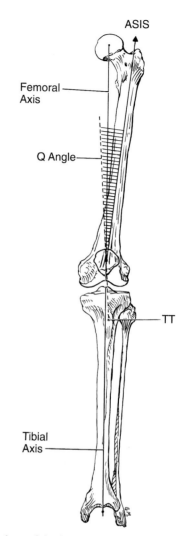

Figure 50.4. Axes of the femur and tibia in the frontal plane. Frontal view of the lower limb in neutral alignment. The femoral mechanical axis is depicted as a *line* from the center of the femoral head to the knee center, and the tibial mechanical axis as a *line* from the knee center to the distal tibial plafond. The diagram shows the usual configuration of the quadriceps-patella ligament mechanism and the Q angle. *ASIS*, Anterior superior iliac spine; *TT*, tibial tubercle.

the joint. Thus a principal aspect of joint dysfunction is loss of cartilage from weight-bearing surfaces, such as evident in OA and even more dramatically apparent in inflammatory diseases like rheumatoid arthritis (RA). Cartilage loss is also a feature of metabolic cartilage disorders (13, 14), crystal-deposition disease (25), or ge-

netic conditions that alter the structure of collagen (3, 49). The interplay of these various mechanical and biologic factors is depicted in Figure 50.8.

In very general terms, attrition of the cartilaginous surfaces in a joint may be likened to a wear process occurring in a mechanical bearing. The assumption here is that some "wear" in the joint is normal, in the sense of reduced thickness or age-related chondromalacic change rather than simple mechanical erosion (19, 73). To take this analogy further, a "wear model" helps to define the interplay of mechanical and biologic factors in the development of joint dysfunction. Thus, when neither factor is aberrant, the wear rate in a joint remains below a critical value (W_{crit}) so that loss of load-bearing tissue (joint space narrowing) over a lifetime of use is

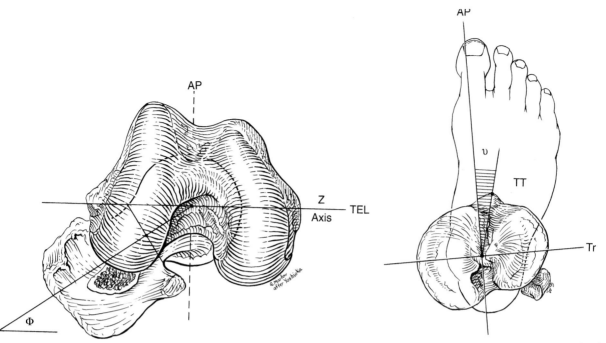

Figure 50.5.   Axes of the femur and tibia in the transverse plane. **A,** Axial view of the distal femur showing a transverse axis (*Z*) that corresponds closely to the transepicondylar line (*TEL*). Superimposed is a view of the proximal femur showing a *line* connecting the centers of the femoral head and neck. Femoral anteversion is the angle (φ) between these two lines. **B,** Axial view of the proximal tibia showing anteroposterior (*AP*) and transverse (*Tr*) axes. *Tr* is a line bisecting the articular surface and running parallel to the anterior margins of the tibial plateau. *AP* is a line running normal to Tr through the knee center. Inclination of the tibial tubercle (*TT*) from AP is indicated (ξ).

not enough to induce major dysfunction (Fig. 50.9, group 1). When aberrant mechanical factors that tend to accelerate the wear rate are present, but biologic factors remain sound, W_{crit} may be exceeded in later years to bring about OA (Fig. 50.9, group 3). At the opposite extreme, very rapid attrition of cartilage occurs when adverse biologic and mechanical factors interact with each other from the outset. An example of this is the genetic condition of alkaptonuria in which W_{crit} may be exceeded very early in life (Fig. 50.9, group 4). Rheumatoid arthritis (RA) is an example of a condition of unsound biologic factors brought on by disease (Fig. 50.9, group 2); the wear rate sharply increases in synchrony with the onset of inflammation, and W_{crit} is rapidly exceeded. However, the pattern in RA is more complex than this because the progressive loss of cartilage destabilizes the joint, leading to deterioration of the biomechanics (unsound mechanical factors) and further acceleration of wear rate. The model predicts that positive influences will help to oppose the effects of negative ones (e.g., healthy cartilage will resist abnormal loading resulting from malalignment), and in the presence of cartilage abnormalities the wear rate will be less when the mechanics are sound. This may help with an understanding of the patterns of joint disease seen clinically. For example, in cases of progressive joint damage without obvious alteration in static biomechanics, adverse factors are likely to be of the dynamic mechanical type, or they may be biologic in origin.

Knee Alignment in Young Healthy Adults

Alignment in the coronal plane was studied in a population of 79 young healthy adult (YHA) volunteers (41 females, 38 males). The means of the parameters (±SD) are shown in Figure 50.10, *A*. There was a clear trend for the knee center to be aligned close to the load axis (mean HKA = −0.97 degrees ±2.81 degrees) (9, 41, 52, 60). Mean angles of condylar valgus and plateau varus were close to 4 and −3.5 degrees, respectively (CH = 4.04 degrees ±2.12 degrees; PA = −3.32 degrees ±2.31 degrees), and the resultant mean angle between the two joint surfaces was less than 2 degrees, converging medially (CP = −1.7 degrees ±1.32 degrees). The small SD for the CP angle indicates relative constancy as might be expected from the apposition of congruent joint surfaces during stance. This was tested by linear regression analysis in which the dependence of overall alignment (HKA) on knee geometry (CH + PA) was measured, treating CP as a constant (see equation No. 1). The high correlation (R square = 0.80, $P<0.001$) indicates that the model is generally applicable (Fig. 50.10, *B*), which implies that there is a developmental trait for "reciprocal balance" to occur in the geometries of the distal femur and proximal tibia, with the effect of producing neutral alignment. Consequently, the lack of reciprocal balance produces malalignment, which in some cases might predispose the individual to arthritis (Fig. 50.10, *C*). Another, perhaps less obvious factor (Fig. 50.10, *A* and *B*)

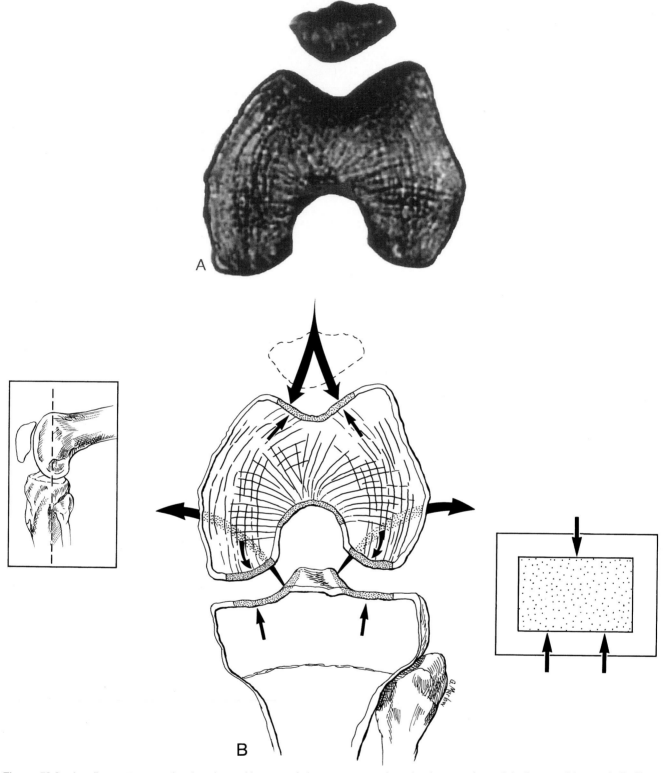

Figure 50.6. Loading patterns and trabecular architecture of the knee. **A,** Computed tomographic scan of a cadaver femur showing a section approximately at the level of the epicondyles. Note the dense subchondral bone of the femoral sulcus and condylar surfaces, linked by an array of linear trabeculae. Oblique and transverse trabeculae emanate from the dense regions of the intercondylar notch. **B,** Simulation of patellofemoral joint loading in flexion. Trabecular orientation is such as to transfer compressive loads between patellar and tibial surfaces, resisting joint reaction forces from the up slopes of the tibial eminence that tend to force the condyles apart.

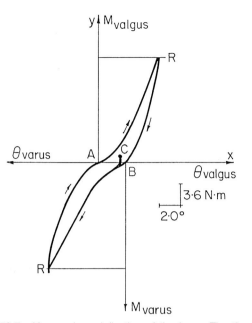

Figure 50.7. Varus-valgus deflection of the knee. The "hysteresis loop" evident when a knee is tested for varus-valgus motion (moment-rotation pattern) at 0 degrees flexion. Tibial varus displacement from center (*C*) (angle varus) shows a cycle of increasing varus tension (moment varus) followed by a cycle of relaxation. A similar moment-rotation pattern occurs in the opposite direction (angle valgus, moment valgus). This pattern is characteristic of the nonlinear load-relaxation response of the collateral and cruciate ligaments.

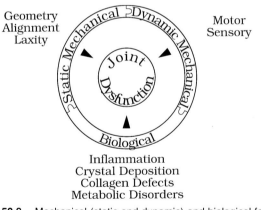

Figure 50.8. Mechanical (static and dynamic) and biological factors that may interact in a potentially synergistic manner to contribute to joint dysfunction.

is that individuals with abnormally large (or small) CH and PA angles may end up with an exaggerated tilt of the joint line even though the HKA angle may be near neutral. This might also be a factor predisposing individuals to arthritis, although longitudinal studies are necessary to test this.

Regarding gender differences, data from this set of volunteers did not substantiate the notion that females tend to have valgus limb alignment (17).

Knee Alignment in Joint Diseases
Signs and Symptoms

A poorly explained feature of commonly seen joint diseases, especially OA, is the lack of correlation between symptoms of pain and dysfunction and the extent of radiographic change (13, 45, 51). This is especially true for the patellofemoral joint, in which symptomatology may dominate in the absence of obvious pathologic conditions (16, 39, 56). Conversely, symptoms may be absent when most expected, such as in the presence of disabling changes in the tibiofemoral compartments together with rotational malalignment (15).

Alignment Changes as Markers of Pathologic Conditions

Because the orientation of the knee weight-bearing surfaces contributes to overall limb alignment, any change in the geometry of these surfaces (e.g., through loss of cartilage) usually shows up as altered alignment. The same principle applies to the settling or collapse of knee replacement components, which may produce sudden large changes of alignment (20, 36). The magnitude of the change in OA is greatest when one compartment of the tibiofemoral joint is affected more than the other. Thus, when loss of cartilage is focussed at the medial side, this compartment collapses during stance, resulting in a more varus alignment (increased negative HKA angle) (Fig. 50.10, *C*). It follows that abnormalities of femorotibial alignment may not be apparent in nonload-bearing situations. In neutral alignment, the load axis passes between the femoral condyles, ensuring that the knee is stable during stance. With a severe loss of joint space (e.g., on the medial side), the knee center shifts to the outer side of the load axis (Fig. 50.10, *C*). If the shift is great enough, the lateral compartment may yawn, introducing instability and a tendency for the knee to buckle laterally (65). This is exhibited clinically as a "lateral thrust." Conversely, a medial thrust occurs with the valgus knee.

Osteoarthritis with Varus Limb Alignment
General Features

For the purpose of classifying OA cases, the definition of varus alignment is a negative HKA angle. In a review of 167 cases that comprised a "symptomatic OA" study group, 128 (76%) were classified as having varus alignment. Bilateral knee involvement was a usual feature of these cases. Males are reported to have this condition more frequently than females in the younger age groups, with the opposite trend in older patients (51). In our outpatient population, the condition appeared to be distributed more or less evenly among the sexes (66 females, 62 males). The alignment parameters of this group are indicated in Figure 50.10, *A*. Compared with the nearly neutrally aligned normal group, a surprising decrease of more than 3 degrees in the valgus angulation at the distal femur (CH angle) (*P*<0.005) contributed to the overall varus alignment. This finding may

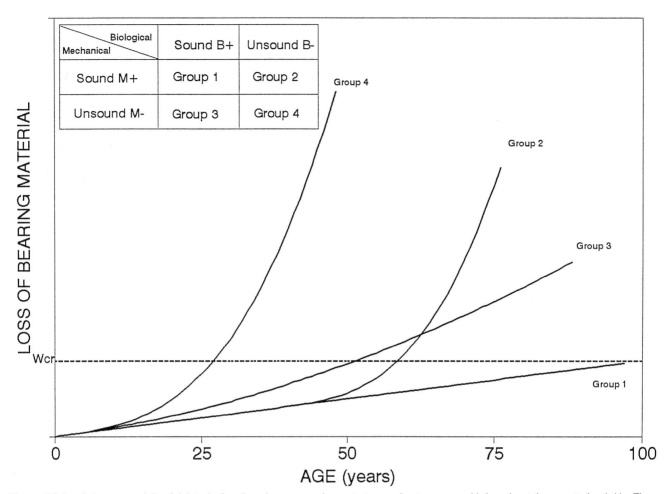

Figure 50.9. A "wear model" of joint dysfunction. In a normal healthy joint the model predicts that the wear rate remains below a critical value (W_{crit}), so a lifetime of use can be sustained without developing arthritis (group 1). When there are adverse factors, broadly distinguishable as mechanical and biological (*inset*), these may oper- ate to accelerate wear and bring about the onset of arthritis. The remaining curves (groups 2 to 4) represent the various combinations of the mechanical and biological factors as indicated. For a full discussion see the text.

indicate a subpopulation with a developmentally abnormal femur that predisposes to OA, or it may reflect disease-induced changes such as a focus of bone erosion at the medial condyle or a bowing of the femur as part of the remodeling response of OA (Kurosaka et al., unpublished observation). A major contribution to the overall varus alignment of the limbs in this group is made by a 3 degrees average increase in the CP angle ($P<0.005$), reflecting a collapse of the medial compartment and (in severe cases) an opening of the lateral compartment. Surprisingly, the mean for the PA angle of the varus group was not significantly different from the YHA (Fig. 50.10, *A*).

The early pathologic characteristics of these varus knee cases typically features a loss of cartilage with damage to underlying bone that tends to be focused at the tibial plateau anteromedially (48, 75). At the femur, early loss of medial condylar cartilage is initially focused on the area loaded within the approximate flexion range of 15 to 40 degrees. This corresponds to the area in which loading is primarily concentrated during the stance phase of gait. During gait, the joint tends to

collapse medially, generating "lateral thrust" as the limb is loaded during stance. When these joints were opened, we noted rupture of the medial meniscus in about half of the cases.

As the disease progresses, a cyclical pattern sets in whereby, with increasing varus deformity, the anteromedial lesion of the tibial plateau extends posteriorly, causing further collapse of the medial compartment and even more varus (48, 75). A commonly associated feature is degenerative change in the patellofemoral joint, which probably arise through maltracking of the patella and progressive damage to the ACL (Fig. 50.11). With further advance of the disease, ACL disruption, probably induced by osteophytic spurs in the intercondylar notch, permits increasing joint shear in the coronal plane and the development of lesions in the lateral compartment. Anteroposterior laxity at this stage (ACL disruption) is seldom obvious, possibly because of the buttressing effect of osteophytes that progressively emerge at the joint margins. The medial collateral ligaments feature contracture or tensioning by the growth of osteophytes around the medial joint space. In advanced

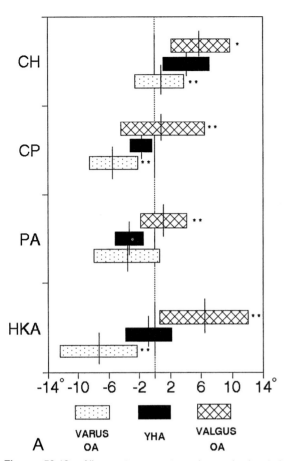

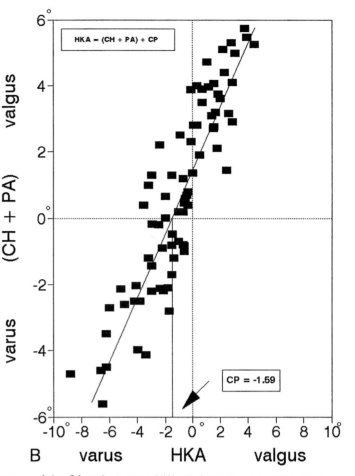

Figure 50.10. Alignment parameters (coronal plane) in young healthy adults with osteoarthritis. **A,** Bar graph showing data for the main parameters of alignment in the coronal plane: *CH,* condylar-hip; *CP,* condylar-plateau; *PA,* plateau-ankle; *HKA,* hip-knee-ankle. *Bars* show standard deviations, and the *vertical lines* through them show the means for the three groups studied: young healthy adults (*YHA*), varus-aligned osteoarthritic (*VARUS OA)* patients, and valgus aligned osteoarthritic *(VALGUS OA)* patients. *Asterisks* denote significance of differences between OA and YHA group parameters from the two-sample *t*-test (**, $P<0.005$; *, $P<0.05$). (The criterion for classification of the OA patients was: $HKA=<0$ degrees varus; $HKA=>0$ degrees valgus.) **B,** Linear regression analysis to show the relationship between the two main sets of variables HKA (limb alignment) and (CH + PA) (knee geometry) in the YHA group. In this analysis CP (joint surfaces angle) is treated as a constant, the value of which corresponds to the intercept (−1.59 degrees). Regression data were: *R* square=0.80; slope=0. 86; *P*<0 001. The data were from 79 young adult volunteers, one knee from each. **C,** Representations of varus, neutral, and valgus lower limb alignment, with associated differences in the Q angle. *ASIS,* Anterior superior iliac spine; *TT,* tibial tubercle.

states of tricompartmental damage, the lateral collateral structures may be stretched. These effects are usually accompanied by progressive loss of joint motion.

Surgery may be indicated at an early stage of the disease when symptoms are severe. For individuals whose demands on their knees are high (by virtue of activity or obesity), a useful strategy is to correct the malalignment by osteotomy. Valgus tibial osteotomy (21, 23, 54, 62) redistributes stresses to the lateral tibiofemoral compartment, retarding the rate of damage to the medial side and providing potential for tissue regeneration (5). High tibial osteotomy (HTO) is the most common approach. A closing wedge is performed between the tibial tubercle and the joint surface (21, 62). Alternatives are a more distal opening wedge osteotomy with bone graft (38) or a high-dome osteotomy, as described by Maquet (53). It is widely (but not universally) agreed that survival of tibial osteotomy for medial compartment OA is favored by overcorrection of the femorotibial angle (66). In a recent study, Coventry et al. (23) reported better survival rates in knees that were overcorrected to at least 8 degress valgus (equivalent to HKA ≥3 degrees). In the same study, low body weight also favored survival of the osteotomies. Another factor favoring survival is relative youth; as many as three-quarters of patients who are 50 years of age or less at the time of osteotomy were reported to be functioning well 11 years afterward (67).

Another consideration is that femoral osteotomies may be appropriate to this group. Our alignment data indicated that, in many patients, a reduced valgus malalignment of the distal femur is a contributing factor. This approach has not, to our knowledge, been fully explored. The orientation of the distal femur may also be important in determining the outcome of correction by tibial osteotomy. This finding was suggested from a

Figure 50.10C.—*(continued)*

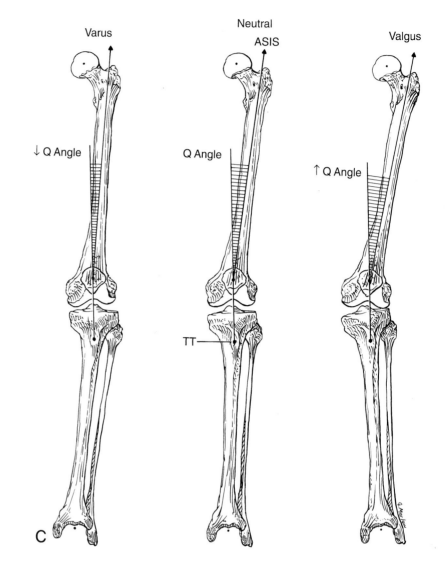

radiographic review of limb alignment following tibial osteotomy cases (more than 1 year after surgery), which showed that the results correlated more with the preoperative geometry of the distal femur (CH angle) than with the degree of tibial correction at surgery (70).

In older patients, especially those in whom the disease is localized medially and the lateral compartment and ACL are in good condition, hemiarthroplasty is a logical option (32, 33, 47). The ultimate measure is total knee replacement (TKR), which usually requires medial soft tissue release and removal of osteophytes. Positioning of the components should be planned so that the outcome is neutral alignment (HKA = 0 degrees) in two-legged stance (i.e., the knee centered on the load axis). This minimizes eccentric loading patterns in the knees to reduce both wear and the risk of component loosening. In general, knee prostheses have poor resistance to varus-valgus displacement, relative to normal joints; thus our recommendation is to position both compo-

nents squarely to the femoral and tibial mechanical axes (CH = 0 degrees; PA = 0 degrees). This helps to minimize shear forces at the joint surfaces (and hence the tendency for subluxation) during weight bearing.

Varus Alignment With Oblique Joint Line

In about 5% of patients attending the clinics in our studies, we encountered a pattern of varus limb alignment with a pronounced inward slope to the joint line in the coronal plane (15). The alignment of this subgroup counters the general trend of the OA varus group because the contributing factors are extreme varus angulation of the tibial plateau combined with excessive valgus angulation of the distal femur. Axial malrotations of the distal femur and proximal tibia, usually in the opposite direction, may accompany the coronal malalignment (Fig. 50.12). In addition to medial compartment OA, these patients show an increased tendency for lateral subluxation of the tibia, probably as the result of

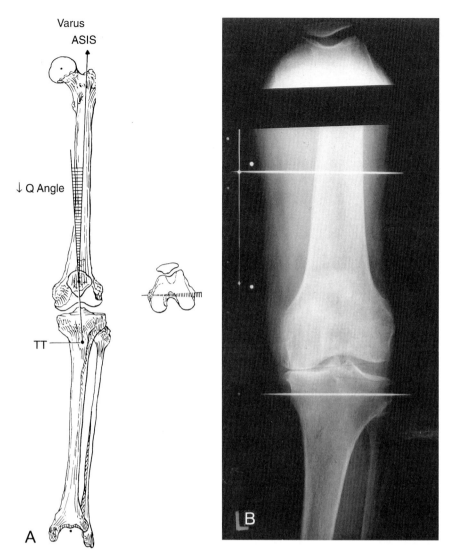

Varus
ASIS

↓ Q Angle

TT

A

Figure 50.11. Varus aligned osteoarthritic knees. **A,** Representation of a varus-aligned lower limb showing the diminished Q angle and illustrating the tendency for medial displacement of the patella that this may induce. **B,** Standardized frontal radiograph of the knee (*below*) and axial view of the patellofemoral joint (*above*) in a patient with a varus osteoarthritic knee. Note the changes in the medial tibiofemoral compartment and medial displacement of the patella. (See also Fig. 50.15.)

shear forces generated at the slanting articular interface. Usually, the tibia is rotated externally, producing lateral displacement of the tibial tubercle, with associated lateralization of the patella and concomitant arthritic degeneration.

It is important to identify these patients because correction by valgus tibial osteotomy alone may yield disappointing results. In selected cases, we used double osteotomies to correct the valgus of the distal femur and the varus of the proximal tibia (15). In advanced cases, TKR is the preferred treatment, with placement of the components to alleviate the malrotations and bring the patellofemoral joint into correct alignment.

Varus Limb Alignment and Inwardly Pointing Knees

This condition may be described as a developmental abnormality in which mild varus limb alignment is accompanied by knees that point inwardly ("in squinting") in normal stance or gait (Fig. 50.13). Typically, patients with this condition are adolescents or active young adults, and complaints center on the patellofemoral joint, with pain imposing a major limitation on functional activity. In about one-third of these cases, we noted a positive apprehension test result; the remainder had secure patellae but showed marked local irritability (Osmond-Clarke sign) (16). The major malalignment observed in these cases was an external rotational deformity of the proximal tibia in the axial plane that contributed to an accentuation of the Q angle. In many cases, especially those that were symptomatic, excessive laxity was manifest in hyperextension of the knee and hypermobility of the patella, both of which may have contributed to the dysfunction.

A number of these cases responded poorly to correction at the level of the soft tissues. All those with major disability responded well to derotation tibial valgus osteotomies, with realignment of the Q angle distally (16). It should be emphasized that femoral osteotomy was inappropriate in these cases in which the malformations

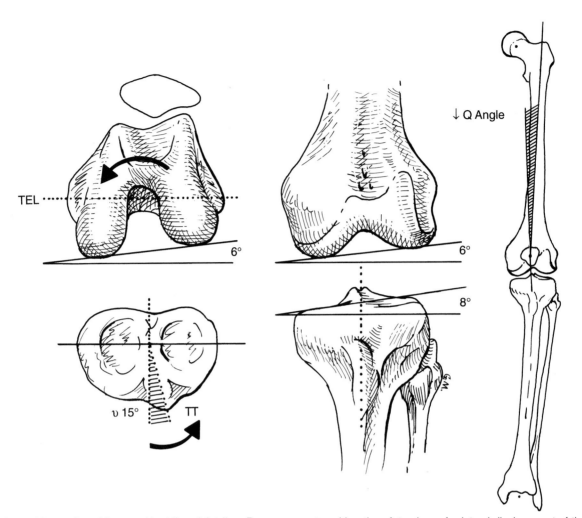

Figure 50.12. Varus aligned knees with oblique joint line. Representation of bone malalignment typically associated with the varus osteoarthritic knee having an oblique joint line. Note the accentuated distal femoral valgus and severe proximal tibial varus that may pro-

mote subluxation. A tendency for lateral displacement of the patella in these knees may best be explained by outward rotation of the proximal tibia.

were traced to problems of axial tibial malalignment. This underscores the importance of thorough radiographic analyses of such cases. The addition of computed tomographic (CT) scans is worthwhile when patterns of axial rotation are still unclear following regular clinical and radiographic examination (42, 77).

Osteoarthritis With Valgus Limb Alignment

Patients with HKA angles of >0 degrees are included in this category. OA cases with valgus alignment were reported less frequently than cases with varus alignment. Our OA study group contained just 39 (23%) of such patients. The condition appeared more often in women than men. Relative to the group of young adults without arthritis (YHA), the mean data for the valgus OA patients indicate an increased distal femoral valgus angle (CH = 5 degrees versus 3.8 degrees; P<0.05), and a tibial plateau almost square to the tibial mechanical axis (i.e., lacking the usual varus angulation) (PA = 0.97 degrees versus −3.5 degrees; P<0.001) (Fig. 50.10, A). The mean

joint angle (CP) was narrow with lateral convergence (CP = 0.61 degrees versus −1.7 degrees; P<0.005), which is consistent with a trend for arthritic collapse of the lateral compartment. However, the large SD (±5.39 degrees) indicates medial compartment collapse in some patients (Fig. 50.10, A). In the axial radiographic view, the tibial plateau may show excessive outward rotation (unpublished observations).

In severe cases of valgus OA that feature a focus of joint space change in the lateral compartment, there may be a yawning of the medial compartment. The Q angle is increased because the knee center is displaced to the inward side of the load axis. This in conjunction with any outward tibial rotation promotes lateral subluxation of the patella (Fig. 50.14). Despite these changes, the range of knee motion is usually well preserved. Also, in contrast to the joint stiffness that typifies the varus knee, soft tissue laxity is not uncommon. Soft tissue contractures, when present, are focused on the lateral side.

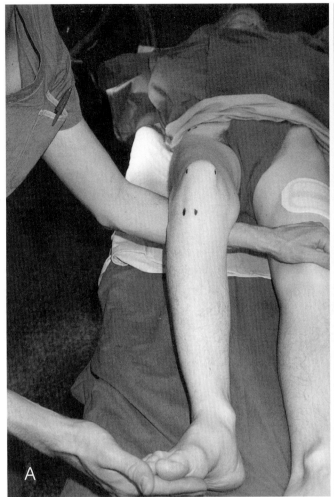

Figure 50.13. In-squinting varus knees. Clinical appearance of a patient with in-squinting knee malalignment. **A,** With feet ahead the knees point inwardly. **B,** With the knee flexion plane aligned sagittally the feet and tibiae are outwardly rotated. Note the lateral position of the tibial tubercle, which accentuates the Q angle.

In our study, there appeared to be a subset of the valgus OA group of patients, typified by polyarticular disease and crystal deposition (usually calcium pyrophosphate dihydrate) (13, 25), suggesting the involvement of both biologically and mechanically inciting factors. RA might also be considered in this category because the developing deformity is usually a valgus one (11) and the pathogenesis is primarily biologic.

Various options for the surgical management of valgus knee deformities have been outlined (22, 57, 71). The most appropriate approach depends on the mechanical and biologic factors that contribute most to the condition. In young or middle-aged patients with high functional demands (and when biologic factors are not in evidence), abnormal geometry may be corrected by osteotomy. In some cases varus tibial osteotomy is appropriate to correct the abnormal valgus geometry of the proximal tibia (22). However, tibial osteotomy alone may have disastrous results in cases in which distal femoral abnormalities coexist and are left uncorrected (22, 71). In such

cases a supracondylar dome-shaped varus osteotomy of the femur may be appropriate, with the aim of adjusting the coronal malalignment and (in the event of axial malrotation) derotating the condyles into neutral alignment. Occasionally, double osteotomy may be needed.

The long-term value of hemiarthroplasty in valgus knee conditions has yet to be demonstrated. In severe valgus deformity with tricompartmental disease, TKR is the treatment of choice. An anterolateral approach may be favored, especially in the event of severe lateral compartment damage with soft tissue contracture (10, 46). Tissues requiring release may include the iliotibial band, lateral collateral ligament, and posterior cruciate ligament. As in the case of varus OA knees, positioning of the components should be planned so that the outcome is neutral alignment (HKA = 0 degrees) during two-legged stance (i.e., the knee centered on the load axis). The aim is to avoid (*a*) eccentric loading patterns in the knees that promote wear, (*b*) the risk of component loosening, and (*c*) the tendency for subluxation.

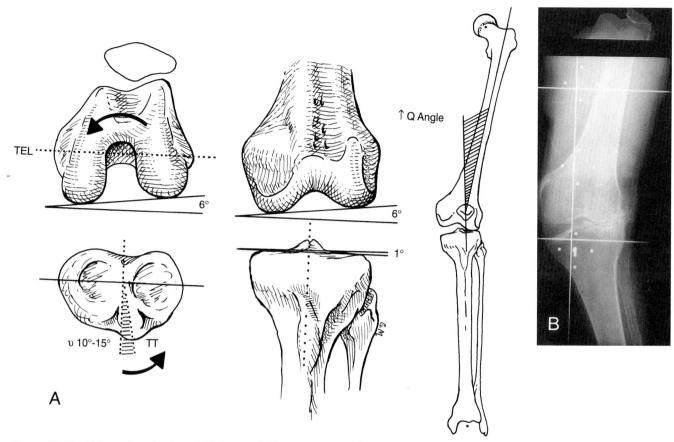

Figure 50.14. Valgus aligned osteoarthritic knees. **A,** Representation of typical bone malalignment evident in valgus knee deformity. Note that the distal femur is somewhat increased in valgus and the proximal tibia is almost square to its mechanical axis; both contribute to excessive loading and osteoarthritis in the lateral compartment. The Q angle is increased as the result of the valgus alignment, and this—together with any outward rotation of the proximal tibia—contributes to lateral displacement of the patella. **B,** Frontal standardized radiograph of a valgus arthritic knee *(below)* and a skyline view of the patellofemoral joint *(above)*. Note the lateral compartment damage, severe patellofemoral joint changes and lateral patellar displacement.

Patellofemoral Joint in Osteoarthritis

Derangements of the patellofemoral joint are extremely common in OA but have received relatively little attention in the literature (56). In the varus-aligned knee, the Q angle diminishes, which creates a vector promoting medial subluxation of the patella in the coronal plane (Fig. 50.11). The reverse occurs in the valgus-aligned knee (i.e., increased Q angle and a vector promoting lateral patellar subluxation) (Fig. 50.14). However, in varus OA cases, we observed medial displacement of the patella in only 20% and lateral displacement in 30%, with the remainder of cases being neutral (35). Obviously, other factors control patellar subluxation, in particular axial malrotations of the femoral condyles and/or proximal tibia (tibial tubercle alignment). External rotation of the condyles may flatten the patellar sulcus. Likewise, outward rotation of the tibial tubercle similarly influences patellar tracking by increasing the Q angle distally (35). Investigation by CT analysis of individual cases may be needed to help devise appropriate treatment.

Special Cases: Traumatic Sagittal Plane Deformities of the Proximal Tibia

We have encountered a small group of cases with major knee dysfunction associated with sagittal plane deformities of the proximal tibia at or above the level of the patellar tendon attachment. In three patients, all adolescents, trauma sustained in hyperextension with axial loading induced compression fractures of the proximal tibia. The resultant deformity was a loss of the normal posterior tibial slope and a functional "back knee" deformity. In one of the three patients, varus was also apparent. All three cases showed significant anteroposterior dysfunctional instability in extension, with features that resembled ACL insufficiency; two had positive pivot shifts. Anterior opening wedge osteotomies were performed in two of the cases, with insertion of iliac crest bone wedges into transverse bone cuts made above the level of the tibial tubercle (Fig. 50.16). The osteotomies resulted in marked functional improvement in both patients, with correction of "back knee" and elimination of the pivot shifts.

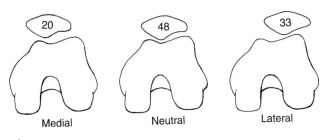

A   Percentage of Varus Knees

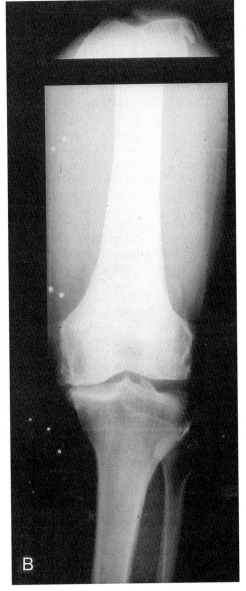

Figure 50.15. Patellar displacement in varus-aligned osteoarthritic knees. **A,** Patellar displacement in patients with varus-aligned osteoarthritic knees. Note that about one-third of cases featured laterally displaced patellae. **B,** Frontal standardized radiograph of a varus arthritic knee *(below)* and a skyline view of the patellofemoral joint *(above)*, featuring a laterally displaced patella.

Summary

The knee is a complex tricompartmental articulation. From the mechanical viewpoint, proper long-term function demands that the principal segments of the limb work together to bring about a stable joint, with appropriate distribution of forces across the bearing surfaces and the supporting soft tissues. From the biological viewpoint, optimal function demands that the various tissues constituting the joint are sound and capable of normal physiologic function and repair.

The corollary of the preceding is that functional deterioration of joints may come about from mechanical factors, biologic deficits, or some combination of these. Currently, the science is inexact for want of systems to collect and integrate data concerning the various static, dynamic, and biologic properties of joints. New developments in techniques for motion analysis that can be applied in conjunction with quantitative radiographic methods are important for further progress (18, 24, 52, 69).

On the assumption that malalignment contributes to

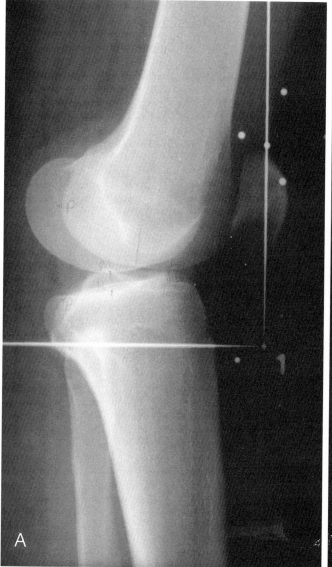
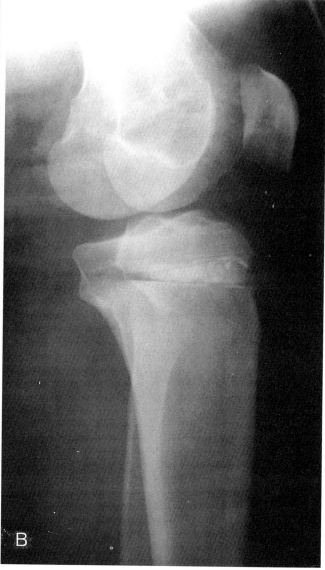

Figure 50.16. Traumatic sagittal deformity of the proximal tibia. Lateral radiographs of a patient before (**A**) and after (**B**) surgical correction of an anterior impaction deformity of the proximal tibia. Insertion of bone wedges into a proximal transverse osteotomy corrected the sagittal plane deformity of the tibia and the associated instability.

abnormal biomechanics, which in turn predisposes patients to arthritis, we would like to know what proportion of the population at large is destined to suffer symptomatic OA by virtue of malalignment. It would be useful, for example, to assess the risk for developing OA in a given case, based on the deviation of alignment parameters from normal values. A definition for normal lower limb alignment can be sought through epidemiological surveys of alignment variables in samples of healthy populations; however, as is shown in this chapter, there are wide standard deviations about the mean values. This makes it difficult to assess the alignment deviations that are tolerable before a joint may be considered to have abnormal biomechanics. A reasonable compromise is to make an arbitrary division between normal and abnormal, taking the view that the further the alignment deviates from the ideal, the greater is the risk for joint damage occurring in later life. We have taken this approach by assigning our OA patients into varus or valgus groups according to the value of their hip-knee-ankle (HKA) angle. The criterion was thus: *varus* = <0 degrees and *valgus* = >0 degrees. We found that, on average, (*a*) the varus group featured abnormal femoral geometry as a major contributing factor to the alignment disorder, with (surprisingly) proximal tibial geometry that did not differ significantly from normal, and (*b*) in the valgus group, geometries of both the femur and tibia were contributing factors. It was not clear to what extent the malalignment predisposed each group to the arthritis or to what extent arthritic degeneration from other causes produced the malalignment. Probably there are complex patterns of interaction in this regard.

In addition to static alignment, there are dynamic factors in the biomechanics of the knee, and these also affect the risk for developing OA (4, 69). Also to be considered are the various negative biologic factors in connective tissue disease that compromise the integrity of the bearing tissues and thus influence outcome. To help understand ways in which biologic and mechanical influences might interact, we devised a "wear model." This provides for a range of conditions represented at the extremes by diseases considered primarily biologic (e.g., RA, genetic collagen defects), and those primarily mechanical (e.g., patellar dysfunction related to axial malformations of the tibia). Even in conditions that are primarily biologic, the model predicts that abnormal knee loading from developing malalignment accelerates the rate of tissue degradation.

In relation to the surgical management of malalignment problems, osteotomy is our recommendation for younger or more active patients with limited joint damage. The knee alignment data for the varus and valgus subgroups of patients with OA are highly relevant in this regard, encouraging a review of the current customary practices of tibial and femoral osteotomy. We recommend that, in each individual case, the factors contributing to the knee disorder (bone geometry and malalignment) be carefully assessed with the aim of a rational surgical plan for correction by osteotomy. Arthroplasty is more appropriate in older patients, especially when joint damage is well advanced. One of the key aims of surgery should be to optimize the distribution of stresses across the knee. This should enhance the opportunity for repair following osteotomy (5) or reduce the risk of premature wear and loosening following TKR (61).

Given the importance of understanding the contribution of alignment factors in the genesis of OA, routine standardized radiography is an excellent means of obtaining quantitative static data for diagnosis and follow-up of individual patients (18).

Further research in this area is necessary. To achieve a fuller understanding of the pathogenesis of alignment and arthritic disorders, the static mechanical data must increasingly be correlated with quantitative motion analysis and documentation of biologic factors that could play a part in the disease process.

Acknowledgments

The authors are grateful to the Human Motion Laboratory of the Clinical Mechanics Group, Queen's University, for allowing us to share their data on knee alignment in the young healthy adults. We acknowledge the valuable advice and assistance of Dr. Jian Li in the preparation and analysis of the data. For the original artwork and the preparation of other illustrations, we are indebted to Greg Marlow, Photographic Services, Department of Academic Affairs, King Faisal Specialist Hospital, Riyadh, Saudi Arabia. To the Clinical Mechanics Group, Queen's University—especially Bryn Fisher and Lorna Spencer—we extend our thanks for assistance in the assembly of background materials and in the preparation of this manuscript.

References

1. Ahlback S, Osteoarthrosis of the knee: a radiographic investigation. Acta Radiol Stockh 1968;277(suppl):7–72.
2. Ahmed A, Burke D, Hyder A. Force analysis of the patellar mechanism. J Orthop Res 1987;5:69–85.
3. Ala-kokko L, Baldwin CT, Moskowitz RW, Prockop DJ. Single base muation in the type II procollagen gene (COL2A1) as a cause of primary OA associated with mild chondrodysplasia. Proc Natl Acad Sci USA 1990;87:6565–6568.
4. Andriacchi TP, Andersson GBJ, Fermier RW et al. A study of lower limb biomechanics during stair climbing. J Bone Joint Surg 1980;62A:749–757.
5. Bergenudd H, Johnell O, Redlund-Johnell I, Lohmander SL. The articular cartilage after osteotomy for medial gonarthrosis. Acta Orthop Scand 1992;63:413–416.
6. Bryant JT, Cooke TDV. A biomechanical function of the anterior cruciate ligament: prevention of medial translation of the tibia. In: Feagin JA Jr, ed. The crucial ligaments: diagnosis and treatment of ligament injuries about the knee. New York: Churchill Livingstone, 1988:235–242.
7. Bryant JT, Cooke TDV. Standardized biomechanical measurements for varus-valgus stiffness and rotation in normal knees. J Orthop Res 1988;6:863–870.
8. Bryant JT, O,Brien JK, Wevers HW, Cooke TDV. Instantaneous centers of rotation in the frontal plane for current prosthetic knee designs. Orthop Trans 1982;7:272.
9. Bryant JT, Cooke TDV, Scudamore RA. The three components of lower limb alignment. In: Transactions of the combined meeting of the Orthopaedic Research Societies of USA, Japan, and Canada, Oct 21–23, 1991, Banff, Alberta, Canada, 1991:265.
10. Buechel FF. A sequential three-step lateral release for correcting fixed valgus knee deformities during total knee arthroplasty. Clin Orthop 1990;260:170–175.
11. Cameron HU and Freeman MAR. Patterns of knee deformity in arthritis. J Rheumatol 1979;6:357–359.
12. Caylor D, Fites R, Worrell TW. The relationship between quadriceps angle and anterior knee pain syndrome. J Orthop Sports Phys Ther 1993;17:11–16.
13. Cooke TDV. Pathogenetic mechanisms in polyarticular osteoarthritis. Clin Rheum Dis 1985;11:203–238.
14. Cooke TDV, Bennett EL, Ohno O. The deposition of immunoglobulins and complement components in osteoarthritic cartilage. Int Orthop 1980;4:211–217.
15. Cooke TDV, Pichora D, Siu D, Scudamore RA, Bryant JT. Surgical implications of varus deformity of the knee with obliquity of joint surfaces. J Bone Joint Surg 1989;71B:560–565.
16. Cooke TDV, Price N, Fisher B, Hedden D. The inwardly pointing knee: an unrecognized problem of external tibial rotational malalignment. Clin Orthop 1990;260:56–60.
17. Cooke TDV, Bryant JT, Scudamore RA, Brittain M. Comparative analysis of static biomechanics in young healthy adults and symptomatic osteoarthritis patients. Trans Orthop Res Soc 1991;16:582.
18. Cooke TDV, Scudamore RA, Bryant JT, Sorbie C, Siu D, Fisher B. Quantitative approach to radiography of the lower limb. J Bone Joint Surg 1991;73B(5):715–720.
19. Cooke TDV, Scudamore RA, Bryant JT. Mechanical factors in the pathogenesis of osteoarthritis. In: Hirohata K, Mizumo K, Matsubara T, eds. Trends in research and treatment of joint diseases. Tokyo: Springer-Verlag, 1992:29–34.
20. Cornwall GB, Cooke TDV, Bryant JT. Role of malalignment in TKR failure: a retrospective analysis of temporal based radiographs and retrieved implants. In: Implant Retrieval Symposium, Society for Biomaterials, September 17–20, St Charles, IL, 1992:68.
21. Coventry MB. Current concepts review: upper tibial osteotomy for osteoarthritis. J Bone Joint Surg 1985;67A:1136–1140.
22. Coventry MB. Proximal tibial varus osteotomy for osteoarthritis of the lateral compartment of the knee, J Bone Joint Surg 1987;69A:32–38.
23. Coventry MB, Ilstrup DM, Wallrichs SL. Proximal tibial osteotomy: a critical long-term study of eighty-seven cases. J Bone Joint Surg 1993;75A:196–201.
24. Deluzio KJ, Wyss UP, Li J, Costigan PA. A procedure to validate three-dimensional dynamic knee assessment systems. J Biomech 1993;26:753–759.
25. Dieppe PA, Doyle DV, Huskisson EC, Willoughby DA, Crocker PR. Mixed crystal deposition disease and osteoarthritis. Br Med J 1978;1:150.

26. Doherty M, Watt I, Dieppe P. Influence of primary generalized osteoarthritis on development of secondary osteoarthritis. Lancet 1983;ii:8–11.

27. Frankel VH, Burstein AH, Brooks DB. Biomechanics of internal derangement of the knee. J Bone Joint Surg 1971;53A:945–962.

28. Fujikawa K, Seedhom BB, Wright V. Biomechanics of the patellofemoral joint. I. A study of the contact and the congruity of the patellofemoral compartment and the movement of the patella. Eng Med 1983;12:3–11.

29. Fujikawa K, Seedhom BB, Wright V. Biomechanics of the patellofemoral joint. II. A study of the effect of simulated femorotibial varus deformity on the congruity of the patellofemoral compartment and the movement of the patella. Eng Med 1983;12:13–21.

30. Fulkerson JP, Shea K. Disorders of patellofemoral alignment. J Bone Joint Surg 1990;72A:1424–1429.

31. Goodfellow JW, O'Connor JJ. The mechanics of the knee and prosthesis design. J Bone Joint Surg 1978;60B:358–369.

32. Goodfellow JW, O'Connor JJ. Clinical results of the Oxford knee: surface arthroplasty of the tibiofemoral joint with a meniscal bearing prosthesis. Clin Orthop 1986;205:21–42.

33. Goodfellow JW, Kershaw CJ, Benson MKA'D, O'Connor JJ. The Oxford knee for unicompartmental osteoarthritis. J Bone Joint Surg 1988;70B:692–701.

34. Grood ES, Suntay WJ. A joint coordinate system for the clinical description of three-dimensional motion: application to the knee. J Biomech Eng 1983;105:136–144.

35. Harrison M, Fisher SB, Griffin M, Cooke TDV. Correlation of patellofemoral arthritis and knee alignment. Paper presented at the Canadian Orthopaedic Research Society meeting, Montreal, Canada, May 30–June 3, 1993.

36. Heck DA, Clingman JK, Kellelkamp DG. Gross polyethylene failure in total knee arthroplasty. Orthopaedics 1992;15(1):23–28.

37. Hernborg JS, Nilsson BE. The natural course of untreated osteoarthritis of the knee. Clin Orthop 1977;123:130–137.

38. Hernigou PH, Medevielle D, Debeyre J, Goutallier D. Proximal tibial osteotomy for osteoarthritis with varus deformity. J Bone Joint Surg 1987;69A:332–354.

39. Hernigou PH, Goutallier D. Patello-femoral joint changes in osteoarthritic varus knees after upper tibial valgus opening osteotomy with bone grafting: a 10 to 13 year follow-up. J Orthop Surg [France] 1987;1:37–41.

40. Hollister AM, Kester MA, Cook SK, Brunet ME, Haddad RJ. Knee axes of rotation: determination and implication. Trans Orthop Res Soc 1986;11:383.

41. Hsu RWW, Himeno S, Coventry MB, Chao EYS. Normal axial alignment of the lower extremity and load-bearing distribution at the knee. Clin Orthop 1990;255:215–227.

42. Hubbard DD, Staheli LT. The direct radiographic measurement of femoral torsion using axial tomography: technique and comparison with an indirect radiographic method. Clin Orthop 1972;86:16–20.

43. Huberti H, Hayes W. Patellofemoral contact pressures. J Bone Joint Surg 1984;66A:715–724.

44. Huberti H, Hayes W, Stone J, Shybut G. Force ratios in the quadriceps tendon and the ligamentum patellae. J Orthop Res 1984;2:49–54.

45. Jorring K. Osteoarthritis of the hip. Acta Orthop Scand 1980;51:523–530.

46. Keblish PA. The lateral approach to the valgus knee. Clin Orthop 1991;271:52–62.

47. Kennedy WR, White RP. Unicompartmental arthroplasty of the knee: postoperative alignment and its influence on overall results. Clin Orthop 1987;221:278–285.

48. Keyes GW, Carr AJ, Miller RK, Goodfellow JW. The radiographic classification of medial gonarthrosis. Acta Orthop Scand 1992;63:497–501.

49. Knowlton RG, Katzenstein PL, Moskowitz RW, Weaver EJ, Malemud CJ, Pathria MN, Jimenez SA, Prockop DJ. Genetic linkage of a polymorphism in the type II procollagen gene (COL2A1) to primary osteoarthritis associated with mild chondrodysplasia. New Engl J Med 1990;322:526–530.

50. Laurin C, Levesque H, Dussault R, Labelle H, Peides J. The abnormal lateral patellofemoral angle: a diagnostic roentgenographic sign of recurrent patellar subluxation. J Bone Joint Surg 1978;60A:55–60.

51. Lawrence JS, Bremner JM, Bier F. Osteoarthrosis: prevalence in the population and relationship between symptoms and x-ray changes. Ann Rheum Dis 1966;25:1–24.

52. Li J, Wyss UP, Costigan PA, Deluzio KJ. An integrated procedure to assess knee joint kinematics and kinetics during gait, using an optoelectric system and standardized x-rays. J Biomed Eng 1993;15:392–400.

53. Maquet P. Advancement of the tibial tuberosity. Clin Orthop 1976;115:225–230.

54. Maquet P. The biomechanics of the knee and surgical possibilities of healing osteoarthritic knee joints. Clin Orthop 1980;146:102–110.

55. Markolf KL, Mensch JS, Anstiutz HC. Stiffness and laxity of the knee: contributions of the supporting structures—a quantitative in vitro study. J Bone Joint Surg 1976;58A:583–593.

56. McAlindon TE, Snow S, Cooper C, Dieppe PA. Radiographic patterns of osteoarthritis of the knee joint in the community: the importance of the patellofemoral joint. Ann Rheum Dis 1992;51:844–849.

57. McDermott AGP, Finkelstein JA, Farine I, Boynton EL, MacIntosh DL, Gross A. Distal femoral varus osteotomy for valgus deformity of the knee. J Bone Joint Surg 1988;70A:110–116.

58. Merchant A, Mercer R, Jacobsen R, Cool C. Roentgenographic analysis of patellofemoral congruence. J Bone Joint Surg 1974;56A:1391–96.

59. Mills OS, Hull ML. Rotational flexibility of the human knee due to varus/valgus and axial moments in vivo. J Biomech 1991;24:673–690.

60. Moreland JR, Bassett LW, Hanker GJ. Radiographic analysis of the axial alignment of the lower extremity. J Bone Joint Surg 1987;69A:745–749.

61. Moreland JR. Mechanics of failure in total knee arthroplasty. Clin Orthop 1988;226:49–64.

62. Morrey BF. Upper tibial osteotomy for secondary osteoarthritis of the knee. J Bone Joint Surg 1989;71B:554–559.

63. Mueller W. The knee: form function and ligament reconstruction. New York: Springer-Verlag, 1983.

64. Nakabayashi Y, Cooke TDV, Wevers HW, Griffin M. Bone hardness and histomorphometry of the distal femur. In: Transactions of the Combined Meeting of the Orthopaedic Research Societies of USA, Japan, and Canada, Oct 21–23, 1991, Banff, Alberta, Canada, 1991:278.

65. Noyes FR, Schipplein OD, Andriacchi TP, Saddemi SR, Weise M. The anterior cruciate-deficient knee with varus alignment. An analysis of gait adaptations and dynamic joint loadings. Am J Sports Med 1992;20:707–716.

66. Odenbring S. Osteotomy for medial gonarthrosis [Dissertation]. Lund, Sweden: University of Lund, 1991.

67. Odenbring S, Tjornstrand B, Egund E, Hagstedt B, Hovelius L, Lindstand A, Luxhoj T, Svanstrom A. Function after tibial osteotomy for medial gonarthrosis below age 50 years. Acta Orthop Scand 1989;60:527–531.

68. Olmstead TG, Wevers HW, Bryant JT, Gouw GJ. Effect of muscular activity on valgus/varus laxity and stiffness of the knee. J Biomech 1986;19:565–577.

69. Prodromos CC, Andriacchi TP, Galante JO. A relationship between gait and clinical changes following high tibial osteotomy. J Bone Joint Surg 1985;67A:1188–1194.

70. Rudan J, Simurda MAS, Cooke TDV. The influence of joint line obliquity on high tibial osteotomy correction. In: Proceedings of the annual meeting of the American Academy of Orthopaedic Surgeons, Atlanta, GA, 1988.

71. Shoji H, Insall J. High tibial osteotomy for osteoarthritis of the knee with valgus deformity. J Bone Joint Surg 1973;55A:963–973.

72. Siu D, Cooke TDV, Broekhoven LD, Lam M, Fisher B, Saunders G, Challis TW. A standardized technique for lower limb radiography: practice, applications and error analysis. J Invest Radiol 1991;26:71–77.

73. Sokoloff L. Aging and degenerative disease affecting cartilage. In: Hall BK, ed. Cartilage, Vol 3, Biomedical aspects. New York: Academic Press, 1983:109–141.

74. Wevers HW, Siu D, Cooke TDV. A quantitative method of assessing malalignment and joint space loss of the human knee. J Biomed Eng 1982;4:319–324.

75. White SH, Ludkowski PF, Goodfellow JW. Anteromedial osteoarthritis of the knee. J Bone Joint Surg 1991;73B:582–586.

76. Woltring HJ, Huiskes R, De Lange A, Veldpaus FE. Finite centroid and helical axis estimation from noisy landmark measurements in the study of human joint kinematics. J Biomechan 1985;18:379–389.

77. Yoshioka Y, Cooke TDV. Femoral anteversion: assessment based on function axes. J Orthop Res 1987;5:86–91.

78. Yoshioka Y, Siu D, Cooke TDV. The anatomy and functional axes of the femur. J Bone Joint Surg 1987;69A:873–880.

51

Nonsurgical Treatment of Knee Arthritis

Agustín Escalante

General Measures
  Education
  Weight Loss
  Psychological Aspects
Nonpharmacologic Treatments

Physical Measures
  Exercise and Physical Therapy
Pharmacologic Treatment
  Topical Therapy
  Nonprescription Drugs

Aspirin and Salicylate Compounds
Nonsteroidal Antiinflammatory
  Drugs
Perioperative Management of the
  Patient on Aspirin or NSAIDS

Systemic Corticosteroids
Disease Modifying Therapy
Conclusion

In most instances, surgery lies at the end of the road in the management of arthritis of the knee. The purpose of this chapter is to provide a tour of the stops along that road, so that the orthopaedic surgeon can become familiar with the many interventions available before the final destination of knee surgery. The roadmap begins with general measures, which include patient education, weight loss, and psychological factors. The next section describes nonpharmacologic treatments such as heat and cold modalities, physical therapy, and exercise. The final portion is an overview of the pharmacologic measures available to treat the different types of arthritis that can affect the knee. Each of these sections could itself be the subject of a textbook. Therefore, this chapter should be viewed as an initial guide, and the references should be consulted for more in-depth discussion.

General Measures

The therapeutic value of the interventions described below in the treatment of arthritis of the knee or any other joint is well established in the literature. Unfortunately, since some of these measures require the investment of time on the part of the physician or allied health personnel, they are often neglected, denying the patient an opportunity for benefit. To complicate matters further, many of the general measures described in this chapter are not directly reimbursed by third-party payers, which places an additional obstacle to their incorporation in routine practice.

Education

The best way to begin the management of arthritis of any joint is to educate the patient (1). This should include information about the diagnosis and nature of the underlying arthropathy as well as about the prognosis and treatment.

A diagnosis of arthritis elicits a number of anxieties and uncertainties in the patient. Questions about pain, deformities, disability, medications, and surgery are often articulated, as are inquiries about types of food to avoid or include in the diet, exercises that may be beneficial or harmful, and travel. If these questions and uncertainties are addressed early in the physician-patient interaction, the patient will be saved from many anxious and sleepless nights.

The value of patient education in the management of arthritis is well established in terms of better understanding of the disease (2) and of decreased disability, pain, and depression (3). Some examples of specific educational interventions for patients with knee arthritis include training in joint protection measures. Simply using high stools for activities requiring prolonged standing, avoiding high-impact activities such as running or jumping, and incorporating rest periods into the daily routine may bring about a decrease in pain and other symptoms. For individuals with chondromalacia patellae, avoiding positions in which the knees are flexed for prolonged periods may have remarkable therapeutic benefits.

It is acknowledged that patient education is time consuming and often difficult, particularly with patients who have limited education, poor English skills, or different cultural values. Excellent resources exist to assist the physician with this difficult but important therapeutic intervention. The Arthritis Foundation is the largest and best-known nonprofit organization that focuses on patient education, and it also funds research in arthritis. It has produced brochures for patient use (available at nominal cost), and it also organizes patient support groups, lectures, and many other activities to increase patients' knowledge about their disease.

Weight Loss

Although there is a relationship between obesity and osteoarthritis of the knee (4, 5), controversy persists about which of these two factors plays the primary role (6). In either case, excessive weight has a detrimental effect on established arthritis of the lower extremities or spine (7). Recent data from the Framingham study has provided further evidence of the deleterious effects of obesity on the knees and has shown that weight loss decreases the risk of developing symptomatic knee osteoarthritis (8). This should reinforce efforts of physicians to motivate patients to lose weight. Perhaps more important for the orthopaedist is the adverse effect of obesity on surgical access to the joints. Obesity has been considered a risk factor for early postoperative complications such as thrombophlebitis (9) and for late complications such as loosening and failure of joint prostheses of the hip (10) and knee (11). In spite of a recent study suggesting that obesity does not place patients at increased risk for complications (12), it is good practice to encourage patients with arthritis of the knee to lose weight. This will have a significant therapeutic effect and will result in improved surgical technique and better results. On occasion the only successful stimulus for weight loss in an obese patient is making it a prerequisite to undergoing joint surgery.

Psychological Aspects

The cardinal symptom of arthritis is pain, an eminently subjective experience. Many factors beyond the pathologic changes in a joint are involved in the genesis of this complex symptom. Joint pain correlates more strongly with psychological factors than with the radiographic severity of arthritis (13, 14). It is important to keep this information in mind when considering the patient as a surgical candidate. When the magnitude and persistence of the complaints are out of proportion to the physical findings or radiographic appearance, the likelihood that a surgical intervention will improve the symptoms is diminished. The more difficult question is how to manage these individuals, and here the importance of a good physician-patient relationship cannot be overemphasized. Prompt referral to a mental health professional may save everyone from a painful and unpleasant experience.

Nonpharmacologic Treatments

Physical Measures

These include a number of modalities used to deliver physical agents, most commonly heat or cold, to the joint. What follows is a brief overview of these modalities. For more in-depth coverage, the reader should refer to several excellent recent reviews (15–17). These interventions are believed to work primarily through reflex pathways involving free nerve endings, vasodilation, and other mechanisms.

Heat Modalities

The application of heat is a time-tried method of producing analgesia, decreasing muscle spasms, and increasing range of motion. Its mechanism of action is complex and may involve free nerve endings and the gamma fibers of the muscle spindles, as well as the physicochemical properties of collagen fibers. However, although it is effective in providing symptomatic relief,

heat does nothing for the underlying progression of the disease (18).

Several modalities for applying heat exist: superficial heat may be delivered by hot packs or simple compresses, heat lamps, and hydrotherapy. Superficial heat has demonstrated systemic effects on the circulation, increasing the cardiac output and metabolic rate. However, it does not penetrate the deep structures and does not raise the intraarticular temperature. In spite of these shortcomings, superficial heat modalities are in widespread use, primarily for treating minor musculoskeletal complaints.

Hydrotherapy consists of the use of warm or hot water baths, usually by immersion of the involved extremity or the entire body. An air blower or whirlpool is commonly added, which can enhance the beneficial effects of this modality. Hydrotherapy is quite beneficial, because it not only delivers superficial heat, but also provides a nearly weightless environment for mobilizing joints against minimum resistance. In addition, the warm bath provides a relaxing and soothing effect on the patient that can be very beneficial.

There are a number of methods that can efficiently deliver heat to deep structures. In order of increasing depth of reach these are shortwave, microwave, and ultrasound. Shortwave and microwaves are capable of reaching only the superficial muscle layers. Ultrasound is the only true deep heat modality. Its absorption by bone makes it particularly useful in heating joints, and it has been shown to be beneficial in relieving flexion contractures. It is safe to use in the presence of metallic implants, but there is evidence that methyl methacrylate, used to cement joint prostheses, may selectively absorb energy from ultrasound and melt (19).

The contraindications to heat modalities are few and intuitive: great caution should be exercised in delivering heat to individuals with impaired sensation or to areas where circulation is compromised. Thus, prior to applying heat to the knee, a thorough examination of pulses and sensory function should be performed. In addition, areas of hemorrhage, edema, severe inflammation, or tumor should not receive heat modalities (20). Patients with pacemakers should not receive treatment with microwaves or short waves.

Cold

Cold is usually applied by means of ice packs or by coolant sprays containing ethyl chloride or fluoromethane. It is particularly useful following acute injuries or hemarthrosis because of its vasoconstrictive effect. In chronic arthritis, it has the metabolic effect of slowing down the activity of collagenase (21) and probably other destructive enzymes. One study has shown that cold applications are better tolerated than heat and produce greater relief of pain and stiffness (22). However, a long-term effect on the development of synovitis should not be expected (23). Coolant sprays of ethyl chloride or fluoromethane are also useful means of inducing analgesia and are widely used as local anesthetics prior to arthrocentesis and in manipulation therapy.

Other Modalities

Various forms of electrical currents are widely used for analgesia in chronic painful conditions. Transcutaneous electrical nerve stimulation (TENS) has been used for treatment of low back pain, although its effectiveness has been questioned (24). This modality has limited application in treating arthritis of the knee.

Exercise and Physical Therapy

The deleterious effect of muscle weakness on knee symptoms is well known. In cases of patellofemoral pain syndrome, one of the most beneficial therapeutic interventions may be strengthening exercises for the knee extensor musculature (25). This improves patellofemoral tracking and greatly relieves pain. Increased muscle strength also has value in other types of arthritis of the knee. In patients with knee osteoarthritis, a fitness walking program can improve functional status without increasing knee pain (26).

The role of physical therapy is also paramount in maintaining range of motion and in preventing or relieving flexion contractures (27). Well-trained physical therapists are valuable assets in the management of patients with musculoskeletal problems. They are able to assist with the evaluation of functional problems, gait, transfers, and the need for assistive devices. In addition, they can implement an exercise program to be carried out at home or can work with the patient in the clinic or hospital with active or passive range-of-motion exercises.

Pharmacologic Treatment

The majority of patients with arthritis of the knee can be managed successfully without surgery. The cornerstone of nonsurgical treatment is provided by pharmacologic measures. Thus, a working knowledge of the pharmacologic agents available to treat arthritis is advisable for all physicians and surgeons who treat musculoskeletal disorders.

The pharmacologic agents available for treating arthritis of the knee can be classified as follows: nonprescription drugs; the salicylates and nonsteroidal antiinflammatory drugs (NSAIDs); corticosteroids, systemic and intraarticular; and, for chronic inflammatory causes of knee arthritis, the so-called remittive agents. A discussion of each of these categories follows.

Topical Therapy

The topical therapy of arthritis of the knee and other joints has been restricted until recently to liniments and ointments containing salicylic acid and various other counterirritants. The mechanism of action of these preparations consists primarily of inducing a mild cutaneous hyperemia, which secondarily produces a sensation of warmth. It is also possible that a small amount of the salicylic acid could be absorbed systemically to produce an antiinflammatory effect. A large number of preparations are available over the counter, and patients commonly use these products without the knowledge of the physician.

A newly available drug is capsaicin, which has been introduced in the United States for topical treatment of various painful conditions. This chemical compound (trans-8-methyl-N-vanillyl-6-nonenamide) is a natural alkaloid derived from the common pepper and is responsible for its "hot" flavor. The mechanism of action of capsaicin is believed to be through depletion from sensory nerve endings of the peptide neurotransmitter known as substance P and inhibition of its reaccumulation (28). Capsaicin has been shown to be safe and effective in the treatment of painful osteoarthritis of the hands (29) and of the knees (30). Patients should be warned of a burning sensation that accompanies the initiation of treatment. They should also avoid accidentally introducing the ointment into conjunctival and mucous membranes. This drug is a promising addition to the armamentarium for conservative treatment of arthritis of the knee and other joints.

Nonprescription Drugs

A number of preparations that are effective in relieving the symptoms of arthritis can be purchased in the United States without a physician's prescription. These products most frequently contain acetaminophen, aspirin, or, more recently, ibuprofen in various proportions. Acetaminophen is an analgesic and antipyretic widely available throughout the world. Its efficacy is well recognized, and it may be equivalent to NSAIDs in treating the pain of rheumatoid arthritis (RA) (31). A survey of British patients with RA revealed that more than half of them were taking simple analgesics such as acetaminophen for relief of pain, and the majority of these were doing so without the knowledge of their doctor (32). This suggests that patients with arthritis view pain relief as one of the most important goals of therapy, a fact often overlooked by their physicians. Thus, physicians who treat arthritis of the knee and other joints should inquire about their patients' use of nonprescription drugs and should keep in mind the effectiveness of these relatively safe and readily available agents in treating arthritic symptoms.

Aspirin and Salicylate Compounds

The salicylates have a venerable tradition in the treatment of rheumatism (33). These drugs have potent antiinflammatory actions, mediated in part by inhibition of prostaglandin synthesis (34). Other mechanisms are probably involved as well (35), a suspicion raised by the fact that low doses of aspirin can suppress prostaglandin synthesis, but much higher doses are needed to suppress inflammation (36). It is useful to separate aspirin, or acetylsalicylic acid, from the nonacetylated salicylates such as salicylic acid, choline trisalicylate, and salsalate. Aspirin irreversibly inhibits cyclooxygenase by acetylation (37), whereas the nonacetylated salicylates are weak cyclooxygenase inhibitors (38). This seemingly subtle pharmacodynamic difference has significant implications for the toxicities of these agents. Although it is not clear whether the therapeutic effects of aspirin and the NSAIDs are related to the ability of these compounds to inhibit prostaglandin synthesis, there is definite evidence that some of their toxicities result from their effects on prostaglandins. Thus, the nonacetylated salicylates have considerably less gastric, renal, or platelet toxicity than do aspirin or other NSAIDs (39).

The analgesic and antipyretic effects of aspirin occur at doses of 2.5 to 3.5 g daily. For antiinflammatory effects to take place, it is necessary to use higher dose ranges. A practical approach is to start at 2.4 g daily (two 300-mg tablets four times daily), and then gradually raise the dose by one daily tablet each week. The dose is raised until tinnitus occurs, or until the serum level reaches 20 to 30 mg/dl. Attempts to start at a higher dose or to raise the dose more rapidly are more likely to result in gastrointestinal toxicity (40). A number of strategies to avoid gastric toxicity have been attempted with variable success, including the use of enteric coated preparations, or the use of preparations containing antacids. Alternatively, H.MDSD/2 blockers, omeprazole, sucralfate, or a prostaglandin analog such as misoprostol can be used to treat or perhaps even prevent gastrointestinal toxicity from aspirin and other NSAIDs (41).

The irreversible effect of aspirin on cyclooxygenase has relevance in the preoperative evaluation. Abnormalities in platelet function can be demonstrated up to 10 days after the administration of aspirin, and in some instances this could result in excessive operative blood loss. One strategy to avoid excessive bleeding during surgery is to switch from aspirin to one of the nonacetylated salicylates such as salsalate, which does not have an antiplatelet effect, 2 weeks prior to surgery (42, 43). This avoids the preoperative exacerbation of symptoms that would result if aspirin were simply discontinued without adding another drug.

Nonsteroidal Antiinflammatory Drugs

NSAIDs enjoy widespread use in the therapy of rheumatic diseases and are indicated in the treatment of nearly all inflammatory and noninflammatory arthritides of the knee. These chemically diverse drugs share many pharmacologic properties, some of which are discussed above. One approach to classification is based on the chemical from which they are derived (Table 51.1) (44). However, it is more practical to remember their pharmacokinetic characteristics, such as half-life and relative toxicities. It is also important to know whether a given drug is available as a generic, given the substantial impact of this factor on cost.

NSAIDs can be used interchangeably in treating the various causes of knee arthritis, as there is no evidence that one agent is superior to another for any specific disease. For example, when faced with a patient with osteoarthritis of the knee, the choice of NSAID depends on the cost of the drug, its half-life (which determines the number of doses per day required to maintain therapeutic blood levels), its relative toxicity, the potential for drug interactions, and the existence of concomitant illnesses, rather than on a purported osteoarthritis specificity. Thus, for the indigent patient without health insurance in whom cost is a significant factor, a generic drug such as

Table 51.1. Chemical Classification of Nonsteroidal Anti-inflammatory Drugs[a]

Chemical Groups	Generic Name	Trade Name
Arylcarboxilic acids		
Salicylic acids	Aspirin	
	Salsalate	Disalcid
	Choline magnesium trisalycilate	Trilisate
	Diflunisal	Dolobid
Anthranilic acids	Mefenamic acid	Ponstel
	Meclofenamic acid	Meclomen
Aryclcanoic acids		
Arylacetic acids	Diclofenac	Voltaren
Arylpropionic	Ibuprofen	Motrin, Advil, etc.
	Ketoprofen	Orudis
	Flurbiprofen	Ansaid
	Naproxen	Naprosyn
	Fenoprofen	Nalfon
Heteroarylacetic	Tolmetin	Tolectin
Indole/indene acetic acids	Indomethacin	Indocin
	Sulindac	Clinoril
Enolic acids		
Pyrazolidinediones Oxyphenbutazones	Phenylbutazone	Butazolidin
Oxicams	Piroxicam	Feldene

[a]Modified from Dudley-Hart F, Huskisson EC. Non-steroidal anti-inflammatory drugs. Current status and rationale for therapeutic use. Drugs 1984;27:232-255.

indomethacin or ibuprofen would be the first choice. In the patient with peptic ulcer disease or a history of gastric intolerance to NSAIDs, it may be best to avoid any of these agents in favor of a nonacetylated salicylate such as salsalate of choline magnesium trisalicylate.

All of these agents, regardless of the chemical group to which they belong, have the property of *reversibly* inhibiting cyclooxygenase. In contrast, aspirin *irreversibly* inhibits cyclooxygenase, while the effect of the nonacetylated salicylates on this enzyme is weak and may not be clinically significant. Cyclooxygenase inhibition explains the most frequent side effects of NSAIDs. Among these, the one that is of the most immediate concern to the knee surgeon is the antiplatelet effect, which can potentially result in excessive bleeding during surgery. The normal process of platelet adhesion begins with the production of prostaglandins by cyclooxygenase. Interference with this process by NSAIDs results in a reversible decrease in platelet adhesiveness (45), the duration of which depends on the half-life of each drug. Normalization of platelet function will occur earlier with drugs such as indomethacin, tolmetin, or ibuprofen, which have short half-lives. When a patient who takes one of these drugs faces surgery, an antiplatelet effect can be avoided by withholding the drug for as little as 24 hours preceding surgery. Longer-acting drugs such as piroxicam or naproxen may require up to 1 week for platelet function to normalize.

Gastric toxicity results from the prostaglandin-dependent ability of the gastric mucosa to impede the backflow of hydrogen ions into the gastric epithelium. When this ability is disrupted, acid injury to the mucosa results (46). Some of the renal effects of NSAIDs are also due to prostaglandin inhibition. In conditions of low cardiac output and low renal perfusion, the glomerular circulation may depend on the vasodilatory effects of prostaglandins to maintain filtration pressure. If prostaglandin synthesis is inhibited in these conditions, a decrease in glomerular filtration follows, with concomitant azotemia (47).

Perioperative Management of the Patient on Aspirin or NSAIDs

The most important surgical issue regarding aspirin or NSAIDs is the effect of these drugs on platelet function, which could interfere with hemostasis during surgery. As discussed above, in the case of aspirin, platelet inhibition lasts for the lifetime of the platelet. Thus, aspirin should be discontinued 2 weeks preoperatively to avoid an antiplatelet effect. For the NSAIDs, the interval between the last dose and surgery should depend on the half-life of the drug (Table 51.2). The question that naturally follows is how to avoid an arthritis flare-up between the time aspirin or one of the long-acting drugs is discontinued and the time of surgery. One option is to substitute a long-acting agent for a short-acting one, and simply discontinue it 24 hours preoperatively. A better choice is to replace aspirin or a long-acting NSAID with a nonacetylated salicylate. As discussed above, these drugs lack an antiplatelet effect and yet are still effective anti-inflammatories.

Systemic Corticosteroids

The discovery of corticosteroids is arguably the most significant development during the 20th century for the treatment of rheumatoid arthritis and other rheumatic diseases (48). These powerful antiinflammatory agents have brought relief to millions of arthritis patients and are prescribed extensively by physicians. Systemically administered, they continue to have a role in the management of all of the inflammatory arthropathies, especially rheumatoid arthritis. Following their introduction in the late 1940s and early 1950s, there was an initial wave of popularity spurred by the mistaken impression that they had a curative effect. It did not take long to realize that these agents were not curative and that when they were used in large doses their side effects were substantial. Two decades of disfavor followed, during which many physicians developed a philosophy of avoiding corticosteroids in RA at all costs (49).

Corticosteroids are generally regarded as having no effect on the progression of bone destruction in RA. This impression stems from early studies that compared prednisolone with aspirin and found that there was no difference between the two drugs in the occurrence of erosions (50, 51). This has remained in the minds of most physicians, despite later studies by the same researchers that concluded that prednisolone does indeed have a suppressive effect on bone erosions (52, 53). More recent experience has shown that, used judiciously, corticosteroids may be among the most valuable drugs available to treat RA (49, 54). A single daily dose of 7.5 mg or less has beneficial effects that are difficult to achieve with any other drug. This is manifested by improved mobility and participation in social activities, and may make the difference between employment and disability. Systemic corticosteroids are commonly used at the beginning of treatment while awaiting the effects of slow-acting drugs, and are essential in the management of vasculitis and other severe systemic complications of RA.

Systemic corticosteroids are less effective in the management of the seronegative spondyloarthropathies (55), although uncontrolled studies have suggested that intravenous supraphysiologic doses of methylprednisolone, the so-called "pulse" therapy, may result in long-term improvement in patients with ankylosing spondylitis (56, 57). In spite of this, "pulse" therapy should be considered experimental while more definitive information is obtained.

While there may be some debate about the beneficial effects of corticosteroids in the treatment of RA and other forms of arthritis of the knee, the side effects of glucocorticoids are indisputable. High doses of corticosteroids for prolonged periods of time produce centripetal obesity (the so-called *Cushingoid syndrome*), hirsutism, glucose intolerance, hypertension, cataracts, depression, insomnia, and steroid psychosis. Furthermore, and of particular interest to the orthopaedic surgeon, the general catabolic effect of these agents on the skin and connective tissue may impair the healing of surgical wounds. Glucocorticoids, through their immunosuppressive effects, also produce a predisposition to infections (58). The osteoporosis that accompanies prolonged therapy with corticosteroids may be more debilitating than the underlying disease itself (59). Finally,

Table 51.2. Dosage of Selected NSAIDs, in Order of Increasing Half-Life

Drug	Dose range (mg/day)	Half-Life (hr)
Diclofenac	100-200	1.25
Ibuprofen	1,500-3,200	1.7
Ketoprofen	150-300	1.7
Tolmetin	600-2,000	2
Fenoprofen	600-3,200	2.7
Meclofenamate	150-400	3
Indomethacin	75-200	4.5
Flurbiprofen	200-400	5
Etodolac	300-600	6.7
Aspirin	1,000-6.000	4-15
Salsalate	1,500-5,000	4-15
Choline magnesium trisalicylate	1,500-4,000	4-15
Diflunisal	500-1,500	7-15
Naproxen	500-1500	13
Sulindac	300-400	16
Piroxicam	10-20	38
Phenylbutazone	200-400	72

these drugs are the most common predisposing cause of avascular necrosis of bone (60). Thus, the decision to use corticosteroids should not be taken lightly, and should be made only when the severity of the underlying disease clearly outweighs the risks that accompany their use.

Perioperative Management of the Patient Receiving Systemic Corticosteroids

Systemically administered corticosteroids in moderate to high doses result in suppression of the hypothalamic-pituitary-adrenal axis (61). This may impair the physiologic increase in the production of ACTH and cortisol in response to the stress of surgery (62, 63). There is a possibility that if such a response is impaired, vascular collapse may occur with potentially disastrous consequences (64). Fortunately, such occurrences can be prevented simply by providing the patient with an exogenous source of corticosteroids equivalent to the amount produced by the normal adrenals under conditions of maximum stress. This amount is equivalent to approximately 300 mg of hydrocortisone intravenously, which can be administered in the 24-hour period during which the surgery takes place. The day following surgery, the preoperative dose of corticosteroids is resumed. Detailed guidelines for perioperative steroid prophylaxis are provided in Table 51.3 (65).

Intraarticular Corticosteroids

The introduction of therapeutic substances directly into the joints by arthrocentesis is a highly effective and safe method of treatment. A number of agents have been tried with variable success (66, 67), but corticosteroids are by far the most often used. Soluble and microcrystalline preparations are both effective, but the soluble preparations are quickly absorbed, and their effect is brief. Thus the microcrystalline preparations are preferred. Of these, triamcinolone hexacetonide is the least soluble and has the most prolonged effect.

The indications for intraarticular corticosteroid injections into the knee include any persistent inflammation

of the joint, provided that infection has been ruled out. In particular, this mode of therapy should be considered in rheumatoid arthritis patients whose disease activity is more prominent in the knees than in other joints. In such patients, one or both knees can be injected simultaneously. This approach can be beneficial even in cases with prominent inflammation in other joints, because a systemic effect is commonly observed in addition to the local effect. During the induction of disease modifying (remittive) therapy, one or more intraarticular injections of corticosteroids can be given as a means of providing a "bridge" while awaiting the effect of slower-acting drugs such as gold or methotrexate. Intraarticular corticosteroids can also be of great benefit in the rehabilitation setting in the patient with prominent knee synovitis with decreased range of motion, who has lost the ability to walk or transfer independently.

Intraarticular corticosteroids are also effective in osteoarthritis of the knee (68, 69), although in this setting, where mechanical factors may be more important than inflammation in the generation of symptoms, improvement may be short-lived. Virtually any other inflammatory arthropathy of the knee has the potential to benefit from intraarticular therapy, including gout, calcium pyrophosphate dihydrate deposition disease, the seronegative spondyloarthropathies, psoriatic arthritis, and systemic lupus erythematosus.

The contraindications to intraarticular therapy are similar to the contraindications to introducing hypodermic needles into other parts of the body: sites where the overlying skin is obviously infected should be avoided, and special precautions should be taken in bacteremic patients. Likewise, injection of corticosteroids into septic joints should probably be avoided. Patients on systemic anticoagulation who require arthrocentesis should be observed carefully following the procedure. However, in the author's experience, hemarthrosis has not resulted from carefully performed injections with a narrow gauge needle in these patients. In patients with coagulopathies, there is a real risk of inducing or worsening a hemarthrosis, so these patients may require coagulation factor replacement prior to arthrocentesis. Patients with badly damaged or destroyed joints may not benefit from intraarticular corticosteroids, unless there is prominent inflammation. In the end-stage joint, if one injection results in short-lived improvement there is no reason to perform repeated injections, as this has been said to result in a Charcot-like picture and may increase the risk of iatrogenic infection.

Excellent reviews of the techniques for arthrocentesis of the knee and other joints exist (70, 71). A careful aseptic technique should be followed, although this does not contraindicate performing the procedure in an office setting (Fig. 51.1). A review of over 200,000 injections in 8,000 patients performed under these conditions demonstrated that infections are extremely rare (72). Most physicians who perform this type of therapy customarily mix the corticosteroid preparation with a local anesthetic such as lidocaine or procaine to provide immediate pain relief. Caution should be used with local anesthetics that contain preservatives such as

---

Table 51.3. Guidelines for Corticosteroid Management in the Patient Undergoing Knee Surgery

Extent of Surgery	Hydrocortisone Dose IV or IM
Total knee arthroplasty	100 mg on call to surgery 100 mg every 8 hr for 24 hr Resume preoperative dose on morning after surgery
Other procedures requiring arthrotomy	100 mg on call to surgery 50 mg every 8 hr for 24 hr Resume preoperative dose in morning after surgery
Arthroscopy	100 mg at the time of surgery Resume preoperative dose on morning after surgery

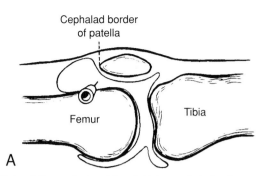

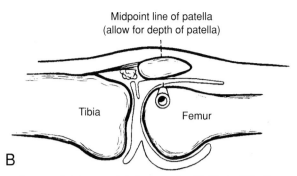

Figure 51.1. Arthrocentesis of the right knee. **A,** Lateral approach to the suprapatellar pouch. **B,** Medial approach under the patella. (Reproduced with permission from Gatter RA. Arthrocentesis tech- nique and intrasynovial therapy. In: McClarty DJ, Koopman WJ. Arthritis and allied conditions. Philadelphia: Lea & Febiger, 1993:712.)

methylparaben, phenol, or others, as these preserva- tives may cause flocculation of the corticosteroid crys- tals, which could explain the finding of corticosteroid "chalk" in some joints (73).

Complications of corticosteroid injections into joints are infrequent. As mentioned above, reports of large numbers of intraarticular injections have described rare infectious complications. Crystalline corticosteroid can cause a corticosteroid-crystal synovitis. Fortunately, this occurs infrequently and is self limited (74).

Disease Modifying Therapy

This designation refers to pharmacologic treatment aimed at modifying the long-term course of the disease in question. In contrast, the modalities discussed above aim to produce an immediate effect on inflammation. Disease modifying antirheumatic drugs (*DMARDs*) are also known as *remittive drugs*, or *slow-acting anti- rheumatic drugs*. Both of these terms reflect the attrib- uted effects and time course of action of these medica- tions. DMARD therapy is used to treat rheumatic diseases that have a systemic inflammatory nature, and this section is included in this chapter in view of the fact that all of these diseases may affect the knees. For each disease, therapy is slightly different; therefore, each disease is discussed separately, beginning with RA, for which DMARD therapy is most developed.

Rheumatoid Arthritis

The concept of DMARD therapy originated with at- tempts to treat rheumatoid arthritis. The oldest of these modalities is chrysotherapy or gold-salt treatment. Other DMARD drugs include D-penicillamine, anti- malarials, and sulfasalazine. Azathioprine and methotrexate are more accurately described as im- munosuppressive agents but are included here in view of the fact that their indications are similar to the other DMARD agents. Drugs such as cyclophosphamide and other alkylating agents and cyclosporine have been studied, but their use is much less widespread. They are reserved for special circumstances and are not dis- cussed here.

Gold Chrysotherapy may be given parenterally or orally. Gold sodium thiomalate and aurothioglucose are

Table 51.4.   Disease Modifying Antirheumatic Drugs

Drug	Indications[a]	Effect on Wound Healing
Gold	RA, PsA	None
Anti-malarials	RA, SLE	None
D-penicillamine	RA	Suspected (76)
Sulfasalazine	RA, AS, Reiter's	None
Methotrexate	RA, PsA, AS, Reiter's	Suspected (90, 91)
Azathioprine	RA, PsA, SLE	Suspected (86)

[a]RA, rheumatoid arthritis; SLE, systemic lupus erythematosus; AS, ankylosing spondylitis; PsA, psoriatic arthritis.

commonly used parenteral preparations, whereas aura- nofin is prescribed for oral administration (75). Par- enteral gold is administered by intramuscular injection weekly or less often according to the therapeutic re- sponse. Initially, a test dose of 10 mg is given to identify hypersensitive patients. If the drug is well tolerated, the dose is raised the next week to 25 mg, and then to the maintenance dose of 50 mg weekly. A response to gold is rarely observed before 6 to 8 weeks of continuous therapy have elapsed, and may it take up to 9 months (76). Common toxicities include rashes, mucosal ulcera- tions, hemocytopenias, and renal side effects. These can be detected early through laboratory monitoring, which should include a complete blood count and a urinalysis, done weekly at the initiation of treatment. Later, if the pattern of response allows it, the frequency of monitor- ing can be relaxed to biweekly or monthly. No concerns have been expressed in the literature about effects of these drugs on wound healing.

D-Penicillamine D-Penicillamine is very similar to the gold compounds in terms of its pharmacodynamics and time course of action, as well as its toxicity spec- trum. It is administered orally at doses starting at 250 mg daily, which is raised by 250 mg every 2 to 3 months until a dose of 750 to 1000 mg daily is reached (77). Toxic effects include dermatitis, hemocytopenias, and proteinuria (78). Rare side effects include autoimmune phenomena such as myasthenia gravis, drug-induced lupus, and polymyositis. Laboratory monitoring is indicated at each patient visit, which should be at least monthly and should include a complete blood count and urinalysis. Since D-penicillamine has the property of inhibiting the formation of disulfide bonds that cross-link collagen chains, a theoretical concern has been raised about its potential for interfering with wound healing. One uncontrolled study found that wound healing is slightly delayed among patients receiving D-penicillamine, to an extent similar to that observed among patients receiving corticosteroids (79). However, pending more definitive studies, at the moment there is no justification for withholding D-penicillamine preoperatively.

Antimalarials The most often used of these agents in the United States is hydroxychloroquine, although chloroquine is also effective. The dose of hydroxychloroquine should not exceed 400 mg daily, or 6.5 mg/kg (80), because with higher doses the incidence of retinotoxicity increases substantially (81). This type of ocular toxicity is due to the deposition of the drug in the pigment layers of the retina (82). The deposits can be detected by ophthalmologic examination before any detectable vision loss occurs. Thus, all patients in whom antimalarial therapy is being considered should have a baseline eye examination by an ophthalmologist and follow-up examinations every 6 months thereafter while taking the drug. The drug should be discontinued immediately at the first sign of retinal deposits. There is no evidence that these agents interfere with wound healing.

Sulfasalazine Sulfasalazine has been more popular in Europe than in the United States, although several recent studies have boosted its popularity in this country (83, 84). The usual dosage is 500 mg four times daily, with a maximum dose of 3000 mg daily. Toxicity most often occurs in the gastrointestinal tract with nausea and vomiting (85). Rashes and hematologic problems appear to be less frequent than with other DMARD agents (86).

Azathioprine Azathioprine, a purine analog, is a powerful immunosuppressant (87) that is effective in reducing inflammation in RA (88). Evidence of a true DMARD effect is weak, and its onset of action is faster than those of the drugs mentioned above. The usual starting dose in RA is 50 mg by mouth daily and can be increased up to 150 mg daily. Major toxicities are bone marrow suppression and gastrointestinal side effects. Laboratory monitoring should include a complete blood count, performed at least monthly, and transaminase levels, determined every 4 to 6 months. Preliminary data has suggested that a slight increase in the incidence of postoperative wound complications may occur among patients with rheumatoid arthritis taking this drug (89). Thus, it may be prudent to discontinue the drug 1 to 2 weeks preoperatively.

Methotrexate Methotrexate is a folic acid antagonist that has potent antineoplastic and immunosuppressive effects. Its introduction for the treatment of rheumatoid arthritis has been a major development in the therapy of this disease, and the drug has enjoyed great popularity since the mid-1980s (90). The drug is administered orally or by intramuscular or subcutaneous injection, in doses starting at 5 or 7.5 mg weekly,

increasing gradually over 6 weeks to 15 to 17.5 mg/week (91). The therapeutic effect of methotrexate becomes evident 3 to 4 weeks after initiation of therapy, which is faster than gold, penicillamine, or the antimalarials. By the same token, a flare of disease follows within a similar interval after stopping the drug. This time course of effect has been believed to reflect its strong antiinflammatory properties, but the evidence of a true DMARD effect is controversial. The major dose-limiting toxicity is gastrointestinal, but bone marrow suppression also occurs. An additional toxicity that has been emphasized in the literature is hepatotoxicity. Thus the drug is contraindicated in alcohol users and in individuals with preexisting liver damage. Laboratory monitoring should include monthly complete blood counts and liver function tests (92).

Perioperative Management of the Patient Taking DMARD Agents At the present time, there is no evidence in the literature that gold, the antimalarials, or sulfasalazine results in an increase in the incidence of postoperative complications. As mentioned above, D-penicillamine may cause slightly delayed wound healing (76), but the clinical significance of this observation is not clear, nor is it known if withholding the drug will correct the problem. In the case of methotrexate, which has definite immunosuppressive effects, retrospective studies have suggested an increased risk of postoperative infections (93, 94), while others have not (89, 95, 96). The preliminary observation of an increased risk of wound complications with azathioprine is also of concern (89). All of these reports are of great interest and have important implications for those who care for patients undergoing reconstructive joint surgery. At issue is the question of how long preoperatively a drug should be withheld to reduce the alleged risk of complications. If the drug is withheld too long preoperatively, surgery will take place in the middle of a flare of disease, whereas if it not withheld long enough, a risk of postoperative complications may exist. At the moment, there are no published prospective studies addressing these questions that could guide therapeutic decisions. Pending completion of more definitive studies, a prudent approach may be to withhold azathioprine or methotrexate 1 or 2 weeks before surgery and to resume treatment 1 week after surgery. Experience suggests that withholding either of these drugs any longer will result in an exacerbation of disease (97), which would probably interfere with postoperative rehabilitation. There is no evidence that any of the other DMARD agents should be withheld prior to surgery.

Seronegative Spondyloarthropathies

Ankylosing spondylitis, Reiter's syndrome, reactive arthritis, psoriatic arthritis, and inflammatory bowel disease-ssociated arthropathy are included under this heading. All of these inflammatory conditions can result in destructive knee pathology. DMARD therapy for these conditions is less developed than it is for RA. Generally, gold, penicillamine, and the antimalarials are ineffective in these diseases, and corticosteroids are also disappointing (98). A number of studies have shown that sulfasalazine is effective (99, 100). Uncontrolled evidence also suggests that methotrexate, alone or in combination with sulfasalazine, is effective in treating these conditions (101).

Crystal-induced Arthropathies

Gout and calcium pyrophosphate dihydrate (CPPD) deposition disease are considered here. DMARD therapy for gout, more accurately described as *uric acid lowering therapy*, consists primarily of the administration of probenecid or sulfinpyrazone as uricosurics, or the administration of the xanthine oxidase inhibitor allopurinol. Additionally, prophylactic administration of colchicine can prevent acute attacks of gout without lowering uric acid levels (102). This may be useful in preventing gouty attacks, which sometimes occur postoperatively.

Therapy for arthritis caused by crystals containing calcium is based on nonpharmacologic modalities, NSAIDs, and intraarticular corticosteroids. Other than addressing factors that predispose to CPPD deposition, such as hyperparathyroidism, no known therapy is effective in eliminating this type of crystal (103).

Conclusion

A variety of pharmacologic and nonpharmacologic interventions available for the treatment of arthritis affecting the knee have been discussed. With the exception of uric acid lowering drugs in gout, none of these modalities are curative. Thus, their beneficial effects are usually temporary and doomed to failure, with surgery lying at the end of the therapeutic road for a large proportion of patients. While the need for knee surgery reflects a failure in our understanding of the mechanisms and causes of knee arthritis, and consequently of the medical methods we use to treat it, the surgical solutions borne of this failure, and discussed elsewhere in this textbook, are among the highest achievements of medical technology.

References

1. Lorig K, Konkol L, Gonzalez V. Arthritis patient education: a review of the literature. Patient Educ Couns 1987;10:207–219.
2. Stross JK, Mikkelsen WM. Educating patients with osteoarthritis. J Rheumatol 1977;4:313–316.
3. Muller PD, Laville EA, Biddle AK, Lorig K. Efficacy of psychoeducational interventions on pain, depression and disability in people with arthritis: a metaanalysis. J Rheumatol 1987;14(Suppl 15):33–39.
4. Anderson JJ, Felson DT. Factors associated with osteoarthritis of the knee in the first National Health and Nutrition Examination Survey (HANES I): evidence for an association with overweight, race, and physical demands at work. Am J Epidemiol 1988;128:179–189.
5. Felson DT, Anderson JJ, Naimark A, Walker AM, Meenan RF. Obesity and knee osteoarthritis. The Framingham study. Ann Intern Med 1988;109:18–24.
6. van Sasse JL, Vandembroucke JP, van Romunde LK, Valkenburg HA. Osteoarthritis and obesity in the general population. A relationship calling for an explanation. J Rheumatol 1988;15:1152–1158.
7. Leach R, Baumgard S, Broom J. Obesity: its relationship to osteoarthritis of the knee. Clin Orthop 1973;93:271–273.
8. Felson DT, Zhang Y, Naimark A, Anderson JJ. Weight loss reduces the risk for symptomatic osteoarthritis in women: the Framingham study. Ann Intern Med 1992;116:535–539.
9. Hume M, Turner RH, Kuriakose TX, Surprenant J. Venous thrombosis after total hip replacement. Combined monitoring as a guide to diagnosis and treatment. J Bone Joint Surg 1976;58A:933–939.
10. Ranawat CS, Atkinson RE, Salvati EA, Wilson PD Jr. Conventional total hip arthroplasty for degenerative joint disease in patients between the ages of forty and sixty years. J Bone Joint Surg 1984;66A:745–752.
11. Insall JN, Ranawat CS, Aglietti P, Shine J. Total condylar knee prosthesis in gonarthrosis. A five- to nine-year follow-up of the first one hundred consecutive replacements. J Bone Joint Surg 1983;65A:619–628.
12. Stern SH, Insall JN. Total knee arthroplasty in obese patients. J Bone Joint Surg 1990;72A:1400–1404.
13. Salaffi F, Cavalieri F, Nolli M, Gerraccioli G. Analysis of disability in knee osteoarthritis. Relationship with age and psychological variables but not with radiographic score. J Rheumatol 1991;18:1581–1586.
14. Hadler NM. Knee pain is the malady—not osteoarthritis. Ann Intern Med 1992;116:598–599.
15. Lehman JF, Warren CJ, Scham SM. Therapeutic heat and cold. Clin Orthop 1974;99:207–245.
16. Lehman JF, DeLateur BJ. Diathermy and superficial heat and cold therapy. In: Kottke FJ, Stillwell GK, Lehman JF, eds. Krusen's handbook of physical medicine and rehabilitation. Philadelphia: WB Saunders, 1990.
17. Tepperman PS, Devlin M. Therapeutic heat and cold. A practitioner's guide. Postgrad Med 1983;73:69–76.
18. Mainardi CL, Walter JM, Spiegel PK, Goldkamp OG, Harris ED Jr. Rheumatoid arthritis: failure of daily heat therapy to affect its progression. Arch Phys Med Rehabil 1979;60:390–393.
19. Lehman JF, Warren CG, Wallace JE, Chan A. Ultrasound: considerations for use in the presence of prosthetic joints [Abstract]. Arch Phys Med Rehabil 1980;61:502.
20. Gerber LH. Rehabilitation of patients with rheumatic diseases. In: Kelley WN, Harris ED, Ruddy S, Sledge CB. Textbook of rheumatology. Philadelphia: WB Saunders, 1985.
21. Harris ED Jr, McCroskery JA. Influence of temperature and fibril stability on degradation of cartilage collagen by rheumatoid synovial collagenase. N Engl J Med 1974;290:1–6.
22. Kirk JA, Kersley GD. Heat and cold in the treatment of rheumatoid arthritis of the knee. A controlled clinical trial. Ann Phys Med 1968;9:270–274.
23. Doewart BB, Hansell JR, Schumacher HR Jr. Effects of cold and heat on urate crystal-induced synovitis in the dog. Arthritis Rheum 1974;17:563–571.
24. Deyo RA, Walsh NE, Martin DC, Schoenfeld LS, Ramamurthy S. A controlled trial of transcutaneous electrical nerve stimulation (TENS) and exercise for chronic low back pain. N Engl J Med 1990;322:1627–1634.
25. Henry JH, Crossland JW. Conservative treatment of patellofemoral subluxations. Am J Sports Med 1979;7:12–14.
26. Kovar PA, Allegrante JP, Mackenzie CR, Petersen MGE, Gutin B, Charlson ME. Supervised fitness walking in patients with osteoarthritis of the knee. A randomized, controlled trial. Ann Intern Med 1992;116:529–534.
27. Swezey RL. Essentials of physical management and rehabilitation in arthritis. Semin Arthritis Rheum 1974;3:349–368.
28. Fitzgerald M. Capsaicin and sensory neurons—a review. Pain 1983;15:109–130.
29. McCarthy GM, McCarty DJ. Effect of topical capsaicin in the therapy of painful osteoarthritis of the hands. J Rheumatol 1992;19:604–607.
30. Deal CL, Schnitzer TJ, Lipstein E, Seibold JR, Stevens RM, Levy MD, Albert D, Renold F. Treatment of arthritis with topical capsaicin: a double-blind trial. Clin Ther 1991;13:383–395.
31. Seideman P, Melander A. Equianalgesic effects of paracetamol and indomethacin in rheumatoid arthritis. Br J Rheumatol 1988;27:117–122.
32. Gibson T, Clark B. Use of simple analgesics in rheumatoid arthritis. Ann Rheum Dis 1985;44:27–29.
33. Goodwin JS, Goodwin JM. Failure to recognize efficacious treatments: a history of salicylate therapy in rheumatoid arthritis. Perspect Biol Med 1981;25:78–92.
34. Ferreira SH, Vane JR. New aspects of the mode of action of nonsteroid anti-inflammatory agents. Annu Rev Pharmacol 1974;14:57–73.
35. Abramson SB, Weissmann G. The mechanism of action of nonsteroidal antiinflammatory drugs. Arthritis Rheum 1989;32:1–9.
36. Crook D, Collins AJ, Bacon PA, Chan R. Prostaglandin synthetase activity from human rheumatoid synovial microsomes. Ann Rheum Dis 1976;35:327–332.
37. Roth GS, Stanford N, Majerus PW. Acetylation of prostaglandin synthetase by aspirin. Proc Natl Acad Sci USA 1975;72:3073–3076.
38. Morris HG, Sherman NA, McQuain C, Goldlust MB, Chang SF, Harrison L. Effects of salsalate (non-acetylated salicylate) and aspirin on serum prostaglandins in humans. Ther Drug Monit 1985;7:435–441.
39. Sheiman JM, Elta GH. Gastroduodenal mucosal damage with salsalate versus aspirin: results of experimental models and endoscopic studies in humans. Semin Arthritis Rheum 1990;20:121–127.
40. Kimberly RP, Plotz PH. Salicylates including aspirin and sulfasalazine. In: Kelley WN, Harris ED, Ruddy S, Sledge CB. Textbook of rheumatology. Philadelphia: WB Saunders, 1989.

41. Simon LS. Toxicities of non-steroidal anti-inflammatory drugs. Curr Opin Rheumatol 1992;4:301–308.
42. Dromgoole SH, Furst DE, Paulus HE. Rational approaches to the use of salicylates in the treatment of rheumatoid arthritis. Semin Arthritis Rheum 1981;11:257–283.
43. Estes D, Kaplan K. Lack of platelet effect with the aspirin analog, salsalate. Arthritis Rheum 1980;23:1303–1307.
44. Dudley-Hart F, Huskisson EC. Non-steroidal anti-inflammatory drugs. Current status and rationale for therapeutic use. Drugs 1984;27:232–255.
45. Crook D, Collins AJ. Comparison of effects of aspirin and indomethacin on human platelet prostaglandin synthetase. Ann Rehum Dis 1977;36:459–463.
46. Miller TA, Jacobson ED. Gastrointestinal cytoprotection by prostaglandins. Gut 1979;20:75–87.
47. Clive DM, Stoff JS. Renal syndromes associated with nonsteroidal anti-inflammatory drugs. N Engl J Med 1984;310:563–572.
48. Hench PS. The reversibility of certain rheumatic and non-rheumatic conditions by the use of cortisone or of the pituitary adrenocorticotropic hormone. Ann Intern Med 1952;36:1–38.
49. Weiss MM. Corticosteroids in rheumatoid arthritis. Semin Arthritis Rheum 1989;19:9–21.
50. Joint Committee of the Medical Research Council and Nuffield Foundation. A comparison of cortisone and aspirin in the treatment of early cases of rheumatoid arthritis. Br Med J 1954;29:1223–1227.
51. Empire Rheumatism Council. Multi-centre controlled trial comparing cortisone acetate and acetyl salicylic acid in the long term treatment of rheumatoid arthritis. Ann Rheum Dis 1955;14:353–368.
52. Joint Committee of the Medical Research Council and Nuffield Foundation. A comparison of prednisolone with aspirin or other analgesics in the treatment of rheumatoid arthritis. Ann Rheum Dis 1959;18:173–188.
53. Joint Committee of the Medical Research Council and Nuffield Foundation. A comparison of prednisolone with aspirin or other analgesics in the treatment of rheumatoid arthritis. Ann Rheum Dis 1960;19:331–337.
54. Million R, Poole P, Kellgren JH, et al. Long term study of management of rheumatoid arthritis. Lancet 1984;1:812–816.
55. Calabro JJ. Seronegative spondyloarthropathies. In: Roth SH, Calabro JJ, Paulus HE, Wilkens RF, eds. Rheumatic therapeutics. New York: McGraw-Hill, 1985.
56. Mintz G, Enriquez RD, Mercado U, Robles EJ, Jimenez J, Gutierrez G. Intravenous methylprednisolone pulse therapy in severe ankylosing spondylitis. Arthritis Rheum 1981;24:734–736.
57. Ejstrup L, Peters ND. Intravenous methylprednisolone pulse therapy in ankylosing spondylitis. Dan Med Bull 1985;32:231–233.
58. Stuck AE, Minder CE, Frey FJ. Risk of infectious complications in patients taking glucocorticosteroids. Rev Infect Dis 1989;11:954–963.
59. Lukert BP, Raisz LG. Glucocorticoid-induced osteoporosis: pathogenesis and management. Ann Intern Med 1990;112:352–364.
60. Fisher DE, Bickel WH. Corticosteroid-induced avascular necrosis. A clinical study of seventy-seven patients. J Bone Joint Surg 1971;53A:859–873.
61. Axelrod L. Glucocorticoid therapy. Medicine 1976;55:39–65.
62. Graber AL, Ney RL, Nicholson WE, et al. Natural history of pituitary-adrenal recovery following long term suppression of corticosteroids. J Clin Endocrinol Metab 1965;25:11–16.
63. Plumpton FS, Besser GM, Cole PV. Corticosteroid treatment and surgery. I. An investigation of the indications of steroid cover. Anesthesiology 1969;24:3.
64. Oyama T. Hazards of steroids in association with anesthesia. Can Anaesth Soc J 1969;16:361–371.
65. White RH. Preoperative evaluation of patients with rheumatoid arthritis. Semin Arthritis Rheum 1985;14:287–299.
66. Neustadt DH, Steinbroker O. Observations on the effect of intra-articular phenylbutazone. J Lab Clin Med 1956;47:284–288.
67. Caruso I, Montrone F, Fumagelli M, et al. Rheumatoid knee synovitis successfully treated with intra-articular rifamycin SV. Ann Rheum Dis 1982;41:232–236.
68. Hollander JL. Intra-articular hydrocortisone in arthritis and allied conditions. J Bone Joint Surg 1953;35A:983–990.
69. Friedman D, Moore MA. The efficacy of intraarticular corticosteroids for osteoarthritis of the knee [Abstract]. Arthritis Rheum 1978;21:556.
70. Steinbrocker O, Neustadt DH. Aspiration and injection therapy in arthritis and musculoskeletal disorders. A handbook of technique and management. Hagerstown, MD: Harper & Row (Medical Department), 1972.
71. Schumacher HR Jr. Arthrocentesis, synovial fluid analysis, and intra-articular injection. Kalamazoo, MI: The Upjohn Company, 1990.
72. Hollander JL, Jesser RA, Brown RR. Intrasynovial corticosteroid therapy: a decade of use. Bull Rheum Dis 1961;11:239–240.
73. Owen DS Jr. Aspiration and injection of joints and soft tissues. In: Kelley WN, Harris ED Jr, Ruddy S, Sledge CB, eds. Textbook of rheumatology. Philadelphia: WB Saunders, 1985.
74. Gray RG, Tenenbaum J, Gottlieb NL. Local corticosteroid injection treatment in the rheumatic disorders. Semin Arthritis Rheum 1981;10:231–254.
75. Auranofin: a new drug for rheumatoid arthritis [Editorial]. Ann Intern Med 1986;105:274–276.
76. Sigler JW, Bluhm GB, Duncan H, et al. Gold salts in the treatment of rheumatoid arthritis: a double blind study. Ann Intern Med 1974;80:21–26.
77. Jaffe IA. The technique of penicillamine administration in rheumatoid arthritis. Arthritis Rheum 1975;18:513–514.
78. Kay A. European League Against Rheumatism study of adverse reactions to d-penicillamine. Br J Rheumatol 1986;25:193–198.
79. Schorn D, Mowat AG. Penicillamine in rheumatoid arthritis: wound healing, skin thickness and osteoporosis. Rheumatol Rehabil 1977;16:223–230.
80. Mackenzie AH. Dose refinements in long-term therapy of rheumatoid arthritis with antimalarials. Am J Med 1983;75(Suppl Jul 18):40–45.
81. Ellman A, Gullberg R, Nilsson E, Rendhl L, Wachmeister L. Chloroquine retinopathy in patients with rheumatoid arthritis. Scand J Rheumatol 1976;5:161–166.
82. Bernstein HN, Ginsberg J. The pathology of chloroquine retinopathy. Arch Ophthalmol 1964;71:238–245.
83. Bax DE, Amos RS. Sulphasalazine: a safe, effective agent for prolonged control of rheumatoid arthritis. A comparison with sodium aurothiomalate. Ann Rheum Dis 1985;44:194–198.
84. Neumann V, Grindulis KA, McConkey B, Bird HA, Wright V. A controlled trial of sulphasalazine in rheumatoid arthritis [Abstract]. Ann Rheum Dis 1982;41:534.
85. Martin L, Sitar DS, Chalmers IM, Hunter T. Sulfasalazine in severe rheumatoid arthritis: a study to assess potential correlates of efficacy and toxicity. J Rheumatol 1985;12:270–273.
86. Pullar T, Capell HA. Sulphasalazine: a "new" antirheumatic drug. Br J Rheumatol 1984;23:26–34.
87. Abdou NI, Sweiman B, Casella SR. Effects of azathioprine on bone marrow-dependent and thymus-dependent cells in man. Clin Exp Immunol 1973;13:55–64.
88. Urowitz MB, Gordon DA, Smythe HA, Pruzanski W, Ogryzlo MA. Azathioprine in rheumatoid arthritis. A double-blind, cross-over study. Arthritis Rheum 1973;16:411–418.
89. Escalante A, Beardmore TD. Disease modifying anti-rheumatic drugs and post operative wound complications [Abstract]. Arthritis Rheum 1991;34(Suppl):B184 S128.
90. Weinblatt ME, Coblyn JS, Fox DA, Fraser PA, Holdsworth DE, Glass DN, Trentham DE. Efficacy of low dose methotrexate in rheumatoid arthritis. N Engl J Med 1985;312:818–820.
91. Tugwell P, Bennett K, Gent M. Methotrexate in rheumatoid arthritis. Ann Intern Med 1987;107:358–366.
92. Health and Public Policy Committee, American College of Physicians. Position paper. Methotrexate in rheumatoid arthritis. Ann Intern Med 1987;107:418–419.
93. Bridges SL, López-Méndez A, Han KH, Tracy IC, Alarcón GS. Should methotrexate be discontinued before elective orthopedic surgery in patients with rheumatoid arthritis? J Rheumatol 1991;18:984–988.
94. West SG, Vogelgesand SA. Methotrexate and postoperative joint infections in rheumatoid arthritis patients undergoing total joint arthroplasty [Abstract]. Arthritis Rheum 1990;33(Suppl):S61 A117.
95. Perhala RS, Wilke WS, Clough JD, Segal AM. Local infectious complications following large joint replacement in rheumatoid arthritis patients treated with methotrexate versus those not treated with methotrexate. Arthritis Rheum 1991;34:146–152.
96. Sany J, Anaya JM, Combe B, Gavroy P, Saker S, Thaury MN. Influence of methotrexate on the frequency of postoperative complications in patients with rheumatoid arthritis [Abstract]. Arthritis Rheum 1991;34(Suppl):S36 21.
97. Andersen PA, West SG, O'Dell JR, Via CS, Claypool RG, Kotzin BL. Clinical and immunologic effects in a randomized, double-blind study. Ann Intern Med 1985;103:489–496.
98. Steven M, Morrison M, Sturrock RD. Penicillamine in ankylosing spondylitis: a double blind placebo controlled trial. J Rheumatol 1985;12:735–741.
99. Dougados M, Boumier P, Amor B. Sulphasalazine in ankylosing spondylitis: a double blind controlled study in 60 patients. Br Med J 1986;293:911–914.
100. McConkey B. Sulphasalazine and ankylosing spondylitis. Br J Rheumatol 1990;29:2–5.
101. Lally EV, Ho G Jr. A review of methotrexate therapy in Reiter's syndrome. Semin Arthritis Rheum 1985;15:139–145.
102. Kelley WN, Fox I. Antihyperuricemic drugs. In: Kelley WN, Harris ED, Ruddy S, Sledge CB. Textbook of rheumatology. Philadelphia: WB Saunders, 1989.
103. McCarty DJ. Calcium pyrophosphate dihydrate crystal deposition disease. In: Schumacher HR Jr, Klippel JH, Robinson DR, eds. Primer on the rheumatic diseases. Atlanta: Arthritis Foundation, 1988:207–210.

SECTION

XI

Non-Total Knee Replacement Surgery for Disorders of Articular Cartilage

52

Synovectomy

Robert B. Salisbury

History of Synovectomy of the Knee

Credit for the concept of surgical synovectomy in the rheumatoid knee is usually attributed to the Viennese surgeon Schuller, who in 1887 described four cases and suggested that cases of hypertrophic villous synovitis were better treated by surgical removal of the synovium than by spa therapy (1). In the same year synovectomy for tuberculous arthritis was described by Volkmann (2). The first complete description of anterior synovectomy coupled with long-term follow-up was that of Mignon, who read his case report before the Surgical Society of Paris in 1900 (3). His indication was chronic proliferative inflammatory reaction of the knee in which the diagnosis of infection had been excluded. Decreases in pain and swelling were reported, and, although some effusion persisted, the procedure was believed to have afforded marked general improvement. Of note is the mention of significant loss of motion after rehabilitation.

In the United States, Goldthwait was the first to report on synovectomy for nontubercular conditions. His operations at the turn of the century were partial excisions, mainly to remove synovial fringes, which he believed blocked joint motion (4). By the 1920s Swett popularized the procedure and established parameters of proper patient selection in anticipation of satisfactory results. He stressed the importance of restricting synovectomy to knees in which pathologic changes were largely or exclusively synovial. The rationale of the procedure at the time was based on manual removal of exudate (mechanical), surgical removal of possible microorganisms, or metabolic stimulation. His original paper demonstrated the feasibility of removing large amounts of synovial tissue without significant postoperative complications (5). Key's 1925 study on rabbit joints after synovectomy provided the surgical community with the assurance that a serviceable membrane

Results of synovectomy during this period were extremely variable, perhaps as a result of inconsistent indications. This essentially led to abandonment of the procedure until the early 1960s, when more encouraging reports began to appear in the literature (7, 8). Marmor's report of 34 synovectomies in which all knees were improved and with no recurrence of disease did much to repopularize the procedure (9). Conaty concluded that of all primary procedures on the rheumatoid knee, excluding total joint replacement, synovectomy was the most successful (10). He stressed proper patient selection and cited good results in patients with minimal articular destruction or deformity.

Not all evaluations of open synovectomy have been positive, however. Studies that specifically questioned whether synovectomy has any effect on the natural history of the disease led to the conclusion that the procedure could not be classified as preventive (11, 12). Several studies of open synovectomy, however, describe excellent long-term results, with decreased pain and swelling and arrested or delayed disease progression (13–15).

The search for a nonsurgical means of ablating diseased synovial tissue has led from installation of caustic substances, such as osmic acid, to intra-articular injections of highly selective radiocolloids. The benefits in terms of cost and patient acceptance are obvious (16). If long-term risks are minimal, the potential for better controlled-outcome studies makes the procedure most exciting.

Equally exciting is the new discipline of arthroscopic surgery, which affords the surgeon a minimally invasive route of access to the knee, enlarged video visualization of the surgical field, and highly specialized instrumentation to accomplish a nearly total synovectomy. The first reports of arthroscopic synovectomy utilizing motorized suction cutting devices begin to appear in the literature after 1984 (17–19).

Results of arthroscopic resection of diseased synovium have uniformly been good to excellent. In early reports of arthroscopic synovectomy, utilizing less effective instrumentation than is currently available, there were no significant differences in results at 2 months than with open synovectomy (20). Efficient motorized instrumentation and improved video optical systems in the hands of experienced arthroscopists have transformed synovial resection from a major surgical undertaking into an outpatient procedure with minimal morbidity and high patient acceptance of the initial and, if required, subsequent operations. Results reported are at least as good as those of open synovectomy (21, 22).

Although the technical approaches to proliferative synovial disease have improved greatly, basic questions have yet to be answered. What is the natural history of each disease that is treated by synovectomy and how does the procedure alter it? Is there an advantage of one method of synovial ablation over others? Are the procedures palliative, curative, or a bit of each? Finally, are the procedures cost effective or effective in improving quality of life?

Surgical Anatomy of the Synovial Membrane

The synovial membrane lines the capsule of the joint and sweeps forward from the posterior capsule to envelop the cruciate ligaments. A small bursa or synovial diverticulum lies between the cruciate ligaments. The posterior cruciate ligament does not have a synovial lining posteriorly. The popliteal synovial recess or bursa lines the popliteal hiatus laterally. The synovial lining is broken medially and laterally by nonsynovial meniscal load-bearing structures that protrude into the joint. Synovium ends at the edge of articular cartilage. In the relaxed knee, synovium of the suprapatellar pouch is redundant in extension and the posterior areas are redundant in flexion (Fig. 52.1).

Surgical Technique

Open Synovectomy

Myriad surgical approaches have been used at one time or another to accomplish synovectomy. In general, early open procedures were anterior synovectomies through longitudinal skin incisions and arthrotomies on either side of the patella. Many surgeons routinely divided both collateral and cruciate ligaments to facilitate posterior exposure (23, 24). A vertical incision in which the patella was split longitudinally, though popular around 1920, was gradually replaced by the anterior longitudinal skin incision with long median parapatellar capsular approach. This approach is well adapted to later arthroplasty. Recommendations regarding treatment of the menisci during open synovectomy have been varied. Allison et al. (25) advised routine excision, while other investigators tended toward preservation unless the menisci or underlying bone was grossly involved (7, 24).

Postoperative Management

Suction or gravity drainage has generally been used for short periods after open synovectomy (26). There has historically been little agreement regarding the initiation of motion postoperatively. Many surgeons believed that early motion was of prime importance (26, 27). Others routinely immobilized the extremity for 1 to 3 weeks and began motion exercises after gentle manipulation under anesthesia (8, 17).

Arthroscopic Synovectomy

The surgical technique of arthroscopic synovectomy has been in evolution since the earliest arthroscopic synovial biopsy in the early 1950s (28). The first attempts at arthroscopic synovectomy were done by avulsing clumps of synovium with large and small rongeurs under direct visualization. Such procedures were arduous, time consuming, and technically demanding. With the evolution of video arthroscopy and highly efficient motorized suction shaver instrumentation, essentially complete synovectomy of the knee can be accomplished by a skilled arthroscopist as an outpatient procedure with minimal postoperative morbidity. This minimal technique has replaced open methods as the surgery option of choice for excision of knee synovium. There are many advantages to arthroscopic synovectomy (Table 52.1). The disadvantages are few and include the need for specialized instrumentation and a surgeon highly skilled in arthroscopic technique.

Rationale of Synovectomy

The purpose behind removal of synovium differs depending on the disease entity amenable to the procedure (Table 52.2). Synovectomy for pigmented villonodular synovitis and focal or posttraumatic synovitis may be curative. Chronic infective synovitis may be eliminated by synovectomy performed in concert with appropriate antibiotic therapy. Synovectomy in synovial chondromatosis and crystalline synovitis is palliative. Removal of the inflamed fragile synovium of hemophiliac arthropathy probably changes the natural history of the disease by reducing the number of bleeding episodes.

The scientific basis of the procedure is less clear in the treatment of rheumatoid disease. The surgical quest to remove or alter tissue that causes pain or cosmetic or functional disability is well served by synovectomy. Inflamed rheumatoid synovium may produce effusions and excess tissue bulk as well as instability and fibroarthrosis.

Cartilage may be destroyed directly, by encroaching synovium or pannus, and indirectly by accelerated mechanical wear that results from destruction of stabilizing structures such as ligaments and menisci. The synovium also transfers acute inflammatory cells into joint fluid and synthesizes antibodies, including rheumatoid factor (29).

Classic teaching has attributed destruction of articular cartilage to synovial encroachment and ingrowth

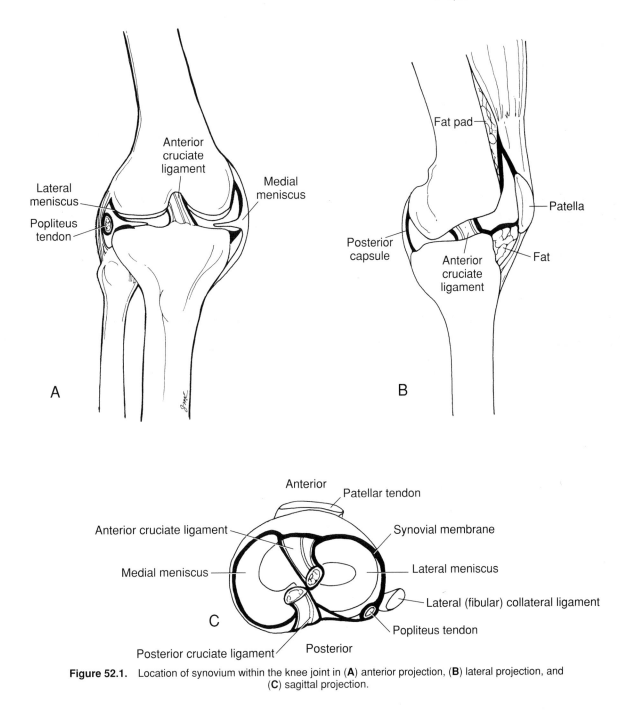

Figure 52.1.   Location of synovium within the knee joint in (**A**) anterior projection, (**B**) lateral projection, and (**C**) sagittal projection.

Table 52.1   Advantages of Arthoscopic Synovectomy

Synovial resection is more complete
Incision is minimal
Quadriceps muscle remains intact
Incidence of infection is decreased
Incidence of hemarthrosis is decreased
Range of motion is maintained or increased
Is cost effective as an outpatient procedure
Postoperative physical therapy is minimal or none
Menisci are spared
Patient acceptance is high

Table 52.2   Synovial Diseases Amenable to Synovectomy

Rheumatoid arthritis
Rheumatoid variants (lupus psoriatic arthritis, Marie-Strumpell arthritis, Lyme disease, etc.)
Pigmented villonodular synovitis
Synovial chondromatosis
Crystalline synovitis
Focal or traumatic synovitis
Hemophiliac synovitis
Chronic infective synovitis

into articular surfaces. The observations supporting this conclusion have come from pathologic specimens or surgical cases in an era when rest and immobilization (rather than active physical therapy and ambulation) were recommended. Arthroscopy of ambulatory seropositive rheumatoid patients suggests, however, that the majority of articular cartilage degradation occurs without pannus invasion (Figs. 52.2 and 52.3). If the form and function of the meniscus are destroyed by pannus, then instability and increased articular cartilage loading lead to accelerated destruction.

These clinical observations are supported by the discovery of antigenic immune complexes in rheumatoid articular cartilage. These complexes probably induce inflammatory immune reactions and in combination with altered joint mechanics erode the rheumatoid cartilage without pannus activity (30, 31). In support of this concept, surgery that ablates articular cartilage (i.e., total joint replacement and fusion) tends to normalize synovium in the joint addressed. In the final analysis, synovectomy for rheumatoid arthritis is probably palliative rather than curative. Further controlled studies should define how the natural history of the disease is affected by synovectomy.

Arthroscopic Operative Technique

Early arthroscopic synovectomies were done with direct-vision, narrow-angle arthroscopes by avulsing synovium with hand instruments. Even these incomplete, interminable, and sodden attempts had recognizable advantages over open synovectomy. The menisci could be stripped of synovial membrane without excision (Fig. 52.4). Postoperative morbidity was minimal. Current video equipment and efficient motorized instrumentation have contributed greatly to the ease with which the procedure may be accomplished.

Basic Arthroscopic Equipment

The preferred system consists of a 4-mm, 30-degree wide-angle arthroscope with a 4.5-mm sheath and obturator system; and a 70-degree arthroscope, light source, camera, and video system.

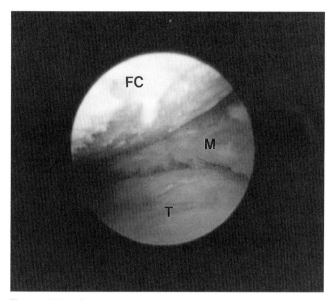

Figure 52.2. End-stage rheumatoid knee without articular pannus encroachment. Pannus has destroyed the meniscus, but femoral condylar and tibial articular cartilage loss has occurred without pannus invasion. *FC,* femoral condyle; *M,* meniscus; *T,* tibia.

Figure 52.3. Kissing sclerosis of articular bearing surfaces in the right knee. Radiographic examination of rheumatoid knees shows increased bone density on point load bearing areas of left knee, a transient sign of functional loss of the meniscus.

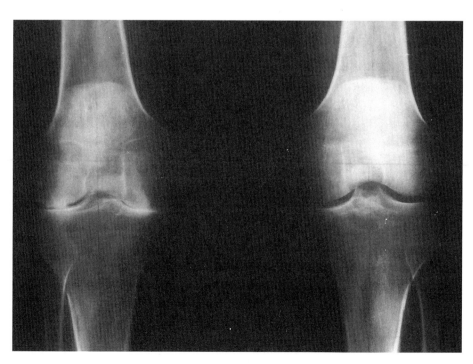

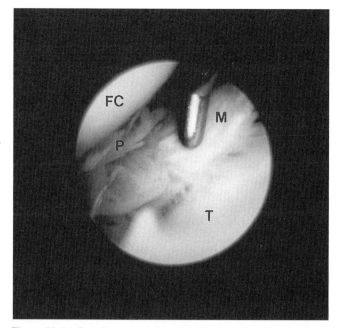

Figure 52.4. Debridement of rheumatoid pannus from meniscal surfaces. Synovectomy without meniscal excision. *P*, rheumatoid pannus; *FC*, femoral condyle; *M*, meniscus; *T*, tibia.

The fluid supply consists of large-bore Y tubing (urologic supply), Ringer's lactate or saline solution in 3-liter bags, and an inflow cannula of at least 3.5 mm diameter.

Table equipment should include a thigh tourniquet and a short kidney rest. The required instruments include a probe, 3.5- and 2.7-mm basket forceps, medium and thin pituitary rongeurs, a motorized suction shaver system with 4.5-mm aggressive resecting heads, and a small curved tendon passing forceps as is used in hand surgery.

Surgical Positions and Methods

Arthroscopic synovectomy and debridement can be accomplished on a standard operating table with a short kidney rest through the use of four basic positions: extended, valgus flexion, "figure four" flexion, and flexion at 100 degrees. Six portals may be required: standard superomedial for inflow catheter, high superolateral, standard inferomedial, standard inferolateral, posteromedial, and posterolateral. Dependable access requires that the tourniquet be placed as proximally as possible. A short kidney rest, secured to the table just lateral to the tourniquet, provides a post for the valgus flexion position.

Examination

A standard arthroscopic examination is performed first through the inferolateral portal with a probe through the inferomedial portal. Inflow through the arthroscopic sheath and outflow through the superomedial cannula are preferable for this phase. A variable-flow stopcock on the outflow cannula regulates the rate of flow and the distention of the knee.

Position I: Extended

Beginning the procedure in the extended position has two main advantages: first, in the knee with proliferative synovium a clear zone is more easily established by resection of tissue in the suprapatellar pouch. The clear zone is an area within the knee that is totally free of synovium. The surgeon may return to it for orientation and for flushing the mechanical system and clearing distention fluid. Although a clear zone may usually be established beneath the medial femoral condyle in the valgus flexion position, resection of anterior and medial synovium can always be accomplished in position I. This establishes the initial clear zone for position II. The second advantage to early anterior resection is better flow in subsequent positions.

The operative procedure begins in the extended position (Fig. 52.5). Inflow is controlled through a large-bore cannula or fenestrated needle, and outflow is controlled via the motorized section shaver system, which is manipulated through either anterior portal. The arthroscope in the high superolateral portal permits visualization of the medial and lateral gutters, the synoviomeniscal junction, the anterior synovium, the patellar fat pad, and the anterior horn of the medial meniscus. The synovial resection tip is introduced through the anterior portals to remove synovium from these areas. Areas of unstable or shedding articular cartilage on the patella and trochlear groove are trimmed with a pituitary rongeur or mechanical shaver system that is manipulated through the inferolateral portal.

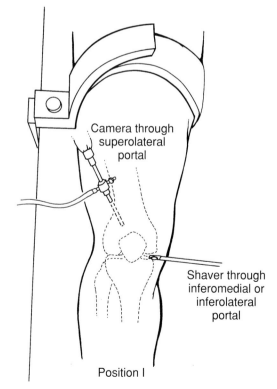

Figure 52.5. Position I: extended. Camera: superolateral portal; shaver: inferomedial or inferolateral anterior portal.

Position II: Valgus Flexion

After the work in position I is completed, the extremity is placed in valgus flexion (Fig. 52.6). The exact amounts of flexion and tibial rotation will vary depending on stability in the area being addressed. A lax knee will occasionally sublux in the stressed or rotated position and close the joint space. Visualization can become difficult and is best improved by gentle traction, instead of valgus stress, in the flexed position. The intercondylar notch is cleared of synovium first. Since the anterior cruciate ligament in the rheumatoid knee may be attenuated or lengthened, care is required during synovial resection. A slight redundancy places the ligament in jeopardy of an aggressive resection blade. Frequent return to the clear zone is in order when operating within the notch area. Articular surfaces are again trimmed with a pituitary rongeur or a mechanical system. While abrasion chondroplasty can be used to grind away areas of proliferative synovial overgrowth on articular cartilage, it should not be used routinely in the rheumatoid knee.

Expansion of synovium over and under the meniscus can erode this essential structure and add a terminal mechanical mode of destruction to the rheumatoid process. Meticulous resection of synovium from the surfaces of the medial meniscus and saucerization of central rim tears are accomplished (Figs. 52.7 and 52.8). The inferior aspect of the medial meniscus in its anterior half can be difficult to clear. It is helpful to switch portals and avulse the synovium with small curved tendon-passing forceps manipulated from the anterolateral portal across the front of the joint. In many rheumatoid knees the posteromedial area may be visualized and synovectomy accomplished from position II.

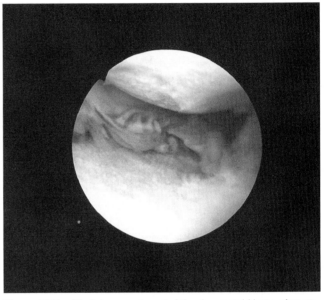

Figure 52.7.   Medial compartment of the rheumatoid knee after creating a clear space but before meniscal debridement.

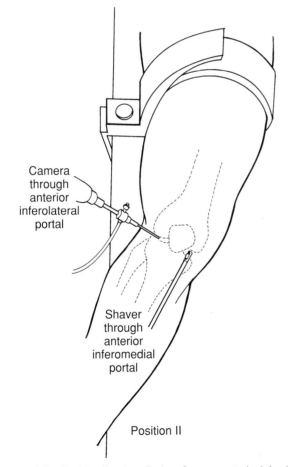

Figure 52.6.   Position II: valgus flexion. Camera: anterior inferolateral portal; shaver: anterior inferomedial portal.

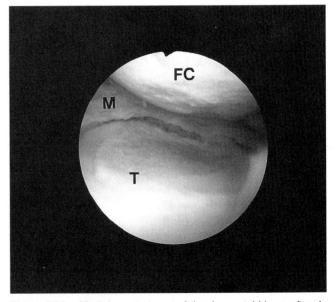

Figure 52.8.   Medial compartment of the rheumatoid knee after debridement of meniscal pannus. *FC,* femoral condyle; *M,* meniscus; *T,* tibia.

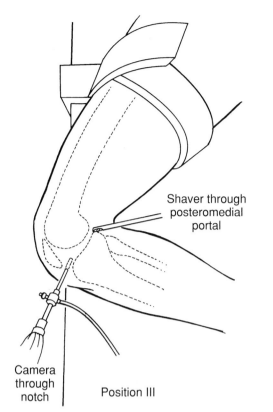

Figure 52.9. Position III: figure four position. Camera: through the notch; shaver: posteromedial portal.

Position III: Figure Four Flexion

Two compartments are addressed from the figure four flexion position (Fig. 52.9). The lateral compartment is apparent from the inferolateral portal; the joint line and menisci may be cleared by instruments positioned in the inferomedial portal. Significant posterolateral clearing may often be done from this position. The figure four position also uses the intercondylar notch approach to visualize the posteromedial area with passage of the arthroscope from the inferomedial portal. With the knee in the figure four position and the tibia internally rotated, the arthroscope is advanced between the medial femoral condyle and the posterior cruciate. The 30-degree wide-angle arthroscope is sometimes adequate, but a 70-degree arthroscope is better. Instrumentation is accomplished through a standard posteromedial joint line portal. This portal is best located by passing a spinal needle into the joint under camera control before making an incision.

Position IV: Flexed

If an adequate lateral compartment synovectomy cannot be accomplished through the anterior portals, access to the posterior capsular area is obtained through the posterolateral portal with the leg parallel to the table and flexed 100 degrees (Fig. 52.10). The portal is placed where lines extended along the inferior border of the iliotibial tract and the fibula intersect. The desired position of the portal is confirmed by inserting a spinal needle while viewing through the notch with a 70-degree arthroscope. This portal is used for instrumentation. An alternative to viewing both posterior areas through the notch is to use high and low posterior portals. Manipulation can be restricted with these, however. The entire joint is inspected prior to closure.

Figure 52.10. Position IV: anterior flexed position. Camera: anterior inferolateral portal; shaver: posterolateral portal.

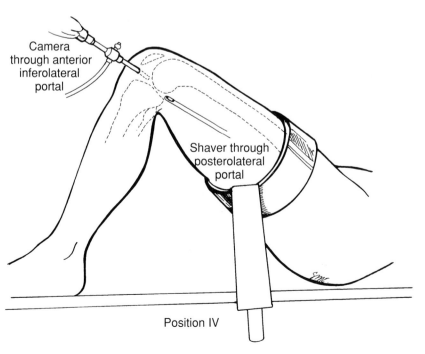

Closure and Dressing

The portals are infiltrated with a mixture of 0.25% bupivacaine hydrochloride (Marcaine) and 1:200,000 epinephrine and are closed without sutures, utilizing surgical tape. A dressing of 4×4-inch sterile gauze pads, several layers of Webril dressing, and an elastic bandage are applied.

Postoperative Care

Patients are discharged from the hospital on the day of surgery and are allowed to resume their preoperative level of ambulation. Patients remove the dressing on the second postoperative day and may apply adhesive bandages to the portals. Oral acetaminophen with codeine (Tylenol 3) is used for postoperative pain. A written protocol for home exercises is prescribed, and formal physical therapy is not required. Patients usually return to their preoperative status within 10 days.

While arthroscopic synovectomy and debridement obviates essentially all of the disadvantages of open synovectomy and can be quite a significant factor in improving the quality of life for patients with rheumatoid disease, it is not curative. Many patients require subsequent procedures at 1- to 3-year intervals. Contrary to the experience with open synovectomy, patients who have had arthroscopic synovectomy often return when symptoms recur, requesting a "repeat clean-out."

Radiosynovectomy

Selected nonsurgical ablation of hypertrophic or diseased synovial tissue is a highly desirable goal. The obvious theoretical advantages are elimination of hospitalization and anesthesia, elimination of surgical complications (infection and embolism), and probably decreased costs.

A chemical that is caustic to one tissue is likely to be caustic to adjacent tissues unless uptake and penetration can be controlled. Chemical synovectomy with agents such as osmium preparations has been supplanted by synovectomy through intra-articular injection of radiocolloids. The ideal agent should provide low total-body radiation dosage, limited leakage from the joint, and tissue penetration limited to the synovium. Results comparable to those of open surgical synovectomy have been reported in a short-term study utilizing yttrium-90 as the radiocolloid (16). An increase in chromosomal abnormalities has been reported in patients after yttrium-90 synovectomy, clarifying the need for long-term controlled-outcome studies (32). Results of radionuclide synovectomy comparable to those of arthroscopic synovectomy have been reported utilizing an injection of dysprosium-165 coupled with ferric hydroxide macroaggregate, a large, relatively inert carrier (33).

Synovial Diseases

Rheumatoid Arthritis

Indications for synovectomy in rheumatoid arthritis are persistent effusion with proliferative synovitis unresponsive to medical management for 6 months. Best results are obtained in early disease without radiologic evidence of joint space narrowing. The best assessment of the joint space can be made by examining a 45-degree posteroanterior flexion, weight-bearing radiograph (34). Contraindications to synovectomy include significant articular involvement, flexion contracture greater than 25 degrees, any varus deformity, and valgus greater than 10 degrees (35).

The efficacy of synovectomy in the rheumatoid knee remains controversial. Most investigators agree that relief of pain and swelling is good to excellent in the short term, especially when synovectomy is done before articular erosions and deformity occur (Figs. 52.11, 52.12, and 52.13). Some long-term studies conclude that synovectomy has little effect on the long-term treatment of

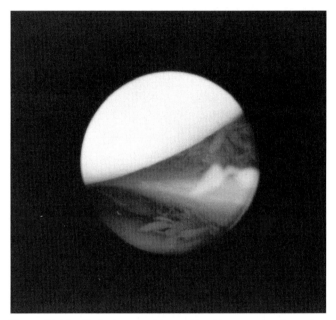

Figure 52.11. Early rheumatoid synovitis without meniscal or articular encroachment.

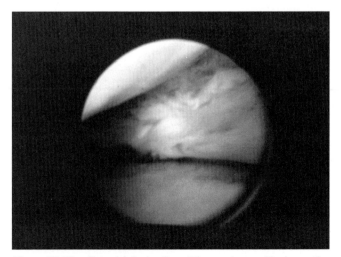

Figure 52.12. Synovial destruction of the meniscus with clear articular surfaces.

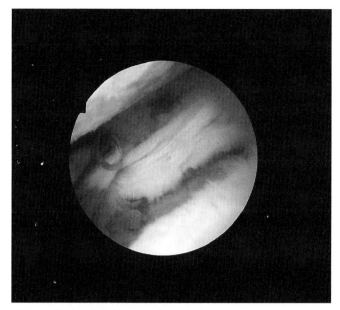

Figure 52.13. Debridement of the meniscus with a suction shaver in an end-stage rheumatoid knee.

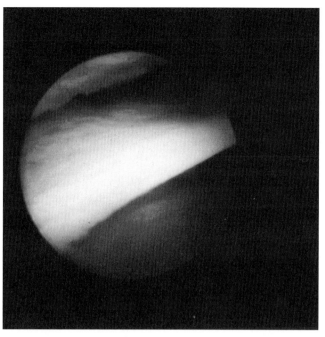

Figure 52.14. Median parapatellar shelf with synovitis.

rheumatoid arthritis and that deterioration of the rheumatoid knee cannot be prevented by early synovectomy (36, 37). These reports are tempered by the results of other long-term studies that suggest that progression of disease may be significantly affected by synovectomy (38). Controlled-outcome studies of radiocolloid or arthroscopic synovectomy in rheumatoid disease have yet to be performed.

Hemophilic Arthropathy

The knee is the most frequent site of hemorrhage in the hemophilic patient. Several episodes of bleeding into the hemophilic knee appear to produce a critical threshold of synovitis and synovial hypertrophy. The friable, hyperemic synovial lining is more susceptible to minor trauma, and this vulnerability imposes a cycle of recurrent hemarthrosis, production of proteolytic enzymes by the synovial cells, and joint deterioration and destruction (39). Synovectomy as a means of interrupting this cycle is an extension of understanding the pathophysiology and the ability to monitor and control the clotting factor deficiencies. The major indication for surgical synovectomy is frequent or persistent hemorrhage with synovial hypertrophy in a knee that does not respond to vigorous nonsurgical management, including aspiration, rest, splinting, and factor concentrate replacement. In 1969, Storti et al. first reported excellent control of recurrent hemarthrosis in hemophiliacs through open synovectomy (40). Subsequently the efficacy of the procedure has been well documented (41–43). Long-term results of arthroscopic synovectomy are generally better than those of open procedures because of retention of motion (44, 45). Arthroscopy has replaced arthrotomy for the hemophilic knee. Radiocolloid synovectomy is a noninvasive alternative.

Meticulous application of universal precautions by the operating team must be emphasized, since the incidence of HIV infection in this patient population is extremely high.

Localized Synovitis

Local hypertrophic synovitis may develop within the knee and mimic meniscal derangement or articular cartilage degeneration. One of the most common areas of local irritation responding to limited synovectomy is the median parapatellar synovial plica. This structure may become symptomatic after minor trauma or increased activity (Fig. 52.14) Anterior massive synovial hypertrophy that is palpably crepitant may also mimic patellar articular degeneration.

Especially in runners, areas of popliteal synovitis may develop, producing lateral knee pain that is related to activity (Fig. 52.15). The pain is virtually indistinguishable from that of a meniscal abnormality or articular degeneration. Arthroscopic removal of this irritated synovium is often curative.

Crystal-Induced Synovitis

Synovial inflammation secondary to the deposition of monosodium urate crystals (gout) and calcium pyrophosphate crystals (pseudogout) may be improved through arthroscopic lavage, steroid wash, debridement of meniscal tears, and local synovectomy (46) (Fig. 52.16). The primary treatment, however, remains nonsurgical.

Synovitis of Degenerative Joint Disease

Although excision of hypertrophic synovial tissue may be part of debridement of the degenerative knee, syn-

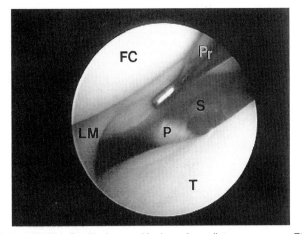

Figure 52.15. Popliteal synovitis in a long-distance runner. *FC,* femoral condyle; *S,* synovitis; *P,* popliteus tendon; *LM,* lateral meniscus; *T,* tibia; *Pr,* probe.

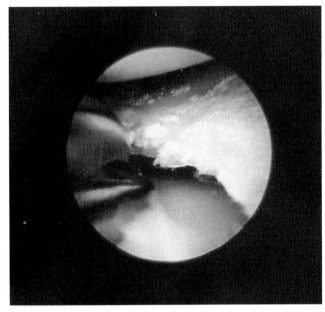

Figure 52.16. Calcium pyrophosphate crystal deposition on the surface and within the substance of the meniscus and articular cartilage.

ovitis secondary to degenerative joint disease is not a recognized indication for synovectomy.

Synovial Chondromatosis

Primary synovial chondromatosis and osteochondromatosis are diseases characterized by the production of discrete bodies of cartilage or cartilage and bone in the synovial membrane by metaplasia of synovial cells. It is a rare monarticular disease characterized by pain, swelling, crepitus, locking, buckling, and often palpable loose bodies. The radiographs may be normal.

Secondary chondromatosis is a more common problem, seen in knees that shed bits of cartilage as in degenerative joint disease. These flakes are engulfed by synovial tissue and may enlarge. The recommended treatments of synovial chondromatosis include simple

arthroscopic removal of loose bodies (47), removal of loose bodies with partial synovectomy (48), and removal of loose bodies and total synovectomy in active stages of the disease (49). Good results are generally reported both long and short term. The major prognostic factor is the condition of articular bearing surfaces at the time of operation.

Infection

Since Volkmann's first report of synovectomy for tuberculous infections of the knee, the procedure has established a niche in the treatment of chronic or acutely infected joints of various etiologies. As an adjunct to pharmacologic treatment, the judicious use of synovectomy may play a primary role in attaining the goals of joint decompression and debridement of nonviable and necrotic tissue (50, 51). In cases of severe fibroarthrosis or flexion contracture in an infected knee, an open procedure may be preferable to arthroscopic debridement and synovectomy.

Pigmented Villonodular Synovitis

Pigmented villonodular synovitis of the knee is typically a monarticular arthritis of unknown cause in young adults. The synovium is usually darkly colored due to hemosiderin deposits and may be locally aggressive. As with other types of chronic synovitis, there are pain and swelling and occasionally mechanical symptoms, such as locking. The abnormal synovium may be in pedunculated, locally nodular, or diffuse forms (Fig. 52.17). The nodular form responds to complete local excision, either arthroscopic or by arthrotomy (52). There is some controversy regarding treatment of the diffuse type of

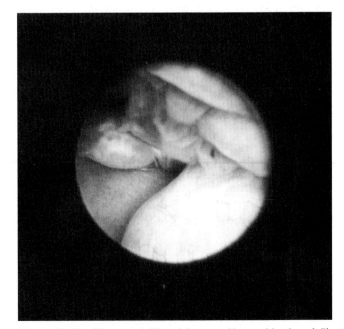

Figure 52.17. Pigmented villonodular synovitis; combination of diffuse and nodular forms.

pigmented villonodular synovitis. Radiation therapy, used in the past, has been abandoned because of systemic side effects and a concern about radiation-induced sarcomas. Intra-articular radiation synovectomy with yttrium-90 has been successful, but long-term outcome studies are needed (53). Prior to the advent of arthroscopy, the most widely accepted treatment was open synovectomy. There is a significant rate of recurrence with this method (54). Excellent long-term results of arthroscopic synovectomy have been reported by Ogilvie-Harris et al. (55).

References

1. Schuller M. Die Pathologie und Therapie der Gelenkentzundungen. Vienna: Urban u. Schwarzenberg, 1887.
2. von Volkmann R. 1877. Quoted by Speed (1924) and Clin Orthop 1964;36:7.
3. Mignon A. Synovectomy du genou. Bull Soc Nat Chir 1900;26:1113.
4. Goldthwait JE. Knee-joint surgery for nontubercular conditions. A report of thirty-eight operations for synovial fringes, injured semilunar cartilage, loose cartilage, coagula, exploratory incision, etc. Boston Med Surg J 1900;143:286–290.
5. Swett PP. Synovectomy in chronic infectious arthritis. J Bone Joint Surg 1923;5:110–121.
6. Key JA. The reformation of synovial membrane in the knee of rabbits after synovectomy. J Bone Joint Surg 1925;7:793–813.
7. Aidem HP, Baker LD. Synovectomy of the knee joint in rheumatoid arthritis. JAMA 1964;187:4–6.
8. Gariepy R, Demers R, Laurin C. The prophylactic effect of synovectomy of the knee in rheumatoid arthritis. Can Med Assn J 1966;94:1349–1352.
9. Marmor L. Surgery of the rheumatoid knee. Am J Surg 1966;111:211–215.
10. Conaty JP. Surgery of the hip and knee in patients with rheumatoid arthritis. J Bone Joint Surg 1973;55-A:301.
11. Arthritis Foundation Committee on Evaluation of Synovectomy in the Treatment of Rheumatoid Arthritis. Multicenter evaluation of synovectomy in the treatment of rheumatoid arthritis. Report at the end of three years. Arthritis Rheum 1977;20:765.
12. Arthritis and Rheumatism Council and British Orthopedic Association. Controlled trial of knee and metacarpal joints in rheumatoid arthritis. Ann Rheum Dis 1977;35:437.
13. Ranawat CS, Desai K. Role of early synovectomy of the knee joint in rheumatoid arthritis. Arthritis Rheum 1975;18:117–121.
14. Ishikawa H, Ohno O, Hirohata K. Long term results of synovectomy in rheumatoid patients. J Bone Joint Surg 1986;68-A:198–205.
15. Marmor L. Surgery of the rheumatoid knee: synovectomy and debridement. J Bone Joint Surg 1973;55-A:535–544.
16. Gumpel JM, Roles NC. A controlled trial of intraarticular radiocolloids versus surgical synovectomy in persistent synovitis. Lancet 1975;1:488.
17. Highenboten CL. Arthroscopic synovectomy. Arthroscopy 1985;1:190–193.
18. Rosenberg TD. An illustrated guide to arthroscopic synovectomy of the knee. Salt Lake City: Dyonics, 1984:1–7.
19. Johnson LL. Arthroscopic surgery principals and practice. St. Louis: CV Mosby, 1986:1269.
20. Shibata T, Shiraoka K, Takubo N. Comparison between arthroscopic and open synovectomy for the knee in rheumatoid arthritis. Arch Orthop Trauma Surg 1986;105:257–262.
21. Ogilvie-Harris DJ, Basinski A. Arthroscopic synovectomy of the knee for rheumatoid arthritis. Arthroscopy 1991;7(1):91–97.
22. Klein W, Jensen K-U. Arthroscopic synovectomy of the knee joint: indication, technique and follow-up results. Arthroscopy 1988;4:63–71.
23. Muller W. Zur frage der operativen behandlung der arthritis deformans und des chronischen gelenkrheumatismus. Arch Klin Chir 1894;47:1–39.
24. Bernstein MA. Synovectomy of the knee joint in chronic arthritis. Ann Surg 1933;98:1096–1108.
25. Allison N, Coonse GK. Synovectomy in chronic arthritis. Arch Surg 1929;18:824–840.
26. Clayton ML. Surgery of the lower extremity in rheumatoid arthritis. J Bone Joint Surg 1963;45-A:1517–1536.
27. Boon-Itt SB. A study of end results of synovectomy of the knee. J Bone Joint Surg 1930;12:853–858.
28. Watenabe M. Arthroscopic clinic of arthrosis deformans and related conditions. J Jpn Orthop Assoc 1954;28:462.
29. Cook TDV. A scientific basis for surgery in rheumatoid arthritis. Clin Orthop Relat Res 1986;208:20–23.
30. Salisbury R, Nottage W. A new evaluation of gross pathologic changes and concepts of rheumatoid articular cartilage degeneration. Clin Orthop 1985;199:242–247.
31. Cooke TDV, Masatoshi S, Masaho M. Deleterious interactions of immune complexes in cartilage of experimental immune arthritis. Clin Orthop 1985;193:235–245.
32. Doyle DV, Glass JS, Gow PJ, Daker M, Grahame R. A clinical and prospective chromosomal study of yttrium-90 synovectomy. Rheum Rehabil 1977;16(4):217–222.
33. Sledge CB, Zukerman JD, Shortkroff S, Zalutsky MR, Venkatesan P, Snyder MA, Barrett WP. Synovectomy of the rheumatoid knee using intra-articular injection of dysprosium-165-ferric hydroxide macroaggregates. J Bone Joint Surg 1987;69_2DA(7):970–975.
34. Rosenberg TD, Paulos LE, Parker RD, Coward DB, Scott SM. The forty-five degree posteroanterior flexion weight-bearing radiograph of the knee. J Bone Joint Surg 1988;70_2DA:1479.
35. Salisbury RB. Arthroscopic evaluation of the rheumatoid knee. Techniques in Orthopedics 1987;2(2):69–72.
36. Doets HC, Bierman BTM, Soesbergen RM. Synovectomy of the rheumatoid knee does not prevent deterioration. Acta Orthop Scand 1989;60(5):523–525.
37. McEwan C. Multicenter evaluation of synovectomy in the treatment of rheumatoid arthritis. Report of results at the end of five years. J Rheumatol 1988;15:765–769.
38. Ishikawa H, Ohno O, Kazushi H. Long term results of synovectomy in rheumatoid patients. J Bone Joint Surg 1968;68-A(2):198–205.
39. Arnold WD, Hilgartner MW. Hemophilic arthropathy: current concepts of pathogenesis and management. J Bone Joint Surg 1977;59-A:287.
40. Storti E, Traldi A, Tosatti E, Davoli PG. Synovectomy, a new approach to haemophillic arthropathy. Acta Haematol 1969;41:193–205.
41. McCollough NC, Enis JE, Lovitt J, Lian E, Niewmann K, Loughlin EC. Synovectomy or total replacement of the knee in hemophilia. J Bone Joint Surg 1979;61-A:69–75.
42. Mannucci, PM, DeFranchis R, Torri G, Pietrogrande V. Role of synovectomy in hemophillic arthropathy. Isr J Med Sci 1977;13:983–987.
43. Pietrogrande V, Dioguarde N, Mannucci PM. Short term evaluation of synovectomy in haemophilia. Br Med J 1972;2:378–381.
44. Klein KS, Aland CM, Kim HC. Long term follow-up of arthroscopic synovectomy for chronic hemophillic synovitis. Arthroscopy 1987;3:231.
45. Wiedel JD. Arthroscopic synovectomy for chronic hemophilic synovitis of the knee. Arthroscopy 1985;1:205.
46. O'Connor RL. The arthroscope in the management of crystalline-induced synovitis of the knee. J Bone Joint Surg 1973;55-A:1443.
47. Dorfmann H, DieBie B, Bonvarlet JP, Boyer T. Arthroscopic treatment of synovial chrondromatosis of the knee. Arthroscopy 1989;5(1):48–51.
48. Coolican MR, Dandy DJ. Arthroscopic management of synovial chondromatosis of the knee. J Bone Joint Surg 1989;71-B: 530–534.
49. Murphy FP, Dahlin DC, Sullivan CZ. Articular synovial chondromatosis. J Bone Joint Surg 1962;44-A:77–86.
50. Torholm C, Hedstrom S, Sunden G, Lidgren L. Synovectomy in bacterial arthritis. Acta Orthop Scand 1983;54:748–753.
51. Smith MJ. Arthroscopic treatment of the septic knee. Arthroscopy 1986;2:30.
52. Rao AS, Vigorita VJ. Pigmented villonodular synovitis and tenosynovitis (giant cell tumor of tendon sheath and synovial membrane). A review of eighty-one cases. J Bone Joint Surg 1984;66-A:76–94.
53. Wiss DA. Recurrent villonodular synovitis of the knee. Successful treatment with yttrium-90. Clin Orthop 1982;169: 139–144.
54. Flandry F, Hughston JC. Current concepts review: pigmented villonodular synovitis. J Bone Joint Surg 1987;69-A: 942–949.
55. Ogilvie-Harris DJ, McLean Jean, Zarnett ME. Pigmented villonodular synovitis of the knee. J Bone Joint Surg 1992;74-A:119–123.

53

Selection of Patients for Surgical Treatment

Michael A. Kelly

History
Physical Examination
Radiographs
Arthroscopy
Surgical Management

Degenerative joint disease (DJD) of the knee may present with a variety of symptoms and disabilities, ranging in severity from mild to crippling. The initial management in the majority of cases will be non-surgical. Medical management may include the administration of nonsteroidal antiinflammatory agents, analgesics as well as the judicious use of intraarticular corticosteroid injections. Medications may be coupled with exercise programs, physical therapy, bracing and ambulatory assist devices such as canes. The individual symptoms may also demand lifestyle changes, possibly affecting activities of daily living, work habits, or recreational athletics. Intolerable lifestyle changes or a poor response to nonoperative management may dictate consideration of surgical treatment. Surgical options vary, and proper patient selection is critical to successful clinical results. This chapter reviews the various criteria involved in surgical decision making in patients with arthritic knees. Assessment of these criteria should allow a more selective approach to surgical management in any given patient. However, despite these criteria, many patients fall into a "gray area" where surgical experience, intraoperative findings, and judgment may dictate the final treatment decision.

History

The selection process begins with a careful patient history. The overwhelming complaint in these patients is pain. Assessment of the knee pain should characterize the severity and duration of complaints. Use of analgesics or antiinflammatory agents should be recorded. Location of pain may be helpful in differentiating relative unicompartmental degenerative disease from more diffuse tricompartmental changes. Pain should be correlated with rest and activity. Rest pain is typically representative of more advanced degenerative joint disease or osteonecrosis. Flexed knee activities such as prolonged sitting, squatting, or stair climbing may be partic-

ularly painful in patients with significant patellofemoral disease. Unilateral versus bilateral knee pain should be noted as well as other joint complaints, particularly the ipsilateral hip.

Closely related to pain is the functional assessment of any given patient (35). The level of severity may range from significant disability in everyday activities to mere difficulty with active recreational sports, such as tennis. Work-related activities should be noted as well. This information, coupled with a patient's desired activity goals after surgery, is extremely important in surgical decision making, particularly in borderline clinical situations where total knee arthroplasty (TKA) may be a consideration. It should be noted that unrealistic patient goals are not uncommon in cases of arthroscopic debridement.

Degenerative joint disease of the knee may affect a broad range of age groups. Although typically presenting in an older population, degenerative changes secondary to previous knee surgery or trauma may appear in a younger patient. Age is clearly a dynamic component in surgical decision making. Precise age restrictions are difficult to define. For example, the emerging excellent long-term clinical results of total knee arthroplasty have particularly affected recent age criteria for total knee arthroplasty (10, 20, 48, 49, 53, 58, 60, 61). Life expectancy, medical history, and employment issues should also be considered. Although age is clearly important, it must be considered in the overall context of the patient.

General medical or neurologic problems in any given patient may affect their ability to tolerate the stress of the proposed surgery or to manage the postoperative rehabilitation program. Preoperative medical or neurologic consultation is important in managing these cases. Any previous knee surgery, osteomyelitis, or joint sepses should be noted as well. This may require additional imaging studies or joint aspiration, particularly when TKA is under consideration.

Physical Examination

Physical examination is the next step in decision making. A patient's height and weight are recorded. A large body habitus or frank obesity may influence surgical decision making, especially considering either uni- or tricompartmental knee arthroplasty. Although the ill effects of obesity seem clear, Stern and Insall have reported successful clinical results with TKA in obese patients with a relatively short follow-up (59).

Examination of the arthritic knee demands particular attention to deformity, ligament laxity, range of motion, and gait (32). Varus or valgus deformities often accompany degenerative disease of the knee. Greater angular deformities are often associated with medial or lateral ligamentous laxity. Severe cases may be associated with a thrusting motion during gait. Osteotomy procedures are typically reserved for less severe deformities with stable ligaments (33). Gait analysis has been used to define the proper candidates for osteotomy (62). Although gait analysis appears to have obvious benefits, the practicality of such evaluations has limited its usefulness.

The integrity of the anterior and posterior cruciate ligaments may be assessed with standard examination techniques. Absence of the anterior cruciate ligament may contraindicate unicompartmental knee arthroplasty (55). Recurvatum deformities of the knee are particularly worrisome and indicate the need for careful neurologic evaluation.

Stiffness may accompany progressive arthritic changes. Limitations of flexion as well as the presence of a fixed flexion contracture should be noted. In general, motion of less than 90 degrees of flexion or a 30 degree fixed flexion contracture are considered relative contraindications to osteotomy procedures (24).

Careful evaluation of the patellofemoral compartment should assess the extent of articular changes and crepitation, local tenderness, and alignment. Rotary signs consistent with meniscal pathology are performed. Related joint complaints are evaluated. Existing degenerative disease or deformity of the hips, particularly the ipsilateral hip, may directly influence surgical indications and the ultimate sequence of hip versus knee surgery. Injection of a painful knee with a local anesthetic may assist in evaluating a problematic knee when the precise source of pain is unclear.

Critical to successful surgical management of any degenerative knee is an adequate vascular supply to the extremity. If any question of vascular adequacy is suspected, preoperative vascular testing should be performed.

Radiographs

Radiographs of the knee are extremely important in the assessment of degenerative joint disease (37). Ahlback emphasized the importance of weight-bearing anteroposterior (AP) radiographs in extension to delineate these degenerative changes (2). He noted increased joint space narrowing in 140 of 161 knees on the weight-bearing views when compared to standard supine views (Fig. 53.1). More recently, Rosenberg and coworkers described the 45-degree posteroanterior flexion weight-bearing radiograph of the knee to further assess suspected arthritic changes (52). Correlating this radiographic view with arthroscopic findings, they noted an increased sensitivity and specificity of this view with conventional standing views in extension.

The 45-degree weight-bearing view should be used in patients whose histories and examinations suggest

Figure 53.1. **A,** Supine anteroposterior x-ray (right knee). **B,** Weight-bearing anteroposterior x-ray right knee of same patient. This demonstrates narrowing of the medial compartment with mild varus deformity.

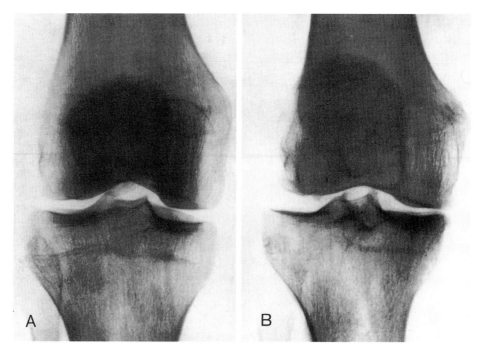

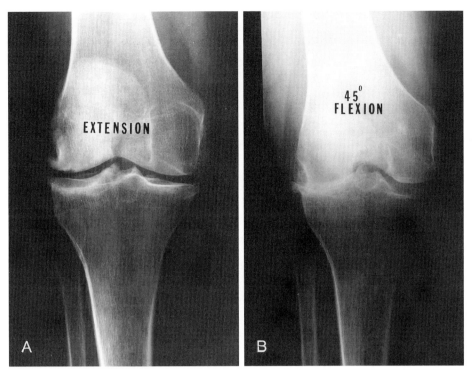

Figure 53.2. **A,** Extension weight-bearing anteroposterior radiograph demonstrating mild lateral compartment degenerative changes. **B,** Forty-five-degree weight-bearing anteroposterior view of the lateral joint space and valgus deformity.

more severe degenerative changes than are apparent on the extension view. I have found this view particularly helpful in evaluating lateral compartment changes and valgus deformities (Fig. 53.2, *A* and 53.2, *B*). This view is useful in preoperative evaluation of borderline patients under consideration for arthroscopic meniscal surgery. Clinical reports suggest inferior results in patients with loss of articular cartilage (18, 28, 39).

Lateral and axial views may demonstrate degenerative changes in the patellofemoral compartment (Fig. 53.3). Additionally, patellar alignment may be assessed (Fig. 53.4). Surgical decisions in patients with relatively isolated patellofemoral arthritis are extremely difficult with less rewarding clinical results.

Three joint views allowing determination of the mechanical axis of the knee are used infrequently in the initial evaluation of the arthritic knee. More commonly, they are reserved for preoperative planning of osteotomy or total knee replacement procedures or evaluating previous fracture malunions.

Historically, bone scans of the knee have been used to evaluate more subtle degenerative changes or suspected osteonecrosis. In practice, these scans are infrequently used today, in favor of magnetic resonance imaging (MRI). These scans are extremely useful in evaluating derangements, such as meniscal tears and osteonecrosis. Extensive degenerative changes on radiographs typically yield an array of MRI findings. Magnetic resonance imaging is more useful in patients with localized pain and with physical findings consistent with meniscal pathology who demonstrate minimal arthritic change on radiographs (Fig. 53.5). Accuracy of MRI in predicting meniscal tears is well documented (31). MRI evidence of a meniscal tear may be useful in selecting

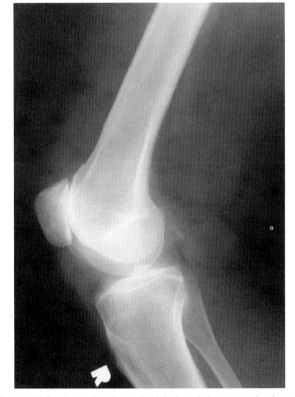

Figure 53.3. Lateral radiograph (right knee) demonstrating loss of patellofemoral joint space and degenerative changes.

Figure 53.4. Axial patellar view. This view demonstrates severe patellofemoral degenerative disease with lateral tilt.

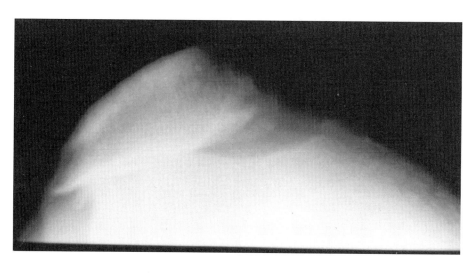

Figure 53.5. MRI sagittal view of the knee demonstrating a grade III signal of the posterior horn medial meniscus consistent with a tear.

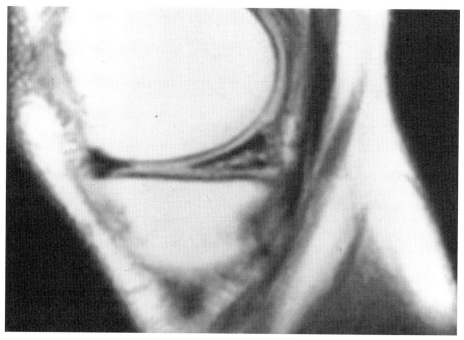

patients for arthroscopic debridement. Additionally, MRI is extremely valuable in diagnosing early osteonecrosis in the older patient, who may otherwise be diagnosed with a degenerative meniscal tear and undergo an unsuccessful knee arthroscopy. Although MRI is clearly a useful adjunct in the evaluation of the arthritic knee, it should *not* replace routine X-rays.

Arthroscopy

In 1974, Jackson described the use of arthroscopy as a diagnostic tool in management of the arthritic knee (25). He felt arthroscopy was particularly applicable to decision making between osteotomy and arthroplasty in borderline cases (Fig. 53.6). Correlation between radiographic evidence of degenerative knee disease and findings at the time of arthroscopy was reported by Lysholm when he described the arthroscopic and radi-

ographic findings in 63 patients with degenerative arthritis (40). Rosenberg also noted this correlation in the flexion contact zones of the knee with the 45-degree weight-bearing posteroanterior view (52).

Although arthroscopy may be a tempting tool for evaluating the arthritic knee and assisting in surgical decision making, the predictive value in patients with relative unicompartmental disease is questionable. Fujisawa, in 1979, reported on 54 patients who underwent upper tibial osteotomy and, later, had arthroscopic evaluation with the evaluation period ranging from 4 months to 6 years and 4 months after osteotomy (15). Based on their findings, they concluded that arthroscopy was of no diagnostic value preoperatively in determining the success of their surgery.

In 1983, Keane and Dyreby evaluated 60 osteoarthritic knees arthroscopically and radiographically prior to upper tibial osteotomy (30). They found that a

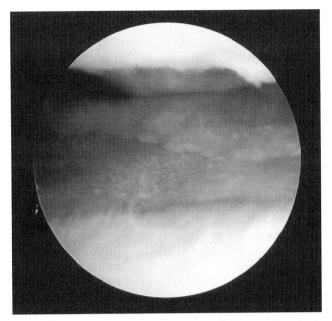

Figure 53.6. Arthroscopic view of the medial compartment after meniscectomy. There is severe loss of articular cartilage and exposed subchondral bone.

postoperative valgus alignment of 5 to 13 degrees correlated with a good or excellent clinical result more closely than the preosteotomy assessment of the lateral compartment, as viewed arthroscopically. It is not clear that arthroscopy serves any predictive role in distinguishing candidates for osteotomy procedures. However, it may be useful in evaluating and treating associated meniscal pathology in selected patients.

Intraoperative assessment of the knee joint may be the final step in surgical decision making, primarily in unicompartmental knee arthroplasty (55). More advanced degenerative changes in either the contralateral or patellofemoral compartment may dictate a tricompartmental arthroplasty.

Surgical Management

The collective data from these evaluations allow further definition of a patient's degenerative knee disease. These changes may be characterized with regard to severity and compartmental involvement. Patients may be broadly classified either into unicompartmental degenerative disease or tricompartmental disease, a more diffuse classification. These categories are further defined as mild, moderate, or severe. Typically, bicompartmental disease is associated with patellofemoral degenerative changes and, if mild, fall into consideration with unicompartmental disease.

Surgical management of advanced tricompartmental disease most commonly involves total knee arthroplasty while decision making in patients with relative unicompartmental degenerative changes is more varied and controversial. Surgical options include arthroscopic debridement, distal femoral or upper tibial osteotomy, unicompartmental arthroplasty, as well as total knee

arthroplasty. The precise criteria for patient selection are poorly defined and may overlap. Personal surgical experience and technical expertise may ultimately dictate surgical treatment.

The limited morbidity and swift postoperative recovery of arthroscopic debridement have popularized this procedure in the treatment of the arthritic knee. The procedure appears particularly well suited to older patients with mild to moderate unicompartmental or tricompartmental degenerative changes. Several investigators have reported successful clinical results with improvement in painful symptoms more common than complete resolution of such complaints (5, 7, 18, 26, 38, 50, 56). It is tempting to expand patient selection for this procedure, but inferior results can be expected in patients with more advanced changes associated with loss of articular joint space, significant angular deformity, and rest pain. Despite this, younger patients with more advanced tricompartmental disease may be considered candidates for arthroscopic debridement as a temporizing procedure. Critical to patient selection is a careful and explicit explanation of the limited goals of such a procedure. Unreasonable patient expectations should serve as a contraindication to arthroscopic debridement. More extensive arthroscopic procedures, such as drilling or abrasion arthroplasty, do not appear to offer additional benefits and should be avoided in the older patient particularly (7, 27, 50).

The clinical success and durability of total knee arthroplasty have altered the indications for corrective osteotomy procedures on the knee over the past decade. Upper tibial osteotomy has been used to treat varus gonarthrosis and distal femoral osteotomy for valgus disease. Historically, tibial osteotomy had been used to correct valgus knees. However, correction of valgus deformities greater than 12 degrees with osteotomy of the upper tibia may produce an obliquity of the joint line leading to incomplete load transfer and possible medial tibial subluxation (24). Therefore, osteotomy of the distal femur is the preferred alternative.

Long-term clinical results have demonstrated that upper tibial osteotomy is a successful operation for varus degenerative disease (11, 12, 13, 17, 21, 23, 30). Notwithstanding these results, studies have also demonstrated deterioration of clinical results with the passage of time and the recurrence of knee pain (23). Patient selection is further complicated by the knowledge that many patients ultimately require total knee arthroplasty. Inferior clinical results and technical challenges have been reported in total knee arthroplasty after upper tibial osteotomy (29, 57, 63). Patient selection in the borderline situation must weigh these factors carefully. Surgical indications vary throughout the orthopaedic community.

Relative contraindications should improve patient selection. Degenerative changes in the patellofemoral compartment often accompany medial compartment arthritis. Clinical history, physical examination, and axial radiographs should provide a careful evaluation. Mild to moderate patellofemoral involvement appears compatible with a successful osteotomy (11, 13, 21, 23,

24). More advanced patellofemoral disease alters the surgical decision making toward total knee arthroplasty. Upper tibial osteotomy does not improve knee flexion and at least 70 degrees of flexion should be present preoperatively. Although minor knee flexion contractures may be corrected with an osteotomy, flexion contractures greater than 20 degrees are considered a relative contraindication to the procedure (24).

Extreme varus deformities are not well suited for upper tibial osteotomy. These deformities are often associated with advanced degenerative changes, bone loss and laxity of the lateral soft-tissue stabilizers. A lateral thrust in gait may be apparent, or lateral tibial subluxation may be present on standing AP radiographs (Fig. 53.7). The precise upper limit of varus deformity suitable for corrective osteotomy is difficult to define. Typically, varus deformities of less than 10 degrees are associated with stable knees and are amenable to good results with a "closing-wedge" upper tibial osteotomy (Fig. 53.8). Greater varus deformities and those associated with lateral subluxation are not generally good candidates for this procedure, although Maquet has reported satisfactory results in these patients with a "barrel-vault" technique (42).

Recently, arthroscopy of the knee has been used with upper tibial osteotomy. Arthroscopic evaluation to assess existing degenerative disease is not of prognostic value. Series by Fujisawa and by Keene did not demonstrate prognostic value of preoperative arthroscopic findings to the eventual clinical result following upper tibial osteotomy (15, 30).

Although age is a dynamic consideration, it remains an important criterion of patient selection. In a recent study of osteotomy results, Insall found that patients over the age of 60 at the time of osteotomy did less well than younger patients. (23). This observation, coupled with the excellent long-term results of total knee arthroplasty, influences patient selection for upper tibial osteotomy toward patients under the age of 60. Other important criteria are activity level, both occupational and recreational, as well as patient weight. Osteotomy is well suited for heavier, more active patients and may be indicated in patients older than 60 years. However, most older patients are better candidates for total knee arthroplasty. This is particularly true of patients with symptomatic bilateral degenerative knee disease.

In summary, upper tibial osteotomy is an excellent surgical procedure for varus gonarthrosis in younger, heavier individuals with varus deformities less than 10 degrees and with reasonable knee motion. This is particularly true for active individuals who may be involved in heavy labor or aggressive athletic activities.

Distal femoral varus osteotomy is useful in the management of valgus gonarthrosis. Healy and coworkers reported 83% good or excellent results in a series of 23 osteotomies followed for an average of 4 years (19).

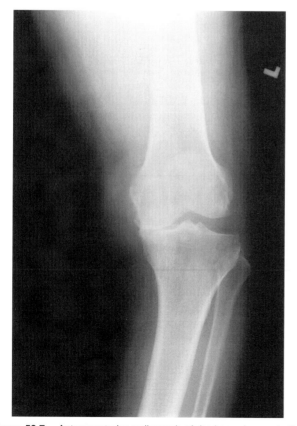

Figure 53.7. Anteroposterior radiograph of the knee demonstrating more advanced degenerative changes associated with a significant varus deformity.

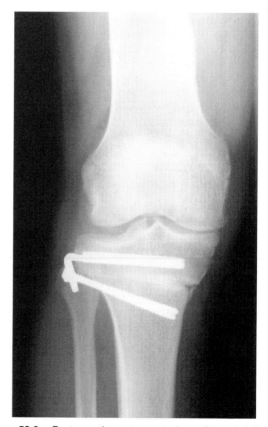

Figure 53.8. Postoperative anteroposterior radiograph following upper tibial osteotomy.

Similar results have been reported by others (6, 44). Edgerton, et al. reported less than satisfactory results with this procedure, noting stable fixation of the osteotomy as a complicating factor (14).

Many decision criteria in selecting patients for supracondylar osteotomy are similar to upper tibial osteotomy. Panarthritis, severe patellofemoral disease, and restricted range of motion contraindicate the procedure. Edgerton noted the severity of existing degenerative disease as a prognostic indicator (14). Similar to the varus knee, advanced valgus deformity may be associated with laxity of the medial soft-tissues, including the superficial medial collateral ligament. This may be detected by noting a medial thrust on gait or medial tibial subluxation on AP standing radiographs. Although there is no clear definition of the upper limit of valgus deformity amenable to osteotomy, instability contraindicates this procedure.

Postoperative rehabilitation after distal femoral osteotomy is more demanding than upper tibial osteotomy and may be particularly difficult for older patients. Again, this procedure is better suited for the younger, active patient who is capable of managing the demanding postoperative rehabilitation that may require prolonged, limited weight-bearing. It should be noted that inflammatory arthritis is a contraindication to any osteotomy.

Despite published clinical success with unicompartmental arthroplasty for unicompartmental disease, the procedure and its indications remain controversial. Early reports by Insall and Laskin noted disappointing results with unicompartmental arthroplasty, but more recent studies have been encouraging (22, 36, 41, 54, 55). From these studies, it is clear that proper patient selection is critical to success. However, there is a lack of consensus regarding patient selection in the literature. The technical demands of unicompartmental arthroplasty and the relative infrequency of the procedure have been named as contraindications to the procedure. Perhaps there is no procedure in the surgical treatment of the arthritic knee for which patient selection is more influenced by individual surgical experience and technical expertise than unicompartmental arthroplasty.

Patients with medial or lateral unicompartmental osteoarthritis or osteonecrosis are considered for unicompartmental arthroplasty (55). Panarthritis, inflammatory arthritis, and crystalline arthroplasty are contraindications. Mild to moderate patellofemoral disease appears to be compatible with a successful result (41, 54). Preoperative knee motion should be good and flexion contractures should be limited to 5 degrees.

Similar to osteotomy, unicompartmental replacement should be limited to moderate angular deformities of approximately 10 to 15 degrees (55). More severe deformities are better suited for tricompartmental replacement (Fig. 53.9). Inferior results with unicompartmental arthroplasty have been reported in heavy patients, and the procedure should be reserved for patients weighing less than 170 pounds (54). The ideal patient age for unicompartmental arthroplasty is debated. Total knee

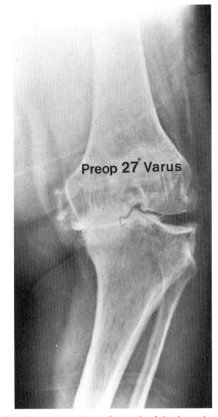

Figure 53.9. Anteroposterior radiograph of the knee in the preoperative angular deformity of 27 degrees varus and advanced DJD. Total knee arthroplasty is the preferred option in this knee.

arthroplasty is a better choice for elderly patients where such a procedure can be expected to last for the life of the patient. Some surgeons have suggested unicompartmental arthroplasty as a conservative procedure for younger patients, for whom later revision will prove easier. This is debatable (46). Relatively sedentary patients in their 60s and 70s with unicompartmental degenerative disease appear to be reasonable candidates for this procedure.

The integrity of both the anterior and posterior cruciate ligaments is essential for successful unicompartmental replacement (55). Additionally, intraoperative inspections of the patellofemoral and opposite compartment allow a final evaluation of the extent of degenerative changes. In cases where degenerative disease is limited to the involved compartment and where ligamentous integrity is present, one may proceed with unicompartmental arthroplasty. If these criteria are not present, a tricompartmental replacement is preferred.

Advanced degenerative disease primarily involving the patellofemoral compartment presents a difficult surgical solution. In the elderly patient, total knee arthroplasty is the most reasonable and most rewarding surgical option. However, many patients presenting with patellofemoral arthritis are younger and active. Prosthetic replacement of either the patella alone or the patellofemoral compartment has been performed (1, 3, 9, 34, 45). Variable results have been reported and these procedures are performed infrequently. Maquet has popularized anteriorization of the tibial tubercle; more recently, Fulkerson advocated an anteromedialization osteotomy of the tubercle (16, 43). These procedures may be considered in specific situations, although precise criteria are difficult to define (4, 8, 16, 47, 51). One should avoid patellectomy.

Total knee arthroplasty is versatile and is the procedure of choice in advanced tricompartmental disease. Advanced degenerative changes, including severe angular deformity, bone loss, flexion contracture, and ligamentous laxity, may be managed with total knee techniques. Older, sedentary patients who are disabled either by advanced unicompartmental or tricompartmental disease are ideal candidates for total knee arthroplasty. However, over the past decade, indications for TKA have expanded to include younger and heavier patients. Selection of these patients is more difficult and commonly requires extreme disability. Successful clinical results have been reported in both obese patients and in patients under 55 years when alternative management is unsuitable (29, 48, 58, 59). Unlike osteotomy and unicompartmental replacement, total knee arthroplasty is indicated in the treatment of inflammatory arthritis of the knee.

Relative contraindications to total knee arthroplasty are few; they include (a) a stable, painless arthrodesis, (b) gross quadriceps muscle weakness, and (c) genu recurvatum. A past history of osteomyelitis or joint sepsis may signal possible increased risk of infection. Joint sepsis, if suspected or proven, may be managed with a staged replacement procedure, provided proper antimicrobial treatment is established. When adequate antimicrobial treatment cannot be achieved, arthrodesis is a better choice. Joint replacement in neuropathic states remains controversial.

To summarize then, successful surgical management of the arthritic knee begins with proper patient selection. Careful preoperative evaluation examining the criteria discussed above allows a more selective approach to the proposed surgical options for the patient. Final decision making is individualized.

References

1. Aglietti P, Insall JN, Walker PS, Trent P. A new patella prosthesis: Design and application. Clin Orthop 1975;107:175–187.
2. Ahlback S. Osteoarthrosis of the Knee: A radiographic investigation (Thesis). Stockholm, Sweden: Karolinska Institutet. 1968;11–15.
3. Arciero RA, Toomey HE. Patellofemoral arthroplasty: A three- to nine-year follow-up study. Clin Orthop 1988;236:60–71.
4. Bandi W. Chondromalacia patellae und femoro-patellare arthrose. Hev Chir Acta (Suppl 11) 1972.
5. Baumgaertner MR, Cannon WD Jr, Vittori JM, Schmidt ES, Maurer, RC. Arthroscopic debridement of the arthritic knee. Clin Orthop 1990;253:197–202.
6. Beaver RJ, Jinxiang-Yu, Sekyi-Otu A, Gross AE. Distal femoral varus osteotomy for genu valgum: A prospective review. Am J Knee Surg 1991;4(1):9–17.
7. Bert JM, Maschka K. The arthroscopic treatment of unicompartmental gonarthrosis: A five-year follow-up study of abrasion arthroplasty plus arthroscopic debridement and arthroscopic debridement alone. Arthroscopy 1989;5(1):25–32.
8. Bessette GC, Hunter RE. The Maquet procedure: A retrospective review. Clin Orthop 1988;232:159–167.
9. Blazina ME, Fox JM, Del Pizzo W, Broukhim B, Ivey FM. Patellofemoral replacement. Clin Orthop 1979;144:98–102.
10. John BT, Krackow KA, Hungerford DS, Lennox DW, Bachner, EJ. Results of total knee arthroplasty in patients 80 years and older. Orthop Rev 1990;19(5):451–460.
11. Coventry MB. Upper tibial osteotomy for gonarthrosis: The evolution of the operation in the last 18 years and long term results. Orthop Clin North Am 1979;10(1):191–210.
12. Coventry MB. Upper tibial osteotomy for osteoarthritis. J Bone Joint Surg 1985;67-A:1136–1140.
13. Coventry MB, Ilstrup DM, Wallrich SL. Proximal tibial osteotomy: A critical long-term study of eighty-seven cases. J Bone Joint Surg 1993;75-A:196–201.
14. Edgerton BC, Mariani EM, Morrey BF. Distal femoral varus osteotomy for painful genu valgum: a 5-to-11-year follow-up study. Clin Orthop 1993;288:263–269.
15. Fujisawa Y, Masuhara, K, Shiomi S. The effect of high tibial osteotomy on osteoarthritis of the knee: An arthroscopic study of 54 knee joints. Orthop Clin North Am 1979;10:585–608.
16. Fulkerson JP. Anteromedialization of the tibial tuberosity for patellofemoral malalignment. Clin Orthop 1983;177:176–181.
17. Harris WR, Kostuik JP. High tibial osteotomy for osteoarthritis of the knee. J Bone Joint Surg 1970;52-A:330–336.
18. Harwin SF, Stein AJ, Stern RE, Kulick RG. Arthroscopic debridement of the osteoarthritic knee: a step toward patient selection. Am. J. Arthroscopy 1991;1(6):7.
19. Healy WL, Anglen JO, Wasilewski SA, Krackow KA. Distal femoral varus osteotomy. J Bone Joint Surg 1988;70-A:102–109.
20. Hungerford DS, Krackow KA, Kenna RV. Cementless total knee replacement in patients 50 years old and under. Orthop Clin North Am 1989;20:(2)131–145.
21. Insall J, Shoji H, Mayer V. High tibial osteotomy: A five-year evaluation. J Bone Joint Surg 1974;56-A:1397–1405.
22. Insall J, Walker, P. Unicondylar Knee Replacement. Clin Orthop 1976;120:83–85.
23. Insall JN, Joseph DM, Msika C. High tibial osteotomy for varus gonarthrosis. J Bone Joint Surg 1984;66-A:1040–1048.
24. Insall JN. Osteotomy. In: Insall JN, Windsor RE, Scott WN, Kelly MA, Aglietti P, eds. Surgery of the knee. 2nd ed. New York: Churchill Livingstone, 1993:635–676.
25. Jackson RW. The role of arthroscopy in the management of the arthritic knee. Clin Orthop 1974;101:28–35.
26. Jackson RW, Silver R, Marans H. Arthroscopic treatment of degenerative joint disease. Arthroscopy 1986;2:14.
27. Johnson LL. Arthroscopic abrasion arthroplasty historical and pathologic perspective: Present stakes. Arthroscopy 1986;2:54–69.
28. Jones RE, Smith EC, Reisch JS. Effects of medial meniscectomy in patients older than forty years. J Bone Joint Surg 1978;60-A:783–786.
29. Katz MM, Hungerford DS, Krackow KA, Lennox DW. Results of total knee arthroplasty after failed proximal tibial osteotomy for osteoarthritis. J Bone Joint Surg 1987;69-A:225–233.
30. Keene JS, Dyreby JR. High tibial osteotomy in the treatment of osteoarthritis of the knee. J Bone Joint Surg 1983;36–42.
31. Kelly MA, Flock TJ, Kimmel JA, Kiernan HA Jr, Singson RS, Starron RB, Feldman F. MR imaging of the knee: Clarification of its role. Arthroscopy 1991;7(1):78–85.
32. Kelly MA, Insall JN. Clinical examination. In: Insall JN, Windsor RE, Scott WN, Kelly MA, Aglietti P, eds. Surgery of the knee. 2nd ed. New York: Churchill Livingstone, 1993;63–82.
33. Kettelkamp DB, Leach RE, Nasca R. Pitfalls of proximal tibial osteotomy. Clin Orthop 1975;106:232.
34. Kolettis GT, Stern SH. Patellar resurfacing for patellofemoral arthritis. Orthop Clin North Am 1992;23(4):665–673.
35. Krackow KA. Patient selection: Indications, assessment, and alternatives. In: Krackow KA, ed. The technique of total knee arthroplasty. St. Louis: C.V. Mosby, 1990;1–48.
36. Laskin RS. Unicompartmental tibiofemoral resurfacing arthroplasty. J Bone Joint Surg 1978;60-A:182–185.
37. Leach RE, Gregg T, Siber FJ. Weight-bearing radiography in osteoarthritis of the knee. Radiology 1970;97:265–268.
38. Livesley PJ, Doherty M, Needhoff M, Moulton A. Arthroscopic lavage of osteoarthritic knees. J Bone Joint Surg 1991;73-B:922–926.
39. Lotke PA, Lefkoe RT, Ecker ML. Late results following medial meniscectomy in an older population. J Bone Joint Surg 1981;60-A:115–119.
40. Lysholm J, Hamberg P, Gillquist J. The correlation between osteoarthrosis as seen on radiographs and on arthroscopy. Arthroscopy 1987;3(3):161–165.
41. Marmor L. Unicompartmental knee arthroplasty: ten- to 13-year follow-up study. Clin Orthop 1988;226:14–20.
42. Maquet P. Valgus osteotomy for osteoarthritis of the knee. Clin Orthop 1976;120:143–148.
43. Maquet P. Advancement of the tibial tuberosity. Clin Orthop 1976;115:225–230.

44. McDermott AGP, Finklestein JA, Farine I, Boynton EL, MacIntosh DL, Gross A. Distal femoral varus osteotomy for valgus deformity of the knee. J Bone Joint Surg 1988;70-A:110–116.
45. McKeever DC. Patellar prosthesis. J Bone Joint Surg 1955;37-A:1074–1084.
46. Padgett DE, Stern SH, Insall JN. Revision total knee arthroplasty for failed unicompartmental replacement. J Bone Joint Surg 1991;186–190.
47. Radin EL. The Maquet procedure—anterior displacement of the tibial tubercle: Indications, contraindications, and precautions. Clin Orthop 1986;213:241–248.
48. Ranawat CS, Boachie-Adjei O. Survivorship analysis and results of total condylar knee arthroplasty: 8- to 11-year follow-up period. Clin Orthop 1988;226:6–13.
49. Ranawat CS, Padgett DE, Ohashi Y. Total knee arthroplasty for patients younger than 55 years. Clin Orthop 1989;248:27.
50. Rand JA. Role of arthroscopy in osteoarthritis of the knee. Arthroscopy 1991;7(4):358.
51. Rappoport LH, Browne MG, Wickiewicz TL. The Maquet osteotomy. Orthop Clin North Am 1992;23(4):645–656.
52. Rosenberg TD, Paulos LE, Parker RD, Coward DB, Scott SM. The forty-five-degree posteroanterior flexion weight-bearing radiograph of the knee. J Bone Joint Surg 1988;70-A:1479–1483.
53. Scott RD, Volatile TB. Twelve years' experience with posterior cruciate-retaining total knee arthroplasty. Clin Orthop 1986;205:100–107.
54. Scott RD, Cobb AG, McQueary FG, Thornhill TS. Unicompartmental knee arthroplasty: 8- to 12-year follow-up evaluation with survivorship analysis. Clin Orthop 1991;271:96–105.
55. Scott RD. Unicompartmental total knee arthroplasty. In: Insall JN, Windsor RE, Scott WN, Kelly MA, Aglietti P, eds. Surgery of the knee. 2nd edition, vol 2. New York: Churchill Livingstone, 1993;805–814.
56. Sprague NF III. Arthroscopic debridement for degenerative joint disease. Clin Orthop 1974;101:61.
57. Staeheli JW, Cass JR, Morrey BF. Condylar total knee arthroplasty after failed proximal tibial osteotomy. J Bone Joint Surg 1987;69-A:28–31.
58. Stern SH, Bowen MK, Insall JN, Scuderi GR. Cemented total knee arthroplasty for gonarthrosis in patients 55-years-old or younger. Clin Orthop 1990;260:124–129.
59. Stern SH, Insall JN. Total knee arthroplasty in obese patients. J Bone Joint Surg 1990;72-A:1400–1404.
60. Stern SH, Insall JN. Posterior stabilized prosthesis: Results after follow-up of 9 to 12 years. J Bone Joint Surg 1992;74-A:980–986.
61. Vince KG, Insall JN, Kelly MA. The total condylar prosthesis: 10- to 12-year results of a cemented knee replacement. J Bone Joint Surg 1989;71-B:793–797.
62. Wang J-W, Kuo KN, Andriacchi TP, Galante, JO. The influence of walking mechanics and time on the results of proximal tibial osteotomy. J Bone Joint Surg 1990;72-A:905–909.
63. Windsor RE, Insall JN, Vince KG. Technical considerations of total knee arthroplasty after proximal tibial osteotomy. J Bone Joint Surg 1988;70-A:547–555.

54

Arthroscopic Treatment of Degenerative Joint Disease

Ralph A. Gambardella

Introduction

The role of arthroscopy in the treatment of degenerative joint disease has been subject to continuous change. The equipment has improved, and arthroscopic techniques continue to be refined. However, the expectations of surgeons and patients have also changed. This chapter reviews the history of arthroscopic surgery in the treatment of degenerative joint disease of the knee, creating an algorithm for the treatment of these patients that is based on published studies.

Historical Review

The use of the arthroscope in the treatment of degenerative joint disease dates back at least to 1934 when Burman, et al. (1) reported on ten patients who were treated with arthroscopic lavage among whom several had improved symptoms. The study was, however, simply a collection of case reports reviewed retrospectively.

Surgical debridement of the degenerative knee originated with Magnuson (2) and Haggart (3) in the early 1940s. Their studies of open procedures revealed good results, because debridement was felt to slow the progression of degenerative disease by eliminating intraarticular mechanical irritants. Haggert reported that 19 of 20 patients were improved, while, in Magnusson's series, 60 of 62 procedures had a "complete recovery." In 1967, Insall (4) reported success with open debridement in 46 of 60 patients.

With the development of operative arthroscopic techniques in the 1970s, it was only logical that people began to investigate the role of the arthroscope in both the evaluation and management of degenerative joint disease (5). Jackson and Abe (6) reviewed 200 consecutive cases in 1972 to determine if diagnostic arthroscopy could help increase the accuracy of diagnosis. They concluded that arthroscopy was useful in over 88% of patients studied. It was felt that diagnostic arthroscopy could be used as a practical and valuable procedure with minimal associated risk and could help to increase accuracy of diagnosis and thereby avoid unnecessary open procedures. In 1990, Dandy (7) reviewed 500 consecutive arthroscopies to examine the impact of arthroscopic surgery on the management of knee disorders. He concluded that arthroscopic surgery had eliminated the need for 96% of the proposed arthrotomies.

As arthroscopic skills improved, several investigators began not only to evaluate but also to attempt to manage degenerative disease with arthroscopic procedures. In the past 10 to 15 years, numerous studies have been published regarding the arthroscopic treatment of degenerative joint disease. These studies may be categorized—as proposed by Burks (8)—according to three indications for arthroscopy in degenerative joint disease:

1. To define pathology and/or assist in planning treatment;
2. To treat specific concurrent problems such as meniscal tears or loose bodies;
3. To prolong use of the knee by generalized treatment such as debridement and/or abrasion arthroplasty.

Role of the Arthroscope in Defining Pathology

The arthroscope has been used in the early detection of arthritis and in biopsies of synovium when laboratory studies have failed to confirm a diagnosis. In 1987, Lysholm, et al. (9) attempted to correlate osteoarthritic changes as seen on radiographs with those seen at the time of arthroscopy. In his study, chondral damage was classified according to a modification of the Outerbridge classification. He found patients with stage II and III chondral changes often had normal radiographic findings. Only in patients with chondral changes on both the tibia and femur did the radiographs usually show joint space narrowing.

Brandt, et al. (10) looked at radiographic grading of the severity of knee osteoarthritis at the time of arthroscopy. In his study, 92 patients with knee pain and mild to moderate osteoarthritis were studied. Each knee was assessed prior to arthroscopy with standing anteroposterior (AP) radiographs. Of 17 patients with normal x-rays, 7 were found to have severe tibial, femoral, or patellofemoral articular cartilage changes at the time of arthroscopy. In addition, measurable joint space narrowing was common on radiographs despite the presence at the time of arthroscopy of normal articular cartilage.

Fife, et al. (11) could not correlate radiographic joint space narrowing and the condition of the articular surface as observed arthroscopically. He evaluated 161 patients with chronic knee pain and found that 33% of the patients who had documented joint space narrowing on standing x-ray analysis were found to have normal articular cartilage at the time of arthroscopic evaluation. In fact, even with greater than 50% medial joint space narrowing, 41% of patients had normal surfaces when visualized arthroscopically.

The ability of the arthroscope to biopsy synovium initiated several investigations of the etiology of osteoarthritis. Myers, et al. (12) in 1990 looked at synovitis in patients with early osteoarthritis and concluded that the severity of cartilage lesions was neither related to the severity of the synovitis nor to the topographical location of the synovitis. Conflicting results were reported in 1987 by Lindblad and Hedfors (13), who performed immunohistologic studies on the synovium of 10 patients with arthritis. They concluded that the inflammatory synovial changes found in osteoarthritis were anatomically restricted but of varied intensity. In addition, they felt that these changes were indistinguishable microscopically from those described in the synovium of rheumatoid arthritis patients.

Meniscal Pathology with Osteoarthritis

Numerous studies from the past 10 years have evaluated the arthroscopic treatment of degenerative joint disease. Several investigators have looked specifically at meniscal disease in patients with osteoarthritis because the two conditions often coexist. In 1978, Casscells (14) reported a cadaveric study and a clinical study of the relationship between the state of the meniscus (torn or degenerative) and degeneration of the adjacent femoral condyle. Of 300 cadaveric knees, 53% had degenerative changes in the femoral condyle despite an intact meniscus. In his clinical study, 40 of 100 knees arthroscoped had intact menisci with chondromalacia of the adjacent femoral condyle. However, 20% of knees had meniscal pathology and normal articular surfaces.

In 1983, Fahmy, et al. (15) examined 115 cadavers. While 57% had degenerative meniscal changes, there was little correlation with adjacent chondral damage. By contrast, In 1989, Zamber, et al. (16) did a prospective review of 200 knees undergoing arthroscopy. He concluded that unstable meniscal tears were significantly associated with destruction of adjacent articular surfaces and also that the medial compartment is especially susceptible to chondromalacic changes.

The role of total meniscectomy in the development of degenerative joint disease has been well reviewed since the articles by Fairbanks in 1948 (17) and Tapper and Hoover in 1969 (18). Others have looked at the results of meniscectomy in older patients and have tried to assess the patients' results after arthroscopic partial meniscectomy.

Lotke, et al. (19) reviewed 101 patients who had an isolated medial meniscectomy after age 45. There was a 10.8-year follow-up. Patients with normal preoperative radiographs had a 90% chance of good or excellent results. However, patients with preexisting x-ray changes had only a 21% chance for a good result. In 1978, Jones, et al. (20) concluded that open, complete medial meniscectomy was usually followed by degenerative changes in the joint.

McBride, et al. (21) were the first to review the results of arthroscopic partial medial meniscectomy in the older patient. In this study from 1984, patients were evaluated at 35-months follow-up. No progressive varus deformity or medial joint space narrowing was observed. While 96% of patients with nondegenerative tears did well, only 65% of those with degenerative tears had satisfactory results at the time of follow-up. The advantages of partial arthroscopic versus complete open meniscectomy were established, especially for the older patient.

One of the most recent studies evaluating arthroscopic meniscectomy in middle-aged to older patients is that of Bonamo, et al. (22) from 1992. All patients were over age 40 and had arthroscopically verified meniscal tears. They were divided into two groups based upon the absence or presence of significant articular cartilage damage (grade III or grade IV Outerbridge changes). Arthroscopic management consisted of partial meniscectomy and limited debridement only. At a mean follow-up of 3.3 years, 60% of patients with significant chondromalacia were significantly improved as compared to 71% of those without chondromalacia at the time of surgery. The results tended to be worse for females and patients greater than 60 years of age, as well as those with grade IV articular lesions and those with moderate or severe preoperative x-ray changes. While obesity and mechanical alignment did not correlate with satisfactory results, satisfaction rates in those patients declined with length of follow-up.

Also in 1992, Covall and Wasilewski (23) reported a 5-year follow-up study of x-ray changes after arthroscopic meniscectomy in patients 45 years or older. In this study of 50 knees, there was 98% patient satisfaction. When compared to the nonoperative limb, 40% showed radiographic progression of Fairbanks' changes, with only 4% of those felt to be significant. One of the largest reviews of arthroscopic management of the degenerative knee in the literature is that of Ogilvie-Harris and Fitsialos (24). In 1991, he reviewed 441 cases of degenerative osteoarthritis treated arthroscopically with debridement, meniscectomy, removal of loose bodies, and osteophyte removal. Overall, 4 years after surgery, 86% of patients felt they had improved from their preoperative status. However, only 53% had no or occasional pain, 59% had no or occasional limitations of their activities, and 21% of patients continued to require analgesic medication. However, despite these limitations, the overall satisfaction rate was 90% when asked if they considered it worthwhile to have the procedure.

In this large study, several factors were evaluated for their predictive value. Patellofemoral disease was not an adverse factor but chondrocalcinosis was. Mechanical alignment was important. 61% of patients with normal mechanical alignment preoperatively were improved at 4-year follow-up, while only 24% of patients with valgus alignment and 47% of patients with varus alignment were improved postoperatively. Patients with severe disease in both medial and lateral femoral condyles did poorly. Patients with unstable flap tears of the meniscus did the best of all groups, with 72% improved 4 years after surgery. By contrast, only 37% of patients with a previous meniscectomy did well with repeat arthroscopic debridement.

Generalized Treatment of Degenerative Joint Disease

The generalized treatment of degenerative joint disease can be further subdivided into lavage, debridement, and abrasion. Studies of these three categories are described below.

Lavage Studies

The effects of isolated lavage of the knee joint in providing temporary relief of symptoms in patients with degenerative joint disease have been studied. Since Burman's, et al. observations in 1934 (1), several authors have noted improvement with this type of treatment. Livesley, et al. (25) reported in 1991 a controlled trial comparing one group of 37 patients treated with lavage and physiotherapy to a control group of 24 patients treated by therapy alone. He found better pain relief in the lavage group, which lasted 1 year postoperatively. However, inflammation of the joint occurred after a 3-month period of time.

Not all surgeons have felt that lavage alone is adequate or optimal. Jackson, et al. (26) compared lavage alone to debridement and reported 68% of patients with permanent improvement with debridement versus 45% permanent improvement with lavage alone.

Debridement Studies

In 1981, Sprague (27) reviewed 68 cases with degenerative osteoarthritis treated by arthroscopic debridement. At a follow-up of 14 months, 74% had good results, 10% fair results with the other 16% rated failures. Jackson, et al. (26) in 1986 reported 68% improvement with debridement at 3.3 years. Shahriaree, et al. (28) in 1982 reported a 7-year follow-up after arthroscopic debridement with 72% success. In 1989, Bert and Maschka (29) reported on arthroscopic debridement in 67 patients with osteoarthritis and grade IV chondromalacic changes. Five years after surgery, 66% good to excellent results were reported.

Baumgaertner, et al. (30) in 1990 studied 59 knees over age 50 with a primary diagnosis of arthritis treated with arthroscopic debridement. Only 52% of results were considered good at a follow-up of 33 months. Chronic symptoms, severe preoperative radiographic changes, and malalignment predicted poor results.

Rand (31) in 1991 reviewed 131 cases with grade III and IV chondromalacic changes that were treated with partial meniscectomy and debridement. He found 80% improvement at 1 year, a rate that fell to 67% at 5 years. Timoney, et al. (32) reported a retrospective study on 109 patients with an average age of 58 years who underwent arthroscopic debridement for osteoarthritis. He found 63% improved at a follow-up of 4 years.

In the 1991 Canadian literature, McLaren, et al. (33) reported the results of arthroscopic debridement in 171 patients with osteoarthritis. A variety of procedures was performed, including meniscectomy, lavage, chondrectomy, removal of loose bodies, and osteophytes. While 65% of patients were satisfied, only 38% had excellent pain relief and only 22% reported improved function. No factors were found to correlate with outcome.

Table 54.1 summarizes the debridement studies of eight authors from 1981 to 1991.

Abrasion Studies

The palliative effects of lavage and debridement are well known in the treatment of degenerative arthritis. However, extensive research has focused on articular cartilage regeneration in an effort to see if degenerative arthritic changes could actually be improved surgically. In 1959, Pridie (34) published a new method of resurfacing osteoarthritic knee joints. This consisted of drilling multiple holes into damaged subchondral bone. Insall (4) reported on this technique performed on 62 knees, with 40 having a good result at 6 years follow-up. Others, including Ficat and Hungerford (35) and Shahriaree (36), have reported similar results with the Pridie open method.

In 1980, Salter, et al. (37) published a basic science study showing that 2 mm holes drilled into cancellous bone led to fibrocartilaginous repair in animals when continuous passive motion was employed.

Arthroscopic drilling of subchondral bone was reported by Richards and Lonergan (5) in 1984, with 80%

Table 54.1. Debridement Studies

Author	Year	Follow-up (months)	Good (%)	Fair/Poor (%)
Sprague	1981	14	74	26
Shahriaree	1982	84	72	28
Jackson	1986	39	68	32
Bert	1989	60	66	34
Baumgaertner	1990	33	52	48
Timoney	1990	48	63	37
Rand	1991	60	67	33
McLaren	1991		65	35

subjective improvement at 2-year follow-up. But even earlier, Mankin (38) had noted the poor wear characteristics of fibrocartilaginous regrowth when compared to normal hyaline cartilage.

The interest in fibrocartilaginous growth led Johnson (39) to advocate arthroscopic abrasion arthroplasty in 1986. After extensive work in the research laboratory, he advocated abrading only the areas of exposed bone that were already denuded of hyaline cartilage. The depth of debridement, felt to be critical, was limited to 1–2 mm into the intracortical layer. Deeper abrasion into the subchondral layer produced poor results. In a 2-year follow-up study of 96 knees treated with nonweight-bearing for two months postoperatively, 74 were improved; however, 15 were worse. He recommended this procedure primarily for patients with normal mechanical alignment, good range of motion, and low activity demands. Contraindications included varus angulation of greater than 10 degrees or valgus angulation greater than 15 degrees as well as evidence of inflammatory joint disease.

In 1985, Salisbury, et al. (40) reviewed the effects of alignment on the result of arthroscopic debridement in degenerative joint disease. They found over 90% of patients had functional improvement with normally aligned knees while only 32% of patients had improvement with varus angulation.

Friedman, et al. (41) reported only 60% improvement with arthroscopic abrasion. His best results were in patients less than 40 years of age; however, over 63% still required medication for pain relief at the time of follow-up. In his study, patients with debridement and abrasion did better than those with debridement alone.

Rand (31), from the Mayo Clinic, compared debridement to abrasion in a study reported in 1991. All patients had grade III and IV chondromalacic changes. Group I (131 patients) was treated with arthroscopic meniscectomy and debridement. Group II (28 patients) was treated with abrasion arthroplasty. Of patients in group I, 80% noted improvement at a 1-year follow-up versus 39% of patients in group II. Group I improvement declined to 67% of patients after 5 years. By contrast, 50% of group II patients did worse with time and underwent total knee replacement at a mean of 3 years postarthroscopy.

Singh, et al. (42) in 1991 also reported on a retrospective study of abrasion arthroplasty for moderate to severe osteoarthritis and found 51% improvement. However, this study involved only a short follow-up. His results were better in the older age group and in patients with normal alignment.

Bert and Maschka (29) in 1989 retrospectively compared debridement alone to abrasion and debridement. All patients had grade IV chondromalacia and follow-up was for 5 years. The abrasion group had 51% good to excellent results compared to 66% for debridement alone. Results were not related to age, previous surgery, weight, or mechanical alignment, but all patients had radiographic evidence preoperatively of joint space obliteration. Certainly one would conclude that, in the face of radiographic evidence of joint space obliteration, abrasion has not been helpful.

Table 54.2. Abrasion Studies

Author	Year	Follow-up (months)	Good (%)	Fair/Poor (%)
Friedman	1984		60	40
Johnson	1986	24	77	23
Bert	1989	60	51	49
Rand	1991	36	50	50
Singh	1991		51	49

Table 54.2 summarizes the abrasion studies of five authors from 1984 to 1991.

Rheumatoid Arthritis Studies

The arthroscope has played an important role in the diagnosis and treatment of inflammatory arthritides. The ease of arthroscopic biopsy has in most cases eliminated open diagnostic procedures. The results of arthroscopic synovectomy have compared favorably to those obtained by open procedures.

Smiley and Wasilewski (43) in 1990 reported on arthroscopic synovectomy in 25 knees with rheumatoid arthritis or psoriatic arthritis. At 2 years, 90% had good results declining to 57% at 4 years. He reported fewer operative complications and decreased postoperative morbidity compared to open synovectomy.

In 1991, Ogilvie-Harris and Basinski (44) reported on 96 patients with rheumatoid arthritis treated with arthroscopic synovectomy. He found only 75% improvement in synovitis and pain at the time of follow-up at 4 years. Range of motion remained unchanged. Arnold (45) in 1992 also reported 75% improvement with arthroscopic synovectomy for rheumatoid arthritis at 2-year follow-up and recommended early treatment to improve long-term results. As reported by Sledge, et al. (46), unanswered questions remain whether this type of mechanical procedure is better or worse than other methods such as radiation or chemical synovectomy,

Arthroscopic synovectomy has also been reported as being successful in the treatment of pigmented villonodular synovitis and chondrocalcinosis. Septic arthritis treated by arthroscopic drainage has been reported by Thiery (47) in 1989. He reviewed 46 cases, noting 78% cures of the septic condition, 10% failures secondary to persistent articular sepsis, and 10% failures secondary to recurrent infection.

Clinician's Algorithm

A reliable algorithm that defines the role of knee arthroscopy in the treatment of degenerative joint disease is difficult to construct. Wouters, et al. (48) in 1992 presented their own algorithm based on a retrospective review of 57 patients over age 50. They found that radiographic findings were the most reliable predictor of the outcome of arthroscopic debridement. Several other authors, including Bonamo, et al. (22) Gross, et al. (49)

Table 54.3. Treatment Algorithm for Arthroscopic Management of Degenerative Joint Disease

Predictors of Success	Predictors of Failure
History	
Males	Females
Onset < 3 months	Pending litigation
Specific twist mechanism	Work injury
Loose bodies	Insidious onset
Mechanical symptoms	
Physical Examination	
Recent effusion	> 10° varus
	> 15° valgus
	ligament laxity
X-Ray Analysis	
Loose bodies	Complete loss of joint space
Normal mechanical alignment	Chondrocalcinosis
Surgical Findings	
Chondral flaps	Grade III & IV chondromalacia
Chondral fractures	
Isolated compartment disease	Grade IV defect > 1 cm
Isolated meniscal tears	Medial and lateral compartment disease
LFC chondromalacia	Combined meniscal tears
Medial flap tears	Tibial chondromalacia
	Degenerative meniscal tears

and Ogilvie-Harris and Fitsialos (24), have tried to correlate preoperative assessment with postoperative findings with varied success.

The following is my algorithm based on the printed literature and 10 years of clinical practice (see Table 54.3). Four categories are considered in the approach to the patient with degenerative arthritis of the knee. They are the following:

History and symptoms
Physical examination
Radiographic analysis
Surgical findings (see Table 54.3).

History and Symptoms

Age alone is not a factor in selecting arthroscopic intervention for the patient with degenerative disease of the knee; however, males may fare slightly better than females (22). Patients with pain of short duration (i.e., less than 3 months) respond better to treatment, especially those with a history of a specific twisting injury and ensuing mechanical symptoms. This is often associated with unstable meniscal tears. Mechanical symptoms may also suggest loose bodies or symptomatic osteophytes, both of which correlate well with good results postoperatively. Patients with pending litigation and work-related compensation claims tend to do poorly.

Physical Examination

The loss of extension preoperatively is not a factor in predicting success, nor is the presence of crepitus. The recent appearance of an effusion correlates with a better result from arthroscopic debridement. Mechanical malalignment correlates with poor results. Thus, a varus angulation greater than 10 degrees or a valgus angulation greater than 15 degrees are relative contraindications to the procedure. Patients with valgus deformities do the worst. Ligamentous instability also correlates with poor results. Obesity is not a factor.

Radiographic Analysis

As mentioned under the section on physical examination, mechanical malalignment as seen on an anteroposterior weight-bearing radiograph correlates with poorer results. Complete loss of joint space on standing x-ray films is also associated with poor results. The presence of loose bodies or osteophytes that correlate with the patient's areas of pain correlate with good results. Chondrocalcinosis correlates with poor results.

Surgical Findings

The presence of more severe chondromalacia (grade III and grade IV) correlates with poor results. grade IV defects greater than 1 cm in diameter also correlate with poor results. Patients with chondral fractures and flaps do better at follow-up than those with diffuse disease. Patients with lateral femoral condyle changes do better than those with medial disease. Patients with chondromalacia in both medial and lateral compartments will do poorly, compared to those with isolated compartment disease. The extent of patellofemoral disease does not correlate with postoperative results. The prognosis is worse if tibial chondromalacic changes are present. Patients with unstable and/or flap tears of their menisci do better than those with degenerative tears. Patients with isolated tears do better than those with medial and lateral tears combined.

Preoperative Assessment

In general, patients who should be considered candidates for arthroscopic management of degenerative joint disease are usually those who have exhausted nonoperative management, including nonsteroidal antiinflammatory medications, physical therapy, analgesics, and/or the possible use of corticosteroid injections.

A complete preoperative assessment includes a comprehensive review of history and symptoms, physical examination, and radiographic analysis.

History and Symptoms

Among the factors to evaluate in the history are the patient's sex, age, onset of pain and/or swelling, and a specific history of the onset of symptoms. Was the onset of problems related to a specific injury or was it more insidious? Is there a history of any mechanical symptoms, which would include mechanical locking and/or episodes of giving way? Attention should also be paid to the patient's activity demands and whether or not these include recreational sport activities. Factors that may be helpful in reviewing the history would include whether the injury was industrially related and/or whether litigation is involved.

One should also try to discover from the patient whether symptoms are related specifically to weight-bearing activities or twisting activities or whether onset of symptoms have any specific pattern and can occur at rest. It should be remembered that often symptoms that occur without a pattern and unrelated to physical demands may be secondary to problems that are present at either the hip or low back area.

Physical Examination

The most effective way to examine the patient's lower extremities is to have the patient wear a pair of shorts or a surgical gown that exposes both lower extremities completely. The patient should be evaluated first in the standing position to evaluate mechanical alignment and to provide a quick assessment of the torsional alignment and weight-bearing attitude of the involved extremity.

In the supine position, range of motion should be assessed and compared to the contralateral limb. Early loss of extension (flexion contracture) is a common finding with more progressive onset of osteoarthritis. An effusion should be noted, and, at this point, it is often best to try to correlate the physical finding of effusion with the patient's perception of the symptoms, particularly of swelling. Often the patient will state that the knee is swollen when in fact there is no palpable effusion present. These patients are more likely describing stiffness rather than a true swelling (i.e., effusion) in the joint. Crepitance can be palpated and should be noted to be present either in relation to the patellofemoral joint or to the tibial femoral joint.

Tenderness is often found on physical examination. The location of the tenderness is often remarkably specific in terms of the involved anatomic structure. In palpating the patellofemoral joint, the tenderness under the medial facet should be differentiated from tenderness along the flare of the medial femoral condyle that may be more associated with osteophytic spurring or chronic changes to the medial plica.

When palpating the medial joint line, it is important to distinguish between posteromedial joint line tenderness and tenderness arising from the posteromedial aspect of the proximal tibia that corresponds with one of the insertional sites of the semimembranosus tendon. Tenderness that seems to be present along the course of the semimembranosus and extending into the pes bursa should not be confused with the tenderness associated with meniscal tears. In addition, specific tenderness along the anteromedial joint line has been associated with a bursitis described by Kerlan and Glousman (50) that responds well to bursal injection. In palpating lateral structures for tenderness, one should try to discern the difference between the lateral joint line, fibular collateral ligament, popliteus tendon, and distal iliotibial band. The presence of instability should be evaluated with Lachman's test, anterior and posterior drawers, and the presence of varus or valgus instability at 30% of flexion.

Radiographic Analysis

Plain x-ray films should include a weight-bearing AP view of both right and left extremities, a lateral of the knee, and bilateral sunrise or Merchant views. Many physicians feel that a standing posteroanterior (PA) film with the knee flexed at 45 degrees should also be obtained. One should try to correlate the presence of specific compartment joint space narrowing and/or the presence of osteophytes with the specific symptoms and specific areas of tenderness as outlined from physical examination. The presence of loose bodies and chondrocalcinosis should be noted and also correlated with patient history and physical examination. If an MRI (magnetic resonance image) scan of the knee has been performed, it is imperative that the specific findings again be correlated with the area of the patient's symptoms and with findings as noted at the time of the physical examination. It should be remembered that many patients will have grade III signal abnormalities of their menisci and that this finding alone is not sufficient to recommend arthroscopic intervention. A bone scan may be helpful in the diagnosis of osteonecrosis.

Other preoperative assessments might include laboratory analysis of sedimentation rate, uric acid level, and, in some cases, more detailed blood work for inflammatory arthritis, including a rheumatoid factor, ANA (antibody to nuclear antigens) and HLA-B-27 (human leukoctye antigen) typing. Joint fluid aspiration for analysis of cell count, protein and glucose levels, mucin test, and crystal analysis for both gout and pseudo-gout may be helpful.

Arthroscopic Technique

Excellent technique is necessary to successfully treat patients with degenerative joint disease as these patients often have tight knee compartments that make access a challenge. Good visualization is mandatory and requires adequate fluid distention, high flow, and an adequate light source. Portal placement is extremely important because this will not only enhance visualization but facilitate instrumentation. I prefer vertical incisions with standard anteromedial, anterolateral, and supramedial portals.

The anteromedial and anterolateral portals are made with the knee flexed 90 degrees. It is my preference to make the incision with a number 11 scalpel blade, with the cutting edge facing proximally to avoid inadvertent incision into the meniscus. A straight Kelly clamp is then used to enlarge the portal, and the arthroscope is introduced using the blunt trochar and sheath, placing the arthroscope into the suprapatellar pouch. The joint is distended with fluid and a supramedial portal is established parallelling skin lines using a large flow cannula. I prefer inflow through the arthroscope to keep debris away from the field of view.

The use of a leg holder is controversial in the older population. Particularly in males, it is not unusual to encounter a varus knee with a tight medial compartment, and, in these instances, a leg holder may help with visualization. However, care must be taken to avoid overzealous distraction which may cause injury to the medial collateral ligament. Assessment of the amount of joint laxity preoperatively and after the induction of anesthesia may help to determine whether or not a leg-holding device is necessary. In general, I prefer a single lateral post to provide valgus stress when needed and, in general, do not require a leg-holding device.

The use of the tourniquet for arthroscopic surgery is also controversial. Bleeding may be minimized by the injection of both the portals and joint with a combination of Xylocaine or Marcaine with epinephrine. Sherman, et al. (51) reported an increased complication rate with arthroscopic surgery associated with the use of the tourniquet for over 45 minutes. However, I prefer the tourniquet as a means to enhance visualization and thereby decrease overall surgical time.

It is important to perform the diagnostic arthroscopic examination systematically to ensure a complete evaluation regardless of the preoperative diagnosis. Failure to inspect each compartment in the same order may result in areas being overlooked. I prefer a sequence of evaluation of the suprapatellar pouch followed by the patellofemoral joint from medial to lateral. Next comes inspection of the medial gutter into the medial compartment followed by visualization of the intercondylar notch area and then inspection into the lateral compartments and finally of the lateral gutter. It may also be possible to visualize the posteromedial and posterolateral compartments through the intercondylar notch.

Accurate knowledge of the patient's specific preoperative complaints and preoperative findings can be extremely helpful in determining whether pathology viewed arthroscopically should be addressed. In general, localized bone spurs are not resected unless they correlate with the patient's specific symptoms and findings.

The improvement in motorized instrumentation and, in particular, the recent introduction of curved meniscal shaver blades have made the removal of degenerative portions of menisci as well as the debridement of chondromalacic changes in the compartments much easier processes to perform. In general, unstable meniscal fragments and unstable tears should be removed and the remaining meniscal rims contoured to leave as much normal tissue as possible. I prefer, when performing chondroplasties, to remove only unstable tissue and/or chondral flaps and to make a specific effort not to be overzealous in the use of motorized instruments. In general, abrasion should not be performed. In most instances, the damaged areas represent large surfaces, and the results from abrasion of large surfaces have been poor. Particularly in compartments of the knee where preoperative symptoms have been minimal, every effort should be made not to further traumatize the compartment.

Postoperative Rehabilitation

Rehabilitation after arthroscopic procedures must be tailored to the individual in consideration of the findings at surgery. In general, patients who require only meniscectomies with minimal debridement will be able to progress more quickly in a rehabilitation program than patients who have had extensive chondroplasties involving multiple compartments. In particular, synovectomies and chondroplasties performed in the weight-bearing portion of the joint or in the patellofemoral compartment can be extremely uncomfortable.

Patellofemoral chondroplasties, in general, result in a reflex inhibition of the quadriceps, muscles which have to be rehabilitated slowly. In the early postoperative period, the patient may complain of instability and giving way. Patients may present at the first visit after synovectomy with a large hematoma that requires aspiration and/or evacuation.

In general, the patient should be encouraged to walk, because bed rest increases the risk of venous thrombosis. A cane or a crutch may be necessary for a few days after surgery to assist with ambulation. The use of analgesics and nonsteroidal antiinflammatory medications should be encouraged as needed for early pain relief. In addition, ice used intermittently can be extremely helpful in reversing early postoperative swelling and pain.

In patients in whom vascular insufficiency may have been noted preoperatively, the use of TED (thromboembolic disease) hose or vascular stockings may prevent venous thrombosis. Intermittent compression devices may also be useful in these high-risk individuals.

It is important to emphasize early range of motion exercises as well as isometric quadriceps strengthening as soon as possible after arthroscopy. Many patients in this age group do best with a supervised physical therapy program for 1 to 3 months. In general, patients who have had meniscectomies and/or removal of loose bodies can expect recovery over a 2-month period. However, patients who have had significant debridements of chondral surfaces and/or synovectomies can expect to wait 3 months postsurgery before seeing progress. There may still be a significant percentage of patients who show gradual improvement from 3-6 months postarthroscopy.

If patients are reluctant or unable to obtain supervised physical therapy, then it is important for the physician to establish an exercise program for them that they can do easily on their own. It is important in the early postoperative period to recommend that patients vary their activity levels, to combine standing, walking, and sitting activities with intermittent rest periods. As swelling subsides and range of motion improves, a strengthening program is begun. In addition to isometric quadriceps strengthening, the patient should be encouraged to perform straight leg raising activities, if possible, with an ankle weight. Associated chronic low back conditions may make straight leg quadriceps exercise difficult, and the patient should be warned against being overzealous. This may create an exacerbation of their low back condition.

If a stationary cycle is available, its use is encouraged, particularly during the first month after surgery. A level walking program can usually be instituted 3 to 4 weeks from surgery, and this program can be advanced to uneven terrain in the 6 to 8 week postoperative period. Most patients can then gradually resume full activities in the second to third month postsurgery.

References

1. Burman MS, Finklestein H, Mayer L. Arthroscopy of the knee. J Bone Joint Surg [Am] 1934;16:255–268.
2. Magnuson PB. Joint debridement. A surgical treatment of degenerative arthritis. Surg Gynecol Obstet 1941;73:1–9.
3. Haggart GE. The surgical treatment of degenerative arthritis of the knee joint. J Bone Joint Surg [Br] 1940;22:717–729.
4. Insall JN. Intra-articular surgery for degenerative arthritis of the knee. A report of the work of the late KH Pridie. J Bone Joint Surg [Br] 1967;49:211–228.
5. Richards RN Jr, Lonergan R. Arthroscopic surgery for relief of pain in the osteoarthritic knee. Orthopedics 1984;7:1705–1707.
6. Jackson RW, Abe I. The role of arthroscopy in the management of disorders of the knee. An analysis of 200 consecutive cases. J Bone Joint Surg [Br] 1972;54:310–322.
7. Dandy DJ. The impact of arthroscopic surgery on the management of disorders of the knee. Arthroscopy 1990;6–2:96–99.Johnson LL.
8. Burks RT. Arthroscopy and degenerative arthritis of the knee: A review of the literature. Arthroscopy 1990;6–1:43.
9. Lysholm J, Hamberg P, Gillquist, J. The correlation between osteoarthrosis as seen on radiographs and on arthroscopy. Arthroscopy 1987;3–3:161–165.
10. Brandt KD, Fife RS, Braunstein EM, Katz B. Radiographic grading of the severity of knee osteoarthritis: Relation of the Kellgren and Lawrence grade to a grade based on joint space narrowing, and correlation with arthroscopic evidence of articular cartilage degeneration. Arthritis Rheum 1991;34–11:1381–1386.
11. Fife RS, Brandt KD, Braunstein EM, Katz BP, Shelbourne KD, Kalasinski LA, Ryan S. Relationship between arthroscopic evidence of cartilage damage and radiographic evidence of joint space narrowing in early osteoarthritis of the knee. Arthritis Rheum 1991;34–4:377–382.
12. Myers SL, Brandt KD, Ehlich JW, Braunstein EM, Shelbourne KD, Heck DA, Kalasinski LA. Synovial inflammation in patients with early osteoarthritis of the knee. J Rheumatol [Canada] 1990;17–12:1662–1669.
13. Lindblad S, Hedfors E. Arthroscopic and immunohistologic characterization of knee joint synovitis in osteoarthritis. Arthritis Rheum 1987;30–10:1081–1088.
14. Casscells SW. The torn or degenerated meniscus and its relationship to degeneration of the weight bearing areas of the femur and tibia. Clin Orthop 1978;132:196–200.
15. Fahmy NRM, Williams EA, Noble J. Meniscal pathology and osteoarthritis of the knee. J Bone Joint Surg [Br] 1983;65:24–28.
16. Zamber RW, Teitz CC, McGuire DA, Frost JD, Hermanson BK. Articular cartilage lesions of the knee. Arthroscopy 1989;5–4:258–268.
17. Fairbanks TJ. Knee joint changes after meniscectomy. J Bone Joint Surg 1948;30-B:664–670.
18. Tapper EM, Hoover NW. Late results after meniscectomy. J Bone Joint Surg [Am] 1969;51:517–526.
19. Lotke PA, Lefkoe RT, Ecker ML. Late results following medial meniscectomy in an older population. J Bone Joint Surg [Am] 1981;63:115–119.
20. Jones RE, Smith EC, Reisch JS. The effects of medial meniscectomy in patients older than 40 years. J Bone Joint Surg [Am] 1978;60:783–786.
21. McBride GG, Constine RM, Hofmann AA, Carson RW. Arthroscopic partial medial meniscectomy in the older patient. J Bone Joint Surg [Am] 1984;66:547.
22. Bonamo JJ, Kessler KJ, Noah J. Arthroscopic meniscectomy in patients over the age of 40. Am J Sports Med 1992;20–2:422–429.
23. Covall DJ and Wasilewski SA. Roentgenographic changes after arthroscopic meniscectomy: five-year follow-up in patients more than 45 years of age. Arthroscopy 1992;8–2:242–246.
24. Ogilvie-Harris DJ, Fitsialos DP. Arthroscopic management of the degenerative knee. Arthroscopy 1991;7–2:151–157.
25. Livesley PJ, Doherty M, Needoff M, Moulton A. Arthroscopic lavage of osteoarthritic knees. J Bone Joint Surg [Br] 1991;73–6:922–926.
26. Jackson RW, Silver R, Marans H. The arthroscopic treatment of degenerative joint disease. Arthroscopy 1986;2:114.
27. Sprague NF III. Arthroscopic debridement for degenerative knee joint disease. Clin Orthop 1981;160:118–123.
28. Shahriaree H, O'Connor RF, Nottage W. Seven years follow-up arthroscopic debridement of the degenerative knee. Field of View 1982;1:1.
29. Bert JM, Maschka K. The arthroscopic treatment of unicompartmental gonarthrosis: a five year follow-up study of abrasion arthroplasty plus arthroscopic debridement and arthroscopic debridement alone. Arthroscopy 1989;5–1:25–32.
30. Baumgaertner MR, Cannon WD Jr, Vittori JM, Schmidt ES, Maurer RC. Arthroscopic debridement of the arthritic knee. Clin Orthop 1990;253:197–202.
31. Rand JA. Role of arthroscopy in osteoarthritis of the knee. Arthroscopy 1991;7–4:358–363.
32. Timoney JM,Kneisl JS, Barrack RL, et al. Arthroscopy update #6.Arthroscopy in the osteoarthritic knee. Long-term follow-up. Orthop Rev 1990;19(4):371–3, 376–379.
33. McLaren AC, Blokker CP, Fowler PJ, Roth JN, Rock MG. Arthroscopic debridement of the knee for osteoarthrosis. Can J Surg 1991;34–6:595–598.
34. Pridie KH. A method of resurfacing osteoarthritic knee joints. J Bone Joint Surg [Br] 1959;41:618.
35. Ficat P, Hungerford D. Disorders of the patellofemoral joint. Baltimore: Williams & Wilkins, 1977.
36. Shahriaree H, ed. O'Connor's textbook of arthroscopic surgery. Philadelphia: JB Lippincott, 1984:263–277.
37. Salter R, Simmonds D, Malcolm B, et al. The biological effect of continuous passive motion on the healing of full thickness defects in articular cartilage. J Bone Joint Surg 1980;62:1232–1251.
38. Mankin H. The reaction of articular cartilage to injury and osteoarthritis, part I. N Engl J Med 1974;291:1285–1292.
39. Johnson LL. Arthroscopic abrasion arthroplasty historical and pathologic perspective: Present status. Arthroscopy 1986;2:54–69.
40. Salisbury RB, Nottage WM and Gardner V. The effect of alignment on results in arthroscopic debridement of the degenerative knee. Clin Orthop 1985;198:268–272.
41. Friedman MJ, Berasi CC, Fox JM, et al. Preliminary results with abrasion arthroplasty in the osteoarthritic knee. Clin Orthop 1984;182:200–205.
42. Singh S, Lee CC, Tay BK. Results of arthroscopic abrasion arthroplasty in osteoarthritis of the knee joint. Singapore Med J 1991;32–1:34–37.
43. Smiley P, Wasilewski SA. Arthroscopic synovectomy. Arthroscopy 1990;6–1:18–23.
44. Ogilvie-Harris DJ and Basinski A. Arthroscopic synovectomy of the knee for rheumatoid arthritis. Arthroscopy 1991;7,en>1:917.
45. Arnold WJ. Arthroscopy in the diagnosis and therapy of arthritis. Hosp Pract Mar 30 1992;27-3A:43–6, 49, 52–53.
46. Sledge CB, Zuckerman JD, Shortcroffs, et al. Synovectomy of the rheumatoid knee using intra-articular injection of Dyprosium 165, ferric hydroxide macroaggregates. J Bone Joint Surg 1987;69-A:970–975.
47. Thiery JA. Arthroscopic drainage in septic arthritides of the knee: a multicenter study. Arthroscopy 1989;5–1:65–69.
48. Wouters E, Bassett FH III, Hardaker WT Jr, Garrett WE Jr. An algorithm for arthroscopy in the over-50 age group. Am J Sports Med 1992;20–2:141–145.
49. Gross DE, Brenner SL, Esformes I, Gross ML. Arthroscopic treatment of degenerative joint disease of the knee. Orthopedics 1991;14–12:1317–1321.
50. Kerlan RK, Glousman RE. Tibial collateral ligament bursitis. Am J Sports Med 1988;16–4:344–346.
51. Sherman OH, Fox JM, Snyder SJ, Del Pizzo W, Friedman MJ, Ferkel RD, Lawley MJ. Arthroscopy—"No-Problem Surgery." J Bone Joint Surg 1986;68A–2:256–265.

55

High Tibial Osteotomy

Arlen D. Hanssen and Edmund Y. S. Chao

Introduction

The use of osteotomy for the treatment of arthritis associated with malalignment about the knee rapidly gained acceptance following the initial introduction by Jackson in 1958 (1). The pathogenesis of degenerative arthritis associated with malalignment and the biomechanical rationale for high tibial osteotomy have been previously described (2). Limb malalignment accentuates the stress on damaged articular cartilage and potentiates further loss of articular cartilage and subchondral bone with subsequent increase in the magnitude of angular malalignment. This vicious cycle of progressive angular deformity and loss of articular cartilage steadily progresses over time. High tibial osteotomy for either varus or valgus knee deformity should provide realignment of the limb to reduce the stress on damaged cartilage and bone and should redistribute the forces to more normal areas of the knee joint.

The goals of osteotomy include relief of pain, improved function, and providing individuals with heavy functional demands the opportunity to continue those activities that would otherwise be precluded by prosthetic joint replacement. The redistribution of these mechanical forces facilitates reparative healing and increases the life span of the knee joint. This distinguishes osteotomy from other treatment for knee arthritis.

Clinical experience over the last three decades has defined the current role of realignment osteotomy about the knee. Careful patient assessment, analysis of prognostic factors, and precise surgical technique enable the high tibial osteotomy with improved and more durable clinical results than initially realized. Recent technological advances have further improved the surgeon's ability to assess and select patients who are candidates for realignment osteotomy. It is important to recognize these clinical and technological advances when evaluating osteotomy: alternative procedures should be compared with osteotomy performed by current standards and not by historical osteotomy controls.

The introduction, refinement, and the present success of total knee arthroplasty as well as the resurgence of enthusiasm for unicompartmental knee arthroplasty have significantly diminished the modern use of upper tibial osteotomy. Although high tibial osteotomy is performed less frequently at our institution, we continue to recommend it because it provides selected patients with a unique opportunity to obtain pain relief and to continue to participate in heavy activities not permitted with prosthetic replacements. (Fig. 55.1). Finally, when evaluating the results of high tibial osteotomy, one should realize that the patients receiving this procedure are usually those patients who have been considered poor candidates for a successful long-term result following a prosthetic replacement.

Indications

Ideal candidates for high tibial osteotomy are in their sixth decade of life with localized, activity-related knee pain, varus malalignment, and medial unicompartmental degenerative arthritis. They have no patellofemoral symptoms, a stable knee, full knee extension, and flexion beyond 100 degrees. In reality, there are many other patients who can benefit from osteotomy, yet fall short of these ideal criteria. However, unfavorable prognostic variables do predict a lower probability of clinical success.

Satisfactory results can be obtained in patients older and younger than the sixth decade of life, in patients with tricompartmental arthritis or with flexion contractures of up to 20 degrees. In general, the lower the patient age, or, if the anticipated activity level will be excessive, the more likely it is that these idealized prognostic factors will not be applied as rigidly. Deviations of selection criteria are acceptable if the final decision has been reached by careful analysis of the patient

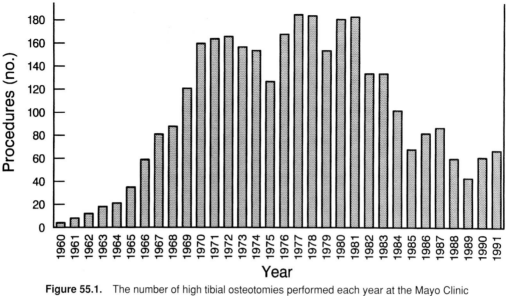

Figure 55.1. The number of high tibial osteotomies performed each year at the Mayo Clinic between 1960 and 1991.

and if they support the fundamental principles of realignment osteotomy. Prognostic factors associated with a satisfactory postoperative result are discussed in this chapter under Results.

Relative Contraindications to High Tibial Osteotomy

Individuals over the age of 65 years are generally better served with a prosthetic joint replacement because of the shorter period of rehabilitation and the more complete pain relief afforded with that procedure. Patients with a diagnosis of osteoarthritis are better candidates than are those with rheumatoid arthritis, and patients with inflammatory arthritis can be considered for prosthetic replacement at a much earlier age (3). Prior medial and lateral meniscectomy probably precludes realignment osteotomy (4).

Obesity has been associated with early clinical failure following high tibial osteotomy, these patients should be counseled that significant weight loss may provide enough symptomatic relief to defer surgery (5). In the young and overweight patient who has exhausted other nonoperative modalities, high tibial osteotomy seems preferable to prosthetic replacement. Skeletal fixation must be rigid in obese patients because excessive body weight and a large, bulbous leg adversely affect postoperative cast immobilization and maintenance of alignment.

Although there is often a mild degree of ligamentous laxity on the concave side of the joint, moderate or severe laxity is a poor prognostic factor for an osteotomy. Symptoms related to knee instability will not be alleviated with high tibial osteotomy alone. In the elderly patient with arthritis and instability, total knee arthroplasty is the treatment of choice. The young, active patient with arthritis and instability requires procedures combining realignment osteotomy and complex soft tissue recon-

struction that are beyond the scope of this discussion. The young patient with degenerative arthritis, extremity malalignment, and knee instability remains a difficult treatment entity deserving considerable investigation.

Excessive malalignment may contraindicate a high tibial osteotomy if the tibial articular surface will be adversely tilted postoperatively (6). Under these circumstances, generally with malalignment of more than 12 to 15 degrees, the location of the osteotomy should be in the supracondylar region of the femur (6). Any distant deformities contributing to extremity malalignment, such as a diaphyseal femoral malunion, are better addressed at the apex of the deformity rather than with a high tibial osteotomy. Surgeons with minimal or occasional experience performing this surgical procedure should seriously consider referral of such patients. The complications of high tibial osteotomy, which may compromise prosthetic replacement, may result from technical problems with the original osteotomy (7).

Evaluation of the Patient

A thorough evaluation should first determine the location and severity of the pain, which should typically be localized to the affected compartment, worsen with activity, and abate with rest. Diffuse pain throughout the knee reduces the chance of a successful outcome following osteotomy. Inspection of the lower limb should reveal axial malalignment. During observation of gait, patients with an excessive lateral thrust may require special consideration for alignment overcorrection (8).

Ipsilateral hip function should be normal. Necessary hip surgery is performed prior to tibial osteotomy to allow appropriate correction of the overall mechanical alignment. Tenderness is usually present along the affected joint line. Range of motion should reveal a flexion arc of more than 90 degrees with less than 10 to 20 degrees of a flexion contracture (9–11). These criteria for joint motion have been established by clinical convention; no study definitively confirms them.

Patellofemoral symptoms should not be the primary cause of the patient's complaints. As a rule, most patients with degenerative arthritis of the medial or lateral tibiofemoral compartments do not have significant patellofemoral symptoms despite significant radiographic evidence of patellofemoral arthritis (11). Mild patellofemoral complaints do not contraindicate realignment osteotomy. The physician should attempt to rule out significant meniscal pathology as the primary source of the patient's symptoms. Any suggestion of mechanical symptoms in the contralateral compartment that will experience higher loading following osteotomy should be addressed prior to, or in conjunction with, the realignment procedure. Symptoms in the compartment to be unloaded will most likely be alleviated following the osteotomy, and treating these symptoms prior to osteotomy is unnecessary (11).

Mild instability, particularly on the concave side of the deformity, is usually detected on examination. Moderate or severe knee instability should not be present. The absence of the anterior cruciate ligament has not adversely affected the postoperative results of high tibial osteotomy in carefully selected patients when the preoperative symptoms could be attributed to an overloading of the degenerative joint compartment (12).

Particular attention should be directed toward evaluation of prior incisions to help plan the intended surgical exposure. Recommendations for placement of incisions are described in the discussion of operative technique.

Radiographic Evaluation

Standing anteroposterior, lateral, intercondylar notch, and skyline patellar views are used to assess the location and severity of the arthritis. Tibiofemoral subluxation, excessive bony erosion, or diffuse arthritic involvement are associated with a higher incidence of unsatisfactory results (3,10). A full-length 51 × 14-inch weight-bearing radiograph is necessary to determine the mechanical alignment of the limb. The mechanical axis is based on a line connecting the center of the femoral head and the center of the tibiotalar joint (Fig. 55.2). The mechanical alignment is more accurate than the anatomic axis when defining the load transmission forces across the knee joint (13). These radiographs are also extremely useful in determining any deformities of the tibia or femur that exist above or below the knee joint. Technetium bone scanning can help assess the location and intensity of bone reaction in the joint, especially in patients with symptoms in the contralateral compartment (11). Not all surgeons consider radionuclide imaging a useful means of patient selection for high tibial osteotomy (14).

Patient Counseling

The patient's activity level and expectations following an osteotomy must be known. The surgeon needs to dis-

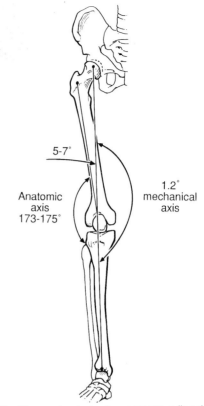

Figure 55.2. The mechanical axis represents a line drawn between the center of the femoral head and the center of the tibiotalar joint and averages 1.2 degrees of varus. The anatomic axis represents the difference between the longitudinal axes of the femur and tibia and averages 5 degrees of valgus in normal individuals.

cuss alternatives to osteotomy, even with an ideal candidate. As with prosthetic replacement, the patient should understand that a surgical procedure will not provide a "normal joint," but is intended to provide pain relief and prolong active knee function. A specific recommendation for a high tibial osteotomy is based on the fundamental concept that high impact and excessive loading activities can be tolerated after osteotomy, whereas these activities are prohibited with prosthetic arthroplasty. Specific activities such as tennis, jogging, occupations requiring heavy labor, or other activities important to the patient need to be assessed prior to a definitive recommendation for either an osteotomy or prosthetic replacement.

The differences of realignment osteotomy with regard to postoperative rehabilitation, pain relief, durability, and long-term results should be compared with the current expectations of prosthetic joint replacement. Patients should expect a longer postoperative recovery period and expect less pain relief following an osteotomy than can be expected with an arthroplasty. These disadvantages need to be weighed against the possible catastrophic complications of prosthetic replacement, which include infection, component wear or failure, and shorter prosthetic survival in the young and active patient.

The patient should be informed that "buying time" with an osteotomy is a viable concept. Many reported series of high tibial osteotomy have revealed a majority of patients with continued satisfactory results 5 to 7 years after a realignment procedure (15–18). After 5 to 7 years, the percentage of satisfactory clinical results appear to significantly diminish (5, 19, 20). These data should be used as an argument rather than a condemnation of realignment osteotomy. Many patients appreciate that there is the real possibility of technological advances with prosthetic replacement over this period of time and, additionally, they can enjoy the benefit of a continuing high activity level until prosthetic arthroplasty is required.

These advantages need to be addressed in conjunction with the expected results of total knee arthroplasty following high tibial osteotomy. Windsor, et al. indicated that patients undergoing total knee arthroplasty following osteotomy had results more comparable with revision knee arthroplasty than patients undergoing primary knee replacement—largely due to the problems of the failed osteotomy (7). Katz, et al. reported that patients treated with total knee arthroplasty after a failed osteotomy have results that approach but do not equal the results of primary total knee arthroplasty (21). Krackow, et al. indicated that prior high tibial osteotomy did not significantly increase the difficulty of a subsequent prosthetic replacement except for those patients who had significant valgus overcorrection (22).

The literature detailing poor results provides the message that osteotomies performed with technical difficulties or osteotomies that suffer complications produce worse results with a subsequent knee arthroplasty. Poor surgical technique, of any type, has the potential for compromising subsequent procedures, but this reality should not be the sole criterion used to abandon a specific operative technique. We have not observed these inferior results and believe that a properly performed high tibial osteotomy does not increase the surgical complexity or significantly affect the clinical outcome when the patient is later converted to a prosthetic arthroplasty (23).

Preoperative Planning

Traditionally, the axial alignment of the limb has been determined by measuring the femoral-tibial (anatomic) angle from standing radiographs and then judging the amount of correction required to normalize, or overcorrect, the limb alignment. The normal anatomic axis measures 5 degrees of valgus (24). The mechanical axis normally averages 1.2 degrees of varus and is more reliable than the anatomic axis when defining lower limb alignment (Fig. 55.2) (13). This is particularly true when there are femoral or tibial deformities away from the knee joint that contribute to the limb malalignment. Standing radiographs have previously been used to measure the anatomic axis and estimate the width of the wedge to be removed in order to correct the extremity malalignment. The length of the base of this wedge has been estimated to be roughly 1 mm per desired degree of angular correction. The primary disadvantage of this

method lies in the fact that the width of the wedge base is significantly altered by the width of the tibia and any distortion caused by radiographic magnification. Coventry has determined that this rule of 1 degree of correction per each millimeter of bone resection applies only when the width of the tibial flare is 56 mm. Use of this method will invariably lead to undercorrection of alignment because the mean tibial width is 80 mm in males and 70 mm in females (25).

An alternative method is based on the determination of the mechanical axis on a full-length standing radiograph and on incorporating radiographic markers to adjust for magnification. The intended wedge is then templated with trigonometric principles and adjusted for radiographic magnification to achieve the desired amount of angular correction.

Recently, it has been suggested that the slope of the distal femoral articular surface will affect the magnitude of alignment correction (26). This slope is determined by measuring the femoral shaft-transcondylar (FS-TC) angle (Fig. 55.3). In their study, patients with FS-TC angles of less than 9 degrees had an increased incidence of angular undercorrection, and they suggest that the FS-TC angle should be considered during preoperative planning.

Regardless of the technique chosen, direct measurement of the mechanical axis with the aid of fluoroscopy at the time of surgery is probably the most accurate method of establishing appropriate alignment. Careful preoperative plans are necessary to estimate the appropriate magnitude of angular correction by determining the location and magnitude of the wedge to be removed. These plans should provide objective criteria to guide the surgeon; however, to be effective, even the most detailed preoperative plans require accurate performance of the surgical procedure.

Osteotomy Analysis Simulation Software (OASIS)

In addition to the mechanical alignment, the effects of soft tissue tension, obliquity of the joint line, and gravity shift of the upper body all affect the tibiofemoral plateau pressure distribution and the ultimately correct location and the correct magnitude of an intended osteotomy. These factors are difficult to assess with visual inspection and manual planning. For these reasons, a software program was developed to provide a comprehensive preoperative assessment of the factors that could assist the surgeon's final determination of the location, magnitude, and type of knee osteotomy most appropriate for the individual patient (13, 27). On the full-length anteroposterior weight-bearing radiograph, the joint centers, the mechanical and anatomic tibiofemoral axes, patella center, joint contour outline, muscle and ligament insertion points, and joint articulating surface contact areas are identified and manually digitized on a translucent, background-lighted electrostatic Scriptel digitizer (Scriptel Corp., Columbus, Ohio 43228) (Fig. 55.4, *A*, *B*). With this analytical model, the muscles, ligaments, and cartilage are represented by a series of lin-

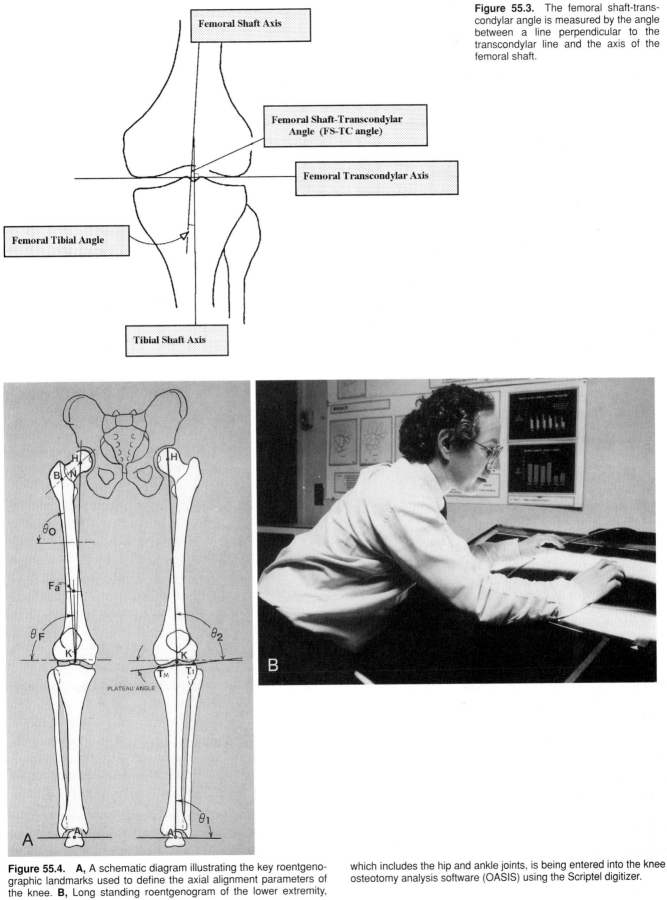

Figure 55.3. The femoral shaft-trans-condylar angle is measured by the angle between a line perpendicular to the transcondylar line and the axis of the femoral shaft.

Figure 55.4. A, A schematic diagram illustrating the key roentgeno-graphic landmarks used to define the axial alignment parameters of the knee. **B,** Long standing roentgenogram of the lower extremity, which includes the hip and ankle joints, is being entered into the knee osteotomy analysis software (OASIS) using the Scriptel digitizer.

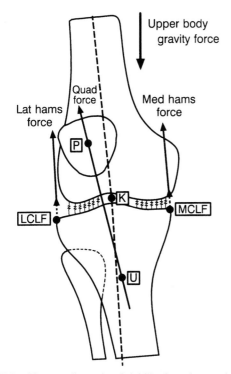

Figure 55.5. The two-dimensional rigid-body spring model (RBSM) used to determine articulating surface pressure and soft-tissue tension in a knee during weight-bearing. Both quadriceps and hamstring muscle groups can co-contract based on assumed conditions. The medial and lateral collateral ligament (MCLF, LCLF) tension is determined based on joint orientation and upper body gravity location.

ear springs while the bony structures are assumed to be rigid bodies (Fig. 55.5).

Simulation analysis input data include body weight, muscle contraction, ligament and cartilage stiffness properties, and the upper body gravity location. Osteotomy simulation parameters for the magnitude and location of the osteotomy wedge can then be performed interactively with immediate tabulation and graphical display of the simulation session. A printout of the upper tibial or supracondylar femoral closing wedge osteotomies at their usual location are provided to the surgeon (Fig. 55.6, A–F). Alternative options of an opening wedge, barrel-vault (also known as the dome) osteotomy at any level of the femur or tibia can also be simulated and made available for the surgeon. The output of the software "OASIS" includes the tibiofemoral angle based on the mechanical and anatomic axes, percent of force passing through the medial plateau, peak plateau pressure, joint shear force, collateral ligament tension, joint line obliquity in degrees from a horizontal line, joint loading axis (a line connecting the hip and ankle joint centers), location in reference to tibial plateau width, and the lower extremity length change. The size of the osteotomy angle, as measured along the bone surface, is also provided to the surgeon. In addition, joint gap in either compartment of the knee can be closed to compensate for weight-bearing effect causing the joint to open in severely deformed knees. It should be realized that this method is a static, two-dimensional

analysis that assumes that an improved redistribution of joint forces in the standing position will be beneficial to the patient during dynamic knee performance. Experimental and analytical studies have been performed to validate this model (28). A large normal data base and clinical case studies have been performed to evaluate the efficacy of this program (13). The value of this method of preoperative planning on the final clinical outcome of patients undergoing osteotomy is being prospectively studied.

Operative Technique

When choosing a specific surgical technique, the surgeon may choose between two fundamental techniques: a wedge osteotomy (opening or closing) or a barrel-vault (dome) osteotomy. These techniques both employ the common characteristic of performing the osteotomy between the knee joint and the tibial tubercle. The advantages of this osteotomy location include a broad cancellous bone surface that heals rapidly, corrects malalignment near the maximal point of deformity, and utilizes the compressive forces of the quadriceps mechanism. The closing wedge osteotomy is inherently the most stable of these techniques as the periosteum and cortex adjacent to the apex of the removed wedge acts as a tether when the osteotomy is closed. For varus malalignment about the knee, most surgeons prefer the lateral closing-wedge osteotomy (11, 19).

A varus closing-wedge osteotomy has been shown to be a reasonable option for valgus malalignment associated with lateral compartment arthritis (6). If the valgus malalignment exceeds 12 degrees or the osteotomy will result in an obliquity of the tibial articular surface of more than 10 degrees, it is preferable to perform a supracondylar femoral osteotomy (6). Some surgeons have preferred a valgus opening-wedge osteotomy with bone grafting for varus malalignment (29). This technique includes the disadvantages of procuring bone graft, dependence on graft healing, and the risk of graft displacement.

The dome osteotomy, popularized by Maquet, incorporates a curved osteotomy whereby the distal tibia is shifted or rotated on the proximal fragment to correct malalignment (30). This type of osteotomy may be preferable for larger degrees of correction, and it also allows anterior displacement of the tibial tubercle to decrease patellofemoral joint reaction forces. To date, there is no evidence that this displacement has been beneficial.

Inherent principles with these techniques include appropriate placement of skin incisions, an accurate osteotomy, and sufficient skeletal fixation. When planning the skin incision, one of the primary concerns should be the consideration of an eventual total knee replacement. Longitudinal, curved incisions on the lateral or medial side of the knee should provide large bridges of skin for any future midline or parapatellar approach. A midline longitudinal incision can be used for the dome osteotomy. Transverse incisions may seem attractive but should be avoided because they may compromise

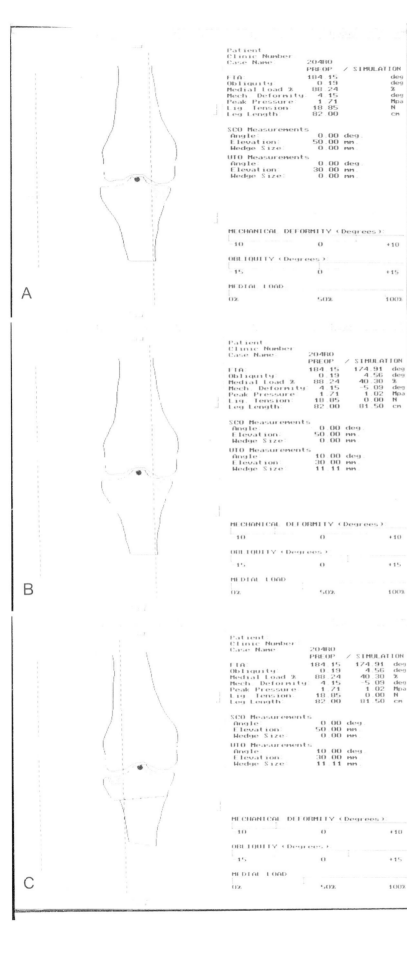

Figure 55.6. The OASIS graphic output for simulated high tibial and supracondylar femoral osteotomies. **A,** A patient with varus deformity of the right knee has 88.24% of the knee joint force passing through the medial plateau. **B,** A 10 degree high tibial osteotomy is proposed that will reduce the medial plateau force to 40.3% of the left knee joint. **C,** The simulated postoperative results and joint pressure distribution.

Figure 55.6. (continued) D, A patient with 7.31 degree varus deformity in his left knee. **E,** Simulated supracondylar femoral osteotomy wedge magnitude and location that reduce the left knee medial plateau force from 91.91% to 47.46% of the entire knee joint force. **F,** Simulated postoperative supracondylar femoral osteotomy pressure distribution.

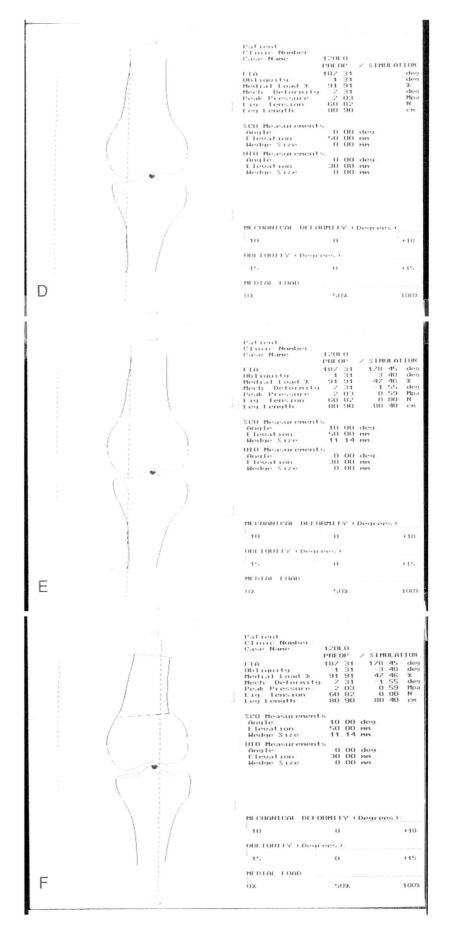

subsequent incisions used for prosthetic replacement. Incisions should be long enough to facilitate exposure and to avoid excessive tension on wound edges during surgical retraction. Poorly placed incisions for the osteotomy may provide catastrophic complications with wound healing and infection at later arthroplasty.

The precision of the osteotomy cannot be overemphasized. Accurate apposition of the osteotomy surfaces facilitates rapid bone healing; the proper orientation and resection of bone ultimately determine the correction of alignment. The use of intraoperative radiographs or fluoroscopy is advised. The use of jigs to assist the placement and orientation of the osteotomy appears to be beneficial and their use is recommended (31–35). This is especially true now when high tibial osteotomy is performed less frequently.

Skeletal fixation should be sufficiently rigid to facilitate bone healing and, if desired, to allow early knee motion. Although many patients have achieved excellent results with an osteotomy and only postoperative cast immobilization, Insall, et al. reported that loss of alignment with a postoperative cast change was one of the factors associated with failure in their patients (10). Postoperative management requires an accurate assessment of the stability achieved at the time of surgery. The reader is referred to the chapter discussing fixation for the high tibial osteotomy.

Valgus Closing-Wedge Osteotomy

This technique was adapted by Coventry (36) from a description of correcting knee flexion contractures in patients with rheumatoid arthritis (37). The patient is placed supine with a sandbag beneath the ipsilateral trochanteric region to provide neutral rotation of the extremity. The operation is performed under tourniquet control with the knee flexed to 90 degrees. The incision courses from the anterior portion of the fibular neck proximally across the joint line in line with the femoral shaft. The iliotibial band is split longitudinally just anterior and parallel to the fibular collateral ligament. The fibular collateral ligament, biceps femoris tendon, and the fibular head are identified while the peroneal nerve is located by palpation only.

The "Y" or conjoined tendon, comprised of the fibular collateral ligament and the biceps femoris tendon, is removed from the fibular head and retracted proximally. The fibular head is excised proximal to the peroneal nerve. Subperiosteal exposure of the tibia extends anteriorly to the patellar ligament and is carried posteriorly across to the medial cortex. Right-angle retractors are placed anteriorly and posteriorly and held by assistants standing on the same side of the operating table as the surgeon. A small capsular incision is created to identify the tibial articular surface.

The proximal osteotomy is placed 2 cm below the joint line and slopes posteriorly 10 degrees. The site of the distal osteotomy is measured distally from the predetermined base of the intended wedge. Placement of Kirschner wires and verification with radiographs or image intensification is helpful to confirm the orientation of the intended osteotomies. The plane of the pins

or osteotomies should converge at the medial cortex of the tibia. An oscillating saw is used to cut approximately three-fourths of the tibial width and then this portion of the wedge is removed. Completion of the osteotomy with a large osteotome can be performed with excellent visibility up to the medial cortex, which is then perforated in several places by a smaller osteotome. Closure of the osteotomy by a valgus force will create a hinge effect with the medial periosteum and soft tissues. Mechanical alignment and osteotomy apposition are then verified radiographically. Step staples are used to stabilize the osteotomy followed by tourniquet release and good hemostasis.

Reattachment of the conjoined tendon with sutures through bone are reinforced with additional sutures in the anterior crural and peroneus longis fascia. The iliotibial band and remaining layers of tissue are closed, and the extremity is placed in a compressive cotton dressing. Resection of the proximal tibiofibular articulation is a reasonable alternative to fibular head resection. This technical alteration is currently used at our institution. The medial one-third of the fibular head and the tibiofibular joint is resected with an osteotome that is oriented parallel to the plane of the joint. If this technique is employed, the surgeon needs to make sure that the fibula does not prevent closure of the osteotomy, and, if so, additional fibular head should be removed. This variation does not allow for direct advancement of the conjoined tendon.

By resecting more bone anteriorly, with a biplanar osteotomy, it is possible to correct a flexion contracture. It should be noted that this correction is accomplished at the expense of changing the normal posterior slope of the tibial articular surface. Recognition of this alteration of the articular surface is important when performing a subsequent knee arthroplasty because more posterior tibial bone will require resection and because retention of a functional posterior cruciate ligament is more difficult in this situation.

Varus Closing-Wedge Osteotomy and Its Technique

For patients with lateral compartment arthrosis and valgus malalignment, varus realignment osteotomy is based upon the same principles as with the more common valgus producing osteotomy (6). Clinical studies have determined that valgus deformity exceeding 12 degrees or if the high tibial osteotomy would create more than 10 degrees of tilt of the tibial articular surface then supracondylar femoral osteotomy is preferred for the valgus knee. The final alignment of the leg with this procedure should be an anatomic axis of zero degrees (6). The technique for this procedure is described as follows: Through a curved incision centered over the medial aspect of the proximal tibia and the medial epicondyle of the femur, the incision is deepened to the posterior aspect of the vastus medialis muscle. Carefully avoid the infrapatellar branch of the saphenous nerve. The tibia is exposed subperiosteally at the anterior edge of the superficial medial collateral ligament. The location and execution of the osteotomy and the wedge removal are similar to the varus osteotomy except for the obvious exclusion of the fibular osteotomy. The osteotomy is stabilized with a step staple.

The medial collateral ligament is usually very lax following this realignment osteotomy, and it is recommended that the ligament be tightened by twisting the ligament. Tightening of the ligament is accomplished by transversely grasping the ligament with a smooth, non-toothed hemostat and then by twisting the hemostat so the ligament is rolled upon itself until the ligament is snug. A nonabsorbable running suture is then used to reef the ligament, the hemostat is removed, and the suture is tightened and tied (6). The wound is then closed, and the extremity placed in a compressive cotton dressing.

Barrel-Vault Tibial Osteotomy

A longitudinal incision over the middle third of the fibula provides for resection of 1 cm of fibular diaphysis (30). A second midline longitudinal incision is made over the patella extending distally below the tibial tubercle. Parallel fascial incisions along the medial and lateral borders of the patellar ligament allow subperiosteal exposure of the proximal tibia. A curved jig is placed beneath the patellar ligament at the superior edge of the tibial tubercle. Jig position is verified radiographically. The anterior cortex is then perforated with multiple drill holes through the jig marker holes. A provisional Steinmann pin is then placed transversely at the junction of the proximal and middle third through the tibia. A second pin is placed in the lateral aspect of the proximal tibia and inserted medially and distally to exit from the medial tibial cortex at the level of the apex of the intended osteotomy. The insertion point and angle of the second pin are determined with the use of a goniometer jig based on the first pin and the desired amount of angular correction. The osteotomy is then performed from anterior to posterior with a thin osteotome or a small saw blade through the previously placed drill holes. Following completion of the osteotomy, the knee is flexed; the distal tibia is then displaced anteriorly 1 cm and then rotated to correct the angular malalignment. At this point, the two pins should be parallel. Appropriate release of the skin surrounding the protruding pins is performed; then the pins are connected and tightened with external fixation clamps and rods. Hemostasis is carefully completed at both incisions, and the wounds are then closed over drains. The clamps usually require retightening in the first several weeks and are removed approximately 8 weeks later.

Arthroscopy

Although the role of arthroscopy prior to realignment osteotomy is controversial, most surgeons have not demonstrated a prognostic value for predicting postoperative osteotomy knee results (38, 39). They documented, with follow-up of 5 to 8.3 years, that prearthroscopy findings did not correlate with post-osteotomy clinical results. Importantly, moderate or severe degenerative changes in the patellofemoral joint observed arthroscopically did not adversely affect the eventual clinical results of high tibial osteotomy.

Several surgeons have demonstrated proliferation of fibrocartilage and regeneration of articular cartilage while comparing arthroscopic findings of the knee visualized preoperatively and in follow-up after high tibial osteotomy (40–42). Only those knees that were overcorrected demonstrated regeneration of cartilage in the previously overloaded compartment (42). These findings support the concept of mechanical realignment to unload the symptomatic compartment of the knee, and they document the reparative capacity of the knee joint once it is unloaded. A small series of patients who had arthroscopic debridement for degenerative arthritis of the knee revealed that debridement may be beneficial for patients with normal extremity alignment, but debridement was unsatisfactory for patients with malalignment (43). It would seem that osteotomy is a better alternative for the malaligned knee with degenerative arthritis when addressing the symptoms present in an overloaded compartment. Intuition would lead one to believe that a few selected patients might benefit from arthroscopic debridement in conjunction with high tibial osteotomy, but this remains controversial. It has been our experience with a valgus-producing, high tibial osteotomy that arthroscopy has not been beneficial if the standing radiograph reveals a well-preserved lateral compartment (44).

Postoperative Management

Traditionally it has been recommended to immobilize the extremity postoperatively with a cylinder or long leg cast for a period of 5 to 8 weeks (19, 36). Immediate crutch walking and quadriceps exercises are encouraged. After cast removal, the patient participates with protected weight bearing, using crutches, and begins joint range of motion exercises. Progressive weight bearing is usually allowed at 8 to 10 weeks when definite evidence of trabeculation is observed at the osteotomy site, and the osteotomy is nontender. In an effort to encourage joint motion and prevent postoperative knee stiffness, some surgeons have used a cast brace for postoperative immobilization to allow immediate knee motion (42, 45). Comparison of patients indicates a shorter period of hospitalization and rehabilitation phase in the patients treated with a cast brace. These surgeons concluded that step-staple fixation provides sufficient fixation to allow early motion with a cast brace (45). Patients treated with a cast brace had better knee motion at a 2-year follow-up than patients treated with cast immobilization (42). Interestingly, there was no difference in the quality or quantity of cartilage repair observed histologically between these two patient groups, providing further evidence of the beneficial results attributed to angular realignment as an independant variable affecting the reparative process. A recent gait analysis study found no difference in any parameter of gait following osteotomy between patients immobilized with a cast for 6 weeks and patients treated with a cast brace and early motion (46). Currently, there is no conclusive evidence to suggest the superiority of either method of immobilization. Other forms of rigid skeletal fixation have been proposed to allow early postoperative motion and are discussed in a subsequent chapter. Excessive body weight adversely affects the ability to immobilize the extremity postoperatively and may influence the choice of skeletal fixation. The final choice of postoperative immobilization should be based on an assessment of skeletal rigidity at the time of surgery, combined with the patients' reliability or their ability to protect the extremity during the rehabilitation period.

Results

Initial clinical experience confirmed the rationale of limb realignment by osteotomy, but results deteriorate over the long term. Many series of high tibial osteotomy have revealed a majority of patients with continued satisfactory results 5 to 7 years after a realignment procedure (11, 15, 16, 18, 47). After 5 to 7 years of follow-up, the percentage of satisfactory clinical results appears to significantly diminish (5, 8, 19, 20). The duration of satisfactory clinical results following high tibial osteotomy seems to be extremely variable when evaluating these series. A recent review of the favorable and unfavorable prognostic factors associated with tibial osteotomy is excellent (44). Multiple factors, such as patient selection and surgical technique, that affect the outcome of high tibial osteotomy have been established over the past 3 decades. The use of historical studies to emphasize the success or failure of high tibial osteotomy is unreasonable. The recent literature suggests that high tibial osteotomy provides durable and satisfactory long-term clinical results if the procedure is accurately performed in appropriately selected patients (48).

Age

Many surgeons have stated that age does not affect the final clinical result following high tibial osteotomy (4, 9, 17, 18). An early report concluded that younger, active males had poorer postoperative results (49). A recent study of 29 patients, with a median age of 42 years and follow-up of 11 years, revealed 24 of these patients still considered themselves improved from their preoperative status (17). A similar study of 45 patients treated with valgus-producing high tibial osteotomy at an average age of 41 years revealed 70% good or excellent results at an average follow-up of 10 years (12). As previously emphasized, these young, active patients do poorly with total joint arthroplasty, and the activity level reported by the patients in the series reporting on high tibial osteotomy would not be expected to be tolerated by patients with prosthetic replacement at follow-up over this period of time.

Underlying Diagnosis

The underlying diagnosis associated with the angular malalignment appears to be an important prognostic factor. Patients with osteoarthritis do better after high tibial osteotomy than do patients with rheumatoid arthritis (3, 50). Patients with a varus deformity do better than patients with a valgus deformity (6). In a group

of young patients with secondary degenerative arthritis, the presence of prior fracture, osteochondritis dissecans, and prior medial menicectomy did not adversely affect the postoperative clinical result (4). All patients who had prior medial and lateral meniscectomies had an unsatisfactory result. If patients with prior medial and lateral menicectomy are excluded, it would seem that younger patients with secondary osteoarthritis, including those with prior medial meniscectomy, can expect results similar to older patients with primary degenerative arthritis.

Patellofemoral Joint

Degenerative arthritis of the patellofemoral joint has been considered to be a major cause of failure following high tibial osteotomy (51). Moderate or severe patellofemoral osteoarthritis was a poor prognostic factor when compared with the result obtained in patients with little or no evidence of patellofemoral disease (26). Conversely, long-term results have shown a very low incidence of patients who had unsatisfactory results due to the patellofemoral joint (29, 39, 52). It is possible that realignment of the extremity may provide a favorable alteration of patellofemoral mechanics. In fact, the dome osteotomy directly addresses this issue by anteriorly displacing the tibial tubercle (30). To date, there have been no carefully controlled clinical series that provide conclusive evidence that high tibial osteotomy is beneficial for the patellofemoral joint.

Postoperative Alignment

One of the single most important factors providing a satisfactory long-term result is the final postoperative extremity alignment. Several surgeons have, perhaps surprisingly, found no association of the postoperative alignment with ultimate clinical outcome (53, 54). Despite these early reports, no recent reports accept this conclusion. Coventry has stressed the need for achieving overcorrection of the normal mechanical axis so that a varus deformity is overcorrected to an anatomic valgus of approximately 10 degrees and that a valgus deformity is overcorrected to a neutral anatomic axis (6, 11). Most recent studies confirm this recommendation for final postoperative alignment (26, 39, 41, 55). At a 2-year follow-up, knees with 5 to 13 degrees of valgus mechanical tibial femoral alignment had significantly better results than those knees with alignment of less than 5 degrees of valgus (38).

At 5-year follow-up, these same patients revealed that, if the alignment was between 7 and 13 degrees of valgus, there were twice as many patients with a satisfactory result when compared with patients who had an extremity with alignment less than 7 degrees of valgus (39). Patients with correction of the anatomic axis to less than 5 degrees of valgus had a 63% failure rate (26). Patients with a final correction of alignment between 6 and 14 degrees of anatomic alignment universally enjoyed a good or excellent clinical result. Hsu demonstrated a significant relationship between the clinical success of the realignment osteotomy and the proper correction of the mechanical axis (41). Cass' and

Bryan's patients had a better long-term result if the anatomic axis was corrected to 10 degrees or more of valgus (56). Survival analysis studies of 40 patients treated with high tibial osteotomy demonstrated earlier clinical failures with postoperative undercorrection or overcorrection (5).

Vainionpaa, et al. have also reported superior clinical results in patients with a postoperative alignment between 5 and 13 degrees of anatomic valgus (57). Proper postoperative alignment was the most important determinate of long-term clinical success in another report (16). At an average of 11.5 years follow-up, patients with a proper mechanical axis remained clinically successful. In contrast, patients with undercorrection or overcorrection of alignment experienced clinical deterioration at an average of 7 years following osteotomy. This paper eloquently emphasizes the importance of proper alignment and long-term clinical success following osteotomy. It is interesting to note that the deterioration of clinical results in patients with improper alignment occurred at an average of 7 years, a finding which coincides exactly with other reports detailing clinical deterioration.

Yasuda, et al. emphasized the need for slight overcorrection of the postoperative femorotibial alignment (58). Actually, the alignment observed at the time of bony union was the most accurate predictor of long-term success in their patients. In patients with appropriate alignment, the clinical result remained satisfactory in 63% of patients beyond 10 years of follow-up. Another study of 39 patients confirmed these excellent long-term results (48). At 12 years follow-up, 59% of the patients had a good or excellent result. The surgeons noted that the 10 patients who were considered failures had the operation prior to the establishment of modern selection criteria and would not now be considered candidates for high tibial osteotomy. If these patients are excluded from their analysis, the overall satisfactory results at 12 years follow-up would be an impressive 79 percent. In 314 patients followed for 10 to 19 years after high tibial osteotomy, there was a significant association with postoperative alignment and eventual clinical failure (47). In the 170 patients who had undercorrection of their alignment, 54 subsequently required additional revision surgery for clinical deterioration. In the 144 patients with a normalized or overcorrected alignment, only 8 patients required surgical revision. Based on this extensive, long-term experience, these surgeons suggest that a properly performed high tibial osteotomy will outlive current prosthetic replacements.

Further support for the continued use of high tibial osteotomy was demonstrated with good or excellent results in 80% of patients at 9 years follow-up (15). Healy, et al. attributed these optimistic findings to careful patient selection and emphasized a precise surgical technique leading to appropriate postoperative alignment. The emergence of these favorable long-term results coupled to careful patient selection, accurate surgical technique, and appropriate postoperative alignment portrays a more favorable outlook on high tibial osteotomy and establishes this procedure as a continued viable option for the active patient.

Recurrent Deformity

Recurrence of the preoperative deformity over time has been correlated with deterioration of the clinical result (8, 11, 16, 19, 39, 57, 59). Several surgeons have correlated the recurrence of deformity with undercorrection of alignment at the time of surgery (16, 41). Stuart, et al., reported that the majority of their patients had some recurrence of varus at a minimum of 5 years follow-up (60). These patients changed from an average of 9.3 degrees of anatomic valgus to 7.8 degrees of valgus over this period of observation. Only 18% of Stuart's patients had more than 5 degrees of progressive return of deformity. In contrast, 83% of his patients had significant progression of lateral compartment degenerative arthritis. Other surgeons have correlated the progression of lateral compartment degenerative arthritis with poor clinical results (61, 62).

Gait Pattern

Andriacci, Galante, and coworkers have examined the relationship between preoperative gait adduction moments and postoperative clinical results (8, 63). In these elegant gait studies, patients were divided into low-adduction and high-adduction gait patterns. At an average follow-up of 3.2 years, good or excellent results were observed in 100% of patients in the low-adduction group, whereas the high-adduction group had only 50% good or excellent results. The only patients who had recurrence of their preoperative deformity were patients with a high-adduction gait pattern. They recommended consideration of overcorrection of alignment in patients with a high-adduction gait pattern. In a follow-up study of these same patients at 3 to 8.9 years follow-up, these findings were amplified (63). All patients with a low-adduction gait pattern had a good or excellent result. Almost all patients with a high-adduction moment had some recurrence of their preoperative deformity. This report indicates the importance of attentive preoperative assessment and appropriate adjustment in the surgical technique.

Alternatives

Currently, the alternatives for treatment of the patient with unicompartmental degenerative arthritis of the knee include arthroscopy with debridement, high tibial osteotomy, unicompartmental arthroplasty, and total knee arthroplasty. For an extensive discussion, the reader is referred to Chapter 53. We have not been pleased with the results of unicompartmental knee arthroplasty (64). Despite initial enthusiasm, the surgeons at our institution have largely abandoned the use of this procedure (Fig. 55.7). In our opinion, the ideal candidate for a unicompartmental prosthesis would be the small patient over the age of 70 with minimal angular malalignment and localized unicompartmental disease. There are currently no properly designed studies that carefully compare the long-term results of high tibial osteotomy and unicompartmental knee replacement. Any study attempting to compare these procedures will need to stratify the patients according to age, activity, and to carefully assess the appropriate preoperative and postoperative prognostic factors.

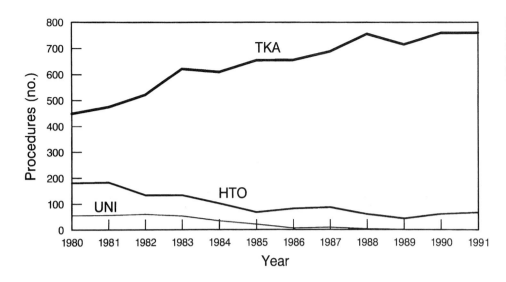

Figure 55.7. The number of total knee arthroplasties, high tibial osteotomies, and unicompartmental knee arthroplasties performed each year at the Mayo Clinic between 1980 and 1991.

Summary

We believe that high tibial osteotomy still possesses a small but significant niche in the knee surgeon's armamentarium. Long-term satisfactory results can be obtained in well-selected patients with unicompartmental degenerative arthritis of the knee associated with malalignment. The success of this procedure is highly dependent on perceptive selection of the patient with appropriate surgical indications. Surgical technique must be precise and based on accurate preoperative planning. High tibial osteotomy, performed with modern technological tools facilitating evaluation and surgical technique, should provide satisfactory long-term clinical results in the majority of patients. If the osteotomy is properly performed, the patient with a high tibial osteotomy can expect a relatively uncomplicated conversion to a prosthetic replacement when knee symptoms require further surgical intervention.

These patients benefit from the pain relief afforded by this procedure and from the ability to continue physically demanding occupations and high activity levels not permissible in patients with a prosthetic replacement. Significant relief of symptoms combined with the ability to continue chosen activities are fundamental characteristics of the high tibial osteotomy that separate this procedure from the other alternatives of treatment available for unicompartmental degenerative arthritis of the knee.

Based on this unique characteristic and the success demonstrated in recent studies, high tibial osteotomy has met original expectations and will continue to be a viable option. In severely deformed knees, single osteotomy at high tibial or femoral supracondylar regions may not be able to correct the alignment and maintain proper joint line obliquity. A complex dual osteotomy may be necessary to achieve proper knee alignment and provide the essential requirements for appropriate pressure redistribution in the knee joint. A computer-aided preoperative planning software package like "OASIS" can help to produce surprisingly positive clinical results for these difficult reconstructive procedures (Fig. 55.8).

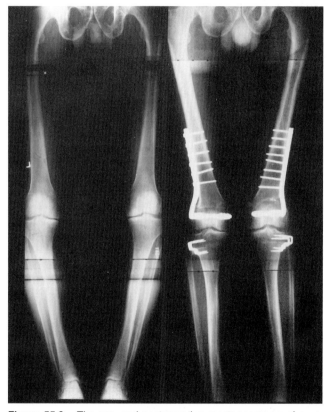

Figure 55.8. The pre- and postoperative roentgenograms of a patient with bilateral knee varus deformities that were corrected using dual osteotomy guided by the OASIS software computer simulation analysis results.

Long-term prospective follow-up studies of patients are required to validate the effectiveness of this preoperative planning scheme and are now in progress. When such methods are properly established, the surgeon should be even more confident in performing osteotomies about the knee for the treatment of unicompartmental knee disease.

References

1. Jackson JP. Osteotomy for osteoarthritis of the knee. In: Proceedings of the Sheffield Regional Orthopaedic Club. J Bone Joint Surg 1958;40B:826.
2. Chao EYS. Biomechanics of high tibial osteotomy. In: American Academy of Orthopaedic Surgeons Symposium on Reconstructive Surgery of the Knee. St. Louis: CV Mosby, 1978:143.
3. Coventry MB. Osteotomy about the knee for degenerative and rheumatoid arthritis. J Bone Joint Surg 1973;55A:23–48.
4. Morrey BF. Upper tibial osteotomy for secondary osteoarthritis of the knee. J Bone Joint Surg 1989;71B:554–559.
5. Matthews LS, Goldstein SA, Malvitz TA, Katz BP, Kaufer H. Proximal tibial osteotomy: Factors that influence the duration of satisfactory function. Clin Orthop 1988;229:193–200.
6. Coventry MB. Proximal tibial varus osteotomy for osteoarthritis of the lateral compartment of the knee. J Bone Joint Surg 1987;69A:32–38.
7. Windsor RE, Insall JN, Vince KG. Technical considerations of total knee arthroplasty after proximal tibial osteotomy. J Bone Joint Surg 1988;70A:547–555.
8. Prodromos CC, Andriacchi TP, Galante JO. A relationship between gait and clinical changes following high tibial osteotomy. J Bone Joint Surg 1985;67A:1188–1194.
9. Muller W, Jani L. Experiences with 75 high tibial osteotomies. Reconstr Surg Traumatol 1971;12:53–63.
10. Insall JN, Shoji H, Mayer V. High tibial osteotomy. J Bone Joint Surg 1974;56A:1397–1405.
11. Coventry MB. Upper tibial osteotomy for osteoarthritis. J Bone Joint Surg 1985;67A:1136–1140.
12. Holden DL, James SL, Larson RL, Slocum DB. Proximal tibial osteotomy in patients who are fifty years old or less. A long-term follow-up study. J Bone Joint Surg 1988;70A:977–982.
13. Hsu RWW, Himeno S, Coventry MB, Chao EYS. Normal axial alignment of the lower extremity and load-bearing distribution at the knee. Clin Orthop 1990;255:215–227.
14. Uematsu A, Kim EE. Role of radionuclide joint imaging in high tibial osteotomy. Clin Orthop 1979;144:220–225.
15. Healy WL, Riley LH. High tibial valgus osteotomy: A clinical review. Clin Orthop 1986;209:227–233.
16. Hernigou P, Medevielle D, Debeyre J, Goutallier D. Proximal tibial osteotomy for osteoarthritis with varus deformity. A 10- to 13-year follow-up study. J Bone Joint Surg 1987;66A:332–354.
17. Odenbring S, Tjorstrand B, Egund N, Hagstedt B, Hovelius L, Lindstrand A, Luxhoj T, Svanstrom A. Function after tibial osteotomy for medial gonarthrosis below aged 50 years. Acta Orthop Scand 1989;60:527–531.
18. Rudan JF, Simurda MA. Valgus high tibial osteotomy: a long-term follow-up study. Clin Orthop 1991;268:157–160.
19. Insall JN, Joseph DM, Msika C. High tibial osteotomy for varus gonarthrosis. A long-term follow-up study. J Bone Joint Surg 1984;66A:1040–1048.
20. Ritter MA, Fechtman RA. Proximal tibial osteotomy: A survivorship analysis. J Arthroplasty 1988;3:309–311.
21. Katz MM, Hungerford DS, Krackow KA, Lennox DW. Results of total knee arthroplasty after failed proximal tibial osteotomy for osteoarthritis. J Bone Joint Surg 1987;69A:225–233.
22. Krackow KA, Holtgrewe JL. Experience with a new technique for managing severely overcorrected valgus high tibial osteotomy at total knee arthroplasty. Clin Orthop 1990;258:213–224.
23. Staeheli JW, Cass JR, Morrey BF. Condylar total knee arthroplasty after failed proximal tibial osteotomy. J Bone Joint Surg 1987;69A:28–31.
24. Kettelkamp DB, Wenger DR, Chao EYS, Thompson C. Results of proximal tibial osteotomy: The effects of tibiofemoral angle, stance-phase flexion-extension, and medial-plateau force. J Bone Joint Surg 1976;58A:952–960.
25. Coventry MB. Upper tibial osteotomy for gonarthrosis: The evolution of the operation in the last 18 years and long-term results. Orthop Clin North Am 1979;10:191–208.
26. Rudan JF, Simurda MA. High tibial osteotomy: A prospective clinical and roentgenographic review. Clin Orthop 1990;255:251–256.
27. Sim FH, Hsu RWW, Chao EY. Mini-symposium: Osteotomy of the knee. Osteotomy. Curr Orthop 1990;4(2):88–94.
28. Ide T, Hara T, An KN, Chao EY. Stability and pressure distribution of joint articulating surfaces. First World Congress of Biomechanics, 1:57, University of California, San Diego, Aug. 31–Sept. 4, 1990.
29. Hernigou P, Goutallier D. Patello-femoral joint changes in osteoarthritic varus knees after upper tibial valgus opening osteotomy with bone grafting. A 10- to 13-year follow-up. J Orthop Surg (Fr) 1987;1:37–41.
30. Maquet P. Valgus osteotomy for osteoarthritis of the knee. Clin Orthop 1976;120:143–147.
31. Hofmann AA, Wyatt RWB, Beck SW. High tibial osteotomy: Use of an osteotomy jig, rigid fixation, and early motion versus conventional surgical technique and cast immobilization. Clin Orthop 1991;271:212–217.
32. Jiang CC, Hang YS, Liu TK. A new jig for proximal tibial osteotomy. Clin Orthop 1988;226:118–123.
33. Mynerts R. The SAAB jig: An aid in high tibial osteotomy. Acta Orthop Scand 1978;49:85–88.
34. Lippert FG, Kirkpatrick GS. A jig for pin insertion in the performance of high tibial osteotomy. Clin Orthop 1975;112:242–244.
35. Odenbring S, Egund N, Lindstrand A, Tjornstrand B. A guide instrument for high tibial osteotomy. Acta Orthop Scand 1989;60:449–451.
36. Coventry MB. Osteotomy of the upper portion of tibia for degenerative arthritis of the knee. J Bone Joint Surg 1965;47A:984–990.
37. Gariepy R. Correction du genou flechi dans l'arthrite. Proc Int Soc Orthop Surg Traumatol 1960;8:884–886.
38. Keene JS, Dyreby JR Jr. High tibial osteotomy in the treatment of osteoarthritis of the knee. The role of preoperative arthroscopy. J Bone Joint Surg 1983;65A:36–42.
39. Keene JS, Monson DK, Roberts JM, et al. Evaluation of patients for high tibial osteotomy. Clin Orthop 1989;243:157–165.
40. Fujisawa Y, Masuhara K, Shiomi S. The effect of high tibial osteotomy on osteoarthritis of the knee. An arthroscopic study of 54 knee joints. Orthop Clin North Am 1979;10:585–608.
41. Hsu RWW: The study of Maquet dome high tibial osteotomy: arthroscopic-assisted analysis. Clin Orthop 1989;243:280–285.
42. Odenbring S, Egund N, Lindstrand A, Lohmander LS, Willen H. Cartilage regeneration after proximal tibial osteotomy for medial gonarthrosis. An arthroscopic, roentgenographic, and histologic study. Clin Orthop 1992;277:210–216.
43. Salisbury RB, Nottage WM, Gardner V. The effect of alignment on results in arthroscopic debridement of the degenerative knee. Clin Orthop 1985;198:268–272.
44. Morrey BF. Upper tibial osteotomy: Analysis of prognostic features: A review. Adv Orthop Surg 1986;9:213–222.
45. Kreigshauser LA, Bryan RS. Early motion with cast brace after modified Coventry high tibial osteotomy. Clin Orthop 1985;195:168–172.
46. Ivarsson I, Larsson LE. Gait analysis in patients with gonarthrosis treated by high tibial osteotomy. Clin Orthop 1989;239:185–190.
47. Odenbring S, Egund N, Knutson K, Lindstrand A, Larson ST. Revision after osteotomy for gonarthrosis: A 10–19-year follow-up of 314 cases. Acta Orthop Scand 1990;61:128–130.
48. Berman AT, Bosacco SJ, Kirshner S, Avolio A Jr. Factors influencing long-term results in high tibial osteotomy. Clin Orthop 1991;272:192–198.
49. Surin V, Markhede G, Sundholm K. Factors influencing results of high tibial osteotomy in gonarthrosis. Acta Orthop Scand 1975; 46 996–1007.
50. Chan RNW, Pollard JP. High tibial osteotomy for rheumatoid arthritis of the knee. Acta Orthop Scand 1978;49:78–84.
51. Insall JN. High tibial osteotomy in the treatment of osteoarthritis of the knee. Surg Ann 1975;7:347.
52. Coventry MB, Bowman PW. Long-term results of upper tibial osteotomy for degenerative arthritis of the knee. Acta Orthop Belgica 1982;48:139–156.
53. Appel H, Friberg S. The effect of high tibial osteotomy on pain in osteoarthritis of the knee joint. Acta Orthop Scand 1972;43:558–565.
54. Ranieri L, Traina GC, Maci C. High tibial osteotomy in osteoarthritis of the knee. Ital J Orthop Traumatol 1977;3:289–300.
55. Jokio PJ, Lindholm TS, Vankka E. Medial and lateral gonarthrosis treated with high tibial osteotomy. Arch Orthop Trauma Surg 1985;104:135–144.
56. Cass JR, Bryan RS. High tibial osteotomy. Clin Orthop 1988;230:196–199.
57. Vainionpaa S, Laike E, Kirves P, Tiusanen P. Tibial osteotomy for osteoarthritis of the knee. A five- to ten-year follow-up study. J Bone Joint Surg 1981;63A:938–941.
58. Yasuda K, Majima T, Tsuchida T, Kaneda K. A 10- to 15-year follow-up observation of high tibial osteotomy in medial compartment osteoarthritis. Clin Orthop 1992;282:186–195.
59. Coventry MB. Upper tibial osteotomy for gonarthrosis. Orthop Clin North Am 1979;10:191–208.
60. Stuart MJ, Grace JN, Ilstrup DM, Kelly CM, Adams RA, Morrey BF. Late recurrence of varus deformity after proximal tibial osteotomy. Clin Orthop 1990;260:61–65.
61. Shoji H, Insall J. High tibial osteotomy for osteoarthritis of the knee with valgus deformity. J Bone Joint Surg 1973;55A:963–973.
62. Tjornstrand B, Hagstedt B, Persson BM. High tibial osteotomy: A seven year clinical and radiographic follow-up. Clin Orthop 1981;160:124–136.
63. Wang JW, Kuo KN, Andriacci TP, Galante JO. The influence of walking mechanics and time on the results of proximal tibial osteotomy. J Bone Joint Surg 1990;72A:905–909.
64. Bernasek TL, Rand JA, Bryan RS. Unicompartmental porous-coated anatomic total knee arthroplasty. Clin Orthop 1988;236:52–56.

56

Fixation in High Tibial Osteotomy

Robert W. Chandler and Dana Seltzer

Introduction

Valgus-producing osteotomy of the proximal tibial (high tibial osteotomy or HTO) is a time-honored treatment of medial compartment arthritis of the knee joint (1–20). The ideal patient is active, under 55 years of age, has a stable varus deformity of less than 10 degrees with primary medial compartment involvement and good bone stock (6, 18). Operative technique is less uniform than are the indications for surgery, and wide variations exist in recommendations regarding planning, preparation, incision, intraoperative measurement, and fixation (4, 9, 12, 16, 21–28). Table 56.1 lists series reported in the literature according to the method of fixation used.

Some surgeons have advocated the use of specific radiographic planning tools, intraoperative cutting jigs, external and/or internal fixation, while others argue in favor of simple estimates of correction angle and limited fixation, such as casting (29–33). Reproducibility of operative outcome, in terms of predictable anatomic correction and functional recovery, must have a high priority (34). Therefore, all techniques contributing to improved reliability of operative results should be considered. This chapter focuses on techniques designed to maximize the reliability of HTO.

Anatomic Goals of Osteotomy

Numerous authors have reported difficulty in producing the desired anatomic result after HTO (Table 56.2). Coventry, more concerned with undercorrection, emphasized overcorrection (4, 9, 35). Bauer, et al. reported 23 of 63 (37%) osteotomies exceeded the desired correction angle (2). Cass reported corrections of 0 to 23 degrees valgus with an average of 14 degrees valgus (3). Matthews reported 25% of his osteotomies exceeded the desired anatomic result with overcorrection in 6 and undercorrection in 4 (range 0 to 30 valgus) and commented that proximal fragment fracture and postoperative alignment errors were "surprisingly common" (18). Similarly, Koshino, Vainionpaa, Hernigou, and Miniacci have noted anatomic outcomes frequently falling outside the desirable range (1, 12, 16, 20).

Studies of results after HTO have often concluded that the success of the procedure correlated well with the (*a*) correction achieved and maintained and (*b*) the degree of the arthritic involvement (Fig. 56.1) (3, 4, 8, 11, 13, 16, 36–40). Typically, good candidates for HTO have mild varus, up to 10 degrees. Final alignments falling within the range of 5 to 15 degrees valgus are cosmetically acceptable and fall within the range recommended by most investigators (See Table 56.3). Valgus greater than 15 degrees may be associated with good function and pain relief, but the cosmetic result is not well accepted by the patient and may require correction. A predictable anatomic result is a goal of osteotomy, although outcome is not totally determined by the final anatomic or mechanical axis (18, 41).

Fujisawa studied 54 patients arthroscopically before and after HTO and found healing of articular ulcerations with corrections that shifted the weight-bearing line to a point 30 to 40% lateral to the transverse midpoint of the knee (Fig. 56.2). Miniacci et al., however, reported difficulty achieving this correction even though their realignment of the anatomic axis was satisfactory (1). In fact, realignment satisfying the Fujisawa criteria may create severe valgus deformity in some patients, particularly those of short stature. Preoperative planning, intraoperative measuring devices and image intensification along with stability of the osteotomy after surgery are important in achieving any set anatomic objective. Realignment of the anatomic axis (femoral tibia angle) to approximately 10 degrees of valgus should be the goal of osteotomy until this more uncertain objective defined by Fujisawa is further analyzed (Table 56.3). This objective allows for 5 degrees of latitude either way for the production of cosmetically and functionally satisfactory outcomes.

Table 56.1   Fixation Used in Literature Series

Ref No	Author	Year	Osteotomy Type	Cast	Staple + Cost	Plate	External Fixation
(14)	Jackson	1969	Ball and socket tubercle	X			X
(44)	Benjamin	1969	Double	X			
(2)	Bauer	1969	Wedge above tubercle	X			
(57)	Gunn	1969	Ball and socket below tub	X			
(26)	Shoji	1973	Wedge above tubercle	X			
(58)	Lamont	1973	Dome	X			
(59)	Hagstedt	1974	Wedge above tubercle	X			
(13)	Insall	1974	Wedge above tubercle	X			
(60)	Gariepy	1975	Wedge above tubercle	X			X
(61)	Seal	1975	Mixed	X			
(17)	Maquet	1976	Wedge/Inverted V above	X	X		
(40)	Tjornstrand	1981	Wedge above tubercle	X			
(36)	Engle	1981	Wedge above tubercle	X			
(11)	Aglietti	1983	Wedge above tubercle	X			
(25)	Putnam	1985	Maquet + Wedge above	X			
(52)	Coventry	1965	Wedge above tubercle		X		
(5)	Coventry	1973	Wedge above tubercle		X		
(62)	Levy	1973	Inverted "V"		X		
(63)	Surin	1974	Wedge above tubercle		X		
(64)	Torgerson	1974	Wedge above tubercle		X		
(65)	Edholm	1977	Wedge above tubercle		X		
(46)	Mynerts	1980	Wedge above tubercle		X		
(24)	Ogata	1983	Interlocking wedge		X		
(18)	Matthews	1986	Wedge above tubercle		X		
(50)	Sundaram	1986	Dome		X		
(41)	Mabrey	1987	Wedge above tubercle		X		
(3)	Cass	1988	Wedge above tubercle		X		
(66)	Odenbring	1989	Wedge above tubercle		X		
(67)	Chapchal	1974	Wedge above tubercle			X	
(68)	Lemaire	1974	Wedge above tubercle			X	
(10)	Fujisawa	1979	Wedge above tubercle			X	
(27)	Sprenger	1979	Wedge above tubercle			X	
(69)	Ha'Eri	1980	Wedge above tubercle			X	
(20)	Vainionpaa	1981	Wedge above tubercle			X	
(12)	Hernigou	1987	Medial opening wedge	X		X	
(16)	Koshino	1989	Wedge above tubercle			X	
(1)	Miniacci	1989	Wedge above tubercle			X	
(21)	Devas	1969	Wedge above tubercle				X
(17)	Maquet	1976	Barrel vault				X
(70)	MacIntosh	1977	Wedge above tubercle				X
(71)	Krempen	1982	Dome				X
(48)	Hsu	1989	Dome				X
Summary				16	14	9	7

Table 56.2   Anatomic Results after HTO

Ref No	Author Varus	Preoperative Valgus	Postoperative	Postoperative Range
(3)	Cass	4	10	2 valgus to 23 valgus
(16)	Koshino	5	13	5 valgus to 26 valgus
(18)	Matthews	6	7	0 to 30 valgus
(1)	Miniacci	3	11	8 valgus to 17 valgus
(25)	Putnam	5	8	0 to 15 valgus
(72)	Rudan	6	9	2 valgus to 26 valgus
(20)	Vainionpaa	5	4	7 varus to 23 valgus
Averages		5	9	7 varus to 30 valgus

Table 56.3   Ideal Final Alignment after HTO

Ref No	Author	Ideal Final Alignment
(3)	Cass	10–12° Valgus
(3–9, 35, 52, 53)	Coventry	5–10° Valgus
(36)	Engle	5–10° Valgus
(37)	Ivarson	3–7° Valgus
(38)	Kettlekamp	>5° Valgus
(16)	Koshino	6–15° Valgus
(39)	Myrnerts	3–7° Valgus

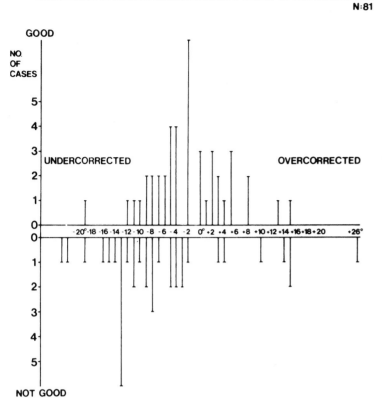

Figure 56.1. Tjornstrand data showing a plot of anatomic results against outcome, illustrating the scatter of anatomic result. (Reproduced with permission from Tjornstrand BA. High tibial osteotomy: A seven-year clinical and radiographic follow-up. Clin Orthop 1981;160(Oct):130.)

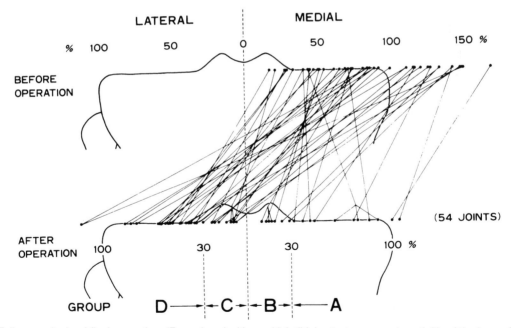

Figure 56.2. Fujisawa criteria of final correction. (Reproduced with permission from Fujisawa Y, Masuhara, K, Shiomi S. The effect of high tibial osteotomy on osteoarthritis of the knee. Orthop Clin North Am 1979;10(3):586.)

Planning for Osteotomy

In practice, the femoral tibial angle derived from standing radiographs has been a reliable angle for the planning of surgery in patients with ligamentous stability. To be accurate for measurement, radiographs must include most of the length of the femur and tibia (12, 36). Koshino et. al. have shown a high correlation between the anatomic and mechanical axes (Fig. 56.3). The use of the mechanical axis is possible in some facilities having the radiographic capabilities of full length standing x-rays, but, in fact, the mechanical axis is more difficult

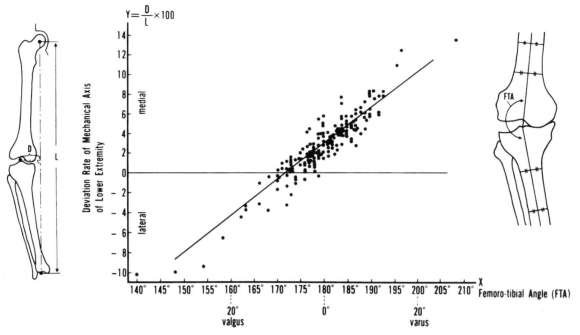

Figure 56.3. Correlation between femorotibial angle and mechanical axis. (Reproduced with permission from Koshino T, et al. High tib-ial osteotomy with fixation by a blade plate for medial compartment osteoarthritis of the knee. Orthop Clin North Am 1989;20(2):237.)

to use in actual practice. However, Korn recently presented data suggesting improved outcome with use of the mechanical axis and the dome technique in 45 HTO patients (42). Preoperative drawings are made showing the correction angle, the level of osteotomy, the location of fixation if used, the size of the wedge, and, finally, the completed osteotomy with final anatomic axis (Fig. 56.4) (36). If possible, the mechanical axis should also be assessed.

Osteotomies in patients with ligamentous instability are more difficult to plan because loading conditions may change the various angles (13). The correction angle should be estimated from the maximum valgus demonstrated with valgus stress (36). Overcorrection in such patients is likely to occur unless stress radiographs, or some other technique, are used to assess ligamentous laxity before surgery. In varus loading situations, medial collateral ligament laxity may escape notice. Operations are typically planned using weight-bearing radiographs that disguise medial instability. Once valgus is produced by osteotomy, the loading conditions change. After correction, a full weight-bearing radiograph will reflect the combined influence of the valgus-producing osteotomy and medial collateral laxity. Any laxity in the medial side becomes apparent as increased valgus during weight bearing and may produce a correction well beyond the desirable range (37).

Intraoperative Tools

Use of an image intensifier during the procedure helps the surgeon assess the location of the joint relative to the osteotomy and internal fixation. Because of its usefulness in assessment, the image intensifier is strongly recommended if available. The operation takes a few minutes longer to set up, but may be completed more expeditiously with the use of radiographic guides. Preoperative planning makes the operator aware of significant landmarks and the length of the lateral cortex (base of the wedge) to be removed. Angle-measuring devices and cutting jigs are available to improve the precision of the angle measurement and intraoperative cuts (Fig. 56.5) (29–33, 43).

If the medial cortex is broken or the osteotomy otherwise destabilized, excessive angulation may result. Displacement may occur due to instability. Special caution will be necessary to maintain the desired correction until union occurs. Medial internal fixation may be desirable in such cases to restore the integrity of the medial cortex, particularly in cases employing tension band principles (1, 16, 27). Table 56.4 lists complications following HTO and includes a relatively high number of secondary displacements (last column).

Arguments for Internal Fixation

Some authorities argue that internal fixation of HTO complicates the procedure and does not affect the result of the operation (9, 44). Ivarsson, Myrnerts, and Gillquist studied patients with HTO treated with staples and casting as compared with internal fixation with a "T" plate. They found no significant benefit in the fixation method and concluded that stapling and casting were preferable (45). On the other hand, Aglietti et al. found more than 10% loss of correction when casting only was used (11). Fixation does, however, add to the technical sophistication required to carry out an already exacting procedure. However, when successfully applied, an internally fixed osteotomy stands a better

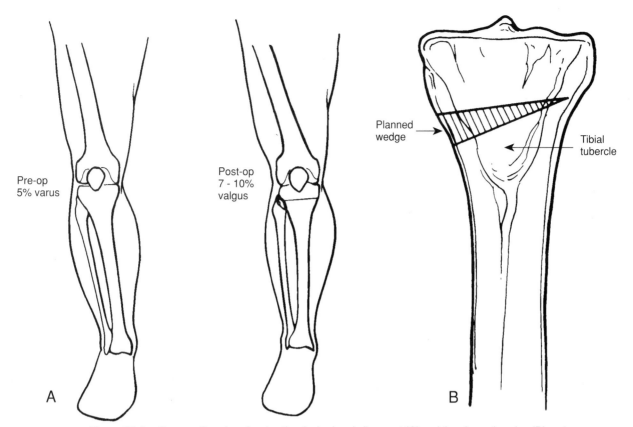

Figure 56.4.   Preoperative plan showing the desired end alignment **(A)** and the planned wedge **(B)**.

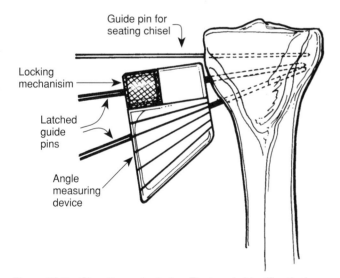

Figure 56.5.   Chandler angle device. The top pin identifies the location of the fixation device, which is appropriately away from the joint.

chance of maintaining the correction achieved in surgery while allowing immediate motion and some weight bearing—both of which are important for arthritic joints (12, 27, 46). In addition, internal fixation allows for immediate motion that may decrease muscular atrophy, decrease stiffness, and reduce overall recovery time.

Stable fixation allows the patient a greater degree of comfort than casting alone or staple combined with casting and may be found to reduce venous complications if continuous passive motion is initiated in the recovery room with active motion started the day following surgery (16). With internal fixation, the patient has access to the skin after wound healing, which favors hygiene and also comfort. We believe these advantages significantly outweigh the disadvantages. Internal fixation of fractures has become routine and very sophisticated in orthopaedic practice; stable internal fixation of HTO is a logical extension of the techniques developed in the management of fractures (47). It should be noted, however, that the superiority of metallic fixation to cast treatment has not been scientifically proven to date in a randomized prospective study.

External Fixation

Casting

The simplest form of postoperative fixation for HTO is application of a well-padded cylinder cast that adheres to the principle of three point fixation. A single well-molded cast may suffice for the entire treatment period, but, more typically, cast changes are necessary as atrophy occurs. Cast changes require care to prevent the change resulting in loss of correction. Cast fixation requires prolonged immobilization of the arthritic knee joint that may lead to stiffness, difficulty in walking, and, in the initial postoperative phase, increased risk of

Table 56.4. Complications of HTO Grouped by Fixation Cast, Staples, Plates, and External Fixator.[a]

Ref No	Author	Year	Net	S.Inf	D.Inf.	Thrmemb	P. Palsy	FxProxFrag	H.Delay	2'Disp
Cast										
(14)	Jackson	1969	70	13		3	8	NDR	3	NDR
(44)	Benjamin	1969	57	0	0	1	NDR	NDR	NDR	NDR
(2)	Bauer	1969	66	NDR	2	4	NDR	6	3	NDR
(57)	Gunn	1969	25	NDR	NDR	2	2	NDR	0	NDR
(26)	Shoji	1973	49	NDR		2	1	2	NDR	NDR
(58)	Lamont	1973	30	NDR	NDR	NDR	NDR	NDR	3	7
(59)	Hagstedt	1974	202	6		6	16	NDR	7	NDR
(13)	Insall	1974	51	0	2	2	NDR	5	1	18
(60)	Gariepy	1975	85		1	1	2	NDR	3	NDR
(61)	Seal	1975	47		1	7	1	0	3	4
(17)	Maquet	1976	25		1	1	5	NDR	NDR	NDR
(36)	Engle	1981	20	0	1	NDR	NDR	2	NDR	1
(11)	Aglietti	1983	139	7	4	7	1	3	10	15
(25)	Putnam	1985	34	0	0	2	NDR	NDR	0	NDR
Staple										
(52)	Coventry	1965	30	2		NDR	1	NDR	NDR	NDR
(5)	Coventry	1973	87	1		3	0	NDR	2	NDR
(62)	Levy	1973	38	3	1	2	1	1	NDR	NDR
(63)	Surin	1974	9	1	1	NDR	3	2	3	NDR
(64)	Torgerson	1974	57	0	1	NDR	4	NDR	1	1
(46)	Mynerts	1980	78	4	1	2	NDR	NDR	3	7
(24)	Ogata	1983	36	0	0	0	2	0	0	NDR
(18)	Matthews	1986	47	NDR	NDR	2	4	8	NDR	7
(50)	Sundaram	1986	105	0	8	6	7	NDR	6	NDR
(41)	Mabrey	1987	72	NDR	NDR	3	3	2	3	NDR
(3)	Cass	1988	86	0	1	2	0	1	2	NDR
Plates										
(67)	Chapchal	1974	92	2		NDR	3	NDR	NDR	NDR
(68)	Lemaire	1974	105	2		1	0	NDR	3	NDR
(27)	Sprenger	1979	45	0	0	0	0	0	2	NDR
(69)	Ha'Eri	1980	71	2	1	2	2	NDR	NDR	NDR
(20)	Vainionpaal	1981	103	2		6	2	1	6	NDR
(12)	Hernigou	1987	93	NDR	2	NDR	1	10	NDR	21
(16)	Koshino	1989	299	1	1	NDR	3	2	3	NDR
(1)	Miniacci	1989	41	0	0	1	NDR	NDR	0	3
External Fixation										
(21)	Devas	1969	28	NDR		NDR	2	NDR	NDR	NDR
(17)	Maquet	1976	182	3	1	4	11	NDR	NDR	NDR
(70)	MacIntosh	1977	136	9	2	11	14	NDR	4	NDR
(71)	Krempen	1982	40		1	NDR	NDR	1	0	NDR
(48)	Hsu	1989	118	8	5	4	7	NDR	1	13
Summary			2983	66	38	87	106	46	72	96

[a]Net, Total number of patients; S.Inf, Superficial infection; D.Inf, Deep Infection; Thrmemb, Thromboembolism; P. Palsy, Phoneal palsy; FxProxFrag, Fracture of the proximal fragment; H.Delay, Healing delay; 2'Disp, Secondary displacements; NDR, No data recorded.

neurovascular compromise due to the circumferential wrap; swelling inside the cast gives rise to elevated pressure, creating a possible compartment syndrome. Later, venous complications may arise because of the cast.

Success with casting alone has been reported by Insall and colleagues (13). Jackson, et al. reported problems with healing that required bone grafting when casting only was used (15). Uniform success with casting alone has not been reported. Myrnerts recommended increasing casting from 6 to 10 weeks with no weight bearing for the same period after discovering loss of correction when using casting alone for a 6 week period (46).

External Fixator

Externally applied metallic fixation has never been embraced as the primary mode of fixation for HTO. External fixation is very flexible in terms of configuration, and a wide range of possibilities exist for frame construction. Advocates point to the advantage of being able to adjust the correction angle after leaving the operating room, if needed. Changing the angle eliminates the compressive effect created with the Charnley external fixator possibly destabilizing the osteotomy. Varisation, in particular, tends to destabilize the construct, perhaps interfering with the healing process or simply delaying an inevitable final "settling" before union. Hsu reported satisfactory results in 85% of 118 patients treated with a Charnley external fixator (48). Of the 118, complications occurred in 39 patients (33%) with recurrent deformity found in 13 (11%), pin tract infection in 13 (11%), common peroneal palsies in 5, and extensor hallucis longus palsies in 2.

The disadvantages of external fixation include the bulkiness of the device, the inconvenience to the patient who must alter clothing, and the relatively high fre quency of pin-related complications in cases where the frames are applied in areas with thick soft-tissue envelopes. Pin tract infections may preclude later conversion to total knee arthroplasty. Thin, wire external fixation (Ilisarov) may be desirable in some cases of severe deformity (more than 20 degrees net) because of ability of this type of device to correct severe deformities gradually. Otherwise, conventional external fixation is best reserved for salvage (union of the fracture, in this instance) following infection or a rare, complex pseudarthrosis (49).

Barrel Vault Osteotomy of Maquet (17)

Maquet's barrel vault osteotomy begins with the removal of a 1-cm section of fibula from the midfibula. A curved jig is used to mark the upper tibia above the tubercle with small Steinmann pins in multiple locations along a curve. Two large Steinmann pins are inserted through the proximal and distal fragments at a correction angle calculated relative to each other in such a way that completion of the osteotomy will achieve parallel alignment of the two pins.

The osteotomy is completed with an osteotome. The distal fragment is rotated into the desired valgus angle and displaced anteriorly to change the force vectors in the patellofemoral joint. The large Steinmann pins are placed into external fixation clamps, creating a frame, and the wounds are closed. Motion is initiated immediately after surgery; the frame is kept in place 6 to 8 weeks. The patient is placed on crutches until full motion returns, and a solid union is present.

Internal Fixation

Staple Fixation

Staples, combined with casting, are probably the most popular form of stabilization following HTO, although Table 56.1 shows a trend toward use of more rigid fixation in recent years. Staple fixation is technically simple, quick and familiar to most orthopaedists. Coventry popularized the step-cut staple designed to accommodate the step-off in the lateral cortex that is produced by the osteotomy and it is a trusted method (35) (Fig. 56.6). In recent years, surgeons using staple fixation have tried to reduce the period of immobilization by shifting the patient from a cast to some type of hinged knee brace prior to bony union.

Staples of various designs are available, but all suffer from the same mechanical deficiency, namely, point concentration of the fixation force. The holding power of staples is not great, and, without the external support

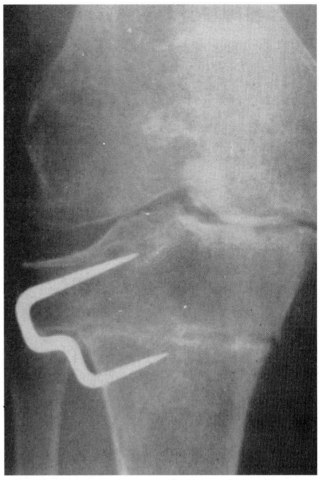

Figure 56.6. Stepped staple of Coventry. (Reproduced with permission from Coventry MB. Stepped staple for upper tibial osteotomy. J Bone Joint Surg [Am] 1969. 51(5):1011.)

provided by casting or some form of orthotic brace, loss of correction can occur. Only a few fixation points are available; they may fail, resulting in compromise of the remaining available cortex.

Sundaram, et al. reported satisfactory outcome in 75% of 105 dome osteotomies fixed with one or two staples. These osteotomies were followed for a minimum of 5 years. Complications recorded in the series included 6 thromboembolic events, 8 infections, 6 delayed unions, 7 peroneal nerve palsies, and 9 instances of painful hardware (50). Slocum and colleagues described 70% satisfactory results after HTO in 51 knees using the Coventry method (51). Mabrey and McCollum obtained 77% satisfactory results with staples alone in 45 HTO's (41).

Coventry Technique

In the Coventry technique (4–9, 35, 52, 53), the skin is divided either by a transverse or a longitudinal incision. The proximal fibula is excised and the fibular collateral and biceps femoris tendon are reattached to the remaining proximal fibula or surrounding soft tissues after completion of the osteotomy. Until the technique is mastered, the Coventry technique recommends expo-

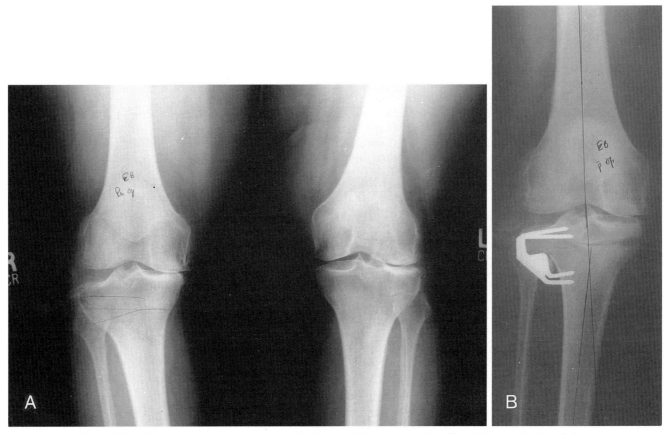

Figure 56.7. Stepped-staple technique used when the available space was insufficient for a tension band plate.

sure of the peroneal nerve. The lateral aspect of the proximal tibia is exposed to the midline posteriorly using subperiosteal dissection. Coventry emphasizes the flexed knee position; this position allows the popliteal contents to hang free, thereby avoiding injury to these vital structures.

Proper positioning is assessed with a guide pin and radiographic control; completion of the osteotomy is done with osteotomes. The medial cortex is not cut entirely, instead it is fractured later by manipulation at the point when the defect is closed and after removal of the wedge of bone. One or two staples are then placed in the lateral cortex to hold the osteotomy closed. A plaster-reinforced, bulky soft dressing is applied and converted to a cylinder cast after wound healing. The cast is applied in full extension and is worn 4 to 6 weeks (Fig. 56.7).

Buttress Plates

Buttress plates were developed for fracture fixation but have been used with and without modification for fixation of HTOs. A limited variety of specially adapted buttress plates are now available for specific use with HTO. Such plates are familiar to orthopaedists, are available from several manufacturers, and are easier to apply than blade plates.

These devices have some theoretical drawbacks. Extensive dissection of the anterior compartment muscu-lature is necessary to accommodate the plate. Plates must be specially and, sometimes, extensively contoured during surgery to compensate for the step-off created in the lateral cortex when a segment of bone is removed. This step-off is variable in size, depending upon the size of wedge removed, the location selected for the osteotomy, and the natural taper of the individual patient's proximal tibia. If the contouring is not precise, adverse mechanical forces will be generated during the tightening of the screws, possibly contributing to delayed union or to nonunion.

The least desirable feature of the buttress plate may be mechanical in nature. After a lateral closing wedge osteotomy, a plate must resist a varus-bending force, not a laterally directed tendency to "collapse," which would be the prime indication for a "buttress" effect in the plate. Postoperative varus/valgus cycling may create toggling of the screws in the plate leading to loosening and possible nonunion or delayed union, or loss of correction prior to union.

Weber Technique

In the Weber technique (27), the fibula is osteotomized first through a separate incision in the upper portion of the middle third of the leg. The tibia is approached through an incision that begins 2 cm proximal to the midlateral joint line. The incision curves anteriorly along the tibial metaphysis to a point just lateral to the tibial tubercle, then extends distally to the upper aspects of the middle third of the leg.

An oscillating saw is used to make the osteotomy cuts as far distally as the patellar tendon insertion will allow. The medial cortex is preserved and the osteotomy is closed manually. The medial cortex is reinforced with a loop of wire tightened around a 6.5 mm cancellous screw in the proximal fragment and a 4.5 mm cortex screw in the distal fragment to prevent failure of the medial cortex during tensioning of the laterally applied plate. A 4-hole "T" or "L" buttress plate is then affixed proximally with 6.5 mm cancellous screws, and the plate is tensioned from its distal screw hole using the AO/ASIF external plate tensioner (Fig. 56.8). Following plate tensioning, the remaining screw holes are filled, and the wound is closed.

Knee motion and quadriceps exercises are initiated immediately with partial weight bearing beginning at 6 weeks. Full weight bearing is permitted according to radiographic signs of union, but generally is allowed at approximately 10 to 12 weeks after surgery.

Two nonunions occurred in 45 patients with this technique, as reported by Sprenger (27). Premature weight bearing was offered as the reason for the nonunions and both healed after bone grafting. Additional complications included two transient peroneal nerve palsies, and an anterior compartment syndrome. Loss of correction was not mentioned.

Hoffman Technique

The Hoffman technique (54) begins with a curved proximal tibial incision made in the form of an inverted "L" and extending for an adequate length from the proximal tibiofibular joint to allow for the plate. The tibiofibular joint is released, and the knee joint is marked with Keith needles. An alignment jig is positioned to touch the Keith needle identifying the level of the joint, and the jig is anchored with two ⅛th-inch drill bits (Fig. 56.9). The upper cut of the osteotomy is made with an oscillating saw; the osteotomy angle guide replaces the alignment jig for the initial cut (Fig. 56.10). The second cut is made according to the preoperative plan.

The wedge is removed, and the osteotomy is closed by tensioning a specially designed "L"-shaped plate that has been fixed proximally with two screws (Fig. 56.11). The closed osteotomy is stabilized by the addition of three cortical screws in the vertical portion of the "L" plate (Fig. 56.12). Motion with a CPM machine is initiated in the recovery room, and weight bearing of 50% is allowed immediately.

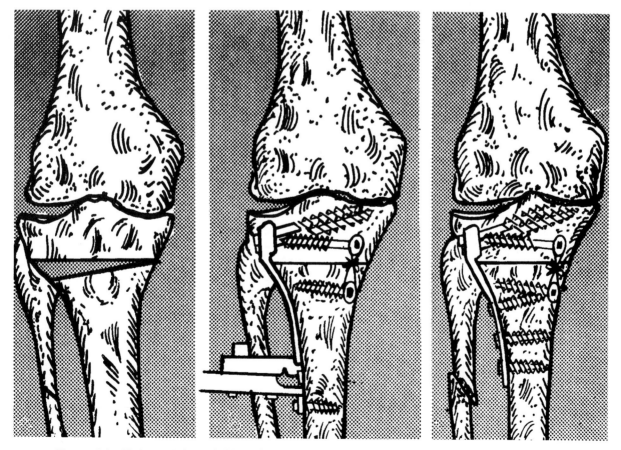

Figure 56.8. T plate technique of Weber. (Reproduced with permission from Sprenger TR, Weber BG, Howard FM. Compression osteotomy of the tibia. Clin Orthop 1979;140(May):104.)

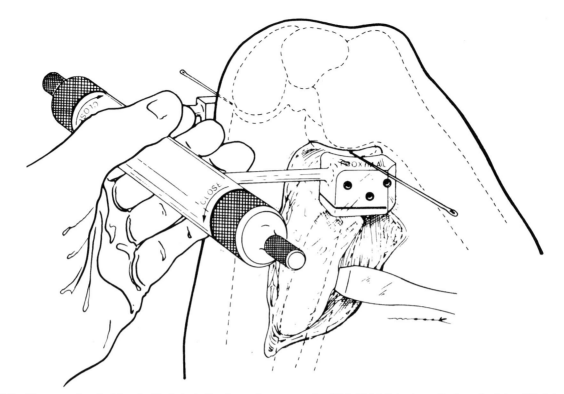

Figure 56.9. The operative incision is illustrated. Small needles identify the level of the joint. The first jig identifies the level of the upper cut. (Reproduced with permission from Hoffman AA. The Inter-medics High Tibial Osteotomy System. Angleton, TX: Intermedics Orthopedics, Inc. 1989:2–7.)

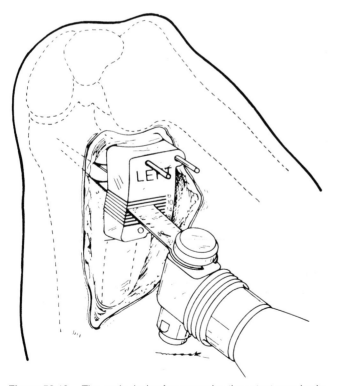

Figure 56.10. The angle device for measuring the osteotomy size is illustrated. (Reproduced with permission from Hoffman AA. The Intermedics High Tibial Osteotomy System. Angleton, TX: Intermedics Orthopedics, Inc. 1989:2–7.)

Hernigou Medial Opening Wedge Technique

In the Hernigou technique (12), a 10 cm incision is made from the medial border of the patellar tendon distally. The pes anserine tendons are divided at their insertions and reflected posteriorly. The tibial collateral ligament is elevated subperiosteally about the osteotomy but remains intact distal to the joint. The tibia is divided with an osteotome proximal to the tibial tubercle, and the osteotomy is opened sufficiently to create the desired angle of correction.

The lateral cortex is preserved. The fibula and tibiofibular joint are left intact. Tricortical iliac crest grafts are placed in the osteotomy and stabilized with flat "T" buttress plate (Fig. 56.13). The pes tendons and tibial collateral ligaments are then repaired and the wound closed. Motion begins immediately after surgery, but weight bearing is postponed an average of 3 months. Originally, no fixation was used; however, plate fixation was later adopted to prevent occasional displacements occurring with lateral cortex fracture.

Of 93 osteotomies, 17 required some form of revision at 5 to 10 years after osteotomy. Best results were obtained in patients having a final mechanical axis of 3 to 6 degrees valgus. Over- and undercorrection were associated with less than optimal outcome. Plate osteosynthesis was thought by the authors of the study to have maintained better corrections than cast fixation.

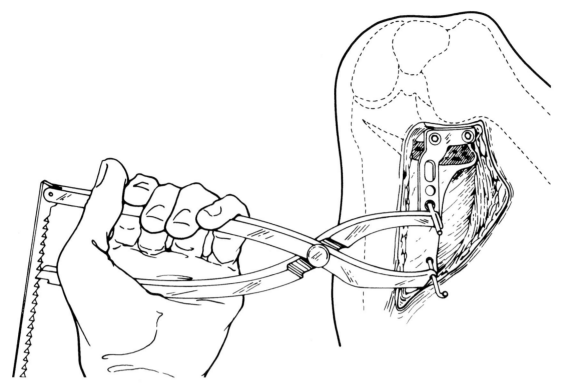

Figure 56.11.   The T plate has been fixed proximally. Using the external tensioning device, the osteotomy is closed and the bone edges are compressed. (Reproduced with permission from Hoffman AA. The Intermedics High Tibial Osteotomy System. Angleton, TX: Intermedics Orthopedics, Inc. 1989:2–7.)

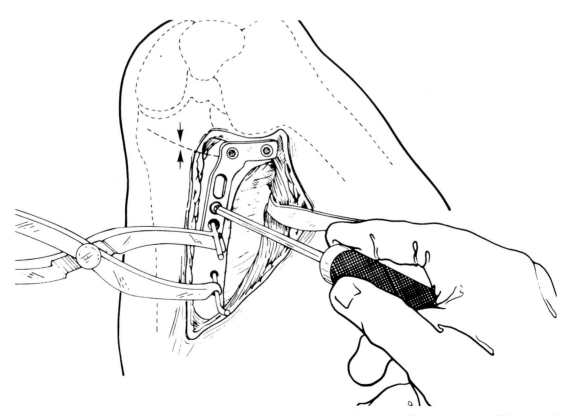

Figure 56.12.   The plate is now fixed distally with cortex screws. (Reproduced with permission from Hoffman AA. The Intermedics High Tibial Osteotomy System. Angleton, TX: Intermedics Orthopedics, Inc. 1989:2–7.)

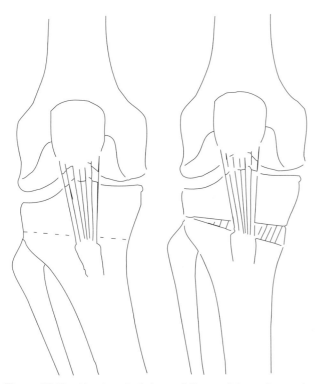

Figure 56.13. Hernigou technique of the medial opening wedge. (Reproduced with permission from Hernigou P, et al. Proximal tibial osteotomy for osteoarthritis with varus deformity. A ten to thirteen-year follow-up study. J Bone Joint Surg 1987;69-A(Mar):335.)

Blade Plates

A transverse metaphyseal blade continuous with a plate running distally across the osteotomy site solves the problem of the "toggle" effect of the buttress plate, discussed earlier, in that the connection between the external cortical portion of the implant and the cancellous portion of the implant is rigid, thus eliminating toggle. The problems of variable lateral cortical step-off and the necessity for extensive soft tissue dissection still remain. The technique of blade plate fixation is very demanding and the requirement for technical sophistication is high (16).

Koshino Technique

Koshino, et al. reported on 13 years of experience with a blade plate developed in 1975 and used at the Yokahama City University School of Medicine (16). Two varieties of Koshino Plate were used: The first was V-shaped with a length of 55 mm twisted posteriorly 30 degrees with a side plate 70 mm in length and with a 15 degree retroversion twist; the second was an inverted U-shaped blade 60 mm long that was twisted posteriorly 15 degrees with a side plate the same length as the first. In both, the side plate accepts three screws that sit in slots to allow for dynamic compression after surgery (Fig. 56.14).

The fibula is osteotomized midshaft prior to tibial osteotomy with removal of a 3.5 cm segment. The tibia is approached through a 15 cm longitudinally curved, lat-

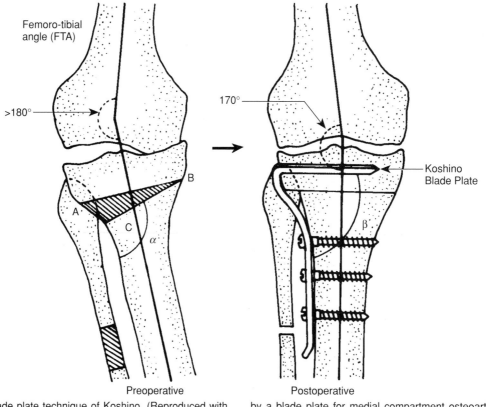

Figure 56.14. Blade plate technique of Koshino. (Reproduced with permission from Koshino T, et al. High tibial osteotomy with fixation by a blade plate for medial compartment osteoarthritis of the knee. Orthop Clin North Am 1989;20(2):228.)

eral incision extending from proximal to the patella to approximately 8 cm distal to the tibial tubercle. This generous incision allows for patellar release of the lateral retinaculum and elevation of the tibial tubercle, a procedure advised by the authors in cases of patellofemoral degeneration. The joint is identified with 3 needles and a guide pin is placed 5mm distal to the joint and directed 30 degrees posteromedially parallel to the joint. A 2.5 mm Kirschner wire is then placed through the guide.

The laterally based tibial osteotomy is then made, creating a proximal segment of 25 mm width on the lateral side. After the wedge is removed the blade portion of the plate is driven across the tibia. If the angle of the side plate and shaft matches that of the osteotomy, the osteotomy is closed and the side plate is fixed to the shaft with three screws. Koshino, et al. note that if the medial side is destabilized, addition of a second small flat (tension band) plate medially is recommended.

Following surgery, the patient is moved immediately with straight leg raising and active knee motion. Partial weight bearing is started in 4 weeks with complete weight bearing in 10 to 12 weeks. A final angle of 10 degrees of valgus is recommended, and casting may be necessary in some cases using two plates, due to "sinking." The authors report on 299 patients treated over a ten-year period during which they were able to review 136 patients (176 knees) with a minimum follow-up of 2 years. The best knee scores were associated with correction to 6 to 15 degrees of valgus. Delayed union with broken plates was encountered in 3 of the 176 knees, all of which healed after plate removal and casting. Two patients developed infection, one of which was superficial and the other deep (16).

Tension Band Plates

The technique of tension band plating is an efficient mechanical technique whereby a relatively small amount of metal can be used to stabilize the osteotomy. Soft tissue exposure or dissection is required only for the completion of the osteotomy and no additional exposure is required. Space, however, is limited, and the placement of the tension band must be precise to work properly. A blade-like device is inserted into the upper tibial metaphysis; the device has attached an area that protrudes from the lateral cortex and is able to accept one or more screws angled distally and medially across the osteotomy site. As the screws are tightened, compression occurs across the osteotomy increasing stability of the construct. Weight bearing further facilitates compression as the stiff metal screw converts tension laterally to compression medially.

Tension band techniques using small blade plates are exacting procedures due to the need to place the implant clear of the joint and the osteotomy. If insufficient bone is available, the technique cannot be used because fixation is so heavily dependent on good bone quality. Failure will occur if the hardware penetrates the joint or the osteotomy. At least 1 cm of bone between the inferior edge of the plate and the upper cut of the osteotomy is necessary to support the blade; success in using this technique depends more on the volume of

bone immediately under the plate than it does on the length of the plate itself.

Weber Semitubular Plate Technique

In this technique of Weber (55), the fibula is sectioned obliquely prior the tibial osteotomy at the level of the junction between the upper and middle thirds. A separate incision is at the level of the third of the fibula. The tibia is approached through a curved lateral incision beginning below the tibial tubercle on the lateral aspect of the leg. The incision goes proximally to the lateral tibial crest, then curves posterior to the level of the proximal fibula. The anterior compartment musculature is partially reflected to expose the proximal tibial metaphysis. The level of the knee joint is determined, but it is not exposed.

Before making the tibial osteotomy cuts, the pilot channel for the blade portion of the device is prepared, as follows: The channel for the blade is made with a straight 4 hole semitubular plate by tapping on one end of the plate with a hammer, driving the plate into the metaphysis to the level of the third hole. Once driven in to the correct level, the plate is then withdrawn using a bone hook. The corrective wedge is then prepared above the tibial tubercle, but its location should be as far below the blade channel as possible. Following removal of the wedge of bone, the plate, now bent between the third and fourth hole of the plate, is reinserted into the channel.

With the plate in the bone channel, the osteotomy is closed manually, taking care not to destabilize the medial side. Weber emphasizes the importance of the integrity of the medial tissues. If medial instability is present, it must be controlled with additional fixation, such as a loop of wire tightened around two screws. Once a stable closure has been achieved, the osteotomy is fixed with a 4.5 mm cortical lag screw placed diagonally across the osteotomy (Fig. 56.15). It is not unusual to require an extra long screw, even as long as 90 mm (Fig. 56.16).

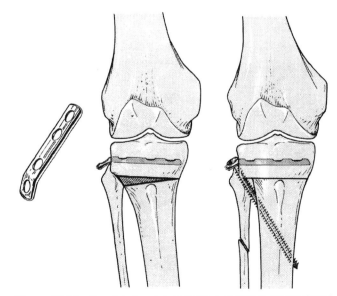

Figure 56.15. Semitubular plate technique of Weber. (Reproduced with permission from Brunner CF, Weber BG. Special techniques in internal fixation. New York: Springer-Verlag,1982.)

Figure 56.16. Weber semitubular plate technique used for bilateral HTO.

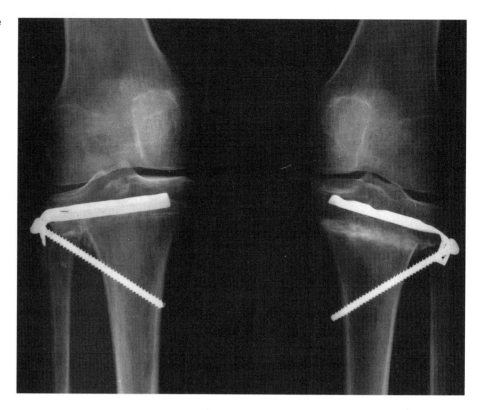

Several modifications of the Weber technique have been developed. Miniacci, et al. have described a modification in which a 5 hole plate is bent so that two screws remain outside the cortex and accept lag screws, thus improving the efficiency of the lag effect and improving distal fixation (1). Proximal fixation, however, still relies on the blade of a semitubular plate (Fig. 56.17) (1). Geibel and others have developed a plate with a wider blade portion giving greater proximal fixation and allowing two-side-by-side lag screws for improved distal fixation (56). A third method, presented in detail below, is our preferred fixation method. It was developed based on the ideas as originally proposed by Weber, but modified for use with an angle guide and guide pin system.

Tension Band Plate Technique

A transverse incision is made from the tibial tubercle to the head of the fibula halfway between the knee joint and the tibial tubercle (Fig. 56.18). The skin should be divided, with extension to the fascia, in one layer without creating a flap. The anterior compartment fascia is released using subperiosteal elevation of the anterior compartment muscles. The proximal tibiofibular joint is exposed anteriorly and released from the tibia by partial excision of the fibula, taking care not to injure the peroneal nerve that is lateral to the fibular neck.

Fluoroscopy is used as necessary during the remainder of the procedure. The plate guide pin should be inserted first in the midlateral plane, parallel to the joint surface, at least 5 to 7 mm distal to the subchondral line and at least 1 cm cephalad to the proximal osteotomy cut. A depth measurement is taken once the guide pin is lodged at a point between the medial tibial spine and the medial cortex. The osteotomy should leave as much bone as possible between the plate and the osteotomy. An angle device is used for locating the osteotomy cuts.

The seating chisel is placed over the plate guide pin, and a pilot channel is prepared (Fig. 56.19). The proximal and distal osteotomy guide pins are shortened with a pin-cutter. Cutting blocks are inserted over each guide pin and seated in the lateral cortex with a mallet (Fig. 56.20). Compensation for mild flexion contractures can be achieved by decreasing the posterior slope of the proximal cutting block, but, in general, the cutting blocks should be perpendicular to the long axis of the tibia. The osteotomy is made between the cutting blocks. The cut wedge of bone is then removed; again, care must be taken to preserve the medial cortex.

After removing the cutting blocks, the plate is introduced over the guide pin into the channel made by the seating chisel. The plate is seated fully using the plate driver and a mallet (Fig. 56.21). Care is necessary to ensure that the plate follows the pin and the chisel tract and that it does not create a new path. The osteotomy is held closed manually, and two lag screws are placed obliquely at about 45 degrees to the long axis to anchor the plate (Fig. 56.22). Motion begins in the recovery room, partial weight bearing starts the day after surgery, and the patient becomes independent of crutches between 6 and 8 weeks following surgery.

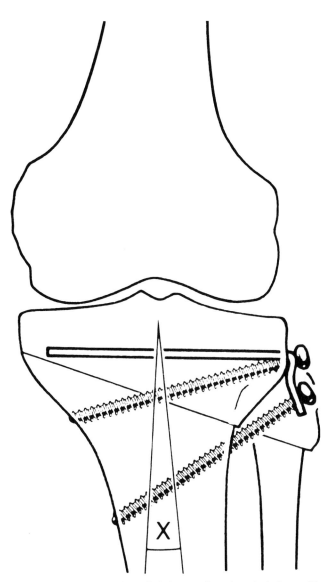

Figure 56.17. Modified semitubular tension plate technique: (Reproduced with permission from Miniacci A, et al. Proximal tibial osteotomy. A new fixation device. Clin Orthop 1989;246(Sep):253.)

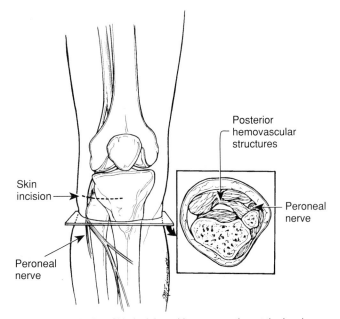

Figure 56.18. Skin incision with cross section at the level of the osteotomy.

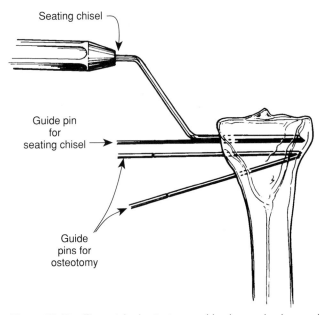

Figure 56.19. The notched osteotomy guide pins are in place as is the guide pin for the seating chisel, which has been partly advanced in the upper tibia.

Conclusions

No large study has been reported comparing a matched, randomly selected series of patients with internal fixation and without internal fixation. Various fixation methods have been described in the orthopaedic literature, but insufficient data exist to conclude beyond a doubt that one technique is clearly superior in all respects. Hernigou made the comment that it became clear that internal fixation was necessary to control the osteotomy as their series progressed (12). Others, no doubt, have had similar experiences, as evidenced by the multiple attempts to develop internal fixation devices for the upper tibia (1, 12, 16, 20, 24, 27, 35).

Complications associated with HTO are presented in Table 56.4. Comparison of articles using different reporting standards for various operative techniques reveals no significant disadvantages for internal fixation. In fact, statistics derived from literature series suggest that lower frequencies of infection, thromboembolism, peroneal nerve palsy, fracture of the proximal fragment, and of healing delay are associated with internal fixation (Table 56.5). In addition, although comparative data are sparse, it appears that internal fixation also decreases postoperative loss of correction.

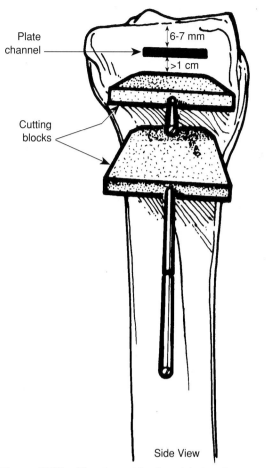

Side View

Figure 56.20. The channel for the plate has been made. Cutting blocks are placed on the osteotomy pins for cutting of the osteotomy between the two blocks.

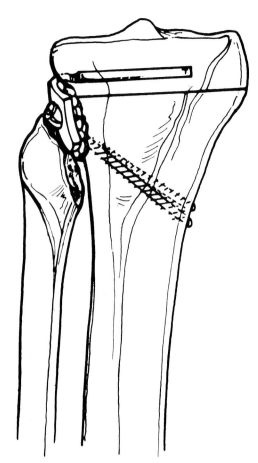

Figure 56.21. The plate has been seated fully in its channel and the osteotomy has been closed. Fixation is provided by two 4.5 self-tapping cortical lag screws.

Preoperative planning, intraoperative measurement following the preoperative plan, and stable internal fixation may ultimately be shown to be superior to casting methods for producing a reliable anatomic outcome. Stable fixation appeals to patients, who usually dislike the inconvenience associated with casting and with external fixation methods. As described earlier, immediate function is possible for the ideal patient after stable internal fixation, with the advantage of initiation of rehabilitation on the day of surgery.

Summary

1. Preoperative planning should use standing, full-length radiographs to measure the femorotibial angle in order to obtain the desired correction angle.

2. Ligamentous laxity should be evaluated and taken into consideration during the planning phase of the operation.

3. A final femorotibial angle of 10 degrees valgus plus or minus 5 degrees is ideal.

Table 56.5 Complications after HTO (Compiled from Table 4)

Fixation	Infection (%)	Thromboembolism (%)	Peroneal Palsy (%)	Fracture of Proximal Fragment (%)	Healing Delay (%)
Cast	4.77	4.47	5.61	4.84	4.41
Staple + Cast	3.93	3.64	3.83	3.75	3.25
Plate	1.53	2.74	1.36	2.41	2.36
External Fixation	6.09	4.36	7.33	2.50	1.70

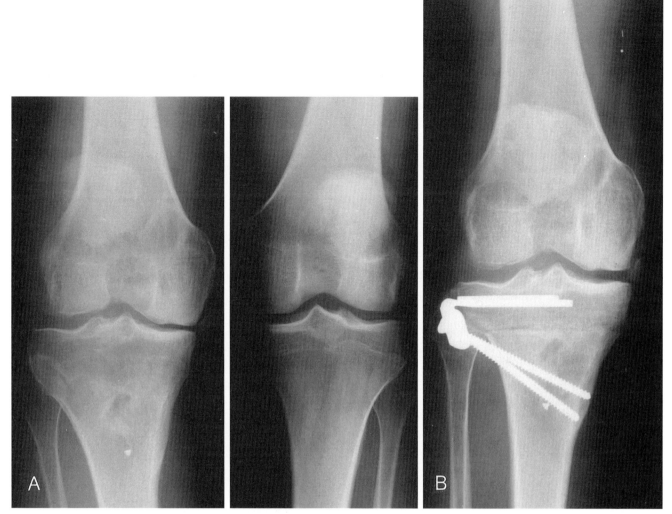

Figure 56.22.   Before **(A)** and after **(B)** radiographs of a patient with posttraumatic medial compartment arthrosis. The tension band plate was used.

4. Internal fixation should improve the reliability of anatomic result.

5. Complications with internal fixation are no more frequent than with external or cast immobilization.

References

1. Miniacci A, et al. Proximal tibial osteotomy. A new fixation device. Clin Orthop 1989;246(Sep):250–259.
2. Bauer GC, Insall J, Koshino T. Tibial osteotomy in gonarthritis (osteoarthritis of the knee). J Bone Joint Surg [Am] 1970;52(2):330–336.
3. Cass JR, Bryan S. High tibial osteotomy. Clin Orthop 1988;230(May):196–199.
4. Coventry MB. Surgery of the hip and knee in patients with rheumatoid arthritis. J Bone Joint Surg [Am] 1973;55(2):301–314.
5. Coventry MB. Osteotomy about the knee for degenerative and rheumatoid arthritis: Indications, operative technique, and results. J Bone Joint Surg 1973;55A:23.
6. Coventry MB. Upper tibial osteotomy. Clin Orthop 1984;182(Jan–Feb):46–52.
7. Coventry MB. Proximal tibial varus osteotomy for osteoarthritis of the lateral compartment of the knee. J Bone Joint Surg 1987;69A:32–38.
8. Coventry MB. Osteotomy of the upper portion of the tibia for degenerative arthritis of the knee. A preliminary report. Clin Orthop 1989;248(Nov):2–8.
9. Coventry MB. Valgus osteotomy for osteoarthritis of the knee. Clin Orthop 1990;249:251–256.
10. Fujisawa Y, Masuhara K, Shiomi S. The effect of high tibial osteotomy on osteoarthritis of the knee. Ortho Clinics North Am 1979;10(3):585–608.
11. Aglietti P, et al. Tibial osteotomy for the varus osteoarthritis knee. Clin Orthop 1983;176:239–251.
12. Hernigou P, et al. Proximal tibial osteotomy for osteoarthritis with varus deformity. A ten- to thirteen-year follow-up study. J Bone Joint Surg 1987;69-A(Mar):332–354.
13. Insall J, Shoji H, Mayer V. High tibial osteotomy. J Bone Joint Surg 1974;56-A:1397.
14. Jackson JP, Waugh W, Green JP. High tibial osteotomy for osteoarthritis of the knee. J Bone Joint Surg 1969;51-B:88.
15. Jackson JP, Waugh W. The technique and complications of upper tibial osteotomy. A review of 226 operations. J Bone Joint Surg [Br] 1974;56(2):236–245.
16. Koshino T, et al. High tibial osteotomy with fixation by a blade plate for medial compartment osteoarthritis of the knee. Orthop Clin North Am 1989. 20(2):227–243.
17. Maquet P. Biomechanics of the knee. New York: Springer-Verlag, 1976.
18. Matthews LS, et al. Proximal tibial osteotomy. Factors that influence the duration of satisfactory function. Clin Orthop 1988;229(Apr):193–200.
19. Tjornstrand B, et al. Ten-year results of tibial osteotomy for medial gonarthrosis. The influence of overcorrection. Arch Orthop Trauma Surg 1991;110(2):103–108.
20. Vainionpaa S, et al. Tibial osteotomy for osteoarthritis of the knee. A five to ten-year follow-up study. J Bone Joint Surg 1981;63-A(Jul):938–946.

21. Devas MB. High tibial osteotomy for arthritis of the knee. A method specially suitable for the elderly. J Bone Joint Surg (Br) 1969.
22. Kettelkamp DB, Leach RE, Nasca R. Pitfalls of proximal tibial osteotomy. Clin Orthop, 1975;136:242–244.
23. Maquet P. Valgus osteotomy for osteoarthritis of the knee. Clin Orthop 1981;120:143–148.
24. Ogata K. Interlocking wedge osteotomy of the proximal tibia for gonarthrosis. Clin Orthop Rel Res 1984;186:129–134.
25. Putnam MD, Mears DC, Fu FH. Combined Maquet and proximal tibial valgus osteotomy. Clin Orthop 1985;197:217–223.
26. Shoji H, Insall J. High tibial osteotomy for osteoarthritis of the knee with valgus deformity. J Bone Joint Surg 1973;55-A:963.
27. Sprenger TR, Weber BG, Howard FM. Compression osteotomy of the tibia. Clin Orthop 1979;140(May):103–108.
28. Soccetti A, Giacchetta AM, Raffaelli P. Domed high tibial osteotomy: The long-term results in tibiofemoral arthritis with and without malalignment of the extensor apparatus. Ital J Orthop Traumatol 1987;13(4):153–162.
29. Odenbring S, et al. A guide instrument for high tibial osteotomy. Acta Orthop Scand 1989;60(4):449–451.
30. Mains DB. Technique of proximal tibial osteotomy using a guide. Am J Knee Surg 1990;3(1):15–22.
31. Mynerts R. The SAAB jig: An aid in high tibial osteotomy. Acta Orthop Scand 1978;49 (1):85–88.
32. Jiang CC, Hang YS, Liu TK. A new jig for proximal tibial osteotomy. Clin Orthop 1988;226:118–123.
33. Lippert FG, Kirkpatrick GS. A jig for pin insertion in the performance of high tibial osteotomy. Clin Orthop 1975;112:242–244.
34. Jakob RP, Murphy SB. Tibial osteotomy for varus gonarthrosis: Indication, planning, and operative technique. Instructional Course Lectures, 1992;61 (chapt 9):87–93.
35. Coventry MB. Stepped staple for upper tibial osteotomy. J Bone Joint Surg [Am] 1969;51(5):1011.
36. Engel GM, Lippert III FG. Valgus Tibial Osteotomy: Avoiding the pitfalls. Clin Ortho Rel Res 1981;160:137–143.
37. Ivarsson I, Mynerts R, Gillquist J. High tibial osteotomy for medial osteoarthritis of the knee. A 5–7 and 11-year follow-up. J Bone Joint Surg 1990;72-B:238–44.
38. Kettelkamp DB, et al. Results of proximal tibial osteotomy. The effects of tibiofemoral angle, stance-phase flexion-extension, and medial-plateau force. J Bone Joint Surg [Am] 1976;58(7):952–960.
39. Myrnerts R. Optimal correction in high tibial osteotomy for varus deformity. Acta Orthop Scand 1980;51(4):689–694.
40. Tjornstrand BA. High tibial osteotomy: A seven-year clinical and radiographic follow-up. Clin Orthop 1981;160(Oct):124–136.
41. Mabrey JD, McCollum DE. High tibial osteotomy: A retrospective review of 72 cases. South Med J 1987;80:975–980.
42. Korn J. A new concept for dome high tibial osteotomy. Orthop Trans 1992;16(1):42.
43. Odenbring S, et al. The angle-measuring device, a practical resource in high tibial osteotomy. Ann Chir Gynaecol 1991;80(1): 54–58.
44. Benjamin A. Double osteotomy for the painful knee in rheumatoid arthritis and osteoarthritis. J Bone Joint Surg [Br] 1969;51(4):694–699.
45. Ivarsson I, et al. Rehabilitation after high tibial osteotomy. Am J Knee Surg 1990;3(1):23–28.
46. Myrnerts R. Failure of the correction of varus deformity obtained by high tibial osteotomy. Acta Orthop Scand 1980;51(3):569–573.
47. Muller ME, et al. Manual of internal fixation. 3rd ed. New York: Springer-Verlag, 1991.
48. Hsu RW. The study of Maquet dome high tibial osteotomy. Arthroscopic-assisted analysis. Clin Orthop 1989;193:280–285.
49. Schatzker J, Burgess RC, Glynn MK. The management of nonunions following high tibial osteotomies. Clin Orthop 1985;193:230–233.
50. Sundaram NA, Hallett JP, Sullivan MF. Dome osteotomy of the tibia for osteoarthritis of the knee. J Bone Joint Surg [Br] 1986;68B(Nov):782–786.
51. Slocum, DB, et al. High tibial osteotomy. Clin Orthop 1974;104:239–243.
52. Coventry, MB. Osteotomy of the upper portion of the tibia for degenerative arthritis of the knee. J Bone Joint Surg 1965;47-A:984.
53. Coventry MB. Upper tibial osteotomy for gonarthrosis. The evolution of the operation in the last 19 years and long-term results. Orthop Clin North Am 1970;10(1):191–210.
54. Hoffman AA. The intermedics high tibial osteotomy system. Intermedics Orthopedics, Inc. 1989;2–7.
55. Brunner CF, Weber BG. Special techniques in internal fixation. New York: Springer-Verlag, 1982.
56. Geibel G, Tscherne H, Daiber, M. Tibial head osteotomy in the treatment of arthrosis of the knee. Orthopaedie 1985;14:144–153.
57. Gunn AL. Results of treatment of painful deformed knee by upper tibial osteotomy. Guy's Hospital Report 1969;118:293–306.
58. LaMont RL, Pasad B. Experience with dome shaped osteotomy of upper tibia for multiplane correction. Clin Orthop 1973;91:152–157.
59. Hagstedt B. The effect of high tibial osteotomy. In: International Congress Rotterdam, 1973. The Knee Joint. Rotterdam, Holland: Excerpta Medica, 1974.
60. Gariepy R, Derome A, Laurin CA. Tibial osteotomy in the treatment of degenerative arthritis in the knee. In: Cruess RL, Mitchell N. Surgical management of degenerative arthritis of the lower limb. Philadelphia: Lea and Febiger, 1975.
61. Seal PV, Chan RNW. Tibial osteotomy for osteoarthrosis of the knee. Acta Orthop Scand 1975;46(141–151).
62. Levy, et al. A high tibial osteotomy: A follow-up study and description of a modified technique. Clin Orthop 1973;93(June):274.
63. Surin V, Markhede G, Sundholm K. Results with high tibial osteotomy with gonarthritis. In: The Knee Joint. International Congress Rotterdam. 1973. Rotterdam, Holland: Excerpta Medica, 1974.
64. Torgerson WJ, et al. Tibial osteotomy for the treatment of degenerative arthritis of the knee. Clin Orthop 1974;0(104):239–243.
65. Edholm P, et al. Knee instability and tibial osteotomy. A clinical study. Acta Orthop Scand 1977;48(1):95–98.
66. Odenbring S, et al. Function after tibial osteotomy for medial gonarthrosis below aged 50 years. Acta Orthop Scand 1989;60(5):527–531.
67. Chapchal G. Osteotomy of the tibia in the treatment of osteoarthritis of the knee. In: The Knee Joint. International Congress Rotterdam, 1973. Rotterdam, Holland: Excerpta Medica, 1974.
68. Lemaire R, et al. High tibial osteotomy for osteoarthritis of the knee joint: A report of 105 cases with blade plate fixation. In: The Knee Joint. Int. Congress Rotterdam. Rotterdam, Holland: Excerpta Medica, 1973.
69. Ha'eri GB, Wiley AM. High tibial osteotomy combined with joint debridement: A long-term study of the results. Clin Orthop 1980;151:153–159.
70. MacIntosh DL, Welsh RP. Joint debridement—A complement to high tibial osteotomy in the treatment of degenerative arthritis of the knee. J Bone Joint Surg 1977;59-A:977–982.
71. Krempen JF. Experience with the Maquet barrel-vault osteotomy. Clin Orthop 1962;168:86–96.
72. Rudan JF, et al. High tibial osteotomy. A prospective clinical and roentgen review. Clin Orthop 1990;255:251–256.

57

Complications of High Tibial Osteotomy

Edgar G. Handal, David R. Morawski, and Richard F. Santore

Introduction

Complications of high tibial osteotomy (HTO) in the treatment of gonarthrosis have been reported in the literature and presented at orthopedic meetings over the past 30 years. These complications can result from problems in preoperative planning, intraoperative technique, or postoperative management. They are often cited by orthopedic surgeons as the main factor in reluctance to perform this operation (27, 104). When successful however, high tibial osteotomy is very effective in *(a)* reduction and/or elimination of pain, *(b)* preservation of functional knee motion and *(c)* postponement or elimination of the need for artificial joint resurfacing. Success is predicated on proper patient selection, the achievement and maintenance of adequate operative correction, and the avoidance of complications.

Unquestionably, HTO has a place in the spectrum of appropriate options in the management of angular knee deformities associated with painful, noninflammatory arthritis, especially in those patients with varus (bow-legged) deformities. Knowledge of the historical frequency and etiology of complications that occur in HTO will increase the attractiveness of this useful operation. The following table (Table 57.1) lists the reported major and minor complications of high tibial osteotomy.

The most significant complications of this osteotomy include peroneal nerve paralysis, undercorrection, excessive overcorrection, intraarticular fracture, nonunion, and loss of correction in the early postoperative period. Less common, although still significant complications include injury to the popliteal artery and vein as well as to the vessels of the trifurcation at the knee, deep venous thrombosis, compartment syndrome, injury to the tibial nerve, hardware failure, and infection, among others. Failure to provide relief of pain, even in the early period following healing of the osteotomy is

appropriately classified as a clinical failure rather than a true complication. However, in certain instances this may represent an error in patient selection.

This chapter first reviews the literature with regard to complications associated with the procedure and discusses specific examples. Most of the text refers to the use of HTO in the patient with varus gonarthrosis. Finally, common errors in patient selection, pitfalls in preoperative planning, and pitfalls in surgical technique are presented. Suggestions on how to avoid these problems are made.

Malalignment

Overview

It is universally agreed that a shift of the mechanical axis (MA) of the lower extremity lateral to the midjoint and an anatomic axis (AA) of at least 5 degrees of valgus are the minimum alignment goals of valgus HTO for varus gonarthrosis. The most frequent complications reported in the orthopedic literature involving high tibial osteotomy are problems of postoperative malalignment related to undercorrection or excessive overcorrection in the coronal plane. Also very important, but less common, is sagittal plane malalignment. This discussion appropriately begins with basic definitions of the terms undercorrection and overcorrection as they apply to final postoperative alignment. With regard to the anatomical axis, most authors concur that a postoperative correction resulting in alignment of 5 degrees of valgus or less is insufficient and is likely to lead to a rapid recurrence of varus. Thus, postoperative alignment of 5 degrees or less of valgus can be referred to as undercorrection.

The use of the term "overcorrection" in considering the correction of a *varus* deformity can be confusing. In most reports, the term "overcorrection" has been used

1153

Table 57.1. Major and Minor Complications of High Tibial Osteotomy

Major Complications	Minor Complications
Malalignment	Infection—superficial
Undercorrection	Skin necrosis
Excessive overcorrection	Skin flap numbness
Flexion deformity	Post-operative instability
Loss of correction and	Post-operative stiffness
recurrent deformity	Delayed union
Neuromuscular injury	Patella infera
Vascular injury	Flare-up chondrocalcinosis
Compartment syndrome	Hardware bursitis
Intraarticular fracture and	
penetration	
Problems of union	
Nonunion	
Malunion	
Deep venous thrombosis	
Pulmonary embolism	
Infection—deep	
Failure of fixation	

to signify the magnitude of additional angular correction created by the surgeon beyond the normal anatomical tibiofemoral valgus for therapeutic reasons. For any given individual, the theoretically "normal" anatomic axis would be that associated with a mechanical axis (the line drawn between the center of the femoral head and the center of the ankle) that passes through or near the center of the knee. In the average male patient, this anatomic axis usually measures 5 to 7 degrees of valgus. To illustrate this point, consider the following situation. If the preoperative standing alignment radiographs indicate an anatomic axis of 4 degrees varus and correction to 10 degrees of valgus is desired, then any valgus that would result in a postoperative anatomical axis greater than the normal 6 degrees would be the amount of overcorrection obtained. Thus, a part of the 10 degrees of postoperative valgus created would represent 4 degrees of overcorrection.

Aglietti, et al. (1), support the rationale of overcorrection of the tibiofemoral (TF) angle by noting the following observations. First, overcorrection of the tibiofemoral angle can overcome the lateral ligamentous laxity and insufficiency of the lateral muscular stabilizing structures that have been theorized to contribute to the evolution of genu varum (76). Secondly, progressive lateral subluxation of the tibia will occur if destruction of the medial compartment continues as a result of undercorrection. Thirdly, those knees corrected to neutral, or undercorrected, have consistently been shown to have poorer results and recurrent deformity as compared to those that were overcorrected. Finally, loads in the medial compartment will not be reduced completely even if neutral or relative varus correction is obtained.

For preoperative varus deformities, a moderate consensus exists that an anatomic axis (i.e., tibiofemoral angle) corrected to a range of 8 to 10 degrees of absolute valgus is desired. This represents 3 to 5 degrees of overcorrection and correlates with a mechanical axis that falls lateral to the midline of the knee in most patients. This alteration in the anatomic and mechanical axes may lead to a change of distribution of load across the knee joint. Reduction in medial compartment load is an essential goal of HTO and, in addition to its biomechanical advantages, may have a beneficial effect on the status of articular cartilage. Fujisawa, et al. (29) arthroscopically evaluated their series of patients pre- and postosteotomy and correlated the extent of medial compartment articular repair with the final position of the mechanical axis. Those cases in which the mechanical axis passed 30 to 40° of the distance from the center of the joint to the lateral margin of the joint, demonstrated the greatest repair.

The definition of excessive valgus is less precise but certainly would pertain to alignments of 15 degrees or more of valgus. There are distinct problems associated with excessive valgus including cosmetic deformity, patellofemoral tracking abnormalities, gait disturbance, excessive bone resection in wedge osteotomies, overload of lateral compartment articular cartilage, and increased difficulty in conversion to total knee replacement (TKA).

Malalignment can result from inaccurate preoperative planning, intraoperative technical errors (i.e., imprecise intraoperative measurements, improper use of instrumentation, errors in performing bone cuts), and failure of fixation of the osteotomy. In addition, each method of osteotomy that has been described has inherent problems that may lead to errors in postoperative alignment. Various types of osteotomies about the tibia for the treatment of gonarthrosis include:

1. Closing wedge
2. Opening wedge
3. Oblique metaphyseal
4. Dome (barrel vault)
5. Corticotomy or Illizarov method
6. Other variations.

Closing wedge osteotomy, originally introduced by Gariepy and utilized by many surgeons today, is vulnerable to error in measurement of the wedge thickness, incomplete closure of the osteotomy site, and unintentional division of the medial cortex and the associated medial periosteal sleeve. When the medial cortex is cut completely, the inherent stability obtained in the closing wedge technique is lost. Undesirable displacement of the proximal and distal fragments can occur during or after internal fixation, thus influencing the net position of the mechanical axis. Postoperative medial collapse into varus resulting in undercorrection is more likely to happen in this scenario. In opening wedge osteotomy, malalignment may result from excessive or insufficient opening at the osteotomy site, resorption or collapse of bone graft used to maintain correction, or displacement of the proximal and distal fragments.

In the case of the dome (barrel vault) osteotomy popularized by Maquet (76, 77) accurate correction of angular deformity and anteromedial displacement of the patellar tendon (which can increase the extensor mechanism lever arm and improve patellofemoral tracking), can be accomplished. The barrel vault procedure requires accurate intraoperative angular measurement that is often difficult to obtain. Vainionpaa, et al. (122), for instance, claim to have abandoned this method since the amount of correction was difficult to estimate at operation, and the preoperative deformity recurred too often during the first 6 postoperative months. While the use of an external fixation device in such procedures has the advantage of allowing modification of alignment postoperatively, accurate readjustment can present problems, especially in the outpatient setting.

Miniaci, et al. (81), described a procedure necessitating an oblique, laterally based closing wedge osteotomy that was fixed with a tubular plate. A disadvantage of this procedure is that it necessitates tibial tubercle elevation since the line of the osteotomy passes through its bed. In addition, shear forces across this osteotomy can lead to instability and poor results with loss of correction in cases in which the medial corticoperiosteal hinge is violated.

Advocates of casting without internal fixation believe that alteration of alignment is possible postoperatively, if satisfactory correction is not obtained intraoperatively. However, this form of treatment may increase the risk for delayed or nonunion and postoperative peroneal palsy. Nevertheless, loss of correction can occur while wearing a cast, as illustrated in 15 of 139 patients in Aglietti's series. Loss of correction with casting has prompted most authors today to rely on some form of skeletal fixation.

Undercorrection

Undercorrection is the most common complication of high tibial osteotomy, with a wide range of frequency from 9.2 to 73% in the larger series (38, 50, 66). It is associated with failure of short-term results and recurrence of varus (Fig. 57.1) (38, 116, 117). Hagstedt et al (33), claimed that there was only a 20% chance for freedom from pain in those patients who were undercorrected. They also found a spontaneous loss of correction of up to 4 degrees in patients corrected to the neutral position immediately postoperation. Insall, et al. (44), cited the surgeon's reluctance to produce a noticeable valgus deformity as the probable major reason for undercorrection. Engel, et al. (27), stated, "the surgeon lacked the courage of his convictions, feeling at the last minute that the measured wedge was too large," a decision leading to undercorrection. Vainionpaa, et al. (122), stated that the tethering effect of the fibula at the proximal tibiofibular joint or shaft may play a role in recurrence or undercorrection. Tjornstrand, et al. (116) found that the degree of articular degeneration in the involved knee varied inversely with the ability to provide lasting pain relief and correction of the mechanical axis. In their series, undercorrection and recurrence of deformity occurred three times more often in cases with ad-

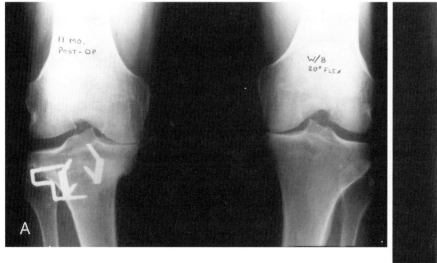
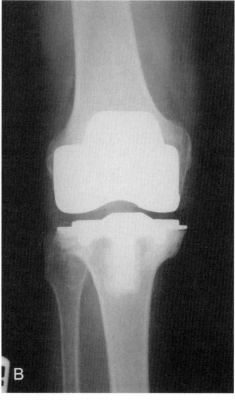

Figure 57.1.   A, This radiograph illustrates undercorrection of the anatomical and mechanical axes of the lower extremity in an otherwise well-performed HTO. **B,** Pain relief was not achieved in this patient, and 2 1/2 years later TKA was required.

vanced stages of arthritis as compared to those with less involvement.

The literature on HTO reflects the controversy surrounding the question of how much is the appropriate amount of correction necessary to give longer lasting good-to-excellent results. Nevertheless, there has been a gradual realization that there exists a narrow zone of overcorrection that will yield such outcomes. Vainionppa found that the best results of valgus HTO were in patients corrected to between 5 to 13 degrees of valgus, and that an anatomical axis of greater than 7 degrees of valgus was the most effective correction in resisting recurrent varus. Insall recommended 10 degrees of postoperative valgus. Keene, et al. (58, 59), showed good to excellent results at 5 years in nearly 70% of patients corrected to between 7 to 13 degrees. Healy and Riley (37), presented the results in 31 consecutive cases of varus gonarthrosis using a closing wedge technique. The average preoperative tibiofemoral angulation was 7 degrees of varus. These knees were corrected to a normal mechanical axis, averaging 5 degrees of postoperative valgus. In spite of the lack of overcorrection in this series, 80% maintained good-to-excellent results at 9-year follow-up.

Coventry, et al. (21), in a long-term follow-up of 87 HTOs for varus gonarthrosis, found a postoperative failure rate of 62% at 5 years and 81% at 10 years if an anatomic axis of at least 8 degrees of valgus was not

achieved at surgery. In this series, the 10-year survival rate of those knees corrected to 8 degrees or more was 94% as opposed to 63% for those corrected to less than 5 degrees of valgus. This illustrates the importance of overcorrection of the femoral-tibial axis to at least 8 to 10 degrees of total anatomic valgus.

Inadequate correction of a varus deformity allows too large a percentage of the body weight to continue to be transmitted to the medial compartment, thus provoking the degenerative process. In 1976, Kettlekamp, et al. (62), predicted from long-standing films that, in a knee with a normal 5 degrees valgus angle, 60% of the load across the knee joint would be borne by the medial compartment and 40% by the lateral compartment. They postulated a proportional decrease in medial loading with increasing valgus realignment.

Johnson and Waugh (53) demonstrated that the dynamic load across the knee joint after HTO differed quite significantly from that predicted by static analysis (Fig. 57.2). Their gait analysis studies revealed that in 20 of 52 knee joints with a valgus anatomical axis greater than neutral, 60 to 100% of the total load was still borne by the medial compartment. In fact, in an earlier study by the same authors (54) it was demonstrated that patients with a valgus deformity, who were candidates for TKA or HTO, developed a compensatory gait pattern that allowed them to load preferentially the medial compartment of the knee joint during walking. Their results indicated that for a valgus tibiofemoral angle of 5 degrees, approximately 75% of the force is located in the medial compartment. In addition, for absolute varus angles of 5 degrees or more, the medial plateau force rapidly approached 100% of the total load. What was most striking was that even at valgus angles of 25 degrees, only a 50% reduction in medial compartment loading occurred. These findings suggest that changes in mechanical axis position and load transference with respect to the knee joint affect the lateral compartment to much lesser degrees than the medial compartment. Furthermore, varus alignment is a potent loader of the medial compartment and valgus realignment can lessen, but not entirely eliminate loads in the medial compartment.

Excessive Overcorrection

Bauer, et al. (4), Insall, et al. (45), Tjornstand, et al. (117), Coventry (13), and Aglietti, et al. (1), all reported that excessive valgus (usually 15 degrees or more) can lead to poor results. Overestimation of the preoperative deformity in knees with increased lateral laxity can lead to excessive overcorrection. Excessive overcorrection may also result from empirical formulas used to determine the amount of desired angular correction. For instance, it has been recommended by some authors that the required valgus "overcorrection" should be normal valgus plus 5 degrees, i.e., 7 + 5 = 12 degrees. In general, this formula leads to greater postoperative valgus than the 8 to 10 degree range supported in the literature and does not take into account the final position of the mechanical axis. Excessive valgus alignment can cause patellofemoral tracking problems and progressive lat-

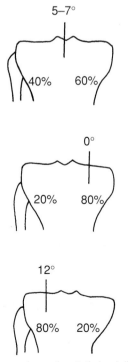

Figure 57.2. This figure shows the static load distribution in the medial and lateral compartments as a function of the anatomical and mechanical axes. Note the asymmetric line of the mechanical axis when the pressure distribution is between 80 and 20% of either compartment. (Adapted from Johnson, et al. Alternative reconstructive procedures. Morrey BF, ed. Joint replacement arthroplasty. New York: Churchill Livingstone, 1991: 1115.

eral compartment degeneration as a result of excessive lateral shift of the mechanical axis. The unsightly appearance of the markedly overcorrected knee is a major cosmetic problem. The patient is forced to ambulate with an awkward wide-based gait.

A secondary consequence that may result from overcorrection is difficulty in conversion of the failed HTO to a total knee replacement (57, 111, 121). This problem is magnified in varus knees that are severely overcorrected due to excessive wedge resection. Windsor, et al. (121), reported up to 25 degrees of valgus and Katz, et al. (57), up to 28 degrees in patients presenting for TKA after failed proximal tibial osteotomy. These authors found that a major factor in the difficulty of conversion to TKA was the change in the length of the extensor mechanism. In Windsor's series, 80% of 41 knees were found to have patella infera as measured from preoperative lateral radiographs using the method of Insall and Salvati. Approximately 50% of the knees with patella infera had pain on walking or stair climbing after TKA. Rinonapoli, et al. (99), reported patella infera in 82% of their cases of HTO. They attributed this to the osteotomy line being behind the tendon, a situation which led to adhesions and contracture during immobilization in extension and encouraged early ROM.

Loss of Correction/Recurrence of Deformity

Loss of correction and recurrence of deformity may occur in 3.0 to 30% as a result of undercorrection, fixation failure, or fracture. Each of these contributing factors are discussed separately below.

Neuromuscular Injury

Injury to the deep peroneal nerve is the most dreaded adverse occurrence in HTO. It ranks as the third most common complication of this procedure after undercorrection and overcorrection, occurring in 2.0 to 13.8% of patients.

Peroneal nerve injury may present as motor weakness in some or all of the muscles supplied by the common peroneal nerve or its divisions. Severe pain and/or sensory loss over the front of the foot and ankle have been described. Most of these injuries are transient in duration, without permanent functional disability; however, some patients are left with permanent deficits (70, 76). The cause of the neural damage has been attributed to numerous etiologic factors including tight postoperative bandages (23), tight plaster casts (11), transient anterior compartment syndrome, direct injury (laceration, retractor placement), or pressure from swelling of the nerve. Osteotomy of the fibular shaft has also been implicated as an etiology of peroneal paralysis after HTO (56). Maquet has reported injury to the peroneal nerve in 16 cases where osteotomy of the fibula was performed in its proximal third (76).

Common Peroneal Nerve

The common peroneal nerve lies close to the fibular head where it is fixed to bone by connective tissue. It is vulnerable during proximal tibiofibular disruption or in techniques that involve partial or total resection of the fibular head. Direct injury from placement of external fixator pins can occur. Jackson (50) reported an occurrence of peroneal palsy of over 40% when an external fixator was used to stabilize the osteotomy. Ogata, et al. (93), noted the absence of further neural complications when using meticulous exposure and performing osteotomy of the fibula cephalad to the superior border of the interosseous membrane (or distal to its midportion).

Maintaining the knee in flexion during the procedure without attempting to visualize the nerve is recommended since exposure and even gentle handling may cause neuropraxia. Careful subperiosteal placement of retractors especially for protection of the vital structures of the popliteal fossa is helpful. Protection from injury in a postoperative cast can be provided with adequate padding and cast splitting. Immobilization of the limb in slight flexion postoperatively will also decrease tension in the nerve.

Deep Peroneal Nerve

Injury to the deep peroneal nerve are the most frequently reported neural injury complicating tibial osteotomy and may manifest itself as an isolated motor neuropathy (foot drop, extensor hallucis longus (EHL) weakness) or combined motor and sensory neuropathy. The anatomy of this nerve is such that the sensory branches of the deep peroneal nerve originate from the nerve distal to the origins of the motor branches. Paraesthesia and pain in the first dorsal web space of the foot can be the presentation of deep peroneal nerve injury if only the sensory branches are involved.

Weakness and paralysis of the EHL muscle is a relatively common occurrence in those patients with reported neural injury during HTO. As an explanation for this finding, Kirgis, et al. (64), noted that the motor branches to the EHL seem to be most at risk for harm during the performance of a double osteotomy of the leg (Fig. 57.3). They performed a human cadaver study to investigate the anatomical levels at which the peroneal nerve and its branches are in greatest peril for injury during HTO. They identified the motor branch to the EHL as being at greatest risk for damage when fibular osteotomy is performed between 68 to 153 mm from the fibular head. The risk is heightened because most of the points of origin of the motor branch were observed in this area. The safe zone for shaft osteotomy was identified as 160 mm or greater from the fibular head. A proximal danger zone extending from 0 to 40 mm from the fibular head was also noted. In this area, fibrous bands were found to tether the motor branches of the tibialis anterior muscle to the fibular periosteum.

Posterior Tibial Nerve

McLaren, et al. (80) found that 15 of 100 patients who underwent high tibial osteotomy had evidence of neurological impairment. What was striking was that 4 of these 15 patients suffered from severe symptomatic pes planus deformity as a result of damage to the posterior tibial nerve (3 out of 4 had deep peroneal injury as well). In these 4 patients, all with preoperative varus gonarthrosis, a Maquet dome technique employing exter-

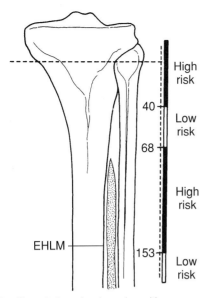

Figure 57.3. Frontal view showing a leg with an accompanying longitudinal scale. The scale illustrates regions that are at high and low risk for intraoperative injury relative to the presence of motor branches from the truncus of the deep peroneal nerve. EHLM, extensor hallucis longus muscle. (From Kirgis A., et al. Palsy of the deep peroneal nerve after proximal tibial osteotomy. J Bone Joint Surg 1992; 74-A: 1185.)

nal fixation and fibular osteotomy was used. Direct surgical trauma or local compression from a hematoma was reported as responsible for posterior tibial nerve injury in this series.

Superficial Peroneal Nerve

Injury to this nerve has been reported as a separate complication in several series and is attributable to causes similar to those mentioned above. The superficial peroneal nerve runs down the peroneal compartment of the leg supplying the peroneus longus and brevis. The dorsal cutaneous branch of this nerve pierces the deep fascia in the lower part of the leg and divides into medial and lateral branches. It is vulnerable to injury during osteotomy at the junction of the middle and distal thirds of the fibular shaft. If it is damaged, numbness on the dorsum of the foot will occur. These injuries can easily be avoided with careful blunt soft tissue dissection and subperiosteal exposure of the fibular shaft. Straying into muscle proximally or into the subcutaneous plane distally will place the superficial peroneal nerve and its branches at risk.

Tourniquet Palsy

Although the literature on HTO does not document a single case of tourniquet palsy, it is likely that some of the unexplained cases of nerve dysfunction that have been reported are attributable to this phenomenon. Paralysis after the use of a tourniquet for the "bloodless field technique" is related to the duration of ischemia and the amount of pressure applied. Despite the considerable decline in the incidence of this complication with the introduction of the pneumatic tourniquet, careful preoperative calibration and intraoperative monitoring of pressures (which generally should not exceed 90 to 100 mm Hg above systolic blood pressure) remains essential.

In tourniquet paralysis, damage to the nerve is most severe in the area where pressure is applied. One experimental investigation demonstrated that the most susceptible portion of the nerve is that lying directly beneath the *proximal* edge of the cuff (100). The authors theorized that this was due to a mismatch in the shapes of the tourniquet (cylindrical) and the thigh (conical) that could allow uneven pressure distribution. The sciatic nerve, in particular its *lateral* division, is especially vulnerable to externally applied pressure. Rorabeck et al., documented the development of five sciatic palsies after the application of a pneumatic tourniquet for knee ligament surgery by electromyographic and nerve conduction studies. Of these patients, 4 recovered fully in 6 months; however, 1 remained with weak dorsiflexion of the foot.

Vascular Injury

Injury to the popliteal artery and vein is a rare (less than 1%) but grave complication of HTO. Despite the surgeon's best efforts to document vascular integrity, the diagnosis of arterial injury may be missed. Reubens et al. (101) reported on the late diagnosis of 2 cases of popliteal artery injury with false aneurysm formation after HTO. In one case, the patient presented with a pulseless, cool foot and a large pulsatile mass in the popliteal fossa 3 1/2 weeks after HTO using staple fixation. In the other case, the diagnosis was made 11 months after surgery, during which time the patient complained of persistent calf pain. A widened popliteal pulse and bruit led to the diagnosis in this patient. The cause of these injuries was more than likely related to operative trauma. Repair in both cases was performed by removing the false aneurysm and reanastamosis with a reversed saphenous vein graft.

Arterial injury proximal to the popliteal fossa has also been reported in HTO. Coventry (12) experienced such a complication in 1 patient with a prior history of arteriosclerosis obliterans and intermittent claudication who underwent HTO. Postoperative thrombosis in the superficial femoral artery occurred and led to irreversible ischemia and damage to the leg necessitating a below-the-knee amputation.

Direct trauma to the popliteal vessels can result from placement of retractors deep in the popliteal fossa. Extraperiosteal dissection of the posterior knee and projection of the oscillating saw blade or osteotomes during the bone cuts may also be responsible. Use of a tourniquet can result in indirect trauma to the intimal layer of the wall of the superficial femoral artery and continued limb ischemia after its deflation (120). Embolic and vascular occlusive events may also transpire with the use of a tourniquet. Manipulation (especially hyperextension) of the knee joint can cause stretching and twisting of the distal portion of the superficial femoral artery about the proximal trunk that is fixed by the tourniquet. Dislodgement and embolization of a loose atheromatous plaque can be a catastrophic consequence of this unpredictable situation (79). Giannestras, et al. (30), reported this complication resulting in occlusion of the tibial artery during routine foot surgery with the application of a tourniquet at a pressure of 500 mm Hg.

Some important observations that have been made in the literature concerning vascular complications in TKA can be applied to HTO. DeLaurentis, et al. (22), have suggested that if there is femoropopliteal calcification in the absence of limb ischemia, omission of the tourniquet during TKA is wise. If femoropopliteal calcification and ischemia or popliteal aneurysm are present, then the danger of arterial thrombosis with the use of a tourniquet is real. They recommend carrying out an arterial bypass first, followed later by TKA without the use of a tourniquet.

Other vascular structures besides the popliteal and superficial femoral vessels are at risk during HTO. These include the anterior tibial, the peroneal, and the lateral geniculate arteries. The anterior tibial artery is vulnerable to injury from proximal tibiofibular joint disruption, osteotomy of the tibia and in the application of pins or screws for rigid fixation. The anterior tibial artery passes forward from the popliteal region just below the lower part of the inferior tibiofibular joint and above the upper edge of the interosseous membrane. The narrow opening of the interosseous membrane is usually at the level of the lower border of the tibial tuberosity. Therefore, the anterior tibial artery is placed in jeopardy if the tibial osteotomy is done below the tuberosity.

Aglietti (1) described an injury to the anterior tibial artery during a tibial osteotomy below the tibial tubercle and an injury to the peroneal artery during exposure of the upper third of the fibular shaft. Both of these required ligation without serious compromise to limb circulation. Bauer and Insall (4) documented severance of the anterior tibial artery during resection of the fibular head in one varus knee without an ensuing circulatory compromise to the limb. These reports underscore the extreme care that is necessary, especially in the area of the interosseous membrane and the fibular head, during bone cuts and proximal disruption of the tibiofibular joint. Finally, the lateral geniculate artery can be injured during placement of drains.

To prevent vascular catastrophe, it is important to evaluate the preoperative vascular status of the limb by clinical history and examination, and, if indicated, by invasive measures in a vascular lab. If arteriographic studies reveal arterial insufficiency, then consultation with a vascular surgeon should be obtained prior to surgery. Risk factors for arterial occlusion and thrombosis, such as calcified atheromatous plaques, and conditions promoting a hypercoagulable state should not be ignored. A red flag should always be raised when heavily calcified vessels are present in the lower extremity on preoperative radiographs. In this situation, exclusion of the tourniquet is wise and should not present major difficulty in the performance of HTO. When the pneumatic tourniquet is used, the minimum effective pressure that

allows a bloodless field should be used. In the lower limb, this has been reported to be 90 to 100 mm Hg above the systolic arm pressure (28).

Intraoperatively, the risk of injury to the popliteal vessels can be minimized by maintaining knee flexion. This allows these vessels to relax and fall posteriorly behind the knee joint for maximal protection from saw blades and other operative instruments. It should be kept in mind that the anterior tibial artery lies just below the inferior edge of the proximal TF joint. Thus, adequate exposure of the proximal tibiofibular joint is important to allow its safe disruption.

Postoperatively, a high index of suspicion and early recognition of tourniquet-induced ischemia, iatrogenic vascular injury, or atheroembolic events is necessary if there is to be any hope for salvage of the arterially deficient limb. In the recovery room, the patient's symptoms of painful ischemia may be obscured by sedation or epidural anesthesia, and easy access to the leg and foot may be prevented by the use of bulky dressings and splints. It is important to reaffirm vascular integrity postoperatively. Once the diagnosis of vascular compromise is made, exploration and arterial embolectomy or vascular grafting and four compartment fasciotomy are indicated to prevent compartment syndrome and loss of limb.

Compartment Syndrome

Anterior compartment syndrome is another infrequent but serious complication of HTO. It is sometimes difficult to separate the clinical picture of compartment syndrome from neural injury. Indeed, there has been a reported case of the disastrous consequence of the late diagnosis of compartment syndrome that was clouded by the presence of a simultaneous tourniquet palsy (74). Thus, a diligent search for compartment syndrome should be made in patients who appear to have only neurologic injury. In addition, the etiology of compartment syndrome and neural injury as a result of HTO may be quite similar. Techniques that include internal fixation with plates and screws all have a higher incidence of hazard with respect to these two complications (18). Lemaire (9), using blade plate fixation, found 1 case of compartment syndrome and 9 peroneal palsies in 207 patients; using compression pins in 201 patients, he reported 1 compartment syndrome and 8 palsies.

Osteotomy of the fibula at the junction of the middle- and upper-third has been implicated in the evolution of anterior compartment syndrome with HTO. Jackson and Waugh reported that transient compartment ischemia accounted for weakness in the muscles of the anterior compartment in those patients with fibular osteotomy at this level. Lemaire recommends that fibular osteotomy should be performed in the lower third of the shaft where the tendinous portions of the anterior compartment musculature are located. He reasons that fibular osteotomy executed at a more cephalad location can cause trauma and swelling of the proximally situated muscle bellies, raising intracompartmental pressures. He also recommends routine prophylactic anterior compartment fasciotomy; he has neither detected compartment syndrome nor has he had major patient complaints of muscle herniation over the last 10 years (Lemaire, personal communication, 1993).

Postoperative hematoma formation can result in increased pressure in the anterior compartment. Gibson, et al. (31) studied the effects of suction drainage on anterior compartment pressures after HTO. They also attempted to establish whether there exists a relationship between weakness of dorsiflexion and elevated anterior compartment pressures. Of 10 knee wounds that were not drained, 7 showed a pressure elevation to over 50 mm Hg, usually with transitory clinical signs of compartment syndrome (swelling, stretch pain, sensory deficit, and weakness of the EHL). Of 10 wounds that were drained, 8 had anterior compartment pressures that remained below 30 mm Hg without clinical signs of compartment syndrome. The accumulation of blood at the operative site was thought to account for the transitory pressure elevation recorded in the undrained group, hence implying a beneficial effect of suction drainage. At follow-up (6 to 14 months), of the 20 patients in this study, 3 had weakness of dorsiflexion. Two patients were in the drained group with normal compartment pressures and only one in the undrained group. On the basis of these findings, it was concluded that permanent weakness of the EHL after HTO was not related to postoperative anterior compartment syndrome.

Fracture

This complication is fully discussed below under the subject of technical pitfalls.

Problems of Union

Delayed Union and Nonunion

There are many potential causes of delayed union (2.6%) and nonunion (2.0 to 4.0%) in HTO. Jackson and Waugh (50) stated that delayed union is likely to occur in patients with an osteotomy performed below the tibial tubercle without the use of internal fixation (i.e., osteotomy immobilized in plaster). Coventry (12) claims that if it is not resected, the fibular head could impact against the proximal tibial fragment during collapse of a closing wedge osteotomy. This would prevent closure of the osteotomy and therefore delay union. Insall, et al. (44, 45) and Harris and Kostuik (35) warned against using power saws for fear of thermal necrosis and subsequent nonunion.

In the closing wedge model of osteotomy, broad cancellous contact surfaces coupled with compression and stabilization via internal fixation promote rapid union and maintenance of proper correction. Flat, well-apposed cuts in the frontal and sagittal planes are essential in achieving this goal. The preservation of an intact medial osseoperiosteal hinge maintains the stability of the osteotomy that is essential for the prevention of delayed and nonunion. Proximal tibiofibular release in the

form of syndesmosis disruption or fibular head resection, judicious employment of fibular shaft osteotomy, and the execution of proper technique of internal fixation help to avoid gaping at the osteotomy site.

It has been recognized that proximal osteotomy of the tibia is associated with a lower rate of nonunion when performed above the tibial tuberosity. The incidence of delayed union in Vainionpaa's series was 3.6% when osteotomy was performed above the tubercle and was 14% when performed below the tubercle. Clearly, there are advantages to the supratubercular osteotomy: first, whether a wedge or dome osteotomy is used, a highly vascular cancellous interface with a large surface area is available for stability and rapid healing; second, compression forces are exerted across the osteotomy through quadriceps contraction and encourage healing (Fig. 57.4) (10); lastly, greater correction is possible at this level since the adjustment of the abnormal anatomical axis is being performed closer to the actual deformity.

When nonunion occurs, bone grafting of the pseudarthrosis with retention of fixation is necessary if alignment has been maintained. However, complete revision and bone grafting of the osteotomy are required if loss of angular correction has also occurred. The use of electrical stimulation may be helpful in cases of delayed union without loss of correction.

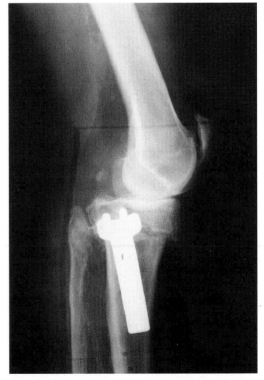

Figure 57.4. This radiograph shows the postoperative appearance of an HTO performed beneath the tibial tubercle. A nonunion with extreme loss of correction developed. Revision of the osteotomy and bone grafting of the nonunion will be necessary.

Malunion

Malunion may occur as a result of the following:

1. Improper osteotomy cuts;
2. Plateau fracture;
3. Failure of skeletal fixation;
4. Failure of casting;
5. Infection with loosening of fixator pins and loss of correction.

These technical sources of malunion are discussed later in this chapter.

Deep Venous Thrombosis/ Pulmonary Embolism

Most authors have listed deep venous thrombosis (DVT) as a complication of HTO. The incidence varies from 1.2 to 13.5%, which is markedly lower than the incidence of 50 to 84% quoted from the literature on TKA (63).

General risk factors involved in the evolution of a venous thrombus apply to patients undergoing HTO. These include major surgery (HTO), general anesthesia, the use of a tourniquet, trauma (e.g., retractor in the popliteal fossa), postoperative immobility, and any other causes of venous stasis (e.g., varicose veins, congestive heart failure, previous partially resolved venous thrombosis (84). Other possible risk factors are age over 70 years, obesity, estrogen use, and the presence of cancer, a presence which has been theorized to lead to a hypercoagulable state. Other prothrombotic states that are present in a small percentage of patients include deficiencies in protein C, protein S, and antithrombin III and the presence of lupus inhibitor. It can be seen that all these risk factors fall under the triad of Virchow— namely, venous stasis, vessel injury, and alteration in blood coagulation.

Use of a tourniquet combined with flexion of the knee intraoperatively may increase the risk of damage to the venous endothelium and the risk of venous stasis in the operated lower extremity. How much the tourniquet plays a role in the evolution of thrombosis is still controversial (71, 107). Nevertheless, tourniquet time should not exceed 2 hours. It has been shown that ischemia for longer periods produces significant swelling in the limb due to increased hyperemia and capillary permeability associated with tissue anoxia (65). Brief rest periods should be allowed in between deflation and reinflation of the tourniquet, and the applied pressure should not exceed 90 to 100 mm Hg over systolic pressure, in order is to minimize the potential risks of its use. It should be made clear that high tibial osteotomy can be performed safely and without significant blood loss even with elimination of a tourniquet altogether.

The proper prophylactic regimen for prevention of DVT is debatable. It is wise to administer prophylaxis, either as pharmacologic agents (e.g., low dose warfarin, aspirin, or low molecular weight heparin) or by mechanical compression of the deep veins (sequential compres-

sion dressings or Venodyne boots). The use of continuous passive motion may also discourage the evolution of deep venous thrombosis, although there are articles in the literature that refute its value. Simple measures may be effective as well. Bauer, et al., attributed a lower incidence (6%) of thromboembolism after HTO to early ambulation, muscle contraction exercises, and straight leg raising.

Pulmonary embolism occurs in approximately 1.2 to 6.1% of patients undergoing HTO. The incidence of fatal pulmonary embolism is between 0.4 to 2.7% and accounted for death in 5 patients reported in Maquet's series of domed HTO. These all occurred in his early experience, and he noted that there were no further deaths with elimination of the use of a tourniquet for intraoperative hemostasis. In comparison, asymptomatic pulmonary embolism occurs in 8.2 to 17% of patients undergoing TKA, symptomatic pulmonary embolism in 0.5 to 3% and death in 0.3%. The lower incidences of both deep venous thrombosis and pulmonary embolism in HTO are probably related to the fact that HTO is a less complicated procedure than TKA.

Infection

The incidence of infection after high tibial osteotomy without the use of external fixation is usually less than 3.0%. Most often, these are superficial wound infections that resolve with wound care and antibiotics, although several cases of tibial osteomyelitis and septic arthritis have been mentioned (66). An infected nonunion or joint infection requires arthrodesis as a salvage procedure (4).

The risk of infection is increases with lack of perioperative antibiotic prophylaxis, arthrotomy (i.e., increased risk for intraarticular infection), and extensive wound exposure. The use of external fixation to maintain osteotomy alignment is associated with an 8.0 to 11% (42, 51) frequency of infection. Debilitated patients, diabetics for example, are at a heightened risk for infection just as in any other operation (66).

When external fixation is chosen, aggressive pin care should be exercised since this has been shown to be effective in the prevention of infection. Pin-tract infection can lead to loosening of fixation and loss of correction; pin loosening may require removal of the fixator and the application of a long leg cast. This jeopardizes the maintenance of correction of the ununited osteotomy. Oral antibiotics can be used for superficial pin tract infections; however, intravenous antibiotics and open debridement are required in deeper, more virulent infections. Patient compliance with fixator precautions and pin care is important, and ample preoperative discussion of this issue with the patient is helpful.

Postoperative Instability

Marked medial or lateral (more than 1 cm subluxation) instability noted at preoperative clinical examination will not resolve with HTO. Appel and Friberg (3) found postoperative instability in 4 cases that were classified as failures (3 of which required fusion). All 4 of these patients demonstrated pronounced lateral instability preoperatively. Mynerts (87) found that patients with a mean increased varus/valgus instability of 2.6 degrees as measured by a three-point radiographic technique (described in Mynerts' study) had a higher chance of a poor result. Those with greater than 5 degrees of instability had incomplete pain relief. Shoji and Insall regard marked instability as a contraindication to HTO and greater than 1 cm of lateral subluxation is generally regarded as unacceptable.

Coventry recommends excision of the fibular head and restoration of tension in the fibular collateral ligament by its reattachment to the shaft after osteotomy of the tibia. He also approximates the fascia lata with horizontal mattress sutures to further strengthen the lateral support of the knee. Other authors feel that these measures are not necessary, and that ligament laxity will diminish after osteotomy (5, 76). Sagittal plane deformity, introduced as a result of inaccurate bone cuts, may accentuate cruciate ligament insufficiency. Excessive posterior slope may create anterior instability, while excessive anterior slope may increase posterior instability. Joint line obliquity introduced by excessive proximal bony resection may result in instability and poor outcome. Lateral subluxation of the tibia on the femur as a consequence of joint line tilt greater than 15 degrees has resulted from varus osteotomy of the tibia to correct valgus gonarthrosis.

Excessive bone loss from the tibial plateau, present preoperatively (teeter effect) or resulting from excessive overcorrection, can produce an unstable knee postoperatively. In these cases, stability and freedom from pain can only be accomplished by prosthetic replacement or arthrodesis (14).

Persistent Pain

Coventry (12), felt that persistent postoperative pain originated from a number of sources such as poor patient selection (e.g., severe preoperative arthritis and obesity), inadequate angular correction, a torn meniscus, osteochondritis dissecans, pyrophosphate disease and tibial subluxation. Perhaps the most important determinant of sustained pain relief is accuracy of correction (38, 45, 78). It has been shown that undercorrection will prevent the reduction of load in the medial compartment and may result in persistent knee pain. As mentioned previously, the best long-term success in pain relief and maintenance of correction has been in those knees that have been overcorrected to an AA of 8 to 10 degrees.

Persistent pain has also been described in patients with a preoperative deformity of greater than 10 to 15 degrees of varus. Reasons why this may be true with such severe deformity include a tendency toward undercorrection, a higher rate of recurrence of varus deformity, and an instability that the osteotomy fails to address (20, 45, 123). Thus, patients with preoperative deformity of such magnitude are not indicated for HTO.

With respect to the stage of osteoarthritis in the involved compartment, the best results with regard to pain relief are in knees with mild to moderate disease (2, 123). Also noteworthy is that those patients who have a high preoperative adduction moment as measured by gait analysis are at higher risk of persistent pain. Fewer of them achieve good or excellent results (95, 118). (See discussion of patient selection below.)

Flare-up Chondrocalcinosis

Coventry (12) reported on the peculiar occurrence of flare-up chondrocalcinosis after HTO, particularly in older patients. It is usually temporary, but painful, and can be treated with intraarticular steroids and NSAIDs. It is interesting to note that in one series of HTO for gonarthrosis, patients having preoperative chondrocalcinosis fared significantly worse at long-term follow-up versus those patients who did not have this disease (52). Another series (117) reported on the failure to relieve pain after HTO in 2 out of 4 patients with pyrophosphate arthritis. Coventry (13) considers this form of inflammatory disease of the knee to be a relative contraindication to the procedure.

Postoperative Stiffness

Postoperative stiffness has been reported in very few series of high tibial osteotomy (with a rate of 3.0 to 9.0%) (1, 5, 7, 32, 75). Scarring and shortening of the patellar tendon may contribute to decreased flexion. As noted by Windsor and Aglietti, patella infera is a very common sequela of HTO and becomes a particularly important consideration when planning TKA.

Skeletal fixation clearly has the advantage of allowing early motion that is not possible with casting. Active assisted, or continuous passive, motion may achieve recovery of mobility prior to discharge from the hospital. In those patients who do not recover satisfactory motion, manipulation under general anesthesia can be attempted only after bony union. One should only expect to recover preoperative range of motion (12).

Wound Problems

It is difficult to identify the main cause of the scattered reports of skin necrosis and wound dehiscence that has complicated the postoperative course following HTO. It was encountered in up to 23% of patients in one series (78). Most often these were minor problems that resolved with local wound care. Contributing factors appear to be the surgical approach, the soft tissue trauma, the type and complexity of the osteotomy, and the duration of the procedure. The extent of skin flaps should be minimized. The combination of the Maquet tubercle osteotomy and the Coventry HTO described by several authors may be complicated by skin necrosis (40, 96). The use of an anterior knee incision as a unitarian one for the index procedure (HTO) and possible future TKA should lessen the likelihood of wound complications. The merits of the anterior approach are discussed later in this chapter.

Avascular Necrosis of the Proximal Fragment

Avascular necrosis of the upper fragment can result from a shallow proximal cut that leaves a thin wafer of bone with insufficient blood supply (15). Maintaining a proximal fragment thickness of at least 15 to 20 mm will help avoid this disaster. Heat necrosis may also occur when performing bone cuts with an oscillating saw. Cool saline irrigation of the bone and blade may help prevent this complication.

Patient Selection for High Tibial Osteotomy

Refined patient selection for HTO based on comprehensive clinical and radiographic examination is essential. The ideal candidate for valgus HTO is generally the younger, active patient with unicompartmental arthritis of mechanical cause. Adequate motion (90 degrees flexion, less than 15 degrees flexion contracture) and less than 1 cm of lateral subluxation of the tibia are also prerequisites. Other preoperative criteria that should be cautiously considered prior to proceeding with surgery include a varus deformity located primarily at the tibia, a competent medial collateral ligament (MCL), a varus stress view showing narrowing of the medial compartment, a valgus stress view showing adequate lateral joint space, and a mechanical axis shift into the medial compartment.

It is imperative to determine on what side of the knee joint the angular deformity originates. Prior to selecting a proximal tibial osteotomy for the operative treatment of valgus gonarthrosis, it should be recognized that joint surface obliquity frequently complicates closing wedge varus osteotomy of the tibia for valgus deformity of significant magnitude (61). This is mainly due to the fact that bone loss occurs from the lateral femoral condyle as well as from the lateral plateau in valgus arthritic deformities. Obliquity is not usually an issue in tibial osteotomy for varus gonarthrosis since the deformity originates mainly on the tibial side with only minor bone loss from the medial femoral condyle.

Excessive obliquity (higher lateral than medial) of the joint line in varus corrections greater than 10 to 15 degrees has historically lead to lateral subluxation of the tibia on the femur and unsatisfactory results (Fig. 57.5) (12, 34, 105). Moreover, varus closing wedge osteotomy of the tibia for valgus deformity will not be successful in the presence of a lax medial collateral ligament. Medial thrust of the femur during stance phase in the presence of an MCL further slackened by the varus osteotomy will produce medial joint opening and recurrent valgus deformity. Finally, correction of severe valgus gonarthrosis with proximal tibial osteotomy puts the peroneal nerve at risk for stretch injury (paresis, paralysis, paraesthesia) that may be permanent. For these reasons, varus supracondylar femoral osteotomy is recommended for significant valgus (12 to 15 degrees) deformities (36).

The evaluation of the MCL is crucial in selecting the appropriate type of osteotomy that will avoid postoperative instability. For instance, a medial *opening wedge*

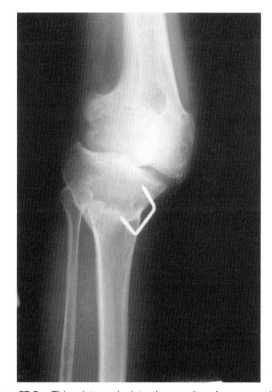

Figure 57.5. This picture depicts the results of a varus-closing wedge osteotomy that was used to correct a knee with a preoperative valgus originating on the femoral side. The true deformity was not addressed, and excess obliquity of the joint line and lateral subluxation of the tibia resulted.

osteotomy is preferred in the patient presenting with posttraumatic varus gonarthrosis, medial bone loss, and a *lax* MCL. This is because a laterally based closing wedge osteotomy may unmask medial knee instability and could lead to lateral subluxation of the tibia. An opening wedge would serve to restore tension in the MCL and stability to the knee joint.

Radiographic evidence of bicompartmental bone loss may prognosticate a suboptimal outcome after HTO. For example, the *teeter effect*, described by Kettlekamp, et al. (61), occurs when simultaneous contact between the medial and lateral tibiofemoral articular surfaces is prevented due to excessive bone loss in one compartment. In this situation, tibiofemoral contact shifts or "teeters" from one side to the other as a function of the relationship of the center of gravity to the center of the knee. Overall limb alignment may then remain in a varus position postoperatively and is therefore a contraindication to the procedure.

Patients suffering from one of the inflammatory arthritides should not be treated with HTO. Chan and Pollard (9) examined the results of high tibial osteotomy performed on 36 rheumatoid knees with either varus or valgus deformity. They found that no patient remained pain free for more than 3 years and that recurrence of pain was not necessarily associated with recurrence of deformity. Failures have been reported in the literature in spite of properly selected, accurately planned, and technically well performed HTOs. This suggests that there are other variables that may play a role in suboptimal outcome and failure. One such variable is dynamic loading of the knee joint during gait.

Prodromos, et al. (95), in 1985, reported that the success of HTO may be related to decreasing the magnitude of the postoperative knee adduction moment as measured by gait analysis. This study was composed of two groups (high and low adduction) who were indistinguishable on the basis of age, weight, preoperative knee score, initial varus deformity and immediate postoperative correction. High tibial osteotomy resulted in reduction of the peak adduction moment in both groups. However, while reduction to statistically normal levels was achieved in the high abduction group, reduction to below normal levels was noted in the low adduction group. At an average 3.2 year follow-up, patients with a low preoperative adduction moment had 100% good or excellent clinical results as compared to 50% in the high adduction group. It was found that the latter group demonstrated a significant recurrent varus deformity.

A 3- to 8.9-year follow-up study (118) of the same group of patients, published in 1990, demonstrated a continued higher incidence of loss of correction occurring in patients with a high preoperative adduction moment (lateral thrust) as compared to those with a low adduction moment. These studies revealed that patients who were in the low adduction moment group walked with a higher than normal *abduction* moment at the knee, a shorter stride, and at a slower speed than did the patients in the high adduction group. In addition, low adductors walked with a toe-out gait which was found to reduce the adduction moment at the knee. In contrast, high adductors walked with a more normal appearing gait. The adaptive gait characteristics of the low adduction group may be a result of proprioceptive signals or subconscious pain, and, if present preoperatively, they may reduce the load transmitted to the medial compartment of the joint. Postoperatively, this modification of gait may continue to protect against recurrence of varus. This may explain why low adductors continued to have a lower recurrence of varus at longer follow-up as compared to the high adductor group, although the results in both groups deteriorated over time to some degree. Keene, et al. (59), documented recurrence of varus deformity in 46 of 51 patients despite adequate postoperative correction. They speculated that this phenomenon may have been related to high preoperative adduction moments undetected in these patients. Johnson, et al. (53), recommend a preoperative gait study for all HTO candidates since it is more accurate in determining the dynamic load borne by the medial and lateral compartments.

Pitfalls in Preoperative Planning

Planning for osteotomy surgery should include a 51-inch long-standing AP film of the entire lower extremity that clearly shows the entire hip-knee-ankle axis. This allows the surgeon to determine both the mechanical and anatomical axes of the lower extremity. It is useful to have some form of magnification marker in the plane of the bone.

Lack of a long-standing AP (anterior-posterior) radiograph can be a significant factor in errors leading to undercorrection or overcorrection. An accurate long-standing AP radiograph of the lower extremity requires full knee extension and neutral rotation of the leg with respect to the x-ray beam. Engel, et al., reported that roentgenograms that are too short lead to an underestimation of the true amount of varus and, thus, to undercorrection. Moreland showed that flexion contracture and external rotation of the limb give the false impression of greater varus deformity and that internal rotation gives the appearance of greater valgus deformity.

Overestimation of the preoperative varus deformity can result from failure to account for lateral laxity. Dugdale and Noyes (25), in a trigonometric analysis of long-standing radiographs of varus arthritic knees, demonstrated that each millimeter of lateral joint separation can cause a 1 degree increase in the apparent varus deformity. To avoid excessive overcorrection, preoperative calculation should include subtraction of the amount of lateral separation from the apparent deformity. This will allow the surgeon to ascertain the true angular malalignment that is due to osseocartilaginous wear and deformity. For example, if there is a 4 mm of lateral joint opening on the AP standing alignment radiograph exhibiting an overall 7 degree varus deformity, approximately 4 degrees would result from lateral laxity. Failure to recognize this may lead to excessive valgus.

In the planning of an HTO, Dugdale, et al. (25) stressed the importance of scrutinizing the position of the mechanical axis after the desired degree of correction of the anatomical axis has been determined. Consideration of only the anatomic axis could lead to a greater than desired shift of the mechanical axis into the lateral compartment. In their study, the average amount of lateral translation of the mechanical axis was determined for each degree of correction intended. In women, average translation measured 3 mm (smaller tibias) and in men (larger tibias), 4 mm. Angular correction of the mechanical axis beyond 186 degrees (anatomic axis of 12 degrees) resulted in a weight-bearing line that fell lateral to their desired position of the medial one-third of the lateral compartment (Fig. 57.6). It was realized that basing overcorrection solely on the anatomic axis could lead to excessive translation of the mechanical axis into the lateral compartment. Lateral unicondylar weight-bearing due to lift-off of the medial femoral condyle, rapid lateral compartment degeneration, gradual medial collateral ligament failure and a progressive valgus deformity were predicted. Thus, these investigators urge that preoperative planning should be based on the final position of the mechanical axis and favor shifting it into the medial one-third of the lateral compartment. This approximates a 183 to 185 degree valgus weightbearing axis.

In the performance of wedge osteotomies, the thickness of the base of the calculated wedge is a critical determinant of the magnitude of correction obtained. It has been suggested that, in general, one degree of cor-

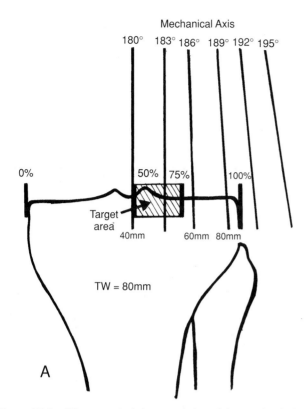

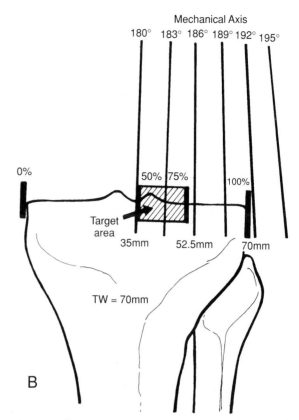

Figure 57.6. Diagrams depicting translation of the mechanical axis as a function of angular correction. Correction beyond 186 degrees results in a weight-bearing line that passes lateral to the desired post-operative position *(target area)* **A,** Represents the average female (smaller tibia); **B,** Represents the average male (larger tibia). (From Lemaire R. Upper tibial osteotomy. Acta Orthop Belg 1982; 48(1): 153.)

rection is obtained for each millimeter of base width that is resected from the upper tibia. However, this rule of thumb is subject to inaccuracies in individuals with very small or large tibias. Slocum et al. (108), demonstrated this point by the use of a series of similar right triangles that varied in width to allow for variation of tibial size. The width of the base of the triangle that corresponds to the base of the wedge to be resected can be calculated by simple geometric mathematics (adjacent/hypotenuse). Accordingly, for any given degree of correction, smaller tibiae require smaller wedges and, thus, smaller base widths as compared to larger tibiae (Fig. 57.7). Rather than "rules of thumb," magnification-controlled x-rays and precise calculation of base widths can help to avoid the component of malalignment error attributable to mistakes in preoperative planning. Also, calculations and techniques need to allow for the amount of bone lost from the cut itself.

Technical Pitfalls

Any breach in technique may lead to inaccuracy of even a few degrees of malalignment.

Fibular Considerations

Failure to perform fibular shaft osteotomy, or to perform a complete syndesmosis disruption and partial fibular head resection, when dealing with larger corrections could result in incomplete closure of the osteotomy site. Bauer, et al., studied the importance of proximal tibiofibular joint release with or without fibular shaft osteotomy. They noted that loss of correction, due to failure of closure or even to an opening of the tibial osteotomy site, occurred in cases with a tethering effect of the fibular if the proximal tibiofibular joint was incompletely disrupted. Fibular osteotomy is not always a benign procedure, especially in the upper third of the shaft. Sundarum reported a 14.3% complication rate associated with osteotomy at this level including weakness of the EHL in 3 cases, paresthesias of the foot in 4, bleeding at the osteotomy site in 3, and continued pain at the osteotomy site in 5 patients. This osteotomy can result in a painful nonunion (Fig. 57.8).

Tibial Bone Cuts

Errors in technique can lead to inaccurate bone cuts, regardless of the type of osteotomy performed (i.e., opening wedge, closing wedge, or dome osteotomy). In particular, when performing a closing wedge osteotomy, failure to achieve flat, well-apposed cuts leads to incomplete closure of the osteotomy site, undercorrection and possible delayed union (Fig. 57.9). Proximal and distal limbs of the wedge osteotomy that are not parallel may lead to sagittal plane deformity (90). This may

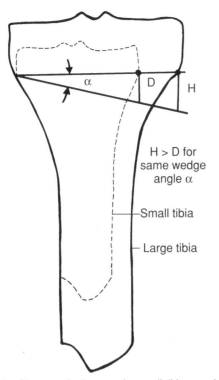

Figure 57.7. Diagram of a large and a small tibia superimposed on each other to show the relationship of wedge-base width and tibial size. Note that the measurement at the base of the wedge shows that *H* (larger tibia) is greater than *D* (smaller tibia), even though the angle of correction is the same. From "Upper Tibial Osteotomy" Acta Orthopeadica Belgica Tome 48 Fasc. 1, 1982 p. 153 (Aci: R. Lemaire)

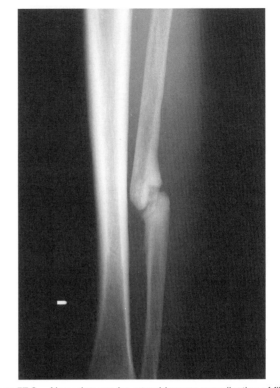

Figure 57.8. Nonunion can be a troublesome complication of fibular osteotomy as it was in this patient who complained of persistent pain at the nonunion site. Excision of the pseudarthrosis without bone grafting relieved symptoms.

manifest as a flexion or recurvatum deformity of the knee (50).

Medial Hinge Violation

Medial cortical and periosteal division may occur during wedge resection and will destroy the medial hinge that is vital for postoperative stability and maintenance of correction (Fig. 57.10). This usually results from poor medial visualization, underestimation of saw blade depth, or the use of excessive force during compression of the osteotomy surfaces. A fluoroscopic AP view of the proximal tibia reveals the angle and depth of the osteotomy intraoperatively (78). In addition to confirming the accuracy of the preoperative plan, it prevents intraarticular penetration.

Difficulty in gently closing the osteotomy should alert the surgeon to a persistent medial bony bridge. Controlled perforation of the medial cortex via multiple drill holes or the edge of a thin osteotome may aid in closure. The position of the foot in relation to the knee is important. If the medial hinge has been completely violated, an external rotational malunion may result, producing patellofemoral problems.

Medial Intraarticular Penetration

Intraoperative fluoroscopic imaging is helpful in averting intraarticular penetration with guide pins, drills, os-teotomes, saw blades, staples, or screws. This is usually due to the extent of the varus slope or comes from insufficient thickness of the osteotomized upper fragment.

In most varus knees, insertion of a guide pin results in a moderate inferomedial trajectory. The surgeon should suspect difficulty whenever the slope of the guide pin is directed superomedially. If the proximal tibial cut is too close to the joint line, then staples or other internal fixation devices may enter the joint—as occurred in 6 patients in Jackson and Waugh's series (50). Intraarticular penetration from staples improperly inserted into the joint has also been reported by Chan and Pollard (Fig. 57.11) (9).

Fracture

The rate of fracture including the tibial plateau is approximately 2 to 4% in most series; however, some authors have related an incidence as high as 11 to 15% (47, 78). These fractures may cause surface irregularities in the joint and instability as well. In general, tibial plateau fractures in HTO result from insufficient proximal fragment thickness, incomplete bony cuts, unintentional superomedial obliquity of saw cuts (in cases of closing wedge osteotomy), a wide medial bony bridge coupled with forceful closure of the osteotomy site, and poor bone quality (e.g., fragile osteoporotic bone). Weight-

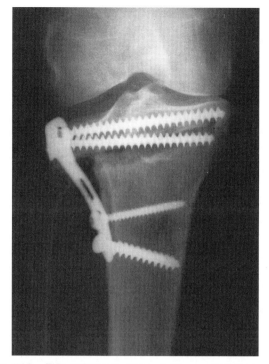

Figure 57.9. This radiograph demonstrates an inability to obtain smooth flat tibial cut surfaces on collapse of the osteotomy. In addition, a thin proximal tibial cut resulted in screw pull-out after a compression device was used in an attempt to collapse the proximal and distal fragments. (From Hsu RWW, Himeno, Shinkichi, Coventry MB, Chao EYS. Normal axial alignment of the lower extremity and load-bearing distribution at the knee. Clin Orthop 1990; 255:215–227.)

bearing and aggressive motion early in the postoperative period may lead to fracture.

Osteotomy closer than 1 cm to the joint line places the plateau at great risk for fracture. Insufficient thickness results from an osteotomy too proximally placed or from an arthritis with a large defect in the medial tibial condyle (4). Harris and Kostuik (35) reported that medial plateau fracture may occur upon collapse of a closing wedge osteotomy if a wide medial bridge is left due to incomplete wedge resection. Osteotomy jigs can lead to a similar situation. Some jigs position an attached blade in a slot created as the proximal portion of the osteotomy. Incomplete osteotomy with a wide medial hinge may theoretically result if the patient's mediolateral, proximal tibial width exceeds that of the jig. By the same token, in smaller tibias, the blade of the jig should not be inserted to its full length since this may cause fracture of the medial cortex and disruption of the periosteal sleeve (Fig. 57.12).

Lateral plateau fractures can occur intraoperatively with the insertion of staples, screws or plates either because of placement too close to one another, too close to the osteotomy site, or from abrupt or excessive application of force with the use of compression devices. A stepped staple was introduced by Coventry in 1969 (11). The plateau may fracture when staples are forcefully malleted into hard cortical bone. Predrilling the proximal and distal fragments at the site of staple entry facilitates uneventful insertion.

In summary, the risk of fracture can be minimized if the width of the proximal fragment is approximately 18

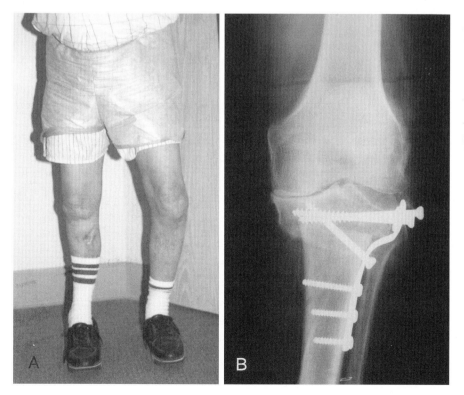

Figure 57.10. A, This clinical photograph demonstrates the postoperative appearance of a patient referred for failed HTO of the left knee (the right lower extremity deformity was a result of previous trauma.) **B,** Intraoperative medial cortical penetration occurred with a loss of medial stability. The distal fragment was drawn laterally by the fixation screws. Further collapse into varus compounded intraoperative undercorrection and led to implant loosening and exaggerated varus deformity.

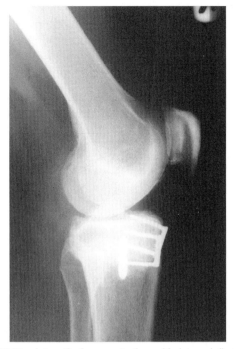

Figure 57.11. Intraarticular penetration with internal fixation may occur during HTO. Careful attention to detail and the use of intraoperative radiographic checks may help avoid this complication.

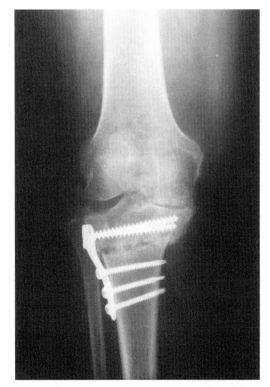

Figure 57.12. This radiograph illustrates medial cortical penetration that may occur when using an osteotomy jig. The blade of the osteotomy jig was placed too far medially in the proximal cut causing it to penetrate the medial cortex. As can be seen from this photo, postoperative loss of correction resulted as the proximal fragment collapsed on the medial edge of the distal fragment.

to 20 mm thick with respect to both its medial and lateral sides. The osteotomy should be carried to the opposite cortex just before reaching the periosteum. Careful direct and indirect (x-ray) visualization of the angle and depth of wedge resection is imperative. In addition, radiographic verification that proximal guide pins have remained parallel to the mediolateral joint line throughout the entire procedure will help prevent intraarticular penetration and fracture. If fracture should occur, accurate open reduction and internal fixation are necessary, with arthrotomy used for verification of correct articular reduction.

Osteotomy Fixation

Stable internal fixation will encourage rapid healing, preservation of correction, restoration of articular function and nourishment, and early resumption of weight bearing. Most forms of fixation of the lateral closing wedge osteotomy rely on an intact medial cortex, which, if violated, may require further stabilization (Fig. 57.13). Staples are still commonly used today, and, although no evidence exists that loss of correction occurs as a result of this method, some authors feel that more stable fixation (e.g., a blade plate, or plate and screws, or external fixator) is required to prevent recurrence of deformity.

Problems with internal and external fixation of the osteotomy are not unique to this procedure. It must be kept in mind that the osteotomy that is created is the equivalent of fracture and that, eventually, without bone healing, there will be implant failure (Fig. 57.14). Screw *cut-out* from proximal fragment and into the osteotomy site due to inadequate proximal fragment thickness can occur, especially if the fragments are compressed using a compression device. Screw loosening and *pull-out* may occur due to excessive loading in the early postoperative period. External fixation risks pin tract infection. Inadequate purchase of fixator pins in osteoporotic or osteopenic bone, stripping, and heat necrosis of the far cortices of the osteotomy fragments during pin insertion, as well as poor patient compliance with fixator precautions may result in pin loosening and resultant loss of correction.

Conclusion

High tibial osteotomy has proven to be a useful, pain-relieving procedure in the treatment of varus gonarthrosis. It can delay or preclude the need for total knee replacement and is an attractive alternative to unicondylar knee arthroplasty in the younger, more active patient. However, complications can occur both during the procedure as well as postoperatively.

Undercorrection or excessive overcorrection are the most common complications of HTO. A postoperative alignment of 8 to 10 degrees of anatomic valgus is desirable for good-to-excellent long-term results. Careful preoperative planning and attention to detail can help achieve this goal. A long-standing 51-inch AP radiograph of the lower extremity, demonstrating the hip-knee-

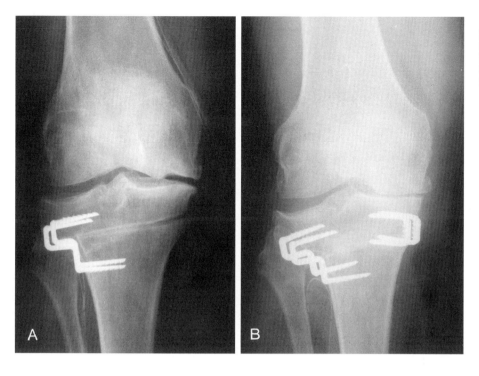

Figure 57.13. A, Unrecognized medial penetration will result in instability and loss of correction if insufficient internal fixation is utilized. **B,** Gaping at the osteotomy site medially was noted, and corrected with medial fixation.

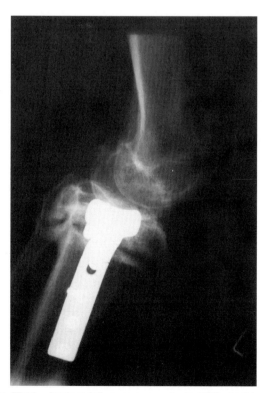

Figure 57.14. Implant failure can complicate HTO. In this photograph, an infratubercular osteotomy was performed which resulted in a nonunion. The plate used in this case has broken at the proximal plate hole.

ankle axis with the presence of a magnification marker, will allow accurate planning of the anatomic and mechanical axes correction of the position, as well as correct determination of wedge size.

Peroneal nerve and vascular injury can be disastrous. Meticulous dissection and careful placement of retractors and other instruments are important in avoiding trauma to the neurovascular bundle. The use of intraoperative fluoroscopy eliminates many of the potential dangers involved in the technical performance of this operation. Intraarticular fracture and improper guide pin placement may be averted with intraoperative radiographs.

While complications in high tibial osteotomy may occur, they can be minimized with careful patient selection, detailed preoperative planning, and meticulous surgical technique. Thus, the orthopedic surgeon should not be discouraged from using this valuable reconstructive procedure in the treatment of varus gonarthrosis.

References

1. Aglietti P, Rinonapoli E, Stringa G, Taviani A. Tibial osteotomy for the varus osteoarthritic knee. Clin Orthop 1983; 176:239–251.
2. Ahlback S. Osteoarthritis of the knee: A radiographic investigation. Acta Radiol. (Suppl 277) 1968.
3. Appel H, Friberg S. The effect of high tibial osteotomy on pain in osteoarthritis of the knee joint. Acta Orthop Scand 1972; 43:558.
4. Bauer GCH, Insall J, Koshino T. Tibial osteotomy in gonarthrosis (osteo-arthritis of the knee). J Bone Joint Surg 1969; 51-A:1545–1563.

5. Beltrami P, Calandriello B, Coli G. Axial deviations of the knee with secondary arthrosis: Correction by high osteotomy of the tibia and fibula. J Italian Orthop Traumatol 1976; 2:163–179.

6. Bourguignon RL. Combined Coventry-Maquet tibial osteotomy: preliminary report of two cases. Clin Orthop 1981; 160:144–148.

7. Cass JR, Bryan RS. High tibial osteotomy. Clin Orthop 1988; 230:196–199.

8. Cassarino A, Pappalardo S. High-domed tibial osteotomy in the treatment of angular deviations of the knee: A new system of surgical instrumentation. Italian J Orthop Traumatol 1985; 11(3)331–339.

9. Chan RNW, Pollard JP. High tibial osteotomy for rheumatoid arthritis of the knee: A one- to six-year follow-up study. Acta Orthop Scand 1978; 49:78–84.

10. Coventry MB. Osteotomy of the upper portion of the tibia for degenerative arthritis of the knee: A preliminary report. J Bone Joint Surg 1965; 47-A:984.

11. Coventry MB. Stepped staple for upper tibial osteotomy. J Bone Joint Surg 1969; 51-A:1011.

12. Coventry MB. Osteotomy about the knee for degenerative and rheumatoid arthritis: Indications, operative technique and results. J Bone Joint Surg 1973; 55-A:23.

13. Coventry MB. Upper tibial osteotomy for gonarthrosis: The evolution of the operation in the last 18 years and long-term results. Orthop Clin North Am 1979; 10:191–210.

14. Coventry MB. Upper tibial osteotomy. Clin Orthop 1984; 182:46–52.

15. Coventry MB. Current concepts review: Upper tibial osteotomy for osteoarthritis. J Bone Joint Surg 1985; 67-A:1136–1140.

16. Coventry, MB. Proximal tibial varus osteotomy for osteoarthritis of the lateral compartment of the knee. J Bone Joint Surg 1987; 69-A:32–38.

17. Coventry MB. Osteotomy about the knee: Principles of treatment. In: Chapman MW ed. Operative Orthopaedics, Vol. 1, Philadelphia: JB Lippincott, 1988:705–712.

18. Coventry MB. Valgus osteotomy of the upper tibia. Tech Orthop 1989; 4:35–40.

19. Coventry MB. The effect of axial alignment of the lower extremity on articular cartilage of the knee. In: Ewing, JW ed. Articular Cartilage and Knee Joint Function: Basic Science and Arthroscopy. New York: Raven Press, 1990: 311–317.

20. Coventry MB, Bowman PW. Long-term results of upper tibial osteotomy for degenerative arthritis of the knee. Acta Orthop Belgica 1982; 48:139–156.

21. Coventry MB, Ilstrup DM, Wallrichs SL. Proximal tibial osteotomy. A critical long-term study of eighty-seven cases. J Bone Joint Surg 1993; 75-A:196–201.

22. DeLaurentis DA, Levitsky KA, Booth RE, Rothman RH, Calligaro KD, Raviola CA, Savarese RP. Arterial and ischemic aspects of total knee arthroplasty. Am J Surg 1992; 164:237–240.

23. Devas MB. High tibial osteotomy for arthritis of the knee. A method secially suitable for the elderly. J Bone Joint Surg 1969; 51-B:95.

24. Dobner JJ, Nitz AJ. Postmeniscectomy tourniquet palsy and functional sequelae. Am J Sports Med 1982; 10(4) 211–214.

25. Dugdale TW, Noyes FR, Styer D. Preoperative planning for high tibial osteotomy. The effect of lateral tibiofemoral separation and tibiofemoral length. Clin Orthop 1992; 274:248–264.

26. Edholm P, Lindahl O, Lindholm B, Myrnerts R, Olsson KE, Wennberg E. Acta Orthop Scand 1977; 48:95–98.

27. Engel GM, Lippert FG, III. Valgus tibial osteotomy: Avoiding the pitfalls. Clin Orthop 1981; 160:137–143.

28. Estersohn HS, Sourifman HA. The minimum effective midthigh tourniquet pressure. J Foot Surg 1982; 21(4):281–284.

29. Fujisawa Y, Masuhara K, Shiomi S. The effect of high tibial osteotomy on osteoarthritis of the knee: An arthroscopic study of 54 knee joints. Orthop Clin North Am 1979; 10:585–608.

30. Giannestras NJ, Cranley JJ, Lentz M. Occlusion of the tibial artery after a foot operation under tourniquet. A case report. J Bone Joint Surg 1977; 59-A:682–683.

31. Gibson MJ, Barnes MR, Allen MJ, Chan RNW. Weakness of foot dorsiflexion and changes in compartment pressures after tibial osteotomy. J Bone Joint Surg 1986; 68-B:471–475.

32. Ha'eri GB, Wiley AM. High tibial osteotomy combined with joint debridement: A long-term study of results. Clin Orthop 1980; 151:153–159.

33. Hagstedt B, Norman O, Olsson TH, Thornstrand B. Technical accuracy in high tibial osteotomy for gonarthrosis. Acta Orthop Scand 1980; 51:963.

34. Harding ML. A fresh appraisal of tibial osteotomy for osteoarthritis of the knee. Clin Orthop 1976; 114:223–224.

35. Harris WR, Kostuik JP. High tibial osteotomy for osteo-arthritis of the knee. J Bone Joint Surg 1970; 52-A:330–336.

36. Healy WL, Anglen JO, Wasilewski SA, Krakow KA. Distal femoral varus osteotomy. J Bone Joint Surg 1988; 70-A:102–109.

37. Healy WL, Riley LH. High tibial valgus osteotomy. A clinical review. Clin Orthop 1986; 209:227–233.

38. Hernigou PH, Medevielle D, Debeyre J, Goutallier D. Proximal tibial osteotomy for osteoarthritis with varus deformity. A ten to thirteen-year follow-up study. J Bone Joint Surg 1987; 69-A:332–353.

39. Hofmann AA, Wyatt RWB, Beck SW. High tibial osteotomy: Use of an osteotomy jig, rigid fixation, and early motion versus conventional surgical technique and cast immobilization. Clin Orthop 1991; 271:212–217.

40. Hofmann AA, Wyatt RWB, Jones RE. Combined Coventry-Maquet procedure for two-compartment degenerative arthritis. Clin Orthop 1984; 190:186–191.

41. Holden DL, James SL, Larson RL, Slocum DB. Proximal tibial osteotomy in patients who are fifty years old or less: A long-term follow-up study. J Bone Joint Surg 1988; 70-A:977–982.

42. Hsu RWW. The study of Maquet dome high tibial osteotomy: arthroscopic-assisted analysis. Clin Orthop 1989; 243:280–295.

43. Hsu RWW, Himeno, Shinkichi, Coventry MB, Chao EYS. Normal axial alignment of the lower extremity and load-bearing distribution at the knee. Clin Orthop 1990; 255:215–227.

44. Insall JN, Joseph DM, Msika C. High tibial osteotomy for varus gonarthrosis. A long-term follow-up study. J Bone Joint Surg 1984; 66-A:1040–1048.

45. Insall J, Shoji H, Mayer V. High tibial osteotomy: a five-year evaluation. J Bone Joint Surg 1974; 56-A:1397–1405.

46. Iversson I, Mynerts R, Gillquist J. High tibial osteotomy for medial osteoarthritis of the knee: A 5- to 7- and an 11- to 13-year follow-up. J Bone Joint Surg 1990; 72-B:238–244.

47. Ivey M, Cantrell JS. Lateral tibial plateau fracture as a postoperative complication of high tibial osteotomy. Orthopaedics 1985; 8(8):1009–1113.

48. Jackson JP. Osteotomy for osteoarthritis of the knee. In: Proceedings of the Sheffield Regional Orthopaedic Club. J Bone Joint Surg 1958; 40-B(4):826.

49. Jackson JP, Waugh W. Tibial osteotomy for osteoarthritis of the knee. J Bone Joint Surg 1961; 43-B(4):746–751.

50. Jackson JP, Waugh W. The technique and complications of upper tibial osteotomy. A review of 226 operations. J Bone Joint Surg 1974; 56-B(2):236–245.

51. Jackson JP, Waugh W, Green JP. High tibial osteotomy for osteoarthritis of the knee. J Bone Joint Surg 1969; 51-B:88–94.

52. Job-Deslandre C, Languepin A, Benvenuto M, Menkes CJ. Tibial valgization osteotomy in gonarthrosis with or without chondrocalcinosis. Results after 5 years. Rev Rhum Mal Osteoartic 1991; 58(7):491–496.

53. Johnson G, Leite S, Waugh W. The distribution of load across the knee. A comparison of static and dynamic measurements. J Bone Joint Surg 1980; 62-B(3):346–349.

54. Johnson F, Waugh W. Evidence for compensatory gait in patients with a valgus knee deformity. Acta Orthop Belg 1980; 46(5):558–565.

55. Jokio PJ, Lindholm TS. The angle-measuring device, a practical resource in high tibial osteotomy. Ann Chir Gynaecol 1991; 80:54–58.

56. Jokio PJ, Lindholm TS, Vankka E. Medial and lateral gonarthrosis treated with high tibial osteotomy: A preoperative study. Arch Orthop Trauma Surg 1985; 104(3):135–144.

57. Katz MM, Hungerford DS, Krackow KA, Lennox DW. Results of total knee arthroplasty after failed proximal tibial osteotomy for osteoarthritis. J Bone Joint Surg 1987; 69-A:225–233.

58. Keene JS, Dyreby JR, Jr. High tibial osteotomy in the treatment of osteoarthritis of the knee. The role of preoperative arthroscopy. J Bone Joint Surg 1983; 65-A:36–42.

59. Keene JS, Monson DK, Roberts JM, Dyreby JR, Jr. The evaluation of patients for high tibial osteotomy. Clin Orthop 1989; 243:157–165.

60. Kettelkamp DB, Chao EYS. A method for quantitative analysis of medial and lateral compression forces at the knee during standing. Clin Orthop 1972; 83:202–213.

61. Kettelkamp DB, Leach RE, Nasca R. Pitfalls of proximal osteotomy. Clin Orthop 1975; 106:232–241.

62. Kettelkamp DB, Wenger DR, Chao EYS, Thompson C. Results of proximal tibial osteotomy. The effects of tibiofemoral angle, stance-phase flexion-extension, and medial-plateau force. J Bone Joint Surg 1976; 58-A:952–960.

63. Kim YH. The incidence of deep vein thrombosis after cementless and cemented knee replacement. J Bone Joint Surg 1990; 72-B:779–783.

64. Kirgis A, Albrecht S. Palsy of the deep peroneal nerve after proximal tibial osteotomy. J Bone Joint Surg 1992; 74-A:1180–1185.

65. Klenerman L. The tourniquet in surgery. J Bone Joint Surg 1962; 44-B:937–943.

66. Koshino T. The treatment of spontaneous osteonecrosis of the knee by high tibial osteotomy with and without bone-grafting or drilling of the lesion. J Bone Joint Surg 1982; 64-A:47–58.

67. Koshino T, Morii T, Wada J, Saito H, Ozawa N, Noyori K. High tibial osteotomy with fixation by a blade-plate for medial compartment osteoarthritis of the knee. Orthop Clin North Am 1989; 20(2):227–243.

68. Koshino T, and Tsuchiya K. The effect of high tibial osteotomy on osteoarthritis of the knee, clinical and histological observation. Internat Orthop 1979; 3:37–45.
69. Krackow KA, and Holtgrewe JL. Experience with a new technique for managing severely overcorrected valgus high tibial osteotomy at total knee arthroplasty. Clin Orthop 1990; 256:213–224.
70. Krempen JF, and Silver RA. Experience with the Maquet barrel-vault osteotomy. Clin Orthop 1982; 168:86–96.
71. Kroese AJ, and Stiris G. The risk of deep-vein thrombosis after operations on a bloodless lower limb. A venographic study. Injury 1976; 7:271–273.
72. Lemaire R. Etude critique de l'ostéotomie tibiale dans la gonarthrose, Acta Orthop Belg 1977; 43:741–766.
73. LeMaire R. Etude comparative dé deux series d'ostéotomies tibialis avec fixation par lame-plaque ou par cadre de compression. Acta Orthop Belg 1982; 48:157.
74. Luk KDK, and Pun WK. Unrecognised compartment syndrome in a patient with tourniquet palsy. J Bone Joint Surg 1987; 69-B:97–99.
75. MacIntosh DL, and Welsh RP. Joint debridement—a complement to high tibial osteotomy in the treatment of degenerative arthritis of the knee. J Bone Joint Surg 1977; 59-A:1094–1097.
76. Maquet PG. Biomechanics of the knee. Berlin: Springer-Verlag, 1976.
77. Maquet, Paul. Valgus osteotomy for osteoarthritis of the knee. Clin Orthop 1976; 120:143–148.
78. Matthews LS, Goldstein SA, Malvitz TA, Katz BP, Kaufer H. Proximal tibial osteotomy: factors that influence the duration of satisfactory function. Clin Orthop 1988; 229:193–200.
79. McAuley CE, Steed DL, and Webster MW. Arterial complications of total knee replacement. Arch Surg 1984; 119:960–962.
80. McLaren CAN, Wootton JR, Heath PD, Wynn Jones CH. Pes planus after tibial osteotomy. Foot Ankle 1989; 9(6):300–303.
81. Miniaci A, Ballmer FT, Ballmer PM, Jakob RP. Proximal tibial osteotomy: A new fixation device. Clin Orthop 1989; 246:250–259.
82. Morrey BF. Upper tibial osteotomy: analysis of prognostic: A review. Adv Orthop Surg 1986; 213–222.
83. Morrey BF. Upper tibial osteotomy for secondary osteoarthritis of the knee. J Bone Joint Surg 1989; 71B(4):554–559.
84. Moser KM. Pathophysiology of venous thromboembolism. Semin Arthroplasty 1992; 3(2):64–71.
85. Mynerts R. The SAAB jig: An aid in high tibial osteotomy. Acta Orthop Scand 1978; 49:85–88.
86. Mynerts R. High tibial osteotomy with overcorrection of varus malalignment in medial gonarthrosis. Acta Orthop Scand 1980; 51:557–560.
87. Mynerts R. Knee instability before and after high tibial osteotomy. Acta Orthop Scand 1980; 51:561–564.
88. Mynerts R. Clinical results with the SAAB jig in high tibial osteotomy for medial gonarthrosis. Acta Orthop Scand 1980; 51:565.
89. Mynerts R. Failure of the correction of varus deformity obtained by high tibial osteotomy. Acta Orthop Scand 1980; 51:569–573.
90. Mynerts R. Optimal correction in high tibial osteotomy for varus deformity. Acta Orthop Scand 1980; 51:689–694.
91. Nguyen C, Rudan J, Simurda MA, Cook TD. High tibial osteotomy compared with high tibial and Maquet procedures in medial and patellofemoral compartment osteoarthritis. Clin Orthop 1989; 245:179–187.
92. Odenbring S, Egund N, Lindstrand A, Tjörnstrand B. A guide instrument for high tibial osteotomy. Act Orthop Scand 1989; 60(4):449–451.
93. Ogata K. Interlocking wedge osteotomy of the proximal tibia for gonarthrosis. Clin Orthop 1984; 186:129–134.
94. O'Neill DF, James SL. Valgus osteotomy with anterior cruciate ligament laxity. Clin Orthop 1992; 278:153–159.
95. Prodromos CC, Andriacchi TP, Galante JO. A relationship between gait and clinical changes following high tibial osteotomy. J Bone Joint Surg 1985; 67-A:1188–1194.
96. Putnam MD, Mears DC, Fu FH. Combined Maquet and proximal tibial valgus osteotomy. Clin Orthop 1985; 197:217–223.
97. Rand JA, Morrey BF, Bryan RS. Patellar tendon rupture after total knee arthroplasty. Clin Orthop 1989; 244:233–238.
98. Ranieri L, Traina GC, Maci C. High tibial osteotomy in osteoarthrosis of the knee: a long term clinical study of 187 knees. So Ital J Orthop Traumatol 1977; 3:289–300.
99. Rinonapoli E, Aglietti P, Mancini GB, Buzzi R. High tibial osteotomy in the treatment of arthritic varus knee. A medium long-term (small) review of 61 cases. Ital J Orthop Traumatol 1988; 14(3):283–292.
100. Rorabeck CH, Kennedy JC. Tourniquet-induced nerve ischemia complicating knee ligament surgery. Am J Sports Med 1980; 8(2):98–102.
101. Ruebens F, Wellington JL, Bouchard AG. Politeal artery injury after tibial osteotomy: report of two cases. Can J Surg 1990; 33(4):294–297.
102. Rudan JF, Simurda MA. Valgus high tibial osteotomy: a long-term follow-up study. Clin Orthop 1991; 268:157–160.
103. Rudan JF, Simurda MA. High tibial osteotomy. A prospective clinical and roentgenographic review. Clin Orthop 1990; 255:251–256.
104. Shea JD. Osteoarthrosis of the knee: Diagnosis and complications of treatment by high tibial osteotomy. South Med J 1973; 66(9):1030–1034.
105. Shoji H, Insall J. High tibial osteotomy for osteoarthritis of the knee with valgus deformity. J Bone Joint Surg 1973; 55-A:963–973.
106. Siegal M. The Maquet osteotomy: A review of risks. Orthopedics 1987; 10:1073–1078.
107. Simon MA, Mass DP, Zarins CK, Bidani N, Gudas CJ, Metz CE. The effect of a thigh tourniquet on the incidence of deep venous thrombosis after operations on the fore part of the foot. J Bone Joint Surg 1982; 64-A:188–191.
108. Slocum DB, Larson RL, James SL, Grenier R. High tibial osteotomy. Clin Orthop 1974; 104:239–244.
109. Soccetti A, Giacchetta AM, Raffaelli P. Domed high tibial osteotomy: the long-term results in tibiofemoral arthritis with and without malalignment of the extensor apparatus. Ital J Orthop Traumatol 1987; 13(4):463–475.
110. Specchiulli F, Laforgia R, Solarino GB. Tibial osteotomy in the treatment of varus osteoarthritic knee. Ital J Orthop Traumatol 1990; 16(4):507–514.
111. Staeheli J, Cass JR, Morrey BF. Condylar total knee arthroplasty after failed upper tibial osteotomy. J Bone Joint Surg 1987; 69-A:28–31.
112. Stuart MJ, Grace JN, Illstrup DM, Kelly CM, Adams RA, Morrey BF. Late recurrence of varus deformity after proximal tibial osteotomy. Clin Orthop 1990; 260:61–65.
113. Stürz H, Rosemeyer B. The isolated loss of extension of the great toe following osteotomy of the fibula. Z Orthop 1979; 117:31–38.
114. Sundaram NA, Hallet JP, Sullivan MF. Dome osteotomy of the tibia for osteoarthritis of the knee. J Bone Joint Surg 1986; 68B:782–786.
115. Surin V, Markhede G, Sundholm K. Factors influencing results of high tibial osteotomy in gonarthrosis. Acta Orthop Scand 1975; 46:996–1007.
116. Tjörnstrand BAE, Egund N, Hagstedt BV. High tibial osteotomy: a seven-year clinical and radiographic follow-up. Clin Orthop 1981; 160:124–136.
117. Tjörnstrand BAE, Egund N, Hagstedt BV, Lindstrand A. Tibial osteotomy in medial gonarthrosis: the importance of over-correction of varus deformity. Arch Orthop Trauma Surg 1981; 99:83–89.
118. Wang JW, Kuo KN, Andriacchi TP, Galante JO. The influence of walking mechanics and time on the results of proximal osteotomy. J Bone Joint Surg., 1990; 72-A:905–909.
119. Wagner H. Indication and technic of corrective osteotomy in post-traumatic authors of the knee joint. Hefte zur Unfallheilkunde 1976; 128:155–174.
120. Williams TA, Baerg RH, Beal WS. Acute arterial occlusion secondary to the use of a pneumatic thigh tourniquet. A case report. J Am Podiatr Med Assoc 1986; 76(8):464–465.
121. Windsor RE, Insall JN, Vince KG. Technical considerations of total knee arthroplasty after proximal tibial osteotomy. J Bone Joint Surg 1988; 70-A:547–555.
122. Vainionpaa S, Laike E, Kirves P, Tiusanen P. Tibial osteotomy for osteoarthritis of the knee. A five to ten year follow-up study. J Bone Joint Surg 1981; 63-A:938–946.
123. Valenti JR, Calvo R, Lopez R, Cañadell J. Long-term evaluation of high tibial valgus osteotomy. Int Orthop (SICOT) 1990; 14:347–349.

58

Distal Femoral Osteotomy

Anthony Miniaci and Larry W. Watson

Introduction

Corrective osteotomy about the knee is a well established treatment for patients with deformities that may or may not be associated with unicompartmental arthrosis. Certainly proximal tibial osteotomies have been used successfully in the treatment of various knee deformities as well as for ligament instabilities.

Valgus knee deformities requiring corrective surgery are uncommon and difficult to manage. The deformity is often, but not always, associated with lateral compartment gonarthrosis. Valgus deformity can be associated with other conditions such as growth abnormalities, trauma, rickets, renal osteodystrophy, polio, or ligament instabilities. Several surgical options have been proposed for the treatment of this condition including proximal tibial varus osteotomy (2, 5, 7, 10, 13), supracondylar femoral varus osteotomies (1–4, 6–8, 14, 16–18, 21–29) and unicompartmental arthroplasty (9, 20) or total knee arthroplasty (12) in the elderly patient with associated lateral compartment arthrosis. Because of the advances in prosthesis design, materials, and surgical technique, knee arthroplasty has become a popular choice for treatment of elderly patients with arthrosis and it has made the role of distal femoral varus osteotomy in this condition uncertain. There are, however, situations where osteotomy becomes an option. Proximal tibial varus osteotomy has been reported as a successful technique (11) to treat valgus deformities; however, results are not consistent and many failures and complications have occurred, so that most physicians choose to correct valgus knee deformities above the level of the knee joint (12, 22, 23). With a valgus knee deformity, the joint line often slopes superolaterally, and this condition cannot be corrected well with a proximal tibial varus osteotomy. Therefore, if the slope of the joint is greater than 10 degrees or if the valgus deformity exceeds 12 to 15 degrees, the osteotomy should be performed in the supracondylar area of the femur.

The goals of the osteotomy largely depend on the patient's complaints, including pain and instability. For patients with pain, correction of the angular deformity theoretically unloads the lateral compartment and can diminish pain. Patients with symptomatic instability often have associated ligamentous insufficiencies. In these situations, correction of the mechanical axis is necessary before ligament reconstruction is considered or performed. In some cases, the symptomatic instability will subside with correction of the deformity and may obviate the need for an additional ligamentous procedure.

It seems, therefore, that distal femoral varus osteotomy is a useful technique for treating disorders of the knee. It can effectively correct the mechanical axis of a valgus knee, transfer the load from the lateral to medial compartment, and correct the valgus tilt of the joint line without interfering with the primary stabilizers of the knee. Clinically, distal femoral osteotomies have enjoyed widespread success in both Europe and North America. This chapter defines the indications, reviews the results and complications, and describes techniques for distal femoral varus osteotomies.

Surgical Indications

Proper patient selection is essential to good results. Surgery is considered for correction of valgus deformity that is greater than 10 to 15 degrees and that may be associated with arthrosis, pain, instability, or a combination of these. Conservative therapy, including physiotherapy, nonsteroidal antiinflammatories, and bracing will have already been tried. Patients should have a relatively good knee motion. Arthrosis and flexion deformities greater than 20 degrees or an arc of motion less than 90 degrees are relative contraindications. We do not find that subluxation and instability are contraindications to osteotomy. Osteotomies that correct mechanical axis deviation can often treat symptomatic instabilities. Tricompartmental arthrosis, inflammatory joint disorders, and poor bone quality are relative contraindications to surgery.

Surgical Results

Several European studies suggest that good results are obtainable in over 80% of patients who have undergone distal femoral osteotomy. However, many of these studies lack objective data in support of their conclusions and involve a relatively short follow-up. Wagner, et al. (28), has published the largest review in the German literature, a review which revealed excellent results. Most of these studies consisted of a medial closing wedge osteotomy with rigid internal fixation.

Maquet (17) has obtained good results with an external fixator and a transverse supracondylar osteotomy performed through a 5 cm medial incision. Four transfixion pins are drilled through the femur, one pair being transcondylar and parallel to the joint and the other pair transdiaphyseal and perpendicular to the diaphysis. After the osteotomy, the pins are made parallel by impaction of the proximal fragment of the femur into the distal fragment. The pins are then fixed by a medial and lateral external compression clamp. The advantages to this technique are the compression that can be applied through the osteotomy site and the ability to adjust the alignment. The disadvantages are that the external fixator is cumbersome, pin tract problems can develop, and the knee may become stiff.

Johnson and Godell (16) were the first to report their experience with corrective supracondylar osteotomies in North America. They reviewed 46 patients who had had 53 corrective medial closing wedge osteotomies for painful genu valgum. These patients were followed for an average of 43.8 months. Clinically, 39 of the 46 patients (85%) were satisfied. The 7 clinical failures included 1 patient with profound knee stiffness, 2 patients who had no relief of their pain, and 4 patients who required conversion to a total knee arthroplasty. Objectively, if one included any patient who required reoperation, had persistent pain, had less than 70 degrees of motion, or had symptomatic loss of leg length, then 30% of the osteotomies were considered to have a poor result. Neither age nor the cause of the pathology affected the results, but those patients with a deformity of 26 degrees or more had a greater than 50% chance of a poor result. Complications included 1 infection, 7 patients with functional loss of knee motion, 7 delayed unions and 3 nonunions. Their conclusions were that medial closing wedge supracondylar osteotomies were a viable therapeutic choice in selected patients, but the surgical procedure was technically demanding and relatively unforgiving.

In 1988, Healy, et al. (11) and McDermott, et al. (18) both presented their experiences with distal femoral varus osteotomies. Healy reviewed 21 patients who had 23 medial closing wedge osteotomies secured with a 90 degree blade plate. The average length of follow-up was 4 years with a minimum of 2 years. Overall, 83% of the knees treated were classified as good or excellent ac-

cording to the Hospital for Special Surgery Knee Score, and 86% were satisfied with their surgery. Of interest was that 93% of the patients who had osteoarthritis had good or excellent results, while all 3 osteotomies in patients with rheumatoid arthritis did poorly. Complications included 2 nonunions, 1 patient who required manipulation under anaesthesia for stiffness, 2 arthroscopies for persistent pain, and 2 total knee replacements in patients with rheumatoid arthritis. The authors concluded that varus osteotomy of the distal femur was a reliable and effective treatment of gonarthrosis associated with valgus deformity due to osteoarthritis or trauma. They confirmed that the procedure should not be recommended in patients with rheumatoid arthritis or in those patients with poor motion.

McDermott, et al. (18) reviewed 24 patients who had degenerative arthritis of the lateral compartment of the knee associated with a valgus deformity. These patients were treated with a medial wedge closing osteotomy and fixation with a 90 degree blade plate. These patients were followed for an average of 4 years with 92% (22 of 24 patients) having a successful outcome. Complications included 1 pulmonary embolus, 1 failure of fixation requiring revision surgery, 1 superficial infection, 1 patient requiring a manipulation under general anaesthesia for persistent knee stiffness, and 1 patient requiring conversion to a total knee arthroplasty for progressive painful arthrosis. The authors concluded this was an effective and reproducible surgical technique.

In 1990, Miniaci, et al. (19) presented a review of 40 supracondylar femoral closing wedge varus osteotomies for valgus knee deformities fixed with either a medial or lateral blade plate. Thirty-five patients were available for clinical and radiographic evaluation at an average of 5.5 years postoperatively with a minimum 2-year follow-up. Of the 35 patients, 30 (86%) had a good or excellent result. In the patients with only a valgus deformity and no arthrosis, 100% had good or excellent results. Twenty-one of 26, or 81%, with associated lateral compartment gonarthrosis, had a good or excellent result using the Hospital for Special Surgery Knee Scoring System. Twenty-five of the 26 patients, or 96%, stated they had significant improvement of their pain. Poor results were associated with a longer time to follow-up and failure to correct the femorotibial angle to 0 degrees. Age of the patient had no clear effect on the final functional results. Complications related to fixation occurred in 4 of the 35 patients (11%), and all occurred when medial plate fixation was used. No device failure occurred in those patients having lateral plate fixation.

The first 14 patients in the study had a closing wedge osteotomy with a 90 degree angled blade plate on the medial femur as recommended by the AO Manual. However, concerns surfaced regarding fixation with the medial plate when two patients had failure of the fixation device and two patients went on to nonunion. As a result of the alarmingly high rate of failure with medial plate fixation (29%), the authors changed to an oblique closing wedge osteotomy with a 7-hole 90 degree condylar blade plate affixed to the lateral side of the femur (Fig. 58.1 and 58.2). This technique was primarily used

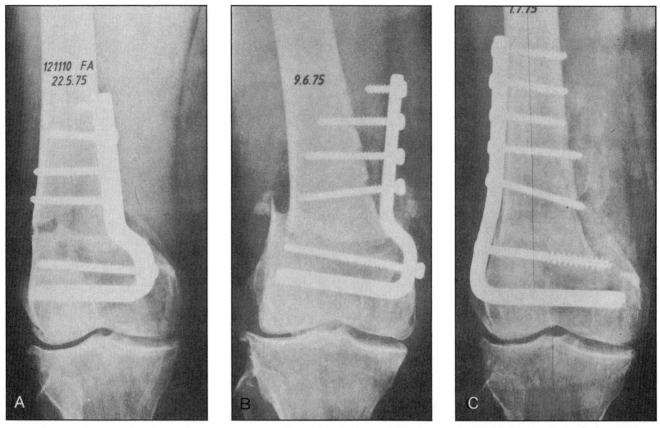

Figure 58.1. **A,** Supracondylar femoral varus osteotomy and medial plate fixation performed for valgus deformity with lateral gonarthrosis in a 64-year-old male. **B,** Subsequently, the medial plate failed as the screws pulled out of the femur. **C,** A second operation with a seven-hole condylar plate on the lateral side resulted in union of the osteotomy. (Reproduced with permission from Miniaci A, Grossmann SP, Jakob RP. Supracondylar femoral varus osteotomy in the treatment of valgus knee deformity. Am J Knee Surg 1990;3:69.)

in the next 21 patients with no occurrence of nonunion or failure of fixation. In addition, the four medial plate failures all had revision surgery using the lateral plate technique, and three of the four went on to uneventful union. The fourth patient had several reoperations for this problem but had persistent pain and had to be converted to a total knee arthroplasty. This accounted for the only poor result in that group.

The failures of fixation medially and the superior fixation by the lateral plate were attributed to violation of the tension band principles with medial fixation (Fig. 58.3). If one considers the normal knee with a valgus femorotibial angle loaded in a single leg stance, then the lateral aspect of the femur is the tension side secondary to the extrinsic varus component of the body weight. In severe genu valgum, the mechanical axis moves laterally so that the medial side becomes subjected to tensile forces; it was for this reason that medial plate fixation has been recommended and utilized. However, when the osteotomy has been performed in the valgus knee, the mechanical axis is moved medially, which again restores the tensile forces to the lateral side of the femur. To act as a tension band, therefore, the plate needs to be applied to the lateral aspect of the femur. Medial plate application places it on the compression side and can potentially lead to nonunion. For this reason, the

authors preference is to fix the osteotomy from the lateral side through a lateral approach. Nevertheless, medial approaches have been used successfully by many surgeons with good clinical results.

In conclusion, supracondylar femoral varus osteotomy is a reliable procedure to realign the knee with valgus deformity. The results are superior in the absence of gonarthrosis, but the procedure still provides over 80% good or excellent long-term results, even when lateral compartment arthrosis is present. Correction of the femorotibial angle to 0 degrees is generally felt to be important to a successful result.

Surgical Technique

Preoperative Planning

Careful preoperative planning is required for a successful osteotomy. Routine standing AP (anteroposterior), lateral, and patellofemoral views of the knee are needed to adequately assess the joint. Full length, hip to ankle, weight-bearing radiographs should be obtained to assess the femorotibial angle and the mechanical axis of the extremity.

The normal femorotibial angle is 5 to 7 degrees of valgus and is formed by the intersection of the lines drawn through the long axis of the femur and tibia. The

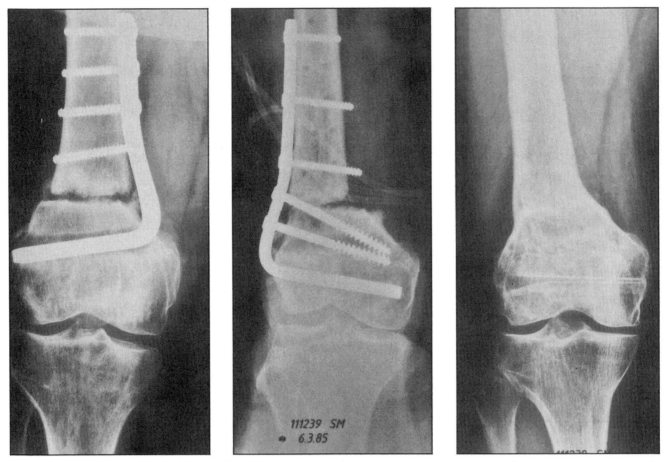

Figure 58.2. **A,** A 46-year-old male with nonunion of the osteotomy. The first operation was the standard, closing wedge, femoral varus osteotomy with a medial right-angled blade plate. **B,** A second operation was necessary because of nonunion. A lateral seven-hole condylar plate was used to provide fixation. An oblique screw across the osteotomy was used to compress the osteotomy. **C,** One year after the second operation, the osteotomy was healed, and the patient had a good result. (Reproduced with permission from Miniaci A, Grossmann SP, Jakob RP. Supracondylar femoral varus osteotomy in the treatment of valgus knee deformity. Am J Knee Surg 1990;3:70.)

normal mechanical axis is 0 and is determined by two lines. One line is drawn from the center of the hip joint to the center of the knee, the second line is drawn from the center of the knee to the center of the ankle joint. These lines should form one straight line in the well-aligned knee. The surgical goal of distal femoral varus osteotomy should be to restore the femorotibial angle to 0 degrees, which represents an overcorrection of 5 to 7 degrees from the usual angle (Fig. 58.4).

Medial Technique

The patient is placed supine on an operating room table that is equipped with a fluoroscope. The knee is draped to allow the surgeon to extend and flex the knee to 90 degrees as needed. A tourniquet is optional. A longitudinal medial incision is standard, but a straight midline incision can be used if future arthroplasty is a consideration. The incision begins just distal to the joint and extends proximally 15 cm. The dissection is carried down to the joint capsule and the fascia of the vastus medialis muscle. The vastus medialis is then dissected from the septum and retracted anteriorly, exposing the

medial femoral cortex and condyle. Blunt retractors maintain the exposure, with care taken to avoid injury of the femoral vessels. Bleeding from the posterior perforating arteries is common and should be controlled.

With the knee flexed 90 degrees, a guide wire is passed from the medial to lateral sides through the medial femoral condyle 2 cm proximal to the joint. A pin should be placed that parallels the femoral articular surface. This pin guides the blade plate seating chisel. A second pin is inserted just proximal to the adductor tubercle and should parallel the first pin. This pin helps guide the osteotomy. A third pin is inserted 3 cm proximal to the medial epicondyle and placed perpendicular to the long axis of the femur. A 90 degree pin guide may help in placement. This pin is proximal to and guides the proximal cut of the osteotomy. All should be parallel in the coronal plane to avoid rotational problems. The position of the pin should be confirmed with fluoroscopy. A medial arthrotomy may be done to confirm placement of the most distal pin or chisel.

Once the pins are in proper position, the seating chisel is inserted. The chisel should be placed in the an-

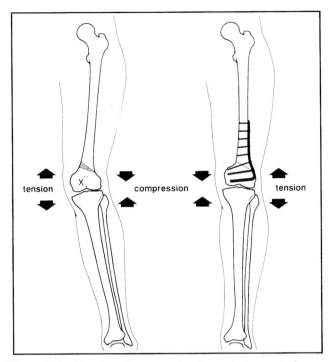

Figure 58.3. Tensile and compressive forces, before and after osteotomy. The plate should be applied to the lateral side to act as a tension band once the osteotomy is performed. (Reproduced with permission from Miniaci A, Grossmann SP, Jakob RP. Supracondylar femoral varus osteotomy in the treatment of valgus knee deformity. Am J Knee Surg 1990;3:72.)

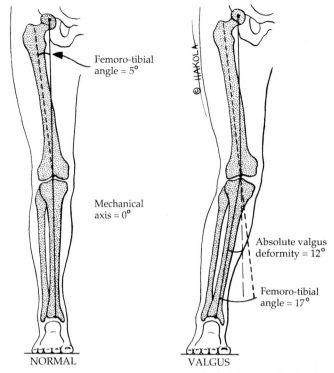

Figure 58.4. Determining valgus deformity. In this example, the true valgus deformity is only 12 degrees. In order to correct the femorotibial angle to 0 degrees, however, a correction of 17 degrees is necessary.

terior one-half of the femur and angled slightly posteriorly. This prevents the blade from exiting the anterior aspect of the lateral femoral condyle and allows it to be flush with the femoral shaft once seated. The chisel should be seated from 50 to 70 mm, depending on the size of the distal femur. The placement of the chisel is checked with fluoroscopy.

Once the surgeon is pleased with the placement of the seating chisel, the osteotomy may be performed with an oscillating saw. The distal cut should follow the second pin, which should be at least 2 cm above the chisel to ensure good fixation and stability distally. The lateral femoral cortex is perforated with a small osteotome to allow better control and prevent lateral translocation proximally. The proximal cut is then made with the oscillating saw, approximately 1 cm above the distal cut. This depends on the size of the medial wedge determined in the preoperative planning. A slightly smaller wedge is recommended to allow impaction of the proximal cortical fragment into the distal cancellous bone to improve stability. The cut should be parallel and distal to the proximal pin. Again, a small osteotome completes the cut on the lateral cortex. The wedge of bone is then removed and saved for graft.

The osteotomy is solidly closed so that the first and third pins are parallel. This ensures a femorotibial angle of 0 degrees. The second pin is removed and can be used to temporarily fix the osteotomy until the blade plate is inserted. A 90 degree blade plate is then se-

lected. The blade plates come in varying lengths and offsets and should be chosen appropriately. The blade plate is seated on the femur, and the distal condylar screw is inserted. Provisional fixation is removed, and the femoral shaft is secured. The first screw placed proximal to the osteotomy should be loaded according to the principles of dynamic compression plating. At least 4 bicortical screws should fix the proximal fragment. The knee should then be moved through a full range of motion and the osteotomy should be checked for stability (Fig. 58.5).

The cancellous bone from the wedge is used to graft the osteotomy. The wound is closed in layers over suction drains. A Jones compression dressing and knee immobilizer are applied in the operating room.

Some additional technical points require discussion. Although blade plates have been traditionally described as the fixation of choice, we prefer the dynamic condylar screw (DCS) because it provides good fixation and is simple to use. A second technical point is a simple method of assuring correction of the femorotibial angle to 0 degrees. This can be achieved easily with the 90 degree fixation device. Because the blade plate or screw and plate are angled at 90 degrees, inserting the screw parallel to the joint after the osteotomy is performed and seating the plate along the medial cortex of the femur automatically eliminates the valgus of the distal femur and makes the femorotibial angle 0 degrees.

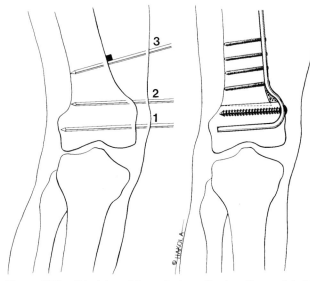

Figure 58.5. Principles of the osteotomy fixed on the medial side. The correction results in a femorotibial angle of 0 degrees.

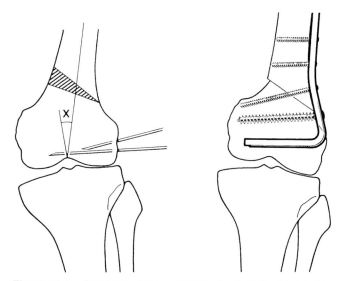

Figure 58.6. Principles of the osteotomy fixed on the lateral side. The correction (X) is required so that the resulting femorotibial angle is 0 degrees. An oblique osteotomy is fixed with a lateral condylar plate. An oblique screw directed through the plate compresses and stabilizes the osteotomy. (Reproduced with permission from Miniaci A, Grossmann SP, Jakob RP. Supracondylar femoral varus osteotomy in the treatment of valgus knee deformity. Am J Knee Surg 1990;3:68.)

Lateral Plate Fixation

The principles of preoperative planning and preparation of the patient are very similar to the medial fixation technique. The patient is supine on the operating table, fluoroscopy is used, and the knee should be free to flex to 90 degrees. Usually, a longitudinal lateral incision is made from just distal to the joint line for approximately 15 to 20 cm proximally. A straight midline incision (for those considering future arthroplasty) can be used but needs to be slightly longer. The iliotibial band is exposed and incised just anterior to the intermuscular septum. The vastus lateralis muscle is identified, dissected from the intermuscular septum, and retracted anteriorly and medially. The joint line and capsule are identified. The perforating vessels are exposed and cauterized.

With the knee flexed 90 degrees, a guide wire is inserted through the lateral femoral condyle 2 cm proximal and parallel to the joint. This positioning should be checked with fluoroscopy. The amount of correction needed to achieve a femorotibial angle of 0 degrees will have been determined preoperatively. A second pin is inserted that makes the angle of desired correction with the first pin (Fig. 58.6). The two pins should meet medially. This second pin guides the blade plate or can be used as the guide wire for the dynamic condylar screw. A third pin can be inserted proximally, parallel to the distal pin. Once the osteotomy is completed and fixed, this pin should be parallel to the screw or blade of the fixation device and the second pin. Finally, the osteotomy cuts are planned. An oblique osteotomy allows a compression screw to cross the site. The osteotomy hinges laterally and should be performed just above the supracondylar ridge approximately 2 to 3 cm proximal to the second pin. With the medial side well exposed, the amount of bone to be resected is marked. The cuts should start in the medial supracondylar area, an area

where one needs to be extremely careful of vascular structures. Good exposure is essential. Before beginning the osteotomy, the blade plate or the screw and plate should be partially inserted. Because the angle of insertion is not parallel to the joint, the 90 degree plate will abut the femur proximally. The osteotomy should be performed from medial to lateral without cutting but only perforating the lateral cortex. Using the plate as a handle, the osteotomy is closed. With the osteotomy closed, the plate should parallel the femur and be capable of being fully seated. It is important to assure that there has been no rotation and that the second and third pins are now parallel. The third hole on the plate is used to insert a compression screw across the osteotomy site. A seven- or eight-hole plate should suffice. Fluoroscopy is used to check the osteotomy and the plate and screws (Fig. 58.7). Bone grafting of the osteotomy with the removed bone is performed, and the wound is closed in the surgeon's preferred manner. Dressing and knee immobilizer are applied in the operating room.

Postoperative Management

Immediately postoperatively, analgesia, compression dressing, and cold therapy are employed. If stable internal fixation has been obtained, immediate knee motion is started. Continuous passive motion is optional. Patients walk with crutches allowing feather touch weight-bearing for a period of 6 to 8 weeks. Radiographic evaluations of union and fixation are necessary to assess progression of healing.

Patients can usually be discharged on the first or second postoperative day. A physiotherapist is consulted for gait training and to initiate quadricep isometric exer-

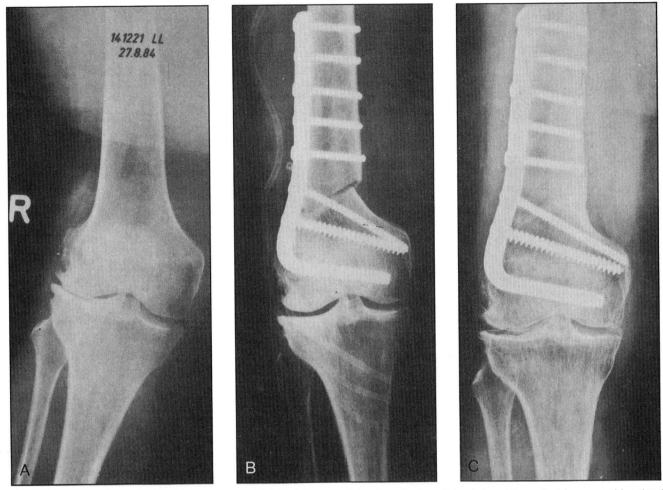

Figure 58.7. **A,** Valgus deformity of the right knee with lateral compartment gonarthrosis in a 63-year-old female. **B,** Following a supracondylar femoral varus osteotomy with a lateral AO condylar plate. The osteotomy has been performed obliquely with a screw through the plate and across the osteotomy to add stability. **C,** Three years later, the osteotomy is healed, and the patient has a good functional result. (Reproduced with permission from Miniaci A, Grossmann SP, Jakob RP. Supracondylar femoral varus osteotomy in the treatment of valgus knee deformity. Am J Knee Surg 1990;3:67.)

cises and straight leg raises. A hinged knee brace is utilized for patient comfort but can be removed for exercises. Once clinical and radiographic union has occurred, progressive weight bearing and resisted exercises are instituted. Functional exercises such as swimming and cycling are encouraged early in rehabilitation. The patient is usually fully weight bearing and independent by 12 weeks postsurgery.

Summary

Fortunately, valgus knee deformities are uncommon; if associated with lateral compartment arthrosis in the elderly, some would suggest that such deformities are best dealt with by unicompartmental or total knee arthroplasty. There are, however, many valgus knee deformities where distal femoral varus osteotomy should be considered. The surgery is technically demanding, but the results can be excellent, if careful attention is given to the principles of patient selection, the technical details of preparation and surgery, and to appropriate rehabilitation.

References

1. Aglietti P, Stringa G, Buzzi R, Pisaneschi A, Windsor RE. Correction of valgus knee deformity with a supracondylar V osteotomy. Clin Orthop 1987;217(4):214–220.
2. Aldinger G. Mittelfristige Ergebnisse der kniegelenksnahen Osteotomie in der Behandlung der Gonarthrose. Z Orthop 1981;119:516–520.
3. Baacke M, Legan H, Luther K. Grenzindikatonen für die suprakondyldre Femurosteotomie zur Behandlung der Gonarthrose. Z Orthop 1974;112:221–229.
4. Coventry MB. Osteotomy about the knee for degenerative and rheumatoid arthritis. J Bone Joint Surg 1973;55-A:23–48.
5. Coventry MB. Proximal tibial varus osteotomy for osteoarthritis of the lateral compartment of the knee. J Bone Joint Surg 1987;69-A:32–38.
6. Gardes JCL. Osteotomie femorale basse de fermeture interne pour correction des gonarthroses avec genu valgum. Rev Chir Orthop 1983;69(suppl 2):110–112.
7. Gekeler J. Knienahe Osteotomien bei Gonarthrose-Planung, Technik und Komplikationen. Orthopadische Praxis 1980;11:961–966.
8. Gorlich W, Albrecht F. Suprakondyldre Varisationsosteotomie bei

Genu valgum unter Verwendung eines Zielgerates. Unfallchirurgie 1980;6(3):171–174.

9. Goutallier D. Arthroplastie femoro-tibiale unicompartimentale et gonarthrose lateralisee. Rev du Rhumatisme 1984;51(7–8):399–404.

10. Harris R, Kostuik JP. High tibial osteotomy for osteoarthritis of the knee. J Bone Joint Surg 1970;52-A(3):330–336.

11. Healy WL, Angler JO, Wasilewski SA, Krackow KA. Distal femoral varus osteotomy. J Bone Joint Surg 1988;70-A(1):102–109.

12. Hernigou PIH, Medeville D, Debeyre J, Goutallier D. Proximal tibial osteotomy for osteoarthritis with varus deformity. J Bone Joint Surg 1987;69-A(3):332–354.

13. Insall JN, Hood RW, Flawn LB, Sullivan DJ. The total condylar knee prosthesis in gonarthrosis. A five- to nine-year follow-up of the first 100 consecutive replacements. J Bone Joint Surg 1983;65-A(6):619–628.

14. Insall JN, Joseph DM, Msika C. High tibial osteotomy for varus gonarthrosis. J Bone Joint Surg 1984;66-A(9):619–628.

15. Jackson JP, Waugh W, Waugh JP, Green JP. High tibial osteotomy for osteoarthritis of the knee. J Bone Joint Surg 1969;51-B(2):88–94.

16. Johnson EW Jr, Godell LS. Corrective supracondylar osteotomy for painful Geun valgus. Mayo Clin Proc 1981;56:87–92.

17. Maquet P. The treatment of choice in osteoarthritis of the knee. Clin Orthop 1985;192:108–112.

18. McDermott AG, Finklestein JA, Farine I, Bognton EL, MacIntosh DL, Gross A. Distal femoral varus osteotomy for valgus deformity of the knee. J Bone Joint Surg 1988;70-A(1):110–116.

19. Miniaci A, Grossmann SP, Jakob RP. Supracondylar femoral varus osteotomy in the treatment of valgus knee deformity. Am J Knee Surg 1990;3(2):65–73.

20. Muller KH, Biebrach M. Korrekturosteotomien und ihre Ergebnisse bei Idiopathischen Kniegelenknahen Achsenfehlstellungen. Unfallheilkunde 1977;80:457–464.

21. Muller ME, Allgower M, Schneider R, Willenegger H. Techniques recommended by the AO Group. In: Manual of internal fixation. 2nd Ed. New York, NY: Springer-Verlag, 1979.

22. Nitsch R, Janssen G. Die Stellung der Suprakondylaren Korrekturosteotomie in der Behandlung der Altersgonarthrose. Z Orthop 1976;114:226–232.

23. Schmitt E, Schmitt O, Mittelmeier H. Indikation, Technik und Ergebnisse der Kniegelenksnahen Umstellungsosteotomie bei hemilateraler Gonarthrose mit der Autokompressionswinkelplatte. Orthopadische Praxis 1984;9–3:913.

24. Scott RD, Santore RF. Unicondylar unicompartment replacement for osteoarthritis of the knee. J Bone Joint Surg 1981;63-A(4):536–544.

25. Teinturier P, Boulleret J, Terver S, Delisle JJ. Les osteotomies supracondyliennes. Rev Chir Orthop 1975;61(2):191–295.

26. Teinturier P, Levai JP, Terver S. Les osteotomies supracondyliennes. Rev Chir Orthop 1975;61(2):191–295.

27. Noesberger B. Osteotomien im Kniebereich. Orthopadische Praxis 1976;2(XII):168–177.

28. Wagner H, Zeiler G, Baur W. Indikation, Technik und Ergebnisse der supra- und infracondylaren Osteotomie bei der Kniegelenkarthrose. Orthopade 1985;14:172–192.

29. Weill D, Jacquemin MC. L'osteotomie cylindrique femorale supracondylienne de varisation dans le traitement chirurgical de la gonarthrose. Acta Orthop Belg 1982;48(1):110–130.

59

Unicompartmental Arthroplasty

Leonard Marmor

Unicompartmental Arthroplasty
Controversy: Osteotomy Versus
    Unicompartmental Arthroplasty
Controversy: Unicompartmental
    Versus Total Knee Replacement

Indications
Contraindications
Patient Selection
Imaging Procedures
Intraoperative Decision

Surgical Techniques
Pitfalls
Complications
Discussion
Conclusion

Unicompartmental Arthroplasty

Unicompartmental disease of the knee was a concept originated by Duncan McKeever (54) in the early 1950s, when he noted that the knee joint could have arthritis involving only the medial or lateral side and that it was not necessary to replace the entire joint. His first unicompartmental tibial prosthesis, which was metallic and had a fin for fixation, was inserted in 1952 (51, 64, 73, 79). Tibial osteotomy for unicompartmental arthritis of the knee was first reported by Jackson and Waugh in 1961 (35). Gunston (24), in 1971, reported his results with the polycentric arthroplasty that introduced the basic concept of cemented knee replacements. The design principles of the prosthesis were later modified by Walker and Shoji (89). The first cemented unicompartmental replacement using the Modular Knee (Richards), a prosthesis based on McKeever's concept, was inserted in the United States in 1972 (Fig. 59.1) (54, 60). The treatment of unicompartmental disease has been controversial: the question posed is whether high tibial osteotomy or unicompartmental arthroplasty is indicated for a patient with unicompartmental disease (18, 27, 50, 58, 67, 68, 76).

A similar controversy exists as to whether a total knee should be utilized in place of a unicompartmental arthroplasty when high tibial osteotomy is not suitable (30, 31, 48). These controversies persist, mainly in the United States. I shall try to present the current status of unicompartmental replacement and point out the fallacies that exist in these concepts.

Some orthopaedic centers in this country believe that only a total knee replacement should be performed if osteotomy is not indicated. However, there have only been a few articles published to date presenting poor results with unicompartmental arthroplasty. These are as follows:

Insall and Walker (31)1976
Laskin (48)1980

Insall and Aglietti (30)1980
Padgett, Stern, Insall (71)1991

In 1976, Insall and Walker (31) reported on 24 unicondylar replacements with a femoral component that had a blunt thick anterior edge, which, if not recessed, could result in patellar impingement producing severe patellar pain (Fig. 59.2). In this small series, there were 15 patellectomies, a number that has never been equalled in any other series with a greater number of cases! They also recommended using the thickest tibial component that could be inserted, which would tend to result in overcorrection of the knee, in turn resulting in failure of the procedure. Their poor results consisted of 5 patients with patellar pain, 2 due to instability from patellectomy, and 1 painful patellar tendon. Of their 8 poor results, 5 were due to extensor mechanism pain or instability. Based on this experience, John Insall stated at the Academy of Orthopaedic Surgeons meeting in 1979 that unicompartmental replacement was not indicated.

Laskin (48), in 1978, reported on 37 unicompartmental knees, with a high incidence of subsidence; however, 35 of the 37 patients were obese. He had 8 revisions; 4 were for degeneration of the opposite side, 2 for patellofemoral pain, 1 for unexplained pain, and 1 for tibial loosening.

The paper by Insall and Aglietti (30) is even more interesting since it includes the previously reported 24 knees from 1976. They reported on a total of 32 unicompartmental replacements in 30 patients from 1972 to 1974. Ten patients were lost to follow-up leaving 22 knees with an average follow-up of 6 years. Only 1 was excellent, 7 good, 4 fair, and 10 poor. Of the 32 knees, 16 required a patellectomy at the time of surgery, and two medial releases were also necessary. It is obvious that these were not properly selected patients based on current criteria for unicompartmental replacement.

Padgett, Stern, and Insall (71) published in 1991 a series consisting of 7 of these original knees and 14 re-

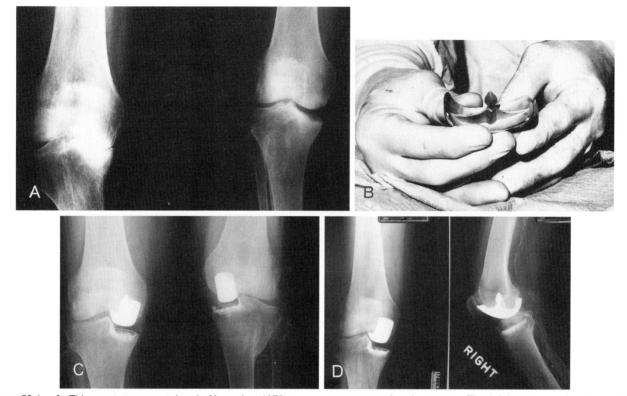

Figure 59.1. **A,** This roentgenogram taken in November 1972 reveals severe osteoarthritis of the right knee with marked loss of the tibial plateau in a 75-year-old woman. This patient was the first unicompartmental replacement with a Modular Knee. **B,** Photograph of the original femoral component that was individually made at that time. **C,** Roentgenogram of both knees January 21, 1974 with uni-compartmental replacements. The left knee is a salvage of a failed tibial osteotomy by a unicompartmental arthroplasty. **D,** Roentgenogram of the right knee November 1980 at 8 years following the surgery in which there is no evidence of loosening of the components or changes in the lateral compartment.

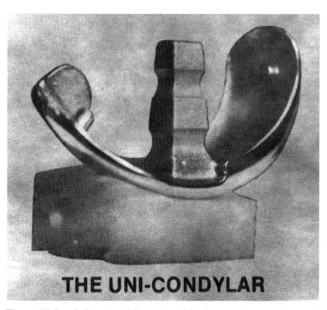

Figure 59.2. A drawing of the unicondylar knee replacement revealing a blunt anterior edge, which, if not recessed, could result in patellar impingement.

ferred patients for a total of only 21 knees, stating that revision of a unicompartmental replacement was difficult and the procedure was not conservative. However, the cases presented were poorly selected, cement was used to fill large defects from the prior surgery rather than bone grafts, and large cancellous defects were created by the previous surgeons with their cement technique. It is important to review these papers critically because they are frequently referred to in discussions, but with their flaws omitted.

Additionally, a vast bibliography on unicompartmental arthroplasty recommends the procedure and presents satisfactory results with long-term follow-up. Christensen (12) in 1991 reported from Sweden on 575 unicompartmental knees with a 9-year follow-up having a revision rate of 3.6%.

The major cause of failure of unicompartmental arthroplasty in the past has been either technical, mechanical, or patient selection (3, 38, 41, 54, 57).

Controversy: Osteotomy Versus Unicompartmental Arthroplasty

Where does osteotomy fit in the picture of unicompartmental arthritis (27, 57)? The ideal patient for osteotomy is:

1. A male patient under 55 years of age, with a high activity level who wants to play running sports or to do heavy labor
2. The patient has less than 10 degrees of varus,
3. The patient has at least 90 degrees of motion.

The complications and morbidity are greater with tibial osteotomy than with unicompartmental arthroplasty. Matthews, et al., (63) in 1988 had a total of 33 complications in 40 patients after high tibial osteotomy. A high complication rate is not unusual with high tibial osteotomy in the literature (5, 19, 34, 42, 43, 67, 81, 82).

The functional results for high tibial osteotomy are 60 to 85% acceptable in short-term follow-up with a durability of 5 to 10 years (Table 59.1) (5, 11, 17, 29, 32, 33, 42, 67, 75). If one compares the long-term results of unicompartmental arthroplasty versus high tibial osteotomy, the results are much better with the arthroplasty (Table 59.2). A review of 7649 unicompartmental arthroplasties with long-term follow-up revealed that the procedure gives good pain relief, excellent range of motion, and few serious complications (44).

A study from Sweden by Knutson, Lindstrand, and Lidgren in 1986 (45) revealed that in patients with osteoarthritis the survival rate with a hinged knee was over 60% and over 90% with a medial compartmental replacement. The survival rate was 96% with the sledge knee and 93% with the Marmor knee (Richards) in over 2300 knees reviewed at 6 years. In my personal series, at a minimum follow-up of 10 years, the Kaplan-Meier

survival rate was 91.6%, when reviewed by Dr. David Heck from the University of Indiana at Indianapolis. A multicenter follow-up by Heck, Marmor, and Gibson (28) of 294 knees at 12 years had a survival rate of 81.6%.

Broughton, Newman, and Baily (9) reported in 1986 in the Journal of Bone and Joint Surgery, on a similar group of knees with osteotomies and unicompartmental replacement followed for 5–10 years and noted a 43% success rate with osteotomy and a 76% rate with unicompartmental replacement.

Karpman and Volz (39) in 1982 reported, "We have discovered at our institution that high tibial osteotomy is a very technical and demanding operation, frequently leading to disabling complications."

Elia and Lotke (21) in 1990 reported, "Our experience confirmed the findings of other long-term follow-up studies that unicompartmental replacement of the knee provides good to excellent results in the majority of patients with unicompartmental arthritis and is more reliable than the long-term results from tibial osteotomy."

There is a place both for osteotomy and unicompartmental replacement based upon the indications and proper selection of patients (91).

Controversy: Unicompartmental Versus Total Knee Replacement

The statement is frequently made that the entire joint should be replaced so it will not be necessary to reoperate later. It seems illogical, however, to destroy normal tissue, for no one can predict the outcome or survival of any operation, and salvage must be possible.

There are many advantages of a unicompartmental replacement over a total knee replacement that are very important to consider in deciding which surgery to recommend for unicompartmental arthritis. The problem of whether to save the posterior cruciate does not arise with unicompartmental replacements because one can save both cruciates allowing better function of the knee joint. Unicompartmental replacement avoids the 4 to 8% patellar complication rate with total knee arthroplasty (13, 74, 83) because the patella is not replaced.

Unicompartmental replacement is the only replacement of the knee joint that can provide a normal gait and near normal postoperative motion (1, 14). Jefferson and Whittle (36) in a comparison of osteotomy, unicompartmental arthroplasty, and total knee replacement noted that the unicompartmental patients had the greatest increase in cadence, velocity, and stride length of the patients studied.

Unicompartmental arthroplasty is a more conservative procedure with respect to the amount of tissue removed and the typical blood loss (Fig. 59.3). I have found that the average blood loss with a unicompartmental replacement is 250 cc and transfusion is not necessary. By contrast, about 1290 cc of blood are lost with a total knee replacement; this usually requires a blood transfusion.

Unicompartmental knee replacement retains an important place in the treatment of unicompartmental

Table 59.1. Long-Term Results of Osteotomy

Name	Number of Osteotomies	Date of Publication	Years Followed	Acceptable Functional, Result (%)
Coventry	31	1987	9.4	77
Hernigou	93	1987	10.0	45
Holden	51	1988	10.0	70
Keene	51	1989	6.2	47
Morrey	33	1989	7.5	73
Ivarsson	65	1990	11.9	43
Rudan	79	1990	5.8	80
Berman	39	1991	8.5	57
Total	442		8.7	61.5

Table 59.2. Long-Term Results of Unicompartmental Replacement

Name	Number	Date	Years	Result (%)
Marmor	60	1988	10.0	70
Mink	75	1989	7.9	92
Page	92	1989	8.0	92
Capra	52	1989	8.3	93
Heck, et al.	294	1992	10.0	91
Knutson, et al.	7,649	1992	15.0	85
Totals	8,232		9.7	87

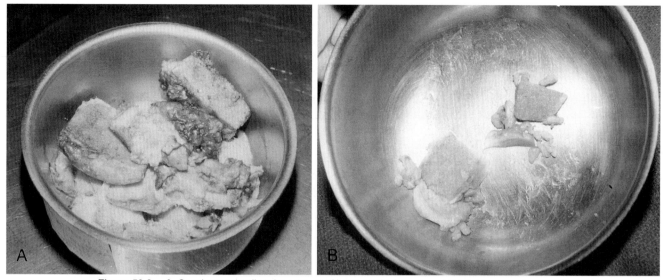

Figure 59.3. **A,** Specimen revealing the amount of bone routinely removed in total knee replacement. **B,** Specimen of bone removed in a unicompartmental arthroplasty.

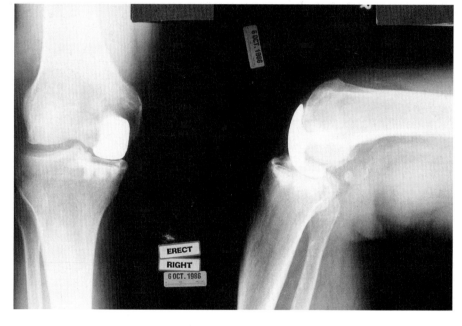

Figure 59.4. Roentgenogram October 6, 1986 of a patient who had a patellectomy 10 years prior to his unicompartmental arthroplasty in May 1975. The roentgenogram revealed no evidence of loosening of the cement or arthritic changes in the lateral compartment. At follow-up 14 years after unicompartmental arthroplasty, the knee was stable anteriorly-posteriorly and he had a range of motion from 0 to 126 degrees.

arthritis. Time has eliminated many of the misconceptions about this procedure.

Indications

The basic indication for unicompartmental arthroplasty is a patient with destruction of the articular surface of the medial or lateral compartment of the knee joint. The three most common diagnoses are osteoarthritis, osteonecrosis, and traumatic arthritis involving one of the above compartments of the knee (56, 57, 88). Patients who have had a prior patellectomy and have unicompartmental disease may do well with a unicompartmen-

tal replacement (Fig. 59.4). Total knee replacement is not necessary in these patients (62).

Contraindications

Patients with inflammatory disease of the knee joint (i.e., rheumatoid arthritis) should not be considered for unicompartmental arthroplasty because of the progressive nature of the disease even though one compartment appears to be involved primarily (3).

Arthroplasty should also be avoided, when possible, in active young patients who are unrealistic in their desires to return to heavy work or sports that require running or jumping that produce undue stress on the implant.

Patients with a recent infection of the knee joint should also be deferred until an adequate time demonstrates resolution of sepsis.

Patient Selection

Selection of the patient is critical in obtaining good results with unicompartmental arthroplasty, and there are a number of important criteria that need to be considered before and during surgery (57, 77).

The ideal patient for a unicompartmental arthroplasty is a patient of average weight who is over 60 years of age and has a moderate or sedentary activity level. Younger patients that have varus deformities over 10 degrees are better candidates for replacement than for osteotomy because patients with 10 degrees or more of varus do not do as well with an osteotomy. Patients with a valgus deformity also should be considered for replacement because varus high tibial osteotomies have a higher failure rate than valgus osteotomies (5, 18, 40, 42, 65, 68).

Age is not a definite contraindication to replacement if patients have severe pain due to unicompartmental disease and are realistic in what they expect to do postoperatively. They will have a good, but not normal, knee joint. It is important that young patients realize that a replacement knee is not normal, but that it will decrease their pain and improve their function.

Weight can also be a factor in selection of the patient. Those over 200 pounds and those with a small tibial plateau create forces on the tibial component that may be excessive and result in subsidence and cracking of the cement. These patients may do better with an osteotomy or total knee replacement.

Physical examination can provide additional information in the evaluation of a patient for a unicompartmental arthroplasty. Patients with a *fixed* varus or valgus deformity over 5 to 10 degrees that cannot be corrected easily without soft tissue releases are not good candidates for unicompartmental replacement. A fixed flexion deformity of 15 degrees is not a contraindication to arthroplasty as this deformity will correct with the replacement (Fig. 59.5). Patients with gross ligamentous instability cannot be stabilized by unicompartmental replacement (Fig. 59.6).

Imaging Procedures

Roentgenograms can provide valuable information if proper views are obtained to evaluate the status of the joint. The most frequent mistake is not to obtain full weight-bearing studies that reveal the true joint narrowing due to loss of the articular cartilage (Fig. 59.7). Prone films will not reveal the narrowing in many patients, and the cause of the patient's pain may not be obvious. It is best to obtain the standing anteroposterior film in about 10 to 20 degrees of flexion as this will reveal the narrowing of the compartment better (Fig. 59.8). The articular cartilage on the distal femoral condyle, shown when the knee is in full extension, is often normal, although with 10 degrees of flexion, the marked erosion is apparent (Fig. 59.9). Ligamentous de-

Figure 59.5.   A, Flexion contracture due to the anterior edge of tibia striking the femoral condyle, thus preventing full extension. **B,** Surgical removal of the anterior edge allows full extension.

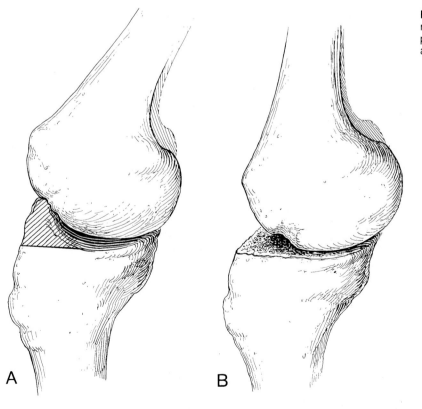

A   B

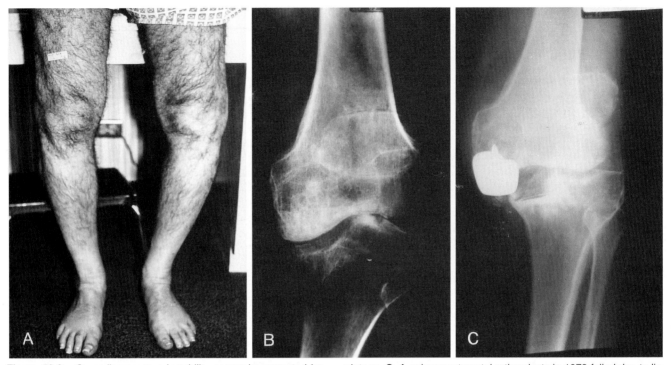

Figure 59.6. Gross ligamentous instability cannot be corrected by unicompartmental arthroplasty. **A,** Patient with bilateral osteoarthritis of the knees with a severe varus deformity of the left knee. **B,** The roentgenogram revealed marked destruction of the medial tibial plateau. **C,** A unicompartmental arthroplasty in 1973 failed due to ligamentous instability with medial subluxation of the femoral component. This patient was a poor choice for this procedure.

Figure 59.7. Roentgenogram of the knee taken at the same examination revealing the marked loss of the articular cartilage of the medial compartment (**A,** nonstanding view; **B,** standing view).

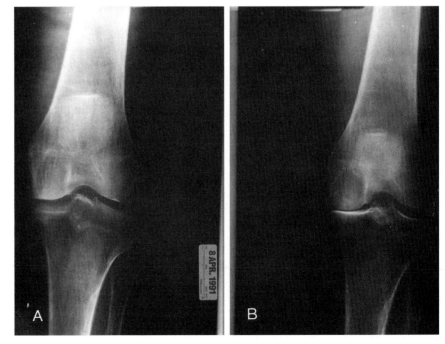

formity may also be more obvious when weight is applied to the joint, and subluxation occurs (Fig. 59.10). Impingement of the tibial spine against the lateral normal compartment can erode an area of the articular cartilage, but this is not a contraindication and can be corrected when the stability of the joint is restored by replacing the medial side. The erosion seen on the lateral condyle will not cause symptoms as it will not bear weight (Fig. 59.11).

The skyline view of the patella can also be very helpful in preoperative planning. If large osteophytes are seen on the condyle opposite to the diseased compart-

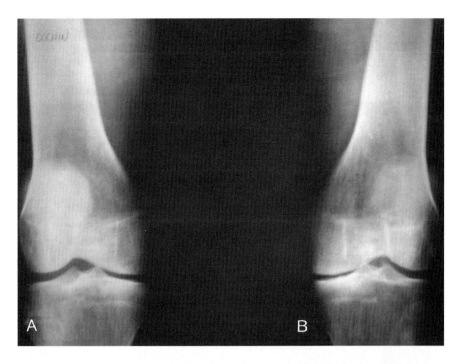

Figure 59.8. Roentgenogram taken in the anterior-posterior view in 10 to 20 degrees of flexion will reveal narrowing of the joint surface that might not be obvious in full extension. Patients with osteoarthritis of the knee tend to walk with a flexed knee and do not wear the articular cartilage on the superior aspect of the femoral condyle. This roentgenogram was taken in 10 degrees of flexion; early narrowing of the medial joint space is seen in the left knee.

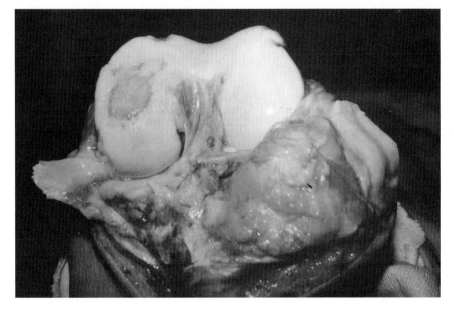

Figure 59.9. A clinical photograph of the patient in Figure 59.8 that clearly demonstrates severe changes in the medial femoral condyle but also shows excellent articular cartilage superiorly. A roentgenogram in full extension would not reveal the joint narrowing.

ment, this should suggest a good deal of arthritis in the apparently normal side. The surgeon should be cautious about the possibility that there may be more disease present in the joint (Fig. 59.12). If severe patellofemoral disease is also present, especially with lateral subluxation of the patella, unicompartmental replacement is not indicated.

A bone scan or an MRI is most helpful in patients with normal-appearing, routine films that have severe knee pain suggestive of osteonecrosis (Fig. 59.13). This diagnosis should be considered in all older patients with the sudden onset of severe knee pain without a history of trauma (70). Degenerative tears of the meniscus are not severely painful, but are often seen on the MRI without being the cause of the patient's symptoms (25, 26, 69, 70). Meniscal tears often lead to unnecessary arthroscopy and no improvement in the patient's symptoms.

Intraoperative Decision

It is at the time of surgery when the joint is inspected that the final decision is made about the choice of the operation to be performed (15). Based on this premise, the surgeon should be prepared to do either a unicompartmental arthroplasty or a total knee replacement; it is important

Figure 59.10. A, Roentgenogram of the same knee without weight-bearing. **B,** Roentgenogram with weight-bearing that reveals gross medial-lateral instability.

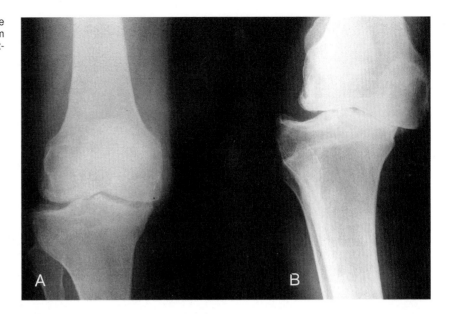

Figure 59.11. Impingement of the tibial spine on the medial aspect of the lateral condyle can cause erosion of the articular cartilage (*arrow*), but it is not a contraindication for a unicompartmental arthroplasty.

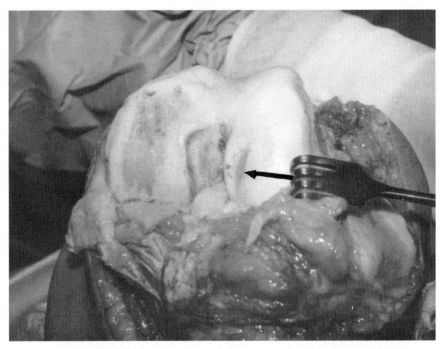

Figure 59.12. Merchant or skyline view of the patella can give additional information in regard to the involvement of the medial or lateral compartment of the knee joint. This roentgenogram reveals severe osteophtyes on the medial femoral condyle (*solid arrow*) and also a large osteophyte on the lateral femoral condyle (*white arrow*).

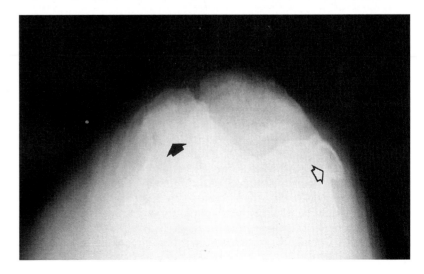

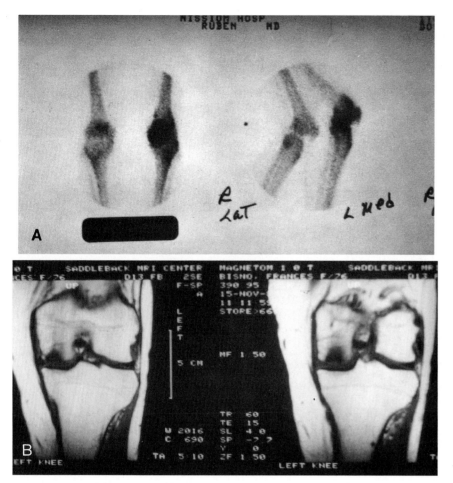

Figure 59.13. **A,** Bone scan of patient with osteonecrosis of the left medial femoral condyle. **B,** MRI of the above patient that reveals a large osteonecrotic lesion of the medial femoral condyle.

that the patient be made aware of this fact and that a signed permission for either procedure be obtained.

Chondromalacia of the patella is very common in elderly patients; it is often severe on the medial or lateral facet, depending on which tibial-femoral compartment is involved (Fig. 59.14). This is definitely not an absolute contraindication and will not cause postoperative symptoms. If the facet is very sclerotic, it can be undercut in a gull-wing fashion with a power bur. Patients with similar roentgenographic studies do not suffer patellar symptoms following high tibial osteotomy.

Keene, et al. (40) evaluated 51 knees in patients with high tibial osteotomy followed for a minimum of 5 years (average of 6.2 years) that had preosteotomy arthroscopic study. It was of marked interest that the number of good and excellent results decreased with time, but this was not related to the preosteotomy condition of the lateral and patellofemoral compartments. The clinical results were compared to the arthroscopy findings of the patellofemoral joint and divided into three groups. Group I had minimal or no articular changes. group II had moderate articular changes, and group III had marked articular changes. The difference between the average clinical scores in the three groups were not statistically significant. They also studied those patients with combined lateral compartment disease and patellofemoral changes and found that there was no significant statistical difference in the clinical scores at 5

years with either minimal or marked degenerative changes in the lateral compartment and patellofemoral joint. This is an important study because many surgeons will not do a unicompartmental arthroplasty if there are minimal degenerative changes in the patellofemoral joint or the lateral compartment. Keene, et al. have shown that the clinical scores are not altered by such findings. This study should correlate as well with unicompartmental replacement as it does for osteotomy.

Osteophytes on the rim of the normal condyle can be removed and are no concern if the weight-bearing surface is normal. Erosion on the medial aspect of the lateral femoral condyle from a "kissing" tibial spine is not a problem, as previously mentioned, and will not cause symptoms. An active synovitis with joint effusion in an osteoarthritic knee is not a contraindication to unicompartmental replacement. During the acute phase of osteoarthritis, there is inflamed synovium that will become quiescent after unicompartmental arthroplasty. The surgeon may also find deposits in the joint from chondrocalcinosis. If these are not severe, unicompartmental replacement can be performed. Christensen (12) has reported a large series from Sweden and has stated that chondrocalcinosis is not a contraindication to unicompartmental arthroplasty. Patients with disruption of the anterior cruciate and arthritic changes due to this instability in one compartment can be salvaged by unicompartmental arthroplasty (12, 53, 54).

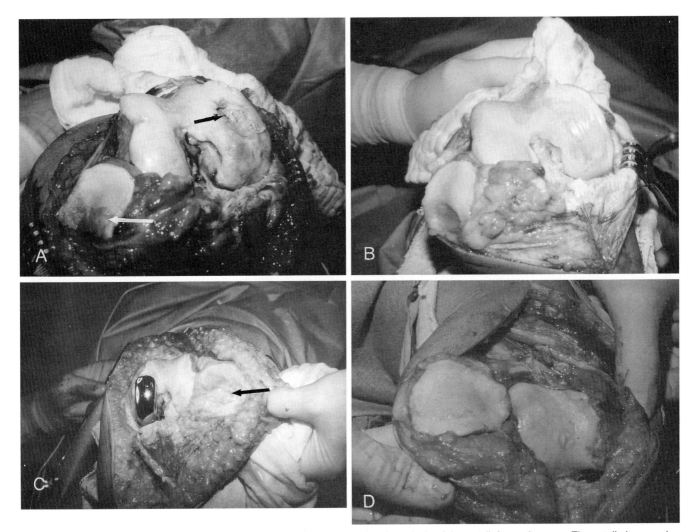

Figure 59.14. Examples of chondromalacia of the patella that are not contraindications for unicompartmental replacement. **A,** This patient had osteonecrosis of the medial femoral condyle (*arrow*). Chondromalacia of the patellofemoral groove is present and severe changes appear in the medial facet of the patella (*white arrow*). **B,** Example of a patient with severe unicompartmental disease and chondromalacia of the patellofemoral groove. The patella has erosion of the articular cartilage down to bone on the medial facet. **C,** This patient has severe involvement of the patella (*arrow*) but has no sequelae following unicompartmental replacement. **D,** This patient has severe changes in the patella and patellofemoral groove but has been asymptomatic following unicompartmental replacement.

It is not possible to see much of the meniscus in the contralateral compartment. If the femoral surface appears normal, one can assume the meniscus is also normal. If the meniscus is torn and has to be removed, then one should be more critical about the appearance of the femoral and tibial surfaces of the opposite compartment. If the surface has advanced changes involving the weight-bearing areas, a total replacement is indicated (Fig. 59.15).

Surgical Techniques

As with any procedure, different techniques have been developed based on the design of the prosthesis and the instruments used for insertion of the components. Rather than discuss one type of prosthesis and the instruments, I shall limit myself to the basic techniques that can be utilized with a variety of prostheses for unicompartmental arthroplasty. One should not transfer the techniques of total knee arthroplasty to unicompartmental replacement. Fixed deformities that require soft tissue releases are a contraindication for unicompartmental arthroplasty.

The operative technique, originally developed in 1972 for the Modular Knee (Richards), was designed to be simple and to require a minimal number of instruments (54, 59). I have continued to use this technique with a few modifications to aid in the placement of the components (Fig. 59.16). The recent tendency has been to develop techniques requiring numerous instruments, a tendency that seems to make unicompartmental arthroplasty much more difficult, and may lead the surgeon to overcorrect the knee joint (7, 80).

There are a variety of prosthetic devices available for unicompartmental arthroplasty, with their own instrumentation. As long as the basic technique is followed, they are all acceptable (7, 22, 23, 52, 59, 80, 85). Although porous implants have been used, they are not recom-

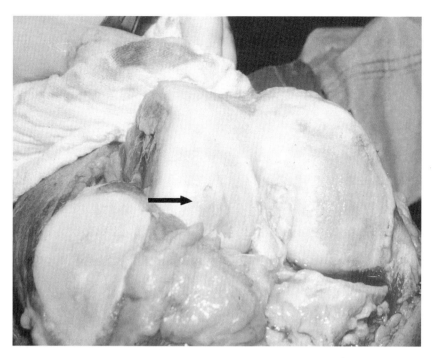

Figure 59.15. This patient had a severe defect on the weight-bearing portion of the opposite femoral condyle (*arrow*), which was a contraindication for a unicompartmental replacement.

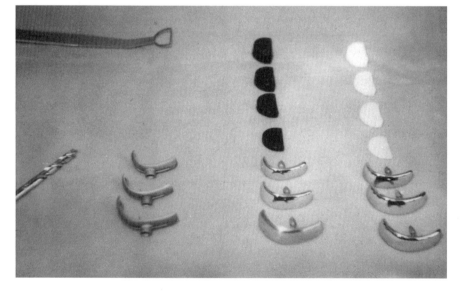

Figure 59.16. The basic instrument set that was developed for the Modular Knee in 1972. There are tibial and femoral templates and trial components available for testing before inserting the final components.

mended at the present time because of the high failure rate due to the lack of ingrowth on the tibial side (6).

A medial parapatellar incision is used, extending from 3 inches above the patellar to the medial side of the tibial tubercle. This is a more cosmetic approach than a straight incision over the front of the knee (Fig. 59.17).

The patella can be everted and the joint visualized to determine the involvement of the joint (Fig. 59.18). The medial or lateral patellar facet may reveal chondromalacia of grade III or IV. This is not a contraindication to unicompartmental replacements nor are small areas of chondromalacia in the opposite compartment. Erosion of the medial aspect of the lateral femoral condyle can occur in medial compartment arthritis from rubbing against the intercondylar eminence with medial-lateral subluxation (Fig. 59.11). This may be corrected by

restoring the medial compartment, and the erosion will not produce any problems.

Soft tissue releases as performed in total joint replacements should not be utilized in unicompartmental arthroplasty. They can produce instability and lead to subluxation. A very limited release will aid considerably in the exposure of the medial compartment. The periosteum and capsule are released along the anterior rim of the tibial plateau to the attachment of the deep medial collateral ligament (Fig. 59.19).

The tibial plateau is removed by an L-shaped cut in to the sclerotic subchondral bone (85). A tibial cutting guide, as used for total knee replacement, can provide a horizontal reference line on the anterior tibial surface for this cut (Fig. 59.20). A power saw cuts the bone and an osteotome can help lift out the piece of plateau (Fig.

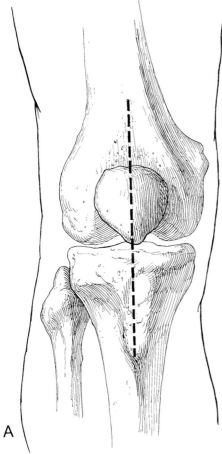

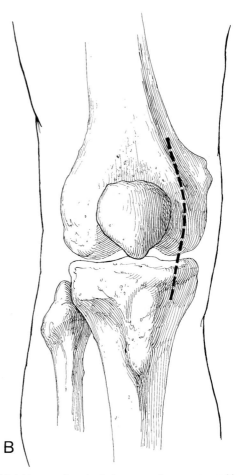

Figure 59.17. Skin Incisions that are utilized for knee arthroplasty. **A,** The commonly used approach for total knee arthroplasty. **B,** The medial parapatellar incision is recommended for unicompartmental and total knee arthroplasty for cosmetic reasons and because it does not interfere with the prepatellar bursa.

Figure 59.18. The patella can be averted and excellent exposure obtained of the lateral compartment from a medial parapatellar approach.

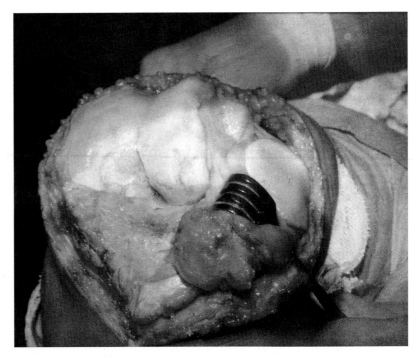

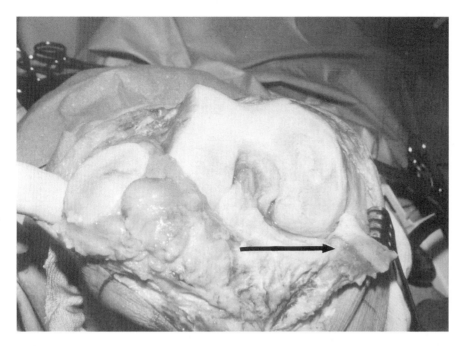

Figure 59.19. Exposure of the medial compartment can be enhanced by a soft tissue release along the tibial rim to the deep insertion of the medial collateral ligament (*arrow*).

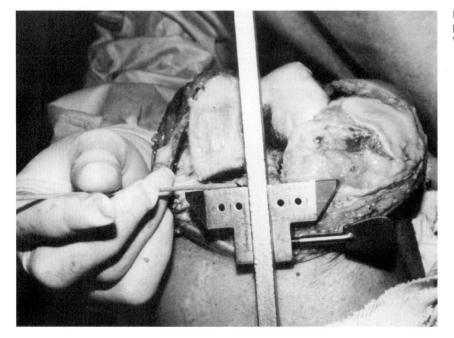

Figure 59.20. The tibial guide is utilized to place a horizontal guide line on the anterior tibia with methylene blue dye.

59.21). Care should be exercised not to fracture the tibial eminence. If this occurs, repair is not necessary as long as it does not displace. It is also possible to remove 2 to 4 mm of the posterior femoral condyle to enhance exposure if desired (Fig. 59.22). The medial meniscus should be excised completely, including the posterior horn, to expose the entire tibial plateau (Fig. 59.23).

If the tibial component has a short fixation stem (to prevent it from sliding posteriorly off the plateau), then the trial that covers the entire surface of the plateau should be selected. I use a marking template and outline the tibial component on the tibial plateau with methyl-

ene blue dye (Fig. 59.24). Then using a 4 or 5 mm carbide bur on its side, I plane down the surface 3 mm and slope it posteriorly about 10 degrees, leaving a posterior bony rim to prevent the trial from slipping backward. It is necessary with either technique to slope the tibial plateau posteriorly and downward to prevent the loss of flexion. If the plateau is high in the back and sloped anteriorly, flexion is limited.

The femoral landmark for placement of the anterior edge of the femoral component can be determined in two ways. I bring the knee to full extension with the tibial trial in place, and, where the anterior edge of the trial

Figure 59.21. The L-shaped cut is made with a power saw as indicated by the dotted lines.

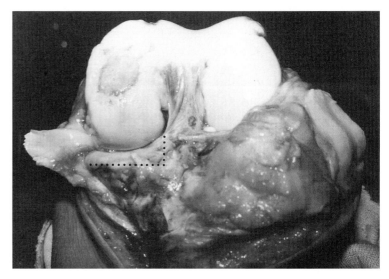

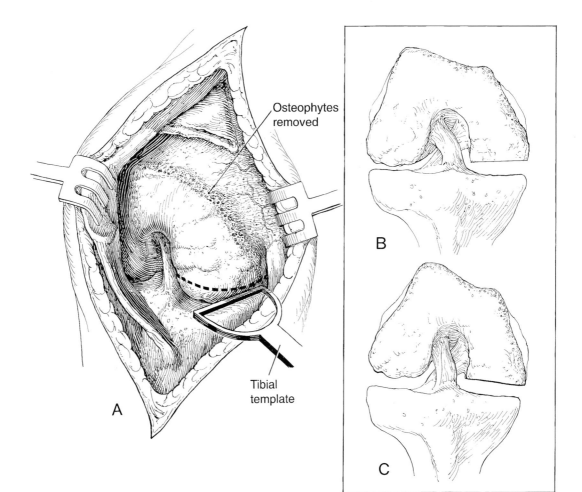

Figure 59.22. Further exposure, if necessary or if preferred, to the L-shaped tibial cut can be obtained on the femoral side. **A,** The dotted line reveals the site of the osteotomy of the posterior femoral condyle that is made with the knee flexed to 90 degree or more. **B,** Only a thin portion of 3–4 mm of the condyle needs to be removed. **C,** The osteotomy should be horizontal or it will tend to cause the femoral template to toe in or out on the femoral surface.

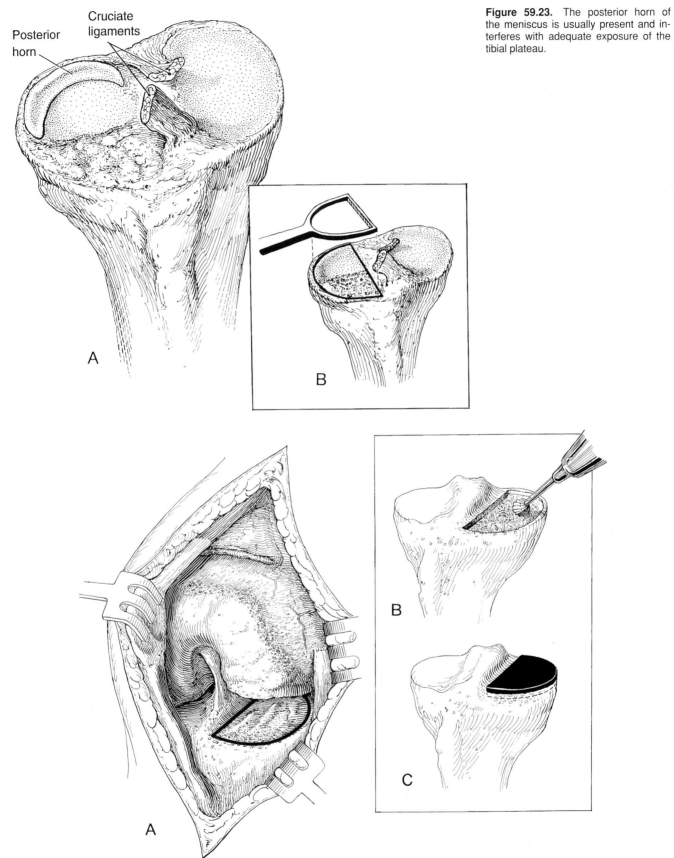

Posterior horn

Cruciate ligaments

A

B

Figure 59.23. The posterior horn of the meniscus is usually present and interferes with adequate exposure of the tibial plateau.

A

B

C

Figure 59.24. Tibial technique utilized for insertion of the trial component. **A,** The tibial plateau is marked with the widest tibial template using methylene blue to leave an outline. **B,** The tibial surface within the outline is deepened 3–4 mm for insertion of the trial. **C,** Trial tibial component locked in place.

strikes the femoral condyle, I make a thin, horizontal methylene blue line on the condyle for my landmark (Fig. 59.25A). Richard Scott (80) uses a technique whereby he marks the junction of the eburnated bone on the condyle with the normal-appearing articular cartilage (Fig. 59.25B). The landmark is essentially the same with either technique.

The femoral condyle is then prepared for the trial prosthesis by using a template that fits on the condyle or by using instruments that make appropriate cuts on the condyle so the trial will fit (Fig. 59.25C, D). The most important concern is that the anterior edge of the femoral component should be recessed below the articular surface to prevent patellar impingement on the anterior

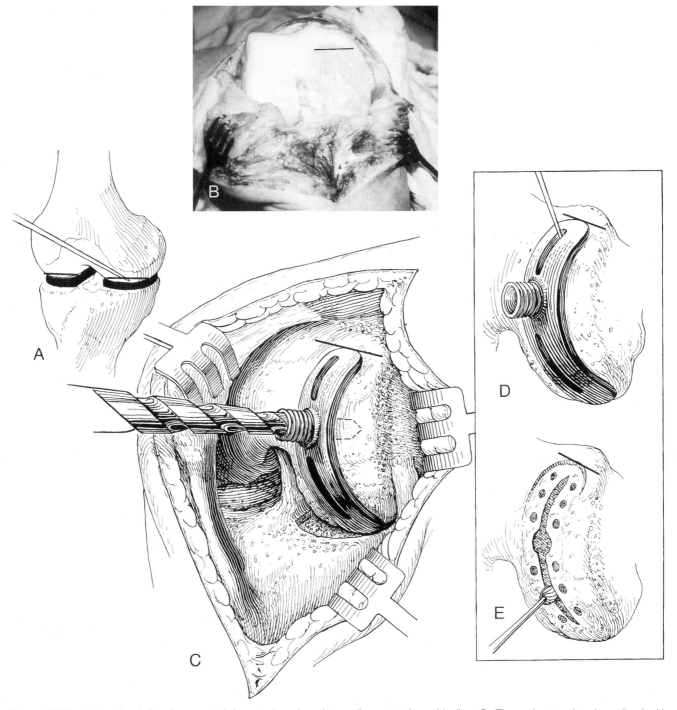

Figure 59.25.   A, Landmark for placement of the anterior edge of the femoral template where anterior edge of the tibial component extends on the femoral condyle. **B,** Scott uses the landmark of the anterior limit of the arthritic change on the femoral condyle (*black line*). **C,** The femoral template of the proper size to fit the condyle is placed adjacent to the guide line. **D,** The entire template is outlined with methylene blue. **E,** A small 1.5 mm bur is used to cut out the area for the fin of the prosthesis, and the entire area within the outline of the template is recessed, especially anteriorly with a 3–4 mm bur.

edge of the femoral component (Fig. 59.25E). If the edge is left protruding upward, impingement may occur (Fig. 59.26). This is one of the major causes of pain and failure of a unicompartmental replacement. The femoral component should fit so that it is flat on the condyle, and it may be necessary to remove some of the condylar surface to accomplish this. The trial should not protrude into the patellofemoral groove in order to prevent patellar impingement problems; it should not extend beyond the bone of the condyle to prevent soft tissue from rubbing on the metallic prominence (Fig. 59.27).

It is important to test for a proper fit of the trial components. This is done by bringing the knee to full extension and testing the medial-lateral stability. If the knee is unstable, a thicker tibial component is inserted to gain stability. It is, however, better not to overcorrect the knee into valgus because this will lead to postoperative pain and to the development of degenerative changes in the opposite compartment (Fig. 59.28).

The next test is to flex and extend the knee. If the tibial component is too thick, it will bind posteriorly and rise anteriorly. A thinner component may be used. If the polyethylene is less that 8 mm thick, however, it is better to deepen the tibial plateau and increase the posterior slope of plateau.

The last check is to observe the tracking of the patella and to see if it clears easily over the anterior edge of the femoral component. It is also advisable to palpate the patella to determine whether catching or grating occurs due to impingement.

If the tests are satisfactory, a series of 3 mm diameter holes are drilled 2 mm deep for cement penetration in the tibial and the femoral condyle (Fig. 59.29). Limiting the depth and diameter of the cement holes preserves the tibial cancellous bone stock.

It is recommended that both components not be cemented at the same time until the technique is mastered because it can be difficult to remove the posterior cement. The final tibial component should be used with the femoral trial compressing both components in extension while the cement is setting. Then the femoral trial prosthesis can be removed as well as the cement from the back of the tibial component. Another batch of cement can be used to cement in the final femoral component. Avoidance of a thick layer of cement on the posterior aspect of the femoral component prevents extrusion posteriorly. It is possible to distract the components after the cement hardens in order to reach the back of the joint with a small Hoke-type of osteotome.

Suction tubes are recommended. When the expansion and capsule have been closed, the knee should be flexed 90 degrees to test the suture line. I prefer the additional strength of #1 suture.

A bulky pressure dressing is used for 24 hours and then removed along with the suction tubes. Early motion begins passively with the continuous passive motion (CPM) machine as well as actively with the physical therapist (16, 88, 90).

Pitfalls

Patient selection for unicompartmental replacement is important. Poor selection leads to poor results. The ideal patient is older with osteoarthritis, osteonecrosis, or traumatic arthritis that involves only the medial or lateral compartment.

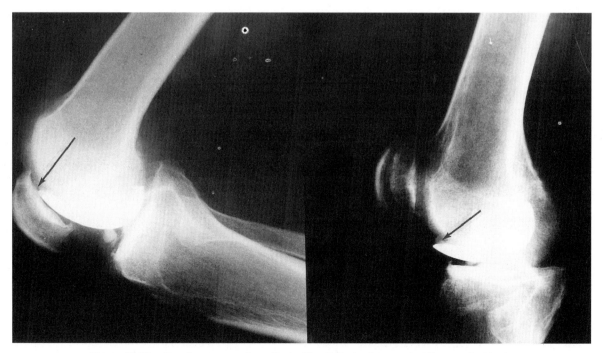

Figure 59.26.   Roentgenogram of a patient with patellar impingement on the prominent edge of the femoral component (*arrows*).

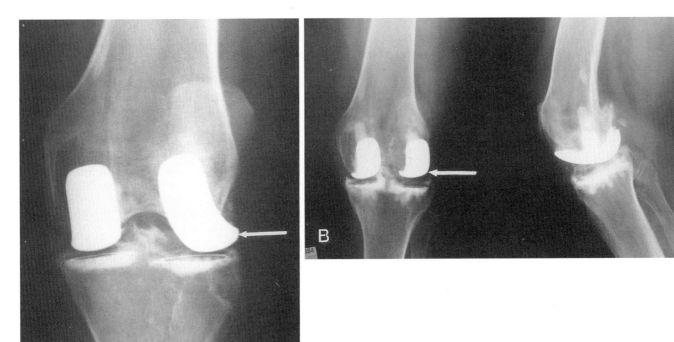
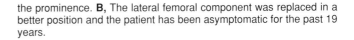

Figure 59.27. Roentgenogram of a patient with a bicompartmental replacement. **A,** The lateral femoral component toes outward off the bone surface (*arrow*) and the soft tissue is painful from rubbing over the prominence. **B,** The lateral femoral component was replaced in a better position and the patient has been asymptomatic for the past 19 years.

Figure 59.28. Roentgenogram of a right knee prior to replacement reveals a varus alignment following unicompartmental arthroplasty; the knee is overcorrected into valgus on the roentgenogram. The tibial component is placed on the cortical surface of the plateau and an inadequate amount of tibial bone has been removed.

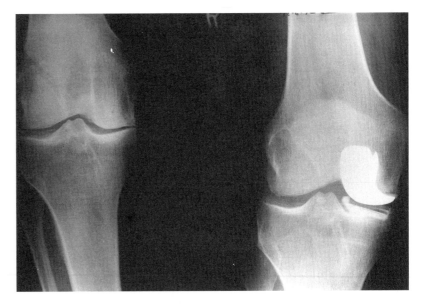

The major problem after unicompartmental arthroplasty is patellofemoral pain, most commonly caused by patellar impingement on the anterior edge of the femoral component (55). This results from failure to adequately recess the anterior edge of the femoral component below the articular surface of the condyle (Fig. 59.30). Therefore, it is extremely important to test for impingement with the trial components in place during the operation as described earlier. If the femoral trial and the final femoral component are dissimilar,

this can also produce the problem. It will only be noted after the component has been cemented in place. The signs of patellar impingement are the following:

1. Pain is noted at 30 to 60 degrees of flexion when the lower pole of the patella strikes the prominent anterior edge of the femoral component.
2. Palpation of the patella may produce grating and catching at 30 to 60 degrees of flexion.

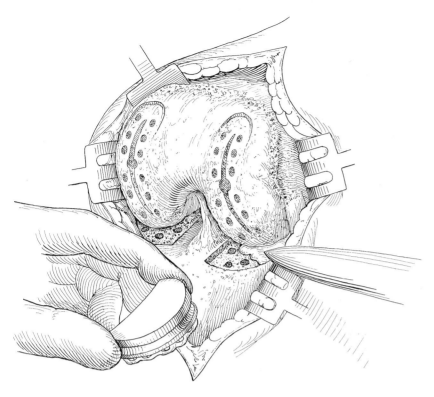

Figure 59.29. A series of small 4 mm holes are drilled into the tibial and femoral surfaces for cement fixation. The depth should only be 2–3 mm to preserve the cortical bone if future surgery is necessary.

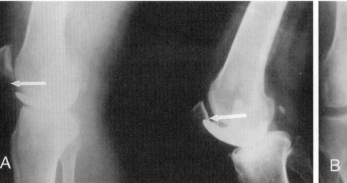

Figure 59.30. Roentgenogram of a patient with patellar impingement. **A,** Lateral view reveals a deep area of destruction of the lower pole of the patella (*arrow*) due to the protrusion of the anterior edge of the femoral component. **B,** The femoral component has been replaced with another component and proper recessing of the anterior edge (*arrow*).

3. Palpation of the femoral condyle may reveal a prominent anterior edge with local tenderness.
4. Pain will improve when the knee is flexed beyond 60 degrees.

A skyline x-ray of the patella may also diagnose this problem after surgery if erosion of the patellar facet is apparent. The treatment of this problem, if noted after surgery, is to revise the femoral component or to undercut the patellar facet that is impinging.

The use of tibial components thinner than 7–8 mm can lead to bending of the plastic and cracking of the cement interface (Fig. 59.31). Most designs have compensated for this problem, but there are still metal-backed tibial components with only a thin layer of polyethylene. They can fail due to destructive wear of the plastic. The femoral component then rubs on the metal tray and produces a synovitis from metal debris.

Overcorrection due to an inordinately thick tibial component or inadequate removal of the tibial plateau will result in pain and failure. It is better to undercorrect the knee with mild laxity than to overcorrect with excessive tension in the knee (Fig. 59.32).

The incidence of tibial component subsidence has decreased with the use of wider components that cover the tibial plateau. The widest component possible should be used, not the thickest.

Finally, avoid deep cement holes that sacrifice the cancellous bone of the plateau. Components with a deep keel on the underside should also be avoided for the same reason. If revision is necessary, it is much easier to do when there is good cancellous bone stock present.

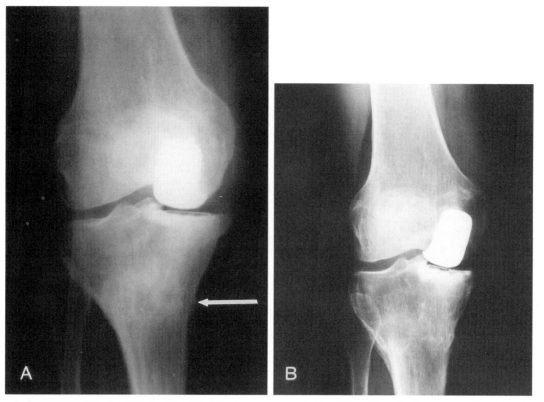

Figure 59.31. **A,** Roentgenogram of a patient with a failed tibial osteotomy (*arrow*) that was followed by a unicompartmental arthroplasty with a 6 mm tibial component. **B,** Roentgenogram 3 years later revealed buckling of the plastic component and breakage of the wire marker around the plastic.

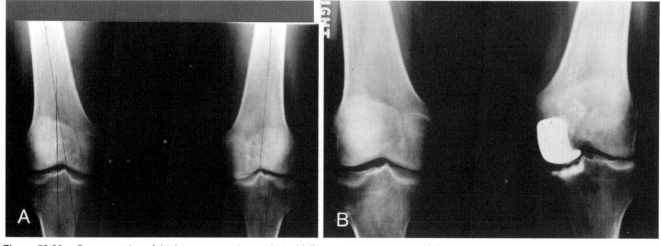

Figure 59.32. Overcorrection of the knee can produce pain and failure of the arthroplasty. **A,** Roentgenogram of patient preoperatively with a varus deformity of the left knee. **B,** Postoperative roentgenogram with inadequate removal of the tibial bone and a valgus deformity.

These pitfalls may be averted by the surgeon who is aware of them.

Complications

The number of major complications reported with unicompartmental arthroplasty have been small. They are generally the result of surgical technique, manufacture method, or design of the prosthesis (2, 4, 6, 12, 20, 24, 31, 37, 38, 41, 47, 49, 61, 78, 84, 86, 92).

Tibial loosening has decreased to less than 10% in 5-year and longer follow-up (10, 12, 20, 28, 45, 46, 66, 72, 78). Avoiding thinner plastic components and using wider components have lowered the loosening rate.

If loosening occurs, the patient will complain of pain when starting to walk, with improvement on walking further. The roentgenogram will reveal lucent lines adjacent to the cement, and sclerosis will occur in the tibial bone beneath the component. These lines tend to radiate distally (Fig. 59.33). Osteolysis can occur gradually, with cystic changes in the cancellous bone due to particulate disease. During the earlier phase, replacement with a thicker tibial component may be all that is required. In the more advanced stage, conversion to a total knee replacement is recommended. Knutson, Lewold, and Lidgren (44) advised in a 1992 study that where revision was indicated, the unicompartmental should be converted to a total knee replacement for most modes of failure. Femoral loosening has not been a frequent problem. If breakage or loosening occurs, total knee arthroplasty is usually required.

Progressive degenerative changes in the unoperated compartment can be limited to about 5% of the cases if overcorrection is avoided and if patients with advanced disease are not selected for unicompartmental arthroplasty.

The infection rate of unicompartmental arthroplasty is less than 1% when performed in a laminar flow room with "space suits."

Discussion

The role of unicompartmental replacement in the treatment of unicompartmental disease of the knee joint is to fill the void between high tibial osteotomy and total knee replacement. It is the logical procedure for the appropriate patient. The combined experience of surgeons using a variety of different prostheses reveals that a cemented unicompartmental knee arthroplasty is a reliable and durable procedure. If revision to a total knee replacement is necessary after a well- performed unicompartmental arthroplasty with minimal bone resection, the results should be similar to those of a primary total knee replacement.

Conclusion

Unicompartmental arthroplasty is an excellent, conservative procedure that can produce satisfactory results with a minimal complication rate in properly selected patients.

References

1. Andriacchi TP, Galante J, Fermier RW. The influence of total knee replacement on walking and stair climbing. J Bone Joint Surg 1982;64-A:1328–1335.
2. Bae KK, Guhl JF, Keane SP. Unicompartmental knee arthroplasty for single compartment disease: Clinical experience with an average four-year follow-up study. Clin Orthop 1983;176:233–238.
3. Barrett WB, Scott RD. Revision of failed unicondylar arthroplasty. J Bone Joint Surg 1987;69–A;1328–1335.
4. Bensadoun JL, Vidal J, Maury P, Salvan J, Shiphorst PT. Unicompartmental arthroplasty. Orthop Trans 1989;13:708.
5. Berman AT, Bosacco SJ, Kirshner S, Avolio A, Jr. Factors influencing long-term results in high tibial osteotomy. Clin Orthop 1991;272:192–198.
6. Bernasek TL, Rand JA, Bryan RS. Unicompartmental porous coated anatomic total knee arthroplasty. Clin Orthop 1988;236:52–59.
7. Bert JM. Universal intramedullary instrumentation for unicompartmental total knee arthroplasty. Clin Orthop 1991;271:79–87.
8. Blunn GW, Walker PS, Joshi A, Hardinge K. The dominance of cyclic sliding in producing wear in total knee replacements. Clin Orthop 1991;273:253–260.
9. Broughton NS, Newman JH, Baily RAJ. Unicompartment replacement and high tibial osteotomy for osteoarthritis of knee. A comparative study after 5–10 years followup. J Bone Joint Surg 1986;68–B:447–452.
10. Capra S, Fehring T. Unicompartmental arthroplasty, a four to fourteen year review. Orthop Trans 1989;13:550.
11. Chillag KJ, Nicholls PJ. High tibial osteotomy, a retrospective analysis of 30 cases. orthopedics, 1984;7:1821–1822.
12. Christensen NO. Unicompartmental prosthesis for gonarthrosis. A nine-year series of 575 knees from a Swedish hospital. Clin Orthop. 1991;273:165–169.
13. Clayton ML, Thirupathi R. Patellar complications after total condylar arthroplasty. Clin Orthop 1982;170:152–155.
14. Cobb AG, Kozinn SC, Scott RD. Unicondylar or total knee replacement. J Bone Joint Surg 1990;72–B:166.
15. Corpe RS, Engh GA. A quantitative assessment of degenerative changes acceptable in the unoperated compartment of knees undergoing unicompartmental replacement. Orthopedics 1990;13:319–323.
16. Coutts RD. Continuous passive motion in the rehabilitation of the total knee patient, its role and effect. Orthop Rev 1986;15:126–134.
17. Coventry MB. Proximal tibial varus osteotomy for osteoarthritis of the lateral compartment of the knee. J Bone Joint Surg 1987;69–A:32–38.
18. Coventry MB. Upper tibial osteotomy for gonarthrosis. Orthop Clin North Am 1979;10:191–208.
19. Curley P, Eyres K, Brezinova V, Allen M, Chan R, Barnes M. Common peroneal nerve dysfunction after high tibial osteotomy. J Bone Joint Surg 1990;72–B:405–408.
20. Eilers VE, Armstrong DT. Unicompartment knee arthroplasty: Long-term results and current concepts. Orthop Trans 1989;13:610.
21. Elia EA, Lotke PA, Ecker ML. Unicondylar arthroplasty for osteoarthritis of the knee. Surg Rounds Orthop 1990;4:17–22.
22. Engelbrecht E. The "sledge" prosthesis: A partial prosthesis for destructions of the knee joint. Chirug (Berlin) 1971;42:510.
23. Goodfellow JW, O'Connor BE. Clinical results of the Oxford knee. Surface arthroplasty of the tibiofemoral joint with a meniscal bearing prosthesis. Clin Orthop 1986;205:21–48.
24. Gunston FH. Polycentric knee arthroplasty. J Bone Joint Surg 1971;53–B:272–277.
25. Hall FM. Further pitfalls in knee arthrography. J Can Assoc Radiol 1978;29:179–184.
26. Hall FM. Osteonecrosis of the knee and medial meniscal tears [Letter]. Radiology 1979;133:828–829.
27. Healy L, Barber TC. The role of osteotomy in the treatment of osteoarthritis of the knee. Am J Knee Surg 1990;3:97–109.

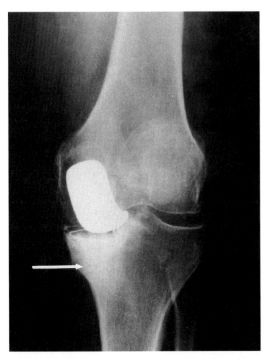

Figure 59.33. Roentgenogram of patient with a loose 6 mm tibial component with severe sclerosis of the tibia below the loose cement due to irritation of the bone.

28. Heck DA, Marmor L, Gibson A. Unicompartmental knee replacement: a multicenter investigation with long-term follow-up. Clin Orthop (In press).
29. Holden DL, James SL, Larson RL, Slocum DB. Proximal tibial osteotomy in patients, fifty years old or less. J Bone Joint Surg 1988;70–A:977–982.
30. Insall JN, Aglietti P. A five- to seven-year follow-up of unicondylar arthroplasty. J Bone Joint Surg 1980;62–A:1329–1337.
31. Insall JN, Walker P. Unicondylar knee replacement. Clin Orthop 1976;120:83–85.
32. Insall JN, Joseph DM, Msika C. High tibial osteotomy for varus gonarthrosis. J Bone Joint Surg 1984;63–A:1041–1048.
33. Ivarsson I, Mynerts R, Gillquist J. High tibial osteotomy for medial osteoarthritis of the knee. J Bone Joint Surg 1990;72–B:238–244.
34. Ivey M, Cantrell JS. Lateral tibial plateau fracture as a postoperative complication of high tibial osteotomy. Orthopedics 1985;8:1009–1013.
35. Jackson JP, Waugh W. Tibial osteotomy for osteoarthritis of the knee. J Bone Joint Surg 1961;43–B:745–751.
36. Jefferson RJ, Whittle MW. Functional biomechanical results of unicompartmental knee arthroplasty compared with total condylar arthroplasty and tibial osteotomy. J Bone Joint Surg 1990;72–B:161–162.
37. Jones WT, Bryan RS, Peterson LFA, Astrup D. Unicompartmental knee arthroplasty using polycentric and geometric hemicomponents. J Bone Joint Surg 1981;63–A:946–954.
38. Jonsson G. Compartmental arthroplasty for gonarthrosis. Acta Orthop Scand 1981;(Suppl)93:52.
39. Karpman RR, Volz RG. Osteotomy versus unicompartment prosthetic replacement in the treatment of unicompartment arthritis of the knee. Orthopedics 1982;5:989–991.
40. Keene JS, Monson DK, Roberts JM, Dyreby JR, Jr. Evaluation of patients for high tibial osteotomy. Clin Orthop 1989;243:157–165.
41. Kennedy WR, White RP. Unicompartmental arthroplasty of the knee: Postoperative alignment and its influence on overall results. Clin Orthop 1987;221:278–285.
42. Kettlekamp DB. A review of proximal tibial osteotomy. JCE Orthopedics 1979;7:11–19.
43. Kettlekamp DB, Leach RE, Nasca R. Pitfalls of proximal tibial osteotomy. Clin Orthop 1975;106:238–239.
44. Knutson K, Lewold S, Lidgren L. Outcome of revision for failed unicompartmental knee arthroplasty for arthrosis. American Academy of Orthopaedic Surgeon Poster Exhibit, Washington D.C., 1992.
45. Knutson K, Lindstrand A, Lidgren L. Survival of knee arthroplasties, a nation-wide multicentre investigation of 8000 cases. J Bone Joint Surg 1986;68–B:795–803.
46. Kozinn ST, Marx C, Scott RD. Unicompartmental knee arthroplasty: 4.5 to 6 year follow-up with metal-backed tibial component. Orthop Trans 1988;21:654.
47. Larsson SE, Ahlgen O. Reconstruction with endo-prosthesis in gonarthrosis. Clin Orthop 1979;145:126–135.
48. Laskin RS. Modular total knee replacement arthroplasty. J Bone Joint Surg 1976;58–A:766–773.
49. Laskin RS. Unicompartment tibiofemoral resurfacing arthroplasty. J Bone Joint Surg 1978;60–A:182–185.
50. Leach RE, Hoaglund FT, Riseborough EJ. Controversies in orthopaedic surgery. Philadelphia: WB Saunders, 1982.
51. MacIntosh DL. The use of hemiarthroplasty prosthesis for advanced osteoarthritis and rheumatoid arthritis of the knee. J Bone Joint Surg 1972;40–A:1431.
52. Mackinnon J, Young S, Baily RAJ. The St. George sledge for unicompartmental replacement of the knee. J Bone Joint Surg 1988;70–B:217–223.
53. Marmor L. Anterior cruciate destruction in osteoarthritis. Comtemp Orthop 1980;2:8.
54. Marmor L. Arthritis surgery. Philadelphia: Lea & Febiger, 1976.
55. Marmor L. Impingement of the patella in total knee replacement. Orthop Rev 1982;XI:93–93.
56. Marmor L. lateral compartment arthroplasty of the knee. Clin Orthop 1984;186:115–121.
57. Marmor L. Patient selection for osteotomy, unicompartmental, replacement, and total knee replacement. Am J Knee Surg 1990;3:206–213.
58. Marmor L. Results of single compartment arthroplasty with acrylic cement fixation. A minimum follow-up of 2 years. Clin Orthop 1977;122;181–186.
59. Marmor L. Surgical technique of unicompartmental replacement. Techn Orthop 1990;5:3–7.
60. Marmor L. The modular knee. Clin Orthop 1973;94:242–248.
61. Marmor L. Unicompartmental arthroplasty of the knee with a minimum ten-year follow-up period. Clin Orthop 1988;228:171–177.
62. Marmor L. Unicompartmental knee arthroplasty following patellectomy. Clin Orthop 1987;218:164–166.
63. Matthews LS, Goldstein SA, Malvitz TA, Katz BP, Kaufer H. Proximal tibial osteotomy, factors that influence the duration of satisfactory function. Clin Orthop 1988;229:193–200.
64. McKeever DC, Elliot RB. Tibial plateau prosthesis. Clin Orthop 1960;18:86–95.
65. Miniaci A, Grossman SP, Jakob RP. Supracondylar femoral varus osteotomy in the treatment of valgus knee deformity. Am J Knee Surg 1990;3:65–73.
66. Mink WF. Unicompartmental knee replacement. Orthop Trans 1989;13:73.
67. Morrey BF. Long-term study of tibial osteotomy in patients under age of forty. Orthop Trans 1988;12:655.
68. Morrey BF. Upper tibial osteotomy: Analysis of prognostic features: A review. Advances Orthop Surg 1986;9:213–222.
69. Noble J, Hamblen DL. The pathology of the degenerate meniscus lesion. J Bone Joint Surg 1975;57–B:180–186.
70. Norman A, Baker ND. Spontaneous osteonecrosis of the knee and medial meniscal tears. Radiology 1978;129:653–656.
71. Padgett DE, Stern SH, Insall JN. Revision total knee arthroplasty for failed unicompartmental replacement. J Bone Joint Surg 1991;73–A:186–190.
72. Page DO. Results in unicompartmental knee arthroplasty. Orthop Trans 1989;13:73.
73. Potter TA. Arthroplasty of the knee with tibial metallic implants of the McKeever and MacIntosh design. Surg Clin North Am 1969;49:903–910.
74. Ranawat CS. The patellofemoral joint in total condylar knee arthroplasty. Clin Orthop 1986;205:93–99.
75. Rudan JF, Simurda MA. High tibial osteotomy. A prospective clinical and roentgenographic review. Clin Orthop 1990;255:251–256.
76. Schmidt RG, Lotke PA, Rothman RH. Tibiofemoral resurfacing arthroplasty utilizing the marmor modular prostheses: a long-term follow-up study. Orthop Trans 1986;10:491.
77. Scott RD, Santore RF. Unicondylar unicompartment replacement for osteoarthritis of the knee. J Bone Joint Surg 1981;63–A:536–544.
78. Scott RD, Cobb AG, McQueary FG, Thornhill TS. Eight-to-twelve-year follow-up results of unicondylar knee replacements with survivorship analysis. Clin Orthop 1991;271:96–100.
79. Scott RD, Joyce MJ, Ewald FC, Thomas WH. McKeever metallic hemiarthroplasty of the knee in unicompartmental degenerative arthritis: Long-term clinical follow-up and current indications. J Bone Joint Surg 1985;65–A:203–205.
80. Scott RD. Robert Brigham unicondylar knee surgical technique. Techn Orthop 1990;5:15–23.
81. Shea JD. Osteoarthritis of the knee: Diagnosis and complications of treatment by high tibial osteotomy. South Med J 1973;66:1030–1034.
82. Skolnick MD, Bryan RS, Persson BM. Non-union after high tibial osteotomy in osteoarthritis. J Bone Joint Surg 1988;60–A:973–977.
83. Soudry M, Mestriner MD, Binazzi R, Insall JN. Total knee arthroplasty without patellar resurfacing. Clin Orthop 1986;205:166–170.
84. Stockelman RE, Pohl KP. The long-term efficacy of unicompartmental arthroplasty. Clin Orthop 1991;271:88–95.
85. Swienckoski J, Page II BJ. Medial compartmental arthroplasty of the knee. Use of the L-cut and comparison with the tibial inset method. Clin Orthop 1990;239:161–167.
86. Tabor OB. Treatment of single compartment osteoarthritis of the knee using modular arthroplasty. Orthopedics 1984;7:979–983.
87. Thornhill TS, Scott RD. Unicompartmental knee arthroplasty. Orthop Clin North Am 1989;20:245–256.
88. Vince KG, Kelly MA, Insall JN, Beck J. Continuous passive motion after total knee replacement. J Arthroplasty 1987;2:281–284.
89. Walker PS, Shoji H. Development of a stabilizing knee prosthesis employing physiological principles. Clin Orthop 1973;94:222–233.
90. Wasilewski SA, Woods LC, Torgerson WR, Jr, Healy WL. Value of continuous passive motion in total knee arthroplasty. Orthopedics 1990;13:291–295.
91. Windsor RE, Insall JN, Vince KG. Total knee arthroplasty after tibial osteotomy: What are the risks? J Bone Joint Surg 1988;70–A:547–555.
92. Wolfgang GL. Unicompartment modular total knee arthroplasty. Orthopedics 1980;3:313–318.

60

Patellofemoral Degenerative Joint Disease

Domenick J. Sisto

The treatment of patellofemoral degenerative joint disease is challenging. The patellofemoral joint degenerates slowly over time and the patient has usually undergone many conservative and operative therapeutic regimens prior to developing arthrosis. The patient is frustrated by the failures of these regimens and frequently has become pessimistic.

The "failure mode" that these patients become accustomed to is the most difficult obstacle in treating patellofemoral degenerative joint disease. The most important factor in treatment is prevention. Patients who initially present with patellar pain and chondromalacia or those with pain and instability with or without chondromalacia must be treated with care and conservatism. The patients are frequently depressed, overweight females with poor self-images of themselves and their bodies. An aggressive surgeon who displays poor judgment may have initiated a series of failed surgeries resulting in a "failure attitude" that is difficult to overcome.

Patients with early patellofemoral disease have to lose weight, improve body mechanics, gain strength, modify activities, and have early psychological counseling to prevent them from being "focused" on their patellae. All of the conservative and operative procedures for patellofemoral degenerative disease are "fair at best" and, therefore, prevention of degeneration is the most important factor in treatment.

Patellofemoral Degenerative Disease

Osteoarthritis is defined as loss of articular cartilage probably resulting from the progression of chondromalacia. Grades I–III chondromalacia of the patella and femoral groove are stages in the degeneration of the cartilage surface of the bone. Grade IV chondromalacia or osteoarthritis is the final stage in this progression (Fig 60.1). Outerbridge (1) has classified grade I cartilage lesions as those with articular cartilage softening only. Grade II lesions have fibrillation of less than ½ inch in diameter. Grade III lesions have fibrillation of more than ½ inch in diameter. Grade IV lesions are eroded to bone. The purpose of this chapter will be to focus primarily on patients with grade IV chondromalacia of the patellofemoral joint, also known as osteoarthritis or patellofemoral degenerative disease.

Symptoms

Degeneration of the patellofemoral joint can occur even when the patients have been carefully treated. The symptoms are pain and catching of the patella on the femoral groove during knee motion. The patients have an aching pain behind the patella, on the medial side of joint occasionally, and, rarely, posteriorly in the popliteal fossa. The pain is exacerbated by activity and most patients cannot negotiate stairs without the aid of a bannister. The patients complain of their knee locking if they keep it in a flexed position as in sitting. They have to "work it back into position" before they can ambulate.

Giving way or buckling is another major symptom of patellofemoral degeneration. Patellar instability can be a major complaint and is usually present in the early stages of the disease. Ficat (2, 3) believes that excessive lateral pressure syndrome is the most frequent cause of patellofemoral degenerative disease. Fulkerson (4) has advanced this concept and believes that patients with patellar tilt and compression will overload the lateral facet of the patella and corresponding femoral groove and that this mechanism is the most common etiology of osteoarthritis. Insall (5) has had a different experience and has found it "unusual for patients with patel-

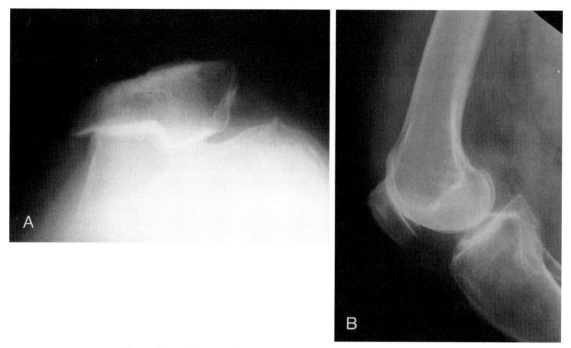

Figure 60.1. **A** and **B,** Severe osteoarthritis of the patellofemoral joint.

lofemoral arthrosis to have experienced patellar dislocation in earlier life." He believes that patellofemoral arthrosis can arise without an apparent cause in a structurally normal joint.

Our experience has revealed two types of patients with advanced patellofemoral degenerative arthritis. The majority of patients do have patellar malalignment with patellar tilt/compression in addition to a history of subluxation and dislocation (Fig. 60.2). These are the patients who have had multiple surgeries, are frustrated, and are frequently depressed. The second group of patients are those who present with patellar pain later in life (50–70 years) and have associated femorotibial

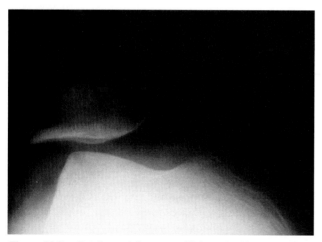

Figure 60.2. Patellar malalignment with lateral subluxation of the patella.

arthrosis. This group includes only those patients with significant patellofemoral arthrosis with minimal femorotibial involvement. These patients do not have patellar malalignment and have usually not had previous surgery. Both groups of patients are difficult to treat and must be meticulously studied because the surgical options depend on the presence of patellar tilt/compression and the severity of the arthritic changes.

Audible "grinding" or crepitus is common and the patients frequently complain of the patella "getting stuck in the flexed position." This occurs secondary to the loss of the normal frictionless glide between the patella and femoral groove resulting from degeneration. The osteophytes and cartilaginous defects on the patellar surface and the femoral sulcus cause uneven and painful tracking. Swelling is frequently present; complaints of medial and lateral joint line pain occur if bicompartmental or tricompartmental disease is present as well.

Physical Examination

The most common signs of patellofemoral degenerative disease are tenderness in the retropatellar space and crepitus. The examination begins by observing the patient in the standing position and evaluating patellar tracking and gait. Lateral patellar tracking can be present, and patellar instability is frequently a problem, as mentioned above. Next, the patient is seated on the examination table in order to observe patellar tracking in this position. Grating or crepitus is frequently present, and catching will be evident in advanced cases of degeneration. There is no need to compress the patella against the femoral sulcus in these patients as this is an extremely painful test and may alienate the patient. The three most important factors in the examination are observation of patellar tracking, determination of severity of patellofemoral degeneration, and evaluation of the medial and lateral compartments. All three of the parameters will be instrumental in selecting the treatment protocol appropriate for the patient.

Radiologic Evaluation

The axial and lateral views are studied with special emphasis given to patellar height, alignment, and patellofemoral congruity. Patellar tilt is evaluated at 30 degree, 45 degree, and 90 degree flexion angles on the axial view. The anteroposterior view must be taken to record the degree of arthrosis of the femorotibial joint and the varus or valgus angulation. Computerized tomography at selected flexion angles may be helpful to evaluate patellar tilt, but this can usually be determined by careful physical examination and by axial view radiograph examination. The bone scan, however, is a vital test used to evaluate the patellofemoral joint as well as to gauge the degree of femorotibial joint arthrosis (Fig 60.3).

Arthroscopy

Arthroscopy is invaluable in determining the degree of patellofemoral degeneration as well as evaluating patellar tracking and femorotibial involvement as well. The majority of these patients have undergone at least one prior arthroscopic examination; it is mandatory for the treating surgeon to evaluate these arthroscopic tapes or photos prior to making future surgical decisions.

Treatment

The surgical treatment of advanced patellofemoral degenerative disease is extraordinarily frustrating. The literature is full of good to excellent results of chondroplasties, tibial tubercle elevations, and patellectomies, yet most surgeons have never achieved these results. There is probably no other area in orthopaedics where the literature more grossly overestimates the beneficial effects of surgery as with that of the surgical treatment of patellofemoral degenerative disease. The most important factor in the treatment of patients with patellofemoral disease is to prevent further degeneration. This is accomplished by weight loss, quadriceps strengthening with particular emphasis on the vastus medialis, orthotics when indicated, McConnell patellar taping when indicated, nonsteroidal antiinflammatory medications, and modifications of activities.

When patients present with documented grade IV chondromalacia or osteoarthritis of the patellofemoral joint, the surgeon always exhausts conservative care. When patients state that they can no longer function with their pain and when they have failed conservative care, the surgeon finally begins to consider a surgical alternative. The surgical options consist of the following:

1. Arthroscopic or open debridement and chondroplasty of the patellofemoral joint with lateral release if indicated;
2. The above combined with a decompression of the patellofemoral joint by a tibial tubercle elevation;
3. Patellectomy;
4. Patellofemoral arthroplasty.

Indications for Surgery

The selection of the proper procedure for the patient depends on the severity of pain, presence of patellar tilt /compression, and the magnitude and location of Outerbridge grade IV lesions of the patellar and femoral groove. Pain symptoms are the least reliable due to their

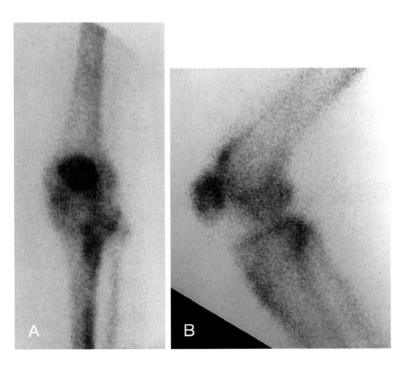

Figure 60.3. A and **B,** Bone scan demonstrating increased focal activity principally involving the patellofemoral joint.

subjective nature, but, obviously, patients with pain on strenuous activities will be treated less aggressively than patients with rest pain. The presence of patellar tilt/compression dictates the need for a lateral release to unload the lateral facet of the patella. The lateral release is usually done in addition to a chondroplasty, tibial tubercle elevation, or patellofemoral replacement, depending on the severity of the degenerative changes. The magnitude and location of the grade IV lesions are the most important findings to determine which surgical procedure is to be performed. Patients with patellar tilt/compression and grade IV lesions of the lateral patellar facet are treated with an arthroscopic lateral release and drilling chondroplasty. Patients with the same malalignment but with more diffuse grade IV lesions of the patella and grade IV changes of the femoral groove are best treated with a tibial tubercle elevation in addition to the lateral release and chondroplasty. Essentially, patellar tilt/compression will always be treated with a lateral release. Also, the grade IV lesions of the patella and femoral groove are always treated with a drilling chondroplasty except in rare cases of patellectomy and, of course, in patients undergoing patellofemoral replacement. The severity and location of the grade IV lesions will determine if a tibial tubercle elevation is to be done or if a patellofemoral replacement is to be selected.

Patients without patellar tilt/compression and minimal grade IV lesions of the patella and no femoral groove lesions are a rare group usually treated with drilling chondroplasty alone. Patients without patellar tilt/compression but with more severe grade IV lesions of the patella and with minimal grade IV lesions of the femoral groove are treated with drilling chondroplasty combined with a tibial tubercle elevation. A grade IV lesion of the femoral groove is a poor prognostic sign and indicates advanced disease. Patients with significant grade IV lesions of the femoral groove usually require a tibial tubercle elevation or patellofemoral replacement in addition to lateral release and/or chondroplasty, if indicated.

The only indication for a patellectomy is a severely comminuted patellar fracture that cannot be reconstructed. This is a rare case, and the surgeon should make every effort to maintain the patella. There is no indication for patellectomy in patellofemoral degenerative disease.

The indications for patellofemoral replacement are among the strictest of all orthopaedic procedures. The patient must have intractable pain, palpable crepitus, and extreme retropatellar tenderness on examination, radiographic evidence of severe patellofemoral degenerative disease on both sides of the joint, and documented arthroscopic evidence of grade IV chondromalacia of the patella and femoral groove. Most of the patients who eventually undergo a patellofemoral replacement have failed previous surgical procedures, and the majority have undergone a failed tibial tubercle elevation. It is difficult to determine if a patient with moderately severe symptoms, radiographic changes on both sides of the patellofemoral joint, and documented grade IV le-

sions on both sides of the joint is best treated with a tibial tubercle elevation or a patellofemoral replacement. In such patients, we usually recommend a tibial tubercle elevation and only recommend a patellofemoral replacement in those patients who have failed a tibial tubercle elevation or who have severe symptoms and severe destruction of the patellofemoral joint. Age and weight are certainly factors, but our median age is younger for patients undergoing a patellofemoral replacement (44 years) as compared to a total knee replacement (69 years). The age disparity is secondary to the malalignment with significant patellar tilt/compression, a condition which results in isolated patellofemoral degenerative disease at a younger age. These younger patients have also had numerous prior surgeries, and this may account for the advanced degeneration as well. Our smaller group of patients with patellofemoral degenerative disease without malalignment who undergo a patellofemoral replacement have a median age of 58 years, which is similar to those undergoing a total knee replacement.

The final determination is to choose between performance of a patellofemoral replacement or a total knee replacement. Younger patients (less that 55 years old) with malalignment and isolated patellofemoral arthrosis are treated with a patellofemoral replacement. A rare group is composed of patients older than 55 years with isolated patellofemoral arthrosis. I recommend patellofemoral replacement in this group, but only after meticulously ruling out the presence of femorotibial involvement that would place them in a total knee replacement group. Younger patients (less than 55 years old) with tricompartmental degenerative disease are best treated with a total knee replacement when indicated.

Lateral Release

The majority of the patients in our practice with advanced patellofemoral degenerative disease has excessive lateral ligamentous tension and patellar tilt/compression. A minimal lateral shift of the patella within the femoral sulcus at 30 degree of flexion decreases the contact surface by 60% (6). The decreased contact surface between the patella and femoral sulcus increases the unit load on the articular cartilage surface and increases the patellofemoral joint reaction forces (7). A lateral tilt of the patella generates significant destructive forces. The loads are concentrated on the lateral facet contact area of the patella. The abnormal cartilage loading leads to failure of normal cartilage secondary to mechanical overload. The cartilage surface breaks down and arthrosis can develop.

Patients with patellar tilt/compression usually present with Outerbridge grade III and IV lesions of the lateral facet of the patella, frequently along the corresponding lateral portion of the femoral sulcus. Chondromalacia of the medial facet of the patella may be secondary to deficient contact and chronic underload that denies the articular cartilage an appropriate mechanism of synovial fluid nutrition (8, 9). The underloaded medial facet is usually not symptomatic.

Fulkerson believes that a lateral release will reduce abnormal tilting of the patella as long as the lateral facet of the patella has not collapsed (10). He also states that a lateral release will be less effective in reducing tilt following collapse of the lateral facet. Huberti and Hayes (11) found that a lateral capsular release will not lead to a "normalization" of contact pressures in the patellofemoral joint. They believe that there was no support for the efficacy of the lateral release procedure for all cases of patellofemoral cartilage degeneration. Others have had similar findings (12). The mediocre results of lateral release in patients with chondromalacia patellae (13, 14) are further evidence of this experimental study.

We agree with Fulkerson, and we reserve a lateral release only for those patients with documented patellar lateral tilt/compression.

The lateral release is an integral part of the surgical treatment of patellofemoral degenerative disease, and it is included in any procedure we perform when there is evidence of patellar tilt. The addition of a tibial tubercle elevation or patellofemoral replacement is based on the severity of the grade IV Outerbridge changes on both sides of the joint. The only patients who do not undergo a lateral release are those rare cases having minimal grade IV changes without patellar tilt who undergo chondroplasty and those patients with advanced patellofemoral degenerative disease without patellar tilt who undergo a tibial tubercle elevation or a patellofemoral replacement.

The technique of lateral release is well described (15), and the complications have been minimized with improved techniques (16). We utilize an electrocautery (17) and complete the distal end of the release with a back-cutting blade, if needed. We prospectively compared 20 patients who underwent a release with a HO:YAG laser with an electrocautery group (Fig. 60.4). The patients were similar in all the usual parameters, and all had lateral tilt/compression with grades I–III Outerbridge chondromalacic changes. The two groups had no differences in their results, including blood loss

as measured by postoperative hemovac drainage, effusions, pain medications, or morbidity. The HO:YAG laser is an effective instrument for performing a lateral release, but has no advantage over the electrocautery.

Chondroplasty

Mankin (18) has shown that a healing response occurs after articular cartilage injury. A superficial cartilage injury causes initial death of the chondrocytes at the margin of injury and is followed by an increased metabolic activity of surrounding chondrocytes (19). The cartilage surface, however, shows no significant change in appearance following the superficial injury. It is recognized, therefore, that a superficial cartilaginous lesion that does not penetrate the tidemark will not repair (20–23). A full-thickness lesion penetrating the tidemark will initiate a vascular response. Mesenchymal cells invade this area forming reparative chondral tissue. Drilling holes into a grade IV Outerbridge lesion appears to stimulate fibrocartilaginous growth (24–27).

The initial reparative chondral tissue is predominantly type I collagen followed by a predominance of type II (articular cartilage) collagen (28). The defects in the articular cartilage are filled in eventually, however, by a fibrocartilage that is high in collagen content and low in proteoglycans. There has been evidence that a decompression of the patellofemoral joint by lateral release or by osteotomy combined with drilling chondroplasty can result in a cartilage repair response more closely resembling articular cartilage and more completely covering the initial defect when compared to chondroplasty or osteotomy alone. Abrasion chondroplasty combined with osteotomy appears to initiate a similar healing response (29). Chondroplasty, if it is to be done on grade IV Outerbridge lesions, must violate the tidemark and initiate a vascular response. There is certainly no role for superficial cartilage shaving in Outerbridge grade IV lesions.

We recommend placing drill holes 2 mm apart and 4 mm deep into the cancellous bone in all patients with grade IV Outerbridge lesions who undergo surgical treatment of patellofemoral degenerative disease (Fig. 60.5). The obvious exception is those patients who undergo a patellofemoral replacement. We believe that there is a sufficient reparative response following drilling procedures to justify its routine use. One has to remember that all of the surgical procedures for advanced patellofemoral degenerative disease give uniformly fair results; drilling chondroplasty certainly falls into this category. There is no single effective procedure for these patients, and the drilling chondroplasty is a "heroic" attempt to stimulate healing and minimize symptoms. We have begun drilling holes into grade IV lesions with varying wavelengths of the HO:YAG laser to increase the reparative response. An advantage of the HO:YAG laser is that there are probes with varying angles to deliver the laser easily on all surfaces of the joint. Our results are preliminary; we cannot recommend the use of the HO:YAG laser for drilling chon-

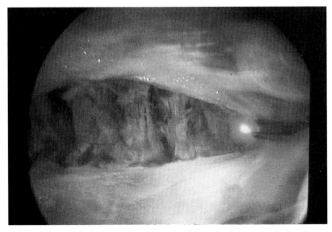

Figure 60.4. Subcutaneous lateral release performed utilizing the HO:YAG laser.

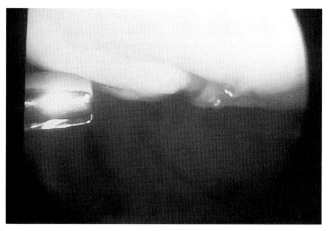

Figure 60.5. HO:YAG laser used to place drill holes into patellar lesion to stimulate a healing response.

droplasty at this time. We do not perform abrasion chondroplasty because the same theoretical benefit can be derived with drilling. The disadvantage of the abrasion arthroplasty is that it is technically difficult and is avoided.

However, chondroplasty is unlikely to be beneficial, if the etiology of the degenerative disease is not addressed. The most common etiology of patellofemoral degenerative disease is patellar tilt/compression with an overload of the lateral facet and corresponding femoral groove. All patients who undergo a chondroplasty will also undergo either a lateral release or a combined lateral release and tibial tubercle elevation. Patients with persistent tilt following lateral release, subluxation, and/or patellar dislocation will also undergo a medial transfer of the tibial tubercle in addition to the elevation. The concept that the mechanical overload must be corrected in addition to performing the chondroplasty cannot be overemphasized.

Osteotomy of the Patella

Some believe that relieving intraosseous hypertension may facilitate articular healing and decrease pain in patients with arthrosis of the knee (30). A simple longitudinal osteotomy of the patella has been reported to give significant relief of pain (31). Nerubay and Katnelson (32) have reported favorable results by performing a coronal plane osteotomy of the patella on patients with patellar pain and malalignment. They believe that the relief of pain was secondary to the reduction of intraosseous pressure and to the mechanical realignment of the patella. Only 1 patient in their group of 15 had a grade IV lesion; this patient was rated fair at follow-up. The role of osteotomy of the patella in patients with patellofemoral degenerative disease is unknown; thus, this procedure cannot be recommended at this time.

Tibial Tubercle Elevation

The patellofemoral joint reaction force and the patellofemoral contact areas are the important parameters in

understanding the biomechanics of the patellofemoral joint in normal and degenerative knees. The patellofemoral joint reaction force is equal and opposite to the resultant of the quadriceps tension ($M1$) and patellar tendon tension ($M2$) (Fig. 60.6) acting perpendicular to the articular surfaces (33). The patellofemoral contact area increases in flexion to compensate for the corresponding increase in patellofemoral joint reaction forces in flexion. This balance must be maintained to prevent excessive joint reaction forces combining with a decrease in contact area. The majority of our patients with patellofemoral degenerative disease have patellar tilt/compression and presumably increased patellofemoral joint reaction forces (34). In advanced cases, a lateral release may be insufficient to decompress this joint adequately when grade IV lesions are present on the patellar and/or femoral sulcus surfaces (34).

Maquet (35) was the first to propose that a decompression of the patellofemoral joint could be achieved by an elevation of the tibial tubercle. The elevation increases the lever arm of the quadriceps and increases the angle formed by the vectors of the quadriceps and patellar tendon that reduces the joint reactive forces (36, 37). He calculated that a 2 cm anterior displacement of the tibial tubercle would reduce the overall patellofemoral articular pressure by one-half. Bandi (38), in an experimental model, demonstrated a one-third reduction of the patellofemoral force by elevating the tibial tubercle 1 cm. Ferguson (39) showed significant reductions in contact pressure with tibial tubercle elevations. These reductions increased with increased tubercle elevation. Most of the reduction occurred at 1 cm elevation; he believed that the smaller additional

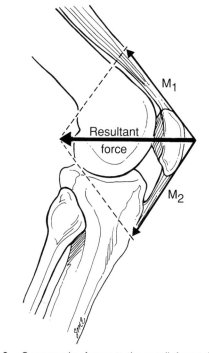

Figure 60.6. Compressive forces to the patellofemoral joint resulting from flexion angles.

reductions at the higher elevations were not justified. Burke and Ahmed (40) confirmed significant load reductions with progressive elevations of the tubercle greater than 1 cm, but they also found migration of the contact area from the distal to the proximal pole of the patella with increasing knee flexion angles. Nakamura, et al. (41) reported progressive decreases and proximal migration of the contact area with increasing elevation of the tubercle. They calculated joint forces and predicted decreasing contact forces with progressive elevation of the tubercle. Hayes, et al. (34) have demonstrated, in a model system, that reductions in patellofemoral contact force and joint contact areas can be obtained with tibial tubercle elevations, but that no consistent reduction in contact pressure occurs with a tibial tubercle elevation. They extrapolated this to a clinical setting, stating that the data provided little evidence to support using a tibial tubercle elevation to decrease contact pressures in chondromalacic patellofemoral joints. They showed that, even though the joint reaction forces could be reduced with a tibial tubercle elevation, this led to a decreased patellofemoral contact area and, therefore, to no overall decrease in contact pressure.

Technique (Tibial Tubercle Elevation)

A lateral parapatellar skin incision (Fig. 60.7) is made extending from the midpatella proximally to 8–10 cm distal to the tibial tubercle. The extensor mechanism is exposed, and a lateral capsular incision is made while being careful not to cut the lateral meniscus. A lateral release is performed in patients with patellar malalignment, and the patella and femoral groove are inspected. Debridement and drilling chondroplasties are performed when indicated. In rare cases without patellar malalignment, arthrotomy and lateral release are not performed. The incision is carried distally, and the interval between the lateral border of the patellar tendon and the anterior border of the anterior compartment musculature is developed. The lateral and medial borders of the patellar tendon are identified, and a retractor is used to protect it at all times. The anterior compart-

ment musculature is carefully dissected off the anterior crest of the tibia from the tibial tubercle distally to the end of the skin incision. A 1-inch, curved, sharp osteotome is used to begin the osteotomy proximally, being certain that the patellar tendon is not violated, but also that no bone is left attached proximal to the tibial tubercle. A 1-inch straight osteotomy is then used to slowly descend down the tibia. The osteotomy plane must be slanted posteriorly to prevent disruption of the anterior cortex, which will necessitate screw fixation of the osteotomy (Fig. 60.8). The osteotomy plane must also be flat in order to prepare a stable bed for the bone graft. Drill holes are not used to outline the osteotomy because they are stress risers that lead to disruption of the anterior cortex. An oscillating saw should not be used because this can increase the possibility of a nonunion. The osteotomy is extended 8–10 cm distally, and the osteotome is rotated within the osteotomy plane to assess the degree of opening of the osteotomy. The medial border of the periosteum is preserved, if possible. The tibial tubercle is levered forward with an osteotome or elevator and held in place by the bone graft. The bone graft is a freeze-dried iliac crest graft that is rigid and is easily contoured (Fig. 60.9) to conform to the plane of the osteotomy. The graft is self-locking and is stable without internal fixation as long as the anterior distal cortex has not been violated. Internal fixation is required if this has occurred. The graft must extend proximally to the tip of the tibial tubercle (Fig. 60.10). Patellar tracking is assessed, and the bone pedicle can be medialized modestly if required. A 3–5 mm medialization is possible and can be maintained by the stability of the bone graft. Medialization greater than 5 mm is not possible with this technique.

A hemovac drain is inserted, and the lateral retinaculum and detached anterior musculature is left open. A pressure dressing is applied. Continuous passive motion (CPM) can begin immediately, since graft stability was achieved at the time of surgery. Protected weight bearing is begun immediately, with the patient wearing a knee immobilizer. Patients are usually full weight bear-

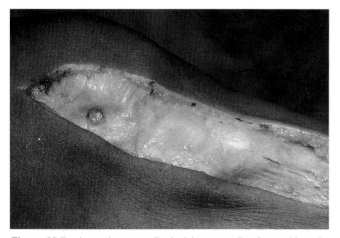

Figure 60.7.   Lateral parapatellar incision extending from midpatella proximally to 8 to 10 cm distal to the tibial tubercle.

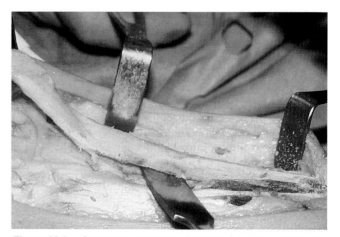

Figure 60.8.   Osteotomy of the tibia should be slanted posteriorly to prevent disruption of the anterior cortex.

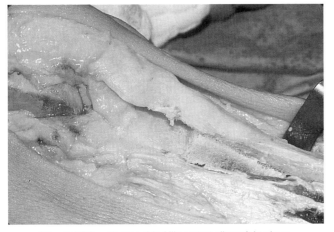

Figure 60.9. Freeze-dried iliac crest allograft in place.

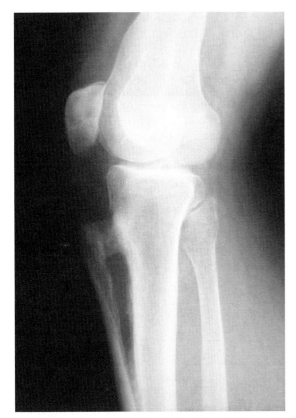

Figure 60.10. Maquet tibial tubercle elevation with iliac crest allograft in place, 5 months postoperative.

ing at 3 to 4 weeks, when they no longer require immobilizer protection.

Fulkerson (42, 43) has advocated the combination of extensor mechanism realignment and anterior placement of the tibial tubercle in patients with patellar arthrosis related to malalignment. He and others (44–46) do not believe that the tibial tubercle elevation alone will correct abnormal patellar tracking. Fulkerson has also been concerned about complications of the Maquet technique and has advocated an anteromedial tibial tubercle transfer without bone graft.

Technique (Fulkerson)

An anterolateral skin incision is made extending from the midlateral patella to a point 5 cm distal to the tibial tuberosity. A lateral release is done; abrasion arthroplasty is performed if indicated. The proximal anterior compartment musculature is released, and the lateral and posterior cortices of the tibia are exposed. The anterior tibial artery and peroneal nerve are protected. The medial and lateral borders of the patellar tendon are identified. The anterior tibial crest is exposed from the tibial tubercle to 7 cm distal. Several 3.2 mm drill holes are made parallel to each other in a plane that extends from the anteromedial tibia in a posterolateral direction, such that the drill tip enters the tibia just medial to the anterior tibial crest and exists just anterior to the posterolateral corner of the tibia. The pins must be parallel; a drill guide is mandatory to maintain the osteotomy plane. The osteotomy plane is tapered distally to preserve 2 to 3 cm of bone at the distal hinge and 5 to 7 cm just distal to the tibial tuberosity. The osteotomy plane must be flat and must be sufficiently oblique to achieve appropriate anteriorization of the tibial tubercle. Osteotomes are utilized to complete the osteotomy through the defined plane. When the osteotomy is complete (Fig. 60.11), the bone pedicle is hinged distally and displaced in an anteromedial direction along the osteotomy plane. Patellar tracking is assessed with the osteotomy maintained in the appropriate alignment. The bone pedicle is fixed with either cortical or cancellous screws with intraoperative radiographs required to check screw length.

The postoperative management is identical to a Maquet osteotomy in which immediate motion and protected weight bearing are encouraged.

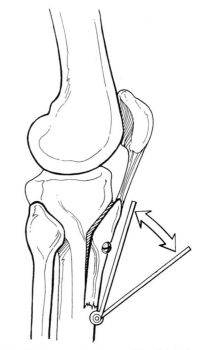

Figure 60.11. Fulkerson osteotomy of the tibial tubercle with bone pedicle hinged distally and displaced in an anteromedial direction.

Results

The literature is full of excellent and good results following a tibial tubercle elevation. Maquet (47) and Bandi (48) have reported good results; Radin and Leach (49) observed good results in 20 of 21 patients with patellofemoral degenerative disease who underwent a tibial tubercle elevation. Many others have experienced similar good results (44, 50–57). Others have had mixed results (58–60). Siegel (61) has reviewed the complications, which include skin necrosis, tibial nonunion, distal tibial tongue fracture, resorption of the tibial bone, pain at the osteotomy site, and a dissatisfaction with the cosmetic appearance of the bump at the tibial crest.

We retrospectively reviewed 54 patients (59 knees) who had undergone the procedure according to the Maquet principle. The preoperative diagnosis was chondromalacia in 30%, patellofemoral arthrosis in 65%, and 5% had had a previous patellectomy. The average age was 32.4 years old (ranging from 15 to 58 years). Ninety-eight percent of the patients had had previous surgery ranging from arthroscopy to patellectomy. Seventy percent had between 2 and 6 previous operations. All patients had a minimum of 24 months follow-up, with the exception of 1 patient who had undergone patellofemoral replacement 15 months after the Maquet procedure. Elevation of the tibial crest was obtained by freeze-dried iliac crest allograft (93%) and harvested autogenous bone graft (7%). The initial amount of elevation averaged 1.5 cm; there was very little settling noted when a freeze-dried iliac crest allograft was used.

There were very few complications. There were no skin complications and no nonunions. One patient developed a fracture at the base of the tubercle elevation and underwent open reduction and internal fixation with union. All of the grafts incorporated, and, of course, there was no graft site morbidity when the allograft was utilized.

Postoperative results were obtained utilizing a rating scale assessing pain, patellar stability, swelling, and function. Good subjective results were obtained in 18%, fair results in 28%, and poor results in 54%. Of the poor results, 68% had moderate to severe grade IV changes of the patellofemoral joint at the time of surgery. Good objective results were obtained in 41%, fair results in 44%, and poor results in 15%. Five patients eventually underwent a patellofemoral replacement.

Our poor results were similar to those reported by Friedman, et al. (59) and Silvello, et al. (58). We are in agreement with Silvello that our poorest results were in the arthritic patients. Silvello, et al. have suggested that their advancement might have been insufficient; they are recommending a 2 cm elevation as initially proposed by Maquet (35). We strongly agree with Friedman that a stringent criterion for a good result may be misleading in evaluating this procedure. Our results were very disappointing, and yet 50% of our patients stated that they were improved, although, in most cases, the improvement was slight. A tibial tubercle elevation is a palliative and end-stage procedure. It probably should not be judged by the same stringent criteria as other procedures.

Because a tibial tubercle elevation is an end-stage procedure, the unpredictability of the result must be completely explained to the patients prior to surgery. Patients must be willing to undergo the procedure with full knowledge that they have a 50% chance of having little or no relief of their symptoms. The complication rate can be minimized by good technique; we had no patients who were worse following the procedure. This likelihood should also be explained to the patient.

The indications for a tibial tubercle elevation are severe pain, the presence of malalignment, and/or significant grade IV chondromalacia changes. The patients we select for a tibial tubercle elevation are those who have either failed a previous lateral release and drilling chondroplasty or who have significant grade IV changes, especially on the femoral side of the joint.

When the patient chooses to undergo a tibial tubercle elevation, we strongly recommend the use of a freeze-dried iliac crest allograft. A 2 cm elevation is recommended, as we agree with Silvello (58) that a smaller elevation may not be adequate in the more severely involved arthritic patients. A Fulkerson osteotomy is recommended in patients with patellar subluxation or dislocation because a medialization is required, which is difficult to achieve with a Maquet procedure. The necessity for fixation of a Fulkerson osteotomy prevents us from routinely using this procedure. Bessette and Hunter (62) have shown that the complication rate is increased when operative fixation is required. An iliac crest allograft without fixation is solid, and immediate motion has not been a problem. It is technically difficult to achieve a 2 cm or greater elevation with a Fulkerson osteotomy; therefore, it is not the best procedure in patients with advanced disease.

Combined Tibial Tubercle Elevation and Proximal Tibial Valgus Osteotomy

The indications for a proximal tibial valgus osteotomy are occasionally limited secondary to the presence of advanced patellofemoral arthrosis. Coventry (63) reported an alleviation of symptoms related to the patellofemoral joint following a proximal tibial valgus osteotomy. Other authors have not had similar results. Maquet (64), Bourguignon (65), and Putnam, et al. (66) have performed a biplane osteotomy and combined the Maquet and proximal tibial valgus osteotomies for the treatment of symptomatic anterior and medial compartmental degenerative disease. Their results are favorable, but contraindicated by Nguyen, et al. (67), who reported that a proximal tibial valgus osteotomy was a good procedure for dual compartment disease for pain relief and that the addition of the Maquet procedure did not improve the results.

Current techniques for proximal tibial osteotomies with fixation devices that allow immediate motion would not be feasible if the osteotomies were combined. The possibility of improving the results by combining the osteotomies must be weighed against the ease and stability of current techniques that allow us to carry out internal fixation and to initiate immediate continuous passive motion.

Tibial Tubercle Elevation After Patellectomy

A patient with a patellectomy requires a 30% increase in quadriceps force to achieve full extension of the knee (68, 36). A tibial tubercle elevation can lengthen the extension movement arm and possibly increase muscle strength. Radin and Leach (49) have reported good results following a Maquet procedure in patients with a failed patellectomy. This approach is reasonable, but may not guarantee pain relief if there are significant grade IV lesions on the femoral groove. A femoral groove replacement may be combined with the tibial tubercle elevation if pain is severe in these patients.

Patellectomy

Patellectomy is a relatively old procedure, but, nevertheless, continues to be controversial. Brooke (69), Hey Groves (70), and Watson-Jones (71) all reported that excision of the patella actually improved the efficiency of the quadriceps muscle. The significance of the patella in quadriceps function, however, has been well documented by both clinical and experimental studies (7, 36, 68, 72, 73). The function is to increase the movement arm of the quadriceps tendon. Maquet (74) has shown that the patellar tendon, without a patella, will fall into the intercondylar groove and will shorten the lever arm of the quadriceps tendon. Kaufer (68) has found that the force necessary to produce full extension after patellectomy was increased by 15 to 30% depending on the type of patellectomy performed. Watkins, et al. (75) utilized a Cybex II isokinetic (dynamometer) to measure quadricep and hamstring function after unilateral patellectomy in 12 patients. Their results revealed that the function of the knee muscles was compromised postoperatively. Their objective findings documented alterations in muscle function that correlated well with the functional limitations of the patients. Steurer (76) found that patellectomy may alter instant centers of rotation and result in plowing forces that could accelerate arthrosis. Benoist and Romadier (77) believe that "the risk of rupture of the extensor mechanism exists after all patellectomies." They attribute this risk to the fact that patellectomy increases the force required from the quadricep mechanism to function properly. Finally, Larson, et al. (78), Lennox, et al. (79), and Bayne and Cameron (80) have all reported a high failure rate in patients who have undergone total knee arthroplasty following patellectomy.

Despite the limitations of function following a patellectomy and the fact that it compromises future total knee arthroplasty, there continues to be support for its role in the treatment of patellofemoral degenerative disease. Haliburton and Sullivan (81), West (82), Boucher (83), Debeyre, et al. (84), Boyd and Hawkins (85), and Baker and Hughston (86) have reported good to excellent results following patellectomy. Other studies have shown quite different clinical results. Scott (87), and Ackroyd and Polyzoides (88) have had poor results, usually secondary to unrelieved pain with weakness and instability. Lewis, et al. (89) had 72% good results and together with Kelly and Insall (90) have emphasized that alternatives to patellectomy should be found.

The objectives of a patellectomy are to:

1. Restore quadriceps strength and continuity;
2. Maintain or improve range of motion;
3. Maintain or improve patellar tendon tracking;
4. Maintain the motor strength of the extensor mechanism.

The creation of a "soft tissue patella" may also be more cosmetically acceptable to the patient. The techniques of Miyakawa (86) and Compere (91) attempt to achieve these goals.

Miyakawa Patellectomy

A lateral parapatellar incision is begun 7½ cm proximal to the patella and is completed at the tibial tuberosity. A medial flap is developed; the quadricep muscle and tendons, and patella are exposed. A medial arthrotomy is made, and the joint is inspected. Appropriate debridement is performed. The patella is removed by sharp dissection; the dorsal patellar aponeurosis is preserved. A superficial quadriceps flap is developed 1 cm above the patellar defect and extended proximally for 8 cm. This superficial flap is developed medially and laterally and is equal to the width of the patella. The flap is divided transversely at its proximal extension. The thickness of the flap is equal to ½ of the thickness of the entire quadricep tendon. The medial and lateral bases of the flap are supported by corner-reinforcing sutures. The flap is reflected distally and sutured into the patellar ligament through a rent developed in the patellar ligament and into the retinaculum. The appropriate length of the flap and the strength of fixation are tested by flexing the knee to 90 degrees (Fig. 60.12). If both flap length and fixation strength are adequate, the quadricep tendon is sutured to the retinaculum proximally to the base of the tongue of the quadricep tendon.

The vastus medialis muscle is advanced laterally to the lateral margin of the defect in the quadricep tendon. The vastus lateralis muscle is advanced medially, and a mattress suture is placed into and through the advanced vastus medialis. It is important to incorporate the underlying quadricep tendon with this mattress suture. The knee is flexed again to 90 degrees to evaluate tension. The knee is flexed, and tension on the suture line is evaluated following each successive suture.

A knee immobilizer is applied and partial weight bearing begun. Active assisted and active range of motion exercises are started immediately. Active assisted flexion greater that 110 degrees is not allowed until 6 weeks postoperatively.

Compere Patellectomy

A transverse skin incision is made, and the patella is exposed. A medial parapatellar arthrotomy is made; then a lateral parapatellar capsular incision is made parallel to the medial incision. The patella is everted and removed by sharp dissection. The dorsal quadricep aponeurosis

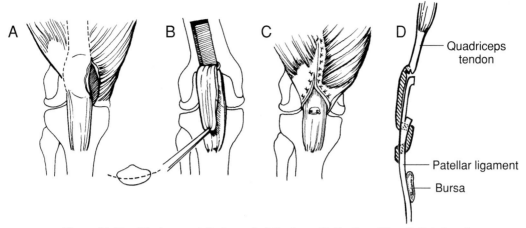

Figure 60.12.   Miyakawa patellectomy. **A,** Arthrotomy; **B,** Fixation of flap; **C,** Suturing of
quadriceps tendon; **D,** Lateral view.

is not violated. When the patella is removed, the medial
edge of the quadriceps aponeurosis is folded underneath and sutured to the lateral edge of the expansion
(Fig. 60.13). This creates a tube of the quadriceps
aponeurosis. The medial capsule is sutured to the tube,
and the vastus medialis muscle is advanced laterally
and distally. The lateral capsule is not sutured to the
tube. The knee is flexed to 90 degrees, so that tension
on the suture line can be evaluated.

The postoperative care is identical to that of the
Miyakawa patellectomy.

Results

In the literature, the clinical results following patellectomy appear good, but it is vital to evaluate and compare the results following a patellectomy performed for
patellofemoral arthrosis with a patellectomy performed
following patellar fracture. Between 1974 and 1990, we
have followed 152 cases of patellectomy performed for
patellofemoral arthrosis and 111 cases of patellectomy
following patellar fracture (Table 60.1).

Of the 152 patients (67.1%) in the patellofemoral
arthrosis group, 102 had surgery following patellectomy.
Of these patients, 67 had surgery that preserved the original concept of patellectomy, i.e., that of a "concept survivor" for whom the patellectomy is still decompress-
ing the patellofemoral joint. (The "concept survivor" is
a patellectomy patient who has not been revised to high
tibial osteotomy, femoral resurfacing, tibial tubercle elevation, arthrodesis, or a total knee replacement.) Twenty-
four cases were secondary to technical error in the original patellectomy, and 11 cases were due to progression of
the arthrosis. Miscellaneous subsequent procedures were
performed on 32 "concept survivors" for reasons unrelated to the original patellofemoral arthrosis. Combining
these 67 cases that had additional surgery unrelated to
patellofemoral joint with the 50 cases that had no further
surgery results in 77% of the 152 cases in this group being
patellectomy "concept survivors."

In the patellofemoral arthrosis group, 33 cases had
further surgery that did not allow for "concept survival"
(23% of the entire patellectomy group). Subsequent

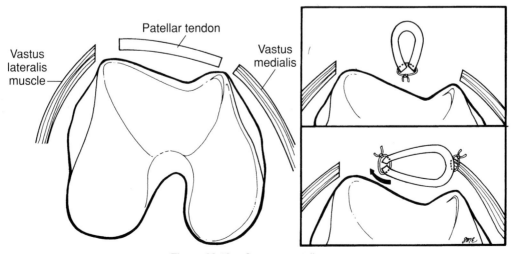

Figure 60.13.   Compere patellectomy.

Table 60.1 Results Following Patellectomy

Diagnosis	Number	Number of Subsequent Surgeries	Number of Subsequent Surgeries for "Concept Survivors"	"Concept Survivors"	Number of Subsequent Surgeries for "Nonconcept Survivors"
Patellofemoral Arthrosis	152	102 (67%)	67	117 (77%)	35 (23%)
Patellar Fracture	111	30 (27%)	27	108 (97%)	3 (3%)

surgery to reestablish the patellofemoral mechanism, which included implanting a patellar prosthesis or resurfacing of the femoral groove, was performed in 13 patients. Total knee replacement was subsequently performed on 22 patients.

In the patellectomy for patellar fracture group, 30 of the 111 patients (27%) required further surgery. Twenty-seven of these patients had surgery that still preserved the patellectomy "concept survivor" principle. Combining these 27 patients with the 81 patients who required no further surgery (108 of the 111 total) resulted in 97.3% of the patellectomy for fracture group being considered "concept survivors."

In the patellectomy group following patellar fracture, 3 cases (2.7% of the entire group) had further surgery that did not allow for "concept survival." Of these patients, 2 underwent a total knee replacement, and 1 patient underwent a subsequent knee arthrodesis.

The patellectomy for patellofemoral arthrosis group had a very high reoperation rate, and the procedure should be regarded as a poor one for end-stage patellofemoral arthrosis. The patellectomy for patellar fracture group had a much lower reoperation rate making patellectomy a satisfactory procedure for irreparable fractures of the patella. Patellectomy for fracture of the patella is a much more satisfactory operation than patellectomy for patellofemoral arthrosis.

Based on our digital results following patellectomy for patellofemoral arthrosis, we recommend this procedure for badly comminuted patella fractures when every effort at reduction and fixation has failed. We recommend patellectomy in the patient with patellofemoral arthrosis only if their disease is too severe to be treated with tibial tubercle elevation and if a patellofemoral replacement or total knee replacement is either unacceptable to the patient or is contraindicated secondary to chronic infection.

Resection Arthroplasty of the Patella

Beltran (92) described a resection arthroplasty of the patella for the treatment of patellofemoral pain caused by osteoarthrosis. In contrast to patellectomy, residual bone is left in this procedure.

Surgical Technique

An arthrotomy is performed, and the peripheral osteophytes are removed. The "true" margin of the patella is identified. An oscillating saw is used to remove the entire surface of the articular cartilage and subchondral bone. A flat cancellous surface is prepared similar to that in a standard patellar resurfacing. Between one-third and two-fifths of the patellar surface are removed. The femoral sulcus is untouched.

Postoperative care includes immediate isometric contractions of the quadriceps and straight leg raising. Knee flexion exercises are begun when the wound has healed.

Results

Beltran reported 33 resection arthroplasties of the patella in 20 patients. Sixty percent of the cases were pain free at 31 months average follow-up. We have no experience with this operation and expect that the long-term results would resemble those of resection arthroplasty in other joints. We do not recommend resection arthroplasty of the patella to our patients.

Patellar Resurfacing

McKeever (93) described a patellofemoral hemiarthroplasty utilizing a Vitallium prosthesis for resurfacing the patella. The patella prosthesis, anatomically shaped with medial and lateral facets, was fixed to the bone with a screw. He had favorable results in 40 knees with no mechanical failures at early follow-up. DePalma, et al. (94) reported utilizing the McKeever prosthesis with good short-term results in 17 patients. Worrell (95) reported favorable results at short-term follow-up in patients undergoing a prosthetic resurfacing of the patella. Harrington (96) reported 17 of 24 patients with good results at 5 years postoperatively. He used a McKeever prosthesis, but augmented the transfixation screw with polymethylmethacrylate in each case. Harrington has stated that his results have been satisfactory and have not deteriorated with time.

Aglietti, et al. (97) believed that patellar resurfacing could be improved by changing the anatomic design to a dome-shaped patella and by using acrylic cement fixation. Insall, et al. (98) reported 2 excellent, 14 good, 3 fair, and 10 poor results with this prosthesis at 3 to 6 years. All of the poor results were attributable to persistent pain. Levitt (99) reevaluated DePalma's original patients with the McKeever prosthesis and found deterioration of the results at longer follow-up. Worrell (100) has reported unsatisfactory long-term results with patellar resurfacing in young patients.

The results with patellar resurfacing are mixed; the procedure is controversial. A patient with osteoarthrosis of the patella severe enough to make him or her a candidate for patellar resurfacing invariably has changes in the femoral sulcus. Successful hemiarthroplasty in a patient with femoral involvement does not seem feasible. The indications for resurfacing are limited to, perhaps limited only to, patients with isolated patellar arthrosis who have failed previous patellar surgeries. We believe that disabled patients, with associated femoral groove involvement, are candidates for a patellofemoral replacement. Older patients with femorotibial arthrosis are candidates for total knee arthroplasty.

Patellofemoral Replacement

The combination of unsatisfactory results in more conservative procedures for severe degenerative patellofemoral disease and the excellent long-term results of total joint replacement encouraged the development of patellofemoral replacement.

Lubinus and Bechtol (101) introduced the patella glide replacement prosthesis in 1979, but did not report long-term results. Blazina, et al. (102) performed 85 patellofemoral arthroplasties in patients with various patellofemoral disorders. They reported results in 55 of 85 patients with an average age of 39 years and average follow-up of less than 2 years. Thirty subsequent procedures were performed in these patients, including realignment of the extensor mechanism or revision of a malpositioned component. The results were disappointing. Blazina and colleagues believed that technical errors were responsible for most of the revisions and that distortion or degeneration of the femoral groove was still best treated by a patellofemoral replacement.

Arciero, et al. (103) reported 18 of 25 (72%) patellofemoral arthroplasties with excellent or good results at 5.3 years average follow-up. The average age at the time of surgery was 62 years, and all 25 knees had roentgenograms demonstrating patellofemoral osteoarthrosis. Five patients had both tibiofemoral and patellofemoral osteoarthritis. The presence of tibiofemoral osteoarthritis adversely affected the outcome, and, with the 5 patients with tibiofemoral osteoarthritis excluded, 17 of 20 patellofemoral arthroplasties (85%) had satisfactory results. Arciero and colleagues reported no mechanical failures and believe that patellofemoral arthroplasty may be indicated for patients with osteoarthrosis limited to the patellofemoral compartment.

Cartier, et al. (104) reported 85% good to excellent results in 72 patellofemoral arthroplasties in 65 patients. The average follow-up was 4 years with a range of 2 to 12 years. In 69 cases, concomitant surgery procedures were performed, including soft tissue realignments, tibial tubercle transfers, and unicompartmental femorotibial replacements. Fourteen complications were noted, 7 related to the implant itself and 7 associated with extrapatellar pathology. They considered age less than 50 years to be a relative contraindication. Patella baja is a

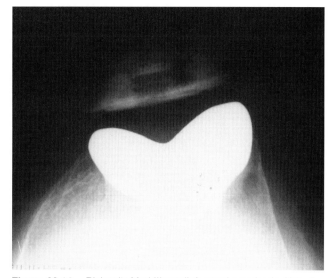

Figure 60.14.   Richard's Mod III patellofemoral prosthesis. Note the deep "retentive" trochlear design.

serious contraindication, secondary to symptomatic "catching" of the components. Cartier and his colleagues believe that patellofemoral replacement surgery is a viable procedure; they recommend it for patients over the age of 50 years with severe patellofemoral arthrosis. They are willing to compromise on this age limit in cases of severe anatomic incongruency.

Prosthesis

The majority of the patellofemoral replacements in all 3 of these series were performed with the Richards Patella II or the Patella Mod III prosthesis. The trochlea component is cobalt chrome and is tongue-shaped. It features a nonanatomic, deep, "retentive" trochlear design (Fig. 60.14). This requires the use of a patellar implant of polyethylene with a prominent ridge that matches the trochlear counterpart. The trochlear component is symmetric and extends quite proximally on the femur. The Richards Mod II features a control peg on the trochlear implant (Fig. 60.15), and the Mod III replaces the central peg with three fine points for fixation. The choice between the two is dependent on the preference of the surgeon and the quality of bone. The patella and trochlea are cemented into position.

Technique (Cartier)

A median parapatellar incision is made and a lateral release is performed if indicated. The fat pad is preserved in all cases. Osteophytes in the intercondylar notch are removed so as to restore normal anatomy. The appropriately sized trochlear drill guide is positioned. The outline of the trochlear trial is drawn on the bone with methylene blue. It is critical that the tip of the guide (and of the final implant) overlie bone and not be allowed to overhang into the notch. Gouges and curettes are used to remove remaining articular cartilage and to create a new trochlear bed. The soft tissues in the area

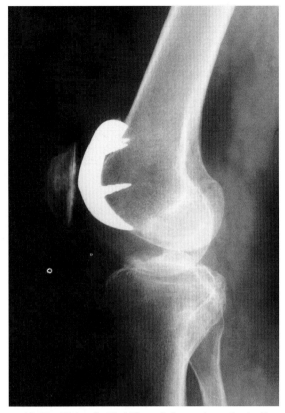

Figure 60.15. Richard's Mod III patellofemoral prosthesis. Note the tongue-shaped trochlear design.

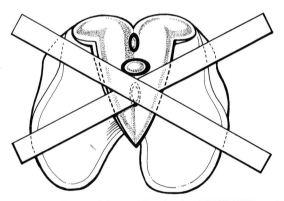

Figure 60.16. The tip of the trochlear implant **MUST NOT** overhang into the intercondylar notch, or impingement will occur.

just above the trochlea are cleared until the lower metaphysis is well visualized. The upper part of the implant will rest on this portion of the femur.

The most distal aspect of the trochlea is deepened until the tip of the trochlear drill guide is flush with the surrounding cartilage. It is important to confirm at this point that the tip of the trochlear drill guide does not overhang the intercondylar notch (Fig. 60.16).

The medial and lateral wings of the implant will ideally lie flush on the condyles. There is often significant dysplasia, however, in which case only one wing will

rest on bone and cement will be needed to fill the gap on the other side. The implant should not be tilted to force contact with bone on both sides.

Three drill holes are made through the trochlear drill guide, which is then fixed with three pins. A microsagittal saw is then used to create the trough for the antirotation blade. The Patella II requires a trochlear drill guide featuring just one hole and a 7 mm drill. The techniques are otherwise identical.

If the position of the drill guide is satisfactory, it is removed and replaced with the trochlear trial. The tibial spines should not impinge on the trochlear implant.

The patella is everted and a conventional cut is made with an oscillating saw. The thickness of the bone removed should approximate the thickness of the implant. The superior and inferior poles of the patella have to be clearly identified, which can be difficult once the patella is everted. The patella should be returned to its normal position (not everted) and K-wires should be inserted through the quadriceps and patellar tendons at the level of the inferior and superior poles. An imaginary line drawn between the two wires should divide the patella in two equal parts. The patella is again everted, and a cautery mark is made on the cut surface of the patella at the level indicated by the K-wires. Again, a line is drawn between the marks and should divide the patella into two parts.

The patellar drill guide is now positioned. The line on the guide should line up with the two cautery marks. The center of the holes in the guide is marked with a cautery. The two marks are then connected with a cautery-drawn line.

The patella is reduced. The line drawn between the two fixation holes should be absolutely perpendicular to the trochlear axis, both in extension and in the first few degrees of flexion. If not, the steps outlined above are repeated with the appropriate adjustments.

The holes for the patella pegs are drilled. The appropriate size for the patella trial is the largest one which overhangs neither at the top nor at the bottom of the patella.

The knee is put through a range of motion. The patellar trial should remain centered throughout, without any tendency to rotate or ride laterally. The patellar trial should track perfectly to the extent that: (a) the ridge on the patellar button should remain perfectly parallel to the trochlear groove throughout the range of motion, and (b) there should be no catching of the component as the knee goes from flexion to extension.

The trochlea and patella are cemented; tracking is assessed a final time. Patellofemoral replacement surgery is not a substitute for realignment surgery. The surgeon must carry out any and all procedures required to assure normal tracking and an absence of tilt throughout a full range of motion.

Postoperative Care

Immediate weight bearing is begun with quadriceps exercises and flexion exercises begun at the surgeon's discretion.

Custom Patellofemoral Prosthesis

The disadvantages of this prosthesis are twofold: it is technically demanding to insert, and it removes considerable femoral bone. Creating a perfect match between the patellar and femoral surfaces is extremely difficult; clicking and catching are not uncommon. There have been no published reports of total knee arthroplasty following failed patellofemoral replacement, but both Insall (105) and Scott (106) have cautioned us on the difficulty of revision surgery of a failed patellofemoral replacement, particularly in younger patients.

Blazina (107) has designed a custom patellofemoral replacement to avoid the disadvantages of the Richards nonanatomic trochlear groove. A software program, developed by Techmedica, Inc. (Camarillo, CA), utilizing the CAT scan allows for the construction of a three-dimensional model of the patient's own femoral groove. This is fabricated into a titanium alloy custom cap that fits exactly over the patient's own femoral groove and trochlear region. The initial design was secured by screws, but screw fretting and synovitis resulted. We now utilize three small fixation pegs on the trochlea and cement the implant in place. In essence, a custom resurfacing prosthesis is made. It eliminates the need to remove bone stock from the femur, impingement in flexion is reduced, and revision to total knee or patellectomy is facilitated later, if necessary.

Technique (Custom-Blazina)

A standard anteromedial incision is made with a medial arthrotomy. A lateral release is performed if indicated. The patella is retracted laterally and the knee is flexed to 60 degrees. Peripheral osteophytes are removed and the custom femoral trial is placed on the femoral groove and held in position. The outline of the trial is made with methylene blue (Fig. 60.17). Gouges and curettes are used to remove remaining articular cartilage, but no bone is removed at any time. The trial is reapplied to the decorticated femoral groove and three drill holes are

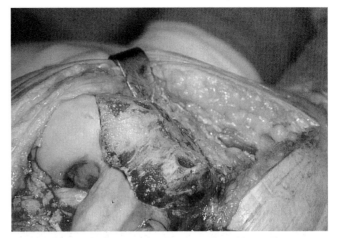

Figure 60.18. Drill holes placed in decorticated femoral groove to accept prosthesis.

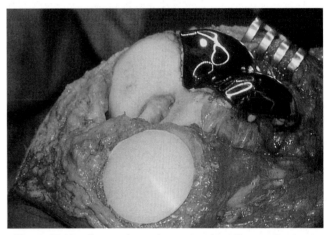

Figure 60.19. Custom femoral groove and patellar prosthesis cemented in place.

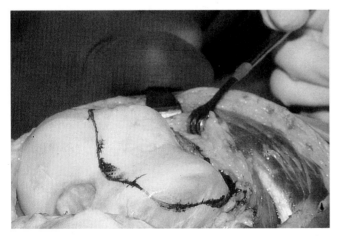

Figure 60.17. Methylene blue outline of femoral groove prosthesis.

made in the appropriate slots in the trial (Fig. 60.18). These holes are countersunk and the final implant is placed into position. The surface of the titanium custom implant is ionized to prolong wear, but caution still has to be shown to avoid violating the surface of the implant.

The patella is everted and is resurfaced with an oscillating saw. A standard dome-shaped polyethylene patella is utilized and the patellar surface is prepared in the usual fashion. The trial patella and the custom implant are inserted; the knee is then flexed fully and extended to 0 degrees. Patellar tracking is assessed, and impingement of the inferior lip of the groove on the inferior pole of the patella is ruled out. The patella and femoral groove are cemented into position (Fig. 60.19).

Postoperative Care

The fixation of the components is solid (Figs. 60.20–60.22) and immediate CPM with full motion is initiated. Full weight bearing is allowed immediately.

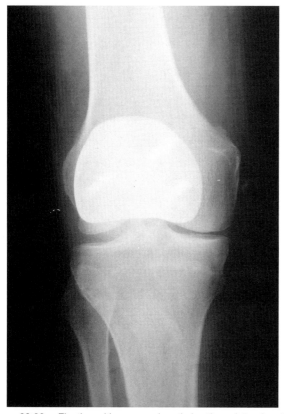

Figure 60.20. Fixation with pegs and methylmethacrylate of custom femoral groove and patellar prosthesis.

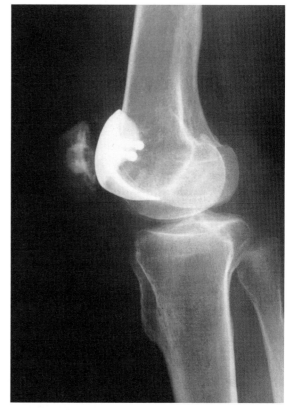

Figure 60.21. Fixation with pegs and methylmethacrylate of custom femoral groove and patellar prosthesis.

Results

We have performed 20 custom, cemented patellofemoral replacements in the last 3 years. The follow-up is preliminary, but the early results are encouraging. We have had no mechanical failures and no revisions.

Between 1974 and 1990 we have followed 131 cases of patellofemoral replacement (Table 60.2). Twenty-nine cases were performed primarily and 102 cases as a subsequent operation. None of these cases had had a prior proximal tibial osteotomy performed. None of these cases had had prior or concomitant knee replacement performed. After the patellofemoral replacement (PFR), 77 of the 131 cases (58.8%) had had further surgery. In the PFR group, 62 cases had had further surgery that allowed concept survival of the PFR principle. Combined with the 54 cases that had no further surgery, 88.5% of the cases in this group were considered concept survivors.

In the PFR concept survivor group, the reasons for reoperation were technical in 29 cases, regressive in 13 cases, and miscellaneous in 20 cases. An example of a reoperation for technical reasons in the PFR concept survivor group is the subsequent removal of a suture granuloma 6 months postoperation PFR. An example of a reoperation for regressive reasons in the PFR concept survivor group is a vastus lateralis release and tibial tubercle transfer 7 months postoperation PFR. An exam-

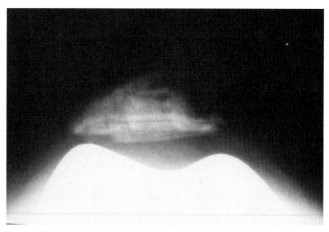

Figure 60.22. Fixation with pegs and methylmethacrylate of custom femoral groove and patellar prosthesis.

ple of a reoperation for miscellaneous reasons in the PFR concept survivor group is a medial meniscectomy performed 3 years following PFR.

In the PFR group, 15 cases had had further surgery that did not allow a "concept survival" (11.5% of the entire group). Four cases were revised to patellectomy, 10 cases were revised total knee replacement and 1 patient underwent a knee arthrodesis.

Table 60.2   Results Following Patellofemoral Replacement (PFR)

Diagnosis	Number	Number of Subsequent Surgeries	Number of Subsequent Surgeries for "Concept Survivors"	"Concept Survivors"	Number of Subsequent Surgeries for "Nonconcept Survivors"
Patellofemoral Arthrosis	131	77 (59%)	62	116 (89%)	15 (11%)

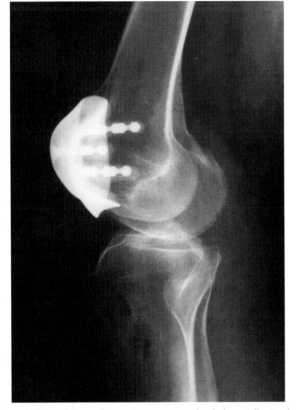

Figure 60.23.   Custom femoral groove prosthesis in patellectomized patient.

Custom Femoral Groove Replacement Following Patellectomy

We have performed a cemented, custom femoral groove replacement in 6 patients who have undergone a previous patellectomy (Fig. 60.23). The indications were persistent pain and tenderness in the femoral groove. All of these patients had severe grade IV changes of the femoral groove. All of these patients had intact extensor mechanisms with only minimal decreases in quadriceps function. A tibial tubercle elevation had been previously performed in 4 of these patients.

Our early results are good and all 6 are satisfied at early follow-up. We recommend the consideration of a cemented, custom femoral groove replacement in all patients with severe femoral groove arthrosis who have had a patellectomy and have failed previous tibial tubercle elevation.

Summary

The surgical treatment of patients with patellofemoral degenerative joint disease is disappointing. All efforts should be made to exhaust conservative, nonoperative care. In selected patients who are disabled, the surgeon should make every effort to perform a single surgery to alleviate symptoms. The patients must be counseled preoperatively about the mediocre results following all surgical procedures and must have reasonable expectations in the postoperative period.

The patellofemoral replacement patients had a very significant reoperation rate (58.8%), but this is a satisfactory end-stage procedure in extensor mechanism surgery (88.5%). Improvements in design will, hopefully, produce even better long-term results.

We recommend a custom, cemented patellofemoral replacement in severely disabled patients with distortion and degeneration of the femoral groove. We try to avoid this procedure in younger patients (less than 50 years), but will not hesitate to perform it when there is no alternative. A possible revision to a total knee replacement is facilitated by the custom femoral groove and noncompromised bone stock. Older patients (greater than 65 years), with truly isolated patellofemoral arthrosis are uncommon and are treated with a total knee replacement.

References

1. Outerbridge RE. The etiology of chondromalacia patellae. J Bone Joint Surg 1961;43B:752–757.
2. Ficat P. La degenerescence du cartilage de la rotule, de la chondromalane a l'arthose. Sem Hop Paris 1974;50:3209–3210.
3. Ficat P, Phillippe J, Cuzacq J. Le syndrome d'hyperpression extreme de la rotule. J Radiol Electrol Med Nual 1972;53:845.
4. Fulkerson JP. Anteromedialization of the tibial tuberosity for patellofemoral malalignment. Clin Orthop 1983;177:176–181.
5. Insall JN. Disorders of the patella. In: Insall JN, ed. Surgery of the knee. New York: Churchill Livingstone, 1984:218.
6. Hungerford DS. Patellar subluxation and excessive lateral pressure as a cause of fibrillation. In: Pickett JC, Radin EL, eds. Chondromalacia of the patella. Baltimore: Williams & Wilkins, 1984:24–42.
7. Goodfellow JW, Hungerford DS, Zindel M. Patellofemoral mechanics and pathology: I. Functional anatomy of the patellofemoral joint. J Bone Joint Surg 1976;58B:287.
8. Fulkerson J, Edwards C, Chrisman OD. Articular cartilage. In: Albright J, Brand R, eds. The scientific basis of orthopaedics. East Norwalk: Appleton & Lange, 1987.

9. Goodfellow JW, Hungerford DS, Woods C. Patellofemoral mechanics and pathology: II. Chondromalacia patellae. J Bone Joint Surg 1976;58B:291.

10. Fulkerson J, Schutzer S, Romsby G, Bernstein R. Computerized tomography of the patellofemoral joint before and after lateral release or realignment. Arthroscopy 1987;3:19–24.

11. Huberti HH, Hayes WC. Contact pressures in chondromalacia patellae and the effects of capsular reconstructive procedures. J Orthop Res 1988;6:499–508.

12. Hille E, Schulitz KP, Henrichs C. Pressure and contact-surface measurements within the femoropatellar joint and their variations following lateral release. Ach Orthop Trauma Surg 1985;104:275–282.

13. Osborne AH, Fulford PC. Lateral release for chondromalacia patellae. J Bone Joint Surg 1982;64B:202–205.

14. Unneberg K, Reikeras O. The effect of lateral retinacular release in idiopathic chondromalacia patellae. Arch Orthop Trauma Surg 1988;107:226-227.

15. Merchant AC, Mercer RL. Lateral release of the patella. Clin Orthop 1974;103:40.

16. Metcalf RW. An arthroscopic method for lateral release of the subluxating or dislocating patella. Clin Orthop 1982;167:9–18.

17. Miller GK, Dickason JM, Fox JM. The use of electrosurgery for arthroscopic subcutaneous lateral release. Orthopedics 1982;5:309–314.

18. Mankin HJ. Current concepts review: The response of articular cartilage to mechanical injury. J Bone Joint Surg 1982;64A:460–466.

19. Ghadially F, Thomas I, Oryschak A, LaRonde J. Long term results of superficial defects in articular cartilage. J Pathol 1977;121:213.

20. Bert JM. The arthroscopic treatment of unicompartmental gonarthrosis: A four year follow-up of abrasion arthroplasty versus arthroscopic debridement. Presentation at Arthroscopy Association of North America, Washington, D.C. 1988.

21. Carlson H. Reactions of rabbit patellar cartilage following operative defects. Acta Orthop Scand (Suppl) 1957;28.

22. Fujisawa MB, Masuhara K, Shiomi S. The effect of high tibial osteotomy on osteoarthritis of the knee; an arthroscopic study of 54 knee joints. Orthop Clin North Am 1979;10:585.

23. Mankin HJ. The reaction of articular cartilage to injury and osteoarthritis, Part I. New Eng J Med 1974;291:1285.

24. Magnusson PB. Technique of debridement of the knee joint for arthritis. Surg Clin North Am 1946;26:249.

25. Meachin G, Roberts C. Repair of the joint surface from subarticular tissue on the rabbit knee. J Anat 1971;109:317–327.

26. Mitchell N, Shepard N. The resurfacing of adult rabbit articular cartilage by multiple perforations through subchondral bone. J Bone Joint Surg 1976;58A:230–233.

27. Pridie KW. A method of resurfacing osteoarthritic knee joints. J Bone Joint Surg 1959;41B:618.

28. Furukawa T, Eyne D, Korde S, Glimcher M. Biochemical studies on repair cartilage resurfacing experimental defect in the rabbit knee. J Bone Joint Surg 1980;62A:79.

29. Tippett JW. Articular cartilage drilling and osteotomy in osteoarthritis of the knee. In: McGinty JB, ed. Operative arthroscopy. New York: Raven Press, 1991:335

30. Lynch J. Venous abnormalities and intraosseous hypertension associated with osteoarthritis of the knee. In: Ingwersen, ed. The knee joint. New York: Americal Elsevier, 1974.

31. Hejgaard N, Arnoldi CC. Osteotomy of the patella in the patellofemoral pain syndrome. The significance of increased intraosseous pressure during sustained knee flexion. Int Orthop 1984;8:189–194.

32. Nerubay J, Katnelson A. Osteotomy of the patella. Clin Orthop 1986;207:103.

33. Fulkerson JP, Hungerford DS. Disorders of the patellofemoral joint. 2nd ed. Baltimore: Williams and Wilkins, 1990:27.

34. Hayes WC, Huberti HH, Lewallen DG, Riegger CL, Myers ER. Patellofemoral contact pressures and the effects of surgical reconstructive procedures. In: Ewing JW, ed. Articular cartilage and knee joint function. New York: Raven Press, 1990:72.

35. Maquet P. Advancement of the tibial tuberosity. Clin Orthop 1970;115:225.

36. Kaufer H. Patellar biomechanics. Clin Orthop 1979;144:51.

37. Maquet P. Mechanics and osteoarthritis of the patellofemoral joint. Clin Orthop 1979;144:70.

38. Bandi W, Brenneald J. The significance of femoropatellar pressure in the pathogenesis and treatment of chondromalacia patellar arthrosis. In: Ingwerson OS, Van Linge B, ed. The knee joint. New York: American Elsevier, 1974:63.

39. Ferguson AB, Brown TD, Fu F, Rutkowski, R. Relief of patellofemoral contact stress by anterior displacement of the tibial tubercle. J Bone Joint Surg 1979;61A:159–166.

40. Burke DL, Ahmed AM. The effect of tibial tubercle elevation on patellofemoral loading. Trans Ors 1980;5:162.

41. Nakamura N, Ellis M, Seedhom BB. Advancement of the tibial tuberosity. J Bone Joint Surg 1985;67B:255–260.

42. Fulkerson JP, Becker GJ, Meaney JA, Miranda M, Folcik MA. Anteromedial tibial tubercle transfer without bone graft. Am J Sports Med 1990;18:490–497.

43. Fulkerson JP. Anteromedialization of the tibial tuberosity for patellofemoral malalignment. Clin Orthop 1983;177:176–181.

44. Hejgaard N, Watt-Boolsen S. The effect of anterior displacement of the tibial tuberosity in idiopathic chondromalacic patellae; a prospective randomized study. Acta Orthop Scand 1982;53:135–139.

45. Noll BJ, Ben-Itzhak I, Rossouw P. Modified technique for tibial tubercle elevation with realignment for patellofemoral pain. Clin Orthop 1988;234:178–182.

46. Miller BJ, LaRochelle PJ. The treatment of patellofemoral pain by combined rotation and elevation of the tibial tubercle. J Bone Joint Surg 1986;68A:419–423.

47. Maquet PG. Biomechanics of the knee. 2nd ed. Berlin: Springer-Verlag, 1984:280.

48. Bandi W. Chondromalacia patellae and femoro-patellae Arthrose Aetiologie, Klinik und Therapie. Helv Chir Acta 1972;39 [suppl]:1.

49. Radin E, Leach R. Anterior displacement of the tibial tubercle for patello-femoral arthrosis. Orthop Trans 1979;3:291.

50. Hirsh DM, Reddy DK. Experience with Maquet anterior tibial tubercle advancement for patellofemoral arthralgia. Clin Orthop 1980;148:136–139.

51. Lund F, Nilsson BE. Anterior displacement of the tibial tuberosity in the treatment of chondromalacia patellae. Acta Orthop Scand 1980;51:679–688.

52. Rozbruch JD, Campbell RD, Insall JN. Tibial tubercle elevation—the Maquet operation: A clinical study of 31 cases. Orthop Trans 1979;3:291.

53. Waisbrod H, Treiman N. Anterior displacement of tibial tuberosity for patellofemoral disorders: a preliminary report. Clin Orthop 1980;153:180–182.

54. Ferguson AB. Elevation of the insertion of the patellar ligament for patellofemoral pain. J Bone Joint Surg 1982;64A:766–771.

55. Sudmann E, Salkowitsch B. Anterior displacement of the tibial tuberosity in the treatment of chondromalacia patellae. Acta Orthop Scand 1980;51:171–174.

56. Mendes DG, Soudry M, Iusim M. Clinical assessment of Maquet tibial tuberosity advancement. Clin Orthop 1987;222:228–238.

57. Heatley FW, Allen PR, Patrick JH. Tibial tubercle advancement for anterior knee pain. Clin Orthop 1986;208:215–224.

58. Silvello L, Scarponi R, Guazzetti R, Bianchetti M, Fiore AM. Tibial tubercle advancement by the Maquet technique for patellofemoral arthritis or chondromalacia. Ital J Orthop Traumatol 1987;13(1):37–44.

59. Friedman MJ. Modified Maquet tibial tubercle elevation. Am J Knee Surg 1990;3:114.

60. Insall JN. Disorders of the patella. In: Insall JN, ed. Surgery of the knee. New York: Churchill Livingstone, 1984:252.

61. Siegel M. The Maquet osteotomy; a review of risks. Orthopedics 1987;10:1073–1078.

62. Bessette GC, Hunter RE. The Maquet procedure; a retrospective review. Clin Orthop 1988;232:159–167.

63. Coventry MB. Osteotomy about the knee for degenerative and rheumatoid arthritis. Indications, operative technique, and results. J Bone Joint Surg 1973;55A:23.

64. Maquet P. Valgus osteotomy for osteoarthritis of the knee. Clin Orthop 1976;120:143.

65. Bourguignon RL. Combined Coventry-Maquet tibial osteotomy; preliminary report of two cases. Clin Orthop 1981;160:144.

66. Putnam MD, Mears DC, Fu FH. Combined Maquet and proximal tibial valgus osteotomy. Clin Orthop 1985;197:217–223.

67. Nguyen C, Rudon J, Cooke TD, Simurda MA. Comparison of Maquet and high tibial osteotomy versus high tibial osteotomy in dual compartment osteoarthritis. J Bone Joint Surg 1989;71B:345.

68. Kaufer H. Mechanical function of the patella. J Bone Joint Surg 1971;53A:1551–1560.

69. Brooke R. The treatment of fractured patella by excision. A study of morphology and function. British J Surg 1937;24:733–747.

70. Hey Groves EW. A note on the extension apparatus of the knee joint. Br J. Surg 1937;24:747–748.

71. Watson-Jones R. Fractures and other bone and joint injuries. Baltimore: Williams and Wilkins;1940.

72. Hungerford DS, Barry M. Biomechanics of the patellofemoral joint. Clin Orthop 1979;144:9–15.

73. Sutton FS, Thompson CH, Lipke J, Kettlekamp DB. The effect of patellectomy on knee function. J Bone Joint Surg 1976;58A:537–540.

74. Maquet PG. Biomechanics of the knee. Berlin: Springer-Verlag, 1984:262.

75. Watkins MP, Harris BA, Wender S, Zarins B, Rowe CR. Effect of patellectomy on the function of the quadriceps and hamstrings. J Bone Joint Surg 1983;65A:390–395.

76. Steurer PA, Gradisar IA, Hoyt WA, Chu M. Patellectomy. A clinical study and biomechanical evaluation. Clin Orthop 1979;144:84–90.

77. Benoist JP, Romadier JO. Luxations et subluxations de la torule (traumatiques exceptees). Rev Chir Orthop 1969;55:89–109.

78. Larson KR, Cracchiolo A, Dorey FJ, Finerman GA. Total knee arthroplasty in patients after patellectomy. Clin Orthop 1991;264:243–254.
79. Lennox DW, Hungerford DS, Krackow KA. Total knee arthroplasty following patellectomy. Clin Orthop 1987;223:220–224.
80. Bayne O, Cameron HU. Total knee arthroplasty following patellectomy. Clin Orthop 1984;186:112.
81. Haliburton RA, Sullivan CR. The patella in degenerative joint disease. A clinicopathologic study. Arch Surg 1958;77:677–683.
82. West F. End results of patellectomy. J Bone Joint Surg 1962;44A:1089–1108.
83. Boucher HH. Patellectomy in the geriatric patient. Clin Orthop 1958;11:33–40.
84. Debeyre J, Levernieux J, Patte D. Gonarthroses traitees pour patellectomie, dans quelques-unes suivies depuis 10 ans. Prosse Med 1962;70:2775.
85. Boyd HB, Hawkins BL. Patellectomy. A simplified technique. Surg Gynec Obstet 1948;86:357–358.
86. Baker CL, Hughston JC. Miyakawa patellectomy. J Bone Joint Surg 1988;70A:1489–1494.
87. Scott JC. Fractures of the patella. J Bone Joint Surg 1949;31B:76.
88. Ackroyd CE, Polyzoides AJ. Patellectomy for osteoarthritis. J Bone Joint Surg 1978;60B:353–357.
89. Lewis MM, Fitzgerald PF, Jacobs B, Insall JN. Patellectomy—an analysis of one hundred cases. J Bone Joint Surg 1976;58A:736.
90. Kelly MA, Insall JN. Patellectomy. Orthop Clin North Am 1986;17:289–290.
91. Compere CLL, Hill JA, Lewinnek GE, Thompson RG. A new method of patellectomy for patellofemoral arthritis. J Bone Joint Surg 1979;61A:714–719.
92. Beltran JE. Resection arthroplasty of the patella. J Bone Joint Surg 1987;69B:604–607.
93. McKeever DC. Patellar prosthesis. J Bone Joint Surg 1955;37A:1074–1084.
94. DePalma AF, Sawyer B, Hoffman JD. Reconsideration of lesions affecting the patellofemoral joint. Clin Orthop 1960;18:63–85.
95. Worrell RV. Prosthetic resurfacing of the patella. Clin Orthop 1979;144:91.
96. Harrington KH. Long-term results for the McKeever patellar resurfacing prosthesis used as a salave procedure for severe chondromalacia patellae. Clin Orthop 1992;279:201–213.
97. Aglietti P, Insall JN, Walker PS, Trent P. A new patella prosthesis. Clin Orthop 1975;107:175–187.
98. Insall JN, Tria AJ, Aglietti P. Resurfacing of the patella. J Bone Joint Surg 1980;62A:933–936.
99. Levitt RL. A long-term evaluation of patellar prostheses. Clin Orthop 1973;97:153–157.
100. Worrell RV. Resurfacing of the patella in young patients. Orthop Clin North Am 1986;17:303–309.
101. Lubinus. Patella glide bearing total replacement. Orthopedics 1979;2:119.
102. Blazina ME, Fox JM, Del Pizzo W, Broukhim B, Ivey FM. Patellofemoral replacement. Clin Orthop 1979;144:98–102.
103. Arciero R, Toomey H. Patellofemoral arthroplasty: A three to nine year follow-up study. Clin Orthop 1988;236:60–71.
104. Cartier P, Sanouiller JL, Grelsamer R. Patellofemoral arthroplasty. J Arthroplasty 1990;5:49–55.
105. Insall JN. Disorders of the patella. In: Insall JN, ed. Surgery of the Knee. New York: Churchill Livingston, 1984:249.
106. Scott RD. Prosthetic replacement of the patellofemoral joint. Ortho Clin North Am 1979;10:129–137.
107. Blazina ME, Anderson LJ, Hirsh LC. Patellofemoral replacement: Utilizing a customized femoral groove replacement. Tech Orthop 1990;5:53–55.

61

Fresh Osteochondral Allografts in Knee Reconstruction

Scott E. Marwin and Allan E. Gross

Fresh osteochondral allografts have been used to reconstruct knee joints with defects produced by trauma, osteochondritis dissecans, osteonecrosis of the femoral condyles, osteoarthritis, and locally aggressive benign bone tumors (1–13). Many of these patients are otherwise young, active, and healthy. The surgical alternatives for these problems in this population may not be appropriate. Partial and total joint replacement may be contraindicated because of the risks of loosening and further bone loss. Arthrodesis of the knee produces a poorly tolerated loss of motion.

The goals of surgery are twofold. First, the affected joint is resurfaced with living, intact articular cartilage. Ideally, the viable chondrocytes will insure the integrity of the cartilage. Second, bone stock is restored in the area of the defect.

Lexer first described allotransplantation of the human knee joint in 1908 and, then again, in 1925 (14, 15). However, the great volume of work done in the field appeared after the contemporary approaches to bone and cartilage banking were reported in the 1940s (16). The early clinical studies done by Parrish (17), Ottolenghi (18, 19), and Volkov (20) reviewed the use of massive frozen osteochondral allografts in limb salvage cases. They reported success rates of 60 to 69%. Articular surface degeneration was a common complication in these studies. The lack of viable chondrocytes was implicated as the cause of cartilage failure.

The desire to include living cartilage on these grafts prompted two trends. First, Mankin and co-workers applied the technique of cryopreservation to the use of massive osteochondral allografts both experimentally and clinically (21–23). Cryopreservation had been successfully used to bank a number of other tissues including spermatozoa, kidney, cornea, and blood (24). Their feline model produced unpredictable chondrocyte viability. They obtained good to excellent results in 66.7% of patients treated with these grafts following tumor resection about the knee. Unfortunately, a high number of these patients required further surgery.

Second, several investigators have championed the use of fresh osteochondral allografts to treat smaller defects about the knee (1–11). The senior author (AEG) has transplanted 204 grafts since 1972, with an average follow-up of 8 years. The remainder of this chapter is devoted to the scientific and clinical data supporting the use of fresh allografts. Pertinent operative techniques are also included.

Terminology

Some confusing terms are defined in this section so that the reader will be better equipped to evaluate the literature. An *autograft* or *autogenous* graft is a transplant from the same individual. An *allograft* or *allogeneic* graft is a transplant between two individuals of the same species. A *xenograft* is a transplant between two individuals of different species.

An *orthotopic* graft is a transplant that is placed into its anatomic position. A *heterotopic* graft is a transplant that is placed in an area different from its position of origin.

Grafts can be characterized by their position in the knee. The patellofemoral joint is typically discussed as a separate entity. A *compartment* refers to either the medial or lateral portions of the tibiofemoral articulation. A *pole* refers to either the femoral or tibial portion of a compartment. Therefore, a graft could be unicompartmental or bicompartmental. It could also be unipolar or bipolar.

Finally, clarification of the banking techniques is warranted. These methods are commonly seen in the literature and are central to any discussion of allograft procedures. *Fresh* grafts are tissues refrigerated at approximately +4°C. *Deep* frozen grafts are tissues maintained at −30 to −70°C. Freeze-drying is not deep freezing. *Freeze-drying* is a process of dehydrating frozen bone (25). Crystalline water (ice) is removed in vacuo from the tissue as vapor, without passing through a liquid phase (25). This is a time-consuming and cumbersome procedure.

Cryopreservation is a technique used to freeze tissue while optimizing cell survival. Freezing and, for that matter, thawing alter the osmotic gradients across cellular membranes (24). Osmotic injury can cause cell death. Cytoprotectants such as glycerol and dimethylsulfoxide (DMSO) stabilize these gradients (24). Treatment of tissues with one of these substances before freezing potentially improves the chance for cell survival.

Tissue Viability

The only valid reason to use fresh grafts in the face of potential histoincompatibility and disease transmission is that these implants serve as a vehicle for living cartilage. Viable chondrocytes help maintain the normal function of the articular cartilage. Chondrocytes are well suited for transplantation. Unlike most solid organs, cartilage is avascular. The cells receive their nutrition by diffusion of synovial fluid through the cartilaginous matrix. There is an ebb and flow to the movement of nutrients because diffusion depends on the periodic motion of the knee joint. The chondrocytes are conditioned to tolerate periods of malnourishment similar to what is seen following harvest.

Unpreserved hyaline cartilage remains 100% viable for 4 to 28 days when stored at +4°C (26–38). Meyers and co-workers have refrigerated fresh canine cartilage in culture media up to 60 days with no change in glycosaminoglycan and collagen content (38). However, cellular viability was decreased significantly at 60 days as measured by autoradiography (38). Shahgaldi et al. suggested that loss of cellular viability of cartilage on implanted fresh grafts in goats occurs with tissue refrigerated over 2 weeks (39).

Other preservation methods have deleterious effects on cells. Deep freezing and freeze-drying kill chondrocytes (25, 40–42). In animal models, cryopreservation can produce 0 to 50% chondrocyte viability (43–45). Enneking and Mindell found necrotic cartilage in six retrieved, cryopreserved, massive human osteochondral allografts that remained in situ 6 to 65 months (40). The cryopreserved cartilage resembled histologically articular surfaces found on two retrieved freeze-dried grafts. Secondary sterilization techniques using irradiation or ethylene oxide also destroy chondrocytes (16).

Long-term cartilage viability for fresh grafts in situ has been demonstrated. Kandel et al. and Oakshott et al. have found living chondrocytes in retrieved, failed fresh grafts as late as 94 months (5, 46). Czitrom et al., using autoradiographic techniques, demonstrated 69 to 99% chondrocyte viability in biopsied functioning grafts as late as 72 months postimplantation (47).

Unlike cartilage, bone is vascular and becomes necrotic following removal from the donor. Few cells survive the transplantation. Fortunately, the bone does not have to be living, because its function is basically passive. The osteoconductive properties of bone remain, and creeping substitution replaces the cancellous scaffolding in as few as 24 months (26, 46, 48). The strength of the graft, particularly before incorporation,

depends on the nonviable matrix. A disadvantage of necrotic bone is that it is unable to repair itself. Accumulated microtrauma to the osseous portion of the graft can lead to subsequent fragmentation and collapse.

Transplantation Biology

Fresh osteochondral allografts are immunogenic (49–54). The major source of alloantigens are living cells that survive the transplant. Remnants of cells are also antigenic. The bone marrow cells have the greatest immunogenicity (55). Bone cells also elicit an immune response (54). Chondrocytes are antigenic but are hidden from the immune system by the cartilage matrix (49). Immunogenicity can be found in the proteinaceous component of the bone and cartilage matrices; however, these are relatively minor contributors (55). Bone banking techniques do have the advantage of decreasing immunogenicity of allografts (56–59).

The following summarizes the immune response as it pertains to allografts. The reader is encouraged to review an excellent synopsis of the topic by Friedlaender (55). The alloantigens responsible for the immunogenicity of fresh grafts are cell surface glycoproteins encoded by the major histocompatibility complex (MHC). Class I alloantigens (HLA A, B, C) are found on all nucleated cells. They function as targets for cytotoxic CD8+ T lymphocytes. Class II alloantigens (HLA D) are found on B lymphocytes and certain activated T lymphocytes. They are also found in high densities on antigen-presenting cells (APC) such as dendritic cells and cells from the macrophage/myeloid lineage. Class II determinants function as targets for regulatory CD4+ T lymphocytes. CD4+ T cells can be divided into TH-1 inflammatory cells and TH-2 helper cells. TH-1 cells participate in a variety of inflammatory processes and secrete important cytokines such as interleukin-2 and interferon-γ. TH-2 cells stimulate B lymphocytes to produce antibodies. In general, the CD4+ T cells play a crucial role in regulating the immune response.

The effector arm of the immune response is a complex series of events. When an osteochondral allograft is implanted, the initial host immune response is nonspecific. This inflammatory reaction is dominated by macrophages and neutrophils. This is a typical foreign body reaction and can last as long as 20 weeks. Eventually, the class I and class II determinants found in the graft stimulate an antigen-specific response by the host. Activated TH-1 T cells secrete interferon-γ, which activates macrophages to secrete interleukin-1. This cytokine amplifies the T cell response. Interleukin-1 also activates host osteoblasts, an osteoinductive activity. However, osteoblasts also stimulate the activity of osteoclasts. CD8+ T cells are activated by class I determinants, and their activity is amplified by interleukin-2 secreted by TH-1 cells. Antibody production is magnified by activated TH-2 cells.

Fresh grafts should elicit an intense response. Acute or chronic rejection, however, rarely occurs. Histologic review of retrieved failed fresh grafts shows no evidence of rejection. Plus, the clinical reality is that these grafts do well almost 80% of the time. The immune system must down-regulate in some fashion. There are several hypotheses for modulation of the immune response. First, the articular cartilage is said to be "immuno-privileged" (49). The cartilaginous matrix protects chondrocytes from the affecter and effector arms of the immune system. These cells are privileged to be isolated from the host response. Second, interferon-γ stimulates osteoblasts through the activities of macrophages. This cytokine has been implicated also in turning down bone resorption. Incorporation is not impeded. Last, transforming growth factor β found in the allograft and released during bone resorption may inhibit osteoclast activity, stimulate osteoblast activity, and dampen the entire T cell response (55).

Because the immune response does not seem to significantly alter the survival of the grafts, tissue typing preoperatively and immunosuppression postoperatively are not done. Stevenson et al. have shown in an animal model that tissue matching may improve the overall performance of massive osteochondral allografts (51, 53). Tissue matching would unnecessarily limit the availability of an already thin supply of fresh tissue.

Disease Transmission

The risk of transmitting disease to a recipient is clearly the greatest problem facing transplantation of fresh allografts (60–66). The American Association of Tissue Banks (AATS) provides strict guidelines and standards for donor selection (60). Donors are chosen on the basis of historical and serologic workup. Of special interest are syphilis, hepatitis B, hepatitis C (non-A, non-B), HTLV I, HIV-1, HIV-2, and cytomegalovirus. Testing for these pathogens is recommended by the AATS. Following these guidelines, the senior author (AEG) has had no cases of disease transmission following the implantation of 204 fresh osteochondral allografts.

Acquired immunodeficiency syndrome (AIDS) is foremost on the minds of recipients who are scheduling elective surgery for a problem that is not life-threatening. One case of HIV-1 transmission following the use of banked bone for spinal surgery and four cases of HIV transmission following bone marrow transplantation have been reported (65, 66). These cases involve tissue donations made before 1985, when initial HIV screening was implemented. Simonds et al. reported on 3 cases of HIV transmission following the use of frozen bone allografts donated by a single individual who tested HIV-negative before tissue harvest (64). This donor, though deceased, had a complete historical workup as well as two HIV antibody tests. Interestingly, other bone taken from this donor, which was subsequently processed (freeze-drying, ethanol extraction) and implanted, did not transmit the virus to the recipients (25 cases). Buck et al. have demonstrated that infected bone remains infected following deep freezing (63). Clearly, meticulous examination of each donor is essential to minimize risk. The accepted risk for a recipient to become infected by a donor testing negative for HIV is less than 1:1 million (62).

Mechanical Considerations

Preserving the mechanical integrity of the allograft is crucial to its longevity. Both the cartilaginous and the osseous portions of the graft contribute mechanically. The articular surface is the load-bearing organ of the joint. It serves two important functions as the load bearer (67). First, it dissipates contact stresses by increasing contact area through deformation. Second, it provides a lubricated surface for opposing bone ends to articulate with minimal friction and wear. Living chondrocytes on the graft insure protection of these functions over time. The bone buttresses the articular surface. It also provides a means of anchoring the graft either through a press-fit configuration or by internal fixation devices (2, 10). Appropriate manipulation of both allograft and host conditions is crucial to the survival of these grafts.

Banking techniques alter the mechanical properties of the graft. Freeze-drying significantly decreases bending and torsional strength of bone, while not affecting compressional strength (68). This technique destroys chondrocytes and dehydrates articular cartilage, thus, rendering the allogeneic joint surface functionally impaired (25, 40). Bone strength is not altered by deep freezing or cryopreservation (68). Cartilage matrix is maintained by these techniques, but chondrocyte function is severely decreased (21, 22, 41, 42). The articular cartilage may function well in the short term, but prospects for prolonged normal function are poor. Fresh grafts retain their original mechanical properties. The viable chondrocytes give the best chance for continued cartilage function.

The size and shape of an allograft contributes to its success. The grafts should be orthotopic (4, 5, 7, 9, 10, 39, 48, 51, 53). This insures maximum congruency of the joint, delaying the degenerative process. Meyers and co-workers, in their series of fresh osteochondral grafts, had three cases of heterotopic implants, all of which failed (9, 10). The fit between graft and host should be precise (4, 5, 7, 32, 51, 53). All efforts should be made to match the size of the donor to the size of the patient. Also, the shape of the graft should match the shape of the recipient bed (5). Oakshott et al. found that 50% of the failed fresh grafts reviewed in his series did not precisely fit the recipient bed (5). There is some controversy surrounding the thickness of the graft. Gross and co-workers believe that the graft should sit flush with the host's joint surface (2, 4, 5, 7). High compressive forces seen at the proud graft are believed to cause failure. Meyers, on the other hand, places the grafts 1 to 2 mm proud, anticipating that the graft will settle, making the joint congruous (9, 10). This contention is supported by Shahgaldi et al. in a goat model using bovine xenografts (39). Grafts less than 5 mm thick are prone to fragmentation (4, 5, 7). The current recommendation is to have a graft thicker than 1 cm (4, 5, 7).

Abnormal mechanical forces secondary to joint instability lead to cartilage degeneration of grafts placed around the knee (9, 10, 69–71). Knee stability may be a prerequisite for resurfacing a joint with a graft. Many patients who require this type of reconstruction have complex injuries involving ligaments as well as joint surface. Meyers recommends that joint stability be restored before the patient with an unstable knee undergoes an allograft reconstruction (9).

Stability at the graft/host junction is required for incorporation (72, 73). The necessary stability can be provided by press-fit fixation or internal fixation. Before 1989, Meyers used press-fit configurations in his fresh grafts successfully (9). Presently, this group is using absorbable pins to secure their femoral condyle grafts (10). Gross and co-workers fix the grafts with two 4.0-mm, partially threaded, cancellous screws with washers (2, 4, 5, 7).

Angular deformity of the affected limb can alter the survival of these grafts. Oakshott et al. showed that 83% of failed fresh allografts occurred in malaligned limbs (5). Zukor et al. found that well-aligned limbs produced fewer failures than poorly aligned limbs (7).

Malalignment is centered at the diseased knee and is often associated with the pathologic defect in the articular surface. Early in their transplant program, Gross and co-workers used the height of the graft to correct a deformity (1). This led to graft failure. Osteotomy about the knee joint is the current recommended realignment procedure (2, 4, 5, 7). This procedure essentially unloads the allograft while correcting the deformity. If the deformity dictates that the osteotomy and the transplantation be done on opposite sides of the joint (one procedure on the femoral side and one procedure on the tibial side), then the procedures could be done simultaneously. If the osteotomy needs to be performed on the same side of the joint as the transplantation (either both on the femoral side or both on the tibial side), then, the realignment should be done 6 to 9 months earlier to allow healing of the osteotomy site.

The most common scenario is a lateral tibial plateau defect with a valgus deformity at the knee. A distal femoral varus osteotomy is performed with a lateral tibial plateau graft (Figs. 61.1 and 61.2). The second most common scenario is a medial femoral condyle defect with a varus deformity at the knee. A proximal tibial valgus osteotomy is performed with a medial femoral condyle graft (Figs. 61.3 and 61.4).

Patient Selection

Appropriate patient selection is tantamount to satisfactory outcome. Gross and co-workers, among others, have identified a number of patient characteristics that are predictive of success.

Diagnoses

McDermott et al. reviewed 100 patients who received fresh, small-fragment osteochondral allografts for articular defects about the knee (1). The diagnoses included osteoarthritis, spontaneous osteonecrosis of the knee, steroid-induced avascular necrosis of the femoral condyles, osteochondritis dissecans, and trauma. Grafts done for posttraumatic changes in the joint did best.

Those done for primary osteoarthritis did poorly. Meyers and co-workers also had poor results with fresh grafts placed into osteoarthritic knees (9, 10). Garrett produced excellent results for patients treated for traumatic defects and osteochondritis dissecans (11). Bell et al. have shown the utility of using fresh osteochondral allografts for the reconstruction of knees following resection of certain giant cell tumors (GCT): those lesions not amenable to curettage because of subchondral bone erosion and pathologic intraarticular fracture or those lesions that recur following adequate curettage (8). It is the opinion of the senior author (AEG) that posttraumatic defects of the knee are the only absolute indication for grafting (1, 2, 4, 5). Osteochondritis dissecans remains a relative indication (1, 2, 4, 5).

Age

Beaver et al., using Meier-Kaplan survivorship analysis, demonstrated that younger patients (< 60 years) in the posttraumatic group had longer-surviving grafts than older patients (> 60 years) in the same group (Fig. 61.5) (3). Actually, the great majority of patients are in their second and third decades.

Site

Unipolar/unicompartmental grafts are the most successful when considering the tibiofemoral articulation (1–5, 7). Meyers et al. obtained satisfactory results in 5 of 7 patellofemoral grafts (9).

Surgical Technique

The senior author's protocol is presented here (2). The reader is encouraged to review the methods of the other authors using fresh grafts for defects of the knee (9, 10, 11).

Procurement

The local organ procurement agency (Multiple Organ Retrieval and Exchange Program of Toronto) identifies potential donors. These donors must meet the criteria outlined by the AATS. Also, donors are always under 30 years of age. This insures that the graft has pristine cartilage and strong bone.

The graft is harvested within 24 hours of the death of the donor, under strict aseptic conditions. The specimen consists of the entire knee joint including an intact capsule. Aerobic, anaerobic, fungal, and tuberculosis cultures are obtained at the time of harvest. The specimen is stored in a sealed container in 1 liter of Ringer's lactate solution with cefazolin (1 g) and bacitracin (10,000 U) added. The container is refrigerated at +4 °C.

Operation

The transplantation is usually performed within 12 hours of harvest and always within 24 hours. The operation is performed in a clean air room with the surgeons wearing body exhaust suits. The patient receives preoperative antibiotics (cefazolin). Two surgical teams work simultaneously: one performs the arthrotomy while the other prepares the graft.

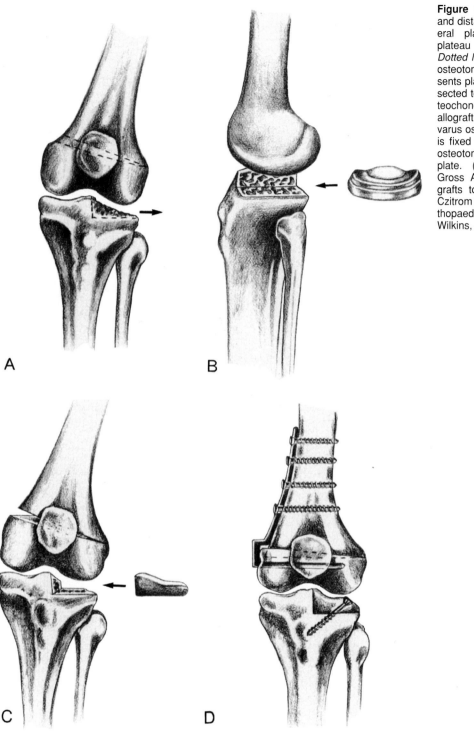

Figure 61.1. Lateral tibial plateau allograft and distal femoral varus osteotomy. **A,** Old lateral plateau fracture with depression of plateau and an associated valgus deformity. *Dotted line* in distal femur represents planned osteotomy. *Dotted line* in proximal tibia represents planned resection. **B,** Lateral plateau resected to healthy cancellous bone with the osteochondral allograft ready for implant. **C,** The allograft is inserted, and the distal femoral varus osteotomy is performed. **D,** The allograft is fixed with two cancellous screws, and the osteotomy is fixed with a 90-degree blade plate. (Reproduced with permission from Gross AE. Use of fresh osteochondral allografts to replace traumatic joint defects. In: Czitrom AA, Gross AE, eds. Allografts in orthopaedic practice. Baltimore: Williams & Wilkins, 1992:69.)

Ideally, the surgical approach is through an anterior, longitudinal incision over the affected knee. This may vary if old surgical scars are present about the knee. The incision is approximately 25 to 35 cm long and is centered over the patella. Proximally, it overlies the quadriceps tendon, and distally, it overlies the tibial tubercle. Minor skin flaps are raised to facilitate later closure. A medial or lateral parapatellar arthrotomy is done, depending on the site of the defect. Excellent access to the affected side of the joint is obtained with these arthrotomies. If a high tibial osteotomy is necessary, the skin incision is carried further distally to allow reflection of the anterior compartment off the proximal and lateral portion of the tibia. There is usually no difficulty doing a standard high tibial osteotomy through this approach. For the femoral osteotomy, the medial aspect of the distal femur is approached through the above skin incision. The fascia over the vastus medialis

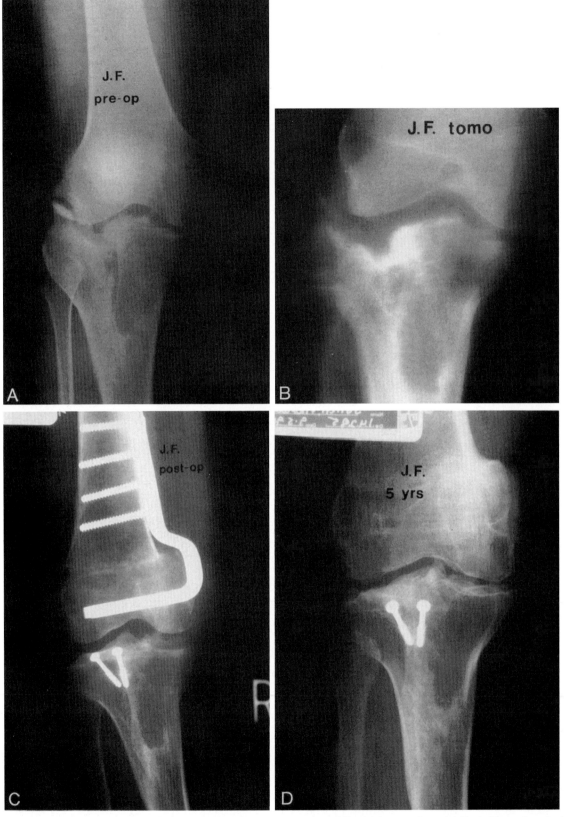

Figure 61.2.   Lateral tibial plateau fracture. **A,** An anteroposterior radiograph of a right knee in a 26-year-old female. **B,** An anteroposterior tomogram. **C,** One-year follow-up anteroposterior radiograph. **D,** Five-year follow-up anteroposterior radiograph. The graft is incorporated, and the joint space is maintained. (Reproduced with permission from Gross AE. Use of fresh osteochondral allografts to replace traumatic joint defects. In: Czitrom AA, Gross AE, eds. Allografts in orthopaedic practice. Baltimore: Williams & Wilkins, 1992:75.)

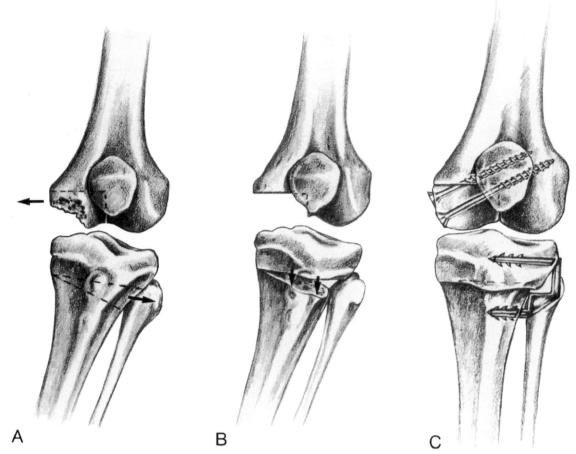

A   B   C

Figure 61.3. Medial femoral condyle allograft and proximal tibial valgus osteotomy. **A,** Traumatic loss of medial femoral condyle and secondary varus deformity. *Dotted line* in distal femur represents planned resection of condyle. *Dotted line* in proximal tibia represents planned osteotomy. **B,** Diseased condyle resected, and proximal tibial osteotomy performed. **C,** Osteochondral allograft inserted and fixed with two cancellous screws. The tibial osteotomy is fixed with two staples. (Reproduced with permission from Gross AE. Use of fresh osteochondral allografts to replace traumatic joint defects. In: Czitrom AA, Gross AE, eds. Allografts in orthopaedic practice. Baltimore: Williams & Wilkins, 1992:71.)

is incised. The muscle is then dissected from the medial intermuscular septum and reflected anteriorly and laterally, exposing the medial portion of the distal femoral shaft and the medial femoral condyle.

Once exposure is obtained, the reconstruction is straightforward and quite conservative. The articular defect is "squared off" with the goal of removing as little bone as possible. The resection is down to bleeding cancellous bone. The graft is machined to accurately fit the recipient bed. As stated earlier, the graft is orthotopic. The articular surface of the graft is made to lie flush with the surface of the host joint. The graft, whether tibial or femoral, is fixed with two 4.0-mm partially threaded cancellous screws. Enough bone must be retained on the graft to accommodate the two screws. For the lateral tibial plateau graft, the screws are directed through the graft's lateral cortical bone inferiomedially into the cancellous bone of the proximal tibia. For the medial femoral condyle, the screws are directed through the graft's medial cortex and directed supero-

laterally into the cancellous bone of the distal femur. In both scenarios, fixation tends to be excellent.

The high tibial osteotomy that is done in concert with a medial femoral condyle graft is a lateral closing wedge osteotomy. The proximal tibiofibular joint is excised. Then, a bone flap is lifted from the anterior aspect of the proximal tibia. It is a rectangular flap that is 3 to 4 cm wide and 5 to 6 cm long. It is left attached to the tibia at its distal end. The flap includes the tibial tubercle. It can slide over the proximal fragment as the osteotomy is reduced. The initial horizontal cut is done at the level of the insertion of the patellar ligament on the tibial tubercle and made parallel to the tibial articular surface. The length of the wedge's base is determined by the amount of varus the limb is in. The senior author likes to correct the limb to a tibiofemoral angle of approximately 10 degrees (valgus overcorrection). The osteotomy is typically fixed with two stepped staples.

The distal femoral osteotomy that is done concurrently with a lateral plateau graft is well described by

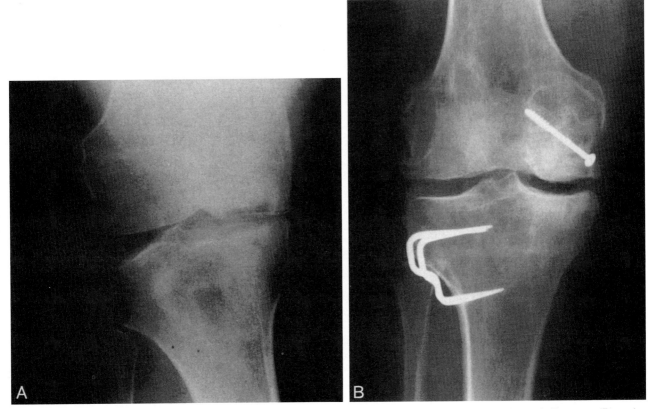

Figure 61.4. Posttraumatic osteonecrosis medial femoral condyle. **A,** Anteroposterior radiograph of the right knee. Posttraumatic osteonecrosis medial femoral in a 32-year-old woman. **B,** Anteroposterior radiograph of the right knee 9.5 years after fresh osteochondral allograft and high tibial osteotomy. Early degenerative changes are seen, but the graft has remodeled without significant collapse, and the joint space is well maintained with good alignment. (Reproduced with permission from Gross AE. Use of fresh osteochondral allografts to replace traumatic joint defects. In: Czitrom AA, Gross AE, eds. Allografts in orthopaedic practice. Baltimore: Williams & Wilkins, 1992:72.)

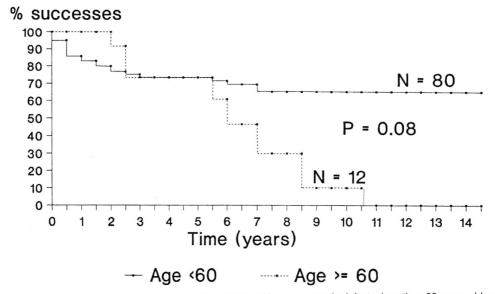

Figure 61.5. Survival of allografts performed in patients with posttraumatic defects, less than 60 years old and 60 years and older (2-tailed P = .08).

McDermott et al. (74). This is a medial closing wedge osteotomy. The first bone cut is made parallel to the transcondylar line of the distal femur. The transcondylar line connects the two distalmost points on the femoral condyles. The base of the wedge is only 5 to 10 mm long. This conservative wedge allows the intercondylar line to become perpendicular to the medial cortex of the femur, producing the desired tibiofemoral angle of zero (varus overcorrection). If the wedge is too small, impaction of the proximal fragment into the distal fragment allows adequate correction. This construct is fixed with a 90-degree blade plate. The blade is placed parallel to the transcondylar line, and the plate is used to reduce the osteotomy as it is fixed to the femoral shaft. The plate forces the transcondylar line to be perpendicular to the medial femoral shaft.

The meniscus at the defect site is inspected and is repaired by direct vision if damaged. However, if the meniscus is irreparable, a meniscal allograft is added to the reconstruction. The use of meniscal allografts is discussed later in the chapter.

Postoperative Regimen

The patient receives postoperative antibiotics for two days (cefazolin). The knee is immediately mobilized in the recovery room with a continuous passive motion (CPM) machine designed to allow varus and valgus adjustments. Early motion facilitates cartilage nutrition and prevents stiffness (75). The patients are carefully protected. They are placed in a long leg, ischial bearing caliper for 1 year. If an osteotomy is done, the patient remains non–weight bearing until signs of radiographic healing are seen. The patient is made partially weight bearing in the caliper if no osteotomy is done or when a osteotomy heals. Physiotherapy consists of active and active/assisted range-of-motion exercises and isometric strengthening exercises. No resistive work is done until the patient is out of the brace and the graft is healed.

Results

Clinical

Zukor et al. reported a 76% success rate for 94 fresh osteochondral allografts with an average follow-up of 4.3 years. These grafts were done for young patients treated for posttraumatic defects of the knee (4, 7). Of the 13 failures, 4 were bipolar grafts, and 6 were poorly aligned limbs. Survival analysis of 99 posttraumatic grafts produced a 75% success rate at 5 years and a 64% success rate at 10 and 14 years (Fig. 61.6) (3). These figures significantly improved when unipolar grafts and young patients were isolated. For instance, the 14-year survival rate for unipolar grafts is 70% (Fig. 61.7). Gender, side (medial or lateral), and anatomic structure (femur or tibia) did not affect results. Meyers had a 77.5% success rate at an average follow-up of 3.6 years in 39 patients who had 40 implants done (9). Garrett et al. had excellent results in 24 of 24 patients with fresh grafts followed more than 2 years (11).

Gross and co-workers have had few complications. These include postoperative stiffness, reflex sympathetic dystrophy, wound hematoma, patellar tendon rupture, and respiratory problems (no pulmonary emboli) (2, 4). Meyers et al. have had two infections (9). Salvage procedures are facilitated by the restoration of bone stock at the graft site. Gross has revised 6 knees to total knee replacements; 3 knees have been fused; 3 have gone on to further allografting; and 1 has been debrided (2, 4). Presently, there are no difficulties with these patients.

Radiological

Union is defined as trabecular bone crossing the graft/host junction or the osteotomy site on x-ray. Enneking suggests that union of the graft to the host can occur with persistent junction lucencies (40). In the

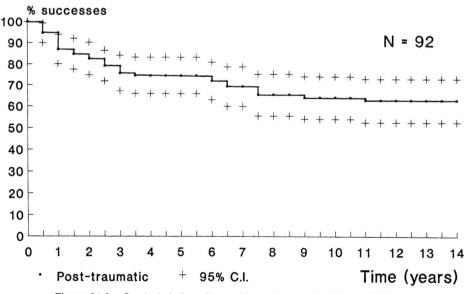

Figure 61.6. Survival of allografts used for posttraumatic defects of the knee.

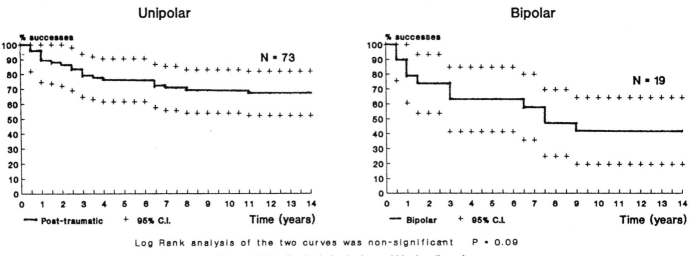

Figure 61.7. Survival of unipolar and bipolar allografts.

posttraumatic group, Gross and co-workers obtained a radiographic union rate of 98% (2, 4, 5, 7). Union appeared 9 to 12 months after transplantation. Complete remodeling of the graft occurs within 2 to 4 years. It has been suggested that the relatively long time to incorporation has immunologic roots (47). The osteotomies usually heal in 6 to 8 weeks.

Some of the radiographic findings are not consistent with the clinical ratings. Although all graphs subside at least 1 to 3 mm, 28% of the grafts subside 4 to 5 mm, and 2% completely collapse (7). The joint space is well preserved or moderately decreased in 74% of patients (7). However, in 26% of the grafts, the joint space was grossly arthritic (7). These radiographic findings do not necessarily indicate bad outcome. The degenerative joints have a lining of suboptimal fibrocartilage that delays the onset of pain. These joints ultimately fail.

Meniscal Transplantation

Arnoczky et al. state that the primary functions of menisci are load bearing, shock absorption, joint stability, and joint lubrication (76). Renstrom and Johnson add that the menisci provide greater congruity to the joint (77). For complex injuries of the knee, the menisci become important stabilizers. Stability of the knee can determine the outcome of these fresh grafts. When a meniscus is irreparable, degenerate, or resected, a meniscal allograft is added to the construct.

Few clinical studies have been done in this area. All involve complex injuries of the knee. Zukor and Gross reported on 54 meniscal allografts transplanted with osteochondral allografts for patients with posttraumatic defects of the knee (78). Ten menisci were examined arthroscopically at an average of 4 years postimplantation. Only minor tears and degenerative changes were demonstrated. No "bucket handle" tears were seen. All were stable peripherally. Garrett et al. had similar results in 6 fresh meniscal transplants (79). Milachowski et al. had good results with deep-frozen menisci but

poor results with freeze-dried menisci (80). Freeze-drying is detrimental to the mechanical structure of the meniscal cartilage.

The senior author's (AEG) technique is as follows. When a tibial plateau is transplanted, its corresponding attached meniscus is implanted with it. After the graft is seated into the recipient bed, the periphery is sewn to host synovial tissue, using 2-0 or 3-0 absorbable sutures. When a femoral condyle is used, the meniscal allograft is implanted separately. The meniscus is placed into its orthotopic position. The anterior and posterior horns are sewn to remnants of the previous meniscus or to synovial tissue, using 2-0 or 3-0 absorbable sutures. The periphery is attached to synovium. Other methods of fixation for isolated meniscal allografts have been suggested. A plausible alternative is the use of press-fit or internally fixed bone plugs at the ends of the implanted meniscus (81).

Summary

The implantation of these fresh grafts is elective surgery for a problem that is not lethal. The benefits of reconstruction with living cartilage must be weighed against the risk of disease transmission. Currently, the risk of infecting a patient when donor selection guidelines are followed is extremely low. Graft survival can be expected if certain principles are adhered to. These principles include

1. Careful patient selection
2. Proper fit of the graft
3. Stable fixation of the graft
4. Restoration of limb alignment
5. Meniscal transplantation when necessary
6. Protected weight bearing postoperatively while maintaining good motion of the joint.

This is not a technically demanding procedure. Obviously, the allogeneic tissue must be available to the surgeon. No bridges are burned when this type of reconstruction is done in the appropriate patient. If the graft fails, at least bone stock is restored, making subsequent revision surgery easier.

References

1. McDermott AGP, Langer F, Pritzker KPH, Gross AE. Fresh small osteochondral allografts. Clin Orthop 1985;197:96.
2. Gross AE. Use of fresh osteochondral allografts to replace traumatic joint defects. In: Czitrom AA, Gross AE, eds. Allografts in orthopaedic practice. Baltimore: William & Wilkins, 1992:67–82.
3. Beaver RJ, Mahomed M, Backstein D, Davis A, Zukor DJ, Gross AE. Fresh osteochondral allografts for post-traumatic defects in the knee, a survivorship analysis. J Bone Joint Surg 1992;74B;105–110.
4. Zukor DJ, Paitich B, Oakshott RD, et al. Reconstruction of post traumatic articular surface defects using fresh small-fragment osteochondral allografts. In: Aebi M, Regazzoni P, eds. Bone transplantation. Berlin: Springer-Verlag, 1989:293–305.
5. Oakshott RD, Farine I, Pritzker KPH, Langer F, Gross AE. A clinical and histological analysis of failed fresh osteochondral allografts. Clin Orthop 1988;233:283–294.
6. Zukor DJ, Gross AE. Osteochondral allograft reconstruction of the knee—part 1: a review. Am J Knee Surg 1989;2(3):139–149.
7. Zukor DJ, Oakshott RD, Gross AE. Osteochondral allograft reconstruction of the knee—part 2: experience with successful and failed fresh osteochondral allografts. Am J Knee Surg 1989;2(4):182–191.
8. Bell RS, Davis A, Allan DG, et al. Fresh osteochondral allografts for advanced giant cell tumors at the knee. J Arthroplasty. In press.
9. Meyers MH, Akeson W, Convery FR. Resurfacing of the knee with fresh osteochondral allograft. J Bone Joint Surg 1989;71A:704–713.
10. Convery FR, Meyers MH, Akeson WH. Fresh osteochondral allografting of the femoral condyle. Clin Orthop 1991;273:139–145.
11. Garrett J. Osteochondral allografts for treatment of chondral defects of the femoral condyles: early results. Proceedings of the Knee Society. Am J Sports Med 1987;15:387.
12. Aichroth PM, Burwell RG, Elves MW, Ford CHJ, Laurence M. Biological and mechanical problems of osteoarticular allografting: the relation to clinical organ transplantation. J West Pac Orthop Assoc 1971;8:25–70.
13. Outerbridge RE. Joint surface transplants—a preliminary report. J West Pac Orthop Assoc 1971;8:1–15.
14. Lexer E. Substitution of joints from amputated extremities. Surg Gynecol Obstet 1908;6:601.
15. Lexer E. Joint transplantation and arthroplasty. Surg Gynecol Obstet 1925;40:782.
16. Friedlaender GE, Tomford WW. Approaches to the retrieval and banking of osteochondral allografts. In: Friedlaender GE, Goldberg VM, eds. Bone and cartilage allografts: biology and clinical applications. Chicago: American Academy of Orthopaedic Surgeons, 1991:185–192.
17. Parrish FF. Allograft replacement of all or part of the end of a long bone following excision of a tumor. J Bone Joint Surg 1973;55A:1.
18. Ottolenghi C. Massive osteoarticular bone grafts: transplant of whole femur. J Bone Joint Surg 1966;48B:646–659.
19. Ottolenghi C. Massive osteo- and osteo-articular bone grafts. Clin Orthop 1972;87:156–164.
20. Volkov M. Allotransplantation of joints. J Bone Joint Surg 1970;52B:49.
21. Schachar NS, Henry WB Jr, Wadsworth P, Castronovo FP Jr, Mankin HJ. Fate of massive osteochondral allografts in a feline model. In: Friedlaender GE, Mankin HJ, Sell KW, eds. Osteochondral allografts: biology, banking, and clinical applications. Boston/Toronto: Little, Brown & Co, 1983:81–101.
22. Mankin HJ, Doppelt SH, Sullivan TS, Tomford WW. Osteoarticular and intercalary allograft transplantation in the management of malignant tumors of bone. Cancer 1982;50:613–630.
23. Power RA, Wood DJ, Tomford WW, Mankin HJ. Revision osteoarticular allograft transplantation in weight-bearing joints: a clinical review. J Bone Joint Surg 1991;73B:595–599.
24. Tomford WW. Cryopreservation of articular cartilage. In: Friedlaender GE, Mankin HJ, Sell KW. Osteochondral allografts: biology, banking, and applications. Boston/Toronto: Little, Brown & Co, 1983:215–218.
25. Malinin TI, Wu NM, Flores A. Freeze-drying of bone for allotransplantation. In: Osteochondral allografts: biology, banking, and applications. Boston/Toronto: Little, Brown & Co, 1983:181–192.
26. Campbell CJ, Ishida H, Takahaashi H, Kelly F. The transplantation of articular cartilage. an experimental study in dogs. J Bone Joint Surg 1963;45A:1579–1592.

27. DePalma AF, Tsaltas TT, Mauler GG. Viability of osteochondral grafts as determined by uptake of S35. J Bone Joint Surg 1963;45A:1565–1578.
28. Lance EM, Fisher RI. Transplantation of the rabbit's patella. J Bone Joint Surg 1970;52A:145–156.
29. McKibbin B. Immature joint cartilage and the homograft reaction. J Bone Joint Surg 1971;53B:123–135.
30. Paccola CAJ, Xavier CAM, Goncalves RP. Fresh immature articular cartilage allografts. A study on the integration of chondral and osteochondral grafts both in normal and in papain —treated knee joints of rabbit. Arch Orthop Trauma Surg 1979;93:253–259.
31. Porter BB, Lance EM. Limb and joint transplantation. A review of research and clinical experience. Clin Orthop 1974;14:249–274.
32. Rodrigo JJ, Sakovich L, Travis C, Smith G. Osteocartilagenous allografts as compared with autografts in the treatment of knee joint osteocartilagenous defects in dogs. Clin Orthop 1978;134:342.
33. Thomas V, Jimenez S, Brighton C, Brown N. Sequential changes in the mechanical properties of viable articular cartilage stored in vitro. J Orthop Res 1984;2:55–60.
34. Craigmyle MBL. An autoradiographic and histochemical study of long term cartilage grafts in the rabbit. J Anat 1958;92:467–472.
35. Pritzker KPH, Gross AE, Langer F, Luk SC, Houpt JB. Articular cartilage transplantation. Hum Pathol 1977;8:635–651.
36. Rodrigo JJ, Thompson E, Travis C. 4°C Preservation of avascular osteocartilagenous shell allografts in rats. Trans Orthop Res Soc 1980;5:72.
37. Wiley AM, Kosinka E. Experimental and clinical aspects of transplantation of entire hyaline cartilage surfaces. J Am Geriatr Soc 1974;25:547.
38. Wayne JS, Amiel D, Kwan MK. Long-term storage effects on canine osteochondral allografts. Acta Orthop Scand 1990;61:539–545.
39. Shahgaldi BF, Amis AA, Heatley FW, McDowell J, Bentley G. Repair of cartilage lesions using biological implants: a comparative histological and biomechanical study in goats. J Bone Joint Surg 1991;73B:57–64.
40. Enneking WF, Mindell ER. Observations on massive retrieved human allografts. J Bone Joint Surg 1991;73A:1123–1142
41. Salenius P, Holmstrom T, Koskinen E, et al. Histological changes in clinical half-joint allograft replacements. Acta Orthop Scand 1982;53:295–299.
42. Simon W, Richardson S, Herman W, et al. Long-term effects of chondrocyte death on rabbit articular cartilage in vivo. J Bone Joint Surg 1976;58A:517–526.
43. Tomford WW, Pugg GP, Mankin HJ. Experimental freeze preservation of chondrocytes. Clin Orthop 1985;197:11–14.
44. Schachar NS, McGann LE. Investigations of low-temperature storage of articular cartilage for transplantation. Clin Orthop 1986;208:146–150.
45. Malinin TI, Wagner JL, Pita JC, Lo H. Hypothermic storage and cryopreservation of cartilage. Clin Orthop 1985;197:15–26.
46. Kandel RA, Gross AE, Gavel A, McDermott AGP, Langer F, Pritzker KPH. Histopathology of failed osteoarticular shell allografts. Clin Orthop 1985;197:103–110.
47. Czitrom A, Keating S, Gross AE. The viability of articular cartilage in fresh osteochondral allografts after clinical transplantation. J Bone Joint Surg 1990;72A:574.
48. Pap K, Krompedier S. Arthroplasty of the knee. Experimental and clinical experience. J Bone Joint Surg 1961;43A:523–537.
49. Langer F, Gross AE. Immunogenicity of allograft articular cartilage. J Bone Joint Surg 1974;56A:297–304.
50. Langer F, Czitrom AA, Pritzker KP, Gross AE. The immunogenicity of fresh and frozen allogenic bone. J Bone Joint Surg 1975;57A:216–220.
51. Stevenson S, Dannucci GA, Sharkey NA, Pool RR. The fate of articular cartilage after transplantation of fresh and cryopreserved tissue-antigen-matched and mismatched osteochondral allografts in dogs. J Bone Joint Surg 1989;71A(9):1297–1306.
52. Stevenson S. The immune response to osteochondreal allografts in dogs. J Bone Joint Surg 1987;69A:573–581.
53. Stevenson S, Li XQ, Martin B. The fate of cancellous and cortical bone after transplantation of fresh and frozen tissue-antigen-matched and mismatched osteochondral allografts in dogs. J Bone Joint Surg 1991;73A:1143–1156.
54. Horowitz MC, Friedlaender GE. Induction of specific T-cell responsiveness to allogenic bone. J Bone Joint Surg 1991:73A(8):1157–1168.
55. Horowitz MC, Friedlaender GE. The immune response to bone grafts. In: Friedlaender GE, Goldberg VM, eds. Bone and cartilage allografts: biology and clinical applications. Chicago: American Academy of Orthopaedic Surgery 1991:85–101.
56. Herndon CH, Chase SW. Experimental studies in the transplantation of whole joints. J Bone Joint Surg 1952;34A:564–578.
57. Chase SW, Herndon CH. The fate of autogenous and homogenous bone grafts. A historical review. J Bone Joint Surg 1952;34A:809–841.
58. Curtiss P, Herndon CH. Immunological factors in homogenous-bone transplantation. J Bone Joint Surg 1956;38A:103–110.
59. Curtiss P, Powell A, Herndon CH. Immunological factors in homogenous bone transplantation: III. The inability of homogenous rabbit bone to induce circulating antibodies in rabbits. J Bone Joint Surg 1959;41A:1482–1488.

60. American Association of Tissue Banks. Standards for surgical bone banking. Arlington, VA: American Association of Tissue Banking, 1987.
61. Muscalow CE. Bone and tissue banking. In: Czitrom AA, Gross AE, eds. Allografts in orthopaedic practice. Baltimore: Williams & Wilkins, 1992:27–45.
62. Buck BE, Malinin TI, Brown MD. Bone transplantation and human immunodeficiency virus: an estimate of risk of acquired immunodeficiency syndrome (AIDS). Clin Orthop 1989;240:129–136.
63. Buck BE, Resnick L, Shah SM, Malinin TI. Human immunodeficiency virus cultured from bone: implications for transplantation. Clin Orthop 251;1990:249–253.
64. Simonds RJ, Holmberg SD, Hurwitz RL, et al. Transmission of human immunodeficiency virus type 1 from a seronegative organ and tissue donor. N Engl J Med 1992;326:726–732.
65. Transmission of HIV through bone transplantation: case report and public health recommendations. MMWR 1988;37:597–599.
66. Atkinson K, Dodds AJ, Concannon AJ, Biggs JC. The development of the aquired immunodeficiency syndrome after bone-marrow transplantation. Med J Aust 1987;147:510–512.
67. Ratcliffe A , Mow VC. The structure, function, and biologic repair of articular cartilage. In: Friedlaender GE, Goldberg VM, eds. Bone and cartilage allografts: biology and clinical applications. Chicago: American Academy of Orthopaedic Surgeons 1991:123–154.
68. Pelker RR, Friedlander GE. Biomechanical considerations in osteochondral grafts. In: Friedlaender GE, Goldberg VM, eds. Bone and cartilage allografts: biology and clinical applications. Chicago: American Academy of Orthopaedic Surgeons 1991:155–162.
69. Entin MA, Alger JR, Baird RM. Experimental and clinical transplantation of autogenous whole joints. J Bone Joint Surg 1962;44A:1518–1536.
70. Entin MA, Daniel G, Kahn D. Transplantation of autogenous half joints. Arch Surg 1968;96:359–368.
71. Kettlekamp DB. Experimental autologous joint transplantation. Clin Orthop 1972;87:138–145.
71a. Lee EH, Langer F, Halloran P, Gross AE, Ziv I. The immunology of osteochondral and massive bone allografts. Trans Orthop Res Soc 1979;4:61.
72. Sauer HD, Schoettle H. The stability of osteosyntheses bridging defects. Arch Orthop Trauma Surg 1979;95:27–30.
73. Schenk RK, Willenegger H. Morphologic findings in primary bone healing. Symp Biol Hung 1967;7:75–86.
74. McDermott AGP, Finklestein JA, Farine I, et al. Distal femoral varus osteotomy for valgus deformity of the knee. J Bone Joint Surg 1988;70A:110–116.
75. Salter RB, Simmonds DF, Malcolm BW, Rumble EJ, MacMichael D, Clements ND. The biological effect of continuous passive motion on the healing of full thickness defects in articular cartilage. J Bone Joint Surg 1980;62A:1232.
76. Arnoczky A, Adams M, DeHaven K, et al. Meniscus. In: Woo SL, Buckwalter JA. eds. Injury and repair of the musculoskeletal soft tissues. Chicago: American Academy of Orthopaedic Surgeons 1987:487.
77. Renstrom P, Johnson RJ. Anatomy and biomechanics of the menisci. Clin Sports Med 1990;9:523.
78. Zukor DJ, Cameron JC, Brooks PJ, Oakshott RD, Farine I, Gross AE. The fate of human meniscal allografts. In: Articular cartilage and knee joint function: basic science and arthroscopy. New York: Raven Press, 1990:127.
79. Garrett JC, Stevensen RS. Meniscal transplantation in the human knee: a preliminary report. Arthroscopy 1991;7:57.
80. Milachowski KA, Weismeier K, Wirth CJ. Homologous meniscus transplantation: experimental and clinical results. Int Orthop 1989;13:1.
81. Siegel MG, Roberts CS. Meniscal allografts. Clin Sports Med 1993;12:59–80.

SECTION

XII

Total Knee Arthroplasty for Disorders of Articular Cartilage

62

Results of Total Knee Arthroplasty

Giles R. Scuderi

Historical Review

Knee arthroplasty dates back to 1861 when Fergusson resected a knee joint and created a pseudarthrosis that he described as a "useful limb" (54). This effort was followed by interpositional arthroplasty, with inconsistent results including stiffness and instability, regardless of the materials used—muscle, fascia, fat, or chromaticized pigs bladder (8, 21, 108, 199). Nevertheless, in the first half of this century there were few alternatives. Allografts of the entire knee joint were attempted as early as 1909, but there was a high incidence of failure (72, 120, 134).

Early attempts to resurface the knee joint utilized prosthetic designs that were anatomically configured to replace only one side of the joint (2, 95, 96, 141). Campbell, in 1940, designed a Vitallium implant for the distal end of the femur (25), while other investigators introduced an acrylic design (105). The results were variable and tended to do poorly over time due to instability and erosion of the tibial articular surface with progressive deformity. At about the same time, resurfacing only the tibial surface was being introduced (40, 123, 131, 198). Although tibial implants were originally designed for unicompartmental replacement, the MacIntosh and McKeever implants were sometimes used to replace both compartments (77, 149). Implantation with the tibial prosthesis allowed retention of both cruciate ligaments, but fixation was a problem. The tibial component was either interposed without fixation or fixed by a phalange, screws, or posts. Similar to the distal femoral replacement, the tibial implant caused erosion of the opposing articular surface and the clinical results were variable.

To maintain stability and resurface both the femur and tibia, constrained prostheses were introduced. This included many hinged designs (17, 71, 117, 118, 138). Walldius originally designed an acrylic prosthesis, which he later modified to Vitallium (204, 205). Wilson reported good results with the Walldius prosthesis even though there was a high incidence of component loosening (208). Further modifications of the hinged knee prostheses were developed by Shiers (178, 179), Young (216, 217), and the Guepar Group in France (130). These hinged prostheses were designed prior to the advent of polymethylmethacrylate and relied on long intramedullary stems for fixation and stability. The early enthusiasm for these hinged implants began to decline in the 1960s as loosening and subsidence became more prevalent. Although there was a short lived resurgence of hinges with the Guepar prosthesis and cement fixation, it became obvious that the early results were not durable. The fixed hinged knee did not allow for rotational movements of the knee, and loosening was common at two years.

Gunston (74, 75) was the first to describe a nonconstrained knee prosthesis with cement fixation. The polycentric knee prosthesis consisted of two metallic semicircular femoral runners inserted into slots into the femoral condyles that articulated with two high density polyethylene tracks cemented in slots on the tibial plateau. Although Gunston reported acceptable results with the polycentric implant, the surgical technique was complex, since four components had to be implanted independently. Further designs were then becoming modifications and improvements of the polycentric knee prosthesis, with more anatomic configurations of the femoral components, broader and better fixed tibial implants, and improved instrumentation (119, 180). All provided the ability to resurface one or both compartments, but none at this time addressed the patellofemoral joint.

Further design modifications linked the separate femoral runners or tibial tracks in order to make implantation of the components less technically demanding. The duocondylar design was reported by Ranawat and Shine in 1973 (155). It linked the femoral runners, but the tibial tracks remained separate (153, 155). The geometric prosthesis (37, 181) linked the two metal femoral runners, while the tibial tracks were connected with a polyethylene bridge. Although originally designed for cruciate ligament retention, the axis of flexion of the geometric prosthesis was incompatible with intact cruciate ligaments, resulting in routine sacrifice of the anterior cruciate ligament. The UCI prosthesis was less constrained than the geometric prosthesis, allowing for more rotation of the limb (206). Still, no prosthesis addressed the patellofemoral joint. It was not until Freeman and Swanson developed the ICLH prosthesis, which had an anterior flange to accommodate the patella, did surgeons begin to consider the influence of the patellofemoral joint on clinical outcome (57, 58, 59).

In order to improve stability and reduce rotational stress at the bone cement interface, some ingenuous designs were developed (139, 140), including the Spherocentric, Herbert, Attenborough (7, 62), Kinematic hinged (203), stabilocondylar, and Sheehan prosthesis (146).

Insall (89, 92, 93) was instrumental in the evolution of designs from unicondylar to a duocondylar/patella-condylar prosthesis, and then to the total condylar. The total condylar prosthesis, with patella resurfacing, had a relatively anatomic metal femoral component, and shallow polyethylene tibial tracks that included a tibial peg for enhanced fixation.

The posterior stabilized knee prosthesis was introduced in 1978 as a modification of the already successful total condylar prosthesis (91). The posterior stabilized prosthesis was designed to improve stair climbing, increase range of motion, and prevent posterior subluxation of the tibia. Originally, the posterior stabilized tibial component was all polyethylene, but it had been demonstrated that metal-backed tibial trays transmit the load better to the underlying bone. November of 1980 marked the first use of the metal-backed tibial components on the Knee Service at the Hospital for Special Surgery, and October, 1981 marked the last use of all polyethylene tibial components. In 1983, the posterior stabilized design was revised to incorporate a deeper patella groove, allowing smoother tracking of the patella. Further design modifications included modularity of components, as introduced by the Insall Burstein Posterior Stabilized II Prosthesis (172) (Fig. 62.1).

The total condylar III prosthesis (TCP III) was developed at the Hospital for Special Surgery as a modification to the total condylar prosthesis. This is a constrained unlinked prosthesis that provides medial and lateral stability by the intimate fit of a high tibial post in a deep femoral box. It is recommended that the constrained condylar prosthesis be implanted when there is severe mediolateral instability with an inability to balance the soft tissues; anteroposterior instability that cannot be corrected by restoring the equal flexion-extension gaps; or severe bony loss with associated instability (78, 164). Donaldson reported satisfactory results with the use of the TCP III in both primary and revision arthroplasty (42).

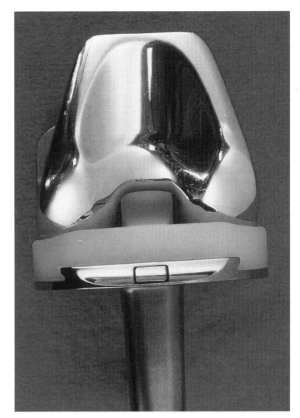

Figure 62.1. The Insal-Burstein Posterior Stabilized II Prosthesis.

Assessment of Results

Clinical studies have always attempted to grade the results of total knee arthroplasty within some numerical rating scale and then to assign a related descriptive rating of excellent, good, fair, or poor result. The problem is that there has not been a universally accepted knee rating system to allow direct comparison of scores. Several knee rating systems have been used, but all have imperfections (14).

The Hospital for Special Surgery (HSS) Knee Score places 10% of its points on quadriceps strength, which may be diminished with rheumatoid arthritis but is unusual with osteoarthritis; the Brigham Knee Score allocates 50% of its points to the subjective category of pain. The Freeman Knee Score assigns 33% of its score to motion with no mention of stair climbing. What is the relative value of pain relief, range of motion, and walking ability? How should descriptive terms such as excellent, good, fair, or poor be ascribed to a numerical total score?

The Hospital for Special Surgery, or HSS, Knee Rating System (88) has been a popular scoring system in use since the early 1970s. This system combines subjective and objective information and is a 100 point system that attempts to get the complete picture of a total knee arthroplasty. The score includes 30 points for absence of pain; 22 points for function; 18 for range of motion; 10 points for muscle strength; 10 points for lack of flexion contracture; and 10 points for stability. From the total score, subtractions are made for walking aids, varus to valgus alignment, and extension lag. An excellent result exceeds 85 points; a good result ranges from 72 to 84 points, a fair result from 60 to 69 points, and a poor result is under 60 points.

The HSS Knee Score was originally introduced when total knee arthroplasty was in its infancy and expectation of results were lower. Because the HSS score also incorporates a functional component, the score tends to decrease as the patient ages or becomes medically infirm, although the knee arthroplasty may remain unchanged.

The Knee Society Clinical Rating System is a dual evaluation of the knee joint itself and also of patient function (it rates the patient's ability to walk and climb stairs) (Fig. 62.2). Patients are initially assigned to one of three categories:

1. Unilateral/bilateral disease;
2. Unilateral with the other knee symptomatic;
3. Multiple arthritis or medical infirmary.

The knee is assessed according to pain, stability, and range of motion. Flexion contracture, extension lag, and malalignment appear as deductions. Therefore, 100 points are obtained by a well aligned knee with no pain, 125 degrees of motion, and negligible instability. The patient function considers only walking distance and stair climbing, with deductions for cane, crutches, or walker. The maximum functional score is 100, which is characterized as a patient who can walk unlimited distances and negotiate stairs normally.

Radiographic Analysis

Postoperatively, radiographic review provides objective data by which to compare results and predict outcome, since component malposition and failure to correct alignment have been associated with poor results. The ideal limb alignment is 5 to 10 degrees of valgus or a mechanical axis of zero degrees. The ideal placement of the tibial component, by classic techniques, is 90 +/-2 degrees to the long axis of the tibial shaft on both the anteroposterior and lateral radiographs. The ideal placement for the femoral component is 7 +/-2 degrees of valgus angulation on the anteroposterior radiograph and 0 to 10 degrees of flexion on the lateral view (172).

Radiolucent lines continue to pose a problem in the assessment of TKA (total knee arthroplasty) (47, 150). They are difficult to quantify and may be obscured by metal-backed components (200).

Patient category
A. Unilateral or bilateral (opposite knee successfully replaced)
B. Unilateral, other knee symptomatic
C. Multiple arthritis or medical infirmity

Pain	Points
None	50
Mild or occasional	45
Stairs only	40
Walking & stairs	30
Moderate	
Occasional	20
Continual	10
Severe	0

Range of motion	
(5° = 1 point)	25

Stability (maximum movement in any position)	
Anteroposterior	
<5 mm	10
5–10 mm	5
10 mm	0
Mediolateral	
<5°	15
6°–9°	10
10°–14°	5
15°	0
Subtotal	—

Deductions (minus)	
Flexion contracture	
5°–10°	2
10°–15°	5
16°–20°	10
>20°	15
Extension lag	
<10°	5
10–20°	10
>20°	15
Alignment	
5°–10°	0
0°–4°	3 points each degree
11°–15°	3 points each degree
Other	20
Total deductions	—

Function	Points
Walking	50
Unlimited	40
>10 blocks	30
5–10 blocks	20
<5 blocks	10
Housebound	0
Unable	
Stairs	
Normal up & down	50
Normal up; down with rail	40
Up & down with rail	30
Up with rail; unable down	15
Unable	0
Subtotal	—

Deductions (minus)	
Cane	5
Two canes	10
Crutches or walker	20
Total deductions	—
Function score	—

Figure 62.2. The Knee Society Clinical Rating System (Reproduced with permission from Insall JN, et al. Rationale of the Knee Society Clinical Rating System. Clin Orthop 1989;248:13–14.)

Figure 62.3. The Knee Society Total Knee Arthroplasty Roentgenographic Evaluation and Scoring System. (Reproduced with permission from Ewald FC. The Knee Society Total Knee Arthroplasty. Roentgenographic Evaluation and Scoring System. Clin Orthop 1989;248:9–12.)

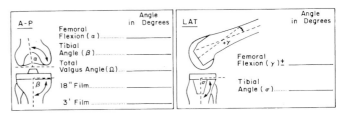

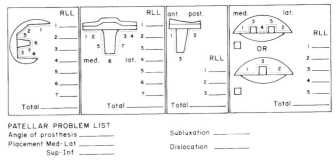

The Knee Society recently recommended an evaluation and scoring system to encourage uniform recording of the radiographic results (51). While no system is ideal, uniformity at least permits comparison. The system measures knee alignment and component position, and it assigns a numerical score to the prosthetic interface in order to assess the quality of fixation (Fig. 62.3). The main advantage of this system is standardization of radiographs for proper position, rotation, and alignment of the knee. The width of the radiolucent lines in each zone is measured for each of the three components. The total widths are added for each of the three components; this generates a score that is rated as follows: 4 or less and nonprogressive is probably not significant, 5 to 9 should be closely followed for progression, and 10 or greater signifies possible or impending failure regardless of symptoms. Additional measurements of the patella should also include patella thickness, prosthetic placement, patella height and alignment.

Fluoroscopically guided radiographs have been shown to position the radiographic beam reliably parallel to the prosthetic bone interface so that the extent of radiolucent lines beneath the tibial component can be measured accurately (135). The Knee Society believes that fluoroscopic evaluation is not mandatory, but, if it is used, that the results be reported.

Roentgen stereophotogrammetric analysis has been used to measure early migration of various designs of TKA. This procedure, although expensive and time con-

suming, can provide very accurate information about only a small number of cases (70).

Survivorship Analysis

Survivorship analysis has been advocated as providing annual and overall failure rates as well as the probability of implant success (100, 174, 196, 197). This technique is easy to apply, because the end point can be specified and will provide a conservative estimate of failure time. It also allows the inclusion of data from patients with short follow-up, those lost to follow-up, and those who died. When survivorship analysis is used, the patient and implant are entered into the series at a different time and followed for different durations. Survivorship analysis is based on the assumption that the outcomes are the same in the patients who are followed and in those who are lost. All patients can be considered in the assessment of results. The second assumption is a clearly defined end point. When the same definition of failure is used, comparison between different prosthesis is possible. The size of the population determines the precision of the estimates; the larger the group, the closer the confidence intervals above and below the estimated survival curve. There are a variety of end points that can be measured, including, but not exclusive to, revision, functional impairment, pain, and radiolucency around the implant. Neilssen (143) defined several endpoints in a recent survivorship analysis:

1. Loosening or revision;
2. Moderate pain at rest and during activity;
3. Severe pain at rest;
4. Relapse to the preoperative pain at rest;
5. Relapse to the preoperative pain with activity;
6. Fair or poor HSS Knee Score.

Patient Outcome Research

With the high number of TKAs being performed in the United States, along with the corresponding decrease in osteotomies, further investigation is being directed toward "patient outcome research" (60). The question to be answered is whether the total knee arthroplasty meets the patient's expected goals within his or her expected time frame. Patient outcome research includes dual data collection, with patients reporting on their physical function, pain, and fatiguability and the surgeon reporting the clinical data. Preoperative baseline data is collected and compared to the postoperative data at follow-up. This research examines regional variations in the number of TKAs and the outcomes associated with them. Mortality, complicating factors, readmission rates, implant failure rates, charges, costs, and length of hospital stay are all of interest. The long-term objective is to determine how much improvement would be expected from a total knee arthroplasty—with emphasis on the patient's expectations. This evaluation concept is new and under investigation.

Current Clinical Experience with Unicondylar Knee Arthroplasty

Changing attitudes and improved designs have allowed unicondylar arthroplasty to evolve from the 1970s when results dissuaded many orthopedic surgeons from implanting unicondylar designs (92, 126, 127). With improvements of design and instrumentation in the later 1980s, unicondylar arthroplasty has become reliable for the carefully selected patient—thin, with unicompartmental degenerative arthritis and minimal deformity or contracture. Kozinn and Scott (101) recommend that patients for this procedure be older than 60 years of age with low demands, that they weigh less than 180 pounds, have minimal rest pain and flex of at least 90 degrees, have a flexion contracture no greater than 5 degrees and angular deformity of less than 15 degrees. Chestnut has described the unicompartmental osteoarthritis protocol that has enabled him to predict appropriate candidates for unicondylar arthroplasty preoperatively in 99% of cases (28). This protocol is based on historical information, physical examination, and radiographic findings; however, the final decision to perform a unicondylar arthroplasty must remain with the operative findings. After arthrotomy, if eburnated bone is noted in the patellofemoral joint or opposite compartment, a total knee arthroplasty should be performed. Patients with osteonecrosis are good candidates for unicondylar arthroplasty as long as there is no major bone loss; while those with inflammatory arthritis, chondrocalcinosis, and synovitis should undergo a total knee arthroplasty. Many believe that both cruciate ligaments must be intact in order for the unicondylar arthroplasty to function properly (48). However, Christensen, in a 9-year follow-up study, noted that absence of the anterior cruciate ligament was not a contraindication to the procedure (29).

Recent clinical results of unicondylar arthroplasty are comparable with those of total knee arthroplasty. Unicondylar arthroplasty has a higher rate of early and long-term success, when compared to osteotomy, and it has fewer complications (35, 36, 90, 101). Another advantage to unicondylar arthroplasty over osteotomy is that bilateral procedures can be performed simultaneously. In patients who undergo osteotomy, the bilateral procedure is usually staged 3 to 6 months apart (101). Broughton reported that 76% of unicondylar arthroplasties had good results at 5 to 10 years compared with 46% of proximal tibial osteotomies (20).

Surgical technique has influenced results of unicompartmental replacements, since improved postoperative limb alignment has been shown to produce better clinical function and improved implant longevity (8, 48, 99, 102, 111). The results of unicondylar arthroplasty depend on careful patient selection. Although Marmor reported 70% of 60 consecutive unicondylar arthroplasties had a satisfactory result at 10 to 13 years, more stringent selection may have improved the results. Still, 87% of patients had continued pain relief at this long-term follow-up (128).

The initial diagnosis influences the outcome. Cartier (27), in a 2- to 10-year follow-up reported 95% good-to-excellent results in osteonecrosis and 93% in osteoarthritis, while other diagnoses had only 76% good or excellent results. The general success of unicondylar arthroplasty has been substantiated by several reports. MacKinnon reported 86% good or excellent results with the St. George-Sledge unicondylar prosthesis at an average follow-up of almost 5 years (124), and Sullivan reported 96% successful results in 107 unicondylar arthroplasties at 5 to 11 years (194).

Christensen, in a 9-year follow-up of 575 unicondylar arthroplasties, demonstrated generally satisfactory results, with the most significant improvement being pain relief (29). However, 7 knees (1.2%) required revision and 14 knees (2.4%) required secondary procedures, including arthroscopy, removal of loose cement fragments, removal of osteophytes, lysis of adhesions, and lateral release for patellar subluxation. Further substantiating the satisfactory results, Rougroff found no difference in loosening between total and unicondylar arthroplasties (165). Survivorship analysis appears, however, to favor TKA over unicondylar arthroplasty (Tables 62.1 and 62.2).

Since unicondylar arthroplasty is performed in knees with minimal deformity, the natural kinematics of the knee is maintained. This may be the reason studies have found patients prefer unicondylar arthroplasty over TKA. Cobb noted that 50% of patients preferred their unicondylar prosthesis, while only 21% preferred the TKA (32). Patients also believed that the unicondylar knee felt more normal (45%) than total knee arthroplasties (14%). Laurencin demonstrated a similar patient

Table 62.1. Unicondylar Arthroplasty Success Rate at 5 and 10 Years of Follow-Up with an End Point of Revision or Loosening

	Success Rate at 5 Years (%)	Success Rate at 10 Years (%)
Unicondylar (101)		83.0
Unicondylar (157)	86.0	68.0
Unicondylar (165)	99.1	92.0
Unicondylar (26)		93.75

Table 62.2. Cemented Total Knee Arthroplasty Success Rate (%) with an End Point of Revision or Loosening[a]

	Success Rate at 3–15 Years of Follow-Up (%)							
	3	5	7	8	10	11	13	15
TCP-APT (174)								90.56
TCP (153)								90.6
TCP (143)					95.0			
TCP MTB (157)					91.0			
TCP (151)						94.1		
TCP (158)								95.0
PC-APT (174)					97.34			
PS MBT (174)			98.75					
PS (170)				93.0				
PS (157)		97.0						
PS (186)							94.0	
AGO (98)	99.0							
AGC (159)					93.4			
KINEMATIC (31)					97.4			
LCS (22)					97.5			

[a]TCP: Total condylar prosthesis; PS: Posterior stabilized prosthesis; AGC: Anatomic graduated component; LCS: Low contact stress; APT: All polyethylene tibia; MBT: Metal-backed tibia.

preference for the unicondylar arthroplasty and believes that the unsurfaced patella may contribute to joint proprioception, giving the knee a more normal feel (115).

Cementless unicondylar arthroplasty has not been used widely. Scott contends that bone ingrowth is not essential to a functionally stable implant interface (101), but a stable fibrous tissue ingrowth interface may provide adequate fixation. Coating the prosthetic surface with hydroxyapatite and using screw fixation to enhance cementless fixation are currently being investigated. Preserving bone stock means insertion of a thinner polyethylene tibial articular surface, especially if it is metal-backed. This thin, flat polyethylene surface is prone to wear. There are a variety of unicondylar implants available, and all are designed to minimize bone resection. Thicker tibial components resect too much proximal tibial bone and make revision to a TKA more demanding (147).

Proximal tibial osteotomy still has a place in young, active patients (35, 36, 90). The ideal candidate for a proximal tibial osteotomy is less than 55 years old, has

unicompartmental degenerative disease, not inflammatory arthritis with synovitis, an arc of motion greater than 90 degrees, a flexion contracture of less than 5 degrees. These criteria are similar to unicondylar arthroplasty except for the age difference, weight, and level of activity. The advantage of osteotomy is that there is no prosthesis, the patient has unlimited activity that includes heavy labor, and the bone stock is not severely compromised. With progression of the degenerative process, revision of the proximal tibial osteotomy to a total knee arthroplasty can be preformed; however, there are technical considerations that make the conversion as complicated as a revision total knee arthroplasty (97, 175, 209).

Current Clinical Experience with Total Knee Arthroplasty

The annual number of TKAs has been rising, so that, in 1990, the National Hospital Discharge Survey reported 129,000 primary and 12,000 revision arthroplasties. Improvement in implant design, surgical technique, bone preparation, and cement technique have made TKA a more predictable procedure (30, 64). In general, the results of revision TKA are not as good as those obtained with primary TKA (87, 156), so it is crucial to implant the prosthesis correctly. A well-positioned arthroplasty has greater than a 90% chance of surviving greater than 15 years (Fig. 62.4) (174).

The controversy regarding retention or sacrifice of the posterior cruciate ligament (PCL), appears to have reached neutral ground. Long-term follow-up has demonstrated that results are satisfactory and comparable whether the PCL was sacrificed or preserved (169, 174, 186). With minimal deformity, the PCL can easily be spared and balanced. However, in fixed angular deformities of the knee, the PCL needs to be recessed or resected in order to balance the collateral ligaments and restore normal alignment. Designs that retain the PCL often require partial release of the PCL in order to maintain a functional ligament. A tight PCL causes excessive rollback, resulting in a stiff and painful knee. If the preserved PCL is lax, the knee will sag posteriorly and not roll back. There have also been concerns about the integrity and function of the retained PCL. Alexiades, in a histologic study, has found that the PCL is involved in the arthritic process with irregularity of the collagen architecture and myxoid degeneration (4). This was especially true with inflammatory arthritis. Biomechanically, Dorr has demonstrated that the PCL in arthritic knees has only 37% of the strength of normal ligaments (44). Yet, there are no reports of spontaneous rupture of the PCL following TKA.

Gait studies have implied that higher interface forces are associated with designs that sacrifice the PCL (43). However, if these higher forces exist, they do not appear to contribute to higher loosening rates as demonstrated by survivorship studies (174). In further support of PCL substitution, the current PCL-retaining designs have flatter, less constrained tibial articular surfaces, which have been shown to have higher wear rates. This

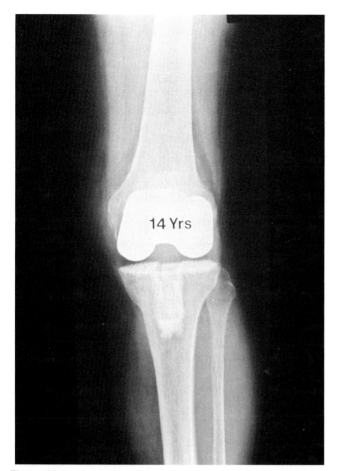

Figure 62.4. A successful, well-fixed cemented total knee arthroplasty at 14 years.

results in polyethylene debris that contributes to implant loosening, as seen in recent reports with longer follow-up.

The total condylar prosthesis was the original modern knee prosthesis. The most recent review of the original Total Condylar Prosthesis at The Hospital for Special Surgery is one of the longest reviews of a prosthesis of modern design (200). At 10 to 12 years, 88% of the knees were still rated good or excellent, 4% fair, and 8% poor. These poor results included 6 knees, 1 due to varus instability, 3 due to tibial loosening and 1 due to femoral component loosening. The sixth, a patient with bilateral replacement had an excellent rating on both knees for 10 years until a cerebrovascular accident affected his right side. Although the arthroplasty remained unchanged, his diminished functional capacity reduced his rating to poor. These results were comparable to earlier reports, since only one new failure, the result of femoral loosening, developed with longer follow-up. The success of this cemented implant supports its continued use.

Despite success with the total condylar prosthesis at the Hospital for Special Surgery, modification introduced the posterior stabilized prosthesis (PS) (91, 172) (Zimmer, Warsaw, Indiana). In the initial report on the

PS knee, 118 knees were followed for 2 to 4 years, 104 (88%) were rated excellent, 11 (9%) good or fair, and 3 (3%) poor (91). These results were maintained after 8 years and longer: 76 (79.2%) excellent; 16 (16.7%) good; 0 fair; and 4 (4.2%) poor (201). Similar results with the PS prosthesis have been reported by Aglietti, who has 90% excellent or good results with follow-up as long as 8 years (1). Scott, et al. (170) reported 98% excellent or good results with the PS knee after follow-up of 2 to 8 years. More recently, a review of 194 PS knees with an all polyethylene tibial component provided the results with follow-up of 9 to 12 years (186). Based on the HSS Knee Rating System, 117 knees (61%) were rated excellent; 51 (25%) good; 12 (6%) fair; and 15 (7%) poor. Although there is a decline of excellent results over time, after 10 years, the overall results remain satisfactory. Looking at the 15 poor results, 14 knees were revised because of failure; this included 5 for infection, 3 for aseptic loosening of the femoral component, and 6 for aseptic loosening of the tibial component. Survivorship analysis showed that the average annual failure rate was 0.4%, and that the overall rate of success at 13 years was 94%. Metal backing of the tibial component has enhanced fixation and reduced aseptic loosening of the tibial component. Since the metal-backed tibial component has been implanted, Scuderi, et al. (174) have reported that none have been revised for aseptic loosening with a 7-year success rate of 98.75%. Finally, the results with the PS prosthesis are comparable with those of the TCP, while the functional outcome appears better (89, 91, 172, 174, 176, 186, 200, 201).

The PCL preserving TKA designs have also been successful. The Kinematic total knee (Howmedica, Rutherford, New Jersey) prosthesis is a cemented posterior-cruciate-preserving design that consists of an anatomic femoral component and a metal-backed tibial tray with a central stem. The results were originally reviewed in 1984. More recently, long-term follow-up has become available, which included later complications (53, 211). At 5 to 9 years following arthroplasty, the function of the reconstructed knees included 90% excellent or good results. The average postoperative knee score for the knees with osteoarthritis was 92, while for the knees with rheumatoid arthritis, it was 88. The later complications included loosening of the patellar component in 5 knees, 1 fracture of the tibial tray with loosening of the patellar component, 1 fracture of the patellar component, and 1 dislocation of the patellar component. Most of the loose patellar components were in patients who had rheumatoid arthritis. However, there was no statistical difference between the rate of patellar loosening in patients with osteoarthritis or rheumatoid arthritis. The patellar problems should not obscure the fact that no femoral or tibial components loosened. Similar to other reports, metal backing of the tibial component has reduced the rate of implant loosening, and, with current design, there is no evidence that loosening across the cement interface will become a problem with longer follow-up.

On the basis of these long-term results and survivorship analyses, cemented TKA has become the "gold

Table 62.3. Cementless Total Knee Arthroplasty Success Rate (%) with an End Point of Revision or Loosening[a]

	% at 3 Years	% at 5 Years	% at 6 Years	% at 9 Years
PCA (137)		84	77	
AGC(98)	88			
TCP (157)		94		
LSC (22)			98	
FS (167)				87

[a]TCP: Total Condylar Prosthesis; PCA: Porous Coated Anatomic; AGC: Anatomic graduated component; LCS: Low Contact Stress; FS Freeman Samuelson.

standard" against which alternative means of fixation are compared (85, 174). A well-positioned cemented TKA has greater than a 90% chance of surviving more than 15 years (165). Concern about the degradation products of PMMA (polymethylmethacrylate), through body wear and deterioration of the bone cement interface, led to the search for alternate means of fixation. The early results of uncemented TKA are limited and inconclusive (41, 45, 81, 83, 110, 162, 163, 192). A comparison of current designs reveals that cemented TKA (Table 62.2) has a longer predicted survival than cementless (Table 62.3). Rosenberg, in a clinical and radiographic comparison of cemented and cementless fixation of the Miller Galante Prosthesis (Zimmer, Warsaw, Indiana), found no cemented failure was due to fixation while 3 cementless failures were due to lack of tibial bone ingrowth (162).

In a comparison of the early results of paired cemented versus uncemented porous-coated anatomic (PCA) knee prostheses (Howmedica, Rutherford, New Jersey), the clinical and functional performance were comparable (41). Yet, cementless designs have shown a precipitous decline in successful results with longer follow-up (3, 137, 138, 142, 177). It seems that the tibial component is usually the site of failed bone ingrowth. Retrieval studies of uncemented tibial components reveal very little bone ingrowth, bringing into question the longevity of these implants (34, 96). Screws have enhanced immediate fixation of the tibia. The "hybrid" TKA (15, 16, 103), an uncemented femoral component with a cemented tibial component, has become popular. The potential advantage of this technique includes decreased operative time and the reduction of polyethylene wear from PMMA debris. In properly selected patients, successful results can be realized with hybrid TKA (103).

Results of Total Knee Arthroplasty in Specific Diagnoses

Most reported series of total knee arthroplasty combine patients with osteoarthritis and rheumatoid arthritis. While some make no mention of comparison, others have looked for differences in the final outcome. Although Insall originally noted a difference in results be-

tween osteoarthritis and rheumatoid knees (92), more recent follow-up and survivorship analysis revealed no difference (174). Moran also found no difference in clinical results between the two diagnostic groups (137). Dennis, in an attempt to clarify this issue, reported on 42 TKAs with an average follow-up of 11 years (39). There were 21 knees with osteoarthritis and 21 knees with rheumatoid arthritis. The clinical results between these two groups at longer follow-up became comparable because the patients with osteoarthritis were older and tended to develop additional functional limitations to other joints. Other studies have found that patients with rheumatoid arthritis do less well (161, 170, 211).

Rheumatoid Arthritis

Rheumatoid arthritis affects a large patient population, 90% of whom have involvement of one or both knees (182). TKAs have been performed in younger patients with rheumatoid arthritis (84, 171). Stuart and Rand found that the major postoperative improvement was pain relief, followed by functional improvement, which tended to be limited because of other joint involvement, including the hips and feet (193).

Kritensen in a 9- to 11-year study of the cemented total condylar prosthesis in rheumatoid arthritis reported a high rate of pain relief and improved walking ability with a survival rate of 89% (107). Goldberg demonstrated similar results noting that the functional ability of all patients decreased between the 4-year and the 9-year follow-up periods (67). This loss of function was most often seen in the aging patient who had difficulty climbing stairs unaided and walking distances.

Laskin, in a 10-year follow-up of 80 cemented TKAs found results less satisfactory in rheumatoid arthritis than in osteoarthritis (112). Although pain relief and range of motion was well maintained over the decade, the HSS knee score deteriorated between the 2- and 10-year follow-up studies—primarily due to multiple joint involvement with rheumatoid arthritis rather than deterioration of the knee itself (112, 114). Nineteen knees had required revision by the end of 10 years, with the main reason for revision being tibial loosening or late infection.

Long-term success with cemented TKA in patients with rheumatoid arthritis had been attributed to low demand and limited functional ability. In a survivorship analysis of 112 TKAs, including 65 with rheumatoid arthritis and 47 with osteoarthritis with an average follow-up of 9.5 years, Ranawat and Boachie-Adjei found that variables such as sex, age, diagnosis, thickness of the cement layer, level of tibial resection, and component alignment did not correlate with radiographic failure (143). The clinical results were excellent to good in 92% of patients. This is similar to the results of Dennis (39) and Schurman (168) who found little difference in the results of patients with rheumatoid arthritis versus osteoarthritis. Dennis reviewed results with the posterior cruciate condylar TKA (which spares the PCL) and found similar results in osteoarthritis and rheumatoid (39). If the PCL is involved with inflammatory disease, as depicted by Alexiades (4), then one would expect less favorable results with cruciate retention. This, however, does not appear to be the case.

Cementless TKA, especially in young patients, has brought some concerns about its application in rheumatoid arthritis where bone quality may be compromised (144). Poor bone quality in patients with rheumatoid arthritis can be attributed to medications, including steroids; direct compromise of the subchondral bone from the invading synovium; bone resorption induced by prostaglandins arising from the synovium; and osteoporosis from disease and limb malalignment (192). Stuchin, et al., in a review of 53 cementless TKAs in patients with inflammatory arthritis, reported satisfactory follow-up at an average of 3.3 years. This study suggests that cementless TKA with appropriate technique can produce early successful results, but further long-term follow-up is needed to make the final decision whether this is an acceptable means of fixation (192). Ebert, et al. found that uncemented TKA can produce results similar to those reported in rheumatoid patients with a cemented TKA (45). The long-term effects of cytotoxic medication on bone ingrowth and cementless fixation is unclear and needs further research.

Osteonecrosis

In contrast to osteoarthritis, osteonecrosis presents the technical problem of poor bone to support the prosthesis. This is, however, only a theoretical problem since recent reports have demonstrated TKA to be a predictable and durable solution for gonarthrosis caused by osteonecrosis. In most instances, the extent of osteonecrosis is limited and the weaker bone is usually resected with standard bone cuts.

Bergman and Rand reported 38 TKAs in 36 patients with osteonecrosis after an average 4-year follow-up (12). In this study, 87% of arthroplasties had excellent or good results, similar to the results of Stern, et al. (188), who reported on 43 TKAs for gonarthrosis caused by osteonecrosis with 86% excellent or good results over an average of 3.8 years. Bergman predicted 85% survivorship at 5 years, similar to Stern. The complications in these series did not differ from those of osteoarthritis, and no failures were related to aseptic loosening of components.

Posttraumatic Arthritis

Periarticular fracture and injuries to the supporting structures about the knee predispose the joint to early arthritic changes and TKA may be required. Soft tissue contractures, poor bone stock, and the possibility of infection often make the procedure as difficult as a revision TKA. Zelicof, et al. (218), in a review of 37 TKAs for posttraumatic arthritis, found generally satisfactory results, yet the average knee score was lower than osteoarthritis with a higher complication rate. The posterior stabilized prosthesis provided greater stability than the total condylar design and yielded 90% excellent or good results. In these 37 knees, there was an infection rate of 6%, probably related to wound complications (including wound drainage with 27%, skin necrosis with 8%, and hematoma with 8%). Postoperative stiffness requiring manipulation occurred with a high incidence (43%) and was attributed to the periarticular soft tissue scarring. Press-fit intramedullary rods and modular augmentation may be required in some cases to enhance fixation (Fig. 62.5).

Similarly, nonunion of fractures about a TKA or associated with an arthritic joint may be troublesome. In a small series of patients with a nonunion of a femoral supracondylar fracture or a proximal tibia fracture, Kress, et al. (106) addressed this problem, utilizing a TKA with an uncemented press-fit intramedullary rod and bone graft. This technique achieved healing of the nonunion by an average of 2 months with none taking longer than 6 months to heal. The average postoperative HSS Knee Score was 78 with 4 excellent, 4 good and 1 poor result, which was associated with a patella fracture.

Hemophilic Arthropathy

Total knee arthroplasty for chronic hemophilic arthropathy is technically demanding due to soft tissue fibrosis, flexion contractures, and poor bone quality. The procedure must be performed under strict hematologic supervision. Complications, including infection, hemorrhage, peroneal nerve palsy, loss of motion, and factor inhibition, are related to both the hematologic problems of hemophilia and the severe deformities. Lachiewicz reported satisfactory results in 87% of 24 knees studied with an average follow-up time of 3.5 years after surgery (109). With 100% factor VIII coverage, there was a lower complication rate. Magone reported 9 knees for an average of 4.3 years and found that the improvement of function was due to correction of deformity and improved motion (125). Figgie, et al. reviewed 19 total knee arthroplasties performed for hemophilic arthropathy, followed for a minimum of 5.5 years and for an average of 9.5 years (55). At last follow-up, 13 knees (68%) had a good or excellent result and 6 knees (32%) were rated as poor. These studies have reported the incidence of radiolucencies ranging from 33% to 72%. They are more prevalent than in other diagnoses and tend to progress, portending failure. Tibial subsidence and component loosening in hemophilic arthropathy have been blamed on the larger tibial resection required to achieve extension, and, secondarily, to the juxtaarticular osteoporosis associated with the disease (55). A metal-backed tibial component that incorporates a longer stem, with adequate proximal tibial coverage, may reduce radiolucency and tibial subsidence. Patella resurfacing should be done routinely in this population in order to decrease the incidence of secondary surgery.

Paget's Disease

Paget's disease (osteitis deformans) will affect 3 to 4% of all individuals older than 40 years of age. Approximately 5 to 10% of these patients are symptomatic with 25% complaining of pain in the hip or knee. The femur and tibia commonly develop deformity. The proximal femur commonly develops the characteristic "shepherd's crook," while the tibia develops anterior bowing.

Figure 62.5. **A,** A previous tibial plateau fracture with depression of the articular surface (*arrows*). **B,** The total knee arthroplasty with tibial wedge augmentation.

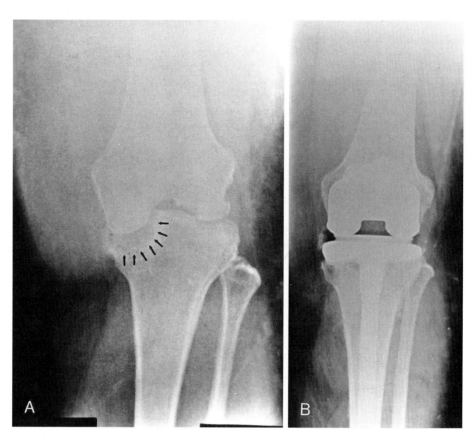

These alterations distort the mechanical axis of the limb. Symptomatic osteoarthritis will develop in the hip in 30 to 50% of these patients and in the knee in 10 to 12%.

Identifying which patient with Paget's disease would benefit from a TKA is sometimes difficult, since the pain may be from the active phase of Paget's disease rather than degenerative arthritis. Pain with weight bearing, in the absence of pain at rest, suggests that the cause is osteoarthritis. For those patients who have rest pain, a diagnostic trial of calcitonin or diphosphonates should identify if pain is from pagetic bone. Intraarticular injection of lidocaine will also differentiate gonarthrosis from Paget's disease (Fig. 62.6).

Paget's disease greatly alters the bony architecture with widening of the bone and thickening of the cortices. Intraoperative difficulties can arise from bone loss, subchondral cysts, contracted collateral ligaments, and abnormal alignment. TKA instrumentation should include extramedullary femoral and tibial guides, because bowing of the long bones makes the use of intramedullary guides difficult. Pagetic gonarthrosis frequently changes the dimensions of the articular surfaces independently, resulting in disproportionate enlargement. For this reason, an implant system should be selected that allows implantation of different sized femoral and tibial components. Malalignment of the knee is exaggerated with Paget's disease, so special attention needs to be given to balancing the collateral ligaments.

There are a few reports of total knee arthroplasty for gonarthrosis associated with Paget's disease. Gabel reported 16 total knee arthroplasties in 13 patients for pagetic gonarthrosis followed for a mean of 7 years (61). Multiple technical difficulties resulted in 63% of the limbs having poor mechanical alignment. Pagetic bone did not, however, affect the amount of blood loss during the operation. At last follow-up, 9 patients had no pain, 3 had mild pain and 1 moderate pain. The median Knee Society Score improved from 42 points preoperatively to 88 points postoperatively, while the functional score increased from 33 to 86 points. Compared to other preoperative diagnoses, there was no increase in clinical or radiographic loosening.

Broberg and Cass concluded, on the basis of 7 arthroplasties, that the results of total knee arthroplasty in patients with pagetic gonarthrosis were comparable to those in patients with osteoarthritis (19). Cameron reported satisfactory results in 2 patients who were followed for 2 years after uncemented total knee arthroplasty for Paget's disease (24).

Psoriasis

Psoriasis vulgaris, a common dermatological disorder, affects 1 to 2% of the population. Patients with this condition may be at greater risk for infection after arthroplasties, because the psoriatic plaques harbor bacterial organisms (5, 129) or because of immunologic compromise (65, 66, 73).

Stern reviewed 27 arthroplasties performed in 18 pa-

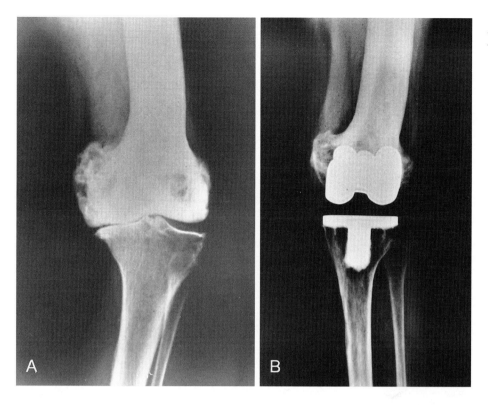

Figure 62.6. **A,** Preoperative radiograph with pagetic gonarthrosis. **B,** Postoperative radiograph of total knee arthroplasty.

tients with established psoriasis (189). The overall deep infection rate on this study was 17%, with an overall revision rate of 21% at an average follow-up of 4 years. This is significantly higher than reported infection rates of 0.7% to 1.9% in other TKA studies. Menon also reported a higher than usual deep infection rate (5.5%) in psoriatic patients undergoing total hip arthroplasty (133).

In contrast, Beyer, from the Mayo Clinic, reported no increased risk of deep infection in patients with psoriasis undergoing a primary TKA (13). The study included 50 primary TKAs performed in 34 patients with known psoriasis. Only one deep infection (2%) occurred 25 months after operation, while there were no superficial wound infections or delay in wound healing. With a potential for infection, it is recommended that the psoriatic lesions in the vicinity of the surgical incision be under the best control preoperatively (13).

Neuropathic Knees

Neuropathic arthropathy has been described in a wide variety of clinical settings including tabes dorsalis and diabetes mellitus. Because the pathophysiology of these disease states differs, the mechanism and degree of joint destruction will also differ. The diagnoses of Charcot and Charcot-like joints have been described to emphasize the variety of clinical presentations (183). The knee is commonly involved because it is a major weight-bearing joint that depends on soft tissue structures for stability. Neuropathic knees usually suffer severe bone loss and abnormal alignment.

Historically, the surgical treatment has been arthrodesis, yet Soudry, et al. have attempted to main-

tain a functioning knee by treating this unique group of patients with TKA. The results of 9 knees at an average of 3 years after arthroplasty were excellent in 8 knees and good in 1 knee. Most knees demonstrated severe ligamentous instability preoperatively due to ligamentous laxity and bone loss. Special care must be taken to reestablish normal alignment with ligamentous balancing, and bone defects can be bone grafted or augmented with metal wedges or custom components (Fig. 62.7).

Poliomyelitis

The knee deformities associated with poliomyelitis include external rotation of the tibia, genu valgum, and genu recurvatum. As patients with poliomyelitis age, they develop gonarthrosis. The weakness of the lower extremity, deformity, and gonarthrosis present a challenge. Patterson and Insall reported their experience in treating 9 such cases (148). All were treated with a cemented TKA and followed an average of 6.8 years. Pain relief was predictably good, and knee stability improved initially. Their surgical approach to multiaxial instability in a weakened lower extremity was to resect less distal femur and to create a 5 to 10 degrees flexion contracture with implantation of a stemmed, constrained condylar prosthesis. Patients with long standing recurvatum may have insufficient quadriceps strength to walk with this degree of flexion contracture and may need to be braced for walking. Three knees in this series required revision. Two were performed for recurrent instability and converted to more constrained implants. The third revision was performed for sepsis and instability. TKA in patients with poliomyelitis is a unique situation with limited supporting literature. Although

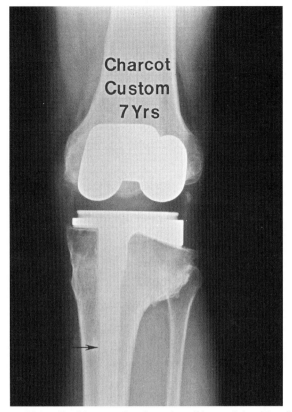

Figure 62.7. Total knee arthroplasty in a Charcot joint. The tibial bony defect was augmented with a wedge.

the procedure relieves pain, the outcome deteriorates with time due to the underlying disease.

Parkinson's Disease

Parkinson's disease is a common geriatric problem with numerous symptoms including tremors, muscular rigidity, gait abnormalities, and characteristic postural and facial expressions. The average age of onset is about 55 years, which is also similar in age to the population that develops painful gonarthrosis. Total knee arthroplasty in this subset of patients does not warrant special considerations.

Oni and MacKenney (145a), reporting on 3 patients, condemned total knee arthroplasty in patients with Parkinson's disease because the rehabilitation of all 3 patients was hampered by inhibition of the extensor mechanism, hamstring rigidity, and poor muscular coordination. The persistent flexion contracture was believed to be induced by hamstring rigidity and inhibition of the opposing quadriceps. They also reported that all three patients died within 6 months of surgery.

Contrary to this previous study, Vince, et al. (199a) reported that, from the results of total knee arthroplasty in patients with Parkinson's disease, TKA is a highly successful procedure with functional improvement. Nine patients with 12 primary total knee arthroplasties and 1 revision arthroplasty with an average followup of 4.3 years were reviewed. All patients had cemented condylar-type resurfacing arthroplasties with deformities corrected by conventional soft tissue balancing techniques. Of the 12 primary arthroplasties, 9 were rated excellent by the HSS knee score system and 3 were rated good. Radiographic assessment revealed the femorotibial alignment to be between 3 and 10 degrees valgus in 11 knees and 1 knee was in neutral alignment. Five arthroplasties had radiolucencies in a single zone, but all were 1 mm or less and nonprogressive. There were no unusual complications in this small group of patients. One patient who fell suffered bilateral patellar fractures that healed without surgery, and another patient required a lateral retinacular release to treat painful patellar subluxation. Although Oni and MacKenney reported avulsion of the quadriceps tendon postoperatively, this was most likely a technical problem with damage to the tendon at the time of arthroplasty. Vince, et al. did not observe this complication in their series.

Although Oni and MacKenney reported a high mortality rate, their patients were older, and the fatalities were influenced by diseases other than Parkinson's disease.

Based on this information, Parkinson's disease is not an absolute contraindication to total knee arthroplasty. Each case should be individualized, taking into account the patient's age and the severity of the disease and its symptoms. The results can be rewarding and similar to routine total knee arthroplasty with relief of pain, correction of deformity, and improvement of function.

Other Factors Influencing the Results of Total Knee Arthroplasty

With the improvement of technique, and the realization that TKA is applicable for a multitude of diagnoses, investigators have reviewed other factors that may influence the clinical result. This includes age, weight, diabetes mellitus, knee deformity, and hip status.

Young Patients

Total knee arthroplasty has become available to younger patients, especially those with juvenile rheumatoid arthritis, posttraumatic arthritis and osteonecrosis. Their activity demands are higher and they may outlive their implants (52).

Ranawat performed 93 total knee arthroplasties with the cemented total condylar prosthesis in 62 patients younger than 55 years of age (average age, 48.7 years) including 76 knees with rheumatoid arthritis and 17 knees with osteoarthritis (154). The clinical and radiographic review included 90 knees (73 with rheumatoid arthritis and 17 with osteoarthritis) with a mean followup of 6.1 years. The average HSS knee score was 87.1 for the entire group and similar for rheumatoid arthritis and osteoarthritis. There were 63 excellent results (70%), 25 good results (27.7%), 1 fair result (1.1%) and 1 poor result (1.1%). Survivorship analysis was also performed using three criteria. Using the criteria of loosening or revision, the success rate was 100% at 10 years; using the end point of clinical or radiographic failure, the success rate was 96% at 10 years; and, using revision for any reason, the success rate at 10 years was 98.4%. The 30% incidence of radiolucent lines—with the majority being less than 1 mm—is similar to other reports. This data supports the successful use of cemented TKA in a young population.

Stuart and Rand reported their results at the Mayo Clinic with 44 patients with rheumatoid arthritis less than 40 years of age (193). They reported 86% good or excellent results at an average follow-up of 5 years with no revisions for component loosening. Ewald and Christie reported excellent results for 95 patients younger than 45 years at almost 4-year follow-up. These two studies included 30 to 50% of patients with juvenile rheumatoid arthritis (JRA). Some believe it is inaccurate to compare these patients to younger patients with either osteoarthritis or rheumatoid arthritis (155), because patients with JRA tend to have more functional limitations, thereby placing fewer demands on the TKA. Reviewing the results of TKA in gonarthrosis in patients 55 years or less, Stern, et al. reported 100% good or excellent results in 68 knees with an average follow-up of 6.2 years (185). The average postoperative HSS Knee score was 90. Rating the knees with the Knee Society Scoring System the average postoperative pain score was 92 points with an average function score of 84 points. The clinical and radiographic evidence is encouraging—suggesting that these results may continue with time.

Cementless fixation became an attractive alternative in total knee arthroplasties especially for younger patients because of concerns about the long-term adverse effects of polymethylmethacrylate. Hungerford reported results of 48 porous-coated anatomic (PCA) TKAs in patients under 50 years of age (82). There was a diversity of diagnoses: 21 knees with osteoarthritis (44%); 18 knees with rheumatoid arthritis (37%); 7 knees with avascular necrosis (15%); and 2 knees with hemophilic arthritis (4%). Overall, 92% of the patients had good or excellent results, 2% fair, and 6% poor at an average follow-up of 51 months. All the fair and poor results were in the osteoarthritis group. Radiographic review demonstrated 31 patients (65%) had no radiolucent lines; 12 patients (25%) had 1 mm or less radiolucency in 2 or fewer zones at the tibial interface; 3 patients had 1 to 2 mm radiolucent lines in 1 to 2 zones on the tibial surface without progression and without symptoms; and 2 knees had complete radiolucent lines with 1 requiring revision.

The 35% incidence of tibial radiolucent lines makes it obvious that bone ingrowth does not occur in all patients. There were no femoral component revisions for loosening. The clinical outcome compares favorably with previous results of cemented total knee arthroplasty in younger patients and with results of cementless total knee arthroplasty in other studies. Yet, there is still concern that the success of cementless fixation will decline with longer follow-up (3, 137, 138, 142, 177).

Obese Patients

Obesity may precipitate degenerative joint disease (DJD), while at the same time the pain and functional limitations of DJD can cause these patients to become overweight. The effect of obesity on TKA is of vital concern to the surgeon, since loading of the joint during gait is complex, and there is concern that excessive body weight will cause aseptic loosening and polyethylene wear. Some investigators have reported adverse effects of obesity (31, 151), while others have found no association (137, 174).

Cobb, in a review of 1943 TKAs, found that women who were overweight had a lower success rate and a higher average annual failure rate, while obesity was not associated with greater failure in men (31). Stern, in a more recent study, demonstrated little difference among knees in various weight groups. Obese patients did experience more patellofemoral symptoms, however (187). Thirty percent of knees in the moderately and severely obese groups had patellofemoral symptoms, whereas the incidence was 14% in the other groups. Patellofemoral reaction forces can exceed more than three times body weight during knee flexion and can cause patellofemoral pain in this group.

Diabetes Mellitus

Diabetes mellitus is the most common metabolic disease and occurs in 2 to 6% of the general population, with an even higher incidence in the aged (56). Several surgical studies have demonstrated that diabetic patients have a higher incidence of superficial and deep infections as well as delayed wound healing (50, 132, 210). England reported on 59 TKAs in 40 patients with diabetes mellitus and noted a deep infection rate of 7%. This is higher than the previously reported rates of 0.7% to 1.9% (50), but is similar to the results of Menon, who reviewed total hip arthroplasty in the diabetic patient (132). England, et al. suggested the use of antibiotic impregnated cement in patients undergoing TKA. Although Wong, et al. reported a higher incidence of wound complications in the diabetic patient (210), England noted a wound complication rate of 12% (including skin necrosis and persistent wound drainage), which is consistent with the 10 to 20% rate in previous TKA studies (46, 67, 91, 93).

There are currently no reports of uncemented TKA in the diabetic patient. Cementless fixation may be compromised since poorly controlled hyperglycemia results in calcium diuresis and secondary hyperparathyroidism (56). This metabolic alteration results in compensatory bone resorption.

Fixed Angular Deformities

Varus deformity is a common finding in patients who have degenerative arthritis and are undergoing TKA. In order to restore normal limb alignment, the surgical technique requires release of the medial structures and balancing of the collateral ligaments (86). The clinical studies, supported by survivorship analysis, have supported the technique of medial soft tissue release for varus deformity with results that are durable and predictable. Vince (200), in reviewing the total condylar prosthesis, had 63 knees with a varus deformity, including 23 with more than 10 degrees of fixed deformity. Stability was maintained at 10 to 12 years with 88% of the knees having good and excellent results. There was one case in which proper balancing was not achieved and varus instability recurred. Although initially rated a good result, this knee deteriorated to a poor result due to progressive instability that required revision. Similarly in a posterior stabilized series, 87% had an excellent or good result, and no prosthesis had to be revised for instability (186). These results are comparable to those of Laskin, who reported on the use of the medial capsular recession to correct varus deformity (113). He found no difference in results when compared to knees of less deformity, and stability did not deteriorate over time. Teeney, however, found slightly dissimilar results (195). Patients with severe preoperative varus deformities had results that approached, but were not equal to, those without a significant angular deformity. He also reported that the postoperative alignment of the varus deformity group tended to be in residual varus. This varus position would be of concern since it has been shown that residual varus alignment tends to fail with time and leads to excessive polyethylene wear.

Valgus deformity presents a special challenge with ligamentous balancing. In a review of 134 total knee arthroplasties with a valgus alignment (all requiring lateral soft tissue release), there were 95 (71%) excellent, 27 (20%) good, 8 (6%) fair, and 4 (3%) poor with an average follow-up of 4.5 years (the range was 2 to 10 years). Several prostheses were implanted, including 118 knees with the posterior stabilized prosthesis, 8 knees with a constrained prosthesis, 4 knees with a total condylar prosthesis and 4 knees with a cruciate retained design (190).

Krackow (104) in a review of 99 knees in 81 patients classified the valgus deformity as follows: type I was defined as a valgus deformity secondary to bone loss in the lateral compartment and soft tissue contracture with the medial soft tissues intact; type II was defined as attenuation of the medial collateral ligament, and type III as a severe valgus deformity with valgus malpositioning of the proximal tibial joint line after overcorrected proximal tibial osteotomy. All of the arthroplasties were performed using the PCA prosthesis (Howmedica, Rutherford, NJ), which is a minimally constrained posterior cruciate sparing design. Type I patients were treated with lateral soft tissue release, and type II patients were treated with medial capsule ligament tightening. Alignment was well corrected in all patients and the knee score for type I and type II were reported as identical. The results were grouped as 72% excellent, 18% good, 7% fair, and 2% poor. These results are similar to those reported by Stern (190). Medial ligament reconstruction remains a controversial issue.

Ipsilateral Hip Fusion

Patients with a hip fusion develop degenerative arthritis in the ipsilateral knee. The extent of involvement is a function of the position of the hip fusion. Biomechanical studies have shown that patients with a fused hip have increased flexion of the ipsilateral knee during the stance phase of gait, and this may lead to degenerative changes (69). Sponseller found that 50% of patients with a hip fusion had ipsilateral knee pain and degenerative changes at an average of 38 years after fusion (184).

Callaghan, et al.(23) reported similar results. Eventually, these patients require a TKA to improve symptoms. At the time of TKA, careful attention must be given to limb alignment, since this is essential to long-term results. When the hip is arthrodesed in an optimal position, maintenance of the fusion still allows a successful TKA. Garvin followed a small series of patients with hip fusions for an average of 7 years, and found that the results of ipsilateral TKA were comparable to other studies without fusion (63). However, flexion was not as good as in those with a functioning hip. Patients who have their hip arthrodesed in a suboptimal position, should be converted to a total hip arthroplasty prior to TKA (18, 160).

References

1. Aglietti P, Buzzi R. Posteriorly stabilized total-condylar knee replacement. Three-to-eight-years follow-up of 85 knees. J Bone Joint Surg 1988;70B:211–216.
2. Albee FH. Original features in arthroplasty of the knee with improved prognosis. Surg Gynecol Obstet 1928;47:312–328.
3. Albrektsson BEJ; Carlsson LV, Freeman MAR, Herberts P, Ryd L. Proximally cemented versus uncemented Freeman-Samuelson knee arthroplasty. A prospective randomized study. J Bone Joint Surg 1992;74B:233–238.
4. Alexiades M, Scuderi G, Vigorita V, Scott WN. A histologic study of the posterior cruciate ligament in the arthritic knee. Am J Knee Surg 1989;2(4):153–159.
5. Aly R, Maibach HD, Madel A. Bacterial flora in psoriasis. Br J Dermatol 1976;95:603–606.
6. Apel DM, Tozzi M, Dorr LD. Clinical comparison of all-polyethylene and metal-backed tibial components in total knee arthroplasty. Clin Orthop 1991;273:243–252.
7. Attenborough CG. The Attenborough total knee replacement. J Bone Joint Surg (Br) 1978;60:333–338.
8. Baer WS. Arthroplasty with the aid of animal membrane. Am J Orthop Surg 1918;16:1–29.
9. Barrett WP, Scott RD. Revision of failed unicondylar unicompartmental knee arthroplasty. J Bone Joint Surg 1987;69A:1328–35.
10. Bartel DL, Bicknell VL, Wright TM. The effect of conformity, thickness and material on stresses in ultra-high molecular weight components for total joint replacement. J Bone Joint Surg 1986;68A:1041–1051.
11. Bartel DL, Burstein AH, Santavicca EA, Insall JN. Performance of the tibial component in total knee replacement. Conventional and revision designs. J Bone Joint Surg 1982;64A:1026.
12. Bergman NR, Rand JA. Total knee arthroplasty in osteonecrosis. Clin Orthop 1991;273:77–82.
13. Beyer CA, Hanssen AD, Lewallen DG, Pittelkow MR. Primary total knee arthroplasty in patients with psoriasis. J Bone Joint Surg 1991;73B:258–259.
14. Binazzi R, Soudrey M, Mestriner LA, Insall JN. Knee arthroplasty rating. J Arthroplasty 1992;7(2):145–148.
15. Bourne RB, Roabeck CH, Nott L. A prospective two year comparison of the hybrid cemented and cementless Miller-Galante total knee replacement in osteoarthritic patients. J Bone Joint Surg 1990;72B:541–542.
16. Bourne RB, Roabeck CH, Lewis P, Nott L. The Miller-Galante knee: A comparison of cemented hybrid and cementless fixation. J Bone Joint Surg 1992;74B(suppl III):287.
17. Brady TA, Garber JN. Knee joint replacement using the Shiers knee hinge. J Bone Joint Surg (Am) 1974;56:1610–1614.
18. Brewster RC, Coventry MB, Johnson EW Jr. Conversion of the arthrodesed hip to a total arthroplasty. J Bone Joint Surg 1975;57A:27–30.
19. Broberg MA, Cass JR. Total knee arthroplasty in Paget's disease of the knee. J Arthroplasty 1986;1:139–142.
20. Broughton NS, Newman JH, Baily RAJ. Unicompartmental replacement and high tibial osteotomy for osteoarthritis of the knee. A comparative study after 5–10 years' follow-up. J Bone Joint Surg 1985;68B(3):447–452.
21. Brown JE, McGraw WH, Shaw DT. Use of cutis as an interposing membrane in arthroplasty of the knee. J Bone Joint Surg (Am) 1958;40:1003–1018.

22. Buechel FF, Pappas MJ. Long-term survivorship analysis of cruciate sparing versus cruciate sacrificing knee prosthesis using meniscal bearing. Clin Orthop 1990;260:162–169.
23. Callaghan JJ, Bran RA, Pedersen DR. Hip arthrodesis. A long-term follow-up. J Bone Joint Surg 1985;67A:1328–1335.
24. Camerson HU. Total knee replacement in Paget's disease. Orthop Rev 1989;18:206–208.
25. Campbell WC. Interposition of Vitallium plates in arthroplasties of the knee. Preliminary report. Am J Surg 1940;47:639–641.
26. Capra SW, Fehring TK. Unicondylar arthroplasty. A survivorship analysis. J Arthroplasty 1992;7(3):247–251.
27. Cartier P. Unicompartmental knee arthroplasty: 2–12 years follow-up. J Bone Joint Surg 1990;72B:941.
28. Chesnut WJ. Preoperative diagnostic protocol to predict candidates for unicompartmental arthroplasty. Clin Orthop 1991;273:146–150.
29. Christensen NO. Unicompartmental prosthesis for gonarthrosis. Clin Orthop 1991;273:165–169.
30. Cloutier J. Long term results after nonconstrained total knee arthroplasty. Clin Orthop 1991;273:63–65.
31. Cobb AC, Ewald FC, Wright J, Sledge CB. The kinematic knee survivorship analysis of 1943 knees. J Bone Joint Surg 1990;72B(3):532.
32. Cobb AG, Kozinn SC, Scott RD. Unicondylar or total knee replacement: The patient's preference. J Bone Joint Surg 1990;72B:166.
33. Cohn BT, Krackow KA, Hungerford DS, Lennos DW, Bachner EJ. Results of total knee arthroplasty in patients 80 years and older. Orthop Rev 1990;19:451–460.
34. Cook SD, Thomas KA, Haddad RJ. Histologic analysis of retrieved human porous-coated total joint components. Clin Orthop 1988;234:90–101.
35. Coventry MB. Upper tibial osteotomy for osteoarthritis. J Bone Joint Surg 1985;67A:1136–1140.
36. Coventry MB, Bowman PW. Long-term results of upper tibial osteotomy for degenerative arthritis of the knee. Acta Orthop Belgica 1982;48:139–156.
37. Coventry MB, Finerman GAM, Riley LH, et al. A new geometric knee for total knee arthroplasty. Clin Orthop 1972;94:171–184.
38. Dannenmaier WC, Haynes DW, Nelson CL. Granulomatous reaction and cystic bony destruction associated with high wear rate in a total knee prosthesis. Clin Orthop 1985;198:224–30.
39. Dennis DA, Clayton ML, O'Donnell S, Mack RP, Stringer EA. Posterior cruciate condylar total knee arthroplasty. Clin Orthop 1992;281:168–176.
40. DePalma AF. Diseases of the knee. Philadelphia: JB Lippincott Co, 1954.
41. Dodd CAF, Hungerford DS, Krackow KA. Total knee arthroplasty fixation comparison of the early results of paired cemented versus uncemented porous-coated anatomic knee prostheses. Clin Orthop 1990;260:66–70.
42. Donaldson WF, Sculco TP, Insall JN, Ranawat CS. Total condylar III knee prosthesis: Long-term follow-up study. Clin Orthop 1988;226:21–28.
43. Dorr LD, Ochsner JL, Gronley J, Perry J. Functional comparison of posterior cruciate retained versus cruciate-sacrificed total knee arthroplasty. Clin Orthop 1988;236:36–43.
44. Dorr LD, Scott RD, Ranawat CS. Importance of retention of the posterior cruciate ligament. In: Ranawat, CS, ed. Total condylar knee arthroplasty. New York: Springer-Verlag, 1985:197–202.
45. Ebert FR, Krackow KA, Lennox DW, Hungerford DS. Minimum 4-year follow-up of the PCA total knee arthroplasty in rheumatoid patients. J Arthroplasty 1992;7(1):101–108.
46. Ecker ML, Lotke PA. Postoperative care of the total knee patient. Orthop Clin North Am 1989;20:55–62.
47. Ecker ML, Lotke PA, Windsor RE, Cella JP. Long-term results after total condylar knee arthroplasty. Significance of radiolucent lines. Clin Orthop 1987;216:151–158.
48. Emerson RH, Head WC, Peters PC. Soft tissue balance and alignment in medial unicompartmental knee arthroplasty. J Bone Joint Surg 1992;74B:807–810.
49. Engh GA, Kwyer KA, Hanes CK. Polyethylene wear of metal-backed tibial components in total and unicompartmental knee prostheses. J Bone Joint Surg 1992;74B:9–17.
50. England SP, Stern SH, Insall JN, Windsor RE. Total knee arthroplasty in diabetes mellitus. Clin Orthop 1990;260:130–134.
51. Ewald FC. The Knee Society total knee arthroplasty roentgenographic evaluation and scoring system. Clin Orthop 1989;248:9–12.
52. Ewald FC, Christie MJ. Results of cemented total knee replacement in young patients. Orthop Trans 1987;11:442.
53. Ewald FC, Jacobs MA, Miegel RE, et al. Kinematic total knee replacement. J Bone Joint Surg 1984;66a:1032–1039.
54. Fergusson W. Excision of the knee joint. Recovery with a false joint and a useful limb. Med Times Gaz 1861;1:601.
55. Figgie MP, Goldberg VM, Figgie HE, Heiple KG, Sobel M. Total knee arthroplasty for the treatment of chronic hemophilic arthritis. Clin Orthop 1989;248:98–107.
56. Foster DW. Diabetes mellitus. In: Isselbacher KJ, ed. Harrison's principles of internal medicine. 9th ed. New York: McGraw Hill, 1980,1741–1755.
57. Freeman MAR, Sculco T, Todd RC. Replacement of the severely damaged arthritic knee by the ILCH (Freeman-Swanson) Arthroplasty. J Bone Joint Surg 1977;59B:64–71.
58. Freeman MAR, Swanson SAV, Todd RC, et al. Total replacement of the knee using the Freeman Swanson Prosthesis. Clin Orthop 1973;94:153–170.
59. Freeman MAR, Todd RC, Bamert P, et al. ICLH arthroplasty of the knee: 1968–1977. J Bone Joint Surg (Br) 1978;60:339–344.
60. Freund DA. Patient outcome research team studies use of knee replacement. Am Assoc Orthrop Surg Bulletin 1992;40(4):12.
61. Gabel GT, Rand JA, Sim FH. Total knee arthroplasty for osteoarthrosis in patients who have Paget's disease of bone at the knee. J Bone Joint Surg 1991;73A:739–744.
62. Gallannaugh C. The Attenborough and Gallannaugh Knee Prostheses for total knee arthroplasty. A comparison and survival analysis. Clin Orthop 1992;281:177–188.
63. Garvin KL, Pellicci PM, Windsor RE, et al. Contralateral total hip arthroplasty or ipsilateral total knee arthroplasty in patients who have a long standing fusion of the hip. J Bone Joint Surg 1989;71A:1355–1362.
64. Gill GS, Mills DM. Long-term follow-up evaluation of 1000 consecutive cemented total knee arthroplasties. Clin Orthop 1991;273:66–76.
65. Gladman DD, Keystone EC, Schacter RK. Aberrations in T-cell subpopulations in patients with psoriatic arthritis. J Invest Dermatol 1983;80:286–290.
66. Glinski W, Obalek S, Langer A, et al. Defective function of T lymphocytes in psoriasis. J Invest Dermatol 1978;70:105–110.
67. Goldberg VM, Figgie MP, Figgie HE III, Heiple KG, Sobel M. Use of a total condylar knee prosthesis for treatment of osteoarthritis and rheumatoid arthritis: Long-term results. J Bone Joint Surg 1988;70–A:802–811.
68. Goodfellow J. Knee prosthesis—One step forward, two steps back. J Bone Joint Surg 1992;74B:1–2.
69. Gore DR, Murry MP, Sepic SB, Gardner GM. Walking patterns of men with unilateral surgical hip fusion. J Bone Joint Surg 1975;57A:759–765.
70. Grewal R, Rimmer MG, Freeman MAR. Early migration of prostheses related to long-term survivorship. Comparison of tibal components in knee replacement. J Bone Joint Surg 1992;74B:239–242.
71. Grimer RJ, Karpinski MRK, Edwards AN. The long term results of stanmore total knee replacements. J Bone Joint Surg 1984;66B:55–62.
72. Gross AE, Silverstein EA, Falk J, et al. The allotransplantation of the partial joint in the treatment of osteoarthritis of the knee. Clin Orthop 1975;108:7–14.
73. Guilhou JJ, Meynadier J, Clot J, et al. Immunological aspects of psoriasis. Dissociated impairment of thymus-dependent lymphocytes. Br J Dermatol 1976;95:295–301.
74. Gunston FH. Polycentric knee arthroplasty. J Bone Joint Surg (Br) 1971;53:272–275.
75. Gunston FH. Polycentric knee arthroplasty. Clin Orthop 1973;94:128–135.
76. Haddad RJ, Cook SD, Thomas KA. Biological fixation of porous-coated implants. J Bone Joint Surg 1987;69A:1459–1466.
77. Hastings DE, Hewitson WA. Double hemiarthroplasty of the knee in rheumatoid arthritis. J Bone Joint Surg (Br) 1973;55:112–118.
78. Hohl WM, Crawford E, Zelicof SB, Ewald FC. The Total Condylar III Prosthesis in complex knee reconstruction. Clin Orthop 1991;273:91–97.
79. Hood RW, Wright TM, Burstein AH. Retrieval analysis of total knee prostheses: A method and its application to 48 total condylar prosthesis. J Biomed Mater Res 1983;17:829–42.
80. Howie DW, Rogers S, et al. Differences in the cell necrosis and release of inflammatory mediators induced by titanium alloy versus cobalt-chrome prosthesis wear particles. J Bone Joint Surg 1992;74B(Supple III):295.
81. Hungerford DS, Kenna RV, Krackow KA. The porous-coated anatomic total knee. Orthop Clin North Am 1982;13:103–122.
82. Hungerford DS, Krackow KA, Kenna RV. Cementless total knee replacement in patients 50 years old and under. Orthop Clin North Am 1989;20(2):131–145.
83. Hungerford DS, Krackow, KA, Kenna RV. Two-to-five years experience with a cementless porous-coated total knee prosthesis. In: Rand Jr, Dorr LD, eds. *Total Arthroplasty of the Knee* Rockville, MD. Aspen Pub 1987,215.
84. Hvid I, Kjaersgaard-Andersen P, Wetherlund JO, Sneepen O. Knee arthroplasty in rheumatoid arthritis. Four to six year follow-up study. J Arthroplasty 1987;2:233–239.
85. Insall JN. Presidential address to the Knee Society: Choices and compromises in total knee arthroplasty. Clin Orthop 1988;226:43–48.
86. Insall JN. Total knee replacement. In: Surgery of the Knee Insall JN, ed. New York: Churchill-Livingstone, 1984;587–695.

87. Insall JN, Dethmers DA. Revision of total knee arthroplasty. Clin Orthop 1982;170:123–130.
88. Insall JN, Dorr LD, Scott RD, Scott WN. Rationale of the Knee Society Clinical Rating System. Clin Orthop 1989;248:13–14.
89. Insall JN, Hood RW, Flawn LB, Sullivan DJ. The total condylar knee prosthesis in gonarthrosis. A five- to nine-year follow-up of the first one hundred consecutive replacements. J Bone Joint Surg 1983;65A:619–628.
90. Insall JN, Joseph DM, Msika C. High tibial osteotomy for varus gonarthrosis. A long-term follow-up study. J Bone Joint Surg 1984;66A:1040–1048.
91. Insall JN, Lachiewicz P, Burstein AH. The posterior stabilized condylar prosthesis: A modification of the total condylar design. Two- to four-year clinical experience. J Bone Joint Surg 1982;64A:1317–1323.
92. Insall JN, et al. A comparison of four models of total knee replacement prosthesis. J Bone Joint Surg 1976;58A:754–765.
93. Insall JN, Scott WN, Ranawat CS. The total condylar knee prosthesis. A report of two hundred and twenty cases. J Bone Joint Surg 1979;61A:173–180.
94. Jones SMG, Pinder IM, Moran CG, Malcolm AJ. Polyethylene wear in uncemented knee replacements. J Bone Joint Surg 1992;74B:18–22.
95. Jones WN. Mold arthroplasty of the knee joint. Clin Orthop 1969;66:82–89.
96. Jones WN, Aufranc OE, Kermond WL. Mold arthroplasty of the knee. J Bone Joint Surg (Am) 1967;49:1022.
97. Katz MM, Hungerford DS, Krackow KA, Lennox DW. Results of total knee arthroplasty after failed proximal tibial osteotomy for osteoarthritis. J Bone Joint Surg 1987;69A:225–233.
98. Kavolus CH, Ritter MA, Keating EM, Faris PM. Survivorship of cementless total knee arthroplasty without tibial plateau screw fixation. Clin Orthop 1991;273:170–176.
99. Kennedy WR, White RP. Unicompartmental arthroplasty of the knee: Postoperative alignment and its influence on overall results. Clin Orthop 1987;221:278–285.
100. Knutson K, Lindstrand A, Lidgren L. Survival of knee arthroplasties. A nation-wide multicentre investigation of 8000 cases. J Bone Joint Surg 1986;68B:795–803.
101. Kozinn SC, Scott R. Unicondylar knee arthroplasty. J Bone Joint Surg 1989;71A:145–150.
102. Kozinn SC, Marx C, Scott RD. Unicompartmental knee arthroplasty a 4.5–6 year follow-up study with a metal-backed tibial component. J Arthroplasty 1989;(suppl 4):S1–10.
103. Kraay MJ, Meyers SA, Goldberg VM, Figgie HE, Conroy PA. Hybrid total knee arthroplasty with the Miller-Galante Prosthesis. A prospective clinical and roentgenographic evaluation. Clin Orthop 1991;273:32–41.
104. Krackow KA, Jones MM, Tenney SM, Hungerford DS. Primary total knee arthroplasty in patients with fixed valgus deformity. Clin Orthop 1991;273:9–18.
105. Kraft GL, Levinthal DN. Acrylic prosthesis replacing lower end of the femur for benign giant-cell tumor. J Bone Joint Surg (Am) 1954;36:368–374.
106. Kress K, Scuderi GR, Windsor RE, Insall JN. Treatment of nonunions about the knee utilizing custom knee replacement with press-fit intramedullary stems. J Arthroplasty 1993;8(1):49–55.
107. Kristensen O, Nafei A, Kjaersgaard-Anderson P, et al. Long-term results of total condylar knee arthroplasty in rheumatoid arthritis. J Bone Joint Surg 1992;74B(6):803–806.
108. Lacheretz M. Traitement des ankylose. Rev Chir Orthop 1953;39:495.
109. Lachiewicz PF, Inglis AE, Insall JN, et al. Total knee arthroplasty in hemophilia. J Bone Joint Surg 1985;67A:1361–1366.
110. Landon GC, Galante JO, Maley MM. Noncemented total knee arthroplasty. Clin Orthop 1986;205:49–57.
111. Larsson SE, Larsson S, Lundkvist S. Unicompartmental knee arthroplasty. Clin Orthop 1988;232:174–181.
112. Laskin RS. Total condylar knee replacement in patients who have rheumatoid arthritis. A ten-year follow-up study. J Bone Joint Surg 1990;72A:529–535.
113. Laskin RS. Soft tissue techniques in total knee replacement. In: Laskin RS, ed. Total knee replacement. New York: Springer-Verlag, 1991,41–54.
114. Laskin RS. Total condylar knee replacement in rheumatoid arthritis. A review of one hundred and seventeen knees. J Bone Joint Surg 1981;63A:29–35.
115. Laurencin CT, Zelicof SB, Scott RD, Ewald FC. Unicompartmental versus total knee arthroplasty in the same patient: A comparative study. Clin Orthop 1991;273:151–156.
116. Lee JG, Keating EM, Ritter MA, Faris PM. Review of the all-polyethylene tibial component in total knee arthroplasty. A minimum seven-year follow-up period. Clin Orthop 1990;260:87–94.
117. Lettin AWF, Kavanagh TG, Craig D, Scales JT. Assessment of the survival of the clinical results of Stanmore total knee replacements. J Bone Joint Surg 1984;66-B(3):355–361.
118. Lettin AW, Deliss LJ, Blackburn JS, et al. The Stanmore hinged knee arthroplasty. J Bone Joint Surg (Br) 1978;60:327–332.
119. Lewallen DG, Bryan RS, Peterson LFA. Polycentric total knee arthroplasty. A ten-year follow-up study. J Bone Joint Surg 1984;66-A:1211–1218.
120. Lexer E. Joint transplantation and arthroplasty. Surg Gynecol Obstet 1925;40:782–809.
121. L'Insalata JL, Stern SH, Insall JN. Total knee arthroplasty in elderly patients. Comparison of tibial component designs. J Arthroplasty 1992;7(3):261–266.
122. Lowe LW, Katz A, Kay AGL. MacIntosh arthroplasty in the rheumatoid knee. J Bone Joint Surg (Br) 1972;54:170.
123. MacIntosh DL. Hemiarthroplasty of the knee using a space-occupying prosthesis for painful varus and valgus deformities. J Bone Joint Surg (Am) 1958;40:1431.
124. MacKinnon J, Young S, Bailey R. The St. George sledge unicompartmental replacement of the knee. A prosective study of 115 cases. J Bone Joint Surg 1988;70B(2):217–223.
125. Magone JB, Dennis DA. Weis LD. Total knee arthroplasty in chronic hemophilic arthropathy. Orthopedics 1986;9:653–657.
126. Marmor L. The modular knee. Clin Orthop 1973;94:242–248.
127. Marmor L. Marmor modular knee in unicompartment disease: Minimum four-year follow-up. J Bone Joint Surg 1979;61A:347–353.
128. Marmor L. Unicompartmental knee arthroplasty 10- to 13-year follow-up study. Clin Orthop 1987;226:14–20.
129. Marples RR, Heaton CL, Kligman AM. Staphylococcus aureus in psoriasis. Arch Dermatol 1973;107:568–570.
130. Mazas FB. Guepar total knee. Clin Orthop 1973;94:242–248.
131. McKeever DC. Patellar prosthesis. J Bone Joint Surg (Am) 1955;37:1074–1084.
132. Menon TJ, Thjellesen D, Wroblewski MB. Charnley low-friction arthroplasty in diabetic patients. J Bone Joint Surg 1983;65B:580.
133. Menon TJ, Wroblewski BM. Charnley low function arthroplasty in patients with psoriasis. Clin Orthop 1983;176:127–128.
134. Meyers MH, Akeson W, Convery R. Resurfacing of the knee with fresh osteochondral allograft. J Bone Joint Surg (Am) 1989;71:704–713.
135. Mintz AD, Pilkington CAJ, Howie DW. A comparison of plain and fluoroscopically guided radiographs in the assessment of arthroplasty of the knee. J Bone Joint Surg 1989;71A:1343–1347.
136. Moeys EJ. Metal alloplasty of the knee joint. An experimental study. J Bone Joint Surg (Am) 1954;36:363–367.
137. Moran CG, Pinder IM, Lees TA, Midwinter MB. 121 Cases in survivorship analysis of the uncemented porous-coated anatomic knee replacement. J Bone Joint Surg 1991;73A:848–857.
138. Moran CG, Pinder IM, Midwinter MJ. Failure of the porous-coated anatomic (PCA) knee. J Bone Joint Surg 1990;72(B):1092.
139. Murry DG. History of total knee replacement. In: Laskin R, ed. Total knee replacement. New York: Springer-Verlag, 1992;3–15.
140. Murray DG. Total knee replacement with a variable axis prosthesis. Orthop Clin North Am 1982;101:155–172.
141. Murray DG, Barranco S. Femoral condylar hemiarthroplasty of the knee. Clin Orthop 1974;101:68–73.
142. Nafei A, Nielsen S, Kristensen O, Hvid J. The Press-Fit Kinemax knee arthroplasty. High failure rate of noncemented implants. J Bone Joint Surg 1992;74B:243–246.
143. Nelissen RGHH, Brand R, Rozing PM. Survivorship analysis in total knee arthroplasty. J Bone Joint Surg 1992;74A:383–389.
144. Nielsen PT, Hansen EB, Rechnagel K. Cementless total knee arthroplasty in unselected cases of osteoarthritis and rheumatoid arthritis. A 3-year follow-up study of 103 cases. J Arthroplasty 1992;7(2):137–143.
145. Nolan JF, Bucknill TM. Aggressive granulomatosis from polyethylene failure in an uncemented knee replacement. J Bone Joint Surg 1992;74B:23–24.
145a. Oni OOA, MacKenney RP. Total knee replacement in patients with Parkinson's disease. J Bone Joint Surg 1985;67-B:424–425.
146. O'Rourke K, Sheehan JM. The Sheehan knee arthroplasty: long-term results. J Bone Joint Surg (Br) 1987;69:488.
147. Padgett DE, Scuderi GR, Windsor RE, Insall JN. Revision arthroplasty of failed unicompartmental knee replacements. Orthop Trans 1989;13(3):558.
148. Patterson BM, Insall JN. Surgical management of gonarthrosis in patients with poliomyelitis. J Arthroplasty 1992:(suppl 7):419–426.
149. Potter TA, Weinfeld MS, Thomas WH. Arthroplasty of the knee in rheumatoid arthritis and osteoarthritis. J Bone Joint Surg (Am) 1972;54:1–23.
150. Railton GT, Albrektsson BEJ, Ryd L, Freeman MAR. Clinical and roentgen stereophotogrammetric analysis (RSA) of the fixation of tibial components in knee. J Bone Joint Surg 1990;72B:935.
151. Ranawat CS, Boachie-Adjei O. Survivorship analysis and results of total condylar knee arthroplasty. Eight- to eleven-year follow-up period. Clin Orthop 1988;226:6–13.

152. Ranawat CS, Insall JN, Shine J. Duo-condylar knee arthroplasty. Clin Orthop 1976;120:76.
153. Ranawat CS, Flynn WF, Saddler S, et al. Long-term results of the total condylar knee arthroplasty: A 15-year survivorship study. J Bone Joint Surg 1992;74B(Suppl III):288.
154. Ranawat CS, Padgett DE, Ohashi Y. Total knee arthroplasty for patients younger than 55 years. Clin Orthop 1989;248:27–33.
155. Ranawat CS, Shine JJ. Duocondylar total knee arthroplasty. Clin Orthop 1973;94:185–195.
156. Rand JA, Bryan RS. Results of revision total knee arthroplasties using condylar prosthesis. A review of fifty knees. J Bone Joint Surg 1981;63A:536–544.
157. Rand JA, Ilstrup DM. Survivorship analysis of total knee arthroplasty. J Bone Joint Surg 1991;73A:397–409.
158. Rinonapoli E, Mancini GB, Azzara A, Aglietti P. Long-term results and survivorship analysis of 89 total condylar knee prostheses. J Arthroplasty 1992;7(3):241–246.
159. Ritter MA, Gioe TJ, Stringer EA. Radiolucency surrounding the posterior cruciate condylar total knee prosthetic components. Clin Orthop 1981;160:149–152.
160. Romness DW, Morrey BF. Total knee arthroplasty in patients with prior ipsilateral hip fusion. J Arthroplasty 1992;7(1):63–70.
161. Rorabeck CH, Bourne RB, Nott L. The cemented kinematic II and the noncemented porous-coated anatomic prosthesis for toal knee replacement. A prospective evaluation. J Bone Joint Surg 1988;70A:483–490.
162. Rosenberg AG, Barden RM, Galante JO. A comparison of cemented and cementless fixation with the Miller-Galante total knee arthroplasty. Ortho Clinic North Am 1989;20:97–111.
163. Rosenberg AG, Barden RM, Glante JO. Cemented and ingrowth fixation of the Miller-Galante Prosthesis. Clin Orthop 1990;260:71–79.
164. Rosenberg AG, Verner JJ, Galante JO. Clinical results of total knee revision using the Total Condylar III Prosthesis. Clin Orthop 1991;273:83–90.
165. Rougraff BT, Heck DA, Gibson AE. A comparison of tricompartmental and unicompartmental arthroplasty for the treatment of gonarthrosis. Clin Orthop 1991;273:157–164.
166. Sambatakakis TW, Newton G. Condylar knee replacement: A 12-Year experience. J Bone Joint Surg 1990;72B(6):1092.
167. Samuelson K, Nelson L. An all-polyethylene cementless tibial component. A five- to nine-year follow-up study. Clin Orthop 1990;260:93–97.
168. Schurman DJ, Parker JN, Ornstein D. Total condylar replacement. J Bone Joint Surg 1985;67A:1006–1014.
169. Scott RD, Volatile TB. Twelve years' experience with posterior cruciate retaining total knee arthroplasty. Clin Orthop 1986;206:100–107.
170. Scott WN, Rubinstein M, Scuderi G. Results after knee replacement with a posterior cruciate substitutive prosthesis. J Bone Joint Surg 1989;70A:1163–1173.
171. Scuderi GR, Insall JN. Knee surgery: Current opinion. Rheumatology 1990;2:160–162.
172. Scuderi GR, Insall JN. The posterior stabilized knee prosthesis. Orthop Clin North Am 1989;20(1):71–78.
173. Scuderi GR, Insall JN. Total knee arthroplasty. Current Clinical Perspectives. Clin Orthop 1992;276:26–32.
174. Scuderi GR, Insall JN, Windsor RE, Moran MC. Survivorship of cemented knee replacements. J Bone Joint Surg 1989;71B:798–803.
175. Scuderi GR, Windsor RE, Insall JN. Observations on patella height after proximal tibial osteotomy. J Bone Joint Surg 1989;71A:245–248.
176. Scuderi GR, Windsor RE, Insall JN. Long-term results of the cemented total condylar knee. In: Total knee arthroplasty. Laskin R, ed. New York: Springer-Verlag, 1991;77–84.
177. Shepherd BD, Goldberg JA, Bruce WJ, Sherry E. The use of the Insall-Burstein cemented total knee replacement in the uncemented mode. J Bone Joint Surg 1990;72B:1098–1099.
178. Shiers LGP. Arthroplasty of the knee. Preliminary report of a new method. J Bone Joint Surg (Br) 1954;36:553–560.
179. Shiers LGP. Hinge arthroplasty for arthritis. Rheumatology 1961;17:54–62.
180. Skolnick MD, Bryan RS, Peterson LFA, et al. Polycentric total knee arthroplasty. A two-year follow-up study. J Bone Joint Surg (Am) 1976a;58:743–748.
181. Skolnick MD, Coventry MB, Illstrup DM. Geometric total knee arthroplasty. J Bone Joint Surg (Am) 1976b;58:749–753.
182. Sledge CB, Walker PS. Total knee arthroplasty in rheumatoid arthritis. Clin Orthop 1984;182:127.
183. Soudry M, Binazz R, Johanson WA, et al. Total knee arthroplasty in Charcot and Charcot-like joints. Clin Orthop 1986;208:199–204.
184. Sponseller PD, McBeath AA, Pepich M. Hip arthrosis in young patients. A long-term follow-up study. J Bone Joint Surg 1984;66a:853–859.
185. Stern SH, Bowen MK, Insall JN, Scuderi GR. Cemented total knee arthroplasty for gonarthrosis in patients 55 years old or younger. Clin Orthop 1990;260:124–129.
186. Stern SH, Insall JN. Posterior stabilized prosthesis. Results after follow-up of nine to twelve years. J Bone Joint Surg 1992;74:980–986.
187. Stern SH, Insall JN. Total knee arthroplasty in obese patients. J Bone Joint Surg 1990;72A:1400–1404.
188. Stern SH, Insall JN, Windsor RE. Total knee arthroplasty in osteonecrotic knees. Orthop Trans 1988;12:722.
189. Stern SH, Insall JN, Windsor RE, et al. Total knee arthroplasty in patients with psoriasis. Clin Orthop 1989;248:108–110.
190. Stern SH, Moeckel BH, Insall JN. Total knee arthroplasty in valgus knees. Clin Orthop 1991;273:5–8.
191. Stockley IN, Smith DC, Lugowski S, Gross A. Trace metal ion release from porous-coated knee prosthesis. J Bone Joint Surg 1992;74B(Suppl III):286.
192. Stuchin SA, Ruoff M, Matarese W. Cementless total knee arthroplasty in patients with inflammatory arthritis and compromised bone. Clin Orthop 1991;273:42–51.
193. Stuart MJ, Rand JA. Total knee arthroplasty in young patients who have rheumatoid arthritis. J Bone Joint Surg 1988;70A:84–87.
194. Sullivan PM, Hugus JJ, Johnston RC. Long-term follow-up of unicompartmental knee arthroplasty. Ortho Trans 1988;12(3):654.
195. Teeney SM, Krachow KA, Hungerford DS, Jones M. Primary total knee arthroplasty in patients with severe varus deformity. Clin Orthop 1991;273:19–31.
196. Tew M, Waugh W. Estimating the survival time of knee replacements. J Bone Joint Surg 1982;64-B(5):579–582.
197. Tew M, Waugh W, Forster TW. Comparing the results of different types of knee replacement. J Bone Joint Surg 1985;67B:775–779.
198. Townley CO. Articular-plate replacement arthroplasty for the knee joint. Clin Orthop 1964;36:77–85.
199. Verneuil AS. Affection articular du genou. Arch Med 1863.
199a. Vince KG, Insall JN, Bannerman CE. Total knee arthroplasty in the patient with Parkinson's disease. J Bone Joint Surg 1989;71-B:51–54.
200. Vince KG, Insall JN, Kelly MA. The total condylar prosthesis: 10- to 12-year results of a cemented knee replacement. J Bone Joint Surg 1989;71B:793–797.
201. Vince KG, Kelly M, Insall JN. Posterior stabilized knee prosthesis: Follow-up at 5 to 8 years. Ortho Trans 1988;12:157.
202. Walker P. Effects of design and technique on the clinical results of total knee replacement. J Bone Joint Surg 1990;72B:169.
203. Walker PS, Emerson R, Potter T, et al. The kinematic rotating hinge: Biomechanics and clinical application. Orthop Clin North Am 1982;13:187–199.
204. Walldius B. Arthroplasty of the knee using an endoprosthesis. Acta Orthop Scand 1957;(suppl)24.
205. Walldius B. Arthroplasty of the knee using an endoprosthesis. Eight years' experience. Acta Orthop Scand 1960;30:137–148.
206. Waugh TR, Smith RC, Orofino CF, et al. Total knee replacement. Clin Orthop 1973;94:196–201.
207. Williams EA, Hargadon EJ, Davies DRA. Late failure of the Manchester Prosthesis. J Bone Joint Surg 1979;61B:451–454.
208. Wilson FC. Total replacement of the knee in rheumatoid arthritis. J Bone Joint Surg (Am) 1972;54:1429–1443.
209. Windsor RE, Insall JN, Vince KG. Technical consideration of total knee arthroplasty after proximal tibial osteotomy. J Bone Joint Surg 1988;70A:547–555.
210. Wong RY, Lotke PA, Ecker ML. Factors influencing wound healing after total knee arthroplasty. Orthop Trans 1986;10:497.
211. Wright J, Ewald FC, Walker PS, Thomas WH, Poss R, Sledge CB. Total knee arthroplasty with the Kinematic Prosthesis. J Bone Joint Surg 1990;72A:1003–1009.
212. Wright TM, Astion DJ, Bansal M, Rimnac CM, Green T, Insall JN, Robinson RP. Failure of carbon fiber-reinforced total knee replacement components. J Bone Joint Surg 1988;70A:926–932.
213. Wright TM, Bartell DL. The problem of surface damage in polyethylene total knee components. Clin Orthop 1986;205:67–74.
214. Wright TM, Rimnac CM, Faris PM, Bansal M. Analysis of surface damage in retrieved carbon fiber-reinforced and plain polyethylene tibial components from posterior stabilized total knee replacements. J Bone Joint Surg 1988;70A:1312–1319.
215. Wroblewski BM. Wear of high density polyethylene on bone and cartilage. J Bone Joint Surg 1979;61B:498–500.
216. Young HH. Use of a hinged Vitallium prosthesis for arthroplasty of the knee. J Bone Joint Surg (Am) 1963;45:1627–1642.
217. Young HH. Use of a hinged Vitallium prosthesis for arthroplasty of the knee: A preliminary report. J Bone Joint Surg (Am) 1965;45:1627–1642.
218. Zelicof, Vince KG, Urs, Scuderi GR, Insall JN. Total knee replacement in post-traumatic arthritis. Ortho Trans 1988;12:157.

63

Wear

John P Collier, Michael B. Mayor, James L. McNamara, Marguerite Wrona, and Victor A. Surprenant

Introduction

As a pioneer in total joint replacement, Sir John Charnley was intensely interested in all facets of the design, performance, and functioning of this novel concept, but especially in "wear" as the confluence of all these facets (7). From the earliest total joint application, the use of polymeric materials mated to metal counterfaces has resulted in concern for the relative rate of wear of the polymeric bearings. Charnley's early experience with the use of polytetrafluoroethylene (Teflon) as a counterface against stainless steel provided insight into the fact that the material of choice for the polymeric bearings was critical to the overall success of the arthroplasty.

Charnley found that the polytetrafluoroethylene bearings wore very quickly, but also that they provided sufficient amounts of polymer debris to cause an aggressive tissue response requiring the removal of all of the bearings. Interestingly, the rate of wear of these components was not difficult to determine, as the linear migration of the femoral head through the full thickness of the polytetrafluoroethylene bearing was easily visualized once the bearing was bivalved. The realization of the unacceptable wear rate of these bearings led Charnley on a search for new materials, a search that ended with ultrahigh molecular weight polyethylene (UHMWPE). Charnley ran his own wear tests, and it was in his laboratory that he concluded that the relative wear rate of UHMWPE was the lowest of any of the polymeric materials that he had tested; as a result of his tests, it became the material of choice then, as it is now, in joint replacement (7).

Charnley continued his research in the measurement of wear of the polyethylene bearings in his patients. Through the use of x-ray data and retrievals, both he and Dr. Wroblewski (31, 32) were able to determine that the wear of the polyethylene in total hip patients ranged from approximately 0.07 to 0.5 mm per year, with an av-

erage of approximately 0.19 mm. These accurate wear rate measurements were possible because of the relatively unchanging resultant force that the abductors put on the hip, resulting in a slow, linear penetration of the femoral head into the polyethylene. This migration occurs due to the gradual removal of successive surface layers of the polyethylene by adhesive wear. Therefore, wear rates can be described as reasonably predictable, slow, and sufficiently determinable so that the effect of patient factors such as age, weight, sex, and activity level, can be assessed.

Charnley found no useful correlation between patient activity level and the overall wear rate (8). While there have been a series of papers over the years assessing the wear rates of acetabular components (9, 24, 25), there are few reliable data for the knee, although rapid wear and associated osteolysis have been reported (3, 5, 6, 14, 28, 29). This chapter describes the mechanisms of wear in the knee and describes the role of design and material.

Wear Mechanisms

It is important to note that there are many different material damage modes that are often grouped under the term wear. The term actually describes the inevitable removal of material that occurs whenever two bodies articulate, with the majority of the material being removed from the softer of the two. When referring to orthopaedic prostheses, the term wear encompasses:

1. Adhesive wear: the successive removal from the surface of the softer material;
2. Third body wear: the removal of material by foreign particles, typically metal, bone, or bone cement;
3. Abrasion: the wear of a rough surface in a bearing, such as a badly scratched metal condyle, an osteophyte, or a cement protrusion against polyethylene;

4. Fatigue: the cyclic loading of a bearing resulting in crack initiation and propagation if the load is too high, the number of cycles too great, or the material properties insufficient to withstand the service.

Wear of prostheses results in characteristic patterns that can be recognized on retrieved components. Normal adhesive wear is characterized by burnishing, which appears as a smooth or shiny area on the articular surface. More aggressive wear usually results from the addition of a third body and leaves a more disturbed-looking surface. The most common form of third-body wear is scratching, recognizable as linear tracks in the AP direction resulting from the entrapment of third-body debris such as particles of metal, bone or bone cement, or from asperities on the metal surface. Abrasion typically results from contact of the polyethylene surface with osteophytes or from overhanging cement giving a shredded appearance to the polyethylene surface (29). Abrasion can be responsible for the release of large amounts of debris. The most destructive forms of damage are the result of fatigue, which is the propagation of cracks from repeated high loads and cyclic stressing in tension and compression. Fatigue damage is more contact stress dependent than adhesive wear and can take the form of: pitting, which is the removal of small chunks of material from the surface; delamination, which is the removal of large sheets of material from the articular surface due to the propagation of subsurface cracks; and cracking, where cracks propagate through the thickness of the component, often resulting in fracture.

Tibiofemoral Articulation

The kinematics of the knee are far more complex than those of the hip. In addition to providing for flexion and extension, the knee must allow for abduction and adduction and for internal and external rotation for a total of three axes of rotation. Knee kinematics also require that the radius of curvature of the femoral component decreases along the posterior femoral condyle. In addition, the contact point of the components must move posteriorly on the tibia to permit flexion beyond 90 degrees. This is commonly referred to as "femoral rollback." A constant radius of curvature on the femoral condyle would result in an "overstuffed" joint with increased flexion resisted by ligamentous tension. If the contact point between femoral and tibial components, which typically begins near the anterior region of the knee, does not move posteriorly, then posterior impingement will typically limit the extent of flexion.

The dual requirements of a change of radius of the femoral component (with the radius becoming increasingly small as the degree of flexion increases) and of a need for translation of the contact area from anterior to posterior, combine to make rolling of the femoral component on the tibial component necessary. Therefore, the motion pattern that the metal components of the knee have relative to the polymeric components is far more complex and difficult to simulate or, in any other way, reproduce. Further, any malposition in the knee,

whether varus or valgus, internal or external rotation, anterior or posterior tilt, or any other sizing or positioning problems can be expected to dramatically change knee kinematics. The resulting change in the contact between the metal and polyethylene surfaces can be expected to significantly affect the wear rate.

The kinematics of the tibiofemoral articulation result in a combination of rolling and sliding of the femoral component against the surface of the tibial component. This can be contrasted with the hip joint in which all relative motion between the femoral head and the acetabular component is pure sliding. The result of adding rolling to sliding in the knee joint articulation produces a variety of wear modes, whereas the pure sliding in the hip results primarily in adhesive wear alone. In pure sliding, the maximum contact stress occurs at the point of contact between the metal and polyethylene surfaces, and the major removal of material occurs by the slow and predictable adhesion of the polymer to the surface of the metal. Rolling, as produced in the knee, results in high subsurface stresses approximately 100 μm to 1 mm below the surface of the polyethylene bearing. The rolling articulation results in cyclic loads, varying between extreme tension and extreme compression, translating across the articular surface of the tibial component. If these subsurface stresses are sufficiently high, cracks may be generated below the surface of the polyethylene in the region of maximum subsurface shear stresses. Over a large number of cycles, these cracks may propagate, connect with one another, and result in pitting, extensive subsurface cracking, and delamination. Thus, the knee, in addition to adhesive wear, is exposed to the additional modes of potential failure from these fatigue mechanisms. Unfortunately, fatigue failure of the polymeric bearings may be rapid, is unpredictable in terms of time of initiation and speed of progression, and, ultimately, may result in catastrophic failure of the bearings themselves.

Patellofemoral Articulation

The patellofemoral articulation is more akin to tibial femoral articulation than it is to the articulation of the hip. While in some knee designs there is near-complete congruency between the patellar component and the anterior flange of the femoral component that would provide pure sliding, this congruency is not typical. Most knee designs produce varying stresses in the patella. These stresses may be the result of a change of curvature through the range of motion or of a change of contact area between the patella and femoral component during flexion, resulting in a transition from contact with the anterior flange to contact with the condylar region of the component. Fatigue failure of patellar components is strongly influenced by implant design and appears to occur with a frequency similar to that of tibial components.

Importance of Design

The most important prosthesis-specific variables that can effect polyethylene damage are design and material.

Stress, both contact and subsurface, can be influenced by implant design and polyethylene thickness. Further, the ability of the polyethylene to resist fatigue is a function of the quality of the polyethylene, as is described later. Factors such as patient weight, activity level, and surgical alignment are beyond the control of the prosthesis designer, but it is crucial that these factors be accounted for in the design of the prosthesis and in the selection of materials.

One of the best ways to prolong the life of the polyethylene components is to design the articular surfaces so that the stresses generated in the tibial component in normal use are well below the yield strength of the material. Yet it is important to remember that there are a number of patient and surgical technique factors that may put the prosthesis in a compromised environment. For this reason, a design must also be able to continue to produce low contact stresses and perform adequately in less than ideal alignment. Another crucial design parameter is the thickness of the polyethylene. Studies (3, 4, 18) have shown that polyethylene bearing surfaces need minimum thickness to avoid the generation of large and potentially catastrophic internal material stresses. Finally, it is important that the materials used be well suited to handle the demands of the environment. This means that, in addition to being strong, durable, resistant to chemical attack and to providing low resistance to sliding, they must be inert to the body both in bulk and particulate form. But beyond concerns about polyethylene wear, a prosthesis must address a host of other concerns such as reproduction of natural kinematics, fixation to host, and ease of insertion. As will be explained, the knee is a complex joint with limited design space. Each critical parameter involves a trade-off that must be considered in order to provide a prosthesis that addresses all of these demands.

Articular Geometries

The three factors that most directly influence contact stress of the tibiofemoral and patellofemoral articulation are positioning, congruency, and thickness of the polyethylene bearings. While positioning is primarily in the hands of the surgeon, a good design with adequate polyethylene thickness will allow a prosthesis to accept small deviations from ideal positioning while still performing normally. Most currently available knees are either fully congruent (where the radius of curvature of the femoral and tibial components, when viewed from both the anterior and sagittal perspectives, have near matching radii of curvature) (4) or moderately congruent. Moderately congruent designs typically have a curved femoral profile on a flat tibial profile when viewed from the sagittal plane. The frontal plane surfaces fall broadly into one of two categories: flat-on-flat, in which the condylar region of the femoral component and the mating tibial articulation are both flat and horizontal to the ground when viewed from an anterior perspective; or curved-on-curved, in which both the tibial and femoral surfaces are curved and generally matching when viewed from an anterior perspective.

As Bartel and Burstein pointed out in their 1985 article, even when the frontal plane profiles are congruent, the relative radii of tibial and femoral curvature when viewed from the lateral perspective are also important (3). However, both flat-on-flat and curved-on-curved geometries typically have nonmatching curvatures in this plane, and only the fully congruent designs match sagittal radii of curvature. Even fully congruent designs only match sagittal plane radii in the first 30 degrees or so of flexion, where the largest radius of curvature of the femoral component is in contact with the tibial bearing. At flexion angles greater than 30 degrees, the radius of curvature of the femoral component decreases, as previously described, and the congruency is thereby lost. If one measures the contact stresses for these three types of configurations, flat-on-flat, curved-on-curved, or fully congruent, using either pressure sensitive film techniques or finite element analysis, it becomes clear that the more congruent the articulating surface geometries are, the lower the contact stresses become.

Patellar geometries also tend to fall into either fully congruent or moderately congruent categories. The fully congruent designs match the condylar geometries of the femoral components in both the sagittal and frontal planes. Moderately conforming patellar designs tend to be dome shaped with profiles that only match the femoral geometry in the frontal plane. As with tibiofemoral designs, patellofemoral designs must balance the benefits of decreased contact stresses through increased conformity with the dangers of overconstraint that typically accompany a more congruent geometry.

Response to Misalignment

Lower contact stresses should result in a lower incidence of fatigue, all other factors being equal. However, not all knees are fully congruent and it is worth assessing why not. Primarily, the degree of difficulty in positioning the components is a factor that must be taken into account in knee design and the extent of congruency. In most cases, the more congruent a pair of articular surfaces is, the more sensitive they will be to some types of misalignment. The three types of misalignment that are most prevalent in the components that have been sent to our laboratory for examination are: posterior tilt, varus-valgus malalignment, and rotational malalignment, comprising the available angular degrees of freedom.

In some implant designs, extensive posterior tilt, especially if combined with even slight flexion of the femoral component, can result in impingement of the anterior surface of the tibial spine of the polymeric component with the intercondylar notch of the femoral component. This is design-specific and far less frequent than the other two types of malalignment.

Varus-valgus malalignment is more critical in flat-on-flat designs, where a slight varus or valgus tilt will result in only the edge of the femoral condyle contacting the tibial surface. This results in dramatically increased contact stress and increases the potential for fatigue failure. From a stress standpoint, curved-on-curved and fully congruent designs are not particularly sensitive to varus-valgus malalignment, as the loss in contact in one compartment can be gained through increased contact of the curved surfaces in the other.

Rotational malalignment does not drastically affect the contact stresses in curved-on-curved or fully congruent geometries as the intercondylar area of the femoral component will engage the tibial spine gently by virtue of the matching curved surfaces on both components. As the components engage in rotation, however, the femoral component will be forced to ride up on the central eminence of the tibial plateau. This will be resisted by the tension in the soft tissues, thus transmitting a rotational force to the tibial component. The result can be high shear stresses at the bone prosthesis interface. The one exception to this rule is the mobile bearing design. In the two configurations of this design, the meniscal bearing and the rotating platform, a fully congruent geometry can be realized without particular sensitivity to malalignment as the bearings are free to move in rotation with the femoral component.

Flat-on-flat geometries are designed to provide little or no resistance to limited rotation. Within limits, the flat-on-flat design allows the femoral component to rotate freely on the tibial component without bone to prosthesis shear stresses and change in tibial contact stresses. At the limit of free rotation, however, when the intercondylar notch engages the tibial plateau, there will be impingement due to the square profiles of the mating geometries. This phenomenon is evidenced by a number of retrieved flat-on-flat components we have observed that show tibial spine damage as a result of impingement from malrotation.

Patellar components have similar trade-offs. The more congruent a patellar component is to its matching anterior flange and condylar region, the more rigorous is the requirement for proper alignment of the component. The typical types of malalignment in the patella are rotational malalignment (only important in congruent designs, not in domes), and proximal or distal placement of the patella, resulting in edge loading of the component. Dome configuration patellae typically are relatively insensitive to proximal or distal positioning and totally insensitive to rotational alignment. However, the lack of congruency between dome-shaped patellae and anterior flanges and condylar regions of the femoral components, can result in high contact stresses. The more congruent the design, the more sensitive it is to position and orientation, but the lower the contact stresses. Again, in this application, the mobile bearing design is less sensitive to rotational alignment than is a fixed bearing component of the same configuration. Interestingly, the mobile bearing design appears to require the mobility only immediately after implantation for alignment purposes. Once the bearing is properly aligned, it does not appear—at least from the 30 or so retrievals we have examined—that the polyethylene rotates relative to its metal backing to any significant degree.

Polyethylene Thickness

The third important characteristic that can control the degree of subsurface contact stress in total knee designs is the thickness of the polyethylene bearing. As demonstrated by Bartel (3, 4) and ourselves (18), contact stress in tibial components dramatically increases below approximately 6 mm, and, therefore, thicker bearings should be used whenever possible. Thicker polyethylene bearings require greater removal of proximal tibial bone, reducing the area of support for the cruciate ligament(s) and providing lower density bone to support the tibial component. While the first concern is valid, the second is of less significance. Recent studies in our laboratory (6) indicate that with depths of resection up to 16 mm, the quality of bone in the proximal tibia does not decrease significantly.

Laboratory Testing and Retrieval Analysis

Tibial Components: Contact Stress Evaluated with Pressure Sensitive Film

Repeated exposure to high contact stresses may put the polyethylene components of total knee prostheses at risk of failing by fatigue. To provide insight into the importance of articular congruency on tibiofemoral contact stresses, Fuji Prescale pressure sensitive film was used to determine the contact stresses of 12 currently marketed knee prostheses. The contact stress for the tibiofemoral articulation was determined at 15 degrees and 90 degrees for each design at an applied load of 3 times body weight (BW).

The prostheses used for this work were selected to represent the varying degrees of tibiofemoral conformity currently available in total knee replacements. They are the Miller Galante I and II and Insall Burstein II (Zimmer), the Natural Knee (Intermedics), the PCA I and II, Kinematic, and Kinemax (Howmedica), and the LCS meniscal bearing and rotating platform (DePuy) (Table 63.1). Components were chosen to be of as near identical size as possible; in general, a medium size was chosen.

Joint force studies have shown that the tibiofemoral force varies from 3 to 4 times body weight for level walking and from 4 to 5 times body weight for activities such as stair climbing and rising from a chair (Table 63.2). Preliminary testing revealed that tibiofemoral loads greater than 4 times body weight tended to saturate the Fuji film, producing contact pressures above the 50 MPa upper detection limit. To simulate physiological loads from daily activities while staying within the

Table 63.1. Grouping of Components by Tibiofemoral Conformity

Fully Conforming	Moderately Conforming Curved-on-Curved	Moderately Conforming Flat-on-Flat
LCS rp[a]	Townley	Miller/Galanté
LCS mb[a]	Kinemax	Miller/Galanté II
Insall/Burstein II	PCA II	PCA I
		Natural Knee
		Ortholoc III
		Kinnematic

[a]rp, rotating platform; mb, meniscal bearing.

Table 63.2. Maximum Compressive Tibiofemoral Joint Forces for Daily Activities

Activity	Morrison 1970	Dumbleton 1972	Ellis 1984	Paul 1976
Walking	$3.4 \times BW$[a]			$3 \times BW$
Up ramp	$4.5 \times BW$		$4.4 \times BW$	
Down ramp	$4.5 \times BW$		$4.4 \times BW$	
Up stairs	$4.8 \times BW$		$4.4 \times BW$	
Down stairs	$4.3 \times BW$		$4.9 \times BW$	
Rise chair		$3.2 \times BW$		
Knee bend			$4.2 \times BW$	

[a]BW, body weight.

limits of the Fuji film, the tibiofemoral components were tested in flexion and extension for an applied load of 3 times body weight (2,130 N).

The components were loaded, using an Instron (Instron Corp. Canton, MA) servohydraulic testing machine, which used specially designed fixtures to hold a set flexion angle while keeping all other alignments neutral. The contact pressure was determined using Fuji Prescale pressure sensitive film. Prescale film consists of two sheets, an A film and a C film. The A film contains a layer of microcapsules of various sizes that burst at different pressure levels releasing a color-forming material. The C film contains a developer that produces a red dot when reacting with the color-forming material released from the A film micro capsules. At higher pressure, more capsules burst, creating a darker image. The color density of the developed pattern can therefore be calibrated as a function of the contact pressure. The film comes in four grades of pressure sensitivity, super low, low, medium, and high. The contact pressures for this work fell within the range of the medium pressure grade with a range of 9.8 MPa to 49 MPa (1420–7110 psi).

The exposed film samples were digitized with a La Cie Silverscanner (La Cie Limited, Beaverton, OR) flatbed color scanner and then analyzed on Image 1.44, a 256 gray scale image analysis system written by The National Institute of Health for the Macintosh. This system has the capability of reading area and pressure for all or part of a contact area as well as for providing information about the histogram distribution (i.e., mean, and standard deviation). From this information, a maximum contact pressure was calculated that corresponds to the pressure in the most highly stressed region of the contact area. The image analysis system was calibrated by producing uniform contact areas of a known contact pressure. When scanned into the computer and assigned pressure values, these standards produce a calibration curve that is applied to scanned images of the test data. Accuracy was checked by integrating the experimentally determined contact pressures over the contact area to back calculate the applied load. This method determined that the results were within the 10% accuracy stated for the film by the manufacturer.

Figure 63.1, A compares the contact pressure for each of the devices tested for an applied load of 3 times body weight at a flexion angle of 15 degrees. At 15 de-grees flexion, the devices with complete conformity produced contact pressures that were substantially lower than the other devices. The majority of the moderately conforming designs produced higher contact pressures that were roughly the same, independent of whether the mating geometry was flat-on-flat or curved-on-curved. At 90 degrees of flexion, (Fig. 63.1, B) no sharp distinctions between the components were observed as a decrease in the femoral, sagittal radii of curvature significantly reduces the conformity of even the highly congruent designs. The Fuji contact stress analysis indicated that each of the prostheses tested produced contact pressures at 3 times body weight and 105 degrees flexion that may exceed the uniaxial yield strength of UHMWPE (21 MPa) (28). Fortunately, walking typically constitutes the greatest cyclic use of the knee, and full flexion therefore constitutes far less of the components' duty cycle than limited (30 degrees) flexion. Also, due to the constraining effects of the surrounding polyethylene, contact stresses in excess of the uniaxial yield strength do not necessarily imply that yielding will occur and should not be used as a failure criterion.

The uniaxial yield strength is the value of the normal stress at failure of a test specimen subjected to pure tension. In the uniaxial state, the shear stress, which is responsible for failure, will be equal to the shear strength of the material. In a three dimensional stress state as encountered in the knee prosthesis, the polyethylene surrounding the contact area will contribute substantial stress components in directions perpendicular to the contact stress. These stresses will increase the hydrostatic stress and decrease the distortional stresses responsible for failure (5). It is therefore possible to produce contact stresses above the uniaxial yield strength while keeping the shear stresses below the yield strength in shear. Conversely, stresses below the yield strength do not necessarily imply safety as fatigue mechanisms can propagate cracks due to voids, notches, or impact loading at stresses well below the yield strength. Failure of tibial components often occurs due to delamination—the result of high subsurface stresses that cannot be determined by contact pressure testing. Finite element analysis, discussed later, provides insight into these stresses and the effect of polyethylene thickness.

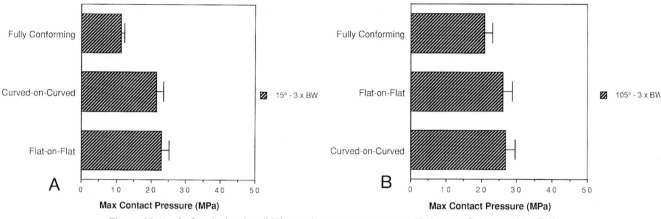

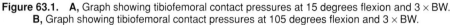

Figure 63.1. **A,** Graph showing tibiofemoral contact pressures at 15 degrees flexion and 3 × BW. **B,** Graph showing tibiofemoral contact pressures at 105 degrees flexion and 3 × BW.

The difference between success and failure for a total knee replacement often depends on the accuracy with which the device has been implanted. Most designs, if aligned correctly and accompanied by proper soft tissue balance, will perform adequately, all other factors being equal. Unfortunately, surgical technique is not always perfect and the ability of the design to accommodate alignment and loading that deviate from the ideal comes into play.

Misalignment or poor balance resulting in varus/valgus component loading can cause load bearing to shift to one condyle with potentially harmful effects. To test the sensitivity of design geometries to varus/valgus misalignment, one design each was selected from the completely conforming, moderately conforming (flat-on-flat), and moderately conforming (curved-on-curved) subgroups. Using Fuji Prescale film, the devices were tested for contact area (rather than contact pressure as the Fuji film was commonly saturated by the abnormal loading) at full extension under a 1 × BW applied load. Contact area measurements were taken of the medial compartment at neutral, 0.4 degrees, 0.7 degrees and 1.4 degrees of varus. The results (Fig. 63.2) indicated that curved-on-curved and fully conforming devices were not particularly sensitive to varus alignment in terms of decreased contact areas. The contact areas for both designs increased steadily with increasing varus, indicating that the medial condyle was able to effectively carry the increased load caused by the change in alignment. The flat-on-flat device, however, actually produced a smaller contact area at 1.4 degrees than 0.7 degrees, indicating a severe stress concentration at the peripheral edge of the flat condyle. This phenomenon has been referred to as edge loading.

Contact pressure testing in rotational misalignment of fully conforming mobile, curved-on-curved, and flat-on-flat devices in rotational alignment subjected each device to a 3 times body weight axial load and to rotational alignments of 0 degrees, 5 degrees, 10 degrees, 15 degrees, and 20 degrees in flexion and extension (Fig. 63.3, *A, B*). The fully conforming, "mobile bearing" implant clearly suffered no ill effects as a result of rota-

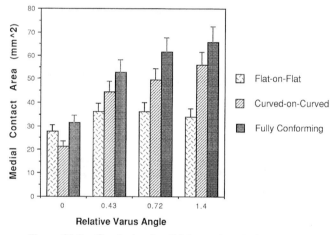

Figure 63.2. Graph showing tibiofemoral contact areas as a function of varus alignment at 1 × BW.

tion. The flat-on-flat device developed a relatively severe increase in stress for rotational angles above 5 degrees at 15 degrees of flexion. At higher flexion angles, the increase in stress with increasing rotational alignment became less severe as the articular geometry became less congruent, thus allowing more laxity. The curved-on-curved device also showed no contact pressure sensitivity to rotational malalignment. This is due to the gentle engagement of the intercondylar notch and the tibial spine, as mentioned previously. While these devices are generally representative of other similar designs, it must be remembered that not all flat-on-flat or curved-on-curved devices will produce the same results. In addition, it must be reiterated that contact stress is only one factor in determining the success or failure of a total knee replacement (TKR); the shear stresses transmitted to the bone-prosthesis interface as a result of the geometry will be of equal importance.

Testing of the same devices in anterior, middle and posterior positions indicated that none were particularly sensitive to alterations in AP position (Fig. 63.4, *A, B*). This is most likely due to the presence of gradually curved lips at the front and back of each tibial insert.

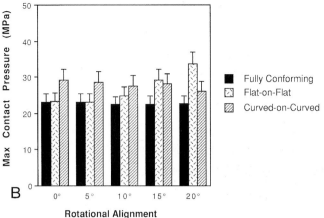
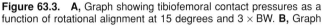

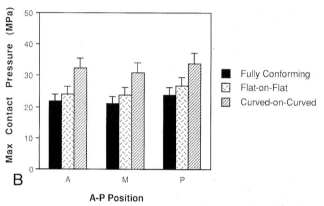
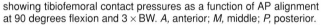

Figure 63.3.   A, Graph showing tibiofemoral contact pressures as a function of rotational alignment at 15 degrees and 3 × BW. **B,** Graph showing tibiofemoral contact pressures as a function of rotational alignment at 90 degrees and 3 × BW.

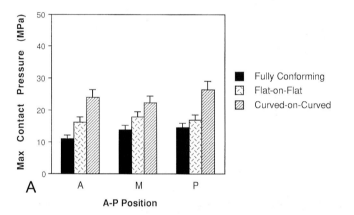
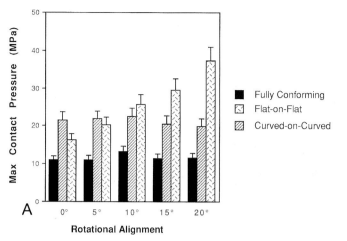

Figure 63.4.   A, Graph showing tibiofemoral contact pressures as a function of AP alignment at 15 degrees flexion and 3 × BW. **B,** Graph showing tibiofemoral contact pressures as a function of AP alignment at 90 degrees flexion and 3 × BW. *A,* anterior; *M,* middle; *P,* posterior.

Tibial Components: Finite Element Analysis

A finite element analysis was used to study the effect of polyethylene thickness on stresses within the tibial component. The analyses were performed on a generic, moderately conforming, curved-on-curved model similar to designs of that category tested for contact area and pressure with Fuji Prescale pressure sensitive film. The analysis made use of gap elements that allow load to be transferred between two separate finite element meshes while also permitting sliding and deformation to take place at the interface. This technique permitted load to be transmitted to the tibia through the mating femoral geometry without presupposing a contact area or pressure distribution.

Due to symmetry, only 25% of the components were modeled to save on computer time. An applied load of 4 times body weight (BW = 160 lbs, 715 N) was quartered and distributed to the top of the femoral component. Tests were performed on models with minimum thicknesses of 2, 3, 4, 6, 8, 10, 12, and 14 mm using the modulus of elasticity of standard UHMWPE (0.9 GPa).

The contact stress results of the finite element analysis agreed with the Fuji Film analysis for a moderately conforming device at the same load and flexion angle (Fig. 63.5). The model predicted that the maximum shear stress would occur at a depth of approximately 0.5 mm from the articular surface. This is consistent with the depth at which most of the fatigue-related damage, such as pitting and delamination, have been observed in retrievals. The moderately conforming model demonstrated a sharp increase in polyethylene stresses for decreases in thickness below 6 mm and no further change in stresses for thicknesses above 10 mm.

The high stresses in thin, polyethylene bearings in noncongruent knee designs are predictable. Further, analysis of retrieved tibial components revealed that the less congruent, higher contact stress-producing devices presented greater wear. Finite element analysis demonstrated that the stress intensity in the polyethylene decreases dramatically with increasing polyethylene thickness. An increase of as little as 4 mm of polyethylene (from 3 mm to 7 mm) reduced the maximum Von Mises

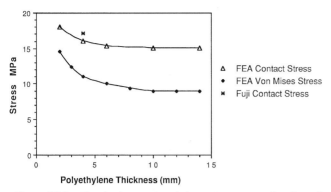

Figure 63.5. Graph of contact and shear stresses as a function of thickness from FEA of a curved-on-curved device at 3 × BW.

stress by as much as 27% and the maximum contact stress by 14%. A similar study by Bartel (3) showed a 26% decrease in contact stress for a 4 mm increase in minimum tibial thickness (from 4 mm to 8 mm). The influence of polyethylene thickness is less prominent for more congruent geometries, such as in the hip, but it is considerable for all knee articulations; even the most congruent must be considered relatively incongruent.

Tibial Components: Retrieval Analysis

Our analysis of failed, metal-backed tibial components indicates that the vast majority of these devices were of a modular type and had been fitted with either the thinnest or one of the thinnest available polyethylene inserts. This is most likely the result of the surgeon's desire to resect as little tibial bone stock as possible, combined with a lack of retrieval data warning against the potential for failure of thin polyethylene inserts. Despite the concern that tibial bone quality diminishes with greater distance from the subchondral area (14), a few additional millimeters should be removed in favor of thicker polyethylene.

Examination of the retrieved prostheses revealed that the fixation of the polyethylene inserts to the metal backing does not eliminate motion between the two and that an additional, initial articulation is provided in many of these modular prostheses. Over time, the polyethylene often creeps significantly; in some components, more than 1 mm of creep into screw holes was seen. While this creep may help the polyethylene to lock in place over time, the extent of creep and the potential for screw/polyethylene contact and fretting wear of the polyethylene raise additional concerns.

The normal tibia transmits the majority of its load through the medial condyle. Therefore, there was an expectation that more wear would occur in the medial compartment than in the lateral. Our examination revealed significant differences between the total wear of the medial versus lateral components and between the anterior and posterior regions of the components. The medial compartment had overall higher total wear scores than the lateral compartment, and the anterior region had overall higher total wear scores than the posterior region.

The benefits of a highly congruent, tibiofemoral configuration were evident from the lack of deep pitting, delamination, or cracking, in the majority of fully conforming meniscal bearing and rotating platform prostheses. Our stress analysis indicated that the maximum stress levels in these designs were approximately one-half of those of the majority of fixed bearing devices. The surfaces of most of these components presented only scratching, burnishing, and very fine (less than 0.5 mm) pits. However, some components with relatively incongruent geometries performed equally well in similar patients for similar durations when retrieved for similar reasons. Detailed examination revealed that there was considerable variation in the degree of consolidation of the polyethylene in knee components (as discussed below), which may be a greater factor in the variation in resistance to fatigue than is design.

Thin polyethylene tibial inserts and low conformity designs increase stresses within the polyethylene that risks fatigue failure. Additionally, surface heat treatment may be a factor in polyethylene delamination. Solutions to the problem of fatigue failure incorporate those guidelines developed by Bartel in his 1986 (3) article: greater conformity and thicker polyethylene bearings. In addition to these earlier guidelines, the apparent increase in extent of delamination of heat-surfaced components suggests that one must weigh that risk versus the undocumented potential benefit of a smoother articulating surface.

Patellar Components: Contact Stress Evaluated with Pressure Sensitive Film

A similar technique to that described for testing tibial components was used to assess patellar components. The prostheses used for this work were selected to represent the varying degrees of conformity currently available. They are the Miller-Galante II (Zimmer, Warsaw, IN), the Kinematic, Kinemax and PCA I & II (Howmedica, Rutherford, NJ), and LCS (DePuy, Warsaw, IN) (Table 63.4). Each prosthesis was chosen in a size which was closest to that of a medium to allow for direct comparison.

Joint studies have shown a more angle-dependent loading profile for the patella (Table 63.5). For normal walking, the patella experiences peak loads of 0.5 to 3 times body weight, while for deeper flexion activities, such as stair climbing and rising from a chair, loads of 2 to 6.5 times body weight can easily be generated at the articular surface. To stay within the range for the Fuji film, loads of 1 times body weight were used at 15 degrees, and 3 times body weight at 90 degrees.

Figure 63.6, A shows the contact pressure as a function of flexion angle for the different load cases. At 15 degrees and a load of 1 times body weight, the dome components produced contact pressures between 31 and 36 MPa. The congruent components produced considerably lower contact stresses around 20 MPa. At 90 degrees and a load of 3 times body weight, the moderately conforming designs produced contact pressures of about 43 MPa, while the more congruent designs produced contact stresses of about 27 MPa (Fig. 63.6, B).

Table 63.3. Evaluation of Wear of Tibial Components

	Overall Wear	Abrasion	Burnishing	Pitting	Cracking	Delamination	Creep	n
Highly congruent	1.7	2.0	2.2	1.6	0.3	0.4	1.1	38
Curve-on-curve	1.9	1.6	1.7	1.8	0.6	1.0	1.3	42
Flat-on-flat	2.0	2.0	2.3	1.5	1.0	0.9	1.1	42

Table 63.4. Grouping of Components by Patellofemoral Conformity

Fully Conforming	Moderately Conforming Dome
LCS	Miller/Galanté II
	Kinematic
	Kinemax
	PCA I
	PCA II

Table 63.5. Maximum Compressive Patellofemoral Joint Forces for Daily Activities

Activity	Morrison 1970	Reilly and Ellis 1984	Martens 1972	Huberti 1984
Walking	$0.7 \times BW^a$		$0.2 \times BW$	
Up ramp	$1 \times BW$			
Down ramp	$2 \times BW$			
Up stairs	$2.8 \times BW$		$1.7 \times BW$	
Down stairs	$2.8 \times BW$		$1.7 \times BW$	
Rise chair		$4.3 \times BW$		
Knee bend		$2 \times BW$		$6.5 \times BW$

^{a}BW, body weight.

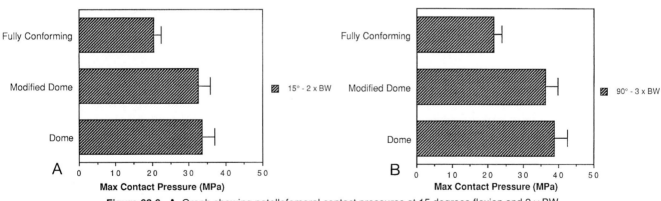

Figure 63.6. A, Graph showing patellofemoral contact pressures at 15 degrees flexion and $2 \times BW$. **B,** Graph showing patellofemoral contact pressures at 90 degrees flexion and $3 \times BW$.

As a group, all the dome-type patellae produced contact stresses in the 30 MPa to 45 MPa range. This level of stress exceeds the 21 MPa yield strength (28) of polyethylene by 40% to 114%. Deformation is therefore expected. The more congruent geometries produced lower contact stresses than other patellae tested. The lowest stresses were at lower flexion angles where there was complete conformity between the femoral and patellar surfaces.

The study of retrieved, patellar components demonstrated that measurable wear, including deformation, was commonly observed. Low congruency, dome-shaped components, with resulting high contact stress, presented the greatest wear while highly congruent designs demonstrated less wear and deformation. Our examination indicates that conformity is beneficial to fatigue resistance, although the ideal positioning of the implant may be difficult to reproduce in surgery. Dome patellae are insensitive to rotational positioning, while "anatomic" or congruent geometries are extremely sensitive to alignment. The rapid fatigue failure of many dome-shaped metal back patellae has led to their abandonment. Of the metal-backed patellar designs, it appears that only the mobile bearing, congruent components are currently being used in any significant numbers.

Contact stress analysis indicates that under loads of 3 times body weight, all but the most congruent designs produce stresses in the polyethylene that exceed its yield strength. The least congruent designs produced more than twice the contact stress of the most congruent designs. Slight deformation of polyethylene patellar components can result in increased conformity and reduced contact stresses, although, if the deformation is too great, cracking at the margins of the component can occur. Whether the deformation or cracking would eventually lead to complete failure of the polyethylene or breakdown of the patella/cement bond remains a possibility that cannot be determined from this study.

Patellar Components: Retrieval Analysis

Our analysis of retrieved patellar components revealed that the bulk of metal-backed, noncongruent components showed evidence of significant wear (wear score of more than 2 out of a possible 3), thus raising the concern for fatigue failure of many of these devices over time. The all-polyethylene components, although too few in number for statistical analysis, generally demonstrated a reduced tendency for severe pitting or delamination of the surface and yet demonstrated creep deformation with a potential for cracking at the margins of the prostheses. In a larger study of all-polyethylene prostheses, Hood, et. al. (16) described deformation in nearly 46% of the 28 patellar components. Further, Wright, et. al. (30) describes the all-polyethylene dome-type patellar loosening rates as being higher than the combined loosening of tibial and femoral components in arthroplasties with a 5–8 year follow-up.

Given the high contact stresses produced by many designs and given the data relating high contact stresses to component failure, it is worth asking why more patellar components don't fail in vivo. There are probably a number of reasons for this. Contact stresses exceeding the uniaxial yield strength of polyethylene do not necessarily equate to the shear stresses responsible for material failure, stresses that are above the material's yield strength in shear. Even if the shear stresses are above yield, yield in polyethylene is characterized by plastic deformation and not by brittle failure. Those components that have been tested in the laboratory are often loaded to points well above the yield strength without any readily apparent catastrophic effects. It is obvious that load on components can produce stresses in excess of the yield stress some finite number of times before noticeable damage begins to appear.

Due to variations in patient activity and gait alteration, it is possible that many components do not experience large, cyclic loads frequently enough to accumulate damage. The loads used in this study were based on studies of healthy subjects. TKR recipients may place less stringent demands on their prosthetic knees by favoring them or using aids such as canes or walkers. They may also limit or aid the deep flexion activities, such as rising from a chair or walking up stairs, that produce higher stresses. Many patients are not capable of flexing beyond 110 degrees. In reality, most prostheses probably experience loads well below 3 times body weight for the majority of their service. It has also been shown that at higher flexion angles, the quadriceps tendon engages the femur and carries almost half of the resultant patellar load, thus reducing the severity of the load on the articular patellar surface (17).

Wear Rate in the Knee

There are significant data on the wear rate of all-polyethylene acetabular components, but little comparable data for wear in the knee. There are a number of factors that make measurement of wear in the knee difficult. First, unlike the hip, in which wear generally occurs in one region in one direction, wear in the knee may occur at random over the entire surface of the tibial component, and the combination of rolling and sliding does not allow for a single resultant force. Further, slight variations in orientation of the component and soft tissue tensioning can significantly vary the location of wear from component to component. Owing to the much greater geometric complexity of the knee, radiographic variables are also much more difficult to control in contrast to that of the hip.

The examination of retrieved components has permitted us to determine that there is greater wear damage medially and anteriorly in tibial components than posteriorly or laterally. However, there was no statistically significant difference in the depth of wear penetration between medial and lateral or between anterior and posterior regions of the component and no well-defined wear troughs, so that an accurate assessment of the wear was impossible. We were confounded in our attempt to measure the wear rate of the tibial components because the wear rates in knees that have not failed due to fatigue appear to be low (on the order of the wear

Table 63.6. Analysis of Retrieved Components

	All Polyethylene	Metal-Backed	Total
Highly-congruent	5	29	34
Less congruent	7	86	93
Total	12	115	127

Table 63.7. Wear of Retrieved Patellar Components by Category

	Overall Wear	Abrasion	Burnishing	Pitting	Cracking	Delamination	Creep	n
Congruent[a]	1.6	1.2	0.6	0.9	0.9	0.9	0.6	34
Noncongruent[b]	2.2	1.4	1.8	1.7	1.1	1.3	1.5	93

[a]LCS, Freeman-Samuelson, and Townley 'Butterfly'
[b]Insall-Burstein, AMK, PCA I (dome and anatomic), Miller-Galante, Ortholoc I & II, Synatomic, and Tri Con

rate in the hip) and, unlike the hip, there is no easily determinable bench mark from which to measure the depth of wear. The majority of retrieved components were revised at periods of less than 5 years; therefore, the wear may be expected to be on the order of a millimeter. Component-to-component variations can account for a large part of this variation in the absence of wear. The manufacturers do not provide data on the original thickness of components nor on what machining tolerances of the components are being held to. Unlike the hip, there is also considerable creep in knee components and, therefore, much of the reduction of thickness of these components may be a function of deformation rather than loss of material. In short, it is unlikely that an accurate measurement of wear rates in metal-backed tibial components will be available in the near future. It may be possible to determine wear rates on the earlier all-polyethylene total condylar type designs. These were more congruent, and the wear pattern may be more focused and easily discernible. Extrapolation of data from this prosthesis to the less constrained metal-backed components, with their thinner polyethylene, may be unreliable.

Wear rates in the knee may parallel wear rates in the hip, if the knee design is not susceptible to fatigue failure. The contact area in the hip varies from 760 mm^2 with a 22 mm head, to 1608 mm^2 with a 32 mm head. In the knee, the contact area varies from 130 mm^2 in the least constrained knees, to 1350 mm^2 with the most conforming knees. Therefore, the contact pressures in some configurations of the two joints are similar. (There is every reason to believe that the surfaces of the knee and hip can be polished to a similar extent, and there is no inherent reason, in the absence of fatigue failure, why rolling/sliding wear must be more aggressive than pure sliding.) As previously described, examination of highly congruent tibial knee components retrieved at periods up to 10 years confirms that the wear rates are low enough to be impossible to measure accurately.

Additional Factors Which May Influence Wear Rate

Third Body Wear Debris

The addition of third body particulate wear to the articulation in the knee can result in dramatically increased wear rates. Third body particles that are as hard or harder than the metal of the femoral component can scratch the component, producing more rapid wear of the polyethylene. Metal debris can come from ablation of the porous coating, impingement of metal components, fretting of screws or other modular metal components, or from the abrasive interaction of instruments used in surgery. Additionally, particles of bone or fine bone dust made at the time of implantation can also cause scratching of the femoral component and a loss of the high polish required for the low wear rates. Manufacturers of porous-coated prostheses have had to be constantly aware of the importance of tightly bonding the porous coating to the components lest particles of the porous coating find their way to the articulating surfaces. Unfortunately, coating is lost from time to time, and the presence of this material at the articulating surfaces can cause severe damage at very short (18 months to 3 years) time periods.

Surface Treatments

To date, UHMWPE articulating against highly polished cobalt chrome alloy is the state-of-the-art in the knee. With good design, elimination of third particle debris, and proper alignment, wear rates on the order of those in the hip are attainable. Reduced wear rates may be attainable by improvements to both the metal of the femoral component and the polyethylene of the tibia. On the femoral side, much effort is being put into providing surfaces that are smoother than those available today. Several alternatives are being investigated. Harder materials are often more easily highly polished than are softer materials; therefore, ion bombardment of cobalt and titanium alloy femoral components in order to increase the surface hardness is being evaluated. The limitation on ion bombardment is that its depth of penetration is quite low; therefore, this process is being used after final polishing in most cases. While the increase in hardness should make the femoral component more resistant to scratching, it is not clear that the surface will necessarily be smoother.

A revisitation of nitriding is also under investigation. Nitriding provides a far thicker hardened layer on the surface of the femoral component, and this process can be done prior to final polishing, resulting in a component that is both smoother and harder. Alternatively, at least some manufacturers are looking at the possibility of ceramic femoral knee components. The current, but conceivably surmountable, limitations of this technique are cost and the lack of toughness of the ceramic. Ceramics are much harder than metals and can be much more highly polished. Ceramic heads have already made their way into hip surgery; ceramic knee components are still in laboratory testing.

There is much concern about the polyethylene against which the metal femoral component articulates. The importance of consolidation and quality control in polyethylene manufacture is discussed below. There are, however, several ongoing efforts to produce polyethylene that has been "enhanced" to improve its performance in a wear mode. While previous attempts to replace polyethylene with other bearing materials have been unsuccessful and the effort to improve polyethylene through the addition of carbon fibers was counterproductive, there is reason to believe that the polyethylene itself may be optimized. One such material, Hylamer, is produced by taking standard UHMWPE and subjecting it to the equivalent of a hot isostatic pressing procedure. The polyethylene, raised to a temperature near its melting point, is subjected to pressures on the order of 10,000 atmospheres for a number of hours. This reorganizes the molecular structure of the material, reducing the number of folds in a given chain length. The developers of this material claim increased resistance to oxidation, reduced creep, increased tensile and yield strengths, and high uniformity. To date, there are few data with which to compare its wear rate or fatigue resistance to standard UHMWPE. Material that has greater resistance to attack in the body and improved fatigue characteristics could result in an improvement in longevity of knee components.

Role of Polyethylene Quality on Wear

The recent observations of fatigue failure and wear damage in ultrahigh molecular weight polyethylene, (referred to below as polyethylene), tibial and acetabular components, and the problems with associated wear debris, have shifted current research to improving the wear characteristics of the polyethylene components. New research includes analysis of the contact stresses between the articulating surfaces, analysis of the integrity of the bone/cement interface or the porous coating/bone interface, and, most recently, analysis of the polyethylene bearing surfaces (19, 20, 25, 26). In the analyses of polyethylene, studies have been conducted to determine the relationship between material characteristics (i.e., consolidation, third body inclusions, oxidation, crystallinity) and implant performance.

As wear behaviors may be influenced by the specific properties of the material, the information regarding the polyethylene components and every aspect of their fabrication is becoming more valuable. Previously, very little documentation was kept regarding the fabrication and use of this material in total arthroplasty. Unlike the metal components used in total joint applications, no record of manufacturing processes and batch properties was kept, nor were any identification numbers given to the components placed in vivo to allow tracing the raw material from which they were made. Few samples were kept for retrospective examination, and only minimal quality control was performed on the material or the components.

As a result, it is very difficult to obtain any information from the orthopaedic manufacturers detailing the history of the components now being analyzed in retrieval studies (i.e., from what grade of polyethylene powder were they made, from what supplier was the polyethylene obtained, when was the component made). This information was not considered important at the time of fabrication and was not recorded. It has since been learned that polyethylene is not all the same and that, in fact, the different "grades" of polyethylene may be responsible for the observed differences in wear. Motivated by these results, several companies are now recording the origin of the polyethylene they use and assembling data on all manufacturing stages. This information may yield insight into the wear damage and failures that have been noted.

Polyethylene Fusion Defects

Previous studies have noted "spots" in polyethylene tibial bearing surfaces examined on retrieval, describing them as "fusion defects" (18, 20, 25). Landy, et al., on examining random components in their laboratory, noted the presence of fusion defects in several components. If a particular type of component exhibited these defects, they examined all other components, used and unused, in their collection from the same manufacturer. Surprisingly, in each case, all other retrieved components from the same manufacturer exhibited similar defects. In addition, no cases of delamination were noted in components that did not possess fusion defects. From their study, Landy, et al. concluded that the fusion defects may be an indication of a weak bonding of intragranular boundaries and of the predisposition for polymer damage (20).

Rose, professor of Material Science and Engineering at the Massachusetts Institute of Technology, and some of his colleagues also noted the presence of fusion defects in several of the components in their studies. From their observations of SEM (scanning electron microscope) micrographs, they reported that cracks and craters formed preferentially at these fusion defects and that crack formation was accelerated by the existence of these particles (25). They concluded that the fusion defects formed in the processing of the polyethylene manifested themselves as surface wear, specifically, as pitting and delamination. They extended the conclusions of Landy, et al. by relating damage directly to the presence of defects, saying the ultimate degree of wear depended on the number and weakness of the defects (25).

Examination of retrieved polyethylene components in our retrieval laboratory has indicated the presence of the fusion defects described previously. These defects, appearing as black or white "spots," have been noted on a macroscopic level in many of the retrieved components examined and scored for wear damage (Fig. 63.7). These observations have generated two main questions: namely, what is the source of these defects and what is their role, if any, in the fatigue failures observed in several retrieved components.

Our original hypothesis, based on early laboratory observations, was that fusion defects were related to in

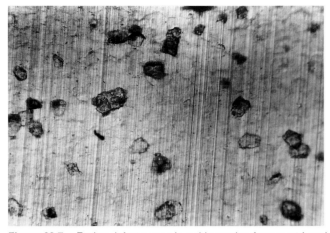

Figure 63.7. Fusion defects seen in a thin section from a retrieved tibial tray. Note the round, cauliflower shape of the defects (63x magnification).

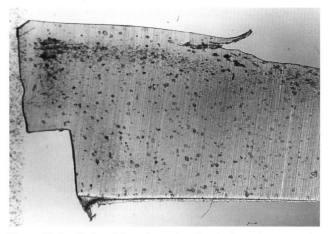

Figure 63.8. Fusion defects located uniformly throughout a section from a retrieved tibial tray (10x magnification).

vivo service. This was based on the finding that none of the examined virgin polyethylene bar stock presented defects and that approximately 20% of the unused components and 60 to 80% of the retrieved components contained defects. This suggested to us that perhaps some mechanism in the fabrication and in the subsequent in vivo use of the material was causing the defects.

However, following an in-depth, microscopic analysis of retrieved components and unused, preprocess polyethylene stock material, we rejected the original hypothesis; we concluded that most fusion defects are a function of the fabrication of the material to bulk form from powder (as will be detailed below). In our more detailed analysis of polyethylene, we determined that some of the unused stock did in fact contain fusion defects. Because this material exhibited defects but had not been exposed to any contact stresses, it became clear that the origins of the defects may be traced back to the original powder and to the forming process of the polyethylene stock.

In addition, if the presence and extent of fusion defects were related to in vivo service, the defects should be present in greater numbers in regions of high stress (i.e., at and just below the articulating surface). This was not the case in the retrieved components we examined; fusion defects were located uniformly through the component, regardless of the stress a particular area was exposed to in vivo (Fig. 63.8).

Thin sections from a subset of several retrieved components were obtained and rated on a 0 to 5 scale for the presence and severity of defects. In any specimen, a "defect rating" of 0 corresponded to a defect-free section, while a rating of 5 corresponded to a section in each specimen filled with the greatest number of defects throughout.

The defect ratings for the loaded and unloaded (stressed and unstressed) regions of the tibial tray components were statistically indistinguishable. In addition, no differences were noted in the extent of defects found in acetabular versus tibial components, despite the fact that these two components have significantly different stress profiles. If fusion defects were a result of in vivo stressing, one would not expect to find similar numbers of defects in both types of components.

Due to the characteristics of the material and the forming processes (detailed below), the possibility of fusion defects in polyethylene bulk material exists. Because ultrahigh molecular weight polyethylene consists of polymer chains that are 10 to 20 times longer than those of high density polyethylene, the material has a high viscosity and thus low flow properties (23); the material never reaches a liquid state, no matter how high the temperature. The ramifications of this property manifest themselves in the forming process of polyethylene components.

Gloor states that compression molding techniques and flow procedures involving large flow channels are the only appropriate methods for fabricating polyethylene (13). In addition, because of the low flow properties, cooling and heating times for these processes can only be approximated from standard heat transfer tables used for other materials. Since the data from these tables are average values and do not take into consideration any phase changes in the polymer during processing, the heating and cooling times necessary to produce well-fused blocks of uniform density material may be up to 50% longer than those predicted by standard tables (13). In support of this, product literature from Hoechst Celanese states that heating and cooling times are variable and can drastically change the integrity of the material (15). If the proper calculations are not made for a specific forming process, the resulting material can be filled with fusion defects.

Rose also noted that total consolidation of polyethylene was not possible, owing to the high processing temperatures required by the high melt viscosity of the material (25, 27). He observed that the polyethylene granules comprising the polyethylene are really assemblages of smaller particles bound together by fibrils. These fibrils, which bridge defects and are thus related to the strength of the material, can be damaged or degraded in processing. This compromises the material's strength. Rose stated that these fibrils are stable at temperatures below approximately 150 degrees C, but are destroyed at higher temperatures.

In addition, it has been shown that temperatures higher than 150 degrees C also cause degradation of the molecular weight due to oxidation of the polymer (25). In the oxidation process, the oxygen radicals cause the polyethylene chains to break by attaching to the hydrogen atoms in the polymer chain. This causes shortening of the molecular chains and loss of molecular weight. As previously stated, the high molecular weight of polyethylene is responsible for its increased wear resistance (25, 26, 27). If molecular weight is decreased, the abrasion resistance, one of the desirable characteristics of polyethylene, is lowered as well (22). This explains the correlations between oxidation and fatigue damage observed by Li, et al. In their studies, Li et al. found high levels of oxidation associated with areas of high damage, specifically pitting, cracking, and delamination (21). To avoid material degradation, and the destruction of fibrils, the processing temperatures of the polyethylene powder should be kept below 150 degrees C. Due to the low (or zero) melt index (a measure of the flow properties of the material), however, the powder particles do not fuse completely when polyethylene is processed below this temperature limit, thus giving rise to fusion defects in the material (25, 27).

There is a clear trade-off between degradation due to oxidation and degradation due to incomplete consolidation of the material. Both compromise the material's properties, but, in order to eliminate one form of degradation, the other is increased. As yet, no fabrication technique balances the two.

The literature and our initial examination of this problem suggested that fabrication played an important role in the consolidation and performance of the material. To understand this problem, it is important to know the fabrication process currently used in producing ultrahigh molecular weight polyethylene for use in total joint components.

Polyethylene Powder Fabrication

There are two companies in the United States, Himont (Wilmington, DE) and Hoechst Celanese (Houston, TX), that produce the ultrahigh molecular weight polyethylene powder from which all orthopaedic components are made. Both companies use the same basic technology to form the powder that they then provide to different companies for commercial use. The polyethylene powder is produced using a Ziegler-Natta catalyst (titanium tetra-chloride ($TiCl_4$) and a cocatalyst. A different cocatalyst, the identity of which is proprietary information, is used by each company. The difference in the cocatalysts results in subtle differences in the powder; the powder supplied by Himont has trace elements (due to their cocatalyst) not found in the powder supplied by Hoechst Celanese (25).

In the powder forming process, ethylene gas is bubbled through a suitable liquid, most often hexane, containing the catalysts. In the reactor where all processing occurs, the ethylene monomers diffuse through the solvent to the surface of the catalyst. At the surface, they migrate to the "growth point" of the polymer chain, where the polymer "grows" out from the catalyst surface, much as a strand of hair grows from its root (22). The result is individual powder particles whose centers contain the catalyst used to cause the chain growth. The catalyst cannot be retrieved from the powder, nor is it thought to bear any effect on the subsequent formation processes of the polyethylene stock material; the majority of it is so deeply "buried" inside the powder particle that the chance it could be liberated, thus having an effect on the polyethylene stock material is very small (25). Any trace amounts of the catalyst present after formation are also unlikely to have an effect on the polyethylene stock material.

Once the molecular chain growth is completed in the reactor, the liquid-slurry phase containing the powder and remaining hexane is removed and centrifuged to remove the hexane. The centrifuging and two drying stages are conducted in a nitrogen environment due to concerns regarding the hexane concentration. After a third drying stage in air, the polyethylene powder is ready to be packaged and shipped to commercial converters. They form the bar or sheet stock polyethylene that is used for several applications; one of the applications is for bearing surfaces for joint replacement, provided that the powder passes the standards indicated by the ASTM Annual Book of Standards (25). One guideline specifies that, if the resulting polyethylene powder has a relative solution viscosity of 2.30 or greater, it can be used in medical grade applications such as total joint replacement (22).

GUR 415

There are three different grades of polyethylene powder that can be acceptable for medical grade applications, Hostalen GUR 415, Hostalen GUR 412, and Himont 1900. The first grade, GUR 415, is one type of polyethylene powder formed by Hoechst Celanese. This powder has a bulk density of 0.4 g/cm^3, an average powder size of 125 μm (range: 60–250 μm), and a yield value within the range 0.3–0.5 N/mm^2, 10 min. This yield value is based on the stress required for 600% elongation of the material in 10 minutes (15).

The GUR 415 powder also contains a corrosion inhibitor, calcium stearate. Calcium stearate accounts for approximately 0.05% of the powder and was originally used years ago to reduce the level of residual chlorine present from the powder-forming process. During the formation of the polyethylene chains, the $TiCl_4$ catalyst undergoes a transformation to $TiCl_3$ in the reactor that leaves residual Cl (approximately 30–40 ppm). In compression molding of bulk polyethylene from the powder, a water-cooled, steel plate molding system is used. The residual Cl, combined with the hydrogen molecules present in water, form HCl, which corrodes the steel plates used in the molding process. Calcium stearate absorbs the excess Cl and thus reduces the incidence of corrosion of the steel molding plates (25). Approximately ten years ago, Hoechst Celanese improved its powder forming process and reduced the amount of residual Cl to only 10–20 ppm. From that time, concern about corrosion of the molding plates lessened, and Hoechst considered removing the calcium stearate from the powder. They hesitated because of concerns about the poor flow properties of polyethylene in the ram extrusion of polyethylene stock from the powder.

Calcium stearate in small concentrations (about .05%) provides lubrication in the extrusion process. Recently, one of the converters of bar stock has been experimenting with GUR 405 powder, a powder produced by Hoechst Celanese that has the same properties as GUR 415, but does not contain calcium stearate. In initial experiments, it has been found that the concerns about lubrication in the ram extrusion process are not as important as originally thought. It also has been found that the polyethylene stock formed from this powder has better fusion characteristics; the stock formed is more completely fused or bonded and thus may be of higher quality.

GUR 412

The second grade of polyethylene powder, GUR 412, is also supplied by Hoechst Celanese. This powder, which contains calcium stearate, is formed by the same method as GUR 415. The differences between GUR 412 and GUR 415 are in the material properties. Like GUR 415, GUR 412 also has a bulk density of 0.4 and an average powder size of 125 μm (range: 60–250 μm). In comparison with GUR 415, it generally has a lower yield strength, 0.20–0.25 N/mm^2, 10 min (15). There is also a difference in the molecular weights of the two powders. GUR 412 typically has a lower molecular weight than GUR 415, which indicates shorter molecular chains in the bulk material. Due to the large range of molecular weights of the individual powder particles as a result of the forming process, some GUR 412 powder particles could have a higher molecular weight than some GUR 415 particles (22). The increased chain length of GUR 415 provides increased strength to the bulk material and increased resistance to wear damage, specifically to abrasion (25, 26, 27). The decreased molecular weight of GUR 412 may explain the differences seen in the wear characteristics of different components.

There are differences in the consolidation of the bulk material made from these two powder grades. Thin sections, approximately 200 μm thick, were taken from samples of both GUR 415 and GUR 412 virgin stock and examined microscopically for the presence and extent of fusion defects. To date, none of the samples of GUR 415 bar stock have presented any defects. The material appeared to be well fused with no "grain boundary" separations at the intersection of the individual powder particles; several of the sections from retrieved components exhibited grain boundaries that appeared to be the intersection of the individual powder particles (Fig. 63.9). The GUR 412 samples, however, contained fusion defects throughout. The extent of defects varied significantly with the type of stock examined (i.e., bar stock, sheet stock). There did not appear to be any particular

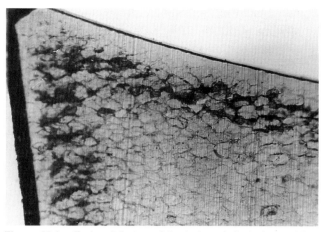

Figure 63.9. Fusion defects and "grain boundaries" observed in a section from a retrieved tibial tray. Note that the size of the fusion defects is roughly equivalent to the size of the individual grains (40× magnification).

location pattern to the defects in either type of the GUR 412 samples; the defects appeared uniformly throughout the entire section in each case.

Representative sections taken from these samples were also examined at higher magnifications to determine the average size of the defects. The size of the defects found in the GUR 412 sections ranged between 40 and 100 μm, which corresponds to the average size of the individual powder particles. This indicates that material grade may, in fact, play an important role in the consolidation of the material.

Himont 1900

The third grade of polyethylene powder is Himont 1900, the powder produced by Himont. The difference between Himont 1900 and the GUR 412 and 415 powders is in the trace elements found in the Himont 1900 powder and in the particle size of the powder. Himont 1900 has an average particle size of 180–190 μm with a much narrower range than the Hoechst Celanese powders. Typically, Himont 1900 has a lower molecular weight than GUR 412 and GUR 415. These differences may also contribute to the differences observed in component performance.

Thin sections from samples of Himont 1900 bar stock, made from Himont 1900 powder, also showed fusion defects throughout. As in the GUR 412 samples, there did not appear to be any preferential location of the defects. The defects were, however, larger than those found in the GUR 412 samples. Their size averaged between 175 and 200 μm, which corresponds quite well with the average size of the individual powder particles.

Taking into consideration the number of defects observed in samples of GUR 412 and Himont 1900, the corresponding differences in the powder itself, and physical appearance of the defects, it seems clear that there is a relationship between powder grade, production technique, and consolidation, as measured by the presence of fusion defects. Specifying GUR 415 extruded bar stock (the only defect-free grade of material we have examined to date) may be enough to ensure that manufacturers are using the best quality material available and that their devices will have the best performance obtainable within the limits of their design and within the limits of the contact stress conditions in vivo. Clearly, more research has to be conducted to determine if all currently produced GUR 415 extruded bar stock is defect free or if, perhaps, there is some other way to ensure defect-free GUR 412 or Himont 1900 polyethylene.

Due to changes in the ASTM guidelines pertaining to the polyethylene powder used for medical grade applications (2) instituted in 1984, the amount of the trace elements allowed in the powder has been reduced to the following: Al—100 ppm, Ti—300 ppm, Ca—100 ppm, and Cl—120 ppm (2). The reduction of the amount of trace elements allowed by the ASTM standard may be yet another step in improving the quality of the polyethylene material used for total joint replacement.

Polyethylene Stock and Component Fabrication

The polyethylene components used in total joint replacement are typically made one of two ways, depending on manufacturer. Components are either formed by machining or by compression molding. In the first case, components are machined directly from either polyethylene sheet or from bar stock supplied from a converter.

In the fabrication of the sheet stock, the powder (generally GUR 412 or Himont 1900), is press molded into sheets from which components are machined. In the press molding process, the powder is placed in a 4-foot by 8-foot mold, leveled with a straightedge, and cold compressed under a pressure of approximately 7–10 MPa for 5 to 10 minutes to expel the air trapped in the powder. The press is then heated to approximately 200 degrees C until the powder is plasticated, or fused, throughout. After the powder is completely fused, the mold is cooled under approximately 7–10 MPa. If this pressure is not maintained, the final bulk material may contain voids or defects (15).

In our studies, the samples of GUR 412 sheet stock that were examined did in fact have fusion defects throughout the entire sample. The extent of defects was widespread; the sections from this material received ratings of 5 on the 0–5 defect rating scale. On the other hand, the GUR 412 bar stock, which did have some defects, had significantly fewer than the sheet stock samples; the sections from the bar stock had an average defects rating of 0.05. We have already indicated that powder grade seems to affect the defect characteristics of the final material. It appears, as Rose suggested, that the actual fabrication process may have an important role as well. The process that forms bar stock may be superior to that used to form sheet stock.

Polyethylene bar stock is formed by ram extrusion. In this process, the powder, generally GUR 415 but also GUR 412 and Himont 1900, is introduced into the cylinder of the ram extruder and compacted by the ram. The compacted material is then passed through a heated zone ranging in temperature between 180 and 200 de-

grees C in order to become plasticated (15). The length of this zone depends on the geometry of the final product; it must be long enough for complete fusion of the material. The length of the zone is important due to the poor melt properties of polyethylene powder. In the ram extrusion process, a perfect cone of material is formed in front of the center of the ram. This cone, opaque in appearance, is made of compacted powder that has not achieved the necessary melt temperature. On the outside of the cone, where the melt temperature has been attained, the material is a translucent gel. When the ram moves through the extruder, there is a delay in the movement of the extrudate. This delay allows the build up of pressure that "moves" the unmelted cone of compacted powder into the gel, where it melts.

Our results have shown that the ram extrusion process is not enough to ensure defect-free material. Sections from Himont 1900 bar stock and GUR 412 bar stock both contained varied amounts of defects. While these samples did not have as many defects as the sheet stock samples, they were not free of defects. Both fabrication and powder grade must be considered when trying to obtain consolidated material.

Compression molding directly from polyethylene powder is the other technique used to manufacture components used in total joint replacement. In this process, the polyethylene powder is placed in a die with the desired component geometry and subjected to a heat and pressure cycle to form the final component. This technique is used primarily in the fabrication of tibial tray inserts. The insert may either be molded directly onto the component's metal tibial tray or it may be formed separately and then inserted into the metal tray (if the design utilizes this feature) at a later time.

Part of our study included an examination of the components formed by machining their final geometry from bar stock versus those formed by the compression molding technique just described. In examining the intact components with transillumination, it appeared that the molded components were fairly defect free and, curiously, exhibited very little damage. Intrigued by this, we included a microscopic analysis of the molded versus machined components. The molded components, as in the macroscopic examination, exhibited very few defects and appeared to be made from completely fused material (Fig. 63.10). The machined components of similar design and contact stress history, exhibited a significantly greater degree of fusion defect and an increased incidence of fatigue-related failure (Fig. 63.11). Although this seems to indicate that molded components are better consolidated and possibly more fatigue resistant than machined components, one must bear in mind the following. In all cases, defect-free material, whether molded or machined, had a relatively low incidence of fatigue-related damage. Perhaps all that is necessary then is defect-free material. To date, no defects have been observed in GUR 415; it appears to be of higher quality. Specifying components machined from this material may lower the amount of fatigue-related damage. Unfortunately, there is no known method of determining through analysis the material grade of a retrieved

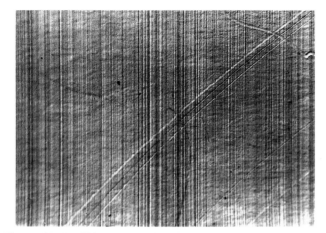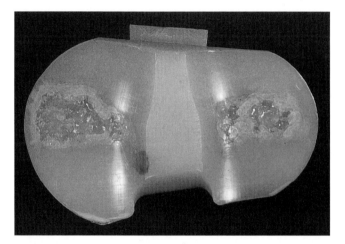

ditions, it may be possible to form higher quality polyethylene components. These components may have better fatigue characteristics, thus eliminating several of the recent concerns regarding the wear of polyethylene components, the subsequent generation of wear debris, and the associated tissue and bone necrosis.

We have also conducted a preliminary investigation of the parameters involved in molding polyethylene. We found that eliminating calcium stearate, decreasing the cooling rate of the molded polyethylene, and processing in an oxygen-free environment, reduced the number of fusion defects. We also noted that in low temperature and low pressure processes, more fusion defects were observed in the samples produced (12). Any defects in the material may act as flaws from which cracks initiate and propagate, increasing the chances of in vivo failure of the component. The exact relationship between the processing parameters, internal defects, and wear damage is still unclear.

Damage Mechanisms

So far, we have established a link between fabrication, powder grade, and fusion defects. While we have not determined the exact source of the defects, continued research should bring us closer to the answer. As of yet, we have not discussed the role of these defects in the performance of total joint components. We have alluded to the relationship between fusion defects and fatigue damage. The question now is, "does such a relationship exist?" Studies by ourselves and others support such a relationship.

The pitting, cracking, and delamination observed in the retrieved tibial components can be associated with the propagation of subsurface cracks. These cracks are propagated by the shear stress that occurs in the component during articulation. In the conforming geometry of the hip, the maximum shear stresses are located at the surface and thus have no effect on the subsurface cracks. In the nonconforming geometry of the knee, however, the maximum shear stresses are located at various depths under the surface, depending on the contact area and the friction coefficient. The depth of these stresses may even be as great as 2 mm below the articular surface, but are generally located between 0.1 mm and 1 mm below the surface. This depth corresponds to the approximate depth of the pits and delaminated areas of polyethylene found in the tibial components (3).

Clearly, fatigue cracking appears to play an important role in the pitting and delamination observed in many of the retrieved polyethylene components that have been studied. At first, this seems confusing given the fact that the ductile polyethylene is highly resistant to crack initiation (11); a mechanism that involves crack propagation should be of little concern. If, however, there are preexisting flaws or defects in the material, then crack propagation does become important. Several authors have hypothesized that fusion defects act as flaws from which cracks initiate and propagate (11, 16, 26). Landy, et al. noted that the severity of the damage observed in their retrieved components was increased by cracks and voids that occurred between inadequately fused gran-

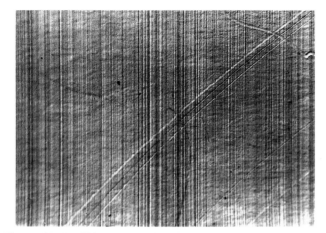

Figure 63.10. Thin section taken from defect-free material. Note that the material is completely consolidated; no defects or grain boundaries are visible (40× magnification).

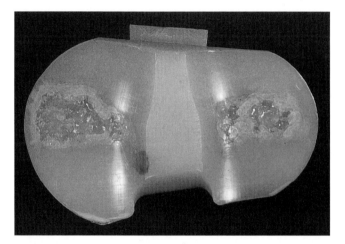

Figure 63.11. Typical fatigue-related damage seen in a retrieved tibial tray. This type of damage, along with cracking, has been correlated to the presence and extent of fusion defects in the polyethylene.

component. Therefore, it cannot be determined whether the defect-free components showing little or no fatigue-related damage were machined from GUR 415. In order to do this, we may have to wait for the retrieval and analysis of (currently in vivo) components that have serial numbers, which will allow the starting batches of the material in question to be traced.

In both machining and compression molding, control of formation parameters for bulk material (for machining) or for molded material is necessary to ensure a homogeneous and defect-free material. If the characteristics of polyethylene, especially its high melt viscosity, are not taken into consideration and if the processing variables are not controlled and adjusted for a specific mold, material weaknesses can be introduced into the final product, giving rise to failure (15). These weaknesses, manifested as a decreased material quality, may be responsible for the wear damage noted in retrieved components. By assessing the different parameters used in manufacture and finding the optimal processing conules (19). Connelly, et al. agreed with this finding, stating that fusion defects may act as stress concentrators and increase the possibility of crack initiation. They concluded that once the failure process starts at these sites, it may take a very short time to reach catastrophic failure of the component (11). They did not, however, give an estimation of time to failure once cracking had begun.

Our studies support the relationship between fusion defects and fatigue damage by correlating the extent of defects in retrieved components with the fatigue damage modes of cracking and delamination and with the total wear observed for each component. The damage modes were rated after Hood, et al. based on the percentage of damage in each of 10 regions in the tibial tray component. We noted that as more defects were observed, more fatigue-related damage was noted. There appears to be a direct relationship between the presence and extent of defects and the occurrence of these damage modes. This indicated that material containing fusion defects does not have all the advantages of fully fused polyethylene in terms of resistance to wear damage.

In this respect there is agreement with the earlier studies by Rose and Landy concluding that fusion defects indicated a compromised material more susceptible to damage, specifically to cracking and delamination (20, 25, 26). Our observation of cracks running through several fusion defects also supports these earlier studies (Fig. 63.12). It was difficult to determine, however, if the fusion defects acted as crack initiation sites as proposed by Landy and Rose; the cracks were noted running through several defects; their origin was unclear. Even though the exact mechanism of crack propagation and the involvement of fusion defects is unclear, the findings of this study support the relationships between fatigue damage and defects proposed by other researchers. These defects or weaknesses, when cyclically stressed in vivo, may be directly related to the cracking and delamination that leads to the fatigue failure of the polyethylene bearings. Defects may be

termed a "marker" for poorly fused material that has a predisposition to these damage modes. The defects may be a measure of an undetermined material characteristic that leads to the formation of cracks in the components and results in the damage observed.

The observation of a new phenomenon, thin section flaking, may extend the findings of Rose and Landy. This damage appeared to be a form of micro-cracking or micro-delamination that occurred approximately 0.5 to 1 mm below all surfaces (including nonarticulating surfaces) of several of the defect-filled components (Fig. 63.13). This damage may begin as single cracks in the material and may increase in number resulting in the micro-cracking or micro-delamination observed in several of the retrieved components we examined for our study. The presence and extent of the thin section flaking may be a measure of differing material characteristics in the sample. Sectioning the sample may highlight these differences; material with thin section flaking may be more prone to micro-cracking and micro-delamination under the shear stresses generated by cutting the section.

This study did prove, however, that the thin section flaking was not solely an artifact of the sectioning processes. If it were, one would expect to find this damage occurring to the same extent in all of the components sectioned. However, thin section flaking was observed to varied degrees in several of the components. It was not observed in any of the sections obtained from the polyethylene stock. At this time, it is unclear how the fabrication parameters relate to this damage, if, indeed, they do at all.

The correlations between fatigue damage, the presence of fusion defects, and thin section flaking indicate that defect-filled material may have a predisposition to failure. These phenomena do not appear to be caused by service and stress in vivo, but rather are characteristic of poorly fused material and related to both the

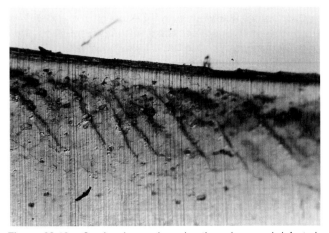

Figure 63.12. Cracks observed running through several defects in a section from a retrieved tibial tray (40× magnification).

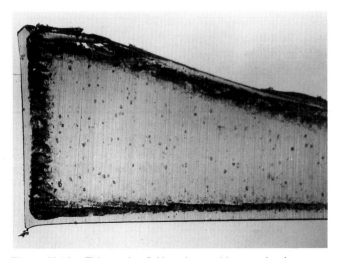

Figure 63.13. Thin section flaking observed in a section from a retrieved tibial tray. Note how the damage is located approximately 0.5 mm in from the edge of the section and follows the contour of the section (10× magnification).

grade of powder and the forming processes used to produce the polyethylene stock and total joint components. This study has demonstrated relationships between fusion defects and both the fabrication technique (i.e., machining from bar stock or sheet stock or compression molding from powder) and the powder grade. Since direct relationships between fatigue damage and the presence and extent of fusion defects were established and corroborated by this and earlier studies, it seems reasonable that, if such relationships exist and can be controlled, it should be possible to fabricate completely fused material that will be less likely to exhibit fatigue failure after service in vivo. Manufacturers should be as concerned with the material characteristics of the bearing surfaces as with every other aspect of the design of these components. Clearly, improving the material's integrity will improve the performance and longevity of the bearing surfaces used in total joint applications. The first step toward this goal is determining the exact relationships between fusion defects, thin section flaking, and the parameters involved in the fabrication of the polyethylene components. Additionally, it may well be that radiation sterilization could have a profound effect on the oxidation of the polyethylene. Studies are currently underway to illuminate the impact of sterilization technique on the fatigue resistance of the polyethylene.

Summary

Wear in the knee is multifactorial and subject to patient age, weight, activity level, component alignment, soft tissue tensioning, implant design, the presence or absence of third body wear debris, smoothness of the articulating surfaces, and quality of the polyethylene, among others. While many of the factors are under the surgeon's control, the design and manufacture of the implants remains a dominant variable. In general, components with lower contact stress should wear more slowly than those with high contact stress. Fatigue failure, the most common source of early polyethylene wear through, can be related directly to contact stress and polyethylene quality. The role of polyethylene quality cannot be underestimated. Even in relatively high contact stress geometries, defect-free polyethylene has been seen to perform quite well. However, defect-filled polyethylene has been seen to fail due to fatigue in even moderately stressed components. Prospects for the future, including more congenial geometries, more durable polyethylene, and greater refinement of bearing surfaces possessing resistance to degradation and improved propensity for wear, promise to leave the functional results of knee arthroplasty more in the hands of the surgeon.

References

1. ASTM designation D4020-81: Standard specification for ultra-high-molecular-weight polyethylene molding and extrusion materials. In: Annual Book of ASTM Standards. ASTM 1991;8(3):317.
2. ASTM designation F648-84: Standard specification for ultra-high-molecular-weight polyethylene powder and fabricated form for surgical implants. In: Annual Book of ASTM Standards ASTM 1991;13(1):201.
3. Bartel DL, Burstein A H, Toda M D, Edwards DL. The effect of conformity and plastic thickness on contact stresses in metal-backed plastic implants. J Biomech Eng 1985;107:193.
4. Bartel DL, Bicknell VL, Wright TM. The effect of conformity, thickness, and material on stresses in ultra-high molecular weight components for total joint replacement. J Bone Joint Surg 1986;68A(7):1041.
5. Bartel DL, Wright T M, Edwards D. The effect of metal backing on stresses in polyethylene acetabular components. In: The hip. Proceedings of the 11th Open Scientific Meeting of the Hip Society. St. Louis: CV Mosby, 1983;229–239.
6. Belec L, Bleday R, Collier JP, Lifrac JT, Mayor MB. Mechanical property distribution in the proximal tibia. Presented at the 60th meeting of the AAOS, San Francisco, 1993.
7. Charnley J, Elson R. Direction of resultant force in total prosthetic replacement of the hip. Med Biol Eng 1968:6(i):19.
8. Charnley J. Rate of wear in total hip replacement. Clin Orthop 1975;112:170.
9. Clarke IC, Black K, Rennie C, Amstutz HC. Can wear in total hip arthroplasties be assessed from radiographs. Clin Orthop 1976;121:126.
10. Collier JP, Mayor MB, McNamara JL, Surprenant VA, Jensen RE. Analysis of the failure of 122 polyethylene inserts from uncemented tibial knee components. Clin Orthop 1991;273:232–242.
11. Connelly GM, Rimnac CM, Wright TM, Hertzberg RW, Manson JA. Fatigue crack propagation behavior of ultrahigh molecular weight polyethylene. J Orthop Res 1984;2:119.
12. Franck K. Effects of fusion characteristics on ultrahigh-molecular-weight polyethylene used in total joint prostheses. ES88 Honors thesis, Dartmouth College, 1992.
13. Gloor WE. Properties and uses of very high-molecular-weight, high-density polyethylene. Mod Plastics 1961;November:131.
14. Goldstein SA, Wilson DL, Sonstegard DA, Mathews LS. The mechanical properties of human tibial trabecular bone as a function of metaphyseal location. J Biomech 1983;16:965.
15. Hoechst Celanese: Company bulletin, Hoechst plastics, 1992.
16. Hood RW, Wright TM, Burstein AH. Retrieval analysis of total knee prostheses: A method and its application to 48 total condylar prostheses. J Biomed Mater Res 1983;17:829.
17. Huberti HH, Hayes WC. Patellofemoral contact pressures. The influence of Q-angle and tendofemoral contact. J Bone Joint Surg 1984;66-A:715.
18. Jensen RE, Collier JP, Mayor MB, Surprenant VA. The role of polyethylene uniformity and patient characteristics in the wear of tibial knee components. Clin Orthop 1994;299:92.
19. Landy M, Walker PS. Wear in condylar replacement knees: A 10-year follow-up. Transactions of the 31st Annual Meeting. The Orthopaedic Research Society, 1985;10:96.
20. Landy MM, Walker PS. Wear of ultra-high-molecular-weight polyethylene components of 90 retrieved knee prostheses. J Arthroplasty 1988;(Oct suppl):S73.
21. Li S, Nagy EV, Wood BA. Chemical degradation of polyethylene in hip and knee replacements. Transactions of the 38th Annual Meeting. The Orthopaedic Research Society 1992;17:41.
22. McCrum NG, Buckley CP, Bucknall CB. Principles of polymer engineering. New York: Oxford University Press, 1988:10–14.
23. Miller RC. UHMW polyethylene. In: Modern plastics. Mid-October Encyclopedia Issue, 1991;67(11):66.
24. Rimnac CM, Wilson PD, Fuchs MD, Wright TM. Acetabular cup wear in total hip arthroplasty. Orthop Clin North Am 1988;19:631.
25. Rose RM, Crugnola A, Ries M, Cimino WR, Paul I, Radin EL. On the origins of high in vivo wear rates in polyethylene components of total joint prostheses. Clin Orthop 1979;145:277.
26. Rose RM, Nusbaum HJ, Schneider H, Ries M, Paul I, Crugnola A, Simon SR, Radin EL. On the true wear rate of molecular-weight polyethylene in the total hip prosthesis. J Bone Joint Surg 1980;62A(4):537.
27. Rose RM, Radin EL. A prognosis for molecular weight polyethylene. Biomaterials 1990;11:63.
28. Stein HL. Ultrahigh molecular weight polyethylenes (UHMWPE). In: Engineering Materials Handbook, Vol. 2, Park City, OH: ASTM International Metals, 1988:161–171.
29. Wright TM, Hood RW, Burstein AH. Analysis of material failures. Orthop Clin North Am 1982;13(1):33–43.
30. Wright TM, Bartel DL. The problem of surface damage in polyethylene total knee components. Clin Orthop 1986;205:67.
31. Wroblewski BM. Direction and rate of socket wear in Charnley Low-Friction arthroplasty. J Bone Joint Surg 1985;67–B:757.
32. Wroblewski BM. Wear and loosening of the socket in the Charnley Low-Friction arthroplasty. Orthop Clin North Am 1988;19:627.

64

Bilateral Total Knee Arthroplasty

Alfred J. Tria Jr., David A. Harwood, and Jose A. Alicea

Introduction

Total knee arthroplasty is recognized as the primary reconstructive procedure for patients with diffuse arthritis of the knee (Figs. 64.1 and 64.2). Several long-term studies have documented its efficacy in relieving pain and improving function (1–4). It is not uncommon for patients to have bilateral disease. Simon et al. reported in 1983 that, of patients undergoing total knee replacement at Brigham and Woman's Hospital, only 2.5% had unilateral disease. Out of 500 knee replacements performed at our institution over the last 10 years, 386 were bilateral.

Bilateral arthritic disease presents a significant problem both for the patient and the surgeon with respect to the timing of the knee replacements. Bilateral total knee replacement can be performed *simultaneously* by two surgical teams, *sequentially* under the same anesthetic, or in a *staged* fashion separated by days, weeks, or months. The decision must consider the type of anesthesia, the amount of estimated blood loss, the potential complications, the length of rehabilitation, and the potential cost of each surgical option.

There are many reports in the literature concerning bilateral total knee replacement (5–13). In 1978, Hardaker was the first to compare the results of simultaneous and staged bilateral replacements. The two groups had similar outcomes, but the cost of the staged procedures was 58% greater (6). Gradillas and Volz reported on sequential versus unilateral procedures in 1979. They indicated that both procedures yielded similar results; however, the sequential group had a higher pulmonary embolism rate (7). In 1985, Soudry evaluated the results of sequential, unilateral, and staged replacements. The three groups had similar knee scores; however, there was a higher incidence of thromboembolism and pulmonary embolism in the staged procedures (8). McLaughlin and Fisher, in 1985, compared simultaneous versus staged procedures and found fewer complica-

tions and shorter hospitalizations in the simultaneous group (9). In 1988, Stein compared simultaneous versus unilateral replacement and reported no difference in the complication rates (13). Morrey reported the largest series in the literature. He concluded that there was no statistical difference in the complication rate between simultaneous and staged procedures and that both groups demonstrated equal clinical results (10). Later studies have reported excellent clinical results with bilateral total knee replacement; however, some suggest the recent advent of intramedullary instrumentation may predispose to a higher incidence of fat embolism during bilateral replacement (14, 15).

At the Robert Wood Johnson Medical School, the preferred surgical approach to patients with bilateral knee arthritis has been simultaneous bilateral total knee replacement (Fig. 64.3). We consider a patient to be a candidate for bilateral replacement if the less symptomatic knee has a strong possibility of requiring replacement within 4 to 6 months of the more symptomatic one. The clinical results of patients undergoing bilateral replacement have been equal to patients undergoing unilateral replacement (16).

Anesthesia

Total knee arthroplasty can be performed under regional or general anesthesia. The choice of anesthesia is equally important in bilateral versus unilateral knee replacement. In the early years of joint replacement, general anesthesia was most commonly chosen, but, by the 1980s, a significant trend toward regional anesthesia emerged. Recent publications have elucidated the advantages of regional versus general anesthesia. Most of the studies emphasize pain control and the incidence of thromboembolic complications. Nielsen stated that patients who received epidural morphine reported a lower level of pain that those who received general anesthesia (17). Mahoney et al. stated that epidural analgesia de-

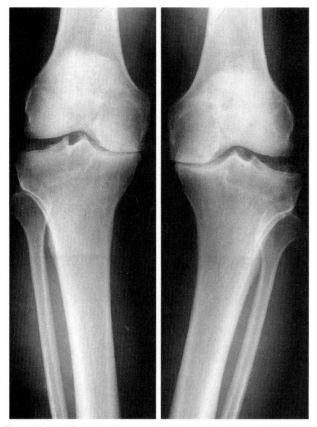

Figure 64.1. Preoperative roentgenogram of a patient with bilateral varus osteoarthritis of the knee.

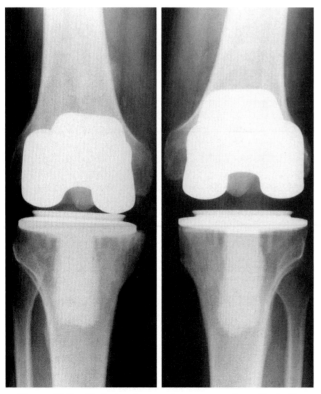

Figure 64.2. Postoperative roentgenograms of a patient with bilateral knee arthroplasties.

creased postoperative pain by 20% compared to the standard general anesthesia approach. However, both the cost and the duration of the operation were increased. These costs were divided between the cost of the catheter, the time to place the device in the operating room setting, and the postoperative monitoring while the catheter was in place (18). McQueen reported a decrease in pain and blood transfusions in the epidural group; however, the patients had significantly increased incidence of urinary retention and pruritis. The authors also suggested that this anesthesia was best followed in a "skilled nursing unit" (acute care environment) after surgery (19).

Both Sharrock and Jorgensen reported a significant decrease in calf vein thrombosis and proximal vein thrombosis in patients undergoing knee arthroplasty under epidural anesthesia as compared to general anesthesia (Table 64.1) (20, 21). Mitchell also reported a decreased incidence of proximal clots with epidural anesthesia (22).

Overall, the advantages of regional anesthesia represent an improvement in pain control and a possible reduction in thromboembolic complication. General anesthesia offers a greater ease of administration, slightly lower cost, and fewer allergic reactions. The choice of anesthesia type should be individualized to each patient, but the increase in pain control and the lower thromboembolic complications seen with epidural anesthesia may be particularly useful in bilateral total knee replacement.

Surgical Approach

Bilateral total knee replacement can be planned as a simultaneous procedure under one anesthesia, a sequential procedure under one anesthesia, or a staged procedure under two separate anesthetics. When the procedure is done simultaneously, the duration of the surgery and anesthesia is less, but the surgery requires two teams of surgeons.

Simultaneous Approach

In our medical center, simultaneous bilateral total knee arthroplasty is performed by two surgical teams working completely independently. Separate sets of instruments are used to avoid interchange of components or size discrepancies. One scrub nurse may be capable of handling both procedures depending upon his or her level of experience and confidence. A single circulating nurse is usually adequate.

Both knees are prepped and draped at the same time. The surgeries are begun at the same time with inflation of the tourniquets staggered by just a few minutes. Standard total knee replacement techniques are observed with ligament balance in flexion and extension with overall valgus alignment. We use intramedullary femoral alignment guides with extramedullary secondary checks. Extramedullary tibia guides are used. The operations proceed in a parallel fashion with simultaneous cementing of the components. The tourniquets are re-

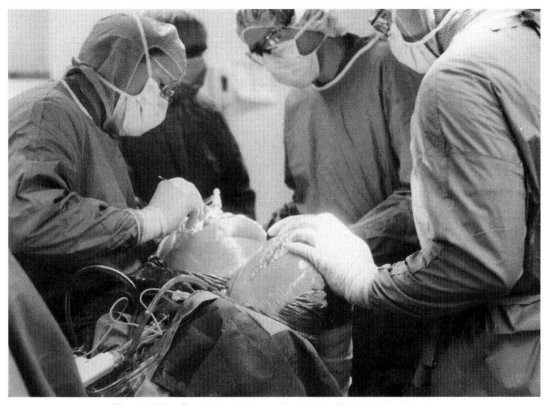

Figure 64.3.   Simultaneous knee arthroplasty with two surgical teams.

Table 64.1.   Comparison of General and Epidural Anesthesia During Knee Replacement

Series Comparison	Epidural (%)	General (%)	P Value
Sharrock, et al. (20)			
Deep Venous Thrombosis	48	64	P<.01
Proximal Clots	4	9	P<.05
Jorgensen, et al. (21)			
Deep Venous Thrombosis	18	59	P<.05
Proximal Clots	12	45	P<.05

leased in a staggered fashion before wound closure for adequate hemostasis.

Sequential Approach

During the planning of the sequential approach, both knees can be prepped initially or separately at the beginning of each procedure. The surgeon must decide if new instruments will be used for each knee surgery. The surgical technique is the same and can be completed by one surgeon with a single assistant.

Staged Approach

Staged bilateral knee arthroplasty can be planned during one or two hospitalizations. Each surgical procedure is performed as an isolated event. The time period

between the surgeries is controversial and extends from days to months.

Operative Data

The total anesthesia time and the surgical time can be significantly shortened by performing the procedure under one anesthetic (Table 64.2). The anesthesia time and surgical time can be decreased even further if the procedure is performed simultaneously; however, the tourniquet time for each knee remains the same. The blood replacement during bilateral knee arthroplasty is not affected by either a sequential or simultaneous approach. The patients require an average of 4 units of blood (Table 64.3). The blood replacement for unilateral arthroplasty is 3 units, thus exposing the patients to 6

Table 64.2.   Comparison of Operative Data in Bilateral and Unilateral Knee Arthroplasty[a]

	Simultaneous	Staged (1) (Same Hospitalization)	Staged (2) (Separate Hospitalizations)
		Operative Time	
		(In Minutes)	
Operating Room Time	280	290	340
Anesthesia Time	230	280	270

[a]From Morrey, BF, et al. Complications and mortality associated with bilateral or unilateral total knee arthroplasty. J Bone Joint Surg 1987;69–A;484–488.

Table 64.3. Comparison of Operative Data and Total Transfusion Data Between Sequential and Simultaneous Bilateral Total Knee Replacements

Operative Section	Sequential	Simultaneous	P value
		Operative Data	
		(in Minutes)	
Tourniquet	94	111	0.11
Surgery	220	166	<.001
Anesthesia	276	224	<.001
Transfusions	4.5 units	4 units	

units for a staged procedure. Most patients participate in the autologous blood program and are able to donate 3 units of their own blood before surgery.

Results

Insall reported on his evaluation of sequential bilateral knee replacement versus unilateral staged replacement and unilateral replacement. The Hospital for Special Surgery (HSS) results at an average of 3½ years after surgery were essentially the same for all three groups. The sequential group had a score of 92, the staged group had a score of 87, and the unilateral group had a score of 88.

Our evaluation of our bilateral replacements regarding alignment and postoperative function using the HSS Knee Score revealed no significant difference between the sequential and simultaneous replacements. At 2-year follow-up, both groups had average scores of 90 and their postoperative alignments were similar, proving that two teams of surgeons can effectively perform the procedure simultaneously without interfering with each other (Table 64.4).

Complications

Bilateral total knee replacement may be considered a reasonable option in patients with bilateral disease if the complication rate is proven to be similar to unilateral knee replacement; however, one might argue that the bilateral surgery involves two knee operations and should be equated with the complications of two unilateral arthroplasties. There are several reports in the literature regarding bilateral total knee replacement and its complications. Most of them emphasize thromboem-

Table 64.4. Comparison of Alignment and 2-year Follow-up HSS Knee Score Between Sequential and Simultaneous Bilateral Replacements

	Sequential	Simultaneous
Post-op Alignment	Valgus 5.0	Valgus 4.8
HSS Score	92	92

bolism and fat embolism as the major perioperative complications of concern.

The Mayo Clinic, in 1987, reported the largest series with 752 knee replacements. Of these, 290 were performed simultaneously or sequentially, 228 were performed staged during one hospitalization, and 234 were performed staged during different hospitalizations. The complication rate for the procedures was not significantly different with 9.3% for the simultaneous or sequential, 7% for the staged during one hospitalization, and 12% for the staged during two hospitalizations (Table 64.5). There was no difference in postoperative surgical complications (i.e., pulmonary embolism, deep vein thrombosis, prosthesis infection or fat embolism) among all groups (Table 64.6). The group of staged procedures with two hospitalizations had a slightly higher complication rate (12%). This may be explained by the fact that the group included patients with increased medical risks who were not felt to be good candidates for bilateral surgery. This brings out the point that some patients are unable to undergo simultaneous surgery because of the cardiovascular demands of the bilateral blood loss.

The concern over increased postoperative medical complications (i.e., urinary tract infections, pneumonia, or cardiopulmonary compromise) after bilateral total knee replacement as compared to unilateral replacement has not been supported in the literature.

In our series, we specifically looked at the difference in complications between simultaneous and sequential replacements during a single anesthetic (16). We found no statistically significant difference between these two groups concerning pulmonary embolism, infection, or mortality. The results of the two groups were not different from those of the unilateral replacements in our experience.

There is considerable concern in the literature regarding the rate of fat and pulmonary embolism during bilateral total knee replacement. Fat embolism with total knee arthroplasty was reported in the early literature with hinged knee devices following intramedullary instrumentation and fixation (14, 23, 24). With the advent of intramedullary alignment guides, there is increased concern that the instrumentation of the medullary canal may increase the risk of fat emboli (9).

Table 64.5. Comparison of Bilateral and Unilateral Total Knee Arthroplasty Complications and Mortality[a]

Procedure	Patient Number	Complications(%)	Reoperation(%)	Mortality(%)
Simultaneous/ Sequential	290	9.3	2.4	5.5
Staged (1)	228	7.0	4.8	0.9
Staged (2)	234	12	8.5	3.8
Unilateral	501	11	5.6	7

[a]From Morrey BF, et al. Complications and mortality associated with bilateral total knee arthoplasty. J Bone Joint Surg 1987;69-A:484–488.

Table 64.6. Comparison % of Complications Between Bilateral Knee Arthroplasty (Simultaneous or Sequential) Under One Anesthetic With Staged Bilateral Arthroplasty and Unilateral Replacement[a]

	SIM/SEQ (Bilateral)	Staged (1) (Same Hospitalization)	Staged (2) (Separate Hospitalizations)	Unilateral
Wound Problems	3	2	3	5
Infection	0.3	1.3	1.3	0.8
Patellar Problems	1.4		1.3	0.6
Loosening	0.3	1.3	1.7	0.2
Instability			1.3	0.2
Fracture	0.7		0.4	1.2
Pain	2	0.4	1.3	2
Thrombophlebitis	0.7	0.4	1.3	2
Pulmonary Embolism	1	0.4		1

[a]From Morrey BF, et al. Complications and mortality associated with bilateral or unilateral total knee arthroplasty. J Bone Joint Surg 1987;69–A:484–488.

Dorr reported a 12% incidence of fat embolism, including 1 death, during bilateral procedures in 65 patients (15). The procedures were performed sequentially under one anesthetic. Eleven patients were hemodynamically monitored, including the patient who subsequently died from sequelae stemming from this complication. This patient demonstrated a sustained increase in the pulmonary artery pressure and pulmonary vascular resistance during inflation and deflation of the tourniquet and also during intramedullary insertion of alignment rods into the tibia and the femur. The preoperative evaluation of the patients did not indicate which individuals were at higher risk for the embolic complications.

Dorr suggested intraoperative Swan Ganz catheter monitoring of patients undergoing *sequential* total knee replacement. He also recommended that the second knee procedure be aborted if there is a sustained elevation of the pulmonary artery pressure or pulmonary wedge pressure following the first procedure. He recommended the use of a fluted intramedullary rod and vent holes during the insertion of alignment devices to decrease the incidence of fat emboli. No hemodynamic guidelines currently exist for *simultaneous* bilateral total knee replacement.

Fahmy considered venting of the medullary canal to be the important factor in "totally" eliminating the hemodynamic changes associated with intramedullary rod insertion and fat emboli. He recommended enlarging the diameter of the insertion hole at least 4.7 mm larger than the diameter of the intramedullary alignment rod (25).

In our published series of bilateral total knee arthroplasties, we had 1 significant clinical case of fat embolism in 54 simultaneous or sequential procedures. This group was studied retrospectively; no specific monitoring was used to detect fat emboli, which certainly can go undetected with the use of simple clinical observation alone. It is our practice to use intramedullary guides for the femur and to vent the femur by enlarging the insertion hole. The tibial cuts are made with extramedullary guides.

The literature concerning fat and pulmonary embolism with respect to simultaneous knee replacement is inconclusive.

Economics

There are several theoretical economic advantages to performing bilateral total knee replacement under one anesthetic. The patient undergoes one anesthetic and one rehabilitation period. Hardaker reported a decreased cost with the simultaneous versus the staged procedure (6). Buscemi studied 26 bilateral replacements in a community hospital over a 52-month period. In his series, patients with bilateral replacement stayed 2 days longer in the hospital than the unilateral knees and the hospital cost was only $2,000 more (26) (Table 64.7). Ritter found an average 20% decrease in hospital cost in simultaneous bilateral replacements when compared with twice that of the unilateral group (11). Brotherton et al. reported an average 18% increase in hospital bills when the procedure was done in a staged fashion as opposed to simultaneously (5). In both of these studies, the patient's hospital stay was more than 46% longer for the staged population. Thus, hospital costs are definitely lower for the bilateral single anesthetic surgery.

The surgeon's reimbursement is another factor. Whether the procedure is completed sequentially with a single surgical attending or simultaneously with two

Table 64.7. Comparison of Cost Factors in Unilateral and Bilateral Arthroplasty[a]

Cost Factors	Unilateral	Bilateral
Length of Stay	10.3 Days	12 Days
Blood Loss	277	419
Hospital Cost	$10,272	$12,315

[a]Data from Buscemi MJ, Jr, et al. Unilateral versus bilateral simultaneous arthroplasties of the lower extremities. J Am Osteopath Assoc 1989;89:1133–1136.

surgical attendings, the reimbursement is commonly equivalent to the reimbursement for 1.5 knee arthroplasties. Thus, surgical fees certainly are higher with the staged approach.

Rehabilitation

Postoperative rehabilitation following total knee replacement can be painful and difficult, especially in patients debilitated from multiple joint involvement. It is certainly reasonable to be concerned about the ability of such patients to undergo rehabilitation following bilateral replacement.

In 1978, Gradillas reported the results of 41 patients who underwent sequential procedures versus 40 who had unilateral replacements (7). He demonstrated that the postoperative rehabilitation and the duration of time before independent walking was not increased in the bilateral group. McLaughlin compared 22 simultaneous versus 46 staged procedures (9). There was no increased difficulty in following the postoperative physical therapy regimen with the simultaneous group. Stanley compared bilateral versus staged procedures in patients with rheumatoid arthritis. Patients who underwent simultaneous bilateral total knee replacement perceived rehabilitation as easier than the patients who had completed the first of a planned staged bilateral procedure. All patients eventually improved function, but the maximum benefit was obtained only after both knees were replaced and was therefore delayed in the staged group (27).

Berman evaluated functional results in terms of gait analysis following either unilateral or bilateral total knee arthroplasty. Functional results improved in both groups of patients. However, the improvement was not as great in patients who underwent unilateral replacement but had radiographic evidence of bilateral disease (28).

Rehabilitation after bilateral total knee replacement under one anesthesia does not appear to be more difficult for the patients and is often perceived as easier than the staged approach.

Summary

Bilateral total knee replacement under one anesthetic is an acceptable approach to treating patients with advanced bilateral knee arthritis. In contrast to patients who undergo the staged approach, the complication rate of both groups is the same, the rehabilitation time for the simultaneous or sequential group is shorter, and the procedure is less expensive. There is no doubt that the problem of fat and pulmonary embolism must be considered. The literature concerning this complication is mixed, with divergent opinions. Our experience with 200 simultaneous total knee arthroplasties has not substantiated the concern for fat and pulmonary embolism. Bilateral total knee replacement does require conscientious surgical planning, but it can be performed safely with distinct advantages to the patient.

References

1. Stern SH, Insall JN. Posterior stabilized prosthesis. J Bone Joint Surg 1992; 74-A(7):980–986.
2. Ranawat CS, Boachie-Adjei, Oheneba. Survivorship analysis and results of total condylar knee arthroplasty. Eight- to eleven-year follow-up period. Clin Orthop, 1988; 226:6–13.
3. Vince KG, Insall JN, Kelly MA. The total condylar prosthesis. Ten to Twelve years results of a cemented knee replacement. J Bone Joint Surg, 1989; 71-B(5): 793–797.
4. Wright J, Edwald FC, Walker PS, Thomas WH, Poss R, Sledge CB. Total knee arthroplasty with the kinematic prosthesis. Results after five to nine years: a follow-up note. J Bone Joint Surg 1990; 72-A: 1003–1009.
5. Brotherton SL, Roberson JR, deAndrade JR, Fleming LL. Staged versus simultaneous bilateral total knee replacement. J Arthroplasty. 1986; 1:221–228.
6. Hardaker WT, Ogden WS, Musgrave RE, Goldner JL. Simultaneous and staged bilateral total knee arthroplasty. J Bone Joint Surg 1978; 60A: 247–250.
7. Gradillas EL, Volz RG. Bilateral total knee replacement under one anesthetic. Clin Orthop 1979; 140:153–158.
8. Soudry M, Binazzi R, Insall JN, Nordstrom TJ, Pellici PM, Goulet JA. Successive bilateral total knee replacement. J Bone Joint Surg 1985; 67-A:573–576.
9. McLaughlin TP, Fisher RL. Bilateral total knee arthroplasties. Clin Orthop 1985; 199:220–225.
10. Morrey BF, Adams RA, Ilstrup MS, Bryan RS. Complications and mortality associated with bilateral or unilateral total knee arthroplasty. J Bone Joint Surg 1987;69-A:484–488.
11. Ritter MA, Meding JB. Bilateral simultaneous total knee arthroplasty. J Arthroplasty 1987; 2:185–189.
12. Wapner JL, Ballas SL, Mallory TM. Rationale for staged versus simultaneous bilateral knee replacements. Ortho Trans 1984; 8:398.
13. Stein A, Shapiro E, Howe JG. Simultaneous bilateral knee arthroplasty. Am J Knee Surg 1988; 1:225.
14. Lachewicz PF, Ranawat CS. Fat embolism following bilateral total knee replacement with total condylar prosthesis. Clin Orthop 1981; 160:1106–1108.
15. Dorr LD, Merkel C, Mellman MF, Klein I. Fat emboli in bilateral total knee arthroplasty. Clin Orthop 1989; 248:112–118.
16. Tria AJ, Alicea JA, Cody RP. Bilateral Total Knee Arthroplasty. Am J Knee Surg 1992; 5:85–90.
17. Nielsen PT, Blom H, Nielsen SE. Less pain with epidural morphine after knee arthroplasty. Acta Orthop Scan 1989; 60(4):447–448.
18. Mahoney OM, Noble PC, Davidson J, Tullos HS. The effect of continuous epidural analgesia on postoperative pain, rehabilitation, and duration of hospitalization in total knee arthroplasty. Clin Orthop 1990; (260):30–37.
19. McQueen DA, Kelly HK, Wright TF. A comparison of epidural and non-epidural anesthesia and analgesia in total hip or knee arthroplasty patients. Orthopedics 1992; 15(2):169–173.
20. Jorgensen LN, Rasmussen LS, Nielsen PT, Leffers A, Albrecht-Beste E. Antithrombotic efficacy of continuous extradural analgesia after knee replacement. Br J Anaesth 1991; 66(1):8–12.
21. Sharrock NE, Haas SB, Hargett MJ, Urguhart B, Insall JN, Scuderi G. Effects of epidural anesthesia on the incidence of deep-vein thrombosis after total knee arthroplasty. J Bone Joint Surg 1991; 73(4):502–506.
22. Mitchell D, Friedman RJ, Baker JD 3d, Cooke JE, Darcy MD, Miller MC 3d. Prevention of thromboembolic disease following total knee arthroplasty. Epidural versus general anesthesia. Clin Orthop 1991; 269:109–112.
23. Bisla, RS, Inglis AE, Lewis, RJ. Fat embolism following bilateral total knee replacement with the Guepar prosthesis: A case report. Clin Orthop 1976; 115:195.
24. Orsini EC, Richards, RR, Mullen JMB. Fatal fat embolism during cemented total knee arthroplasty: A case report. Can. J Surg 1986; 29:385.
25. Fahmy N, Chandler HP, Danylchuk K, Matta EB, Suncer N, and Siliski JM. Blood-gas and circulatory changes during total knee arthroplasty. The role of the intramedullary alignment rod. J Bone Joint Surg 1990; 72A:19–26.
26. Buscemi MJ JR, Page BJ, Swienckowski J. Unilateral versus bilateral simultaneous arthroplasties of the lower extremities. Am Osteopath Assoc 1989; 89:1133–1136.
27. Stanley D, Stockley I, Getty CJ. Simultaneous or staged bilateral total knee replacements in rheumatoid arthritis. A prospective study. 1990; 72-B:772–772.
28. Berman AT, Zarro VJ, Bosacco SJ, Israelite C. Quantitative gait analysis after unilateral or bilateral total knee replacement. J Bone Joint Surg 1987; 69-A:1340–1345.

65

Blood Conservation in Arthroplasty

Steven T. Woolson

Risks of Homologous Transfusion
Legal Issues in Blood Transfusion
History of Autotransfusion
Predeposit Autologous Blood
Postoperative Blood Salvage
Combination of Predeposited and

Salvaged Autologous Blood
Surgical Technique
Criteria for Homologous Blood
 Transfusion After Knee
 Arthroplasty

Total knee arthroplasty is a relatively bloodless procedure because of the use of a tourniquet with an average intraoperative blood loss of less than 200 ml. However, the loss of blood after knee arthroplasty can be significant, since raw cancellous bone surfaces and extensive soft tissue dissection can cause prolonged bleeding. Numerous authors have measured the blood loss from wound drainage tubes that occurs after cemented total knee arthroplasty at 500 to 1000 ml (1–6) (Table 65.1). However, blood loss estimates solely determined from postoperative wound drainage are an underestimation of the actual total postoperative blood loss volume; the actual total also includes the unevacuated hematoma remaining within the joint and a considerable volume of blood that dissects into the soft tissues around the knee.

Other authors have calculated higher postoperative blood loss estimates from knee arthroplasty preoperative and postoperative hematocrit (or hemoglobin) values (7, 8). These studies estimated that the blood loss after cemented knee arthroplasty averages 1000 to 1500 ml and that the actual total blood loss is about three times the measured drainage tube volume. Several of these studies have also shown that the postoperative blood loss for patients who have an uncemented knee implant is greater than for patients who have cemented knee implants (2, 5). Bone cement evidently prevents a significant portion of the postoperative cancellous bone bleeding that is not restricted by a knee prosthesis. Using calculated estimates, the postoperative loss from uncemented total knee arthroplasty may be as high as 2000 ml.

If the average blood loss after cemented knee arthroplasty is between 1000 and 1500 ml, this is 20 to 30% of the total blood volume (5000 ml) of a 70 kg patient who has an average body habitus. Other studies have corroborated this by showing a 20% drop in the hematocrit after unilateral knee replacement when transfusions are not given (9, 10). As expected, the postoperative losses

from bilateral procedures are double that of unilateral procedures. In the elderly patient, an acute reduction in blood volume of 20% or more is not tolerated without considerable strain on cardiovascular reserves and blood transfusion is routinely needed to prevent complications of acute anemia. This makes it mandatory to plan for postoperative blood transfusion and/or blood salvage in all knee arthroplasty patients, especially for those undergoing bilateral procedures.

Risks of Homologous Transfusion

Having established that significant postoperative blood loss routinely occurs after total knee arthroplasty, blood conservation should be considered by the surgeon from the perspective of options for lowering the risks associated with transfusing these patients with homologous blood. Eliminating the use of homologous blood prevents the transmission of viral disease (HIV, hepatitis, Epstein-Barr, cytomegalus, human T-cell leukemia [HTLV-1] and retroviruses), and other blood borne diseases including syphilis, malaria, brucellosis, toxoplasmosis, and trypanosomiasis. Transfusion reactions and potentially fatal errors of ABO compatibility are also avoided. However, the frequency of each of these risks should be quantified so that surgeons and patients have accurate data with which to make informed decisions on the type of blood transfusion to be given after knee surgery.

Hepatitis is still the viral disease most commonly transmitted by blood transfusion. In the 1970s and early 1980s the risk of non-A, non-B hepatitis from homologous transfusion was estimated at 5 to 18% (11, 12). At the time of this writing, the risk of hepatitis has been markedly reduced due to stringent screening of donors for elevation of alanine aminotransferase, for antibody to the hepatitis B core antigen, and, more recently, for antibody to hepatitis C virus (the new term for parenterally transmitted non-A, non-B hepatitis). With the use of

Table 65.1. Blood Loss After Knee Arthroplasty

Author/Reference	Number Knees	Average Measured Total Blood Loss (ml)	Average Calculated Total Blood Loss (ml)
Mylod, 1990 (2)	11 Cemented	600	
	27 Uncemented	1400	
Hays, 1988 (5)	21 Cemented	1036	
	16 Uncemented	1598	
Cushner, 1991 (3)	82 Cemented	805	
	30 Uncemented	976	
Marmor, 1991 (8)	68 Knees		1397
Lotke, 1991 (7)	121 Cemented		1518

all these screening tests, the current risk of transmission of posttransfusion hepatitis C from homologous blood is estimated at 1 per 3300 units (0.03%) transfused (13) and 1 per 250,000 units for hepatitis B (14). The frequency of human T-cell leukemia is about the same as for hepatitis C, or 1 per 4800 units (15).

The risk of HIV transmission from homologous blood is about 1 per 40,000 units (14). However, despite reduction of the risk of transmission of the HIV virus by blood screening, there are still individuals with HIV risk factors who donate blood to determine their HIV status, in effect, gaining a free HIV test by blood donation. Eradication of all donors with transmissible viruses is probably impossible. It is likely that an extremely low risk of contracting disease from a transfusion will always persist.

Legal Issues in Blood Transfusion

Orthopaedic surgeons have a legal responsibility to give adequate informed consent to patients when ordering homologous blood transfusions because of the above-mentioned risks, especially that of AIDS. There are three claims of negligence, each of which can lead to recovery of damages from physicians by patients who develop transfusion-related illness (16). The physician becomes liable in any of the following three circumstances:

1. Negligently determining that a blood transfusion should be given;
2. Negligence in treatment that creates a necessity for transfusion that would not normally be needed;
3. Negligence by failure to use available or easily obtainable autologous blood.

Several states, including California, have laws in place requiring that patients undergoing elective surgery be informed of their option to use autologous blood to lower or eliminate the need for homologous blood. Informed consent received prior to the transfusion of homologous blood is recommended in order to educate patients about the risks and to protect the surgeon from lawsuits that result from late complications.

History of Autotransfusion

The use of autologous blood for knee arthroplasty takes form in two types of transfusion: predeposit autologous blood donation and perioperative salvage of autologous blood.

The predonation of autologous blood in preparation for elective orthopaedic surgery has been reported extensively in the literature, but the first presentation of the technique to the orthopaedic community was in 1968 by Turner at the American Academy of Orthopaedic Surgeons annual meeting (17). He documented a series of 28 patients who had elective orthopaedic procedures, half of which were posterior spinal arthrodeses, using predeposited blood. Many articles on predeposit autologous blood for total joint replacement patients have followed (1, 18–31). Intraoperative red cell salvage became safe and practical in 1976 with the introduction of the Haemonetics Cell Saver (Haemonetics Corporation, Braintree, MA), which allowed the recovery and reinfusion of washed red cells during surgery. Recently, the salvage and reinfusion of shed blood that has not been washed has been advocated as an alternative to the washed cell technique.

Predeposit Autologous Blood

This technique involves the preoperative collection from donor-patients of 1 or more units of blood that are stored in a liquid or frozen state for perioperative use. Liquid storage is the preferable means of storage for reasons of economy and convenience. The most common anticoagulant used for liquid blood storage is adenine citrate-phosphate dextrose (ACD), which allows for a 35 day outdate period. Six weeks of storage is possible for packed red blood cells using Adsol (Baxter Health Care, Fenwal Division, Deerfield, Ill) for anticoagulation. Red blood cells may be frozen at −80 degrees C while being stored in 2,3 diphosphoglycerate (2,3 DPG). Thawing of frozen cells, however, requires time for the cells to be washed and resuspended in a balanced electrolyte solution, and, after thawing, they must then be infused within 24 hours. Allowing for these inconveniences, frozen red cells may be stored for indefinite time periods; thus, frozen storage allows the greatest flexibility for the timing of donations. However, the cost of freezing blood is at least twice that of liquid storage.

The recommended interval between the donation of each autologous unit is a minimum of 5 to 7 days and the last donation should be made no less than 3 days prior to the day of surgery. One unit of autologous blood (450 ml) removes approximately 9% of an average patient's total blood volume. Patients weighing less than 50 kg may predonate autologous units that are smaller in volume, using collection bags containing proportionately less anticoagulant.

All patients who donate predeposit autologous blood should take supplemental oral iron, preferably ferrous sulfate or gluconate, at a dosage of 325 mg, 2 or 3 times daily. Donor-patients who have conditions causing preoperative chronic anemia may benefit from the use of recombinant human erythropoietin that can enhance red cell production, especially when more than 1 unit is required (32, 33). Erythropoietin is particularly useful for small-statured female patients who have a small total blood volume.

Advanced age (over 65 years) is not a contraindication to autologous donations, since the frequency of donor reactions is no different in the older population than in younger donors (34). Patients who have cardiac conditions may require written consent from a physician in order to participate in a predeposit program. Unstable angina, severe aortic stenosis, and uncontrolled hypertension usually contraindicate blood donation, and, of course, patients who have an active infection should be deferred until resolution to avoid possible bacteremia. Autologous blood that tests positively for hepatitis may be safely reinfused, but blood banks generally will not store autologous blood from HIV positive donors because of the slight, but highly dangerous risk of reinfusion to the wrong recipient. Unused autologous and directed-donor blood is also routinely discarded by most blood banks, despite negative screening tests, and does not enter the general blood bank pool.

There are potential problems with any predeposit autologous program that relate to the patient and to logistical planning. Poor venous access may make it impossible to obtain blood. Preoperative anemia (a hematocrit less than 33) may disqualify the patient from predonating, and, if adequate time is not allowed between the donation(s) and surgery, predeposit donation may result in an iatrogenic preoperative anemia and hypovolemia. Postponement of the knee surgery can cause outdating of liquid units unless they are converted to the frozen state. The predeposit units may have to be donated at blood bank facilities distant from the hospital where the surgery is to be performed and then transported in a timely fashion prior to the procedure.

Aside from these problems, there are only two major risks of autologous transfusion: bacterial contamination of the blood during collection and clerical errors resulting in transfusing the wrong unit of blood. Both of these risks are also possible when transfusing homologous blood; however, autologous blood completely avoids the additional risks of disease transmission from homologous blood transfusion.

Although predeposit autologous blood is much preferable to homologous blood, it is important to understand that the donation of excessive amounts of predeposit blood units can be wasteful. This is because hospital transfusion committee guidelines normally recommend against the transfusion of any blood, even autologous, unless the patient's postoperative hematocrit falls below 30. Therefore, the collection of 3 units of predeposit blood for an uncomplicated primary cemented knee arthroplasty may result in the eventual discarding of 1 or 2 of these units, which is a considerable waste of resources.

The efficacy of predeposit autologous transfusion for total knee arthroplasty was studied by this surgeon in a consecutive series of patients who had 110 knee arthroplasties including 22 one-stage bilateral and 66 unilateral procedures (1). An average of 2 units was predonated by 82% of the patients who had bilateral procedures, and 73% of the patients who had unilateral surgery donated an average of 1.3 units. Postoperative red cell salvage was also used successfully for 44% of the procedures for an average savings of 290 ml of blood per patient. In this series, the frequency of homologous blood transfusion for patients who predonated blood was only 3% compared to 35% for patients who did not predonate autologous blood. Overall, the use of predeposit blood and postoperative salvage reduced the frequency of receiving homologous blood to 11% of these patients. This low frequency occurred because ¾ of all the patients predonated blood for surgery and because 19% of the patients was allowed to be discharged despite a hematocrit of less than 30. This study suggests that the predonation of 1 or 2 units of blood for unilateral procedures and of 2 to 4 units for bilateral procedures is the appropriate amount. When cementless knee arthroplasty is planned, the upper limits of these ranges should be collected.

In summary, with adequate preoperative planning, an effective predeposit autologous blood program should reduce the risk of exposure to homologous blood to less than 15% of knee arthroplasty patients, even without considering perioperative blood salvage.

Postoperative Blood Salvage

Intraoperative blood salvage is not a practical technique for unilateral total knee arthroplasty because of the use of a tourniquet. Even if the tourniquet is released for a short period prior to wound closure for purposes of hemostasis, the blood loss during this time is not sufficient to warrant attempts at salvage. It is, however, feasible to use intraoperative salvage for bilateral knee arthroplasty when the procedures are done sequentially, since the salvage of shed blood from the drainage tubes of the first knee can be done while the other procedure is being performed. However, in unilateral cases, postoperative salvage is the only option.

Two techniques are available for postoperative salvage, namely, washed or unwashed red cell salvage (35).

Washed red cell salvage or semicontinuous flow centrifugation involves the aspiration of blood from the drainage tubes by conventional vacuum suction and anticoagulation of this blood with heparin. Washing this shed blood with saline and using centrifugation to concentrate the red cells are done prior to reinfusion. Unwashed cell salvage entails the collection of blood from the drainage tubes within a sterile plastic container and reinfusion of this blood without cell washing or concentration of the blood. The use of a blood filter to remove particulate debris is mandatory when transfusing either washed or unwashed cells.

There has been considerable interest among surgeons in the relative risks and effectiveness of these two forms of blood salvage. The major advantage of cell washing is the removal of a large percentage of the contaminants of the knee joint drainage fluid including methyl methacrylate monomer, antibiotic from the irrigation fluid, free hemoglobin, fat, and bacteria. The blood that is salvaged after cell washing has a hematocrit of approximately 50%, which is higher than that of unwashed shed blood (25 to 35%). Adverse reactions to washed autologous red cells have been rarely reported. On the other hand, cell washing is expensive; the cell washing device and a dedicated technician or nurse to perform the washing are costly. In addition, a considerable volume of drainage (a minimum of 400 ml) must be available in order to make it cost-effective.

The collection of blood in a simple sterile reservoir separate from the cell washing device itself is indicated for knee procedures in which the bleeding may prove insufficient to make cell washing feasible. By using this system of reservoir collection, the expense of the cell washing device and the technician can be avoided in cases where the amount of drainage is insufficient for cell washing; in such a case, the small amount of shed blood would be discarded. Since a cell washing device can realistically be operated only in the operating room or recovery room, it has the additional disadvantage of being usable only for a short (2 to 3 hour) postoperative period, whereas the unwashed collection devices can be used for 6 hours.

The efficacy of washed cell salvage following unilateral primary total knee arthroplasty has been demonstrated by several studies that have shown the average volume of cells salvaged at 200 to 300 ml (36–38) (Table 65.2). However, this surgeon found that cell washing was successful in recovering sufficient amounts of blood for reinfusion in only 42% of unilateral knee arthroplasty patients compared to an 89% success rate in patients who had bilateral knee arthroplasty (1). Washed cell salvage in bilateral knee replacement results in an average savings of 400 to 500 ml of blood during surgery and in the recovery room (1, 36).

The use of unwashed cell salvage systems for unilateral total knee arthroplasty is successful in providing autologous transfusion in over 80% of the cases (39). This method is a much less expensive technique than cell washing. Because shed blood can be collected and reinfused up to 6 hours after surgery, the vast majority of all knee wounds will have had over 300 ml of drainage in that time period, thus making the technique efficient. The literature indicates that between 200 to 400 ml of shed blood may be salvaged for unilateral cemented arthroplasty and 800 ml for unilateral uncemented procedures (38–42) (Table 65.3). Bilateral arthroplasty can yield 500 to 1100 ml per patient (39, 42).

Although there are no major concerns about the safety of washed cells, some surgeons have expressed a

Table 65.2. Blood Salvage After Knee Arthroplasty Washed Cell Salvage

Author/Reference	Number Unilateral Knees	Unilateral Salvage Volume (ml)	Number Bilateral Knees	Bilateral Salvage Volume (ml)
Bovill, 1986 (37)	28	300		
Semkiw, 1989 (36)	13	339	6	579
Clements, 1992 (38)	9	193		
Woolson, 1993 (1)	20	210	16	383

Table 65.3. Blood Salvage After Knee Arthroplasty Unwashed Cell Salvage

Author/Reference	Number Unilateral Knees	Unilateral Salvage Volume (ml)	Number Bilateral Knees	Bilateral Salvage Volume (ml)
Groh, 1990 (40)	22	461		
Gannon, 1991 (42)	32	152	26	501
Clements, 1992 (38)	12	475		
Martin, 1992 (39)	153	829	44	1131

fear that patients may develop adverse reactions from the reinfusion of unwashed cells. The frequency of febrile responses during reinfusion of unwashed red cells has been reported at 2 to 10%; this frequency increases if collection and reinfusion is delayed for over 6 hours (39, 41, 42). Occasional episodes of transient hypotension were reported from one series of patients, which was probably related to the use of ACD anticoagulant in the collection device (38). Anticoagulation with ACD was considered necessary to prevent clotting of shed blood when these devices were first introduced. At the present time, the use of anticoagulants in unwashed cell recovery devices is not recommended, since the blood shed from the knee joint has been defibrinated and does not normally clot.

Studies have been done to determine the concentrations of methyl methacrylate monomer, plasma free hemoglobin, coagulation factors and fibrin-degradation products within shed blood from knee joint drainage tubes. Although methyl methacrylate monomer is detectable in this blood, the levels are low and dissipate over a period of several hours and, therefore, do not appear to be a risk to the patient (43). Cell washing dramatically reduces the concentration of all other extraneous contaminants, although their levels in unwashed shed blood are probably not harmful to the patient unless large volumes are reinfused (44).

Free fat globules are present in drainage from all knee arthroplasty procedures and are not removed by standard 40 micron microaggregate filters. Fat has the potential to cause pulmonary embolism and is probably the most dangerous contaminant of salvaged blood. This surgeon feels that it is prudent to prevent the infusion of fat in unwashed salvaged blood, and that the best way to do that is to prevent the infusion of the top layer of drainage fluid from the collection reservoir. Some unwashed cell salvage systems are designed to protect the patient from intravascular free fat by not allowing 100 ml of the supernatant layer of fluid in the collection reservoir to be transfused.

Cell washing produces a safer, less contaminated product of autologous blood that is more concentrated than when collected. However, the logistical restraints and expense of cell washing make it cost-effective only for bilateral arthroplasty or for a unilateral complex revision procedure. Unwashed cell salvage is the only practical method of postoperative blood salvage available for routine unilateral cemented knee arthroplasty. If unwashed cell collection is limited to no more than 6 hours postoperatively and if ACD anticoagulant is not used, the risks of this form of autologous blood appear to be minimal.

It is difficult to determine how effective the use of postoperative blood salvage is by itself in reducing the requirements for homologous transfusion after knee arthroplasty. This is because all studies of red cell salvage have also utilized predeposit autologous transfusion as another source of autologous blood. However, several studies that compared patients who had postoperative unwashed cell salvage to control groups reported lower overall transfusion rates (for both homolo-

gous and autologous blood) when red cell salvage was performed (40, 42). There is no question that red cell salvage decreases the amount of blood loss after surgery by returning a portion of the losses to the patient. One must assume that any reduction in blood loss should reduce the need for homologous transfusion.

Combination of Predeposited and Salvaged Autologous Blood

If predeposit transfusions are efficacious in reducing the frequency of homologous transfusion in total knee patients and if red cell salvage is effective in recovering some of the blood that is lost postoperatively from knee arthroplasty, then the combination of both these techniques should have an additive effect in reducing the need for homologous transfusion in these patients. However, one may question the cost-effectiveness of using both techniques for all patients. This question leads to a second question: namely, whether there are circumstances for which one technique should be emphasized over the other. Three examples of typical knee replacement patients illustrating the different emphases of these techniques follow:

Example 1
Situation: A patient with a large blood volume and good iron stores undergoing a procedure with a relatively small blood loss
Patient: 65-year-old man with osteoarthritis
Preoperative hematocrit: 48
Weight: 100 kg
Estimated total blood volume: 7500 ml
Procedure: Unilateral cemented total knee arthroplasty
Estimated total blood loss: 1500 ml
Preoperative plan for blood conservation:
   1. Predeposit blood: 1 unit donated 2–4 weeks preoperatively and postoperative unwashed cell salvage
OR
   2. Predeposit blood: 2 units donated 4–5 weeks preoperatively without postoperative cell salvage
Expected postoperative hematocrit: 35–40

Example 2
Situation: A patient with a low blood volume and poor iron stores undergoing a procedure with a high estimated blood loss
Patient: 45-year-old woman with rheumatoid arthritis
Preoperative hematocrit: 34
Weight: 50 kg
Estimated total blood volume: 3500 ml
Procedure: Bilateral cemented total knee arthroplasty
Estimated blood loss: 2500 ml
Preoperative plan for blood conservation:
   1. Predeposit blood: 4 units
   1st unit (frozen) donated 3 months preoperatively
   2nd unit (frozen) donated 2 months preoperatively
   3rd unit (liquid with Adsol) donated 6 weeks preoperatively
   4th unit (liquid with ACD) donated 4 weeks preoperatively

2. Oral iron supplementation and consideration of recombinant erythropoietin during donation period
3. Intraoperative washed cell salvage continued through entire recovery room stay
4. Unwashed cell collection for initial 6 hours on orthopaedic floor

Expected postoperative hematocrit: 25–30

Example 3
Situation: A patient with a normal blood volume and iron stores undergoing a procedure with moderate blood loss
Patient: 55-year-old man with posttraumatic arthritis
Preoperative hematocrit: 40
Weight: 70 kg
Estimated total blood volume : 5000 ml
Procedure: Hybrid (uncemented femoral and cemented tibial) components
Estimated blood loss: 1800 ml
Preoperative plan for blood conservation:
  1. Predeposit blood: 2 units (liquid with ACD) donated 4–5 weeks preoperatively
  2. Postoperative unwashed cell salvage for 6 hours starting after wound closure
Estimated postoperative hematocrit: 30–35

In general, patients expected to have large postoperative blood losses should always have red cell salvage as well as predeposit blood. Bilateral knee patients can have either washed or unwashed cell salvage in the operating and recovery rooms. However, until there is evidence that postoperative blood salvage is effective in reducing the risk of homologous blood transfusion in these patients by itself, predeposit blood should remain the most important technique to avoid homologous blood transfusion for knee arthroplasty. Perioperative salvage should be considered as an adjunctive technique especially helpful for patients who have difficulty in predonating sufficient amounts of predeposit blood and for patients for whom bilateral procedures are planned.

Surgical Technique

There are several technical aspects of knee arthroplasty that may affect the blood loss and that have stirred controversy. These factors are the timing of tourniquet release, when to begin the use of continuous passive motion (CPM), and whether or not to use a surgical drain.

Tourniquet release prior to wound closure for establishing hemostasis has been advocated by many who feel that this reduces postoperative blood loss. However, two randomized studies of patients who had tourniquet release either prior to or after wound closure definitively concluded that intraoperative tourniquet release does not lower the blood loss and actually may increase it. Newman, et al. (4) found a statistically significant increase in the blood loss after procedures during which the tourniquet was released for hemostasis prior to closure compared to procedures during which the tourniquet was released after the surgery was completed. The patients in this study received low dose heparin for anticoagulation prophylaxis. In a more recent study, Lotke, et al. (7) found no significant difference in the calculated blood loss of patients randomized to either tourniquet release or no release, when continuous passive motion (CPM) was not begun in either group until the second postoperative day. However, there was a significantly increased blood loss in patients who had tourniquet release prior to wound closure, when the CPM was begun in the recovery room.

These two studies should serve to reassure surgeons of the safety of maintaining tourniquet control until the procedure is completed. However, if the tourniquet is not released prior to wound closure, hemostatic control of the geniculate branches of the popliteal artery (especially the superior lateral branch) must not be neglected during the surgical procedure. If one of the geniculate branches may have been divided during a lateral retinacular release, it must be identified and ligated or electrocauterized prior to closure in order to avoid substantial postoperative hemorrhage from the drainage tubes. If the surgeon is not sure that adequate control of this vessel has been accomplished, the tourniquet should definitely be released in order to establish hemostasis of that one bleeder. Of course, all knee procedures that are prolonged for more than 90 minutes should have tourniquet release to prevent ischemic damage to the lower extremity, and, if this is prior to wound closure, hemostatic control can then be accomplished. However, this surgeon believes that overall blood losses will be minimized and the surgery expedited by maintaining tourniquet control until wound closure in all uncomplicated procedures.

The use of CPM in the recovery room has been shown to increase the postoperative blood loss by several studies (7, 45). This is undoubtedly because early knee motion prolongs bleeding from cancellous bone. Because of this, some surgeons feel that if CPM is to be used, it is prudent to delay its initiation until the first or second postoperative day.

The ultimate solution for the reduction of blood loss after knee arthroplasty is to eliminate *all* postoperative losses by omitting the use of a surgical drain. Although contrary to a basic principle of surgery, namely, the prevention of hematoma formation, it has been tested in two studies (46, 47). These studies found no difference in wound healing, persistent drainage, or other clinical parameters such as knee range of motion between knees that had drainage tubes and tubes without drains. Regarding the blood loss with or without drainage tubes, one would intuitively expect the same initial drop in the postoperative hematocrit when no drain was used unless the use of a drain produces a larger postoperative blood loss by preventing the tamponading effect of a knee hemarthrosis. Of course, most surgeons worry that in not draining a total knee wound, prolonged drainage from the incision will occur from the intraarticular hematoma and that this will result in a higher incidence of sepsis or will interfere with the normal progress of physical therapy. Further randomized studies of the omission of drains should be done on total knee patients prior to considering this to be a safe technique.

Criteria for Homologous Blood Transfusion After Knee Arthroplasty

Despite all of the techniques for blood conservation after surgery discussed in this chapter, the most important determinant of whether patients receive a homologous transfusion or not is the lowest hematocrit that can be tolerated by each particular patient without requiring homologous blood. Guidelines for transfusion of homologous blood in the perioperative period in the past have been based on empirical grounds rather than from controlled clinical studies. At the present time, most hospital transfusion committee guidelines do not question homologous transfusions given to patients with a hematocrit below 30. However, there is no scientific evidence indicating that all patients should be transfused at this threshold. The NIH held a Consensus Development Conference on Perioperative Red Cell Transfusions (47) in 1988. The consensus concluded that mild to moderate anemia does not cause postoperative morbidity, such as poor wound healing or a higher infection rate, nor does it contribute to a longer hospital stay or delayed functional rehabilitation. Therefore, the decision to transfuse homologous blood should be based on numerous other factors including the patient's age, the potential for further bleeding, and coexisting medical conditions, such as impaired pulmonary function, poor cardiac output, myocardial ischemia, or cerebrovascular insufficiency, rather than on the hematocrit alone. The consensus also recommended that autologous blood transfusion and intraoperative blood salvage should be encouraged to reduce the use of homologous blood and its risk of viral disease transmission.

Orthopaedic surgeons performing total knee arthroplasty should be aware of these consensus findings and modify their decision-making to limit the amount of homologous transfusions in these patients. An effective autologous blood program combining predeposit donation and postoperative salvage should lower the risk of exposure to homologous blood to less than 10% of patients, if enough time is allowed for an adequate amount of predeposit blood to be collected and if postoperative blood salvage is used in all patients at high-risk for bank blood transfusions.

References

1. Woolson ST, Pottorff G. Use of preoperatively deposited autologous blood for total knee replacement surgery. Orthopedics 1993;16(2):137–142.
2. Mylod AG, France MP, Muser DE, Parsons JR. Perioperative blood loss associated with total knee arthroplasty. J Bone Joint Surg 1990;72-A:1010–1012.
3. Cushner FD, Friedman RJ. Blood loss in total knee arthroplasty. Clin Orthop 1991;269:98–101.
4. Newman JH, Jackson JP, Waugh W. Timing of tourniquet removal after knee replacement. J Royal Soc Med 1979;72:492–494.
5. Hays MB, Mayfield JF. Total blood loss in major joint arthroplasty. A comparison of cemented and noncemented hip and knee operations. J Arthroplasty 1988;(suppl):S47–S49.
6. Page MJ, Shepherd BD, Harrison JM. Reduction of blood loss in knee arthroplasty. Aust N Z J Surg 1984;54:141–144.
7. Lotke PA, Faralli VJ, Orenstein EM, Ecker ML. Blood loss after total knee replacement. Effects of tourniquet release and continuous passive motion. J Bone Joint Surg 1991;73-A:1037–1040.
8. Marmor L, Avoy DR, McCabe A. Effect of fibrinogen concentrates on blood loss in total knee arthroplasty. Clin Orthop 1991;273:136–138.
9. Pattison E, Protheroe K, Pringle RM, Kennedy AC, Dick WC. Reduction in haemoglobin after knee joint surgery. Ann Rheum Dis 1973;32:582–584.
10. Erskine JG, Fraser C, Simpson R, Protheroe K, Walker ID. Blood loss with knee joint replacement. J Royal Coll of Surg of Edinburgh 1981;26:295–297.
11. Grady GF, Bennett AJ. Risk of posttransfusion hepatitis in the United States. A prospective cooperative study. JAMA 1972;220:692–701.
12. Koziol DE, Holland PV, Alling DW, et al. Antibody to hepatitis B core antigen as a paradoxical marker for non-A, non-B hepatitis agents in donated blood. Ann Intern Med 1986;104:488–495.
13. Donahue JG, Munoz A, Ness PM, et al. The declining risk of post-transfusion hepatitis C virus infection. N Engl J Med 1992;327:369–373.
14. AuBuchon JP, Busch M, Epstein JS, et al. Increasing the safety of blood transfusions. Washington, DC: American Red Cross, 1992.
15. Anonymous, Centers for Disease Control: Human T-lymphotropic virus type 1 screening in volunteer blood donors—United States, 1989. MMWR 1990;39:915–924.
16. Stevens D. Negligence liability for transfusion-associated AIDS transmission. An update and proposal. J Leg Med 1991;12:221–241.
17. Turner RS. Autogenous blood for surgical autotransfusions. J Bone Joint Surg 1968:50-A:834.
18. Mallory TH, Kennedy M. The use of banked autologous blood in total hip replacement surgery. Clin Orthop 1976;117:254–257.
19. Marmor L, Berkus D, Robertson JD, Wilson J, Meeske KA. Banked autologous blood in total hip replacement. Surg Gynecol Obstet 1977;145:63–64.
20. Thomson JD, Callaghan JJ, Savory CG, Stanton RP, Pierce RN. Prior deposition of autologous blood in elective orthopaedic surgery. J Bone Joint Surg 1987;69-A:320–324.
21. Woolson ST, Marsh JS, Tanner JB. Transfusion of previously deposited autologous blood for patients undergoing hip-replacement surgery. J Bone Joint Surg 1987;69-A:325–328.
22. Woolson ST, Watt JM. Use of autologous blood in total hip replacement. J Bone Joint Surg 1991;73-A:76–80.
23. James SE, Smith MA. Autologous blood transfusion in elective orthopaedic surgery. J Royal Soc of Med 1987;80:284–285.
24. MacFarlane BJ, Marx L, Anquist K, Pineo G, Chenger J, Cassol E. Analysis of a protocol for an autologous blood transfusion program for total joint replacement surgery. Can J Surg 1988;31:126–129.
25. Lorentz A, Schipplick M, Gmehlin U, Osswald PM, Winter M. Präoperative Eigenblutspende mit Flussiglagerung bei kunstlichem Gelenkersatz. Anaesthetist 1989;38:480–489.
26. Haugen RK, Hill GE. A large-scale autologous blood program in a community hospital. A contribution to the community's blood supply. JAMA 1987;257:1211–1214.
27. Eckardt JJ, Gossett TC, Amstutz HC. Autologous transfusion and total hip arthroplasty. Clin Orthop 1978;132:39–45.
28. Wilson WJ. Intraoperative autologous transfusion in revision total hip arthroplasty. J Bone Joint Surg 71A:8–14, 1989.
29. Turner RH, Capozzi JD , Kim A, Anas PP and Hardman E. Clin Orthop 256:299–305, 1990.
30. Cowell HR. Editorial: Prior deposit of autologous blood for transfusion. J Bone Joint Surg 69A:319, 1987.
31. Stanisavljevic S, Walker RH and Bartman CR. Autologous blood transfusion in total joint arthroplasty. J Arthroplasty 1986;1(3):207–209.
32. Goodnough LT, Rucnick S, Price TH, et al. Increased preoperative collection of autologous blood with recombinant human erythropoietin therapy. N Engl J Med 1989;321:1163–1168.
33. Thompson FL, Powers JS, Graber SE and Krantz SB. Use of recombinant human erythropoetin to enhance autologous blood donation in a patient with multiple red cell allo-antibodies and the anemia of chronic disease. Am J Med 1991;90:398–400.
34. Pindyck J, Avorn J, Kuriyan M, Reed M, Iqbal MJ Levine SJ. Blood donation in the elderly. Clinical and policy considerations. JAMA 1987;257:1186–1188.
35. Anonymous, Guidelines for blood salvage and reinfusion in surgery and trauma. Arlington, VA: American Association of Blood Banks, 1990:1–12.
36. Semkiw LB, Schurman DJ, Goodman SB, Woolson ST. Postoperative blood salvage using the cell saver after total joint arthroplasty. J Bone Joint Surg 1989;71-A:823–827.
37. Bovill DF, Moulton CW, Jackson WST, Jensen JK, Barcellos RW. The efficacy of intraoperative autologous transfusion in major orthopedic surgery: A regression analysis. Orthopedics 1986;9:1403–1407.
38. Clements DH, Sculco TP, Burke SW, Mayer K, Levine DB. Salvage and

reinfusion of postoperative sanguineous wound drainage. J Bone Joint Surg 1992;74-A:646–651.

39. Martin JW, Whiteside LA, Milliano MT, Reedy ME. Postoperative blood retrieval and transfusion in cementless total knee arthroplasty. J Arthroplasty 1992;7:205–210.

40. Groh GI, Buchert PK, Allen WC. A comparison of transfusion requirements after total knee arthroplasty using the solcotrans autotransfusion system. J Arthroplasty 1990;3:281–285.

41. Faris PM, Ritter MA, Keating EM, Valeri CR. Unwashed filtered shed blood collected after knee and hip arthroplasties. A source of autologous red blood cells. J Bone Joint Surg 1991;73-A1169–1178.

42. Gannon DM, Lombardi AV, Mallory TH, Vaughn BK, Finney CR, Niemcryk S. An evaluation of the efficacy of postoperative blood salvage after total joint arthroplasty. A prospective randomized trial. J Arthroplasty 1991;1:109–114.

43. Healy WL, Balerio M, Hallack G, Pfeifer BA, Valeri R, Wasilewski SA. Methyl methacrylate monomer and fat content in shed blood following total joint arthroplasty. Presented at American Academy of Orthopaedic Surgery Annual Meeting, Feb 25, 1992, Washington, DC.

44. McCarthy JC, Turner RH, Renten JJ, Valeri CR, Ragno GM, Korten KW. The effect of cell washing on the quality of shed blood in major reconstructive surgery. Trans Ortho Res Soc 1992;17:335.

45. Romness DW, Rand JA. The role of continuous passive motion following total knee arthroplasty. Clin Orthop 1988;226:34–37.

46. Beer KJ, Lombardi AV, Mallory TH, Vaughn BK. The efficacy of suction drains after routine total joint arthroplasty. J Bone Joint Surg 1991;73-A:584–587.

47. Ritter MA, Keating EM, and Faris PM. Closed wound drainage in total hip or total knee replacement. A prospective, randomized study. J Bone Joint Surg 1994;76-A:35.

66

Surgical Exposure in Total Knee Arthroplasty

Steven H. Stern

Introduction

It has been a maxim handed down through generations of surgeons that excellent visualization of the operative region is a prerequisite to consistently achieving successful results. As with all surgical procedures, knee arthroplasty commences with exposure of the relevant anatomic structures. In addition, most surgical approaches are designed so that dissection is carried through regions where the chance of significant neurovascular injury is minimized. Knee surgery, specifically knee arthroplasty, is in no way an exception to these basic tenets. There are several unique aspects of knee arthroplasty that place extra emphasis on surgical exposure and handling of the soft tissues. First, the knee is a relatively superficial joint compared to the hip, which is the other anatomic structure most commonly involved in reconstruction. Thus, the knee's soft tissue envelope is not as extensive as that surrounding the hip. Second, the knee arthroplasty surgeon is faced with the twin goals of obtaining soft tissue healing and maximizing knee motion. Therefore, skin problems, especially skin necrosis, are a definite concern in knee surgery (2, 11, 12). This further raises the need for specific attention to surgical exposure and proper handling of soft tissues in knee arthroplasty.

The surgical approaches most commonly favored by implant surgeons are designed to allow easy access to the knee joint and surrounding tissues. Exposure needs to be accomplished while minimizing excess skin and soft tissue tension. As in all surgical exposures, several general principles apply. Generally, extensile exposures are favored so that dissection can be extended, as needed, either proximally or distally to enhance visualization. One long incision is preferred to several shorter incisions. However, it is widely accepted that prior transverse skin wounds can be successfully crossed at right angles by new longitudinal incision (2, 11, 26). If possible, previous vertical incisions should be incorpo-

rated into current skin incisions, and parallel incisions should be avoided. On occasion, prior vertical incisions are in areas that make inclusion of them in a current longitudinal approach impractical. In these cases, it may be necessary to make a second vertical incision, leaving as wide a soft tissue bridge between the two wounds as possible. Finally, the possible need for future surgical procedures should always be considered by the implant surgeon at the time of skin incision.

Primary Procedures

A standard midline anterior approach remains the most common method utilized to achieve exposure of the knee. However, there are certain circumstances that require, and certain surgeons who prefer, alternative methods of exposure in knee arthroplasty. In revision surgeries, or with ankylosed knees, it is often necessary to perform either proximal soft tissue releases or distal bone osteotomies in order to enhance visualization (1, 18, 20, 23, 25, 27, 29). There has also been recent interest in other methods of obtaining adequate knee exposure in index arthroplasty (3, 9). This is partially related to continued problems and concerns with the knee's extensor mechanism after total knee arthroplasty (4, 19, 21, 28). The standard anterior approach with a midline or medial parapatellar arthrotomy dissects directly through the extensor mechanism. Because of this disruption, some authors advocate either a "subvastus" or "trivector retaining" approach for total knee replacements (3, 17).

Anterior Approach for Knee Arthroplasty

The anterior approach is extensile, allowing access to both distal femur and proximal tibia. Patellar eversion permits excellent visualization of all compartments of the knee. An anterior knee approach can be used for fractures, arthroplasty, arthrodeses, and extensor mechanism procedures. Multiple procedures can be per-

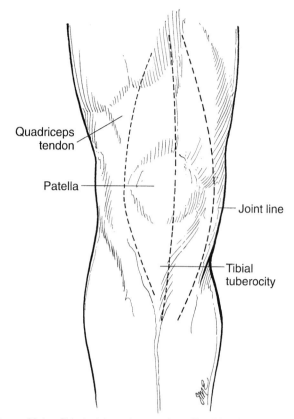

Figure 66.1. Skin incisions that can be utilized for the anterior approach to the knee.

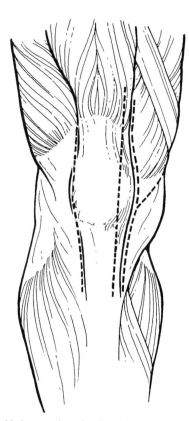

Figure 66.2. Various options for the retinacular capsular incision in knee arthroplasty. These include the subvastus medial parapatellar, midline, and lateral parapatellar incisions.

formed through the same incision with excellent visualization of both medial and lateral structures and minimal neurovascular injury. While the basic philosophy behind all anterior exposures is similar, there are slight variations in technique. Skin incisions can be made directly midline, or with slight medial or lateral curves (Fig. 66.1). Some surgeons believe there is a theoretical benefit to wound healing with a curved medial parapatellar skin incision (12). Others favor a compromise with a straight or very gently curved incision, made slightly medial to midline. Lateral skin incisions associated with medial arthrotomies are normally not encouraged because of the extensive skin flaps they require.

Dissection is then carried down through the subcutaneous tissue in order to expose the quadriceps and patellar tendons. After adequate exposure of the extensor mechanism, most surgeons perform a medial retinacular arthrotomy. This allows eversion of the patellar laterally and exposure of the knee joint proper. Retinacular incisions can be curved or straight (Fig. 66.2). Insall advocates a straight medial retinacular exposure (10). This is carried along the medial aspect of the quadriceps tendon, over the medial aspect of the patellar, and distally onto the anterior tibial cortex. The quadriceps expansion including the periosteum is sharply dissected from the medial patella with less damage to the distal insertion of the vastus medialis. This is preferred over a curved retinacular incision, which transects the insertion of the vastus medialis into the patella (11). Insall

feels that repair of the extensor mechanism with this approach is not as strong as with a midline retinacular incision.

Others advocate a medial parapatellar retinacular incision (2, 15), where the retinacular incision is medial to the patellar through the anteromedial knee capsule. The incision then curves back to the medial aspect of the patellar tendon and distally along its medial margin. This allows for a thicker cuff of soft tissue for closure at the level of the patellar bone.

After the arthrotomy is performed, the knee is flexed and the patellar everted. This should be accomplished without placing excessive tension on the patellar tendon. In revision surgery or in obese patients, it may be necessary to extend the dissection further proximally to help facilitate patellar eversion. In rare cases, it may be impossible to evert the patella. However, in these instances it may still be possible to perform a knee arthroplasty by retracting the extensor mechanism and patellar laterally. The knee arthroplasty can then be carried out in the standard fashion, depending on the alignment of the knee and the types of components to be implanted.

During closure, great care is taken in positioning the initial sutures in order to minimize patellar baha, which is known to be associated with prior knee procedures (24). The author attempts to minimize the baha formation by placing the initial suture in a specifically angled manner (Fig. 66.3). The arthrotomy and subcutaneous

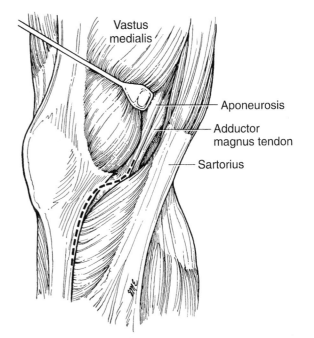

Figure 66.4.   Subvastus technique. Note that with this technique the extensor mechanism is preserved. The approach proceeds below the inferior edge of the vastus medialis obliquus muscle belly.

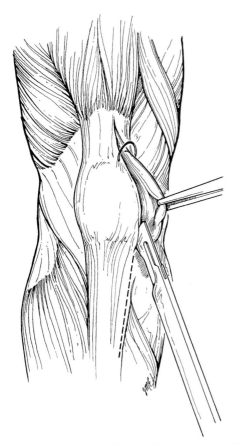

Figure 66.3.   Placement of the initial retinacular suture during closure to minimize postoperative patella baha complications.

tissue can be approximated in a number of ways depending on individual surgeon's preference.

Subvastus Approach for Knee Arthroplasty

There has been a recent interest in the use of the subvastus knee approach for knee arthroplasty. This approach was first described by Erkes in 1929, but fell out of favor over the next several decades (7). One advantage of the subvastus technique is that it preserves an intact extensor mechanism (8). Advocates of this approach believe that it results in less postoperative pain and a stronger extensor mechanism. The procedure also preserves the vasculature to the patella and quadriceps expansion. It is now being used by surgeons for both unicompartmental replacements and total knee arthroplasties in selected individuals (8, 9, 14, 22) (Fig. 66.4). Theoretically, preservation of the extensor mechanism allows the surgeon to more accurately judge patellar tracking in knee arthroplasty. Also, the integrity of the soft tissue envelope decreases the chance of wound dehiscence.

Advocates of this approach stress its limitations (9). Specific relative contraindications include revision total knee arthroplasty or previous arthrotomy. In addition, obese patients, especially those weighing more than 200 pounds, represent a relative contraindication to this method, because of the difficulty in everting the patella.

Procedure

The patient is positioned in a standard supine fashion on the surgical table. The subvastus approach to the knee commences with the knee flexed to at least 90 degrees. A direct anterior skin incision is made. The anterior portion of the incision is made 4 fingerbreadths above the patella and carried to a point 1 cm distal and slightly medial to the tibial tubercle. A slightly longer incision is made than with the standard midline approach. This is done in order to minimize skin tension. Dissection is carried through deeper levels until fascial layer 1 is identified proximally. It is incised in line with the skin incision down to the level of the patella. In the patella region, dissection is carried slightly medially. After incising the fascial layer, blunt dissection is used to raise this layer off the underlying vastus medialis. Dissection is meticulously carried down the fascial layer of the vastus medialis to its insertion site. This continues until the inferior edge of the vastus medialis is clearly identified. After identification of the inferior edge, the vastus medialis obliquus (VMO) muscle belly is bluntly dissected free of the periosteum and intramuscular septum. This dissection is carried for a distance approximately 10 cm proximal to the adductor tubercle. During this approach, blunt dissection minimizes risk to the underlying neurovascular structures.

The vastus medialis muscle is continually retracted anteriorly in order to clearly identify its musculotendinous insertion onto the medial capsule (Fig. 66.5). When dissection allows clear visualization, the insertion is transversely incised at the level of the midportion of

Figure 66.5. Anterior retraction of the VMO and blunt dissection allows identification of the region for the capsular incision. (Photo courtesy of William Brien, M.D., Los Angeles, California.)

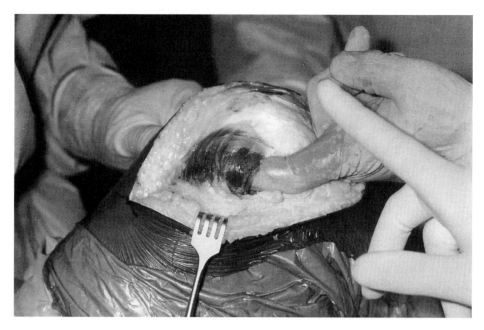

Figure 66.6. Knee arthrotomy performed with the subvastus technique. (Photo courtesy of William Brien, M.D., Los Angeles, California.)

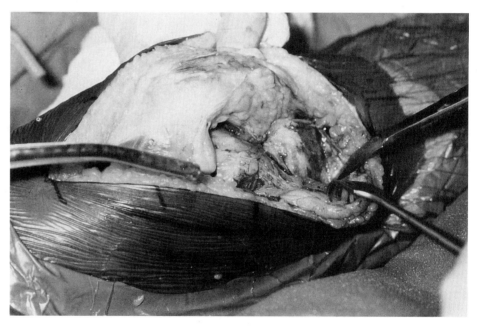

patella (Fig. 66.6). The arthrotomy is continued distally in a curvalinear manner with the incision carried down, in a standard fashion, along the medial aspect of the patella and patella tendon to the region of the tibial tubercle. The patella is then everted and dislocated laterally (Fig. 66.7). The knee is slowly flexed with continued blunt dissection of the vastus medialis muscle belly off the intermuscular septum. In this approach, the bulk of the vastus medialis remains attached to the patella and quadriceps tendon.

At this point, adequate visualization of knee should allow placement of the knee components in a standard fashion. Patellar tracking is assessed through the arthrotomy. If the patellar does not track in an accept-

able manner, a lateral retinacular release is performed. This can be done in an outside to inside fashion with the knee in full flexion. In an attempt to minimize injury to the anterior tibial, as well as the lateral geniculate vessels, the release is made at least 1.5 cm lateral to the patella (13, 17).

After the surgery is finished, the wound is closed in a routine manner. The vertical limb of the incision, as well as the proximal horizontal limb, are closed with interrupted sutures. The distal arthrotomy is closed with interrupted sutures. No reattachment of the vastus muscle belly to the intermuscular septum is needed.

Kim described a slight modification of the subvastus technique in his report on a quadriceps dislocating me-

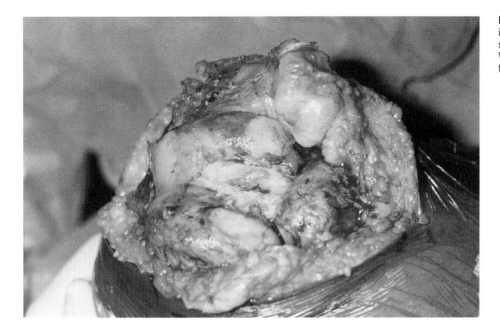

Figure 66.7. Patella eversion and satisfactory exposure achieved with the subvastus technique. (Photo courtesy of William Brien, M.D., Los Angeles, California.)

dial knee approach (14). This surgical approach is essentially a subvastus technique with some minor modifications. He advocates a straight longitudinal skin incision commencing from the medial lower third of the thigh running anteriorly and distally. The incision is carried to a level just distal to the tibial tubercle. Utilizing this superficial exposure, it is possible to make a straight incision through the underlying synovium, conjoined retinaculum, and medial capsule after retraction of the muscle. This results in a subvastus type approach with the retinacular incision in line with the skin wound.

Results with Subvastus Approach

Kim analyzed 200 knees undergoing total knee arthroplasty with different operative approaches (14). Eighty-one had a lateral capsular incision approach, 61, a medial capsular incision approach, and 58, a quadriceps dislocating medial approach (subvastus approach). Of the 142 patients with the medial or lateral capsular incisions, 6 developed skin sloughs. This is in contrast to no wound problems in the 58 patients in the quadriceps dislocating medial approach. (p < .05). Subluxation of the patella was noted in 13% with the medial approach, 1% with the lateral approach and 0% with the subvastus approach. The authors felt that traditional anterior skin incisions led to increased skin tension in flexion, which caused the higher incidence of skin sloughs with these methods. Conversely, with the quadriceps dislocating medial approach, they felt that skin tension was negligible, even in full flexion. This was because the skin incision was on the medial aspect of the joint. In addition, they felt that undermining of the skin was minimized with this approach.

Ritter, et al. compared results achieved with a vastus medialis-sparing approach to those found with a standard midline exposure (22). They examined 28 patients

undergoing simultaneous bilateral total knee arthroplasty. In each patient, one knee was randomly chosen for exposure utilizing the vastus medialis-sparing approach (study group), while the contralateral knee received a standard medial parapatellar arthrotomy (control group). All knees were implanted with Anatomic Graduated Components (AGC) (Biomet, Warsaw, IN). Lateral retinacular releases were required in 52% of the study group, and 48% of the control group. Postoperatively, all knees were evaluated by a physical therapist who was unaware of the surgical approach utilized. The authors felt that they encountered increased difficulty with dislocating and retracting the patella in the knees exposed with the subvastus technique. In this series, the average range of motion at discharge was from 4 to 82 degrees for both groups. At both 6 months and 1 year, the subvastus group had motion from 2 to 99 degrees. This was similar to the average motion of 2 to 101 degrees seen in the control group. There were no significant complications, infections, or thrombophlebitic events in either group. The authors concluded that they could find no correlation between postsurgical recovery and morbidity related to the surgical approach employed. They did, however, feel that the vastus medialis-sparing method was more technically demanding and made exposure more difficult. Thus, they expressed their continued preference for a medial parapatellar arthrotomy.

Trivector Retaining Arthrotomy Technique for Knee Arthroplasty

Bramlett, et al. have proposed a "trivector-retaining arthrotomy technique" as an alternate method of knee exposure (3). They advocate its use in both primary and revision total knee replacement procedures. Theoretically, this method spares the anatomic trivector arrangement of the quadriceps (vastus medialis, vastus intermedius, vastus lateralis, and rectus femoris) insertion into the patellar. Advocates of this technique feel that it is reproducible and combines advantages of both the standard medial parapatellar arthrotomy with those inherent to the subvastus approach. They feel that these benefits are achieved while reducing disadvantages intrinsic to both methods. The trivector approach is similar to the subvastus method in that both minimize disruption of the vastus medialis insertion and the vascular supply to the patellar. However, advocates of the trivector approach feel that it allows for a more extensile exposure of both the lateral and posterolateral knee compartments than does the subvastus technique. Thus, this method can theoretically be used in revision arthroplasty and in obese patients.

Procedure

The trivector technique begins with a routine midline skin incision. This is carried both above and below the patellar for a distance of approximately 4 fingerbreadths. Dissection proceeds down through the fascial tissue until the triangular tendon insertion of rectus intermedius and the three separate vastus muscle groups can be easily identified. The knee is then flexed to 90 degrees, and a straight arthrotomy is performed. The arthrotomy begins at a point approximately 3 fingerbreadths above the superior pole of the patellar and 1.5 centimeters medial to the medial border of the quadriceps tendon. The arthrotomy proceeds directly through the vastus medialis oblique (VMO) muscle. It is extended distally in a straight line running one centimeter medial to the patellar and carried distally to the level of the tibial tubercle. (Fig. 66.8). Once the trivector arthrotomy technique has been performed, patellar eversion and posterior lateral exposure are easily obtained.

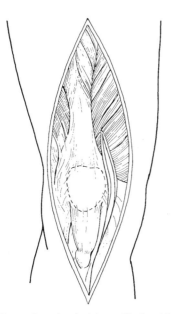

Figure 66.8. The retinacular incision with the trivector retaining arthrotomy technique extends directly through the anterior fibers of the vastus medialis. (Drawn from photo courtesy of Kenneth W. Bramlett, M.D., Birmingham, Alabama.)

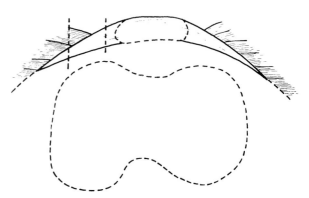

Figure 66.9. Cross section of the quadriceps tendon showing the inferior extension of the tendon below the muscle belly fibers. (Drawn from photo courtesy of Kenneth W. Bramlett, M.D., Birmingham, Alabama.)

Advocates of this technique feel that it is acceptable to incise the distal portion of the VMO fibers. They feel that there is a medial extension of the common quadriceps tendon that underlies the oblique anterior VMO muscle fibers (Fig. 66.9). It is this underlying tendon that provides for a secure arthrotomy closure. Bramlett, et al. feel that, with this technique, the remaining VMO function plus contributions from the nonviolated quadriceps muscles prevent unopposed lateral pull on the patella. They feel that the increased anatomic pull of these remaining muscles helps minimize the need for lateral retinacular releases.

Results with Trivector Retaining Arthrotomy Technique

Bramlett, et al. have reported on 148 total knee arthroplasties performed over a 21-month period during which this particular technique was utilized (3). Surgical procedures included 103 index total knee arthroplasties, 26 unicondylar replacements, and 19 knee revisions. There were no patella tendon ruptures nor patella evulsions in their series. Only one "V-Y" turndown was necessary; this turndown became necessary in a knee undergoing a third revision procedure. All patients were able to initiate physical therapy on the first postoperative day. There were no wound complications nor infections in this cohort of patients, but one patient underwent reoperation for closure of a synovial fistula. In addition, they did not find any patella fractures, patella component loosening, or tendon unit failures. Finally, in utilizing this approach, they found no evidence of recurrent dynamic patella subluxation or patella dislocation.

Lateral Approach for Knee Arthroplasty

Keblish (13a) advocates a lateral approach for knee arthroplasty when performing the procedure on knees with a fixed preoperative valgus deformity. He feels the standard medial approach has significant technical limitations and disadvantages, resulting in an increased incidence of patellar maltracking and extensor mechanism problems. This is because the medial exposure requires lateral displacement and eversion of the extensor mechanism, which is accomplished with external tibial rotation. Thus, this technique indirectly approaches the most severely involved lateral pathologic anatomy, while the external tibial rotation further retracts the knee's posterior-lateral corner away from the operative field. Additionally, the medial exposure usually requires an extensive lateral release in valgus knees, thereby violating the blood supply to the extensor mechanism on both the medial and lateral sides.

Keblish developed the lateral approach in an attempt to deal with these problems and utilizes it when correcting a valgus deformity during total knee arthroplasty. He believes that advantages of this technique include a more direct approach to the pathologic lateral anatomy. A lateral retinacular release is routinely performed as an integral part of the exposure. Medial displacement of the extensor mechanism causes internal rotation of the tibia, further exposing the posterior-lateral corner. Vascularity is preserved because the extensor mechanisms medial blood supply is undisturbed. Finally, he feels that adequate tracking of the patellar is easily achieved via the self-centering mechanism of the retained extensor mechanism.

Keblish does concede that the lateral technique is technically more demanding than the traditional medial approach. Orientation is reversed, and the anatomy is less familiar to most surgeons. Finally, medial eversion and displacement of the extensor mechanisms is more difficult.

Procedure

The lateral approach to the knee commences with a long longitudinal incision. This is made just lateral to the midline, and is carried distally to a point 1 to 2 cm lateral to the lateral aspect of the tibial tubercle. As with other knee approaches, previous longitudinal incisions should be utilized whenever possible to minimize wound problems. The lateral retinacular arthrotomy originates proximally along the lateral border of the quadriceps tendon and extends distally 1 to 2 cm lateral to the lateral patellar border. The arthrotomy courses along the medial border of Gerdy's tubercle, ending distally in the anterior compartment fascia at a point approximately 2 cm lateral to the lateral patellar tendon border (Fig. 66.2). Care must be taken during the exposure not to violate the fat pad as the preservation of its blood supply is necessary for soft tissue closure.

After the arthrotomy is performed, Keblish advocates testing the limb in extension in order to evaluate the degree, if any, of iliotibial band contracture. This is accomplished by applying a varus stress to the extremity while it is held in full extension. If the knee cannot be brought to an acceptable anatomic alignment, the iliotibial (IT) band is released proximally at a point approximately 10 cm proximal to the joint line. If release of the IT band is necessary, it is exposed utilizing blunt finger dissection carried from proximal to distal. Care is taken to palpate and protect the peroneal nerve. Exposure can be enhanced by placing a long instrument from anterior to posterior behind the IT band. While there are several techniques for effecting an IT band release, Keblish ad-

vocates performing multiple small punctures. This is done while an assistant applies a constant varus stress to the extremity. In this way, he feels that he is able to titrate his release to the extent necessary to achieve acceptable limb alignment. If physiological valgus cannot be achieved with this method, then further posterior lateral release is required.

It may be noted that other surgeons (3a) favor a distal IT band release in knees with severe fixed valgus deformities, as opposed to the proximal technique outlined above. Advocates of distal releases normally perform this step after medial displacement of the extensor mechanism with the joint exposed in flexion. The distal release can include elevation of Gerdy's tubercle with a sleeve of anterolateral fascia. In addition, fibular head resection can be added to minimize stress on the peroneal nerve.

The next step with the lateral approach is mobilization of the fat pad and capsule in order to maintain an adequate soft tissue envelope. Because correction of a valgus knee leads to a lateral retinacular gap, it is necessary to mobilize the soft tissues in order to provide an adequate envelope for closure. Keblish advocates sharp dissection along the underside of the patellar tendon. This is carried to the medial extent of the intermeniscal ligament, which is then incised to bone. This allows the composite of fat pad, capsule, intermeniscal ligament, and rim of lateral meniscus to be mobilized laterally. Care is taken not to dissect through the fat pad, especially along its lateral aspect, which is the region for its blood supply.

The next step involves preparation for medial translocation of the extensor mechanism. An osteoperiosteal sleeve is elevated off the lateral tibial tubercle with an osteotome. This is done in a meticulous and careful manner to allow for a gradual peel of the lateral 50% of the patellar tendon. At this time, patellar eversion and medial patellar displacement can be accomplished. This is slightly more difficult than with the traditional lateral displacement techniques, but Keblish believes it can be performed safely and adequately. A varus moment is applied to the flexed knee, while the patellar is everted medially. The patellar tendon attachment is observed at all times during this maneuver. If needed, adhesions or large patellar osteophytes are resected to achieve eversion. Patellar resection, which is part of prosthetic resurfacing, can be accomplished at this time to ease eversion, if desired. Keblish believes that, once medial patellar displacement has been achieved, the tibia will rotated internally, enabling direct visualization and a more accurate analysis of the posterior-lateral corner and arcuate complex.

If necessary, a posterior lateral release can be performed at this point in the exposure. This osteoperiosteal release is carried out along the femur after all osteophytes are excised. This is carefully titrated to minimize the amount of soft tissue stripping necessary to achieve an anatomic valgus limb alignment.

The posterior medial compartment is the most difficult to visualize with this lateral exposure. Curved retractors can be placed over the posterior-medial corner and the tibia rotated back to a neutral position in order to improve visualization. At this point, it should be possible to perform the proximal tibial cut, as well as the rest of the bone cuts in a relatively straightforward and standard manner.

After component insertion, patellar tracking is assessed. Keblish believes that the extensor mechanism more naturally adjusts to the midline with this lateral approach, thereby minimizing the tendency for lateral patellar subluxation commonly seen with the traditional medial exposure. In addition, a lateral retinacular release has already been routinely performed as part of the initial approach. Closure of the arthrotomy includes utilization of the previously developed lateral soft tissue composite (lateral meniscus, capsule and fat pad) to fill any gap in the lateral retinaculum. Significant expansion of the fat pad can be achieved, while preserving its vascularity, by making transverse relaxing incisions in line with the retained lateral meniscal rim. This composite can then be sutured to the proximal capsular flap, helping to restore a soft tissue retinacular envelope. Final closure of this composite to the border of the lateral extensor mechanism is accomplished with the knee flexed. Closure of the skin incision and postoperative rehabilitation are carried out in a standard manner.

Results with Lateral Approach

Keblish (13a) has reported his results on 53 knees having greater than 2-year follow-up, in which the lateral approach was utilized. Valgus deformities ranged from 12 to 45 degrees (mean: 22 degrees). The vast majority of the knees were implanted with a Low Contact Stress (LCS) (DePuy, Warsaw, IN) knee prosthesis. Cement fixation was used in 12 knees. 94% of the knees scored in the good to excellent range utilizing the New Jersey Orthopaedic Hospital rating scale. Range of motion improved from an average of 85 degrees preoperatively to 115 degrees postoperatively. Complications included 5 nonfatal pulmonary embolisms, 2 subcutaneous hematomas that healed uneventfully, and 1 wound dehiscence requiring debridement and secondary closure. Intraoperative problems included 3 minor split type fractures, and 1 failure of an uncemented patellar component requiring revision to a cemented component. Finally, 1 meniscal-bearing tibial component placed in a knee with a complex deformity was felt to be malpositioned; it required reoperation 1 week after surgery. Both 1 transient sensory and 1 transient motor peroneal nerve palsy resolved uneventfully by 6 months. The authors reported no patellofemoral maltracking problems.

Exposure in Revision or Difficult Knees: General

Routine patella eversion and adequate knee exposure cannot always be easily achieved, especially in knees that have undergone prior surgical procedures, in those with severe flexion contractures or malalignment, or in knees in obese patients. In these instances, it is often possible to improve visualization with some basic techniques. These include extending the quadriceps incision proximally, performing a lateral retinacular release, and, externally, rotating the tibia. External rotation of the tibia enhances medial subperiosteal dissection along the proximal tibia. If patellar eversion and adequate exposure cannot be achieved with these methods, the surgeon must consider alternative techniques (25).

Exposure enhancement normally falls into one of two categories. Some surgeons advocate proximal soft tissue techniques in order to allow retraction of the extensor mechanism laterally and distally (1, 18, 23, 25). Others advocate a distal tibial tubercle osteotomy, letting the extensor mechanism and tibial tubercle retract laterally and superiorly (6, 27, 29). Advocates of proximal soft tissue techniques feel this method minimizes the rate of major mechanical complications that have been reported with tubercle osteotomy (29). They acknowledge the theoretical jeopardy to the extensor mechanism blood supply with proximal soft tissue methods, but feel that this has not been a clinical problem (25). Advocates of tubercle osteotomies believe that an appropriately sized osteotomy will minimize complications. It would also permit bone-to-bone healing, which they postulate is superior to soft tissue healing.

Basic Techniques

The principles of surgical exposure in revision total knee arthroplasty are documented in a short article by Windsor and Insall (28). They describe techniques that were developed on the Knee Service at the Hospital for Special Surgery and successfully applied to over 250 revision knee arthroplasties. This means commencing revision procedures by using the prior skin incision. They suggest that prior midline longitudinal incisions can be lengthened proximally and distally. Undermining the medial and lateral skin flaps should be minimized and carried only to the extent needed to expose the quadriceps tendon, patella, and patellar tendon. They advocate blunt dissection techniques, minimal retraction of the skin flaps, and minimal soft tissue undermining to minimize the risk of skin necrosis. If more than one longitudinal incision is already present, the more lateral of the approaches should be selected. This is based on the belief that the better blood supply is on the medial aspect of the knee.

With adequate exposure of the extensor mechanism, the medial retinacular incision can be made. If possible, a straight longitudinal retinacular incision is performed. A medial parapatellar, retinacular incision can also be done if this will minimize undermining of the skin flaps. Care must be taken not to cut across the proximal extension of the quadriceps tendon. At this point, they recommend careful subperiosteal elevation of soft tissue over the medial tibial cortex, extending to the posterior margin of the tibial plateau. They emphasize the need for a full posterior medial exposure, including the need for sharp dissection of the insertion of the semimembranosus muscle. Care must be taken to leave the medial collateral ligament and medial soft tissues in an intact sleeve.

The next step is the removal of scar tissue, usually found in abundance in the medial and lateral gutters. These adhesions are normally dissected with a combination of sharp and blunt techniques. Patellar eversion is the next step and can usually be accomplished with the knee flexed to 90 degrees. This must be done carefully to minimize patellar tendon disruption. Certain maneuvers can facilitate patella eversion.

First, moving the tibia anteriorly, while rotating externally, will move the extensor mechanism laterally (8). It may be possible to use a bent Hohman or other retractor to pull the extensor mechanism further laterally. This will allow adequate exposure of the knee without eversion of the patella. A lateral retinacular release can also increase exposure of the knee and will, in many instances, facilitate patellar eversion. However, if adequate exposure is not obtained, proximal soft tissue techniques or distal tubercle osteotomies will be necessary (see below).

After adequate exposure of the femur and tibia, Windsor and Insall recommend a "femoral peel" in which the posterior capsule and scar surrounding the distal femur are dissected from bone with a large curette. The scar is "peeled" away, effectively skeletonizing the distal femur in a single layer. The medial and lateral collateral ligaments should be preserved. Severe flexion contractures may necessitate further posterior capsular dissection.

Proximal Soft Tissue Techniques

Coonse and Adams

Coonse and Adams originally described the patellar turndown approach in 1943 as an alternative method for exposure of the knee (5). They described an inverted "Y" incision. In their original method, the quadriceps tendon was split down the middle, beginning at the tendon's proximal pole. This incision was carried to a point 0.25 to 0.5 inch superior to the bony patella. Two limbs were then extended distally from the end of the midline incision, traveling both medially and laterally to the patella (Fig. 66.10). This soft tissue technique allowed the patella and the patellar tendon to be reflected distally and adequate visualization of the knee obtained. The authors emphasized that this method practically eliminated the need for soft tissue retraction, thereby minimizing trauma to the surrounding knee structures. They felt that this technique would be applicable to fractures, synovectomies, and internal derangements of the knee joint. However, because of the extensive dissection inherent in this method, it never achieved widespread, routine use.

There were some specific difficulties with the method originally devised by Coonse and Adams with regard to knee arthroplasty. The original procedure, like all proximal soft tissue procedures, required a broad-based distal flap in order to maintain an adequate blood supply for the extensor mechanism (29). Thus, the surgeon was obliged to choose whether or not to use this technique before beginning the operation. Since the original method could not be converted from a routine exposure, Insall modified their procedure to a more accommodating "patellar turndown."

Patellar Turndown

The patellar turndown approach (modified Coonse-Adams) described by Insall (11) offers several advantages over the original Coonse-Adams technique. Insall's modification may be used at any stage of the operation,

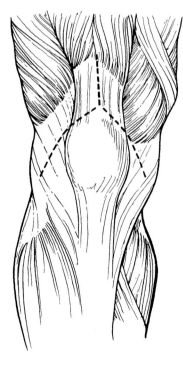
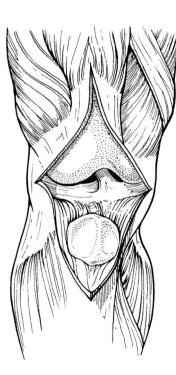

Figure 66.10. The original Coonse-Adams V-Y turndown technique.

Figure 66.11. The modified Coonse-Adams patellar turndown approach as described by Insall (11). Note that this method commences with the use of a routine midline retinacular arthrotomy. The second quadriceps incision is inclined approximately 45 degrees inferiorly and can be performed at any point if it is needed to enhance exposure.

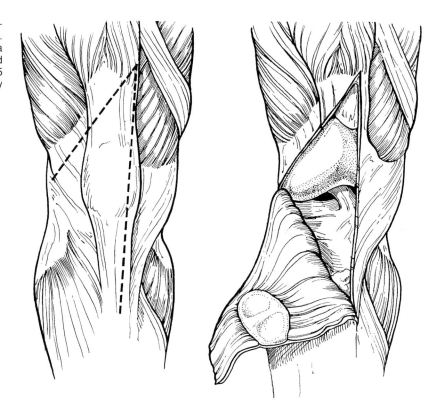

which commences with a straight anterior skin incision (11). The capsular knee incision is made vertically over the medial aspect of the patella, as in the standard anterior approach (Fig. 66.11). If the surgeon encounters quadriceps tightness or is unable to obtain adequate exposure, a second quadriceps incision is made, inclined approximately 45 degrees to the apex of the first. It is extended laterally and distally through the vastus lateralis and upper portions of the iliotibial tract. Insall describes it as stopping short of the inferior lateral geniculate artery in order to preserve the blood supply. During wound closure, the vertical or medial incision is always repaired. However, the portion of the incision that extends laterally can be left open, if needed, to enhance patella tracking.

Rectus Snip

The patella turndown approach was later modified to a "rectus snip" procedure (26). It was Insall's intent to reduce destruction of the proximal soft tissue envelope. As with the modified Coonse-Adams approach, the initial approach to the knee is made with a standard midline arthrotomy (10). The initial medial arthrotomy is extended distally over the medial aspect of the patella and medial to the patella tendon. If exposure is difficult, it can be enhanced with the "rectus snip" technique (Fig. 66.12). The apex of the quadriceps retinacular incision is extended laterally across the superior portion of the quadriceps tendon into the distal aspect of the vastus lateralis. Lateral mobilization and retraction of the patella and quadriceps tendon can then be accomplished. The arthrotomy is closed with a standard technique after insertion of the components, and a new, normal postoperative therapy can be instituted.

Results with Proximal Soft Tissue Techniques

Scott and Siliski reviewed the experience at Boston's Brigham and Women's Hospital with the modified V-Y turndown (23). They used this technique in 7 index knee arthroplasties in ankylosed knees. The average preoperative arc of motion was 15 degrees, which improved to a postoperative average of 67 degrees. Postsurgery, the mean flexion contracture was 8 degrees. In this series, only 1 wound complication occurred: a small skin dehiscence in a patient with hemophilia. The wound was resutured and healed. There was 1 poor result in a patient status post five prior lower extremity joint replacements who became nonambulatory after placement in a nursing home.

Aglietti, et al. from Florence, Italy reported their experience with the modified V-Y approach in 1991 (1). They reviewed 16 knees implanted with a posterior cruciate substituting design in which a patellar turndown was utilized. Of the 16 surgeries, 3 were revision procedures, while another 5 were status post prior knee surgery. The average follow-up was 5.5 years. Evaluation of the knees with the Hospital for Special Surgery rating system revealed 6 excellent, 4 good, 5 fair, and 1 poor result. The poor result developed from a late, deep infection. Preoperatively, the arc of knee motion averaged 43 degrees and increased to 74 degrees postsurgery. Flexion contractures decreased from a preoperative average of 25 degrees to a postoperative value of 5 degrees. Extensor lags were seen in 7 cases (47 per-

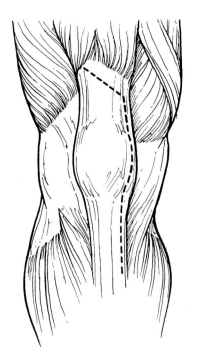 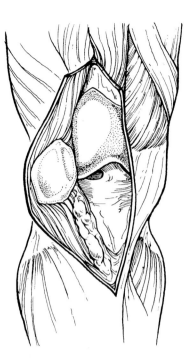

Figure 66.12. The rectus snip approach. As with the modified Coonse-Adams turndown, this also commences with a routine midline retinacular incision. However, in this approach, the quadriceps retinacular incision is extended laterally across the superior border of the quadriceps tendon in an oblique fashion. As with the modified Coonse-Adams approach, this can be undertaken at any point in the procedure.

cent), and averaged 10 degrees. The authors found no complications that they attributed directly to the V-Y technique. There were no patellar fractures or wound dehiscences. One knee with many previous incisions had skin necrosis that required a graft. Aglietti and colleagues expressed a preference for the V-Y turndown in difficult knees, because of its success rate and minimal complications. Trousdale, et al. reported on their results with a V-Y quadricepsplasty in 16 total knee arthroplasties (25). There were 10 revision and 6 primary arthroplasties. The average postoperative active range of motion was from 4 to 85 degrees. This represented a mean increase of 12 degrees. Biomechanical testing was carried out in 9 patients. They found a statistically significant weakness in extension in knees with the V-Y quadricepsplasty compared to a normal contralateral knee. When the V-Y quadricepsplasty knees were compared to contralateral knees in which a medial parapatellar incision had been made for arthroplasty, the extensor weakness was still apparent in the V-Y group, but to a lesser degree. They concluded that a V-Y quadricepsplasty would produce near-normal, active extension with moderate weakness. They did not encounter any extensor mechanism necrosis or patella fractures. Because of the low complication rate, satisfactory motion and strength, the authors felt that this technique was safer than tibial tubercle osteotomy for knees that required extraordinary methods of exposure.

Miller, et al. reported on the Hospital for Special Surgery results with the modified Coonse and Adams quadricepsplasty (18), utilizing this technique in 12 revision and 3 primary knee arthroplasties. Follow-up averaged 4 years, when 14 of 15 knees had normal, or 4 of 5, quadriceps strength. They devised a quadriceps score for their knees, finding that 87% of the knees achieved

good or excellent results at follow-up. Extension lags averaged 6 degrees. The authors felt that the arthroplasty results were not compromised by this method of exposure.

Osteotomy of the Tibial Tubercle

Some surgeons advocate osteotomy of the tibial tubercle as a method of achieving surgical exposure in difficult knees. This is especially useful in situations where previous scarring makes eversion of the patella difficult. However, there is concern over the technical difficulties and complications associated with this procedure (24). Conversely, osteotomy offers the potential of bone-to-bone healing and, theoretically, does not jeopardize the patella blood supply. It also offers superior exposure compared with proximal soft tissue techniques.

Procedure

Knees in which a tibial tubercle osteotomy is to be performed are exposed in a standard manner, using previous skin incisions when possible. The tubercle is exposed on both sides (Fig. 66.13). Screw holes that are predrilled facilitate later osteotomy repair (Fig. 66.14). A general attempt is made to retain an adequate lateral periosteal hinge (Fig. 66.15). In Wolff's, et al. report, the length of the osteotomy ranged from 2 to 9 cm (24). However, it is generally felt that a larger tubercle fragment is beneficial. Oscillating saws or osteotomes can be used for the actual osteotomy.

Most surgeons recommend a slight modification in postoperative physical therapy, but range of motion, including use of a continuous passive motion machine, can be instituted. Active extension is avoided for six weeks. The patients wear a knee immobilizer with ambulation or other weight bearing activities.

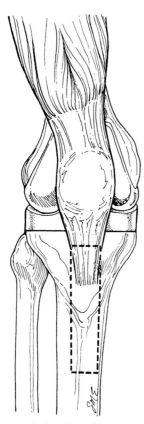

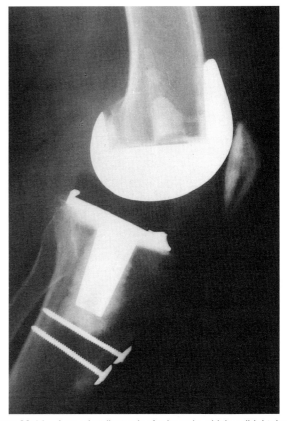

Figure 66.13. Schematic detailing of the area of exposure needed to perform a tibial tubercle osteotomy.

Figure 66.14. Lateral radiograph of a knee in which a tibial tubercle osteotomy was performed with screws utilized for fixation. (Photo courtesy of Richard Wixson, Northwestern University, Chicago, Illinois.)

Figure 66.15. Intraoperative photograph of a tibial tubercle osteotomy. Notice that the osteotomized bone is hinged laterally to aid in exposure. (Photo courtesy of William Brien, M.D., Los Angeles, California.)

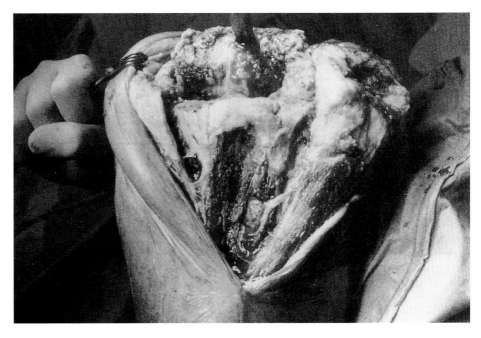

Results with Tibial Tubercle Osteotomy

In 1983, Dolin reported on his results with a tibial tubercle osteotomy in 30 patients (6). In his original reports, the osteotomy was approximately 45 mm in length. The tibial tubercle was reattached using a 36 mm cortical screw inserted with a lag effect into a threaded hole in the tibial bone cement. The only complication was a partial perforation of the anterior proximal tibial cortex because of excessive thickness of the osteotomy. He stated in his report that the technique allowed early physical therapy to be administered. In addition, all patients could move the knee and bear weight within a week of surgery. He did not report any failures of fixation or nonunions.

Wolff, et al. reported on the results with a tibial tubercle osteotomy in 26 knees (6). They found complications in 35% of the knees. Six knees (23 percent) had major nonmechanical complications ranging from superficial skin necrosis to deep infections or deep wound necrosis requiring a gastrocnemius flap. Fifteen percent of knees (note: 1 knee had both mechanical and nonmechanical complications) had major mechanical complications ranging from displacement of the osteotomized segment to patellar tendon rupture. The complication rate was higher in patients with rheumatoid arthritis. The authors found higher rates of osteotomy union with two cortical lag screws and recommended long osteotomy segments to minimize stress concentrations in the osteomized bone.

Whiteside and Ohl reported on tibial tubercle osteotomy for difficult knee replacements in 71 knees (27). This included 54 revisions, 10 procedures for lysis of adhesions, 3 for primary total knees in patient status post patellectomy, and 4 for exposure of primary total knee arthroplasty in patients with quadriceps contracture. Their technique requires careful attention to detail. They stressed the need to take a long, thick segment of the anterior tibial crest, which was elevated with the tubercle. They further suggested an oscillating saw to transect the tibial crest between 8 and 10 cm below the tubercle. A curved osteotome was used to separate the crest and tubercle finally from the underlying host tibial bed. The lateral periosteal and muscular attachments should remain fixed to the elevated bone. The bone was reattached with two heavy gauge cobalt chromium wires that were passed through the lateral edge of the tibial tubercle fragment and through the medial tibial cortex. Early motion and full weight bearing were allowed within the first week of surgery. The authors reported no failures with this technique. None of their tibial tubercles fractured or pulled loose. In significant contrast to the report from Wolff, et al., Whiteside and Ohl concluded that the higher success rate of their patients was the result of the longer fragment of osteotomized bone in their series. They pointed out that the failures in Wolff's series involved smaller tibial tubercle ostomies. Whitesides and Ohl preferred the osteotomy technique to proximal soft tissue releases, because secure fixation could be achieved with heavy wire loops passed through bone. They contrasted this to repair that is achieved with proximal procedures, in which sutures are passed through soft tissue to resist tension failure.

Osteotomy and Transfer of the Tibial Tubercle

An alternative method of a tibial tubercle osteotomy has been suggested by Masini and Stulberg wherein the osteotomized tubercle is actually transferred medially and placed in a new bone bed (16). Proponents of this technique feel that it can be utilized for distal realignments or difficult exposures in either complex primary or revision knee arthroplasties. In their technique, thick medial and lateral soft tissue flaps must be preserved. A fixation of the long strip of tibial crest is achieved with bone staples that do not penetrate the graft.

A standard midline or medial parapatellar approach may be used for this technique. Dissection is extended distally along the tibial crest to approximately 15 cm inferior to the tubercle. Great care is taken to maintain full thickness soft tissue sleeves. On the medial side, the subperiosteal dissection is carried to the posterior margin of the tibia. Laterally, the full thickness soft tissue sleeve is extended to the lateral margin of the tibial tubercle.

At this point, a standard medial retinacular incision is made, as well as a complete lateral release. The lateral retinacular is released from outside to inside. The region for a rectangular osteotomy is then defined along the anterior tibial cortex. The osteotomized bone should be a 1.5 by 10 cm rectangle created with a drill and osteotome or an oscillating saw. The medial tibia is decorticated with a high speed burr to create a cancellous bone bed that will accommodate the osteotomized fragment.

After the arthroplasty is accomplished, the tibial tubercle is transferred into the medial cancellous bone bed. The osteotomized bone segment is secured with multiple staples (16 by 10 mm) implanted with a power stapler. Care is taken to place the staples over, but not into, the osteotomy segment. After stable fixation is ensured, the soft tissue flaps are reattached via sutures passed either through drill holes or anchored into bone, utilizing Mitek or Statak. Advocates of this technique feel that excellent soft tissue coverage can be obtained because the bone segment is inset into a cancellous bone bed and not elevated as with a Macquet procedure. Cast immobilization is recommended for 6 weeks postsurgery to reduce complications. One case been reported with this technique.

References

1. Aglietti P, Buzzi R, D'Andria S. Quadricepsplasty with the V-Y incision in total knee arthroplasty. Ital J Orthop Traum 1991;17(1):23–29.
2. Boiardo RA, Dorr LD. Surgical approaches for total knee replacement arthroplasty. Contemp Orthop 1986;12:60.
3. Bramlett KW. Trivector arthrotomy for total knee arthroplasty. American Academy of Orthopaedic Surgeons, Poster Exhibit. San Francisco, CA, February, 1993.
3a. Buechel FF. A sequential three-step lateral release for correcting fixed

valgus knee deformities during total knee arthroplasty. Clin Orthop 1990;260:170.

4. Cameron HU Fedorkow DM. The patella in total knee arthroplasty. Clin Orthop 1982;165:197.

5. Coonse K, Adams JD. A new operative approach to the knee joint. Surg Gynecol Obstet 1943;77:344.

6. Dolin MG. Osteotomy of the tibial tubercle in total knee replacement. J Bone Joint Surg 1983;65A:704.

7. Erkes F. Weitere Erfahrungen mit physiologischer Schnittfuhrung zur Eroffnung des Kniegelenks. Bruns' Beitr zur Klin Chir 1929;147:221.

8. Gustke KA. Southern approach for total knee replacement. Florida Orthop Soc J 1989;31.

9. Hoffman AA, Plaster RL, Murdock LE: Subvastus (Southern) approach for primary total knee arthroplasty. Clin Orthop 1991;269:70.

10. Insall JN. A midline approach to the knee. J Bone Joint Surg 1971;53A:1584.

11 Insall JN. Surgical approaches to the knee. In: Surgery of the Knee. New York: Churchill Livingstone, 1984:41 .

12. Johnson DP, Houghton TA, Radford P. Anterior midline or medial parapatellar incision for arthroplasty of the knee. A comparative study. J Bone Joint Surg 1986;68B:812.

13. Kayler DE, Lyttle D. Surgical interruption of patellar blood supply by total knee arthroplasty. Clin Orthop 1988;229:221.

13a. Keblish PA. The lateral approach to the valgus knee: Surgical technique and analysis of 53 cases with over two-year follow-up evaluation. Clin Orthop 1991;271:52.

14. Kim JM. Orthopedic surgery in Korea. Quadriceps dislocation medial approach for intra-articular and medial structures of the knee. Orthopedics 1991;14:1147.

15. Krakow KA. The technique of total knee arthroplasty. St. Louis: CV Mosby, 1990:168-197.

16. Masini MA, Stulberg SD. A new surgical technique for tibial tubercle transfer in total knee arthroplasty. J Arthroplasty 1992;7(1):81-86.

17. Merkow RL, Soudry M, Insall JN. Patellar dislocation following total knee replacement. J Bone Joint Surg 1985;67:1321.

18. Miller DV, Insall JN, Urs WK, Windsor RE. Quadricepsplasty in total knee arthroplasty. Orthop Trans 1988;12(3):706.

19. Mochizuki RM, Schurman DJ. Patellar complications following total knee arthroplasty. J Bone Joint Surg 1979;61A:879.

20. Mullen JO. Range of motion following total knee arthroplasty in ankylosed joints. Clin Orthop 1983;179:200.

21. Rand JA, Morrey BF, Bryan RS. Patellar tendon rupture after total knee arthroplasty. Clin Orthop 1989;244:233.

22. Ritter MA, Keating EM, Faris PM. Comparison of two anterior medial approaches to total knee arthroplasty. Am J Knee Surg 1990;3(4):168.

23. Scott RD, Siliski JM. The use of a modified V-Y Quadricepsplasty during total knee replacement to gain exposure and improve flexion in the ankylosed knee. Orthopaedics 1985;8(1):45-48.

24. Scuderi GR, Windsor RE, Insall JN. Observations on patellar height after proximal tibial osteotomy. J Bone Joint Surg 1989;71(2):245-248.

25. Trousdale RT, Hanssen AD, Rand JA, Cahalan TD. V-Y quadricepsplasty in total knee arthroplasty. Clin Orthop 1993;286:48-55.

26. Vince KG. Revision arthroplasty technique. Instructional course lectures. In: Heckman J, ed. Total Joint Arthroplasty. Rosemont IL: American Academy of Orthopaedic Surgeons, 1993:325-339.

27. Whiteside LA, Ohl MD. Tibial tubercle osteotomy for exposure of the difficult total knee arthroplasty. Clin Orthop 1990;260:6-9.

28. Windsor RE, Insall JN. Exposure in revision total knee arthroplasty: The femoral peel. Techn Orthop 1988;3(2):1-4.

29. Wolff AM, Hungerford DS, Krackow KA, Jacobs MA. Osteotomy of the tibial tubercle during total knee replacement. A report of twenty-six cases. J Bone Joint Surg 1989;71A:848.

67

Instrumentation

Kim C. Bertin

Through each step in the evolution of total knee arthroplasty design, instrumentation has played an important role. Indeed, reviewing the results of each design shows that the results achieved with any prosthesis are directly proportional to the accuracy with which it has been implanted. Therefore, surgical technique is the single most important variable that surgeons can control to obtain good results. Today, as designs become more and more alike, surgical technique with instrumentation is the deciding factor for success or failure of a total knee arthroplasty.

Historically, instrumentation for total knee replacement was rudimentary. The first designs of knee replacements had intramedullary stems that were used not only for fixation but also to help the surgeon obtain appropriate alignment of the prosthesis. In these early days of knee arthroplasty, almost all surgery was done without any organized instrumentation. As implants evolved in design, instruments continued to be rudimentary. Most surgery was done with eyeball judgment using a saw, osteotome, or rongeur.

Probably the earliest attempts at providing organized instruments for implantation came with the total condylar knee. These instruments were very basic and had some intramedullary guides for femoral component positioning and an extramedullary guide for preparation of the tibia. As results with unlinked implants were reviewed, it became clear that alignment and soft tissue balancing were extremely important to the success of the procedure. To improve the surgeon's ability to achieve correct alignment and balance the soft tissues, Freeman developed the tenser (4). Using this instrument to assist with ligament release and obtaining correct alignment, the results of knee replacement progressively improved. The next significant step in instrumentation came with the use of complete instrument systems. These third-generation instruments allowed accurate cuts on the femur and tibia to provide for consistent correct alignment and implant placement. Today, these complete systems of instruments have both intramedullary and extramedullary references and have been simplified to the point that surgeons can routinely achieve the desired results, which have become expected.

Principles of Surgical Technique

To achieve the desired results, designers of total knee instrument systems have based their instrument design on two important principles: (*a*) flexion and extension gaps must be equal in size and (*b*) accurately placed implants allow better fixation and reproduction of knee function. The designers of most total knee implants have created prostheses that have the same femoral component thickness in extension and in flexion. When an implant with this thickness articulates with a tibial component in flexion and extension, the knee is stable and functions well. Therefore, the surgeon must create equal-sized flexion and extension gaps while making bone cuts to prepare for implantation of the prosthesis. This matching of flexion and extension gaps can be achieved in one of two conceptually different ways. A tenser can be used or measured resections can be made from the femur in flexion and extension.

The use of a tenser to equalize flexion and extension gaps works well for those who developed this technique. The recommended sequence in using a tenser begins with a conservative flat resection of the proximal tibia. The posterior condyles of the distal femur are then resected. The resection is usually the same thickness as the prosthesis that will be used to replace the condyles. The surgeon then inserts the tenser into the space created by the posterior condylar resection and tibial resection, with the knee in flexion. The tenser is then used to expand the space and tighten the soft tissues with the knee in flexion. This space is measured, and the tenser removed. The knee is then extended, and the tenser placed back into the knee. The tenser is then tightened, and the soft tissues become tight with the knee in extension. An alignment rod is used to check the alignment to make sure the mechanical axis of the lower extremity is straight. If there is a contracture on the medial or lateral sides prohibiting straight mechanical alignment, the soft tissues are released until the correct alignment is obtained. At this point in the procedure, the tenser is still equally tight in the medial and lateral compartments of the knee, and a straight line from the center of the femoral head to the center of the knee extends to the center of the ankle. If extensive soft tissue release has been done, the surgeon should remeasure the flexion gap, using the tenser while tightening the soft tissues in flexion again. This measurement taken in flexion is then transferred into extension. With the knee in extension, the tenser is again tightened, and the space measured from the cut surface of the tibia proximally. This distance, which was first measured in flexion, is now transferred into extension, and a cut is made on the distal femoral condyles to create an extension gap equal in size to the flexion gap. The surgeon has thus created an equal space in flexion and extension for the prosthesis, balanced the soft tissues to have appropriate ligament tension resisting varus and valgus stresses, and achieved good limb alignment.

Although the tenser was used successfully by individuals familiar with its application, in practice, the tenser has fallen into disfavor among many surgeons. There are a number of reasons for this. The instrument is very cumbersome to use and conceptually somewhat difficult to understand. Furthermore, it is difficult intraoperatively to know the exact location of the center of the femoral head. This difficulty in locating the landmark for the mechanical axis makes use of the system somewhat arbitrary. Furthermore, it is impossible to check ligament stability in any degree of flexion other than 90 degrees. Therefore, a surgeon who wants to assess varus or valgus stability in 20 or 30 degrees of flexion has no accurate way to perform this test.

Because of the technical and conceptual difficulties in using a tenser, most surgical techniques have evolved into a system of measured resections (1). With a tenser, the static alignment of the knee (i.e., the bone cuts) is determined *indirectly* as a result of the ligament balance, but in fact, regardless of the preoperative deformity, the angle of the bone cuts should be what is necessary to restore a neutral mechanical axis.

The principle of measured resections allows the surgeon to anatomically replace the knee surfaces that are removed during the operation. Instrument systems are designed so that in preparing the femur and tibia each bone can be prepared independently. The femoral cuts remove the same amount of bone from the distal, anterior, and posterior femur as will be replaced by the implant. These measured resections thus allow the surgeon to prepare the distal femur and proximal tibia and then insert a trial prosthesis. With the trial prosthesis in place, the surgeon uses the implants to tense the soft tissues and determine whether any releases are needed.

If asymmetrical soft tissue tension exists between the medial and lateral compartments, releases can be made on the tight side. This corrects the deformity and provides symmetrical soft tissue tension. This tension can be assessed in full extension or any degree of flexion, because the implant itself is being used, and the knee can be observed directly wherever the surgeon positions it. Furthermore, the surgeon can assess both anterior-posterior stability and varus-valgus stability. Using the techniques based on measured resection, either intramedullary or extramedullary instruments can be designed to prepare the femur and tibia.

The accuracy of each bone cut has also been addressed. This is important obviously on the distal femur and proximal tibia, where cuts determine the eventual weight-bearing alignment of the extremity. Additionally, excellent apposition of the prosthesis against the bone is necessary if bone ingrowth is desired for stabilization of the prosthesis. To obtain ingrowth fixation, the surgeon must prepare surfaces that are accurately opposed to the prosthesis. Thus, for alignment and fixation reasons, instrument designers have tried to achieve ever more accurate methods of preparing bone surfaces. Instruments have evolved that guide saw blades. These include slots or saw-capture mechanisms. Additionally, planing or machining-type instruments have been developed to make absolutely flat cuts for improved prosthesis fixation.

Preoperative Planning

It is important to determine preoperatively the unique anatomic specifics of each patient. To accurately cut the correct amount of valgus into the distal femur, the offset between the femoral mechanical and anatomic axes must be known if intramedullary instruments are being used. The intramedullary rod will establish the femoral anatomic axis in surgery, and the surgeon can then select an angle based on that reference to make to distal femoral cut perpendicular to the femoral mechanical axis. This offset between mechanical and anatomic axis can vary from two to ten degrees. In addition to naturally occurring variation, the presence of a hip prosthesis or prior femoral fracture can change the expected difference.

To most accurately evaluate the femur, a 36- or 51-inch radiograph centered on the involved knee can best show the whole femur. Standard radiographs (AP, lateral, and sunrise) are useful for prosthesis selection. The approximate size needed can be determined, and any potential need for augmented implants established. In performing these functions, markers to correct for magnification are crucial.

Surgical Technique Issues by Anatomic Location

The specific unique considerations for femoral, tibial, and patellar instrumentation must be addressed individually. Their interrelationships are presented below.

Femoral Instrumentation

Surgical instrumentation to prepare the distal femur is extremely important because the orientation and positioning of the femoral component determine total knee kinematics and function. The proximal-distal position of the prosthesis determines the joint line, and the inclination of the prosthesis determines the extremity alignment during weight bearing.

The most important cut on the femur is the distal resection, which determines the valgus position of the knee. The surgeon has two general choices in this regard. If, for example, the anatomic axis of the knee is to be 6 degrees postoperatively and the surgeon is going to cut the tibia at 90 degrees to its mechanical axis, the femur should be cut in 6 degrees of valgus. If, on the other hand, the surgeon decides to cut the tibia in 3 degrees of varus, the femur must be cut in 9 degrees of valgus. These two different options will both leave the knee with a 6-degree anatomic axis after the replacement is complete and the soft tissues are balanced.

The choice of 6 degrees for the anatomic axis is based on the normal population (5). Indeed, some in the normal population have different lower extremity anatomy. In patients with coxa valga or in patients who have a total hip arthroplasty with a high-angle femoral neck, the knee anatomic axis could be from 2 to 5 degrees. Others with coxa vara or a broad pelvis may have an increased offset between the femoral mechanical and anatomic axes. This requires being in slightly more valgus than usual to obtain a straight mechanical axis after reconstruction. This straight mechanical axis from the femoral head to the knee to the ankle is important to transfer weight correctly across the prosthesis. To achieve this in a variety of situations, an instrument system must allow the surgeon to make various selections in cutting the distal femur. The surgeon must be able to choose the amount of valgus to cut into the distal femur so that the final limb alignment is correct.

A further important decision in resecting the distal femoral condyles is the amount of resection. If the joint line is to be preserved and not moved proximally or distally, the amount of bone that will be replaced by the prosthesis should be removed. Proximal migration of the joint line can cause problems with knee kinematics. Therefore, accurate positioning of the femoral component is imperative. Most knee instrument systems, therefore, provide a measured resection of the distal femur. To measure this resection, bony landmarks are referenced. The usual landmark for reference is one of the femoral condyles. Some instrument systems always measure from the distal portion of the medial femoral condyle. Others choose the most prominent distal femoral condyle, measure proximally from there, and orient the cut at the desired amount of valgus. Both techniques work well if the surgeon remembers that the instruments are indeed measuring for a certain depth of resection. The surgeon must make sure that this measurement does not result from a defect in one of the condyles. If this happens, an excessive amount of distal femoral resection can be made, so that the extension gap does not match the flexion and the knee will be too tight in flexion. This most commonly occurs in instrument systems consistently measuring from the medial femoral condyle, and if a varus knee with a defect in the

medial femoral condyle were replaced, an excessive amount of resection could be made on the distal femur.

The second most important consideration in preparing the distal femur is the anterior-posterior dimension chosen for the prosthesis and the amount of bone resected to accommodate that selection.

Currently, there are two approaches to this step in the operation. The first approach initially cuts the anterior condyles flush with the femoral shaft and then measures the distance from that cut to the articular surface of the posterior condyles. The femoral component size selection is based on this measurement. The goal here is to resect the same amount of bone from the posterior condyles that will be replaced by the prosthesis. If the measurement from the cut anterior condyles to the remaining articular surface of the posterior condyles falls between two sizes of femoral components, the correct approach is to downsize to the smaller-sized femoral component. This slightly decreases the anterior-posterior dimension of the new articulation. This small compromise eliminates the possibility of overreplacing the anterior-posterior dimension of the distal femur. If a larger-size prosthesis were chosen and the posterior condyles pushed further posteriorly, the knee would become excessively tight in flexion, and it would not bend normally without releasing ligaments or recutting bone. This approach obviously requires an adequate inventory of femoral sizes in the AP dimension. With an adequate number of sizes, the compromises that must be made are infrequent and small. Because the knee is normally slightly more lax in flexion than in extension, this 1- to 3-mm compromise in AP sizing is well tolerated, does not leave the patient with any functional instability, and allows the knee to flex well.

The second approach to anterior-posterior sizing begins after the distal condyles are cut. Measurement is then made from the intact articular surface of the posterior condyles toward the front of the femur. It is planned to do an exact resection of the posterior condyles, corresponding to the amount of metal that the femoral prosthesis will provide. The distance is measured over the intact anterior condyles to the distal portion of the femoral shaft. The compromise here is choosing between two sizes of implants when the measurement does not exactly correspond to that of one of the available femoral components. In this scenario, choose the next larger-size femoral component to prevent notching of the distal femur. If the smaller-size prosthesis is chosen, a cutting guide will be selected that will reference the posterior condyles and resect an anatomic amount of the posterior condyles and then the measured resection anteriorly. Because this measured selection is less than what exists in the patient, a notch will be created in the distal femur anteriorly, proximal to the prosthesis. This puts the distal femur at high risk for fracture. This increased risk of fracture makes it more appropriate to avoid the notch and select a slightly larger prosthesis. There is another compromise in selecting a slightly larger prosthesis: the larger prosthesis will not anatomically replace the anterior condyles and will provide more prosthesis in the anterior aspect of the knee than the patient's ligaments and muscles were used to. The problem arises when the patient flexes the knee and the quadriceps tendon proximal to the patella is tented over this more prominent anterior condyle. This can potentially cause problems with patellar tracking by pulling the patella laterally and also limit flexion of the knee. Posterior-oriented measurement also requires an adequate inventory of sizes of femoral components. If the size graduations are too large, the compromise made anteriorly will be excessive, and limited flexion and more patellofemoral complications will occur routinely.

Another consideration in making the anterior and posterior cuts for the prosthesis is the flexion-extension orientation of the implant. It is crucial to have the implant oriented in the correct flexion attitude to allow the normal kinematics of the knee and to prevent impingement on the tibial component and full extension of the knee. If this impingement occurs, knee extension will be limited and/or excessive polyethylene wear will occur on the tibial component during each cycle of flexion and extension. Thus, the prosthesis must be oriented in a neutral position as far as flexion and extension is concerned. Extension of the prosthesis causes two other problems: (*a*) the anterior flange will potentially notch into the distal femur, increasing the risk for fracture, and (*b*) the posterior condyles of the prosthesis will not provide the normal radius of curvature for the ligaments to function, and the condyles will end before adequate flexion can occur. With all of these considerations, instrument designers have based the flexion-extension of the prosthesis on the distal cut. Since the distal cut is usually based on an intramedullary alignment rod, this intramedullary rod will also give the correct flexion-extension position of the distal cut and the correct valgus position. With the flexion-extension position determined and set usually at 90 degrees, the cutting guides for the anterior and posterior cuts are placed flush on this distal cut, and the anterior and posterior cuts oriented appropriately.

Rotational position of the femoral component is likewise important. The rotational positioning of the guides that make the anterior and posterior cuts determines the rotational position of the prosthesis. This position must correspond to the surgeon's desire to either make equal resections from both posterior femoral condyles or to externally rotate the femoral component 3 degrees to remove more bone from the medial femoral condyle and less from the lateral femoral condyle. This 3 degrees of external rotation is selected to balance the soft tissue tension in flexion when a 90-degree cut was made on the tibia (Fig. 67.1). If equal resection is made from the posterior condyles and a 90-degree cut is made on the proximal tibia, there will be asymmetrical tension in the posterior compartment, with more laxity on the lateral side because of more resection of the lateral tibial condyle than of the medial condyle. This is usually not a clinical problem, but if desired, it can be addressed by slightly externally rotating the femoral cutting guides. Another advantage of externally rotating the femoral component involves patellar tracking (7). Slightly better patellar tracking occurs with the femoral component externally rotated 3 degrees. (Patellar tracking is further discussed in the section on patellar preparation.) If the surgeon decides to externally rotate the femoral component 3 degrees and cut the tibia at 90 degrees, a 6-degree valgus cut on the femur should be made. If, on the other hand, the surgeon decides to keep the femoral component in a neutral rotation with equal resection from both femoral condyles and cut the tibia in 3 degrees of varus, the distal femur must be cut in 3 additional degrees of valgus. This would be a 9-degree valgus cut on the distal femur, which achieves the same overall anatomic alignment (6 degrees) as the above-described 90-degree tibial cut and 6-degree valgus cut on the femur.

The final consideration in femoral instrumentation involves medial lateral positioning of anchor holes for the femoral component. Usually, the femoral component is centered on the distal femur. The prosthesis must **not**

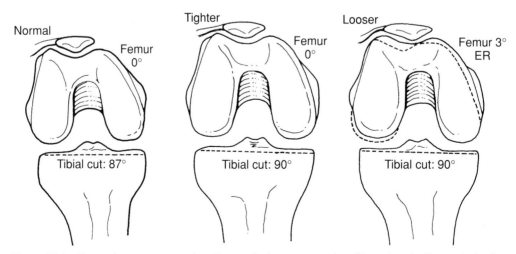

Figure 67.1. Femoral component rotation effect on flexion space tension. (Reproduced with permission from Axial rotation of the femoral knee component. Curr Top Orthop Technol 1991;5(6).)

be too medial because this increases the tension in the patellar retinaculum, which would lead to lateral subluxation of the patella. Alternatively, if possible, positioning the prosthesis 2 or 3 mm laterally may be helpful in the unusual case in which problems cannot be rectified in another way with patellar tracking. Be careful in this lateral positioning to avoid having the ligaments interfere with the femoral component. Ligament impingement could occur in the intercondylar notch, with the medial femoral condyle interfering with the posterior cruciate ligament, or on the lateral side of the knee where the popliteus and lateral collateral ligament could impinge on the lateral surface of the femoral component. The accepted standard is to position the femoral component in a neutral position, and if problems exist with patellar tracking, to do a lateral retinacular release and balance the soft tissues.

Tibial Preparation Technique

The preparation of the upper tibia is extremely important. The orientation of this cut directly affects the alignment of the knee and tibial component fixation. Since alignment and tibial fixation are the most important factors in long-term success with total knee arthroplasty, this part of the surgical technique deserves special attention.

The tibial cut can be oriented either 90 degrees to the axis of the tibia or inclined 3 degrees medially. The 3-degree medial inclination is the more anatomic replacement of the proximal tibia (5). It is based on the fact that the upper tibial surface is inclined 3 degrees medially. It is postulated that this 3-degree inclination results from the 3-degree divergence of the vertical axis from the mechanical axis of the lower extremity during normal gait and the fact that the ankles are closer together than the hips, which brings the mechanical axis in 3 degrees at the ankle. Having the medial portion of the tibia inclined downward by 3 degrees puts the transverse axis of the knee parallel with the floor. This eliminates sheer stresses at the joint surface during gait. Stresses all become normally directed across the surface. The mechanical axis is still a straight line from the center of the hip to the center of the knee to the center of the ankle, but the whole axis is slightly inclined. Some think that this more normal gait pattern does not exist in older patients or those who develop arthritis. They are thought to have a wider-based gait so that this 3-degree inclination of the mechanical axis disappears. Therefore, the second school of thought is that the tibial cut should be made 90 degrees to the axis of the tibia, so that the mechanical axis parallels the vertical axis, and the transverse axis of the knee will continue to be parallel with the floor in the gait pattern with a wider base at the ankle. A second reason for making the resection at 90 degrees is the ease of orientation of cutting guides. If surgeons attempt to make a 3-degree medial inclination to the cut, the cut is frequently inclined 4 to 6 degrees medially, and the overall limb alignment is negatively affected (6). This leads to component loosening. A cut at 90 degrees is more predictable and easier to perform

and, therefore, leads to better long-term results. Either technique accurately performed should provide the desired result, but if a 3-degree medial inclination is chosen, an appropriate adjustment of the femoral cut into 3 degrees more valgus must be made. This additional valgus on the femoral side maintains the relationship between the femoral shaft axis and the tibial shaft axis and keeps the mechanical axis from the center of the hip to the center of the ankle going through the center of the knee (Fig. 67.2).

The two options for tibial preparation, cut at 90 degrees or a cut at 87 degrees to the tibial axis, give surgeons three distinct choices of flexion alignment (Fig. 67.1). The first approach could be called the conventional approach, in which the tibial cut is made at 90 degrees and in flexion is associated with a femoral component positioned in neutral or with no external rotation. The second approach makes the tibial cut at 90 degrees, and the femoral component is externally rotated 3 degrees. In the third approach, the tibial cut is made at 87 degrees, and the femoral component is positioned in neutral or with no external rotation.

The conventional approach has been standard for many years. It removes slightly more bone on the lateral tibial plateau than on the medial tibial plateau when a 90-degree cut is made. When the femoral cuts are made

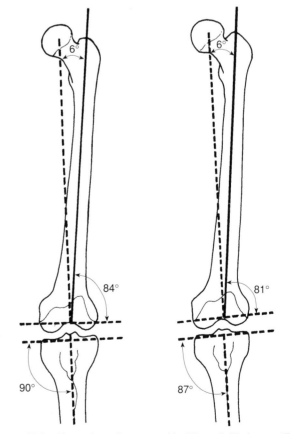

Figure 67.2. Extension alignment with 87- and 90-degree tibial cuts. (Reproduced with permission from Axial rotation of the femoral knee component. Curr Top Orthop Technol 1991;5(6).)

with neutral orientation of the femoral component, equal amounts of femur are removed from the medial and lateral condyles. When the knee is at 90 degrees of flexion and the soft tissues are distracted, the joint space is slightly trapezoidal in shape. When the implants are positioned, this results in minor asymmetrical collateral ligament tension, with approximately 3 degrees of laxity in the lateral compartment in flexion. Occasionally this is associated with a slightly tighter lateral retinaculum and may affect patellofemoral tracking.

The second constellation of events occurs with the tibial cut made at 90 degrees and the femoral cuts made in 3 degrees of external rotation. This compensates for the difference in the flexion gap by slightly raising the medial femoral condyle and lowering the lateral femoral condyle. This external femoral rotation makes the gaps equal when the joint is distracted in flexion, and a rectangular space will exist. This eliminates the laxity on the lateral side and may have a beneficial effect on patellar tracking. One concern with this method of preparation is the difficulty in determining the 3 degrees of rotation on the femoral component. It is a very small amount of rotation, and the bony landmarks make it difficult to judge this small change. The femoral component rotation can be based on slightly rotating the femoral cutting guides to have more bone exposed medially than laterally. Another way to achieve this small external rotation of the femoral component is to make the 90-degree tibial cut first. The joint is then distracted, and the femoral cutting guide is placed and rotated until it is parallel with the cut surface of the tibia. A cut in this position should approximate the 3 degrees of external rotation and will create a rectangular flexion gap.

The femoral component must not be internally rotated. This not only accentuates the difference between the medial and lateral flexion gaps but also compromises patellofemoral tracking. Furthermore, excessive external rotation of the femoral component should be avoided. This causes laxity on the medial side of the knee and limits rollback and flexion because of excessive tightness on the lateral side. It could also create a notch on the anterior lateral aspect of the femur and potentially cause patellar subluxation because the lateral edge of the implant is rotated lower and would not provide the normal resistance to patellar subluxation. Of special note is the condition that exists in a varus knee where a significant amount of medial release is anticipated. In this knee, the femoral component should not be externally rotated because after soft tissue release, the flexion space on the medial side will be increased, and if the femoral component is externally rotated, the knee will not have the desired stability on the medial side in flexion.

The third approach is to prepare the tibia with a cut 87 degrees to the axis of the tibia and remove equal amounts of bone from the medial and lateral posterior femoral condyles. Thus, the femoral component will be in neutral or have no external rotation, and the tibial cut is 87 degrees. This replicates normal anatomy. The gaps on the medial and lateral sides will be equal in flexion, and the collateral ligament tension will not be altered.

The sagittal orientation of the proximal tibial cut is equally important. Anatomic studies verify the posterior inclination of this surface in normal subjects. This posterior slope is usually between 6 and 12 degrees, with the variation resulting more from the method of measurement than from the actual amount of slope. If one considers the normal forces on the tibial surface, the highest forces occur at heel strike. In this part of the gait cycle, the knee is usually flexed approximately 10 degrees. Thus, with 10 degrees of knee flexion, the 10 degrees of posterior slope on the upper tibia will allow the forces to be transmitted perpendicular to that surface and eliminate any sheer forces that might exist during high loading. For this same reason, it is important to place the tibial component in a posteriorly sloped position. This allows the interface forces between the prosthesis and bone to be absorbed without any sheer component. Thus, the cut on the upper tibia should be inclined 6 to 10 degrees posteriorly, which parallels the anatomic surface of the tibia. By orienting bone removal parallel to the anatomic surface, bone can be conserved. Excessive resection of the anterior tibia while making a cut that is perpendicular to the tibial shaft exposes bone for tibial fixation that has less strength than normal bone. This could be associated with tibial subsidence anteriorly in making this cut without a posterior slope. The cutting guide must be placed directly anteriorly. If the cutting guide is positioned incorrectly toward the medial side of the tibia, a slope will be cut into the posterior lateral corner of the tibia rather than directly posteriorly. This can also affect the frontal plane position of the tibial component. Indeed, cutting the posterior slope at the wrong rotation cuts varus or valgus into the tibial cut, which can result in knee malalignment.

The next consideration in tibial resection is the amount of bone that should be removed from the tibial surface in preparing for implantation. To preserve the best bone for tibial fixation, a very conservative or minimal cut of the tibia is suggested. As the cut becomes thicker, the stronger bone of the upper tibial surface is removed, and weaker bone is exposed. Indeed, cuts that are more than a centimeter thick expose quite inadequate bone for tibial fixation. Another important consideration in this regard is polyethylene thickness. The less bone that is removed from the tibia, the thinner the overall polyethylene will have to be. If the polyethylene gets too thin, it can wear and fracture at an unacceptable rate. Therefore, the surgeon must compromise and remove enough bone to allow adequate tibial component thickness while preserving as much bone as possible for long-term fixation strength. Further consideration must be given to handling defects in the tibia. If these defects are significant, rather than the cut to the bottom of the defects, the surgeon may chose to be more conservative in most of the resection and fill the defect with either bone graft or an augmented type of tibial component. If, on the other hand, the defects are small, the surgeon may elect to simply resect below them and have a surface without augmentation that allows slightly thicker polyethylene to compensate for the difference.

Many implants today have been designed to retain the posterior cruciate ligament (PCL). If the surgeon desires to have the PCL function optimally after replacement, special consideration must be given to maintaining the ligament insertion onto the posterior aspect of the tibia. The PCL inserts on the upper portion of the tibial plateau in a small fossa in the posterior aspect of the tibial plateau. A resection greater than 6 or 8 mm begins to compromise this insertion site. It becomes necessary to leave an island of bone in this area to keep 100% of the PCL intact. Many surgeons therefore suggest that routinely this island of bone should be left intact so that the PCL is not inadvertently lengthened or compromised in the process of cutting the tibial plateau.

This island of bone can be predictably maintained by paying special attention to surgical detail. If the cutting guide is positioned in front of the tibia in the desired position for frontal and sagittal alignment of the cut and the depth of resection has been determined, the surgeon can then make the cut. The lateral plateau is cut from the medial side of the cutting guide, and the medial plateau from the lateral side of the cutting guide. This leaves a triangular island of bone in the posterior aspect of the knee uncut. The surgeon can then use a reciprocating saw to cut down on the sides of this island to remove the segments of bone medially and laterally (Fig. 67.3). The island of bone can then be contoured with a rongeur to decrease its size until the tibial component fits without impinging into the plateau. This maintains the island of bone completely and keeps the PCL intact. As this technique becomes a routine part of the surgeon's practice, it becomes apparent how frequently the posterior cruciate insertion would be compromised if this island of bone were not maintained.

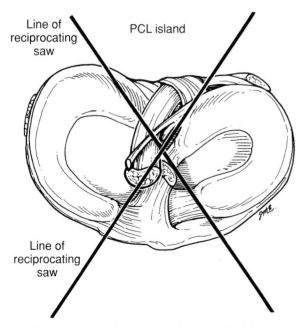

Line of reciprocating saw

PCL island

Line of reciprocating saw

Figure 67.3. Technique for maintaining PCL island.

The next issue that arises is balancing the PCL so that its tension is correct. This is easiest to accomplish during the trial reduction with the femoral and tibial component trials in place. If, during flexion and extension of the knee, the femur hinges back on the tibial component and does not roll back normally, the PCL is too tight. This booking open of the knee posteriorly can be relieved by lengthening or releasing the PCL (8). Other signs of excessive tightness of the PCL include lifting of the anterior portion of the tibial baseplate with the knee in flexion during the trial reduction. The femoral component may also be pushed off the distal femur if the knee is too tight in flexion. The surgeon can palpate the PCL and see whether the ligament tension in flexion is excessive. All these signs of excessive ligament tightness in flexion must be addressed if the kinematics of the knee are to be correct. Furthermore, if the knee is too tight in flexion, with an overly tight PCL, there will be excessive wear of the tibial polyethylene in the posterior aspect of the knee and also excessive stress on the tibial fixation interfaces, with a tendency to rock the tibial component down posteriorly and up anteriorly with stressful activity such as rising from a chair or going up and down stairs.

When the PCL is excessively tight, it can be balanced by releasing it subperiosteally from its tibial insertion site or from its femoral origin. It is also possible to Z lengthen the posterior cruciate and repair it. The results of these techniques have not been reported, and they may defunctionalize the PCL. If the ligament is released from a bony attachment site, reattaching it to one of these bony attachment sites may achieve better function than allowing it to reattach itself without surgical attention.

Different types of cutting guides have been devised for making the tibial resection, based on either intramedullary positioning or extramedullary landmarks. Both methods of preparation have advantages and disadvantages. The best results are most likely when a surgeon selects one method of preparation, becomes very familiar with it, and recognizes its limitations.

Extramedullary guides for tibial resection are based on positioning the guide in the center of the tibial plateau proximally and then localizing the center of the guide distally so that it points to the center of the talus. Extramedullary guides have been used since the early days of knee replacement, and surgeons are very familiar with their use. The proximal positioning of the guide needs some special attention. It must be oriented on the very anterior aspect of the tibia and not rotated toward the medial side. This is occasionally difficult because of the patellar tendon. If the tendon is adequately retracted laterally, the guide can be placed in the front of the tibia without problems. The guide must also be centered in the proximal aspect of the tibia. The center of the tibia can be found either by measuring it with a ruler or by centering the guide by eye.

After the guide is centered and placed anteriorly, it can be preliminarily secured. Positioning the distal portion of the extramedullary tibial cutting guide seems to give the most trouble. It is moderately difficult to locate the landmarks of the distal tibia, to find the center of the talus. It had been thought that by centering the guide over the medial and lateral malleoli, it would point at the center of the talus. It is now clear that this puts the guide approximately 1 cm lateral to the center of the talus and, therefore, puts some varus inclination to the cut on the proximal tibia. If surgeons recognize that the intermalleolar center point is located laterally, they can compensate by positioning the distal portion of the guide approximately 1 cm medial to this point.

Another fairly accurate landmark is the subcutaneous border of the tibia, approximately 6 cm above the ankle. This point is routinely on a direct line with the center of the talus, and a guide positioned to point to this landmark will align distally with the center of the talus. Surgeons must be cautious in draping patients for knee replacement because excessive drapes make the landmarks over the ankle difficult to palpate, and the guide impossible to position. If the center of the knee and the center of the ankle can be accurately identified and the guide positioned to correspond to these two landmarks, the correct frontal-plane cut will be made on the upper tibia.

The flexion and extension position of the guide must also be reckoned with. The guide must be positioned so that the cut has the correct posterior inclination. This position is usually parallel with the anterior crest of the tibia between the tibial tubercle and the ankle joint. The instrument designers build the desired amount of posterior slope into the cutting platform of the guide if the body of the guide is parallel with the shaft of the tibia. Any bow in the tibia is bypassed as the guide bridges from the center of the knee to the ankle. Bow in the tibia can be neglected as the mechanical axis of the tibia is the important feature for orienting the tibial component correctly.

Intramedullary tibial cutting guides are favored by some surgeons (1). Accuracy is based on starting the guide in the center of the tibia proximally and then allowing the intramedullary rod to obtain a position in the isthmus that will orient the cutting platform of the guide proximally. This technique gained favor because of its simplicity and because it may require slightly less exposure around the upper surface of the tibia, but disadvantages of the technique have arisen and dissuaded many surgeons from its continued use. Approximately 25% of normal tibias have a bow. This angular deformity in the tibia inaccurately positions the intramedullary rod and forces the cut on the upper surface of the tibia to be inclined into valgus or varus. The usual malalignment leads to a valgus inclination to the tibial cut. Because crooked tibias occur commonly, many intramedullary systems now include an extramedullary checking option to make sure the alignment is correct (Fig. 67.4). These systems then become an intramedullary stabilization with an extramedullary alignment system, which allows correction when the tibia is bowed. Other surgeons liked the intramedullary guide because it begins a hole in the tibia for subsequent placement of a stemmed tibial component. This likewise has fallen into some disfavor because of the common occurrence of an offset

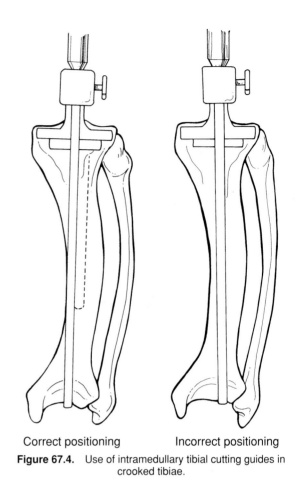

Correct positioning   Incorrect positioning

Figure 67.4. Use of intramedullary tibial cutting guides in crooked tibiae.

between the center of the medullary canal of the tibia and the center of the tibial plateau at the joint level. Thus, a centrally located stem put down the medullary canal of the tibia will offset the tibial prosthesis, and the implant will overhang the tibial plateau border. Therefore, intramedullary tibial cutting guides seem to be less attractive than they were at one time.

Patellar Preparation

Patellar preparation is currently central in discussion of the technical considerations regarding knee replacement. Approximately half of the complications that arise in total knee arthroplasty concern the patella, and many think that surgical technique plays a direct role in these complications. It is anticipated that correct technique can minimize subluxation, dislocation, tilting, abnormal prosthetic wear, patellar fracture, etc. (3). To obtain these desired results, correct component positioning is crucial, not only of the patella but the femur and tibia as well.

Femoral component position errors that negatively affect the patella include excessive valgus position, internal rotation, anterior displacement, and proximal displacement. Excessive valgus of the femoral component must be avoided. It tends to move the tibial tubercle laterally and increase the Q angle at the knee. This causes increased stress laterally on the patellofemoral joint and tends to lead to subluxation and dislocation. Internal rotation of the femoral component also adversely affects the patellofemoral articulation. It raises the lateral flange anteriorly and causes increased tension in the lateral retinaculum. This tends to pull the patella laterally. Anterior displacement of the femoral component likewise causes increased tension in the extensor mechanism. This increases the pressure in the patellofemoral joint, limits flexion, and causes tendencies for increased wear and lateral subluxation. Proximal displacement of the femoral component is also a problem. Proximal migration of the joint line increases patellofemoral complication and changes the instant center of the knee.

The tibial component can also be malpositioned and cause problems with the patella. If the tibial component is internally rotated, the tibia distal to the prosthesis will be relatively externally rotated. This increases the Q angle, causes the patella to have increased lateral forces, and tends to cause subluxation and dislocation. If the tibial component is shifted medially, there is an increased Q angle and lateral movement of the tibial tubercle. This likewise causes a negative effect on the patellofemoral articulation.

Patellar component positioning itself is crucial. The overall thickness of the patellar composite must not be increased after replacement. Thus, the depth of resection is crucial. If an inadequate amount of patellar bone is removed and then replaced with a patellar prosthesis, there will be increased tension on the extensor mechanism, and the tendency to cause lateral subluxation increases. The depth of resection is also important because removing excessive bone weakens the remaining patellar bone, and the risk for fracture increases. Leave at least a 10-mm bone fragment after resection to eliminate this risk. The amount of bone removed must equal the thickness of the prosthesis.

Medial-lateral positioning of the patellar component is important. The normal patella has a central ridge that is located toward the medial side. Thus, the lateral facet is wider and shallower than the medial facet. If the patella is going to be replaced by an axi-symmetric prosthesis (a central dome-type implant), it is important to realize that the central ridge is located medially and that the center of the patellar component should be offset toward the medial side to keep the ridge medially offset after replacement. Moving the ridge toward the center forces the patella toward the medial side of the knee during tracking and increases tension on the lateral retinaculum. This can likewise lead to lateral subluxation or increase stresses in the lateral aspect of the patellofemoral joint. The lateral facet of the patella is normally thin, and most patellar resections do not remove much bone from the lateral facet. Replacing the most lateral portion of the patella with a 6- or 8-mm thick prosthesis will also overtighten the lateral retinaculum and tend to cause patellar tilting.

After the patellar resection is completed and the prosthesis appropriately oriented on the bony remnant, a trial reduction is necessary. It is important to ascertain whether there is any tilt or subluxation tendency during this maneuver. If there is, it is imperative that a lateral retinacular release be performed.

There is also an interest in insetting patellar components into the patellar bone. This technique tends to replace the central eminence and preserve a peripheral rim of bone. There have not been any studies that would indicate that this is a significantly better approach. The same considerations of overall patellar thickness, ridge location, and appropriate fixation apply (9).

Instrumentation for Revision Total Knee Arthroplasty

The technique for revision total knee arthroplasty puts special demands on instrumentation. After the prosthesis and cement are removed, there is always less bone left to work with than there is in a primary total knee arthroplasty. This bone deficit results in difficulty in attaching or securing instruments as well as implants. Thus, special instruments are needed in the femur and in the tibia.

Femoral instrumentation in revision total knee surgery relies on obtaining some type of fixation in the medullary canal of the femur. After the medullary canal has been identified and instruments inserted, it can be used as a reference point for alignment and for fixing other instruments, too. The bone surfaces can then be prepared to receive the augmented implants necessary to compensate for defects on the femur.

To prepare the tibia for a revision implant, an extramedullary tibial cutting guide is very useful. Frequently, there are enough defects in the medullary canal to make a small intramedullary guide ineffective. A larger intramedullary guide can also be an effective reference point for the tibial anatomic access. The minimal resection necessary on the tibia can then be performed.

Complications Caused by Instrumentation

Problems can arise during total knee arthroplasty. Many of them are inherent risks of the procedure and can be anticipated. Occasionally, problems arise because of the use of instrumentation. Possibly the most significant of these is the occurrence of fat embolism syndrome secondary to placement of intramedullary rods or reaming (2). Insertion of intramedullary rods, particularly into the femoral canal, is thought to be associated with fat embolism syndrome. Therefore, when rods are used for alignment on either the femoral or tibial side, it is important to remove the fluid contents of the canal with suction before insertion of the rod. It is also important to vent the canal through either an enlarged hole at the surface of the knee or some other technique, to decompress the canal during insertion of the rod. If these principles are followed, this potential complication should be eliminated.

Another potential complication associated with instrumentation is avulsion of the patellar tendon from the tibial tubercle. This can occur with excessive retraction of the extensor mechanism or forward subluxation of the tibia. It can also result from inappropriate placement of the tibial cutting guide and transection of the patellar tendon with either a saw or the guide itself. This devastating complication should be avoided, as repair is almost impossible.

Neurovascular injury has also been reported as a complication of surgical technique. In placing instruments around the knee, special attention must be given to protecting the neurovascular structures. The same is true for other ligaments around the knee. The medial collateral ligament can be at particular risk and should be protected with a retractor so that it is not cut with the saw during the preparation of the proximal tibia or the posterior femoral condyles.

Bone Preparation for Fixation

After all the bone surfaces have been prepared for implantation, some special instruments exist to help prepare the knee to accept the cement, based on preparing the bone surfaces to allow cement to interdigitate with cancellous bone. Special lavage techniques provide pulsatile irrigation of the cancellous bone. After thorough drying of the surfaces, the bone cement can interdigitate and obtain a three-dimensional interlock with the cancellous bone before insertion of the prosthesis.

Future of Instrumentation

The goal of instrument design is to improve the accuracy and reproducibility of the preparation of the bone surfaces to accept the implant. Great progress has been made in this direction, and further improvements will require new technology. To obtain success with cementless implantation, very accurate bone cuts are imperative. Indeed, cementless tibial fixation may have failed because surgeons could not routinely obtain a surface flat enough for a porous implantation. If better surface appropriation could be obtained, more reproducible bony ingrowth and long-term fixation might be achieved.

To obtain smoother, flatter surfaces for implantation, the future may hold special machining devices that will actually mill the bone surfaces in a manner similar to that used for machining implants. This may provide surfaces that are absolutely flat and smooth, or the surfaces could be contoured in different geometric shapes. This would allow bone conservation on the femoral side as the surfaces were curved to correspond to the curves of the prosthesis. Improved fixation may also be obtained through these milling techniques as more complex surfaces are easily machined and more rigid initial fixation is obtained with implantation of the prosthesis. Furthermore, as the machining is driven by more refined instruments, the error introduced by intersurgeon variation could be minimized. If the variation from human error were kept to a minimum, the desired results might be achieved more frequently.

Summary

The surgical technique of total knee arthroplasty is the single variable over which surgeons have control. If instruments can be designed to provide accurate and reproducible preparation of the distal femur, proximal tibia, and patella, successful total knee arthroplasty can be accomplished. The surgeon must understand how this is done and be aware of potential errors that can occur during the surgical procedure.

References

1. Bertin KC. Intramedullary instrumentation for total knee arthroplasty. In: Goldberg VM, ed. Controversies in total knee arthroplasty. New York: Raven Press, 1991:175–183.
2. Fahmy NR, Chandler HP, Danylchuk K, Matta EB, Sunder N, Siliski JM. Blood-gas and circulatory changes during total knee replacement, role of the intramedullary alignment rod. J Bone Joint Surg 1990;72A:19–25.
3. Figgie HA, Goldberg VM, Heiple KG, Moller HS, Gordon NH. The influence of tibial-patellofemoral location on function of the knee in patients with the Posterior Stabilized Condylar Knee Prosthesis. J Bone Joint Surg 1986;68A:1035–1040.
4. Freeman MAR, Sculco TP, Todd RC. ICLH total knee arthroplasty in severely damaged knees. J Bone Joint Surg 1977;59B:64–71.
5. Moreland JR, Bassett LW, Hanker GJ. Radiographic analysis of lower extremity axial alignment. J Bone Joint Surg 1987;69A:745–749.
6. Rand JA, Bryan RS. Alignment in porous coated anatomic total knee arthroplasty. In: Dorr LD, ed. The knee. Baltimore: University Park Press, 1985:111–115.
7. Anouchi US, Whiteside LA, Kaiser AD, Milliano, MT. The effect of axial rotational alignment of the femoral component on knee stability and patellar tracking in total knee arthroplasty. Clin Orthop 1993;287:170–177.
8. Ritter MA, Faris PM, Keating EM. Posterior cruciate ligament balancing during total knee arthroplasty. J Arthroplasty 1988;3(4):323–326.
9. Gomes LSM, Bechtold JE, Gustilo RB. Patellar prosthesis positioning in total knee arthroplasty: a roentgenographic study. Clin Orthop 1988;236:72–81.
10. Axial rotation of the femoral knee component. Curr Top Orthop Technol 1991;5(6).

68

Cruciate Ligament Retention in Total Knee Arthroplasty

Aaron A. Hofmann and Thomas B. Pace

The role of the cruciate ligaments in the functioning total knee arthroplasty is controversial. In some cases, the disease process necessitating arthroplasty has destroyed the posterior cruciate ligament (PCL), although most of the time it is present (1). The contribution of the cruciate ligaments to a "balanced" knee post arthroplasty and the surgical technique for preserving the PCL is the subject of this chapter.

Cruciate Ligament Anatomy and Function

The anatomic and functional aspects of the cruciate ligaments are described in detail by Girgis (2). The PCL is attached to the posterior part of the lateral surface of the medial condyle of the femur; it is oriented vertically and attaches to the posterior aspect of the proximal tibia. The posterior cruciate, with an average length of 38 mm and an average width of 13 mm, is narrowest in the middle portion. The fibers are attached to the tibia in a lateromedial direction and to the femur in an anteroposterior direction.

The tibial attachment is to a depression behind the intraarticular upper surface of the tibia extending approximately 2 cm distal to the posterior joint line (Figs. 68.1 and 68.2) (3). The attachment extends for a few millimeters onto the adjoining posterior surface of the tibia. Above its tibial attachment, there may be a fibrous band posterior to the PCL that blends with the posterior horn of the lateral meniscus (ligament of Wrisberg). The anterior fibers of the PCL may be accompanied by another fibrous band that extends from the medial femoral condyle to the posterior horn of the lateral meniscus (ligament of Humphrey). The ligaments of Humphrey and Wrisberg are present 70% of the time (2).

As shown in Figure 68.1, the anterior cruciate ligament (ACL) attaches to the posterior part of the medial surface of the lateral femoral condyle and courses obliquely to insert just medial to the anterior tibial spine. The femoral attachments of both cruciate liga-

ments and the tibial attachment of the posterior cruciate ligament are behind the axis of flexion while only the tibial attachment of the anterior cruciate ligament is in front of it. The attachment of the anterior cruciate ligament is not on the anterior tibial spine but over an area just medial to it. The course of the anterior cruciate ligament is more oblique in the anteroposterior plane than is that of the PCL (2).

It is important to note that the fibers of each ligament are not all taut at the same time. The bulk of the fibers of the anterior cruciate ligament are loose in flexion, although a band of the anteromedial fibers remain taut in 120 to 130 degrees of flexion. The opposite is true for the PCL, which remains tightest in flexion and loose in knee extension.

Interactive Function of Knee Ligaments

There is an interactive function between the anterior cruciate ligament and the posterior cruciate ligament. On knee flexion, both ligaments are twisted around their longitudinal axes in opposing directions. The direction of the torsion is toward the center of the joint and various portions of each ligament are tense at any point in time depending on the amount of flexion or extension of the knee (4).

The PCL prevents posterior displacement of the tibia with knee flexion by being directly tensed and prevents posterior tibial displacement by holding the femur down against the tibia in the model proposed by Biden (5). The relative attachments of the PCL, medial collateral ligament (MCL), ACL, and lateral collateral ligament (LCL) affect the relative motion of the articulating surfaces of the femur and tibia. The PCL is also felt to be a secondary stabilizer to varus and valgus laxity (normally between 2 to 10 degrees) (6–8). The axis of tibiofemoral motion is posterior to the center line of the tibial plateau in flexion. Maintaining this position is a primary goal after arthroplasty; achievement of this goal requires an understanding of the factors that affect tibiofemoral kinetics.

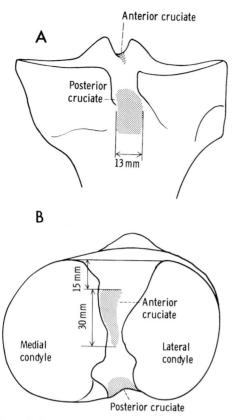

Figure 68.1. **A,** Posterior surface of the tibia and **B,** the upper surface of the tibial plateau showing average measurements and relations of the tibial attachments of the anterior and posterior cruciate ligaments. (Reproduced with permission from Girgis FG, et al. Clin Orthop 1975;106:222.)

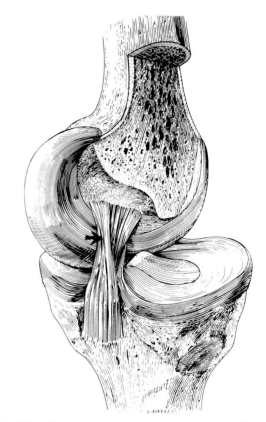

Figure 68.2. Dissected specimen showing the area of insertion of the posterior cruciate ligament. (Reproduced with permission from Girgis FG, et al. Clin Orthop 1975;106:223.)

Femoral Rollback in Knee Flexion

The positional changes that occur with knee extension and flexion are primarily affected by the interaction of the anterior and the posterior cruciate ligaments. Their function is often described as a four-bar linked chain (Fig. 68.3). The representation shown in Figure 68.3 is by no means a true representation of a functioning knee for three important reasons: ligaments are not rigid; various portions of the ligaments are tight at different times through knee motion; and the ligament attachments occur over a broad area. This four-bar linked chain system is often used to introduce the concept of femoral rollback which can be described as posterior displacement of the femur on the tibia as a normal positional change in knee flexion. While some suggest that knee flexion allows "rolling back" of the femur on the tibia both in the normal knee and in the knee arthroplasty with an intact posterior cruciate ligament, others contend that the radiologic appearance of rollback in the normal knee is due to the concomitant occurrence of axial tibial rotation and the cam shape of the femoral condyles (5, 7). Knee motion in flexion is probably a combination of rolling, gliding, and rotation of the femoral condyles. It is the goal of knee arthroplasty to match the normal kinematics in the best possible way (Fig. 68.4).

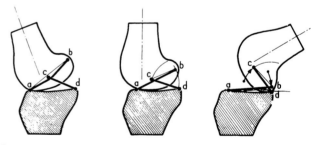

Figure 68.3. Diagrammatic representation of the mechanism of the knee showing the cruciate ligaments acting as two links in a four-bar chain. (Reproduced with permission from Kapandjii A. Physiology of the joints. In: Lower Limb. 5th ed. New York: Churchill Livingstone, 1987:120.)

Acquisition of Full Flexion After TKA

Prerequisites

Knee flexion of at least 90 degrees is considered the minimum required for activities of daily living. More than 90 degrees are required in at least one leg in order to rise from a chair. This degree of flexion and more is usually achieved after knee replacement. Factors affecting postoperative range of motion (ROM) were studied by Shoji, et al. in 197 total knee arthroplasties (TKA) (9). Factors associated with postoperative motion (of less

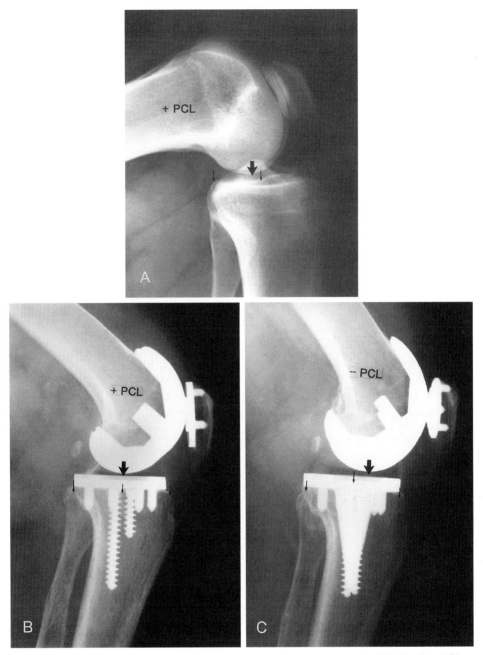

Figure 68.4. Radiograph demonstrating femoral rollback normally **(A)**, with PCL functional **(B)**, and no rollback without PCL **(C)**.

than 90 degrees) were the following: elevation of the joint line; increase in patella thickness more than 20%; and lack of aggressive early physical therapy. PCL retention or excision did not significantly affect flexion (9).

Common Variables

The work of Walker and Garg using a computer generated model based on an average of 23 anatomic specimens looked at knee flexion affected by several independent variables. Noting that an excessively tight PCL was restrictive to knee flexion, several factors were shown to accommodate PCL function within its maxi-

mal allowable strain (15%) and yet result in increased flexion. All of the following resulted in increased flexion with an intact PCL compared to the "normal" model: sloping the tibial surface posteriorly (to match the normal 5–8 degrees), using a flatter, less conforming tibial surface, maintaining a tibial component centered posterior to the central axis of the tibia, and translating the femoral component 2.5 mm anterior to the central axis of the femur (Figs. 68.5–68.8). The most important variable allowing maximal flexion with an intact PCL was the posterior slope of the tibial component in the sagittal plane (4).

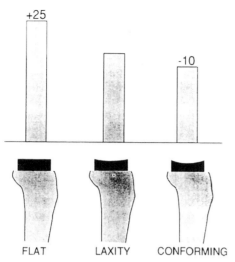

Figure 68.5. Bar graph showing the effect of tibial component geometry on maximum knee flexion, relative to the surface of laxity. (Reproduced with permission from Walker PS, Garg A. Clin Orthop 1991;262:232.)

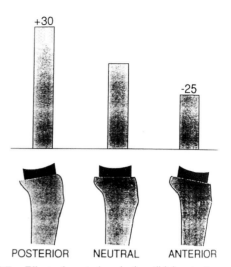

Figure 68.7. Effect of posterior sloping tibial osteotomy on maximum knee flexion. (Reproduced with permission from Walker and Garg A. Clin Orthop 1991;262:232.)

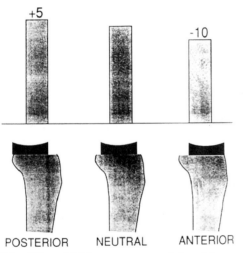

Figure 68.6. Effect of tibial component translation of 5 mm on maximum knee flexion. (Reproduced with permission from Walker PS, Garg A. Clin Orthop 1991;262:232.)

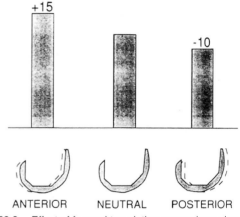

Figure 68.8. Effect of femoral translation on maximum knee flexion. (Reproduced with permission from Walker PS, Garg A. Clin Orthop 1991;262:233.)

Functional Stability

Posterior Cruciate Ligament Retention or Excision

Proponents of PCL retention note that the PCL is the strongest ligament in the knee and it may direct the forces generated by most common activities. The quadriceps produces a posteriorly directed force on the fully flexed knee. Andriacchi has shown that by maintaining the increased quadriceps lever arm with a stabilized posterior tibiofemoral contact axis, patients with PCL-preserving arthroplasties have better function in stair climbing (Fig. 68.9) (7). Certain prosthetic configurations of the femoral condyle are designed to maximize the kinematic role of the quadriceps mechanism and patella by maintaining a deeper and more normal

trochlea groove (10). Also, the subvastus surgical approach to knee replacement may well facilitate the extensor mechanism function by decreased scarring of the extensor mechanism and by enhanced visualization for patella alignment intraoperatively (11). It has been proposed that the retained PCL, as a secondary stabilizer to varus and valgus stress, helps prevent lateral lift off and stress loading of the medial compartment as the knee assumes a more adducted position in the stance phase of walking (Fig. 68.10) (7).

Accommodating Prosthetic Designs

It is postulated that the absence of the PCL would produce greater shear forces to the articulating surfaces of the arthroplasty and to the implant-bone-cement interface. While these surfaces tolerate compressive forces better than shear forces, review of 100 cemented TKA

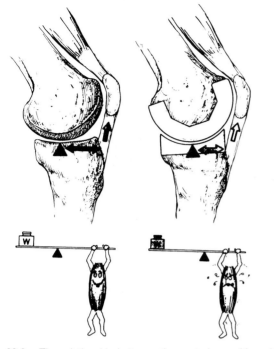

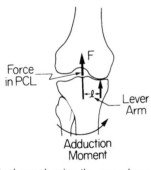

Figure 68.9. The relationship between the posterior position of the tibial component and the effect on the quadriceps lever arm. (Reproduced with permission from Andriacchi TP, Galante JO. J Arthroplasty 1988;(Oct suppl):S-17.)

Figure 68.10. The knee showing the normal varus thrust or adduction moment that occurs during walking and the stabilizing effect of the PCL. (Reproduced with permission from Andriacchi TP, Galante JO. J Arthroplasty 1988;(Oct suppl):S-17.)

with PCL excision by Ranawat and Hansraj did not show any adverse effect on the implant-bone-cement surfaces at 15-year follow-up (12). In reviewing 30 cases of bilateral-paired cruciate retaining and cruciate substituting total knee arthroplasties, Becker concluded that there was no difference in the function of either knee (13). Buechel, reporting on the survivorship rate of a mobile-bearing knee prosthesis system noted essentially equal results (98%) in comparing posterior cruciate retaining and posterior substituting components (14). In theory, the patella strain should be greater in the knee without the PCL acting to stabilize the tibial component; however, Reuben, et al., in reviewing cadaveric knees with and without PCL retention, was not able to demon-

strate any significant effect on patellar strain (15). Performing total knee arthroplasty on knees with deficient PCLs as well as with deficient patellae can be challenging. Our preference in this situation is to use an ultra congruent semiconstrained tibial insert (Fig. 68.11 A) to help stabilize the femoral condyles in flexion and to suture the extensor mechanism into a tube. This thickens and mechanically assists the quadriceps mechanism. A knee without a patella but with a functional PCL can have successful arthroplasty with this procedure (Fig. 68.11 B).

Advocates of PCL excision in TKA point to the work of Door, Freeman, and others showing that gait analysis on level ground and on stairs is the same in the presence or absence of the posterior cruciate ligament (6). Freeman proposes that the benefits of a posteriorly placed tibial component can be achieved with a more constrained roller-in-trough component design, excision of the PCL, and adequately tensed soft tissues in flexion and extension. Furthermore, he suggests that the increased motion at the articulating surfaces results in an increased tibiofemoral contact area and may diminish the eventual polyethylene wear rate (16). The roller-in-trough design can, however, make flexion beyond 90 degrees difficult to achieve (17).

Whiteside reviewed the effect a posterior tibial component rim on varus, valgus, and rotatory laxity of the knee using cadaveric specimens. He concluded that, while flexion was restricted, the constrained rim improved stability in the range of 45 to 90 degrees of flexion (6).

Accommodating Surgical Techniques

Saving the posterior tibial spine with the PCL offers several advantages: less likelihood of inadvertently cutting the PCL with the tibial osteotomy, avoiding attrition and wear from cement or the posterior border of the metal tibial tray, and facilitating the proper PCL tension in full knee flexion by not shortening its excursion (18). Prior to tibial osteotomy, the posterior tibial spine can be protected with a 1/4-inch osteotome placed just anterior to it (Fig. 68.12). Because of the broad insertion of the PCL along the posterior proximal tibia, some surgeons resect the posterior tibial spine with the tibial osteotomy. The PCL can be protected with an appropriately shaped retractor placed anterior to the ligament at its uppermost insertion along the proximal posterior tibia. Due to the caudal extension of the tibial insertion of the PCL, this can be consistently accomplished, even with a posteriorly sloping tibial osteotomy. This is consistent with reports showing that tibial cuts parallel to the articular surface (as opposed to cuts perpendicular to the axis of the tibia) result in stronger supporting bone, facilitate intraoperative soft tissue balancing, and lessen the frequency of anterior subsidence of the tibial plate (19). The tibial base plate can be further stabilized by autologous bone paste under the surface of the tibial plate (20, 21).

Ritter, et al. have described a technique of balancing the PCL surgically to assure satisfactory flexion gap ten-

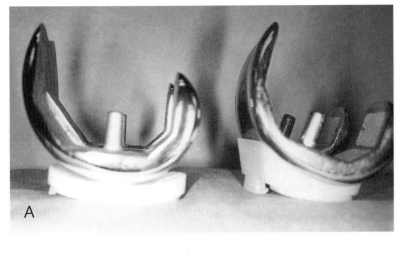

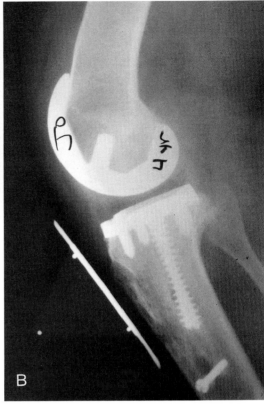

Figure 68.11.   **A,** Standard tibial insert (*left*) and "ultra-congruent" insert (*right*). **B,** Radiograph of patella deficient knee with functional PCL and "tubularized" patella after TKA.

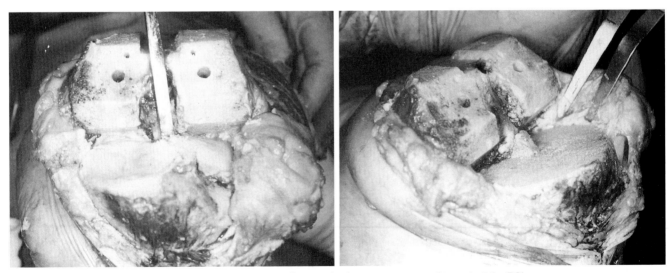

Figure 68.12.   Intraoperative photograph of an osteotome used to protect the PCL during tibial osteotomy of TKA.

sion in TKA (3). The surgical technique involves testing stability of the knee with trial femoral and tibial components and partially releasing the more proximal fibers of the broad insertion of the PCL on the tibia. While assessing the knee in flexion with the trial components in place (no pegs on the undersurface of the tibial plate) if there is anterior subluxation, superior tilting, or posterior hinging of the tibial trial, then subperiosteal recession of the PCL is performed. The tibial insertion fibers of the PCL are released in 2–3 mm increments followed

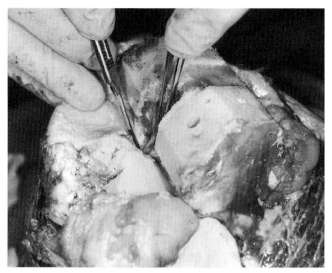

Figure 68.13. Intraoperative photograph of surgical recession of PCL.

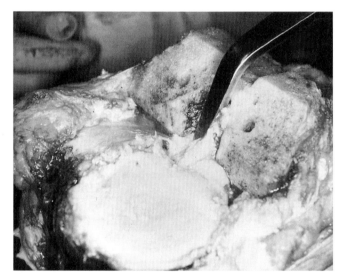

Figure 68.14. Intraoperative photograph showing a Homan retractor protecting the substance of the PCL.

by reassessment of PCL tension with the trial components.

We prefer the routine release of some of the more proximal fibers of the PCL inserting on the upper posterior tibia (Fig. 68.13); then we use a large, dull, angled knee retractor that is placed through the substance of the PCL while displacing the tibia forward during tibial osteotomy (Fig. 68.14). If the PCL is absent or nonfunctional, we prefer to slightly overfill the tibia 2 mm sizes larger than the level of cut (i.e., cut 7 mm and use a 9 mm tibial polyethylene insert). The terminal 5 to 10 degrees of extension is lost intraoperatively, but will be regained by eventual stretching of the posterior capsular structures (10). "A test drive" of the functional limits of the posterior cruciate ligament with trial components in place intraoperatively is recommended. This is done by

preforming a posterior drawer test on the knee as well as attempting hyperextension. If the posterior cruciate ligament is only marginally functional and if there is a reasonable chance of its disruption after surgery, it is better to appreciate this inadequate PCL function intraoperatively and to make appropriate changes using a slightly oversized tibial component or semiconstrained tibial component. In the absence of the PCL, the MCL works in conjunction with the LCL to maintain tibiofemoral position; therefore, care should be taken not to overrelease the collateral ligaments to obtain an excessively oversized tibial polyethylene component.

Additional Effects of Retaining the PCL

Technical Considerations

Arguments are sometimes made that the retained PCL makes surgical exposure technically challenging by restricting forward displacement of the tibia from the femur during tibial component preparation. Tibial exposure is facilitated by reflecting the medial and lateral capsular sleeves posteriorly from the tibia and transecting all remaining anterior cruciate fibers from their insertion on the tibial spine. Removal of osteophytes from the posterior femur (Fig. 68.15) and removal of the posterior horns of both menisci facilitates exposure as does using various retractors to displace the tibia forward.

Effect on Component Stress Forces

Studies assessing the effect of TKA with PCL sacrifice have not shown adverse effects on the bone-cement interface in cemented TKA (8). There is the theoretical benefit of relieving component stress forces by having the retained PCL absorb some of the anteroposterior shear forces, and of reducing patellofemoral stress by reducing posterior displacement of the tibia in the flexed knee after arthroplasty (22), although there is no conclusive data to confirm this.

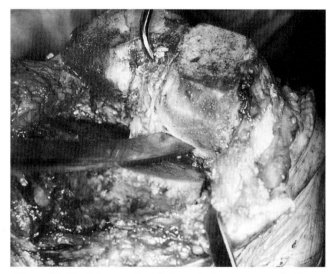

Figure 68.15. Intraoperative photograph showing removal of large posterior femoral osteophytes.

Anterior Cruciate Ligament Retention

The reports by Buechel of the mobile (moveable) bearing arthroplasty comparing bicruciate retaining, posterior retaining alone and bicruciate sacrificing prostheses showed over 98% survivorship for each group at twelve years (14). While this study did not address patient satisfaction with each cruciate retaining design, some surgeons contend that patients with retained anterior cruciate ligaments feel that the arthroplasty is like "their own knee." This may be a reflection of preservation of the proprioceptive function of the anterior cruciate ligament. The role of sparing the anterior cruciate ligament in cases where it is present and functional remains to be defined, although the early reports are encouraging. The work of Cloutier, utilizing the nonconstrained, bicruciate retaining prosthesis, reports 91% excellent or good results with postoperative flexion and stair climbing capabilities (23).

Summary

Posterior cruciate retention in the well-balanced knee arthroplasty may improve stress transfer and kinematics. The debate remains lively on both sides of the issue. There is general agreement, however, that inappropriate PCL tension can compromise prosthetic function. The excessively tight PCL can restrict flexion, and the PCL that is too loose in flexion may allow anteroposterior instability, compromise the quadriceps moment arm, and/or increase the anterior tilting moments on the tibial component. The role of anterior cruciate retention is under study with mobile bearing designs.

Whether the PCL is sacrificed or retained in total knee replacement, appropriate soft tissue tension must be achieved in flexion and in extension. The posterior position of the tibial component should be maintained, while not compromising knee flexion or altering functional tibial-patellofemoral mechanics. In most cases, with attention to the other related factors, this can be achieved while preserving the posterior cruciate ligament. The question of posterior cruciate retention is not an isolated one and must be approached from the perspective of a balanced knee considering the relevant bone, soft tissue and implant components involved.

References

1. Scott RD, Volatile TB. Twelve years' experience with posterior cruciate-retaining total knee arthroplasty. Clin Orthop 1986;205:100–107.
2. Girgis FG, Marshall JL, Monajem AA. The cruciate ligaments of the knee joint: Anatomical, functional and experimental analysis. Clin Orthop 1975;106:216–231.
3. Ritter MA, Faris PM, Keating M. Posterior cruciate ligament balancing during total knee arthroplasty. J Arthroplasty 1988;3(4):323–326.
4. Walker PS, Garg A. Range of motion in total knee arthroplasty, a computer analysis. Clin Orthop 1991;262:227–235.
5. Freeman MAR. Total arthroplasty of the knee. In: Dorr L. Proceedings of the Knee Society, 1985–1986. Rockville, MD: Aspen Pub, 1987:3–22.
6. Whiteside L. Total arthroplasty of the knee. In: Dorr L. Proceedings of the Knee Society, 1985–1986. Rockville, MD: Aspen Pub, 1987:57–74..
7. Andriacchi TP, Galante JO. Retention of the posterior cruciate in total knee arthroplasty. J Arthroplasty 1988;3(Oct suppl):13–19.
8. Newman A, et al. Postoperative return of motion in MCL/ACL injuries: The effect of MCL rupture location. Am J Sports Med 1993;21(1):20–25.
9. Shoji H, et al. Factors affecting postoperative flexion in total knee arthroplasty. Orthopedics 1990;13(6)643–649.
10. Hofmann AA, Murdock LE, Wyatt RWB, Alpert JP. Total knee arthroplasty—two-to-four-year experience using an asymmetric tibial tray and a deep trochlear-grooved femoral component. Clin Orthop 1991;269:78.
11. Hofmann AA, Plaster RL, Murdock LE. Subvastus (southern) approach for primary total knee arthroplasty. Clin Orthop 1991;269:70.
12. Ranawat CS, Hansraj KK. Effect of posterior cruciate sacrifice on durability of the bone-cement interface. Ortho Clin North Am 1989;20(1)63–69.
13. Becker MW, Insall JN, Faris PM. Bilateral total knee arthroplasty, one cruciate retaining and one cruciate substituting. Clin Orthop 1991;271:122–124.
14. Buechel FF. Long-term survivorship analysis of cruciate-sparing versus cruciate-sacrificing knee prostheses using meniscal bearings. Clin Orthop 1990;260:162–169.
15. Reuben JD. Effect of patella thickness on patella strain following total knee arthroplasty. J Arthroplasty 1991;6(3)251–258.
16. Freeman MAR. Should the posterior cruciate ligament be retained or resected in condylar nonmeniscal knee arthroplasty? J Arthroplasty 1988;3(Oct suppl):3–12.
17. Insall JN. Surgery of the knee. New York: Churchill Livingstone, 1984:601.
18. Scott RD, Volatile TB. Twelve years experience with posterior cruciate-retaining total knee arthroplasty. Clin Orthop 1986;205:100–107.
19. Hofmann AA, Bachus K. Wyatt RWB. Effect of the tibial cut on subsidence after total knee arthroplasty. Clin Orthop 1991;269:63–69.
20. Hofmann AA, Bloebaum RD, Rubman MK, et al. Microscopic analysis of autograft bone applied at the interface of porous-coated devices in human cancellous bone. Int Orthop (SICOT) 1992;16:349–358.
21. Bloebaum RD, Rubman MH, Hofmann AA. Bone ingrowth into porous-coated tibial implants with autograft bone chips, analysis of ten consecutively retrieved implants. J Arthroplasty 1992;7:483–493.
22. Figgie HE, Goldberg VM, Heiple KG, et al. The influence of tibial-patellofemoral location of function of the knee in patients with the posterior stabilized condylar knee prosthesis. J Bone Joint Surg 1986;68A:1035–1040.
23. Cloutier J-M. Results of total knee arthroplasty with a non-constrained prosthesis. J Bone Joint Surg 1983;65-A:906–919.

69

Sacrificing the Posterior Cruciate Ligament with and without Substitution in Total Knee Arthroplasty

Jonathan P. Garino and Paul A. Lotke

Historical Overview of PCL
   Sacrifice/Substitution in TKR
Biomechanics and Kinematics of
   the PCL in the Normal Knee and
   TKR

Intraoperative Advantages of PCL
   Resection
Results of Posterior Cruciate
   Sacrificing/Substituting TKA
Summary

The treatment of the posterior cruciate ligament (PCL) in total knee arthroplasty is currently one of the significant controversies surrounding prosthetic designs. This is, in part, due to the excellent results reported by experiences with retaining (1–3), sacrificing (4, 5), and substituting (6, 7). The ability of a surgeon to choose between these designs requires a fundamental knowledge of the role of the cruciate ligament in normal and arthritic knees, and its subsequent impact on total knee arthroplasty. This chapter delineates the technical and survivorship aspects of posterior cruciate sacrifice in prosthetic replacement of the knee.

Historical Overview of PCL Sacrifice/Substitution in Total Knee Replacement

The discovery of high molecular weight polyethylene as a bearing surface and the subsequent evolution of highly constrained hinged prostheses into the unlinked designs of the early 1970s began a new period of total knee arthroplasty. The designs were, for the most part, of two types: those that sought to totally replace the proximal tibia and distal femur and those that sought to replace only the pathologic articular cartilage, while maintaining as much of the original anatomy as possible. Early successes and failures of both types eventually led to the PCL-sacrificing and PCL-sparing prostheses. These designs have many features in common.

The Freeman-Swanson (8), the ICLH (9) and the Total Condylar (10) (Fig. 69.1) knee replacements were among the most widely used and, hence, most thoroughly examined and analyzed of the PCL-sacrificing designs. The Freeman-Swanson and ICLH knees were essentially roller-in-trough designs with a relatively high level of constraint. The Total Condylar knee, the prototype of modern total knee replacements, more closely resembles the anatomy of the distal femur, with separate symmetrical condyles. Sagittal plane stability was

provided by the conformity of the polyethylene articulation of the tibia. A median intercondylar eminence was the main stabilizer in the coronal plane. These original designs had few sizes and an all-poly tibial component.

The virtues of the PCL in normal knee kinematics became increasingly clear with further study of the complex geometry and motion of the normal knee. Subsequently, Insall, one of the designers of the Total Condylar knee, in conjunction with Burstein, developed a posterior-substituting prosthesis (11). This design uses a cam on the femoral component, which engages a polyethylene spine on the tibial component (Fig. 69.2). Over the ensuing 15 years, the prosthetic components of total knee arthroplasty have continued to evolve. Multiple sizes, metal backing of the tibia, porous ingrowth fixation, and modularity are among the most common additions to modern total knee systems (Fig. 69.3).

Biomechanics and Kinematics of the PCL in the Normal Knee and TKR

The knee is one of the most complex joints in the human body. Originally considered as a simple hinge, careful analysis of its kinematics has revealed an elaborate interdependence of menisci, bone, and ligaments, with multiple degrees of freedom. Because of the unconstrained geometry of the bony structures, the knee depends highly on the collateral and cruciate ligaments for stability. These relationships should be thoroughly examined before deciding whether to sacrifice the posterior cruciate ligament at knee arthroplasty.

There is significant asymmetry between the medial and lateral articulations of the knee. The medial femoral condyle is larger, and the medial tibial plateau is considerably more dished, than their lateral counterparts. This asymmetry allows external rotation of the tibia about its long axis and "rollback" of the femur, particularly the lateral condyle, during flexion (12). In addition, as the knee flexes, the insertion point of the PCL on the lateral

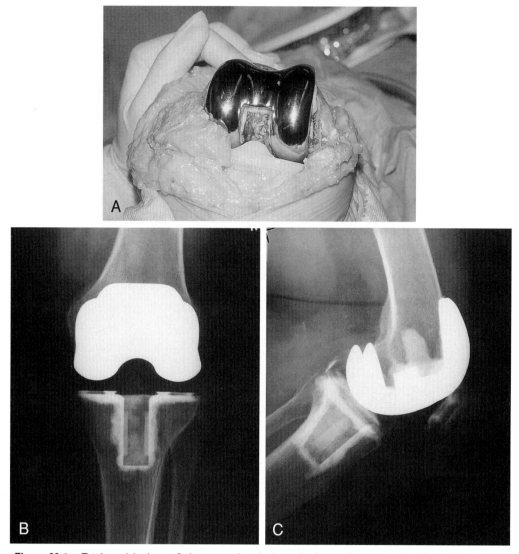

Figure 69.1. Total condylar knee. **A,** Intraoperative photograph of a newly cemented total condylar knee. Fifteen-year follow-up anteroposterior (**B**) and lateral (**C**) radiographs of a total condylar knee.

aspect of the medial femoral condyle begins to displace anteriorly, increasing tension in the PCL. As flexion continues, the insertion point would continue to proceed anteriorly, but the PCL checks this motion, causing a posterior displacement, or rollback, of the femur on the tibia with increasing flexion. Tension in the ACL, conversely, displaces the femur anteriorly during extension, reversing the rollback of flexion. This combination of external rotation and rollback of the lateral femoral condyle permits flexion approaching 140 degrees. Without this mechanism, impingement of the soft tissues of the knee between the posterior rim of the tibia and the posterior aspect of the femur would limit flexion to between 90 and 105 degrees (Fig. 69.4) (13). An additional benefit of femoral rollback is the increase in the quadriceps lever arm and subsequent increase in quadriceps force (Fig. 69.5) (14).

The configuration of the cruciate ligaments provides most of the anterior-posterior stability. The posterior

and anterior cruciate ligaments restrain posterior and anterior displacement, respectively, of the tibia on the femur. The relationship of these two ligaments has been described mechanically as a four-bar link (15). The motion of the normal knee in the sagittal plane is defined by the rigid cruciates and the bone that separates their origins and insertions (Fig. 69.6). The shape of this linkage constantly changes throughout the range of knee motion. The geometry of the linkage allows flexion and extension of the femur and tibia while the cruciates remain isometric. This demonstrates why the bones can move relative to one another within an allowable range without ligament strain or cartilage indentation (15).

The tibial plateau is a relatively flat surface. The menisci increase the conformity of the articulating surfaces and subsequently distribute the load across the joint and decrease point-contact stresses. The menisci, however, are not held rigidly to the tibial plateau, but rather, slide posteriorly and anteriorly with flexion and

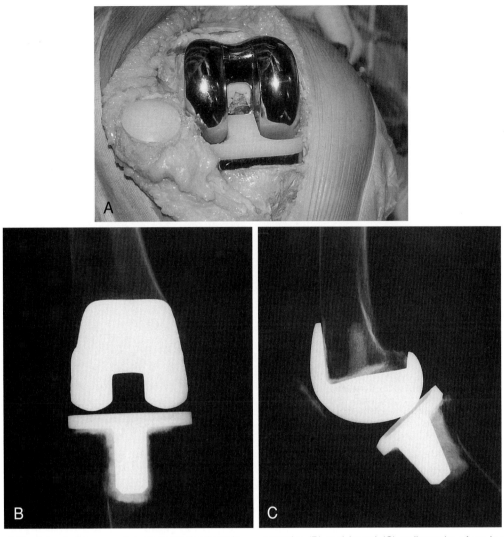

Figure 69.2. Insall-Burstein. **A,** Intraoperative photograph of newly cemented Insall-Burstein (IB-I) total knee. Ten-year follow-up antero-posterior (**B**) and lateral (**C**) radiographs of an Insall-Burstein total knee.

extension, to maintain this high degree of conformity while minimizing point-contact stresses during femoral rollback (16).

In total knee replacement, there is significant controversy over whether the PCL should be retained, sacrificed, or substituted. The preceding discussion outlined the importance of femoral rollback for increased flexion and increased quadriceps strength. Achieving a similar situation in a total knee is also desirable. Since this rollback phenomenon is the primarily the result of PCL function within the confines of the four-bar linkage, it is logical to save it. However, if the same action can be achieved by substituting for the PCL within the design of the prosthesis itself, this holds many theoretical/actual advantages.

The anatomy of the normal knee is not, for the most part, recreated by total knee arthroplasty. It represents an adequate functional replacement for the relief of pain in a variety of arthritic conditions. Many successful prosthetic designs have symmetrical medial and lateral condyles. These total knees are created as such to standardize the surgical technique and to minimize inventory. The ACL is normally sacrificed if it is intact at the time of arthroplasty. These accepted deviations from the normal situation, by definition, alter the kinematics and subsequent function of prosthetic knees. The PCL, along with the ACL, contributes to the "screwhome mechanism" of the knee. The anatomy of the meniscofemoral ligaments of Wrisberg and Humphrey reveals the intimate relationship between the PCL, the popliteus muscle, and the lateral meniscus (17). There is a disruption of the four-bar linkage that defines motion in the sagittal plane. Not surprisingly, patients receiving total knee replacements have significant alterations in their gait compared with age-matched controls (18). With certainly two, and perhaps three, components of the four-bar linkage replaced by a prosthesis, maintaining the PCL as a lone survivor of the linkage mechanism does not make intuitive sense.

Although the virtues of a posterior position of the femur on the tibia are clear, whether or not there is any advantage to femoral "rollforward" during extension

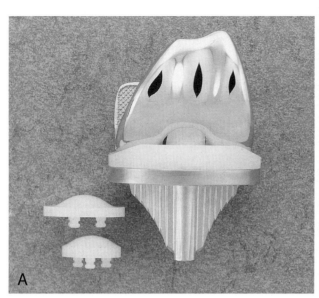

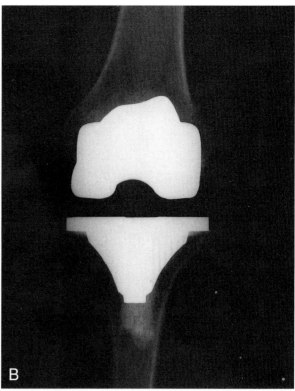

Figure 69.3. Osteonics knee. **A,** Photograph of new-generation posterior-stabilized total knee. These devices have increased modularity over earlier designs and allow the intraoperative addition of tib- ial and femoral wedges and stems to the basic components. Three-month follow-up of Osteonics Series 7000 total knee. **B,** AP radiograph of Osteonic knee.

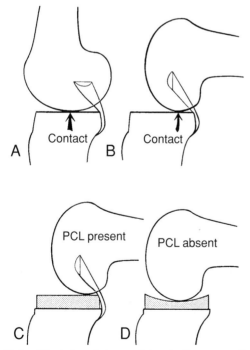

Figure 69.4. Effect of posterior cruciate retention on prosthetic design. To allow rollback with an intact PCL, the tibial surface must be flat. However, more conforming or "dished" tibial components can be used once the PCL is sacrificed. Conflicts in the kinematics can result if tibial components designed for PCL sacrifice are used when the PCL is retained. (Reproduced with permission from Insall JN, ed. Surgery of the knee. New York: Churchill Livingstone, 1984.)

must be considered. The prime force in the anterior displacement of the femur on the tibia during extension is the ACL, which is resected in most knee replacement systems. Anteroposterior displacement of the medial and lateral femoral condyles in Kinematic knees, in which the PCL is retained, is only 2.2 mm (19). This small displacement suggests that ACL resection disrupts the four-bar mechanism, resulting in uncontrolled "skidding" of the femur over the tibia rather than controlled rollback and rollforward (20).

Functional retention of the PCL requires a flattened tibial articular surface to allow the rollback that a more constrained surface would prevent. As such, sliding and rolling both occur during flexion of a PCL-retaining device. To stay within the manufacturer's recommended limit of stress on the polyethylene, it has been calculated that the femoral condyle and tibial articulating surface should have matching radii of curvature of at least 24 degrees over the entire range of flexion (20). This degree of conformity would render femoral rollback difficult, if not impossible. Conversely, sufficient mismatch of the bearing surfaces to smoothly allow rollback may create excessively high point-contact stresses (Fig. 69.7) (21, 22) and has been implicated as a causative factor in polyethylene wear (23). High point-contact stresses coupled with an unrecognized tight PCL may be responsible for significant posterior wear in some long-term follow-ups (24).

Femoral rollback also shifts the contact points with

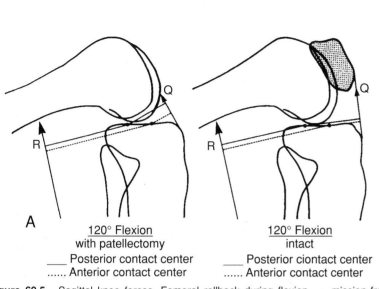
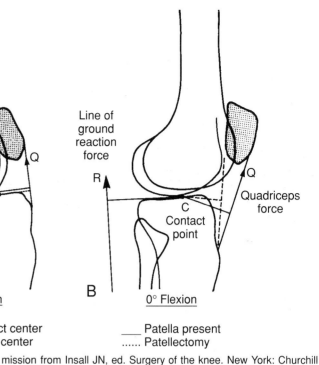

Figure 69.5. Sagittal knee forces. Femoral rollback during flexion increases the moment arm of the quadriceps. This results in approximately a 30% increase in quadriceps strength. (Reproduced with permission from Insall JN, ed. Surgery of the knee. New York: Churchill Livingstone, 1984.)

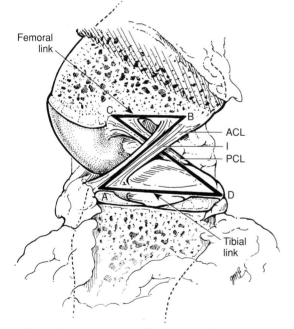

Figure 69.6. Four-bar linkage. The four-bar linkage of the knee. Each cruciate and the bone between their respective origins and insertions act like four rigid structures during knee motion.

Figure 69.7. Contact stresses. Increased conformity between the tibial and femoral components decreases the contact forces on the polyethylene. Higher stresses exist in the flat tibial component used by PCL-retaining designs than in the more "dished" component used in PCL-sacrificing and PCL-substituting total knees. (Reproduced with permission from Insall JN, ed. Surgery of the knee. New York: Churchill Livingstone, 1984.)

the tibia posteriorly. This anterior-to-posterior shifting of the contact forces with flexion and extension of the knee results in a rocking of the tibial component, which may lead to loosening (Fig. 69.8). A central fixation peg has enhanced fixation of the tibial component and excellent survivorship has been reported in both PCL-sac-

rificing and PCL-retaining designs with this type of fixation. The PCL-substituting prosthesis, however, has its resultant force vector always pointing along the tibial peg, minimizing this seesaw effect (Fig. 69.9). Although not shown clinically to have a superior loosening rate, this secondary benefit of the posterior-stabilized design may represent some insurance for those instances when less than ideal tibial alignment takes place.

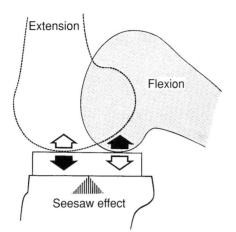

Figure 69.8. Seesaw effect on tibial surface. Femoral rollback moves the contact point between the tibia and femur posteriorly. The constant shifting of this contact point from anterior to posterior during flexion may create loosening over time. (Reproduced with permission from Insall JN, ed. Surgery of the knee. New York: Churchill Livingstone, 1984.)

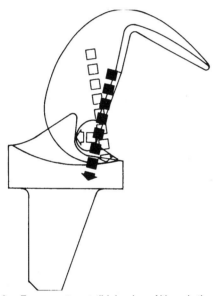

Figure 69.9. Force vector at tibial spine. Although the cam of the posterior-stabilized knee causes femoral rollback, the resultant vector of the forces about the cam pass through the fixation peg, eliminating the seesaw effect that occurs in PCL-retaining designs. (Reproduced with permission from Insall JN, ed. Surgery of the knee. New York: Churchill Livingstone, 1984.)

Clearly, the PCL is critical to the normal knee. These kinematics must be considered when contemplating total knee arthroplasty. However, substitution of this structure within the prosthetic design has far more biomechanical advantages than disadvantages. There are intraoperative advantages as well.

Intraoperative Advantages of PCL Resection

The ability to achieve exposure, particularly of the posterolateral aspect of the tibia, is very important to consistent proper placement of the tibial component. Only

good visualization of the proximal tibial anatomy, which may require excessive osteophyte resection, will regularly prevent posterior and medial component overhang. Because the tibia is difficult to sublux, this wide proximal tibial exposure may be difficult to achieve with an intact PCL. Although the PCL is present in a very high percentage of knees undergoing total knee replacement (25), histologically it is definitely involved in the arthritic process (26). The arthritic PCL is tight, contracted, attenuated, or destroyed. The intact PCL restricts access to the posterior aspect of the knee, particularly if it is tight. Loose bodies tend to accumulate in the posterior recesses of the knee and may go unnoticed or be difficult to remove with an intact PCL (Fig. 69.10).

Knee balancing is a critical step in total knee arthroplasty. Measuring the flexion and extension gaps after initial resection of distal femur and proximal tibia and subsequently adjusting either the soft tissues about the knee or the bone cuts to equalize these two dimensions are among the most important aspects of successfully implanting a prosthesis. Preserving the PCL in the face of flexion contractures and large deformities, particularly valgus, makes precise soft tissue balancing very difficult. If the PCL is resected, balancing only the medial and lateral soft tissue structures is technically easier than balancing medial, lateral, and posterior soft tissues. During the assessment of flexion and extension gaps and the process of soft tissue balancing, the tight or scarred PCL may not allow an accurate reconstruction, by maintaining a tight flexion gap. In these circumstances, recession of the PCL may be required to appropriately balance a PCL-retaining device.

Recession, or selective cutting, of some PCL fibers, is a flawed technique. Weakening the structure upon which a particular prosthetic design is based is not an ideal way to adjust the soft tissue envelope about the knee. There is a report of postoperative avulsion of the PCL with subsequent decreased function in PCL-retaining devices (27). The flexion gap, on which such cases are originally based, becomes significantly larger, resulting in instability in flexion. Routine recession, in addition, may lead to an overlengthened or nonfunctional PCL. This phenomenon may also result from overly aggressive proximal tibial resection, disrupting, to varying degrees, the origin of the PCL. In one cadaver study, the PCL failed at an average of 8.6 mm of proximal tibia resection under physiologic loads (26). Systems that incorporate a slight posterior tilt into the tibial resection guide increase the risk of weakening the PCL origin during proximal tibial resection.

Substituting for the PCL requires creating a box for the polyethylene tibial spine within the intercondylar region of the femoral component. To accommodate the prosthesis, a small block of bone (in the range of 5 to 8 cm^3) must be resected from the intercondylar notch of the distal femur (Fig 69.11). The femoral component must fit tightly into this area, but inadequate bone resection and subsequent hammering of the component into place could result in an intercondylar fracture. This bone resection is often criticized as excessive, but no additional problems specific to bone removal in this

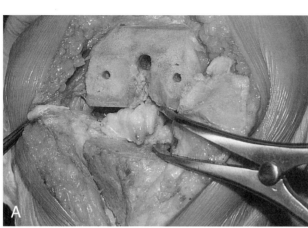
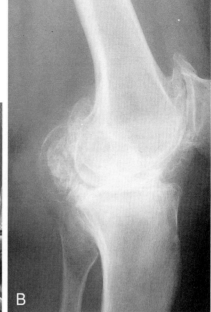

Figure 69.10. **A,** Photograph of large loose body in posterior aspect of the knee. **B,** Lateral x-ray film demonstrating large posterior osteophyte. The increased posterior exposure afforded by resection of the PCL facilitates balancing and joint debridement. Here a large osteo-phyte (**A**) is being excised from the posterior aspect of the knee. The dimensions of this osteophyte can be better appreciated in the lateral x-ray view (**B**).

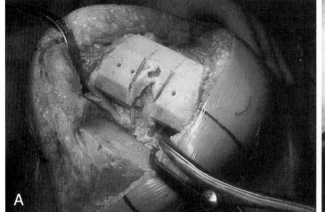
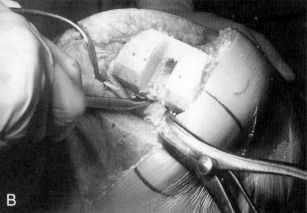

Figure 69.11. **A,** Photograph of intercondylar bone retention in PCL-retention design. **B,** Photograph of intracondylar bone resection with PCL-substituting design. The distal femur before (**A**) and after (**B**) bone resection in the intercondylar notch necessary for PCL substitution.

area have been identified. Fractures can be avoided with good surgical technique. In addition, this cutout within the femoral component has "stem-like" benefits by increasing the bone-cement interface and by providing increased resistance to femoral shear forces.

Prosthetic knees are available in a finite number of sizes. Thus, properly adjusting a knee so that it has maximal function for a "best-fit" size often requires small compromises. The ability to easily add or remove millimeters of polyethylene, to minimize bone defects or improve the balance of gaps by resecting additional bone, and to remove large posterior loose bodies or osteophytes are among the most compelling intraopera-tive reasons to resect the PCL routinely during total knee replacement.

Results of Posterior Cruciate Sacrificing/Substituting Total Knee Arthroplasty

One clear theoretical advantage of PCL-retaining devices is the absorption of shear forces by the PCL (13). In prostheses that resect the PCL, these forces are transferred to the bone-cement interface. However, this theoretical concern has not been supported by a significantly lower loosening rate in the clinical setting.

Long-term results and survivorship analyses of the total condylar knee, a cruciate-sacrificing device, have been reported by numerous investigators. Rinonapoli had an 82% good-or-excellent rating at an average of 9.5 years, with a predicted 15-year survivorship of 95% (28). Vince reported 87% good or excellent at 10 years (29). Only five patients required revisions in this series, four of which were related to initial varus malalignment. Ranawat had a clinical survivorship of 98.9% in his first 112 knees at 10 years (30). Scuderi reviewed 224 total condylar knees and found over 90% survival at 15 years (31).

Posterior-stabilized designs have also fared well over the long term. Scuderi demonstrated that the posterior-stabilized knee with an all-polyethylene tibia had a 10-year success rate of 97%, with an average annual failure rate of 0.27% (31). The metal-backed counterpart was equally successful, with 98% and 0.19% success rate and annual failure rate, respectively. Infection caused most failures, and none of the metal-backed components have yet failed for aseptic loosening. The femoral loosening rate of the posterior-stabilized design was 0.3%, which represented a significant improvement over the 0.9% rate of the total condylar. Rand reported a similar success rate, 97%, at 5-year follow-up (32). Cruciate-retaining designs fared equally well, with a 5-year success rate of 98%.

The most recent long-term follow-up by Stern and Insall demonstrated a similar success pattern for the posterior-stabilized knee up to 13 years (33). Of the 194 knees available for examination, 168 (87%) were rated as good or excellent. Survivorship analysis revealed a 0.4% average annual rate of failure and a 94% overall success rate at 13 years. Fourteen knees were revised, 5 for infection, 3 for femoral loosening, and 6 for tibial loosening (all-poly tibias). Patellofemoral symptoms were present in 12% of patients (11% grade I and 1% grade II). In addition, 7 patella fractures were identified, all of which were asymptomatic at long-term follow-up.

Several functional comparisons of PCL-substituting and PCL-retaining devices have been performed. Figgie did an x-ray study of 15 Insall-Burstein and 15 Miller-Galante, a design that retains the posterior cruciate (34). Only knees with excellent clinical results were selected for testing. The retaining designs maintained a more normal instant center of rotation and joint velocity throughout the 0 to 90 degrees of flexion tested. The instant center of rotation shifted anteriorly, and joint velocity was reduced in the Insall-Burstein knee. Gait analysis of these two designs revealed less range of motion and a forward lean during stair climbing, suggesting quadriceps weakness, in the posterior-stabilized knees (35, 36). However, these objective differences are not evident clinically (37). In fact, one third of patients preferred the posterior-stabilized and one third preferred the cruciate-retaining knee. One third of patients had no preference.

A study at the University of Pennsylvania compared the clinical results of 77 PFC total knees with posterior cruciate excision, 80 PFC posterior cruciate–retaining total knees, while 85 Insall-Burstein total knees were compared (38). Using the Knee Society score, no significant differences in any of the groups were found, except in range of motion. The PCL-retaining and PCL-sacrificed groups averaged 102 and 103 degrees of motion, respectively. The Insall-Burstein knee averaged 112 degrees of motion and was the only group where the lower 95% confidence limit exceeded 90 degrees of flexion.

Summary

As outlined above, resection and substitution for the PCL in total knee arthroplasty is superior, at least technically, to cruciate-retaining devices. The large degree of "fiddle-factor" in appropriate soft tissue balancing and creation of equal flexion and extension gaps in instances of cruciate retention can be problematic and at times, as in the presence of large deformities, warrants the resection of the PCL. This may be a concern for those who perform a limited number of knee replacements.

In terms of survivorship, PCL-retaining and PCL-substituting designs boast equivalent success without a demonstrable difference. As follow-up lengthens, polyethylene wear may prove to be a much larger concern than issues regarding mechanical stress. Unlike PCL-retaining prostheses, the increased component conformity of the posterior-stabilized devices may keep wear, and subsequently, failures to a minimum.

References

1. Scott RD, Volatile TB. Twelve year's experience with posterior cruciate-retaining total knee arthroplasty. Clin Orthop 1986;205:100–107.
2. Cobb AC, Ewald FC, Wright RJ, Sledge CB. The kinematic knee survivorship analysis of 1943 knees. Proceedings of the Annual Meeting of the British Orthopaedic Association. J Bone Joint Surg 1990;72-B:542.
3. Ritter MA, Campbell E, Faris PM, Keating EM. Long-term survival analysis of the posterior cruciate condylar total knee arthroplasty: a 10-year evaluation. J Arthroplasty 1989;4:293–296.
4. Ranawat CS, Boachie-Adjel O. Survivorship analysis and results of total condylar knee arthroplasty: eight to eleven year follow-up period. Clin Orthop 1988;226:6–13.
5. Vince, KG, Insall JN, Kelly M. The Total Condylar Prosthesis. Ten to twelve year results of a cemented knee replacement. J Bone Joint Surg 1989;71-B:793–797.
6. Scott WN, Rubenstein M, Scuderi G. Results after knee replacement with a posterior-substituting prosthesis. J Bone Joint Surg 1988;70-A:1163–1173.
7. Scuderi GR, Insall JN. The posterior stabilized knee prosthesis. Orthop Clin North Am 1989;20:71–78.
8. Freeman MAR. A three to five year follow-up of the Freeman-Swanson arthroplasty of the knee. J Bone Joint Surg 1977;59B:64–71.
9. Freeman MAR, Todd RC, Bamert P, Day WH. ICLH arthroplasty of the knee: 1968–1978. J Bone Joint Surg 1978;60B:339–344.
10. Insall JN, Ranawat CS, Scott WN, Walker P. Condylar knee replacement: preliminary report. Clin Orthop 1976;120:149–154.
11. Insall JN, Lachiewicz PF, Burstein AH. The posterior stabilized condylar prosthesis: a modification of the total condylar design. Two to four year clinical experience. J Bone Joint Surg 1982;64A:1317–1323.
12. Soudry M, Walker PS, Reilly DT, Kurosawa H, Sledge CB. Effect of total knee replacement design on femoral-tibial contact conditions. J Arthroplasty 1986;1:35–45.
13. Sledge CB. Arthroplasty of the knee. In: Evarts CM, ed. Surgery of the musculoskeletal system. New York: Churchill Livingstone, 1990:3603–3644.
14. Sledge CB, Walker PS. Total knee replacement in rheumatoid arthritis. In: Insall JN, ed. Surgery of the knee. New York: Churchill Livingstone, 1984:697.
15. O'Connor J, Shercliff T, Fitzpatrick D, Bradley J, Daniel DM, Biden E,

Goodfellow J. Geometry of the knee. In: Daniel DM, Akeson W, O'Connor J, eds. Knee ligaments: structure, function, injury, and repair. New York: Raven Press, 1990:163–199.

16. Brantigan OC, Voshell AF. The mechanics of the ligaments and menisci of the knee joint. J Bone Joint Surg 1941;23A:44–66.

17. Van Dommelen BA, Fowler PJ. Anatomy of the posterior cruciate ligament. Am J Sports Med 1989;17:24.

18. Andriacchi TP, Galante JO, Fermier RW. The influence of total knee-replacement design on walking and stair-climbing. J Bone Joint Surg 1982;64A:1328.

19. Kurosawa H, Walker PS, Abe S et al. Geometry and motion of the knee for implant and orthotic design. J Biomech 1985;18:487.

20. Freeman MAR, Railton GT. Should the posterior cruciate ligament be retained or resected in condylar nonmeniscal knee arthroplasty? The case for resection. J Arthroplasty 1988;3(suppl):3.

21. Wright TM, Bartel DL. The problem of surface damage in polyethylene total knee components. Clin Orthop 1986;205:67.

22. Landy M, Walker PA. Wear in condylar replacement knees: a 10 year follow-up. Trans Orthop Res Soc 1985;10:96.

23. Maily T, Scott WN. Posterior stabilized knee arthroplasty. In Rand JA (ed) Total knee arthroplasty. Raven Press, New York, 1993.

24. Scott RD. Personal communication. Closed meeting of the Knee Society, 1993.

25. Scott RD. Duopatellar total knee replacement: the Brigham experience. Orthop Clin North Am 1982;13:89.

26. Alexiades M, Scuderi G, Vigorita V, Scott WN. A histologic study of the posterior cruciate ligament in the arthritic knee. J Bone Joint Surg 1989;71A:153.

27. Ochsner JL, McFarland G, Baffes GC, Cook SD. Posterior cruciate avulsion in total knee arthroplasty. Orthop Rev 1993;22:1121.

28. Rinonapoli E, Mancini GB, Azzarra A, Aglietti P. Long-term results and survivorship analysis of 89 total condylar knee prostheses. J Arthroplasty 1992;7:241.

29. Vince KG, Insall JN, Kelly M. The total condylar prosthesis. Ten to 12 year results of a cemented knee replacement. J Bone Joint Surg 1989;71B:793.

30. Ranawat CS, Boachie-Adjel O. Survivorship analysis and results of total condylar knee arthroplasty. Eight to 11 year follow-up period. Clin Orthop 1988;226:6.

31. Scuderi GR, Insall JN, Windsor RE, Moran MC. Survivorship of cemented knee replacements. J Bone Joint Surg 1989;71B:798.

32. Rand JA, Ilstrup DA. Survivorship analysis of total knee arthroplasty: cumulative rates of survival of 9200 total knee arthroplasties. J Bone Joint Surg 1991;73A:397.

33. Stern SH, Insall JN. Posterior Stabilized Prosthesis: results after follow-up of nine to twelve years. J Bone Joint Surg 1992;74A:980.

34. Figgie HE, Goldberg VM, Shea K, Davy D, Singerman RB, Salwan P. A clinical kinematic comparison and a mechanical correlation of posterior or cruciate retaining versus posterior cruciate-substituting total knee prostheses. 58th Annual Meeting of the American Academy of Orthopaedic Surgeons, Anaheim, CA, March 7–12, 1991.

35. Andriacchi TP, Galante JO, Dragnich LF. Relationship between knee extensor mechanism and function following total knee replacement. In: Dorr LD, ed. The knee. Baltimore: University Park Press, 1985.

36. Andriacchi TP, Galante JO. Retention of the posterior cruciate in total knee arthroplasty. J Arthroplasty 1988;3(suppl):s13.

37. Becker-Fleugel MW, Insall JN. Bilateral total knee replacement: one cruciate-retaining and one cruciate substituting. Presented at the Annual Meeting of the Knee Society, New Orleans, LA, February 11, 1990.

38. Hirsch HS, Morrison LD, Lotke PA. The posterior cruciate ligament in total knee surgery: save, sacrifice, or substitute? Presented at the 61st Annual Meeting of the American Academy of Orthopaedic Surgeons, New Orleans, LA, February 24–March 1, 1994.

70

Constrained Knee Arthroplasty

Adolph V. Lombardi, Jr., Thomas H. Mallory, and Robert W. Eberle

Recreation of the complexities of the knee joint, concomitant with the reestablishment of its proper function, has been the primary goal of designers of prosthetic knee devices. Early attempts to substitute for the diseased knee joint were interpositional designs that did not integrate joint mobility and stability (1). This dilemma was addressed by the rigid-hinge devices that provided excellent stability but only one degree of freedom (2–4). These devices yielded promising early relief of the adverse symptoms; however, orthopaedic surgeons were confronted with a high rate of failure and ultimately recurrence of the painful syndrome (5–21). In understanding knee joint mechanics, much has been learned about the simultaneous interactions of both the soft tissues and the contoured surfaces of the knee joint (22–27). Knee motion occurs in multiple planes. Within the normal ranges of knee joint flexion/extension; varus/valgus angulation, anterior/posterior translation, rotation, rolling, and gliding all occur. With an understanding of these kinematic principles and biomechanical observations, a wide array of prosthetic devices has been developed to alleviate pain and restore stability and function. The evolution of knee prosthetic devices has led to an excess of loosely defined nomenclature by which prosthetic components are identified (28, 29). Therefore, a standard classification of design and the specific indications for each classification need to be established.

History

A complete review of the literature defines a distinct path of evolution with respect to knee prosthetic designs. The earliest attempts at articular resurfacing involved surgical interposition of soft tissues (30) and produced discouraging results. The principles of mold hip arthroplasty were extended to prosthetic replacement of the knee (31–36). McKeever designed metallic condylar inserts with modestly satisfactory results (34).

Simple mechanical principles were then used to develop rigid-hinge prostheses intended to restrict, direct, and stabilize the joint surfaces. Short-term results were reduction of knee pain and increased joint mobility. Unfortunately, these unidirectional prosthetic devices did not dampen rotational joint forces about the knee, leading to failures from limited motion, patellar pain, bone resorption, loosening, adjacent bone fractures, deep infection, and generation of patellar wear debris (5–21).

Rotational stresses were alleviated by the rotating-hinge devices (24, 37–41). The union of a ball and socket at the articulation answered the constraint imposed by rigid-hinge components. While the early rotating hinge devices showed promise, complications still arose from the surgical technique. Large amounts of bone needed to be sacrificed for implantation, thus complicating revision procedures as a result of bony deficiency.

Nonlinked knee devices were developed coincident with linked prostheses. The Charnley low-friction total hip arthroplasty promoted the use of ultra high molecular weight polyethylene (UHMPE) and polymethylmethacrylate (PMMA) as well as concepts of decreasing stresses at the prosthetic cement and cement bone interfaces (42). Gunston, who had worked with Charnley, introduced the four-part Polycentric Total Knee Arthroplasty System (Howmedica, Inc., Rutherford, NJ) in the early 1970s. Bicompartmental Knee Replacement Systems, such as the Geomedic (Howmedica, Rutherford, NJ) and the Duo Condylar (Johnson & Johnson Orthopaedics, Raynham, MA) soon followed. The persistence of patellofemoral pain following these arthroplasties led to the development of tricompartmental total knee arthroplasty systems. Two schools of tricompartmental arthroplasty developed: favoring preservation of the posterior cruciate ligament and substitution for the posterior cruciate ligament. Within the posterior cruciate substituting designs, yet another strategy was introduced, which added varus/valgus stabilization to the anterior-posterior stabilization.

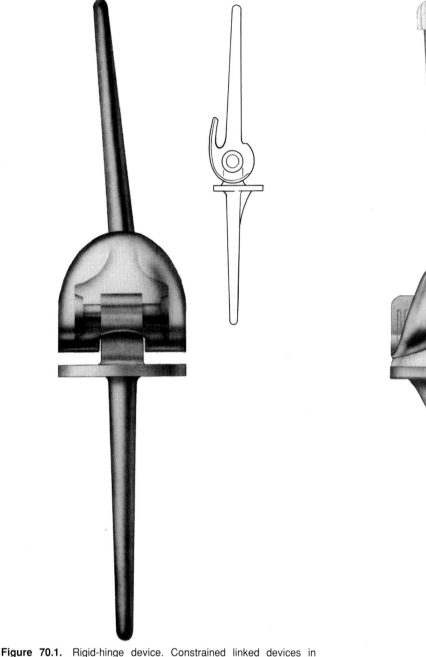

Figure 70.1. Rigid-hinge device. Constrained linked devices in which motion is restricted to flexion and extension.

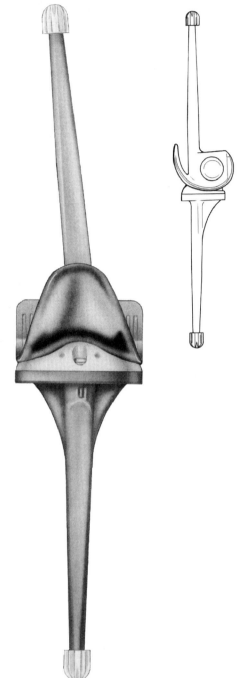

Figure 70.2. Rotating-hinge device. Constrained linked devices that allow minimal rotation within the flexion/extension axis of the knee.

Table 70.1. Prosthetic Knee Devices by Category

Linked	Nonlinked
Rigid hinge	Constrained condylar
Rotating hinge	Posterior stabilized
	Conforming condylar
	Posterior cruciate retaining

Numerous knee arthroplasty designs have evolved, but the classifications are loosely defined. Two major categories, *linked* and *nonlinked* exist (Table 70.1). Two subgroups of linked devices exist. The first is the *rigid-hinge* (Fig. 70.1). Examples include, but are not limited to, the Guepar (Howmedica, Rutherford, NJ), the St. Georg (Waldemar Link GmbH & Co., Hamburg, Germany), and the Walldius (Howmedica, Rutherford, NJ). The second subgroup is the *rotating-hinge* (Fig. 70.2). Current designs include the Finn Knee System (Biomet,

Table 70.2A.   Rotating-Hinge Total Knee Systems—Femoral Components

Company	BIOMET	Howmedica	Joint Medical Products	Link America
Design	Finn Knee System	Kinematic Rotating Hinge	Noiles S-ROM Modular Hinge	Endo Model Rotating Hinge
Ti 4Al V6 CoCr	X	X	X	X
Modular Monolithic	X	X	X	X
Anatomic profile Universal profile	X	X	X	X
Fixation Cement Cementless	X	X	X	X
Sizes (mm)	Resurfacing & Replacement One Size	Standard	XS-62 M/L 58 A/P S-66 M/L 62 A/P M-71 M/L 66 A/P	S-60 M/L M-65M/L L-75M/L
Femoral IM stems				
Straight	X (89)	X	X (Fluted & slotted)	X
Bowed	X (152)		X (150 mm)	X
Valgus angle (degrees)	7			6
Lengths (mm)	89	140–300 mm (Special orders)	100–150 mm	140, 195 (Special orders)
Diameters	89 mm 10, 11, 12, 14, 16, 18, 20, 22	11 mm—Standard	11, 13, 15, 17	12-A/P 10-M/L 13-A/P 11-M/L 15-A/P 13-M/L
	152 mm 11, 12, 13, 14, 15, 16 (Segmental)	11–14 mm Special orders		
Fixation Cement Cementless	X	X	X	X X (Fluted)
Ti 4Al V6 CoCr	X	X	X	X
Femoral augments				
Distal & posterior (comb/mm)	Segmental (cm) 10, 12, 14, 16, 18, 20, 22, 24		Sleeves M/L 20, 31, 34, 40, 46	10, 20, 30, 45, 55, 65
Distal (mm) Posterior (mm)		5, 10		
Bolt/screw Peg Cement	Morse taper bolt		Sleeves (taper) X	X X

Inc., Warsaw, IN), the Kinematic Rotating Hinge (Howmedica, Rutherford, NJ), the Link Endo Model Rotational Knee (Waldemar Link GmbH & Co., Hamburg, Germany), and the Noiles Modular Rotating Hinge Knee (Joint Medical Products Corporation, Stamford, CT) (Table 70.2, *A–D*).

The first type of nonlinked devices is the *constrained condylar* device (Fig. 70.3) that provides varus/valgus anterior-posterior stability. The Coordinate System (DePuy, Warsaw, IN), the Insall-Burstein Constrained Condylar (Zimmer, Warsaw, IN), the Kinemax Plus Super Stabilizer (Howmedica, Rutherford, NJ), the

Maxim Posterior Stabilized Constrained (Biomet, Inc., Warsaw, IN), the PressFit Condylar Constrained (Johnson & Johnson Orthopaedics, Raynham, MA), PressFit Condylar, Total Condylar III (TC-III) (Johnson & Johnson Orthopaedics, Raynham, MA), the Series 7000 PS III (Osteonics, Allendale, NJ), and the Total Condylar III (Johnson & Johnson Orthopaedics, Raynham, MA & Zimmer, Warsaw, IN) are the current and original designs within this group (Table 70.3, *A–D*).

The second type of nonlinked devices is the *posterior stabilized* prosthetic knee device (Fig. 70.4). Within this group are the DePuy Anatomic Modular Knee Posterior

Table 70.2B.   Rotating-Hinge Total Knee Systems—Tibial Components

Company	BIOMET	Howmedica	Joint Medical Products	Link America
Design	Finn Knee System	Kinematic Rotating Hinge	Noiles S-ROM Modular Hinge	Endo Model Rotating Hinge
Fixation				
Cement	X	X	X	X
Cementless				
Sizes baseplate (ML/AP)	67, 71, 75, 79, 83	One size (43) 100–200 mm length	M/L 66, 71, 76, 81, 87	S-60 mm M-65 mm L-75 mm
Ti 4Al V6				
CoCr	X	X (polyethylene and metal)	X	X
UHMWPE		X (All polyethylene)		
Sizes (mm)	Small & standard	S-64 M/L 43 A/P M-69 M/L 47 A/P	XS, S, M	M/L 60, 65, 75 mm
Thickness (mm)	10, 12, 16, 20	11–21 mm	12, 16, 21, 26, 31	8 mm
Tibial IM stems				
Size	Custom only		(Fluted & slotted)	S, M, L
Length (mm)	89	100, 200 Metal-encapsulated only	100, 150	145
Diameter	10, 11, 12, 14, 16, 18, 20, 22	Taper (11–8 mm)	9, 11, 13, 15	Taper (AP/ML) 10.5/10.5 13.0/11.5
Fixation				
Cement	X	X		X
Cementless			X	X (Fluted)
Ti 4Al V6	X		X	
CoCr		X		X
Tibial augments				
Blocks (mm)			Sleeves M/L 37, 45, 53, 61	5, 10, 15, 25
Wedges (degrees)			Blocks 4, 8, 12	
Medial		X	X	
Lateral		X	X	
Fixation				
Bolt/screw			Screw & taper (sleeves)	
Cement		X	X (blocks)	X
Tibial locking mechanism	Locking pin	Self-locking	Nonlocking rotating post	Pin/screw

Stabilized (DePuy, Warsaw, IN), the Genesis Posterior Stabilized (Smith & Nephew Richards, Inc., Memphis, TN), the Insall-Burstein II Posterior Stabilized (Zimmer, Inc., Warsaw, IN), the Kinemax Plus Stabilizer (Howmedica, Rutherford, NJ), the Kinematic II Stabilizer (Howmedica, Rutherford, NJ), and the Maxim Posterior Stabilized (Biomet, Inc., Warsaw, IN).

The third group contains the *conforming condylar* prosthetic knee devices (Fig. 70.5). Posterior subluxation is prevented in these designs by a roller-in-trough design and by tensing the collateral ligament systems. The Total Condylar Prosthesis (Johnson & Johnson Orthopaedics and Zimmer) is the original design in this group.

The final group is the *posterior cruciate retaining knee* design (Fig. 70.6). The many devices in this category include but not limited to the Anatomically Graduated Components (AGC, Biomet, Inc., Warsaw, IN), the Anatomic Modular Knee (AMK, Depuy, Warsaw, IN), the Genesis (Smith & Nephew Richards, Inc., Memphis, TN), the Maxim Knee, the Miller-Galante Total Knee Arthroplasty Systems (MG, Zimmer, Warsaw, IN), the Natural Knee (Intermedics, Austin, TX), the Porous Coated Anatomical system (PCA, Howmedica, Rutherford, NJ), the Pressfit Condylar (PFC, Johnson & Johnson Orthopaedics), and the Whiteside Ortholoc Modular Knee System (Dow Corning Wright).

The orthopaedic surgeon has many choices. Knowing the categories of devices assists the surgeon in selecting systems that will achieve the maximum outcome.

Table 70.2C. Rotating-Hinge Total Knee Systems—Patellar Components

Company	BIOMET	Howmedica	Joint Medical Products	Link America
Design	Finn Knee System	Kinematic Rotating Hinge	Noiles S-ROM Modular Hinge	Endo Model Rotating Hinge
Patella				
Dome (M/L)	S, M, L	S, M, L	30, 32, 35, 38	S-30 M-35 L-40
Offset (M/L)				30, 35, 40
Inset			X	X
UHMWPE	X	X	X	X
Metal-backed	X			
Pegs (#)	1	1	3	1
Tracking				
Deepened groove	X		X	
Shallow groove				X
Funnel-shaped groove				
Lateral rise			X	

Table 70.2D. Rotating-Hinge Total Knee Systems—Component Mechanics

Company	BIOMET	Howmedica	Joint Medical Products	Link America
Design	Finn Knee System	Kinematic Rotating Hinge	Noiles S-ROM Modular Hinge	Endo Model Rotating Hinge
ROM				
Flexion/extension (degrees)	0/135	–5/unlimited	–6/120	–3/165
Rotation				
Internal (degrees)	20	15	Limited by soft tissue	30
External (degrees)	20	15	Limited by soft tissue	30

Indications

The primary goals of total knee arthroplasty involve relief of pain, restoration of function, and provision for stability. While these are the definitive goals, the surgeon must remember the concepts of prosthetic longevity and durability (43). Generally, the least prosthetic constraint required to accomplish these goals should be used. Walker has emphasized the overwhelming success of the condylar-type designs; however, sometimes designs of increasing constraint must be used (44). The joint replacement surgeon must be cognizant of these specific indications.

Rigid-Hinge Prosthetic Devices

There are few current indications for rigid-hinge devices, as a consequence of unsatisfactory results in both primary and revision total knee arthroplasty (5–21). Collateral ligament incompetence with weakness or deficiency of the extensor mechanism is the major current indication for a rigid-hinge device (37, 38, 41). These devices are restricted to patients whose only other option is arthrodesis or resection arthroplasty. Limb salvage procedures for malignancy may represent the largest number of patients within this category of prosthetic knee devices (45).

Rotating-Hinge Prosthetic Devices

Dampening the rotational torque stress inherent in *rigid-hinge* knee arthroplasty was the major objective of *rotating-hinge* knee arthroplasty designs (24, 37, 38, 40, 41). Very few patients are candidates for *rotating-hinge* knee arthroplasty. They generally have deficiencies of both collateral ligaments but still retain a satisfactory extensor mechanism. Patients whose knee arthroplasty involves the use of a large segmental distal femoral allograft in the treatment of tumor or osteopenic periprosthetic distal femoral fracture can be effectively managed with a long-stem *rotating-hinge* device (46, 47). Patients identified for reconstructive arthroplasties complicated by extreme imbalance of flexion/extension gaps may be candidates for arthroplasty with a *rotating-hinge* design (Fig. 70.7). Dislocation of *constrained condylar* designs supports the use

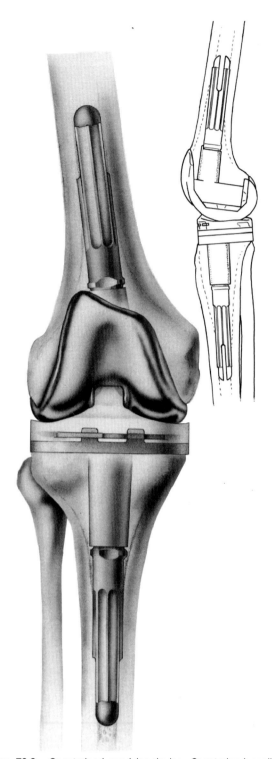

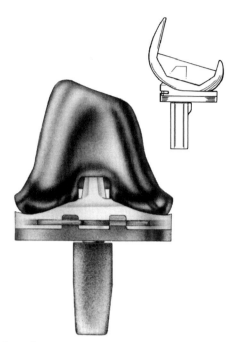

Figure 70.4. Posterior stabilized device. Nonlinked devices that substitute for the posterior cruciate ligament by means of a polyethylene spine that articulates within a femoral cam.

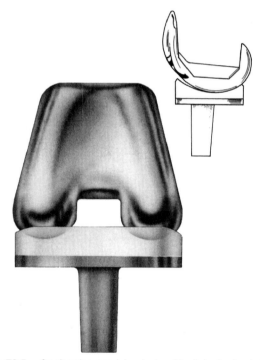

Figure 70.3. Constrained condylar device. Constrained nonlinked devices that provide varus/valgus stability as well as anterior/posterior stability.

Figure 70.5. Conforming condylar device. Nonlinked roller-in-trough design that depends on appropriate tension of the collateral ligament systems to prevent posterior subluxation.

Table 70.3A. Constrained Condylar Total Knee Systems—Femoral Components

Company	BIOMET	DePuy	Howmedica	J & J	J & J	Osteonics	Zimmer
Design	Maxim Posterior Stabilized Constrained	The Coordinate System	Kinemax Plus Super Stabilizer	PressFit Condylar Constrained	PressFit Condylar: Total Condylar III	Series 7000 Posterior Stabilized III	Insall-Burstein Constrained Condylar
Ti 4AI V6 CoCr	X	X	X	X	X	X	X
Modular Monolithic	X	X	X	X	X	X	X
Anatomic profile Universal profile	X	X	X	X	X	X	X
Femorotibial Interchangeability							
Full Limited	X	X	X	X	X	X	X
Fixation Cement	X	X	X	X	X	X	X
Cementless				X	X	X	
Sizes (ML/AP)	60/43, 65/49 70/53, 75/57	61/52, 68/58 74/64, 81/70 86/76	S 65/57 M 70/62 L 75/66	1-50/54 2-55/60 3N-51/63 3-61/88 4-65/71 5-69/73 6-74-78	1-50/54 2-55/60 3-61/88 4-65/71 5-69/73	3-51/54 5-55.5/59 7-60/64 9-64.5/69 11-69/74 13-73.5/79	60/42, 65/46.2, 70/50.5
Femoral IM stems							
Straight Bowed	X X (160 mm)	X	X	X	X	X	X X (150 mm)
Valgus offset (degrees)	7	6	7	5, 7, 9, (90, 130) 7 (125, 175)	5, 7, 9, (90, 130) 7 (125, 175)	7	5
Lengths	80, 120, 160 >15 mm OD (Slotted and fluted)	50, 70, 95, 110, 140 (Fluted and smooth)	40, 80, 155 80, 155 (Fluted)	90, 130 125, 175 (Fluted)	90, 130 125, 175 (Fluted)	115, 165 (Fluted)	25, 40, 75, 150 (Fluted)
Diameters	80 mm 10, 12, 13, 14, 15, 16, 17, 18, 19, 20, 22, 24 120/160 mm 12, 14, 16, 18, 20, 22	8, 10, 12, 14, 16, 18, 20, 22, 24, 26	15.5–7.5 mm (Taper) 13, 14, 15, 16, 17, 18,19, 20, 21, 22, 23 (Fluted)	13, 15 10, 12, 14, 16, 18, 20, 22, 24 (Fluted)	13, 15 10, 12, 14, 16, 18, 20, 22, 24 (Fluted)	10, 12, 14, 16, 18, 20, 22, 24	25/40/75 mm 10, 12, 13, 14, 15, 16, 17, 18, 19, 20, 22, 24 150 mm 10, 13, 15
Cement	80 (11, 13, 15 OD)	X	X (Taper)	X (13, 15 OD)	X (13, 15 OD)		
Cementless	X	X	X	X	X	X	X
Ti 4A1 V6	X			X	X		X
CoCr		X	X			X	
Femoral augments							
Distal & posterior (combined/mm)			4 (S, M, L)	4, 6, 8	4, 6, 8	D:8 P:4	5.5, 10.5
Distal (mm)	6, 10	4, 10	S, M, L	4, 6, 8	4, 6, 8, 12, 16	4, 8	5, 10
Posterior (mm)	6, 10	4, 8	S, M, L	4, 6, 8	4, 6, 8	4	
Fixation Cement		X	X	X	X		
Bolt/screw	X	Peg		Snap	Screw/snap	X	X

Table 70.3B. Constrained Condylar Total Knee Systems—Tibial Components

Company	BIOMET	DePuy	Howmedica	J&J	J&J	Osteonics	Zimmer
Design	Maxim Posterior Stabilized Constrained	The Coordinate System	Kinemax Plus Super Stabilizer	PressFit Condylar Constrained	PressFit Condylar: Total Condylar III	Series 7000 Posterior Stabilized III	Insall-Burstein Constrained Condylar
Baseplate sizes (ML/AP)	59/38, 63/41 67/43, 71/46 75/48, 79/51 83/53, 87/56 91/58	63/43, 66/46 72/48, 73/50 76/53, 81/55 83/57, 86/60 90/62	S 65/41 M 70/45 L 76/48	2-64/43 3N-87/45 3-71/47 4-78/51 5-83/55 6-89/59	1-58/38 2-64/43 3-71/47 4-78/51 5-83/59	3-40/60.4 5-43.5/65.7 7-47/71 9-50.5/76.3 11-54/81.6 13-57.5/86.9	59/44, 64/48 70/52, 75/56 81/60
Ti 4Al V6	X			X	X		X
CoCr		X	X			X	
Polyethylene Thickness (mm)	10, 12, 14, 16 18, 20, 22, 24	10, 12, 14, 16, 18 20, 22, 24, 26	10, 12, 15, 18, 21, 25	10, 12.5, 15, 17.5, 20, 22.5, 25, 30	10, 12.5, 15, 17.5, 20, 22.5, 25, 30	8, 10, 12, 15, 18, 21, 24	10, 12, 15, 18, 21
Tibial locking mechanism	Locking bar	Pin & clip	Slide & snap	Slide & snap	Slide & snap	Self-locking	Locking clip with dovetail
Reinforced tibial post		X	X	X	X	X	X
Tibial IM stems							
Length	80, 120 (Fluted) ≥15 (OD) (Slotted) 80 mm-cement 11, 13, 15	50, 70, 95, 110, 140 (Fluted and smooth)	40, 80, 155 80, 155 (Fluted)	30, 60 75, 115, 150 (Fluted)	30, 60 75, 115, 150 (Fluted)	105, 155	25, 40, 75, 150 (Fluted)
Diameter	80 mm 10, 12, 13, 14, 15, 16, 17, 18, 19, 20, 22, 24 120 mm 12, 14, 16, 18, 20, 22	8, 10, 12, 14, 16, 18, 20, 22, 24, 26	15.5-7.5 mm (Taper) 13, 14, 15, 16, 17, 18, 19, 20, 21, 22, 23 (Fluted)	13, 15 10, 12, 14, 16, 18, 20, 22, 24 (Fluted)	13, 15 10, 12, 14, 16, 18, 20, 22, 24 (Fluted)	10, 12, 14, 16, 18, 20, 22, 24	10, 12, 13, 14, 15, 16, 17, 18, 19, 20, 22, 24 150 mm 10, 13, 15 (Fluted)
Cement	80 (11, 13, 15 OD)	X	X (Taper)	X (13, 15 OD)	X (13, 15 OD)		
Cementless	X	X	X	X	X	X	X
Ti 4Al V6	X			X	X		X
CoCr		X	X			X	
Tibial augments							
Blocks (mm)	6, 10, 16	4, 10	10, 20, 30, 40 S, M, L (7.5 mm thick)	10, 15	10. 15	4, 8	5, 10
Wedges (degrees)	10	5, 10, 15 (nonmodular)		10, 15, 20	Full, 10, 15, 20	5, 10	7, 13, 16, 20, 26
Medial	X	X	X	X	X	X	Half/full
Lateral	X	X	X	X	X	X	Half/full
Fixation							
Cement		X	X	X	X	X	
Bolt/screw	X				X		X

of *rotating-hinges* when extreme imbalance of flexion/extension gaps exist (48). Finally, patients whose surgical exposure is performed by the "femoral peel approach" as described by Windsor and Insall may require a *rotating-hinge* design (49, 50).

Constrained Condylar Prosthetic Devices

Constrained condylar prosthetic devices differ from the *rigid-hinge* devices and *rotating-hinge* devices in being nonlinked. These designs incorporate an intracondylar notch in the femoral component and an ex-

Table 70.3C. Constrained Condylar Total Knee Systems—Patellar Components

Company	BIOMET	DePuy	Howmedica	J&J	J&J	Osteonics	Zimmer
Design	Maxim Posterior Stabilized Constrained	The Coordinate System	Kinemax Plus Super Stabilizer	PressFit Condylar Constrained	PressFit Condylar: Total Condylar III	Series 7000 Posterior Stabilized III	Insall-Burstein Constrained Condylar
Concentric round dome	30, 32, 34, 36	32, 34, 38, 40		25, 28, 32, 28, 32, 35, 38, 41	25, 28, 32, 28, 32, 35, 38, 41	5-35 7-38 9-41 11-44	32, 34, 36, 38, 40
Offset dome			36, 40, 44 (9, 9.5, 10 mm thick)			7-38 9-41 11-44	
Inset	25 only			X (25, 28, 32, 28, 32, 35, 38, 41)	X (25, 28, 32, 28, 32, 35, 38, 41)	X (5-35, 7-38 9-41, 11-44)	X (32, 34, 36, 38)
UHMWPE	X	X	X	X	X	X	X
Metal-backed		X				X (Inset)	X
Pegs (#)	1	Concentric grooves	3	1	1	3	3
Tracking (groove) Deepened	X	X		X	X		
Shallow							
Funnel-shaped	X		X			X	
Lateral rise	X	X				X	

Table 70.3D. Constrained Condylar Total Knee Systems—Component Mechanics

Company	BIOMET	DePuy	Howmedica	J&J	J&J	Osteonics	Zimmer
Design	Maxim Posterior Stabilized Constrained	The Coordinate System	Kinemax Plus Super Stabilizer	PressFit Condylar Constrained	PressFit Condylar: Total Condylar III	Series 7000 Posterior Stabilized III	Insall-Burstein Constrained Condylar
Range of motion Flexion/extension (degrees)	−7/130	−5/120	−5/130	−5/115	−5/115	−5/135	−5/120
Rotation Internal (degrees)	2	2		1.5	1.5	2	3
External (degrees)	2	2		1.5	1.5	2	3

tended tibial spine on the tibial component. The articulation of the tibial spine within the intracondylar notch affords stability with reference to anterior/posterior, varus/valgus, and rotation (51–58). The Total Condylar III knee arthroplasty system is the original design within this category (Fig. 70.8). There are several *constrained condylar* designs. Modularity, multiple stem options, wedge options, augments, and an increasing number of sizes characterize these arthroplasty systems. These prosthetic systems are effectively summarized in Table 70.3, *A–D*. Collateral ligament deficiency is the most notable indication for the *constrained condylar* systems in both primary and revision total knee arthroplasty (58–60).

Knee arthroplasty complicated by severe preoperative deformity, bony deficiency, and ligamentous instability (Fig. 70.9) may require a constrained condylar device (Table 70.3, *A–D*). The surgeon has many options for effectively customizing the prosthetic device during surgical intervention. Severe deformity is treated by appropriate ligamentous release, and stability is provided by the constrained articulation. Bony deficiency is addressed with the use of a combination of stems, wedges, and augments. Recent reports of posterior dislocation of posterior stabilized arthroplasties lend consideration to the use of the *constrained condylar* devices in which there is imbalance of flexion/extension gaps (Fig. 70.7) (61–66). Furthermore, patients with a type II valgus de-

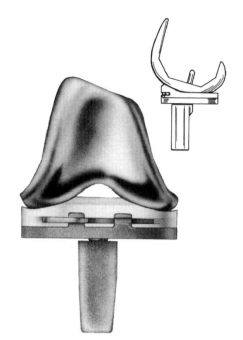

Figure 70.6. Posterior cruciate retaining device. Nonlinked resurfacing devices.

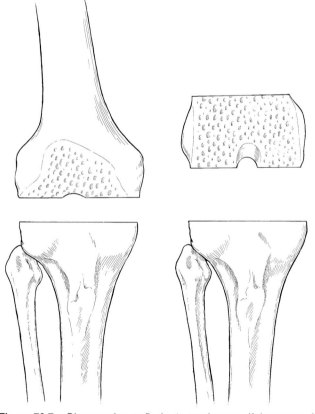

Figure 70.7. Disproportionate flexion/extension gap. If the cause of a disproportionate flexion/extension gap is bony deficiency, then this should be treated by augmentation of the posterior femoral condyles. However, if the cause is ligamentous incompetency, then a *rotating-hinge* device should be considered.

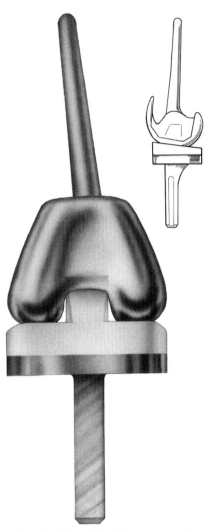

Figure 70.8. The Total Condylar III represents the original *constrained condylar* design.

formity (medial collateral ligament instability) as described by Krackow may be effectively treated with a *constrained condylar* prosthetic device (Fig. 70.10) (67). The two other options available for these patients are a medial collateral ligament advancement, which requires modification of the postoperative physical therapy and rehabilitation program (67) (Fig. 70.11), or ligamentous balancing with an excessively thick tibial component, which significantly alters the patellotibial femoral dynamic (23) (Fig. 70.12) and also is associated with a higher incidence of peroneal palsy.

Posterior Stabilized Devices versus Posterior Cruciate Retaining Devices

Considerable controversy exists about the posterior cruciate ligament (49, 68, 69). Some support routine sacrifice of the posterior cruciate ligament, arguing that this ligament is part of the deforming force and noting that it is extremely difficult to appropriately tense this ligament through the full range of motion while per-

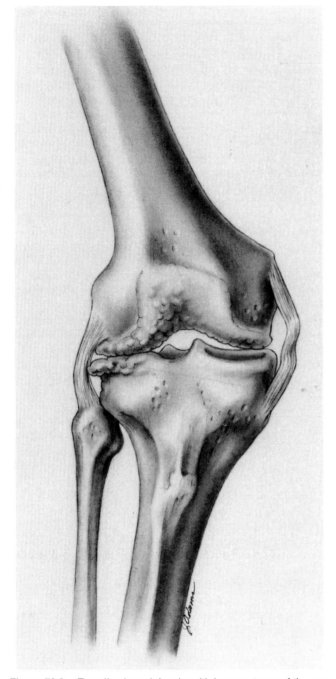

Figure 70.9. Type II valgus deformity with incompetency of the medial collateral ligament.

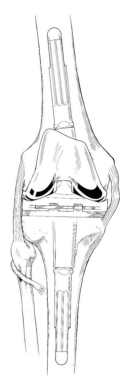

Figure 70.10. Type II valgus deformity treated with a *constrained condylar* device. Note maintenance of the joint line.

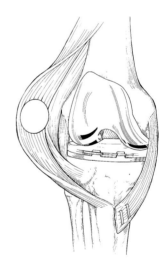

Figure 70.11. Type II valgus deformity treated with advancement of the medial collateral ligament.

forming the arthroplasty (70). Others argue for preservation of the posterior cruciate ligament in all situations, noting its function in promoting femoral rollback and, thus, enhancing flexion. They further emphasize that it is one of the strongest ligaments in the body and, therefore, is a significant stabilizing structure within the knee (71).

Laskin has suggested that there are specific situations in which the posterior cruciate ligament is best preserved or sacrificed (72). Patients with significant angular deformity and flexion contractures are candidates for sacrifice of the posterior cruciate ligament and use of a posterior stabilized device. Patients with minimal deformity can be effectively treated with a posterior cruciate retaining device.

Conforming Condylar Devices

The *conforming condylar* devices are roller-in-trough designs such as the Total Condylar. Stability is afforded by tension of the collateral ligament systems. In light of

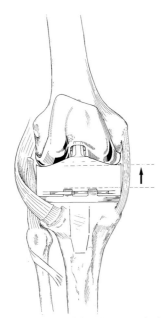

Figure 70.12. Type II valgus deformity treated with a *posterior stabilized* device and a thick polyethylene insert. Note alteration of the joint line as well as the possibility for stretch palsy of the peroneal nerve.

the advantages of the posterior stabilized arthroplasty as documented by Insall et al. (73–75), the conforming condylar devices are rarely indicated or used (76).

Surgical Technique

A thorough assessment of the preoperative status of the patient will help the surgeon select the proper prosthetic device. In degree of preoperative deformity, the status of the ligamentous structures about the knee and the extent of bony deficiency are of paramount importance in the decision. Minimally deformed knees may be addressed with posterior cruciate retaining devices. Knees with combined varus or valgus deformity and flexion contractures can be appropriately treated with posterior cruciate substituting devices. Knees with combined deformities, deficiencies of the collateral ligament systems, and bone loss can best be handled with *constrained condylar* designs. When there is total loss of the collateral ligament systems, then *rotating-hinge* arthroplasty is considered, and in extreme salvage situations, *rigid-hinge* arthroplasty (Table 70.4).

The surgical technique must restore knee kinematics and biomechanics. Constrained arthroplasty systems are capable of enhanced fixation with medullary stems. This provides the additional necessary fixation and restores alignment in that the stems are attached at a 5 to 7 degree valgus angle for the femoral component and at a 90 degree angle for the tibial component. There is a trend toward the use of stems in a press-fit cementless fashion (77). The impetus for press-fit stems has been to avoid stress shielding and facilitate revision. Successful knee arthroplasty must restore the anatomical joint line. To accomplish this, the *constrained condylar* devices provide augmentation of the distal as well as the poste-

rior femoral condyles. The normal joint line is approximately 1.5 cm distal to the medial femoral epicondyle (78). Therefore, surgeons reconstructing knees in the face of bony deficiency can use distal femoral augments to reestablish the femoral joint line. There is extreme difficulty in utilizing bone grafts or polymethylmethacrylate to augment the posterior femoral condyles. Some of the *constrained condylar* systems offer the surgeon the ability to augment the posterior femoral condyle. Reestablishment of the anterior/posterior femoral dimension assists in the development of the correct flexion gap and, therefore, in the ultimate balance of the flexion/extension gaps.

The difficult arthroplasty that requires a constrained implant may pose special problems of surgical exposure, component removal (in the case of revision surgery), and reconstruction of bone defects. Since constrained devices use medullary stem fixation, the femoral and tibial canals are identified and reamed to appropriate depth and diameter. The femoral and tibial resection must be performed with the concept of restoration of the joint line. The average thickness of currently available femoral components is approximately 1 cm, as is the relative thickness of the tibial base plate of the polyethylene insert. Therefore, resections of approximately 1 cm for the tibia and femur should each be approximately 1 cm from the original joint line. With intramedullary alignment systems, the tibial resection is carried out perpendicular to the tibial axis and the femoral resection at 5 to 7 degrees valgus, as indicated by the prosthetic device being considered. In the case of revision knee arthroplasty with significant bony deficiency, the principles of reestablishment of the original femoral and tibial joint lines and the subsequent effect on patellar positioning must be considered. Ranawat has noted that the femoral joint line should be established 1.5 cm distal to the medial femoral condyle (78). Also, Insall and Salvati reported that the tibial joint line is a relative distance proximal from the patellar tendon insertion and that this distance is approximately one-half the length of the patellar tendon (96). With these concepts in mind, the surgeon can assess the extent of augmentation required for the distal femur and proximal tibial plateau.

Appropriate-size implants for the femur and tibia must be selected. Most systems have guides to assist in the selection of the appropriate-size implant in primary situations. However, in revision situations, consideration of the size of the prosthetic implant removed and review of the preoperative roentgenograms to assess the level of posterior condylar resection performed at the time of primary arthroplasty will help the physician select the proper-size femoral component. In certain prosthetic devices, the proximal tibial dimension dictates the size of the femoral component. Other systems have full and complete interchangeability, and therefore, the size of the tibial component has no bearing and no influence on the size of the femoral component (Table 70.3, *A–D*). Once the size selection has been made and the appropriate anterior/posterior chamfer and intracondylar resections are executed, a trial reduction can be performed with the prosthetic devices. With

Deformity

Bone loss

Contracture

Ligamentous instability

Osteopenia

Table 70.4. Distribution of Prosthetic Devices by Classification

Minimal	Moderate	Severe	Salvage
Posterior Cruciate Retaining	Conforming Condylar	Constrained Condylar	Rotating-Hinge
			Rigid-Hinge
	Posterior Stabilized	Stems	
		Wedges	
		Augments	

respect to the femur, the surgeon should assess the degree of fit of the stem with the intramedullary canal and the appropriateness of augmentation of the distal and/or posterior femoral condyles. With respect to the proximal tibia, again, the surgeon must assess the degree of fixation of the intramedullary stem and the fit of the augmentations if they have been used. I prefer to use the rectangular block tibial augments as opposed to wedge augments, because there is a plethora of literature describing an increased incidence of loosening with varus or valgus malalignment (97–104). Furthermore, Fehring et al. recently reported that "block augmentation appears to stress the proximal tibia more uniformly than wedge augmentation" (88).

Once the trial implants have been seated, the surgeon must assess the competency of the medial and lateral collateral ligaments. I prefer to evaluate ligamentous stability with a posterior stabilized trial insert rather than the posterior stabilized constrained insert. This will offer the surgeon a better assessment of the competency of the collateral ligaments. Release of the contracted side should be performed and balanced, bearing in mind the concepts of preservation of the joint line as previously described. Then appropriate tibial polyethylene thickness is selected to effectuate a stable prosthetic complex. The next step is implantation of the prosthesis. There still exists a significant controversy as to whether these prosthetic units should be inserted with or without polymethylmethacrylate. The hybrid technique in which the surfaces of the distal femur and proximal tibia are coated with polymethylmethacrylate and the stems are placed with press-fit fixation has been described in the literature (77) and remains my choice.

The final step in the surgical exercise is a standard closure. If a Coonse-Adams or a modified V-Y quadricepsplasty (Fig. 70.13) was used, then closure should be performed with the knee slightly flexed, as described by Sculco and Faris (92). A tibial tubercle osteotomy must be repaired as described by Whiteside (94). If either of the above have been used for the operative approach, postoperative physical therapy and rehabilitation must be modified accordingly.

Results of Constrained Total Knee Arthroplasty

Multiple complications of rigid-hinge arthroplasty, including septic and aseptic loosening; patellar subluxation, dislocation, and fracture; femoral fracture; tibial

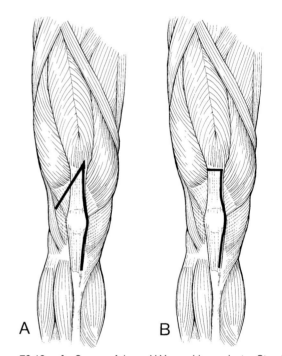

Figure 70.13. **A,** Coonse-Adams V-Y quadricepsplasty. Standard medial peripatellar arthrotomy is performed. The dissection is then carried across the quadriceps tendon into the lateral retinaculum. **B,** Rectus snip. Standard medial peripatellar arthrotomy. Approximately four finger breadths proximal to the superior pole of the patella. The transverse incision in the quadriceps tendon is made to effectuate a fractional lengthening.

fracture; and implant failure, have been reported (5–21). With follow-up ranging from 1 to 7 years, revision rates have been noted to be from 6 to 22% (Tables 70.5 and 70.6). Rigid-hinge arthroplasty has been recommended in a select group of salvage knee arthroplasties when arthrodesis represents the only other effective alternative. Favorable results with the St. Georg rigid-hinge arthroplasty and the Link Endo model rotational arthroplasty, however, are reported by Englebrecht and Heinert (37). They promote a philosophy of varying the degree of constraint to accommodate various patient profiles. Significant complication and revision rates have been reported with rotating-hinge devices (Tables 70.7 and 70.8). As with *rigid-hinge* arthroplasty, most

Table 70.5. Rigid Hinge Devices (Primary)

Author	Component	n	Follow-Up (years)	Good–Excellent (%)	Fair (%)	Poor (%)	Average Survival (%)	Post HSS[a]
Bargar (5)	GUEPAR	39	2–4	–	–	–	87	–
Cameron (7)	GUEPAR II	8	1–7	–	–	–	–	–
Deburge (8)	GUEPAR	92	2	–	–	–	–	–
Engelbrecht (37)	St. Georg	1154	10	–	–	–	–	–
Freeman (9)	Walldius	80	–	78	16	6	88	–
Grimer (10)	Stanmore	83	7 (max)	–	–	–	80	–
Habermenn (11)	Walldius	18	1–3.5	–	–	–	89	–
Hoikka (12)	GUEPAR	55	5	–	–	–	75	–
Hui (13)	GUEPAR	77	3.3	–	–	–	76	–
Insall (14)	GUEPAR	45	2–3.5	69	22	9	96	72.5
Jones (15)	GUEPAR	108	1–3	61	10	29	90	–
Jones (16)	Walldius	45	1–7	–	–	–	93	–
Oglesby (1)	Walldius	90	6	–	–	–	91	76
Phillips (18)	Walldius	67	3.5	–	–	–	81	–
Wilson (20)	Walldius	42	6	–	–	–	90	–

[a]HSS, Hospital for Special Surgery.

Table 70.6. Rigid Hinge Devices (Revision)

Author	Component	n	Follow-Up (years)	Good–Excellent (%)	Fair (%)	Poor (%)	Average Survival (%)	Post HSS
Bargar (5)	GUEPAR	17	2–4	–	–	–	24	–
Cameron (7)	GUEPAR II	21	1–7	–	–	–	–	–
Deburge (8)	GUEPAR	11	2	–	–	–	–	–
Karpinski (17)	Stanmore	52	4	23	48	29	90.4	–

Table 70.7. Rotating Hinge Devices (Primary)

Author	Component	n	Follow-Up (years)	Good–Excellent (%)	Fair (%)	Poor (%)	Average Survival (%)	Post HSS
Engelbrecht (37)	ENDO Model	1074	6	–	–	–	–	–
Finn (24)	Finn	25	1	–	–	–	92	–
Kaufer (108)	Spherocentric	82	4	–	–	–	95	–
Matthews (109)	Spherocentric	58	8	–	–	–	85	–
Murray (110)	Herbert	35	–	–	–	–	85	–
Rand (39)	Kinematic	15	2–6	33	–	–	80	–
Shindell (40)	Noiles	18	5	33	11	56	78	–
Sonstegard (41)	Spherocentric	25	2–3	–	–	–	100	–

authors recommend that *rotating-hinge* devices be used in patients with significant soft tissue deficiency.

A number of reports on results of the Total Condylar III prosthesis are outlined in Tables 70.9 and 70.10. This prosthetic device has been used in both primary and revision arthroplasty. We, as well as others, have reported and described the specific indications for the use of this design, as outlined in this manuscript. Our results and those of others are somewhat inferior to results with the less-*constrained condylar* devices. However, the patients who require this prosthesis have significant preoperative deformities and significant ligamentous defi-

Table 70.8.   Rotating Hinge Devices (Revision)

Author	Component	n	Follow-Up (years)	Good–Excellent (%)	Fair (%)	Poor (%)	Average Survival (%)	Post HSS
Rand (39)	Kinematic	23	2–6	70	–	–	57	–

Table 70.9.   Constrained Condylar (Primary)

Author	Component	n	Follow-Up (years)	Good–Excellent (%)	Fair (%)	Poor (%)	Average Survival (%)	Post HSS[a]
Chotivichit (51)	TC-III	9	2–8	89	11	0	100	77.0
Donaldson (52)	TC-III	17	5	100	0	0	100	82.5
Hohl (53)	TC-III	6	6.1	66	–	–	100	73.3
Kavolus (54)	TC-III	5	5	100	0	0	100	93.4
Kraay (47)	TC-III	14	4	36	50	14	86	OA:69 RA:82
Lombardi (57)	TC-III	65	3–10	98	2	0	100	88.0

[a]HSS, Hospital for Special Surgery.

Table 70.10.   Constrained Condylar (Revision)

Author	Component	n	Follow-Up (years)	Good–Excellent (%)	Fair (%)	Poor (%)	Average Survival (%)	Post HSS[a]
Chotivichit (51)	TC-III	18	4	78	17	5	–	74
Donaldson (52)	TC-III	14	2–8	50	7	43	64.0	51.2
Kavolus (54)	TC-III	11	4.2	45	45	10	–	84
Kim (59)	TC-III	14	2–6	–	–	–	100	81
Kraay (47)	TC-III	17	4	65	11	24	82.4	OA:80 RA:70
Lombardi (56)	TC-III	64	2–5	74	11	15	92.0	78.4 in situ
Rand (105)	TC-III	21	4	50	25	25	–	73
Rosenberg (60)	TC-III	36	3.8	69	17	11	91.7	77
Wilde (111)	TC-III	11	2.7	73	27	0	91.0	83.3

[a]HSS, Hospital for Special Surgery.

ciencies. As outlined, current modifications of the Total Condylar III involve the incorporation of a large size inventory, press-fit noncemented intramedullary stems, and metallic augments and wedges. Montgomery et al. (77) and Rand (105) propose that the use of these newer designs will yield improved results with the *constrained condylar* systems.

With respect to our personal experience, from 1980 to the present, 4233 total knee arthroplasties have been performed at our institution, representing 3510 primary and 723 revision total knee arthroplasties. The type of arthroplasty performed according to prosthetic device is outlined in Table 70.11. Review of this information will reveal a bias toward the *posterior stabilized* prosthesis. *Constrained condylar* devices, *rotating-hinge* devices, and *rigid-hinge* devices have been used in both

Table 70.11.   Joint Implant Surgeons, Inc. Total Knee Arthroplasties Performed by Category

Category	Primary	Revision
Linked		
Rigid hinge	0	4
Rotating hinge	15	103
Nonlinked		
Constrained condylar	205	279
Posterior stabilized	2366	319
Conforming condylar	0	0
Posterior cruciate retaining	924	18
Total	3510	723

Figure 70.14. **A,** Survival analysis for primary total knee arthroplasty. **B,** Survival analysis for revision total knee arthroplasty.

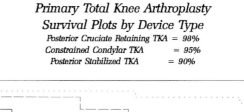

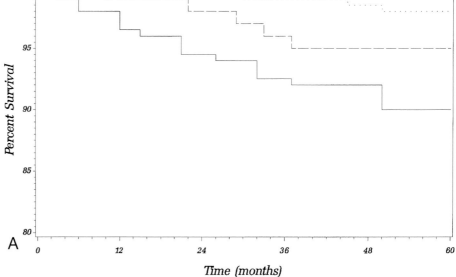

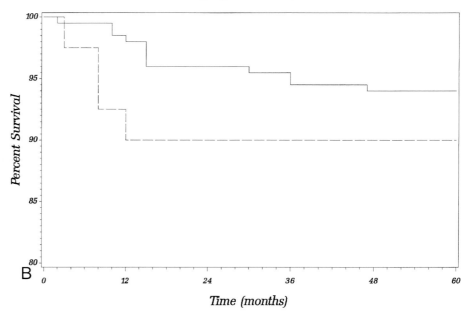

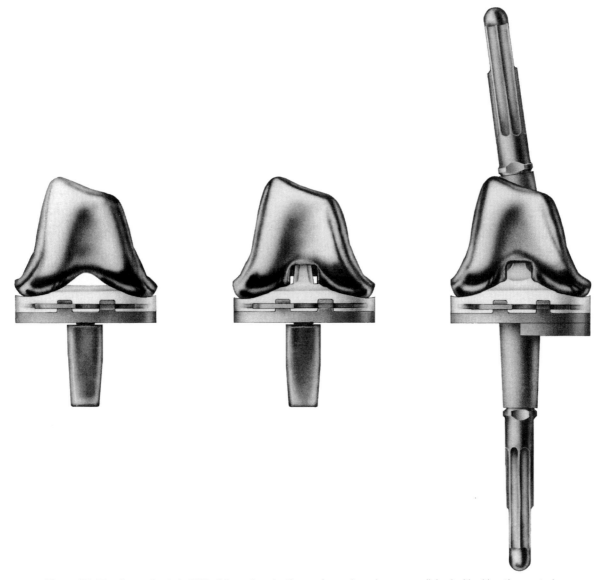

Figure 70.15.   Approximately 99% of the arthroplasties performed can be accomplished with either the *posterior cruciate retaining* design, the *posterior stabilized* design, or the *constrained condylar* design.

the primary and revision situation, in accordance with the indications outlined in this chapter. Survival analysis is provided in Figure 70.14, *A* and *B*.

Conclusion

With the inevitable graying of America, the number of total knee arthroplasties performed annually continues to increase. Our present practice of total knee arthroplasty represents the current combination of evolution in concepts and designs (Fig. 70.15). Condylar total knee arthroplasties of the posterior cruciate retaining and posterior stabilized designs have recently been reported

to have 12-year survivorship above 90% (106, 107). Although most arthroplasties can be performed with either of these two devices, a number of complex primary and revision arthroplasties still require constrained devices. In light of the complexities confronted in this patient population, results with constrained knee arthroplasty tend to be somewhat inferior to those of nonconstrained arthroplasty. However, in patients with compromised bone and soft tissue anatomy, the patient and the surgeon have limited options. Using the concepts presented in this chapter, the surgeon can effectively match the patient with the appropriate prosthetic device and thus maximize the results of total knee arthroplasty.

References

1. Oglesby JW, Wilson FC. The evolution of knee arthroplasty. Clin Orthop 1984;186:96–103.
2. Jones GB. Arthroplasty of the knee by the Walldius prosthesis. J Bone Joint Surg 1968;50-B(3):505–510.
3. Merryweather R, Jones GB. Total knee replacement: the Walldius arthroplasty. Orthop Clin North Am 1973;4(2):585–596.
4. Phillips RS. Shiers' alloplasty of the knee. Clin Orthop 1973;94:122–127.
5. Bargar WL, Cracchiolo A, Amstutz HC. Results with the constrained total knee prosthesis in treating severely disabled patients and patients with failed total knee replacements. J Bone Joint Surg 1980;62–A(4):504–512.
6. Besser, MIB. Bilateral Attenborough total knee replacement as a single procedure. Arch Orthop Trauma Surg 1983;101:271–272.
7. Cameron HU, Jung YB. Hinged total knee replacement: indications and results. Can J Surg 1990;33(1):53–57.
8. Deburge A, GUEPAR. Guepar hinge prosthesis: complications and results with two years' follow-up. Clin Orthop 1976;120:47–53.
9. Freeman PA. Walldius arthroplasty: a review of 80 cases. Clin Orthop 1973;94:85–91.
10. Grimer RJ, Karpinski MRK, Edwards AN. The long-term results of Stanmore total knee replacements. J Bone Joint Surg 1984;66-B(1):55–62.
11. Habermann ET, Deutsch SD, Rovere GD. Knee arthroplasty with the use of the Walldius total knee prosthesis. Clin Orthop 1973;94:72–84.
12. Hoikka V, Vankka E, Eskola A, Lindholm TS. Results and complications after arthroplasty with a totally constrained knee prosthesis (GUEPAR). Ann Chir Gynaecol 1989;78:94–96.
13. Hui FC, Fitzgerald RH, Jr. Hinged total knee arthroplasty. J Bone Joint Surg. 1980;62-A (4):513–519.
14. Insall JN. Total knee replacement. In: Insall JN, ed. Surgery of the knee. New York: Churchill Livingstone, 1984:587–695.
15. Jones EC, Insall JN, Inglis AE, Ranawat CS. GUEPAR knee arthroplasty results and late complications. Clin Orthop 1979;140:145–152.
16. Jones GB. Total knee replacement—the Walldius hinge. Clin Orthop 1973;94:50–57.
17. Karpinski MRK, Grimer RJ. Hinged knee replacement in revision arthroplasty. Clin Orthop 1987;220:185–191.
18. Phillips H, Taylor JG. The Walldius hinge. J Bone Joint Surg 1975;57-B(1):59–62.
19. Roscoe MW, Goodman SB, Schatzker J. Supracondylar fracture of the femur after GUEPAR total knee arthroplasty: a new treatment method. Clin Orthop 1989;241:221–223.
20. Wilson FC, Fajgenbaum DM, Venters GC. Results of knee replacement with the Walldius and Geometric prostheses. J Bone Joint Surg 1980;62–B(4):497–503.
21. Wilson FC, Venters GC. Results of knee replacement with the Walldius prosthesis: an interim report. Clin Orthop 1976;120:39–46.
22. Dorr LD, Boiardo RA. Technical considerations in total knee arthroplasty. Clin Orthop 1986;205:5–11.
23. Figgie HE, Goldberg VM, Heiple KG, Moller HS, Gordon NH. The influence of tibial-patellofemoral location on function of the knee in patients with the posterior stabilized condylar knee prosthesis. J Bone Joint Surg 1986;68–A(7):1035–1040.
24. Finn HA, Kneisl JS, Kane LA, Simon MA. Constrained endoprosthetic replacement of the knee. [Abstract] 6th International Symposium on Limb Salvage. Montreal, Quebec, Canada, September 10, 1991.
25. Ranawat CS. The patellofemoral joint in total condylar knee arthroplasty: pros and cons based on five- to ten-year follow-up evaluations. Clin Orthop 1986;205:93–99.
26. Ranawat CS, ed. Total-condylar knee arthroplasty. New York: Springer–Verlag, 1985.
27. Riley LH. Total knee arthroplasty. Clin Orthop 1985;192:34–39.
28. Laskin RS. The spectrum of total knee replacement. In: Laskin RS, Denham RA, Apley AG, eds. Replacement of the knee. New York: Springer-Verlag, 1984:11–45.
29. Scott, NW. Constraint in total knee arthroplasty. In: Goldberg VM, ed. Controversies in total knee arthroplasty. New York: Raven Press, 1991:19–25.
30. Verneuil A. De la creation d'une fausse articulation par section ou resection partielle de l'os maxillaire inferieur, comme moyen de remedier a l'ankylose vraie ou fausse de la machoire inferieure. Arch Gen Med 1860;15(Ser. 5):174.
31. Aufranc OE. Arthroplasty: constructive hip surgery with Vitallium mold arthroplasty. A report of 1000 cases of arthroplasty of the hip over a fifteen-year period. J Bone Joint Surg 1957;39A:237–248. In: Petty W, ed. Total joint replacement. Philadelphia: WB Saunders, 1991:7.
32. Campbell W. Arthroplasty of the knee. J Orthop Surg 1921:3:430. In: Petty W, ed. Total joint replacement. Philadelphia: WB Saunders, 1991:3–18.
33. Jones WN, Aufranc OE, Kermond WL. Mould arthroplasty of the knee. J Bone Joint Surg 1967:49-A(5):1022. In: Petty W, ed. Total joint replacement. Philadelphia: WB Saunders, 1991:11.
34. McElfresh E. History of arthroplasty. In: Petty W, ed. Total joint replacement. Chap 1. Philadelphia: WB Saunders, 1991:3–18.
35. Moore AT. Hip joint surgery: an outline of progress made in the past forty years. Columbia, South Carolina, 1963. In: Petty W, ed. Total joint replacement. Philadelphia: WB Saunders, 1991:9.
36. Smith-Petersen MN. Evolution of mould arthroplasty of hip joint. J Bone Joint Surg 1948:30-B:59–75. In: Petty W, ed. Total joint replacement. Philadelphia: WB Saunders, 1991:7.
37. Engelbrecht E, Heinert K. Experience with a surface and total knee replacement: further development of the model St. Georg. In: Niwa S, Paul JP, Yamamoto S, eds. Total knee replacement. Tokyo: Springer-Verlag, 1988:257–273.
38. Nieder E. Rotationsprothese, rotatiosknie und scharnieprothese Modell St. Georg und Endo-Modell: differentialtherapie in der primaren kniegelenkalloarthroplastik. Orthopade 1991;20:170–180.
39. Rand JA, Chao EYS, Stauffer RN. Kinematic rotating-hinge total knee arthroplasty. J Bone Joint Surg 1987;69-A(4):489–497.
40. Shindell R, Neumann R, Connoly JF, Jardon OM. Evaluation of the Noiles hinged knee prosthesis: a five-year study of seventeen knees. J Bone Joint Surg 1986;68-A(4):579–585.
41. Sonstegard DA, Kaufer H, Matthews. Biomechanical testing and clinical trials. J Bone Joint Surg 1977;59-A(5):602–616.
42. Charnley J, ed. Friction arthroplasty: theory and practice. New York: Springer-Verlag, 1979.
43. Stulberg BN, Hupfer T. Indications and preoperative planning for total knee arthroplasty. In: Petty W, ed. Total joint replacement. Philadelphia: WB Saunders, 1991:3–18.
44. Walker PS. Requirements for successful total knee replacements: Design considerations. Orthop Clin North Am 1989;20(1):15–29.
45. Sim FK, Chao EYS. Prosthetic replacement of the knee and large segment of the femur or tibia. J Bone Joint Surg 1979;61-A(6):887–892.
46. DiGioia AM, Rubash HE. Periprosthetic fractures after total knee arthroplasty. Clin Orthop 1991;271:135–142.
47. Kraay MJ, Goldberg VM, Figgie MP, Figgie HE. Distal femoral replacement with allograft/prosthetic reconstruction of supracondylar fractures in patients with total knee arthroplasty. J Arthrop 1992;7(1):7–16.
48. Sydney SV, Mallory TH. Dislocation of a constrained knee prosthesis: two case reports. Complications Orthop 1989;4(3):93–97.
49. Andriacchi TP, Galante JO. Retention of the posterior cruciate in total knee arthroplasty. J Arthrop 1988;(suppl):S13-S19.
50. Windsor RE, Insall JN. Exposure in revision total knee arthroplasty: the femoral peel. Techniques Orthop 1988;3(2):1–4.
51. Chotivichit AL, Cracchiolo A, Chow GH, Dorey F. Total knee arthroplasty using the total condylar III prosthesis. J Arthrop 1991;6(4):341–350.
52. Donaldson WF, Sculco TP, Insall JN, Ranawat CS. Total Condylar III knee prosthesis: long-term follow-up study. Clin Orthop 1988;226:21–28.
53. Hohl WM, Crawford E, Zelicof SB, Ewald FC. The total Condylar III prosthesis in complex knee reconstruction. Clin Orthop 1991;273:91–97.
54. Kavoulus CH, Faris PM, Ritter MA, Keating EM. The total Condylar III knee prosthesis in elderly patients. J Arthrop 1991;6(1):39–43.
55. Kraay M, Goldberg VM, Figgie MP, Figgie HE, Fisher DA. Technical factors influencing the results of total condylar III knee arthroplasty. Am J Knee Surg 1988;1(2):125–133.
56. Lombardi AV, Mallory TH, Troop JK, Vaughn BK. Total condylar III prosthesis in revision total knee arthroplasty. [Abstract] Mid-American Orthopaedic Association. Hilton Head Island, South Carolina, April 28 to May 2, 1993.
57. Lombardi AV, Mallory TH, Vaughn BK, Pruis DT, Troop JK. The total condylar III prosthesis in complex primary total knee arthroplasty: a three–to-ten year clinical and radiographic evaluation. [Abstract] The Ninth Combined Meeting of the Orthopaedic Associations of the English-Speaking World. Toronto, Ontario, Canada, June, 1992.
58. Sculco TP. Total condylar III in ligament instability. Orthop Clin North Am 1989;20(2):221–226.
59. Kim YH. Salvage of failed knee arthroplasty with a total condylar III type prosthesis. Clin Orthop 1987;221:272–277.
60. Rosenberg AG, Verner JJ, Galante JO. Clinical results of total knee revision using the total condylar III prosthesis. Clin Orthop 1991;273:83–90.
61. Cohen B, Consyant CR. Subluxation of the posterior stabilized total knee arthroplasty: a report of two cases. J Arthrop 1992;7(2):161–163.
62. Galinet BJ, Vernace JV, Booth RE, Rothman RH. Dislocation of the posterior stabilized total knee arthroplasty: a report of two cases. J Arthrop 1988;3(4):363–367.

63. Gebhard JS, Kilgus DJ. Dislocation of a posterior stabilized total knee prosthesis: a report of two cases. Clin Orthop 1990;254:225–229.
64. Lombardi AV, Mallory TH, Vaughn BK, Krugel R, Honkala TK, Sorscher M, Kolczun M. Dislocation following primary posterior stabilized total knee arthroplasty. J Arthrop 1993;8(6):633–639.
65. Sharkey PF, Hozack WJ, Booth RE, Balderston RA, Rothman RH. Posterior dislocation of total knee arthroplasty. Clin Orthop 1992;278:128–133.
66. Striplin DB, Robinson RP. Posterior dislocation of the Insall/Burstein II posterior stabilized total knee prosthesis. Am J Knee Surg 1992;5(2):79–83.
67. Krackow KA, ed. The technique of total knee arthroplasty. St. Louis: CV Mosby, 1990.
68. Dorr LD, Ochsner JL, Gronley J, Perry J. Functional comparison of posterior cruciate-retained versus cruciate sacrificed total knee arthroplasty. Clin Orthop 1988;236:36–43.
69. Freeman MAR, Railton GT. Should the posterior cruciate ligament be retained or resected in condylar nonmeniscal knee arthroplasty? The case for resection. J Arthrop 1988;3(suppl):S3-S12.
70. Corces A, Lotke PA, Williams JL. Strain characteristics of the posterior cruciate ligament in total knee replacement. [Abstract] American Academy of Orthopaedic Surgeons. Las Vegas, Nevada, February 9–14, 1989.
71. Aglietti P, Buzzi R. Posteriorly stabilized total-condylar knee replacement: three to eight years' follow-up of 85 knees. J Bone Joint Surg 1988;70–B(2):211–216.
72. Laskin RS, Rieger M, Shchob C, Turen C. The posterior stabilized total knee prosthesis in the knee with severe fixed deformity. Am J Knee Surg 1988;1:199–203.
73. Insall JN, Kelly M. The total condylar prosthesis. Clin Orthop 1986;205:43–48.
74. Insall JN, Ranawat CJ, Aglietti P, Shine J. A comparison of four models of total-knee replacement prostheses. J Bone Joint Surg 1976;58-A(6):754–765.
75. Insall JN, Scott WN, Ranawat CS. The total condylar knee prosthesis: a report of two-hundred and twenty cases. J Bone Joint Surg 1979;61–A(2):173–180.
76. Insall JN, Lachiewicz PF, Burstein AH. The posterior stabilized condylar prosthesis: a modification of the total condylar design. J Bone Joint Surg 1982;64–A(9):1317–1323.
77. Montgomery WH, Haas SB, Insall JN, Becker MS, Windsor RE. Revision total knee arthroplasty for aseptic failure using metal-backed tibial and custom implants. [Abstract] The Knee Society: Scientific Meeting. Washington, D.C., February 23, 1992.
78. Ranawat CJ. Personal communication, 1991.
79. Lotke PA, Wong RY, Ecker ML. The use of methylmethacrylate in primary total knee replacements with large tibial defects. Clin Orthop 1991;270:288–294.
80. Ritter MA. Screw and cement fixation of large defects in total knee arthroplasty. J Arthrop 1986;1:125–129.
81. Brooks PJ, Walker PS, Scott RD. Tibial component fixation in deficient tibial bone stock. Clin Orthop 1984;184:302–308.
82. Dorr LD, Ranawat CS, Sculco TP, McKaskill B, Orisek BS. Bone graft for tibial defects in total knee arthroplasty. Clin Orthop 1986;205:153–165.
83. Gross AE, McKee NH, Pritzker KPH, Langer F. Reconstruction of skeletal deficits at the knee. Clin Orthop 1983;174:96–106.
84. Windsor RE, Insall JN, Sculco TP. Bone grafting of tibial defects in primary and revision total knee arthroplasty. Clin Orthop 1986;205:132–137.
85. Brand MG, Daley RJ, Ewald FC, Scott RD. Tibial tray augmentation with modular metal wedges for tibial bone stock deficiency. Clin Orthop 1989;248:71–79.
86. Laskin RS. Total knee arthroplasty in the presence of large bony defects of the tibia and marked knee instability. Clin Orthop 1989;248:66–70.
87. Walker PS, Greene D, Reily D, Thatcher J, Ben-Dov M, Ewald FC. Fix-
ation of tibial components of knee prostheses. J Bone Joint Surg 1981;63-A:258–267.
88. Fehring T, Peindl R, Frick S, Humble R. Augmentation wedges versus blocks for deficient bone stock in total knee arthroplasty. [Abstract] Second Annual Meeting of the Association for Arthritic Hip and Knee Surgery. Dallas, Texas, November 13–15, 1992.
89. Craig SM. Soft tissue considerations. In: Scott NW, ed. Total knee revision arthroplasty. Orlando: Grune & Stratton, 1987:99–112.
90. Coonse K, Adams JD. A new operative approach to the knee joint. Surg Gynecol Obstet 1943;77:344.
91. Nichols DW, Dorr LD. Revision surgery for stiff total knee arthroplasty. J Arthrop 1990;5(suppl):S73-S77.
92. Sculco TP, Faris PM. Total knee replacement in the stiff knee. Techniques Orthop 1988;3(2):5–8.
93. Vince KG, Insall JN, Kelly MA. The total condylar prosthesis: 10- to 12-year results of a cemented knee replacement. J Bone Joint Surg 1989;71–B(5):793–797.
94. Whiteside LA, Ohl MD. Tibial tubercle osteotomy for exposure of the difficult total knee arthroplasty. Clin Orthop 1990;260:6–9.
95. Firestone TP, Krackow KA. Removal of femoral components during revision knee arthroplasty. J Bone Joint Surg 1991;73-B(3):514.
96. Insall JN, Salvati E. Patella position in the normal knee joint. Radiology 1971;101:101–104.
97. Aglietti P, Rinonapoli E. Total condylar knee arthroplasty: a five-year follow–up study of 33 knees. Clin Orthop 1984;186:104–111.
98. Cooke TDV, Pichora D, Siu D, Scudamore RA, Bryant JT. Surgical implications of varus deformity of the knee with obliquity of joint surfaces. J Bone Joint Surg 1989;71-B(4):560–565.
99. Elia EA, Lotke PA. Results of revision total knee arthroplasty associated with significant bone loss. Clin Orthop 1991;271:114–121.
100. Krackow KA, Jones MM, Teeny SM, Hungerford DS. Primary total knee arthroplasty in patients with fixed valgus deformity. Clin Orthop 1991;273:9–18.
101. Lombardi AV, Mallory TH, Pruis DT, Troop JK, Vaughn BK. Total condylar III prosthesis in complex primary total knee arthroplasty: a three-to-ten-year clinical and radiographic evaluation. [Abstract] 59th Annual Meeting of the American Academy of Orthopaedic Surgeons Washington, D.C., February 20–25, 1992.
102. Lotke PA, Ecker ML. Influence of positioning of prosthesis in total knee replacement. J Bone Joint Surg 1977;59-A(1):77–79.
103. Rose HA, Hood RW, Otis JC, Ranawat CS, Insall JN. Peroneal-nerve palsy following total knee arthroplasty: a review of the Hospital for Special Surgery experience. J Bone Joint Surg 1982;64-A(3):347–351.
104. Teeny SM, Krackow KA, Hungerford DS, Jones M. Primary total knee arthroplasty in patients with severe varus deformity: a comparative study. Clin Orthop 1991;273:19–31.
105. Rand JA. Revision total knee arthroplasty using the total condylar III prosthesis. J Arthrop 1991;6(3):279–284.
106. Gill GS, Mills DM. Ten to sixteen year follow-up of cemented total knee arthroplasties (TKA). Second Annual Meeting of the Association for Arthritic Hip and Knee Surgery. Dallas, Texas, November 13–15, 1992.
107. Stern SH, Insall JN. Posterior stabilized prosthesis: results after follow-up of nine to twelve years. J Bone Joint Surg 1992;74-A(7):980–986.
108. Kaufer H, Matthews LS. Spherocentric arthroplasty of the knee: clinical experience with an average four-year follow-up. J Bone Joint Surg 1981;63–A(4):545–559.
109. Matthews LS, Goldstein SA, Kolowich PA, Kaufer H. Spherocentric arthroplasty of the knee: a long-term and final follow-up evaluation. Clin Orthop 1986;205:58–66.
110. Murray DG, Wilde AH, Werner F, Foster D. Herbert total knee prosthesis: combined laboratory and clinical assessment. J Bone Joint Surg 1977;59–A(8):1026–1032.
111. Wilde AH, Schickendantz MS, Stulberg BN, Go RT. The incorporation of tibial allografts in total knee arthroplasty. J Bone Joint Surg 1990;72–A(6):815–824.

71

Roentgen Stereophotogrammetric Analysis (RSA) of Knee Prostheses

Leif Ryd

Bone reacts to the presence of foreign material such as prosthetic implants, and this reaction is inherently connected to the problem of implant fixation. Hence the question of whether an implant will stay fixed and function over long periods of time or whether it will loosen is largely a question of how the bone reacts. This reaction occurs in the interface between the two materials, and in the living patient, this reaction can only be studied by indirect radiographic methods such as plain radiography, scintigraphy, and more recently, CT and MR.

Using such methods, a radiolucent zone can be seen between the bone and the foreign cement, prosthetic metal, or polymer (1, 2). Histologically, this zone consists of soft tissue ranging from loose or even necrotic fibrous tissue to highly organized fibrocartilage (3–8). This membrane was noticed previously by Walldius (9) who named it the "para-prosthetic" membrane, alluding to the parodontic membrane that bonds teeth to the jaws. He suggested that it should be regarded as a natural reaction of the bone to the new demands of the foreign material. By dissipating peak stresses, Walldius even thought it was beneficial for fixation, a notion supported by others (10). Other studies, however, have shown that this membrane is weak, that rifts and hemorrhages occur, and that prostheses often loosen through a breakdown of this membrane (3, 6, 11). The bone can also, under certain conditions, react in much the opposite way and integrate the implant in a very secure bond that has been termed "osseointegration" (12, 13). This type of reaction has been studied extensively in dentistry and formed an entire concept that is in clinical use and gives almost 100% success after 10 years if the implant has become fixed.

The interface is defined as the two-dimensional film that initially separates the bone from the foreign material. In terms of mechanical loosening and its prevention, the reactions in the bone underneath the "interface" is of greater interest. Therefore, a better working definition of the interface should be the three-dimensional

soft tissue membrane and an additional amount of bone that penetrates to an arbitrary depth into the prosthetic bed. This entire interface "reacts" to the implantation of a prosthesis by forming different kinds of soft tissue in a healing and maturation process not unlike that of fracture healing (14, 15).

Loss of fixation implies motion. Studies of fixation should include investigation of motion. Such motion could occur in response to forces, in which case the results correspond directly to the question of bond strength as a function of time, i.e., migration. Migration involves a biologic process that alters the prosthetic bed without indicating how loose the prostheses is at a particular moment in time.

Motion of prosthetic implants in response to cyclic load can be reproduced in the laboratory. Numerous such reports have been published (16–22). To study the biologic processes in conjunction with migration, in vivo studies become a necessity, and radiographic methods are called for. Conventional radiography, however, has an accuracy, or resolution, of only 2 to 3 mm (7, 23–25), inadequate for these studies. Attempts to increase the accuracy by external calibration frames (26) and other methods have been made (27), but only with true stereogrammetry did the accuracy became sufficient. Of a number of such systems (28–30), perhaps the best known is that of the Swedish physician and engineer, the late Goran Selvik.

Selvik Roentgen Stereophotogrammetric Analysis (RSA)

The RSA system combined the principles of bone markers for exact identification of landmarks, stereophotogrammetry for three-dimensional data, and high-precision digitizing with rigid-body kinematics to describe the motion between the two objects of interest. These techniques had been used individually in the past. Bone markers had been used in studies of the spine (31);

stereogrammetry was attempted shortly after the discovery of roentgen rays (32) and further developed by Hallert (33). Rigid-body kinematics is even older (34). With modern microcomputers they formed together a formidable instrument, applicable to almost any part of the skeletal system.

After attempts with rod-shaped markers and different materials, notably stainless steel, Selvik settled for spherical markers of tantalum to establish landmarks. Tantalum has the advantage of being a heavy metal (atomic number, 73) that gives distinct images on radiographic films. Under certain conditions, the tantalum markers can be implanted into other metal objects (i.e., prosthetic implants), and by choosing proper radiographic exposure data, these markers can be "seen" within the prosthesis. Furthermore, tantalum is inert in body fluids, resulting in "osseointegration" (35).

To date, several tens of thousands of markers have been implanted in almost any part of the body in living patients without adverse reactions. It is imperative that the markers are deposited in such a way that they are firmly seated and cannot move within the bone (see below). To achieve this, the markers are introduced into the bone, usually during surgery, by using heavy cannulas and a spring-loaded piston. In this way, precision can be achieved without hammer blows or the like. In reality, the cannulas are heavy enough to penetrate cancellous bone. Thus, percutaneous insertion into the metaphyses of the long bones, the pelvis, or vertebral bodies is possible under local anesthesia (and fluoroscopy, when necessary).

In each object of interest (e.g., bone and prosthetic component, two bones), at least three noncolinear markers must be inserted to allow kinematic analysis. To safeguard against unstable markers and for redundancy, four to six, up to nine, markers may be used in each object of interest. For maximum accuracy, the markers should be spread out to make the intermarker distances as large as possible.

In polyethylene prosthetic components, the markers are usually introduced into slightly undersized holes created with a dental drill, or the markers are included in the manufacturing process. As pointed out above, titanium objects can often be marked by inserting tantalum balls into the titanium (36, 37) (Fig. 71.1), while chrome-cobalt or steel objects usually must be marked by metal protrusions (38) (Fig. 71.2). Recently, wear of polyethylene bearing surfaces has caused considerable problems, especially in knee prostheses, raising the possibility that insertion of markers in the polyethylene may decrease its wear resistance. A recent finite element analysis (FEM) has shown that stresses increase in the polyethylene immediately surrounding the bead (39). A marker should not be placed directly under the point of load; placement at least 5 mm away from this area is quite safe.

The RSA system consists of two alternatives; a biplanar and a convergent-ray mode (for larger body segments). The radiographic exposures are obtained by discharging two x-ray tubes simultaneously. For practical purposes, this can be done by using one ceiling

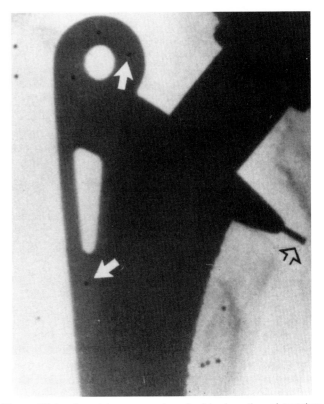

Figure 71.1. A metal component marked by insertion of tantalum markers within the core metal, in this case a thin lateral flange of chrome-cobalt. Usually, only titanium implants can be marked this way. (Reproduced with permission from Wykman A, Selvik G, Goldie I. Subsidence of the femoral component in the noncemented total hip: a roentgen stereophotogrammetric analysis. Acta Orthop Scand 1988;59:635–637.)

mounted unit and one bedside unit, discharged by one trigger button each. In specially arranged RSA laboratories, two generators can be controlled by the same trigger for perfect coordination. The RSA examination involves exposure of both the patient and a calibration object, usually taken simultaneously.

In the biplanar mode, which yields slightly better accuracy especially in depth, and which is usually sufficient for a knee examination, the exposures are obtained with the knee inside a calibration cage (Fig. 71.3). In the hip, simultaneous calibration can be obtained using an object behind the examination top (Fig. 71.4). In situations where the cage is too confined (e.g., when bending or motion is required), the calibration can be done with reference planes between the cage and the cassettes. The cage is removed after calibration, and the reference planes of plexiglass with tantalum markers are retained to refer the subsequent patient examinations to the proper set of calibration films. When separate calibration films are used, the radiographic setup (i.e. the x-ray tubes and the cassette holder with the reference planes) must not be moved during the subsequent patient examination.

The calibration objects have markers of exactly known position in two planes for each focus. The markers in the plane adjacent to the film—fiducial marks—

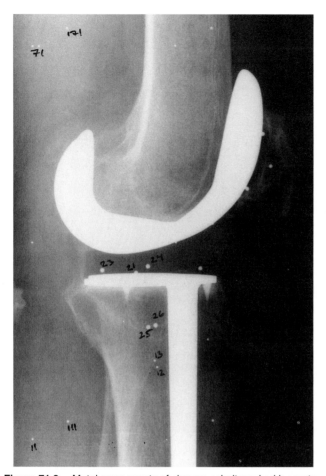

Figure 71.2. Metal components of chrome-cobalt marked by protrusions from the core metal.

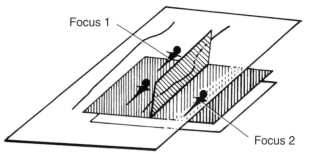

Figure 71.4. The convergent-ray setup of RSA. The fiducial marks are positioned in the plane above the two radiographic films. The control points are situated in the vertical plane and are exposed on both radiographic films. With this calibration object, simultaneous calibration and patient examination can be performed also with the convergent-ray alternative. Simultaneous calibration safeguards against accidental motion within the radiographic setup during the investigation.

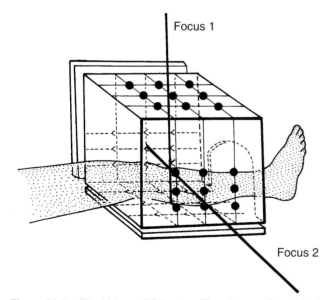

Figure 71.3. The biplanar RSA setup. The planes adjacent to the film cassettes contain the fiducial markers defining the cage coordinate system. The planes distant to the film cassettes contain the control points by which the position of the foci are determined.

define the laboratory coordinate system; the markers in the distant plane—control points—are used to determine the position of each x-ray focus. A film-focus distance of 100 cm with the central beam centered on the center marker for each focus is preferable but not critical. Indeed the rays sometimes have to be oblique to avoid interference with other metal objects in the examined area, notably prosthetic implants.

The exposure characteristics are chosen to give a low absorbed radiation dose, i.e., the kV is set high. This gives radiographs of rather low quality, which is of little importance as long as the images of the tantalum markers are distinct. In RSA studies of inducible displacement or those using film-exchanger technique, a considerable number of radiographs are obtained during one examination. Measurements during stress examinations for inducible displacement (see below) have shown the absorbed dose (mean 15 radiographs) to be about 80% of that during a routine knee examination (40).

The position of the body segment in the laboratory coordinate system (i.e., the orientation of the axes) is determined at the first examination, and the extremity should be aligned as parallel to the long axis of the cage as possible. Since this is often a postoperative examination with a patient in discomfort, correct alignment can be difficult. Should the alignment be judged to be excessively out of order, a "rotate" subroutine in the RSA system reorients the coordinate system to achieve proper alignment.

Analysis of the radiographs starts by assigning each marker image an identification number, which should correspond on both stereoradiographs. This is not always achieved initially, and corrections may be required later in the computations. Subsequently the images are digitized using any high-precision digitizer with precision better than 10 to 20μm, and the x and y coordinates are stored in a PC-clone microcomputer (AT version with a math coprocessor and a minimum of 1 Mb RAM) (Fig. 71.4).

Using the control points in the calibration objects, the positions of the foci are calculated, and the subsequent measurement of the patient marker images defines two points on a straight line (the computed focus and the measured image of the marker on the radiographic film). Given two foci, two such lines will intersect at the 3-D position of the patient marker. Because of measurement and other errors, the crossing lines will not intersect perfectly, and the coordinates of the midpoint of the shortest intercrossing line vector is provisionally chosen to represent the marker position, and all possible combinations of crossing lines 1000 μm are stored in a reserve file. By feeding a number of sets of 3-D coordinates from different time points into the program KINEMA and using Euler rigid-body kinematics (34), motion of the prosthesis is derived and expressed relative to the reference object (30). This last stage also involves "solving of the rigid body," i.e., ascertaining the proper numbering of the markers at each time point and the proper combination of crossing lines.

Since the mathematics of rigid-body kinematics depend on rigidity, this factor is meticulously controlled in the system. This is done by minimizing the "mean error of rigid body fitting" (ME) according to the formula:

$$ME = \sqrt{(a^2 + b^2 + c^2 + \ldots n^2)/n}$$

where a, b, $c \ldots n$ represent the residual 3-D vectors of the individual markers after optimizing the rotation matrix and subtracting the rigid body displacement, using a least-squares method. This "solving of the rigid body" may sometimes be extremely laborious, and software (KINERR) has been designed to assist in the proper numbering of the markers and to find the correct coupling of crossing lines (41). "Solving of the rigid bodies" is always possible, but sometimes unstable markers must be excluded to reach a reasonably small ME. Occasionally, all or most markers are found to be unstable and the whole case has to be excluded. In the final analysis, however, the RSA system is adequately safeguarded against the possibility that data presented as motion between two bodies in reality are due to unstable markers moving within one of these bodies.

Motion of the object of interest is presented relative to the reference object as rotations about, and translations along, the three cardinal axes defined by the cage coordinate system or according to the screw, or helical, axis system. In the cardinal axes coordinate system, the results are presented as rotations and translations of the center of gravity of the rigid body (representing the object studied) relative to the reference segment (segment motion) or as translations of individual markers (point motion) (Fig. 71.5). To characterize pure tilt into varus of a tibial component in the knee, for example, segment motion would report rotation about the sagittal axis and nothing else. Point motion would report cranial translation of the lateral markers and caudal translation of the medial ones. According to the usual nomenclature (42), this would not be reported as subsidence, even though the medial condyle of the prosthesis translates downward into the tibia. To simplify reporting the magnitude of the migration, the maximum total point motion (MTPM), i.e., the 3-D motion vector of the marker in the studied segment which moved the most,

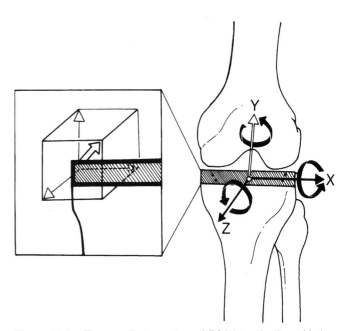

Figure 71.5. The coordinate system of RSA investigations. Motion pertains either to the geometric center of the prosthesis (rotation and translation, 6 degrees of freedom) or to each tantalum marker (translation only, 3 degrees of freedom). The orientation of the axes has been chosen so that the x-axis is transverse and the + direction is medial, the y-axis is vertical and the + direction upward, and the z-axis is sagittal with a + translation directed anteriorly. The directions of rotation were chosen according to the screw-axis convention.

has been used. Contrary to segment and point motion, the MTPM value does not have a direction.

Occasionally, the motion of particular anatomical points or parts of a prosthesis, not specifically marked, is sought. In a tibial component, for example, this can be the anterior, posterior, medial, and lateral extremes, which cannot be marked because the femoral component and metal rods within the polyethylene obscure the markers (43). These points of interest can be marked on the two films from one stereo investigation and digitized with the rest of the tantalum markers. The midpoint of the shortest distance between crossing lines (the intersection will in this case occur at a relatively large distance because the measured point is fictive and can usually not be marked on exactly corresponding sites on the two radiographs) will determine the approximate (within ~1 mm) position of the point of interest, which (by a POINT TRANSFER subroutine) can be transferred to all other stereo investigations for that patient.

The accuracy of RSA depends on a number of different factors such as size configuration of the rigid bodies, number of markers, quality of the radiographic films, precision of digitizing table, and RSA setup. Therefore, the accuracy should be determined for each application separately. For knee arthroplasty, the accuracy has been determined to 0.3 degrees for rotations and 0.2 mm for translations at the 95% confidence limit (42).

Using RSA, migration (i.e., motion over time) and inducible displacement (i.e., cyclic motion in response to forces applied to the knee) of prosthetic components have been studied. For migration, a postoperative reference examination is usually done before the patient has put any weight on the operated limb. Subsequent examinations can be done at random intervals, usually 6 to 12 weeks, 6 months, and yearly. For inducible displacement, examinations are performed in the weight-bearing, vertical position after an initial supine exposure. In the weight-bearing position, external forces such as abduction-adduction, shear, rotation, and flexion can be applied (42, 44, 45). Truly dynamic investigations have also been carried out using RSA. By exposing films in a setup consisting of two angiographic film exchangers set at two to four frames per second, motion of a knee going through a flexion-extension arc has been measured (46, 47).

RSA Investigations on Migration

Before the development of precise radiographic methods such as RSA, it was generally thought that motion over time of a prosthetic component was equivalent to loosening (48–51). Conceptually, loosening was considered to be a sudden rupture of the hitherto sound fixation, analogous to falling through thin ice. With increased accuracy, these concepts could be explored and tested. The first knee prosthesis was marked for RSA at the Department of Orthopedics in Lund in 1978. At that time the prostheses used were the unicompartmental Marmor knee and the Total Condylar total knee, both types having exclusively polyethylene tibial components. Both types were cemented.

Much to our surprise, all 51 clinically successful prostheses migrated. The migration followed a distinct pattern: rather rapid initial migration leveled off at about 1 year (Fig. 71.6). After 1 year, the prostheses could be subdivided into two groups: those that showed no further migration and those (approximately 1/3 of the total number) that showed continuous migration, with large differences in rate between the individual cases (Fig. 71.7). Furthermore, at 1 year, those in the continuously migrating group had migrated significantly more than the prostheses that later turned out to remain stable. The migration was about 0.5 mm (MTPM) for the stable group and between 1 and 4 mm (MTPM) for the prostheses that migrated continuously. The direction of the migration was erratic. There was some varus and valgus tilting, with downward migration of one condyle often combined with a corresponding liftoff of the other side. True subsidence (segment motion) was found only occasionally. No correlation with pre- or postoperative alignment was found. Most of the migration occurred about the vertical axis, and most of the Total Condylar prostheses rotated in a toe-out fashion relative to the tibia (24, 42, 52). Tibial component migration was corroborated by a simultaneous and independent study in which all 14 Total Condylar prostheses (12 of which were clinically loose) migrated up to 5.8 mm (53).

Based on experimental and analytical studies using finite element methods (FEM) (21, 54–56), a metal tray underneath the polyethylene was introduced in the late 1970s. RSA tests of different metal-backed, cemented designs such as the Kinematic, the PCA, and a unicom-

partmental Prototype design have failed to find any effect of the metal tray (40, 44, 57). These findings have been corroborated by independent studies using stemmed and nonstemmed versions of the Tricon-M design (43).

In the early 1980s, noncement fixation, pioneered by Freeman (58), Galante (59), and Hungerford (60), became increasingly popular. It was natural to study these patients with RSA. Studies on the the Porous Coated Anatomic (PCA) knee have revealed considerable migration (Fig. 71.6), all during the first 6 months. After 1 year, the migratory behavior resembled that of cemented cases. Most uncemented prostheses stabilized after 1 year and remained stable over periods approaching 10 years (61). In this series, a significant correlation was found between alignment of the knee and position of the tibial component on the one hand and continuous versus initial migration on the other. Thus, knees that were less well aligned and positioned more often exhibited continuous migration. Finally, significant subsidence (~1 mm) was a regular finding, and the fast initial migration could be largely explained by impaction of the prosthesis into the bone during the early postoperative period (44).

An almost identical migratory pattern was found for the Freeman-Samuelson knee with the "magic peg" for noncement fixation without bone ingrowth. This prosthesis also showed considerable subsidence in the early postoperative period with stabilization after 6 months to 1 year (62), that was corroborated by Broström et al. in an independent study (63). Based on, among other things, the somewhat large inducible displacement (see below) for the Freeman-Samuelson prosthesis, a metal base-plate and a long intramedullary stem were added to the tibial component. The idea was that this stem would engage the endosteal diaphysis and prevent tilt. RSA studies convincingly showed that this happened; varus-valgus and anteroposterior tilt were significantly reduced and migration stopped totally after 6 months in all cases with stems (64).

A second-generation noncemented device has been tested; the Miller-Galante prosthesis uses four screws through the tibial baseplate to achieve initial fixation and has a titanium-mesh porous surface designed for bony ingrowth. The migratory pattern of the Miller-Galante tibial component differed markedly from that of the previously mentioned noncemented designs. Some initial migration occurred, but much less, actually even less than with cemented components (Fig. 71.6). Subsidence was virtually nonexistent, and all components stabilized by 1 year (65). Nilsson et al. have partly corroborated these results in a recent publication (66). In 34 Miller-Galante knees, randomized between cemented and noncemented fixation, small initial migration was found, slightly larger for the noncemented cases. Some continuous migration occurred in both groups and also some subsidence, about 0.6 mm after 1 year (66).

RSA Investigations on Cyclic Motion

The most direct way to determine how well bonded a prosthesis is to bone is to apply a "stress-strain" line of

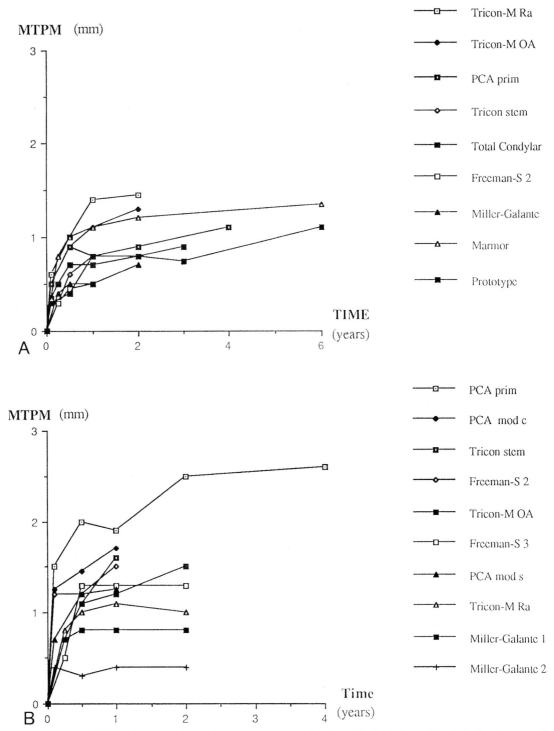

Figure 71.6. A, Migration (MTPM) of cemented prostheses. The Tricon-M in OA and Ra cases (43), the PCA primary (44), the Tricon stem (66), the Total Condylar (52), the Freeman-S "2" with a 110-mm stem (38), the Miller-Galante prosthesis (84), and the Marmor and the Prototype prostheses (57). **B,** Migration (MTPM) of noncemented prostheses. The PCA primary (44), the PCA modular with a cooled saw blade (102), the Tricon stem (66), the Freeman-S "2" in with a 110 mm stem (38), the Tricon-M in osteoarthritic patients (43), the Freeman-S "3" with an 80-mm stem (139), the PCA modular with a standard saw blade (102), the Tricon-M prosthesis in rheumatoid patients (43), the Miller-Galante "1" prosthesis (84), and the Miller-Galante "2" prosthesis (76).

reasoning. This was done in the laboratory studying how prosthetic implants move in response to forces brought to bear on them (17, 18, 20–22, 55, 67–70). With the high resolution of RSA, such studies can now be performed in vivo. The term given this type of motion,

inducible displacement, implies motion induced by reproducible forces of external or internal origin.

In the beginning, these studies were done about 1 year after the arthroplasty. At 1 year, the interface is a very complex structure, with a highly irregular shape

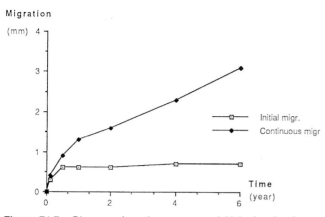

Figure 71.7. Diagram of continuous versus initial migration for cemented prostheses of the Total Condylar, Kinematic, Marmor, Prototype, and PCA primary prostheses (n = 106).

depending on how cement happened to protrude into the cancellous bone in the individual patient. Furthermore, the mechanical behavior of the different tissues in the interface is only slightly known (71). Based on the assumption that in this situation motion could occur at different magnitudes in different directions, a "stress series" was designed (42) to study inducible displacement in every direction. This resulted in a rather cumbersome procedure, tiresome for both patient and investigator. Since the rotatory forces consistently produced the largest displacements, the investigations were eventually scaled down to include (a) a supine reference examination with careful alignment of the limb parallel to the cage, (b) weight-bearing, (c) weight-bearing with a 10-Nm torque applied in the externally rotating direction to a rotating plate on which the patient stands, (d) as position (c) with the torque acting in the opposite direction, and (e) the patient squatting to about 60 degrees of knee flexion. Position (e) was added only recently (45).

These in vivo studies can only be qualitatively compared with true laboratory studies. Many factors are not well controlled, notably those acting across the joint. Added to the applied external forces are always muscle forces of much greater magnitude (72, 73), acting in unknown directions. The direction of the inducible displacement (with some occasional exceptions possibly explained by the "irrelevant" internal forces mentioned above) has always corresponded to the forces applied, and therefore, only the magnitudes of the displacements (MTPM) have been reported. The MTPM concept implies that all other portions of the prosthesis moved less, some parts probably not at all. Assuming that those processes, mechanical or biological, leading to loosening because of motion, occur most readily at the point of maximum strain, the MTPM value was judged to be adequate.

Tested this way, all-polyethylene tibial components, both Total Condylar and Marmor design, displaced a mean 0.4 mm (range 0.2 to 1.0 mm) 1 year after the arthroplasty (42, 52, 57). Again, addition of a metal base-

plate did not change this pattern; inducible displacement was still of the same magnitude (40, 44). In noncemented fixation, the PCA showed mean inducible displacement of 0.7 mm (0.4 to 1.3 mm) after 1 year. Two years postoperatively, the displacements were the same, indicating a stable situation after a mature interface had been reached. This amount of inducible displacement was considered incompatible with bony ingrowth, a conclusion later corroborated using histologic techniques (74, 75).

Studies of the Freeman "magic peg" concept revealed considerably more inducible displacement: a mean 1.9 mm (0.5 to 5.0 mm). In one case, the prosthesis moved 5 mm and twisted considerably, as seen by distortion of the rigid body, during rotatory stress. The patient did not feel pain, and when the force was released, the prosthesis regained its original position (62). As mentioned above, these results, along with other considerations, led to the addition of a metal baseplate and a 110-mm long tapered stem designed to engage the endosteal bone in the distal tibial diaphysis. Significantly less inducible displacement was found for this design (64).

Finally, the Miller-Galante design showed significantly less inducible displacement in six of seven components tested, between 0 and 0.3 mm; the seventh component moved 1.7 mm during stress (Fig. 71.8). Considering that bone is elastic and deflects under load, minute inducible displacement, measurable by RSA, may occur despite sound mechanical coupling in the interface proper (45). The results from the Miller-Galante study may be compatible with bony ingrowth in some cases (76).

These investigations of the interface, done 1 to 2 years after the arthroplasty, clearly reflect the mechanical situation after postoperative tissue differentiation has altered the operative fixation considerably. They represent a way to characterize, in vivo, the *result* of a particular fixation concept or even the fixation achieved in a particular patient. To determine whether motion also occurred postoperatively, when it could have a *causative* effect on the development of the interface, stress investigations using RSA were performed during the first 2 months after operation (45). Inducible displacement was found: about 0.4 mm for cemented tibial components and 0.7 mm for noncemented ones. In that investigation, the squatting position (position (e) above) was included for the first time. This position, mimicking everyday activities like rising from a chair and climbing stairs, proved to be the most revealing, and a consistent posterior rollback during flexion often resulted in posterior tilt of the component (45) (Fig. 71.9).

Dynamic Investigations Using RSA

The in vitro motion pattern of the normal knee has been studied by Blankenvoort et al. using RSA (77). They defined the outer limits for tibial rotation, which were rather consistent and relatively unaffected by outer forces. Interestingly, they were unable to find any end rotation of the tibia upon extension ("screw-home

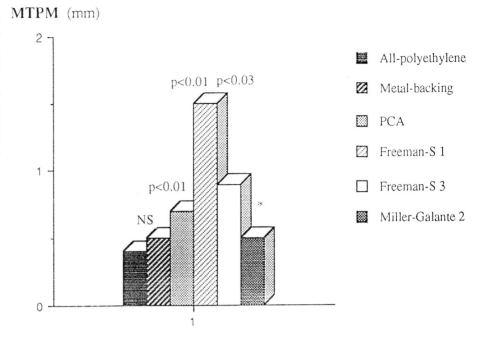

Figure 71.8. The mean inducible displacements of five different types of prosthetic fixation (Σ N=67): All-polyethylene Total Condylar cemented prosthesis (52), the metal-backed Kinematic prosthesis (40), the noncemented PCA primary prosthesis (44), the noncemented Freeman-Samuelson prosthesis (62), the noncemented Freeman-Samuelson prosthesis with a 110-mm stem (64), and the noncemented Miller-Galante prosthesis (76). * Indicates significantly less inducible displacement for the Miller-Galante prosthesis than for all other noncemented devices at P .01.

mechanism") in their passive model using intact knee specimens and concluded that the screw-home effect is due more to active stabilization by muscles and external forces.

Nilsson et al. studied the kinematics in vivo after total joint replacement with the Tricon M knee prosthesis, which sacrifices both cruciate ligaments, using the film exchanger technique. They found abnormal patterns in translation (Fig. 71.10), rotation, and varus-valgus tilt, which they attributed to the configuration of the articulating surfaces and the absence of the cruciate ligaments (47). Later, they studied kinematics of the Miller-Galante and the New Jersey LCS knees. They found almost normal screw-home for both prostheses. Most significantly, they found a distinctly larger posterior translation (about 20 mm) of the tibia on flexion in both prostheses than in the normal knee (46). The authors could only partially explain this extraordinary finding.

Most recently, Nilsson and co-workers reported on the kinematics of the Tricon-M and the Miller-Galante knees in the weight-bearing situation when the patient ascended and descended a platform placed 40 cm above the floor (66). In this situation the prosthetic knees displayed a large posterior translation with flexion. Moreover, the screw-home mechanism was less pronounced than in the non-weight-bearing situation. They also found more sliding and less rolling motion of the femur on the tibia, a finding that has considerable bearing on the problem of polyethylene wear (78), a source of great concern in recent years (79). Nilsson et al. also used the helical axis mode of describing the motion, an option available in the RSA system. These kinematic studies indicate abnormal motion between the femur and the tibia after joint replacement, induced by forces that are carried by the interfaces.

Clinical Significance of Micromotion

As previously mentioned, two distinct migratory patterns have been identified. In most cases, migration is found only during the first year. After ½ to 1 year, the prostheses stabilize, and no additional migration seems to occur for up to 10 years (80). For a smaller group of less stable prostheses, initial migration exceeds that of the stable group during the first year. Moreover, migration in this group continues after the first year, at different rates for individual cases.

The RSA studies in Lund have always included enough prostheses to eventually have a number fail by mechanical loosening. At the time of this writing, 13 tibial components have been revised for mechanical loosening in the RSA material analyzed in Lund from 2 to 12 years after surgery. This group included one Marmor prosthesis and four PCAs, all cemented. The remaining eight were Freeman-Samuelson prostheses, one cemented and seven noncemented. Each case belonged to the continuously migrating group of prostheses. An additional case, a noncemented prosthesis of a modified ICLH design, migrated continuously during a 2-year period. Two years later, the patient started to experience clinical symptoms of loosening, which was subsequently verified during revision surgery (63).

In Umeå, Sweden, three cases have been revised for mechanical loosening after having been assessed by RSA. One cemented Tricon-M tibial component was revised for mechanical loosening after 21 months. At this time the prosthesis had migrated continuously and reached an MTPM value of 2.4 mm after 18 months, significantly above the mean migration for that group of prostheses (81). Two more patients were revised after 6 months (hydroxyapatite-coated Tricon-II) and 2 years (cemented Tricon-M). Both had migrated continuously

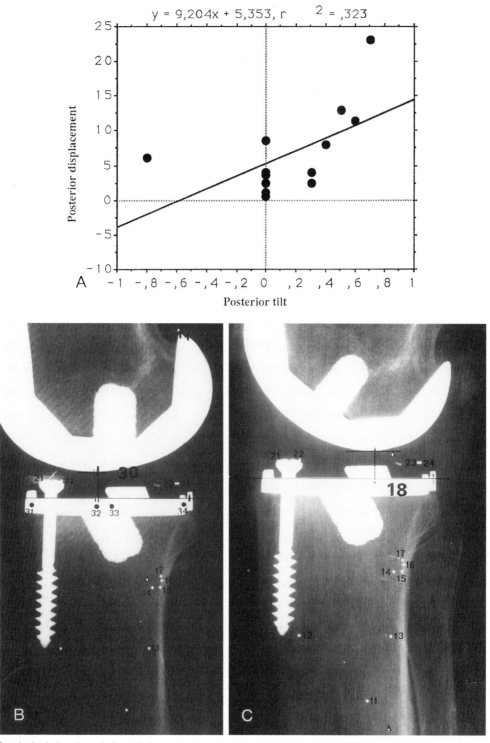

Figure 71.9. **A,** Graph depicting the relationship between posterior tilt of the tibial component and posterior displacement of the femoral component on the tibial one when the knee moves from the extended position (**B**) to a position of approximately 60 degrees of flexion (**C**).

and significantly more than the remainder in their group (66).

In all, 17 identified cases of mechanical loosening have been followed by RSA. All belonged to a group that in the total RSA material actually constitutes a minority. The statistical probability for this to be spurious is neg-

ligible (P < .0001). One must conclude that a precise radiographic technique can identify a subpopulation of cases that are at high risk of becoming loose, while the remaining cases are likely to function adequately, from the point of view of fixation, for long periods of time. Moreover, this subpopulation can be identified within 2

Figure 71.10. Translation of a central point of the tibial component in the prosthetic knee and the tibial eminence in the normal knee during active flexion and extension (*dashed line*, normal knee; *solid line*, Tricon-M prosthesis). (Reproduced with permission from Nilsson KG, Karrholm J, Ekelund L. Knee motion in total knee arthroplasty. A roentgen stereophotogrammetric analysis of the kinematics of the Tricon-M knee prosthesis. Clin Orthop 1990;256:147–161.)

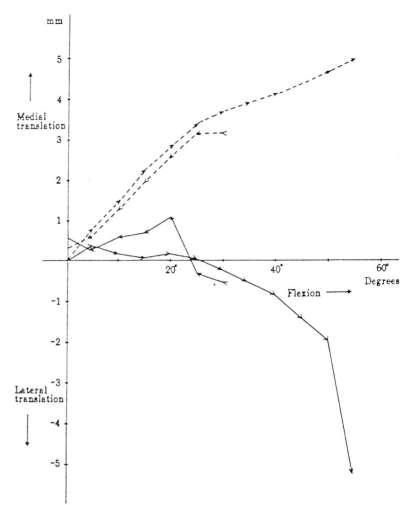

years of surgery, and in most cases, *before they become symptomatic*. This finding has considerable practical and theoretical implications.

Clinical Implications of Precise Radiographic Techniques

RSA studies have shown that much inducible displacement occurs when physiologic forces, representing everyday activities, are applied. In noncemented cases, this motion is too large to permit bony ingrowth, and sparse ingrowth is found histologically. Clinically, this situation has been reported to translate into more pain, especially "first-step pain" (82). The predicted positive effect of stems and/or screws is borne out by less cyclic motion in vivo, and histologically, better ingrowth has been found for such devices, which clinically fare quite well. There may, therefore, be reason to heed these findings in choosing a prosthesis or fixation concept. There is clinical relevance to the sequential evaluations by laboratory testing, in vivo mechanical follow-up by RSA, and the eventual clinical outcome. This connection has been reported for large groups (25, 83) and also seems valid in the individual case. A number of laboratory investigations have shown that a stem and/or screws re-

duce micromotion; in the RSA material, stemmed (64) or screwed (76, 84) implant reduces continuous displacement. In one study, cemented components of the Tricon-M design showed significantly more continuous migration than the noncemented controls (66). However, this latter finding could not be corroborated for other prostheses (44, 52) and may not be widely applicable.

Joint replacement surgery represents a considerable portion of the work of any orthopaedic unit. Since deterioration of the interface with destruction of the bone stock sometimes occurs asymptomatically, some kind of follow-up protocol, including plain radiography, is usually instituted. This follow-up of large numbers of patients may be superfluous; with more precise techniques, most patients can be identified as not subject to failure from interface breakdown. This large subgroup of joint replacement recipients may be excluded from further investigations, and limited resources can be concentrated on the smaller subgroup subject to continuous migration.

The number of different prosthetic systems available on the commercial market is vast and grows every year. For each system, the final proof of success is the clinical track record, which takes at least 10 years and many operations to accumulate. With a more precise method, the results of RSA indicate that the clinical efficacy of a particular design can be assessed within a few years and with significantly fewer patients.

Theoretical Implications from the Point of View of Fixation

Conceptually, finding that all mechanical loosenings belong to a subgroup of arthroplasties that migrate pathologically from the start implies that loosening of prosthetic components (at least the tibial component in the knee) is a slow process that begins in the early postoperative period. The clinical entity of loosening is thus not a sudden occurrence, like "falling through the ice," but rather, a slow process that starts immediately after the operation. The patient, by analogy, walks out on "quicksand and starts to sink." Any models we envisage to explain the processes leading up to loosening must be reconciled with these very distinct findings.

The process of loosening is clearly multifactorial. Important factors for fixation by osseointegration are (a) material compatibility, (b) the implant surface, (c) state of the host bed, (d) surgical technique, (e) implant design, and (f) loading conditions (13). Contemporary arthroplasties, irrespective of anatomic location, do not aim at osseointegration, but these factors may be applicable to fixation of the joint implants of today, with or without cement.

Regarding material compatibility, some materials are clearly more biocompatible than others. Commercially pure titanium is considered by some the material of choice (85), but because of poor mechanical properties, titanium alloys containing aluminum and vanadium, are often used. Possible side effects from leakage of potentially harmful ions from such alloys into the tissue have been discussed (86), but no data exist to show this to be a clinical problem. Chrome-cobalt, because of its excellent corrosion resistance and mechanical properties, is the most commonly used alloy. Concerns about toxicity and sensitivity to one or more of the included metals (chrome, nickel, and cobalt) (87) and even carcinogenesis (88) have been raised. As of today, no causal relationships have been proven, and chrome-cobalt implants are regarded as relatively well tolerated (89). The relatively poor corrosion characteristics of stainless steel make it a poor choice in implant surgery (90). Despite the success of PMMA bone cement in arthroplasty, cement has been blamed for a number of adverse effects in the interface, such as toxicity (91), heat necrosis during curing (92, 93), and macrophage activation (94, 95). In the final analysis, it is hard to see how any effect of these materials per se could explain the results found by RSA, in which the migratory patterns were similar, irrespective of whether PMMA, polyethylene, chrome-cobalt or titanium alloy faced the bone. Most importantly, polyethylene wear particles, of imminent concern in loosening, because they elicit an intense macrophage response upon phagocytosis (11, 79, 96, 97), are probably not present at this early stage.

The surface energy of the implant, defined as the extent of unsatisfied bonds at the surface of the metal may have a role in the fixation of uncemented implants. Such factors, studied mostly in the context of dental implants aiming at osseointegration (13), may also play a role in fixation of joint implants. They could hardly, however, have a bearing on the RSA findings, in which identical implants behave differently.

The state of the host bed and surgical technique address the same problem: bone should be strong and viable when the implant is inserted. Weak bone is often present in osteoporosis and rheumatoid arthritis. Such bone weakness per se has, however, not been linked to inferior clinical results (98), and prostheses in rheumatoid patients as a group do not migrate differently by RSA (38, 47). The bone should be handled delicately and precisely during surgery, to obtain optimal conditions for fixation. Recent work has shown that temperatures high enough to cause bone necrosis are consistently reached during cutting (99). By the use of a cooled saw blade, these high temperatures could be perfectly controlled (100, 101), and by RSA, a cooled saw blade resulted in a significantly stiffer interface and a tendency for less migration in a randomized series of patients receiving a noncemented knee implant (102). This indicates that surgical handling may indeed be a significant factor in the individual case. New bone cannot bridge gaps between bone and prosthesis to any large extent, and voids as small as 0.35 mm can impede ingrowth (103). Gaps exceeding 1 mm between the tibia and the tibial component are the rule rather than the exception (104) and may be of importance for noncement fixation. They could not, however, explain the identical migratory pattern for cemented prostheses in which the cement acts as a grout to fill all crevices between prosthesis and bone. Surgical technique also involves postoperative alignment, and RSA investigations have shown an influence of alignment on the migratory pattern, i.e. continuous versus initial migration (44). Alignment touches on the sixth and last factor, namely the mechanical situation.

Implant (macro-) design and loading conditions address the mechanical situation across the interface, where stresses caused by gravity and muscle forces will always produce strains in the tissue and materials involved.

Motion in the interface exceeding 100 to 150 μm inhibits bone ingrowth into porous noncemented devices (105, 106). Motion of this magnitude occurs readily in the normal intact bone (107), and extirpation of the subchondral bone plate significantly increases these motions (108, 109). Indeed, differences in moduli of elasticity and Poisson ratios will produce interfacial shear of about 150 μm (110). The weak and surgically compromised tibial metaphysis allows cyclic motion. As suggested by Hvid (111), repetitive fatigue fractures may be one pathway by which large and continuous migration occurs.

Several biomechanical investigations have shown that prosthesis design influences the amount of micromotion, indicating the importance of the fixation surface facing the bone (18, 19, 21, 67–69). In recent studies, an intramedullary stem on the tibial component seemed beneficial, and the addition of screws further stabilized the prosthesis during the early stages (18, 19). Less interfacial motion occurs with cement, because of the grouting effect of PMMA, although stress and corresponding strain, occurs in the materials adjacent to the interface, i.e., the bone itself (45, 112, 113). In addition to the design of the parts of the prosthesis facing the bone, the geometry of the articulating surfaces affects the stability of the prosthesis. Constraint has been discussed extensively. Excessive constraint caused loosening of hinged prostheses. However, prostheses with too little constraint may run the risk of edge loading, with deleterious effects on the fixation (68, 69). The optimum tradeoff regarding constraint from the point of view of force transmission is probably not known at this time. In addition, the issue of constraint addresses the problem of wear, presently perhaps the most imminent cause for concern in knee arthroplasty. Thus for at least two reasons, the search for the anatomic knee prosthesis, i.e., unconstrained prostheses, (114) may have gone too far.

Depending on the prosthetic design and postoperative alignment, preoperative bone quality, muscular capability, choice of fixation, and other factors, a unique mechanical situation will develop in each case, and the stresses and strains across the individual interface may well explain the RSA findings (Fig. 71.11). Certainly, this mechanical situation fulfills one important criterion: it is established from the very start and acts in the postoperative period.

During the operation, surgical trauma inevitably occurs; some cells die and some are sensitized, with the release of cytokines such as growth factors, etc. Weeks later, a granulation phase begins, and connective tissue is formed in the interface. This phase evolves into a callous phase, when, between 4 weeks and 3 months, the interface tissue develops along different pathways according to local conditions (15). At this stage, the patient is walking and the mechanical conditions are established. Such mechanical stimuli are potent signals for bone and tissue adaptation (115–117). Even if the immediate fixation prevents relative motion between materials (i.e. interfacial micromotion), strains within the materials will, by the laws of mechanics, always occur when the stresses of everyday activities are applied. Recent work has suggested that the biologic signal may be the strain induced rather than the primary stresses themselves. Loading cells in compression or shear yields profound differences (16). Thus, according to Carter and co-workers, loading in hydrostatic compression will not induce any changes in the shape of the cells, which will differentiate along a cartilaginous pathway to produce (fibro)cartilage, while loading in shear will produce spatial changes in the cells, which will respond by the development of fibrous tissue (16). Given the ideal conditions of no relative motion (106, 118, 119) and a state of compressive stress in the bone (120), bony ingrowth in noncement fixation or bone "apposition" on the cement (121, 122) may occur.

Histologic studies of the interface of tibial components support the mechanical predictions. Available data from laboratory investigations, finite element analyses, and RSA show that the preconditions for an interface of "ingrown" or "ongrown" bone are not good regarding the tibial component in the knee. Laboratory studies show that considerable motion occurs in tension and shear (19, 21, 67–69), and FEM studies add additional support. Thus, the tangential motion in the upper tibia caused by cyclic expansion of the metaphysis may amount to 150 μm (110), and interference pegs seem to preclude ingrowth into the tibial tray (123). These findings are supported by the RSA findings of inducible displacement in the postoperative period of 200 to 300 μm (45). Using the dynamic RSA method, prosthetic knees show considerably altered kinematics in rotation and translation between the femoral and tibial components, with abnormal forces that have to be carried by the interface (46). These findings translate into histologic findings of mainly soft tissue. In an early series on 90 tibial components of various designs, only one third showed any significant ingrowth, never exceeding 10% (74, 75). A second-generation noncemented prosthesis with screws has been shown to give more bony ingrowth (124, 125), corresponding to the improved mechanical behavior of such components, as measured in the laboratory (19) and by RSA (76, 84).

Most studies on the interface originate from hip arthroplasties, where fibrous tissue, oriented parallel to the implant surface and often in combination with osteolytic activity, is usually found in the interface (6, 11, 126–128). In the knee, three cemented unicompartmental arthroplasties of the Marmor design, showing RSA findings of initial migration only, showed highly differentiated fibrocartilage in the interface adjacent to the

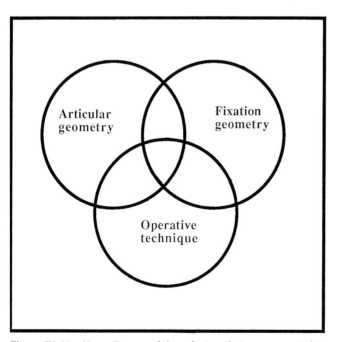

Figure 71.11. Venn diagram of three factors that are suggested to affect the interface in a decisive way. The interface of a prosthesis in the central "position" develops favorably, yielding initial migration only.

tibial component (8), and such an interface was also reported for another design (7). These findings illustrate the different mechanical conditions in the hip and knee and support the theories of Carter and co-workers (16). They show that a tibial component, loaded predominantly in compression, may have a benign-looking interface compatible with the long-term integrity found for most cases by RSA. Indeed, such a soft-tissue interface has been considered advantageous by some (10). While readily found in the fibrous interface, blood vessels, macrophages and inflammatory cells, and wear debris were virtually absent in the cartilaginous portion of the interface of the Marmor prostheses (8).

Wear debris, especially of UHMW polyethylene, is today perhaps the most commonly cited cause of mechanical loosening. While rather innocuous in the bulk form, small particles of polyethylene cause an intense inflammatory reaction, with the release of cytokines capable of inducing bone resorption (96, 97, 129–132).

As stated above, wear particles alone cannot explain the RSA findings of immediate and large migration for cases that eventually loosen. However, a pathway linking the biology of wear particles to factors of mechanical origin may be envisaged. RSA (44) and laboratory studies (19) indicate that the soft tissue interface should probably be regarded as an open compartment, where (joint-) fluid is squirted in and out with every step. By such a mechanism, wear particles gain access to the interface and can be found long distances from the joint (11, 133). It is conceivable that soft tissue of different composition (i.e., fibrocartilage versus fibrous tissue) responds differently to such wear particles. Thus, fibrocartilage may itself be a barrier to wear particles (134), which, in the absence of blood vessels, may generate a less intense reaction. In a fibrous interface with blood vessels and macrophages, possibly induced by the presence of cement (126), wear particles may provoke a more deleterious response. In the RSA material, although not bonded by bony ingrowth, a smaller proportion of noncemented prostheses tend to migrate continuously than of cemented prostheses. In one series this tendency was statistically significant (66).

Other Components

So far, only the problem of tibial component fixation has been addressed in this chapter. This is not unreasonable since the femoral component causes very little problem in terms of loosening, and the vast majority of studies, laboratory and clinical, have been done on the tibia. Regarding the femoral component in the knee, in one RSA study on noncemented Freeman knees the femoral component was marked, and "subsidence" was found, in the cranial direction, of a magnitude approximately equal to that of the tibial components in the same study (63). Essentially the same findings have been made for the Miller-Galante prosthesis (135).

Whether the findings on the clinical importance of continuous migration in the knee apply to the hip is unclear. In studies of both the femoral and acetabular components in the hip, a pattern of fast initial migration and subsequent stability or slow migration after 1 year has been reported (136). The migration was not as consistent as in the knee, but symptomatic and eventually loose cases have been reported to migrate continuously (36, 136–138).

Summary

The application of a precision radiographic system has shown patterns of migration that correlate strongly with clinical outcomes. Thus, components that migrate continuously risk eventual loosening, while no loose prosthesis has been found in the group that migrates only initially. These migratory patterns can be distinguished as early as 1 or 2 years in the individual case, long before those with eventual loosening are symptomatic. In some series, improvement of design factors, based on laboratory studies, give the predicted results, as measured by inducible displacement in vivo and favorable migratory patterns during the first years.

These findings have clinical implications because they link preclinical testing of prosthetic devices with RSA results and actual clinical outcomes. Prosthetic systems and fixation concepts can be chosen before the clinical trial, and once under way, the results of such trials can be assessed as early as a couple of years.

Conceptually, the findings indicate that loosening starts in the early postoperative period and slowly progresses until clinically apparent mechanical loosening with symptoms necessitates revision surgery. Two proposed pathways of loosening are discussed: (a) continuous migration because of fatigue fractures of the tibial metaphysis and (b) tissue differentiation in the interface along different pathways governed by mechanical stimuli, where cellular responses, with or without the additional effects of wear products, play important roles.

References

1. Mintz AD, Pilkington CAJ, Howie DW. A comparison of plain and fluoroscopically guided radiographs in the assessment of arthroplasty of the knee. J Bone Joint Surg 1989;71-A:1343–1347.
2. Ahlberg A, Linden B. The radiolucent zone in arthroplasty of the knee. Acta Orthop Scand 1977;48:687–690.
3. Willert HG, Ludwig J, Semtlisch M. Reaction of bone to methacrylate after hip arthroplasty. J Bone Joint Surg 1974;56-A:1368–1382.
4. Vernon-Roberts B, Freeman MAR. Morphological and analytical studies of the tissue adjacent to joint prostheses: investigation into the causes of loosening of prostheses. In: Schaldach M, Hohmann D, eds. Advances in artificial hip and knee technology. Berlin: Springer-Verlag, 1976:148–186.
5. Charnley J. The reaction of bone to self-curing acrylic cement. J Bone Joint Surg 1970;52-B:340–353.
6. Johanson NA, Bullough PG, Wilson PD, Salvati EA, Ranawat CS. The microscopic anatomy of the bone-cement interface in failed total hip arthroplasties. Clin Orthop 1987;218:123.
7. Blaha JD, Insler HP, Freeman MAR, Revell PA, Todd RC. The fixation of a proximal tibial polyethylene prosthesis without cement. J Bone Joint Surg 1982;64-B:326–335.
8. Ryd L, Linder L. On the correlation between micromotion and histology. J Arthroplasty 1989;4(4):303–309.
9. Walldius B. Arthroplasty of the knee joint using endoprosthesis. Acta Orthop Scand 1957;24(suppl 19).
10. Tibrewal SB, Grant KA, Goodfellow JW. The radiolucent line beneath the tibial component of the Oxford meniscal knee. J Bone Joint Surg 1984;66-B:523–528.
11. Willert HG, Bertram H, Buchhorn GH. Osteolysis in alloarthroplasty

of the hip. The role of ultrahigh molecular weight polyethylene wear particles. Clin Orthop 1990;258:95–106.

12. Albrektsson T, Breanemark P-I, Hansson H-A, Lindstrom J. Osseointegrated titanium implants. Acta Orthop Scand 1981;52:155–170.
13. Albrektsson T, Albrektsson B. Osseointegration of bone implants. A review of an alternative mode of fixation. Acta Orthop Scand 1987;58:567–577.
14. Frost HM. The biology of fracture healing, an overview for clinicians. Clin Orthop 1989;248:283–309.
15. Johansson CB. On tissue reactions to metal implants [Thesis]. Gothenburg, University of Gothenburg, 1991.
16. Carter DR. Mechanical loading history and skeletal biology. J Biomech 1987;20(11/12):1095–1109.
17. Dempsey AJ, Finlay JB, Bourne RB, Scott MA, Millman JC, Rorabeck CH. A comparison of anchorage systems for fixation of tibial knee components. Trans 35th Annual ORS. Las Vegas, 1989:374.
18. Miura H, Whiteside LA, Easley JC, Amador DD. Effects of screws and a sleeve on initial fixation in uncemented total knee tibial components. Clin Orthop 1990;259:160–168.
19. Volz RG, Nisbet JN, Lee RW, McMurtry MG. The mechanical stability of various noncemented tibial components. Clin Orthop 1988;226:38–42.
20. Walker PS, Ranawat CS, Insall J. Fixation of the tibial components of condylar replacement knee prostheses. J Biomech 1976;9:269–275.
21. Walker PS, Greene D, Reilly D, Thatcher J, Ben-Dov M, Ewald FC. Fixation of tibial components in knee arthroplasty. J Bone Joint Surg 1981;63-A:258–267.
22. Whiteside LA, Pafford J. Load transfer characteristics of a noncemented total knee arthroplasty. Clin Orthop 1989;239:168–177.
23. Herrlin K, Selvik G, Pettersson H. Space orientation of total hip prosthesis. A method for three dimensional determination. Acta Radiol 1986;27(6):619–627.
24. Ryd L, Boegard T, Egund N, Lindstrand A, Selvik G, Thorngren K-G. Migration of the tibial component in successful unicompartmental knee arthroplasty. A clinical, radiographic and roentgen stereophotogrammetric study. Acta Orthop Scand 1983;54:408–416.
25. Albrektsson BEJ, Herberts P. ICLH knee arthroplasty. A consecutive study of 108 knees with uncemented tibial component fixation. J Arthroplasty 1988;3(2):145–156.
26. Cooke TD, Pichora D, Siu D, Scudamore RA, Ryant JT. Surgical implications of varus deformity of the knee with obliquity of joint surfaces. J Bone Joint Surg 1989;71-B:560–565.
27. Ilchmann T, Franzen H, Mjoberg B, Wingstrand H. Measurements accuracy in acetabular cup migration. J Arthroplasty 1992;7(2):121–127.
28. Lippert FG, Hartington RM, Veress SA, Fraser C, Green D, Bahniuk E. A comparison of convergent and bi-plane x-ray photogrammetry systems used to detect total joint loosening. J Biomech 1982;15(9):677–682.
29. Hunter JC, Baumrind S, Genant HK, Murray WR, Ross SE. The detection of loosening in total hip arthroplasty: description of a stereophotogrammetric computer assisted method. Invest Radiol 1979;14(4):323–329.
30. Selvik G. A roentgen stereophotogrammetric system for the study of the kinematics of the skeletal systems [Thesis]. University of Lund, Sweden, 1974. Reprinted in: Acta Arthop Scand 1989;60(suppl 232) 1974:1–51.
31. Lysell E. Motion of the cervical spine. Acta Orthop Scand 1969;40(suppl 123).
32. Davidson M. Roentgen ray and localization. An apparatus for exact measurement and localization by means of roentgen rays. B Med J 1898;1:10–13.
33. Hallert B. X-ray photogrammetry. Basic geometry and quality. Amsterdam: Elsevier, 1970
34. Euler L. Formulae generales pro translatione quaqunque corporum rigidorum. In: Novi commentarii academie scientiarum Petropolitanae. Orell Füssli Turici. Basel 1968;9:84–98. ed. 1776:180–207. (Blanc C, ed. Reprinted in: Leonhardi Euleri Opera Omnia—series secunda;vol 20).
35. Alberius P. Bone reaction to tantalum markers. A scanning electron microscopic study. Acta Anat 1983;115:310–318.
36. Wykman A, Selvik G, Goldie I. Subsidence of the femoral component in the noncemented total hip: a roentgen stereophotogrammetric analysis. Acta Orthop Scand 1988;59:635–637.
37. Karrholm J. Roentgen stereophotogrammetry. A review of orthopedic applications. Acta Orthop Scand 1989;60(4):491–503.
38. Albrektsson BEJ, Carlsson LV, Freeman MAR, Herberts P, Ryd L. Proximally cemented versus Uncemented Freeman-Samuelson Knee arthroplasty. J Bone Joint Surg 1992;74-B:233–238.
39. Sathasivam S, Walker P. Personal communication.
40. Ryd L, Lindstrand A, Rosenquist R, Selvik G. Tibial component fixation in knee arthroplasty. An in-vivo roentgen stereophotogrammetric study of cemented metal-backed devices. Clin Orthop 1986;213:141–149.

41. Nystrom L. Algorithms and program system for roentgen stereophotogrammetric analysis [Thesis]. Umea University, 1990.
42. Ryd L. Micromotion in knee arthroplasty. A roentgen stereophotogrammetric analysis of tibial component fixation. Acta Orthop Scand 1986;57(suppl 220).
43. Nilsson KG, Karrholm J, Ekelund L, Magnusson P. Evaluation of micromotion in cemented vs. uncemented knee arthroplasty in osteoarthritis and rheumatoid arthritis. Randomized study using roentgen stereophotogrammetric analysis. J Arthroplasty 1991;6:265–278.
44. Ryd L, Lindstrand A, Stenstrom A, Selvik G. PCA tricompartmental tibial components; relation between prosthetic position and micromotion. Clin Orthop 1990;251:189–197.
45. Ryd L, Toksvig-Larsen S. In-vivo measurements of the stability of tibial components in the postoperative phase. J Orthop Res 1993;11(1):142–148.
46. Nilsson KG, Karrholm J, Gadegaard P. Abnormal kinematics of the artificial knee. Roentgen stereophotogrammetric analysis of 10 Miller-Galante and five New Jersey LCS knees. Acta Orthop Scand 1991;62(5):440–446.
47. Nilsson KG, Karrholm J, Ekelund L. Knee motion in total knee arthroplasty. A roentgen stereophotogrammetric analysis of the kinematics of the Tricon-M knee prosthesis. Clin Orthop 1990;256:147–161.
48. Schneider R, Freiburger RH, Ghelman B, Ranawat CS. Radiologic evaluation of painful joint prostheses. Clin Orthop 1982;170:156–167.
49. Kaufer H, Matthews LS. Spherocentric arthroplasty of the knee. J Bone Joint Surg 1981;63-A:545–559.
50. Harris WH. Advances in total hip arthroplasty, The metal backed acetabular component. Clin Orthop 1984;183:4–11.
51. Boegard T, Brattstrom H, Lidgren L. Seventy-four Attenborough knee replacements for rheumatoid arthritis. Acta Orthop Scand 1984;55:166–171.
52. Ryd L, Lindstrand A, Rosenquist R, Selvik G. Micromotion of all-polyethylene prosthetic components in total knee replacements. A stereophotogrammetric analysis of migration and inducible displacement. Arch Orthop Trauma Surg 1987;106:82–88.
53. Green DL, Bahniuk E, Liebelt RA, Fender E, Mirkov P3. Biplane radiographic measurements of reversible displacement (including clinical loosening) and migration of total joint replacements. J Bone Joint Surg 1983;65-A:1134–114.
54. Bartel DL, Burnstein AH, Santavicca EA, Insall JN. Performance of the tibial component in total knee replacement, conventional and revisional design. J Bone Joint Surg 1982;64-A:1026–1033.
55. Bargren JH, Day WH, Freeman MAR, Swanson SAV. Mechanical tests on the tibial component of non-hinged knee prostheses. J Bone Joint Surg 1978;60-B:256–261.
56. Reilly D, Walker PS, Ben-Dov M, Ewald FC. Effects of tibial components on load transfer in the upper tibia. Clin Orthop 1982;165:272–282.
57. Ryd L, Lindstrand A, Stenstrom A, Selvik G. The influence of metal-backing in unicompartmental knee arthroplasty. An in-vivo roentgen stereophotogrammetric study on prosthetic fixation. Arch Orthop Trauma Surg 1992;111:148–154.
58. Freeman MAR, Blaha JD, Brown G, Day W, Insler HP, Revell PA. Cementless fixation of a tibial component for the knee. Trans 27th Annual ORS. Las Vegas, Nevada, 1981;7:154.
59. Galante J, Rostoker W, Lueck R, Ray RD. Sintered fiber metal composites as a basis for attachment of implants to bone. J Bone Joint Surg 1971;53-A:101–114.
60. Hungerford DS, Kenna RV, Krackow KA. The Porous Coated Anatomic total knee. Orthop Clin North Am 1982;13(1):103–122.
61. Ryd L, Albrektsson BEJ, Carlsson L, Toksvig-Larsen S, Herberts P, Lindstrand A. The clinical significance of micromotion. Trans 39th Annual ORS 1993;246.
62. Ryd L, Albrektsson B, Herberts P, Lindstrand A, Selvik G. Micromotion in uncemented Freeman-Samuelson knee prostheses. Clin Orthop 1988;229:205–212.
63. Broström L-A, Goldie I, Selvik G. Micromotion of the total knee. Acta Orthop Scand 1989;60(4):443–445.
64. Albrektsson BEJ, Ryd L, Carlsson LV, et al. The effect of a stem on the tibial component; a roentgen stereophotogrammetric analysis of stemmed and non-stemmed, uncemented tibial components in clinically successful Freeman-Samuelson knee arthroplasties. J Bone Joint Surg 1990;72-B:252–258.
65. Carlsson L, Ryd L, Herberts P. An in vivo roentgen stereophotogrammetric analysis of the Miller-Galante tibial component. Trans 37th Annual ORS 1991;16:168.
66. Nilsson KG. Kinematics and fixation of total knee arthroplasties. University of Umea, Sweden, 1992.
67. Bourne RB, Finlay JB. The influence of tibial component intramedullary stems and implant-cortex contact on the strain distribution of the proximal tibia following total knee arthroplasty. Clin Orthop 1986;208:95–99.
68. Branson PJ, Steege JW, Wixson RL, Lewis J, Stulberg SD. Rigidity of

initial fixation with uncemented tibial knee implants. J Arthroplasty 1989;4:21–26.

69. Kaiser AD, Whiteside LA. The effects of screws and pegs on the initial fixation stability of an uncemented unicondylar knee replacement. Clin Orthop 1990;259:169–178.

70. Volz RG, Wilson RJ. Factors affecting the mechanical stability of the cemented acetabular component in total hip replacement. J Bone Joint Surg 1977;59-A:501–504.

71. Hori RY, Lewis JL. Mechanical properties of the fibrous tissue found at the bone-cement interface following total joint replacements. J Biomed Mater Res 1982;16:911–927.

72. Morrison JB. Bioengineering analysis of force actions transmitted by the knee joint. J Biomed Eng 1968;April:164–170.

73. Maquet P, Simonet J, de Marchin P. Biomecanique du genou et gonarthrose. Rev Chir Orthop 1967;53:111–138.

74. Cook SD, Thomas KA, Haddad RJ. Histologic analysis of retrieved human porous-coated total joint components. Clin Orthop 1988;234:90–101.

75. Hainau B, Reimann I, Dorph S, Rechtnagel K, Henschel A, Kragh F. Porous-Coated knee arthroplasty. A case report concerning bone ingrowth. Clin Orthop 1989;239:178–184.

76. Ryd L, Carlsson L, Herberts P. Micromotion of a noncemented tibial component with screw fixation. An in vivo roentgen stereophotogrammetric study of the Miller-Galante prosthesis. Clin Orthop 1993;295:218–225.

77. Blankenvoort L, Husikes R, deLange A. The envelope of passive knee joint motion. J Biomech 1988;21:705–720.

78. Blunn G, Walker PS, Joshi A, Hardinge K. The dominance of cyclic sliding in producing wear in total knee replacements. Clin Orthop 1991;273:253–260.

79. Goodman S, Lidgren L. Polyethylene wear in knee arthroplasty. Acta Orthop Scand 1992;63(3):358–364.

80. Ryd L, Albrektsson BEJ, Carlsson L, Toksvig-Larsen S, Herberts P, Lindstrand A. On the clinical significance of micromotion of joint implants. Trans 39th Annual ORS 1993;246.

81. Nilsson KG, Bjornebrink J, Hietala SO, Karrholm J. Scintimetry after total knee arthroplasty. Prospective 2-year study of 18 cases of arthrosis and 15 cases of rheumatoid arthritis. Acta Orthop Scand 1992;63(2):159–165.

82. Lindstrand A, Stenstrom A, Egund N. The PCA unicompartmental knee: a 1–4 year comparison of fixation with or without cement. Acta Orthop Scand 1988;59:695–700.

83. Grewal R, Grimmer MG, Freeman MAR. Early migration of prostheses related to long-term survivorship. Comparison of tibial components in knee replacement. J Bone Joint Surg 1992;74-B:239–242.

84. Nilsson KG, Karrholm J. Increased varus-valgus tilting of screw fixated knee prostheses. J Arthroplasty 1993;8(5)529–540.

85. Albrektsson T. The response of bone to titanium implants. In: Williams DF, ed. Critical review in biocompatibility. Boca Raton, FL: CRC Press, 1984:53–84. vol 1.

86. Woodman JL, Jacobs JJ, Galante JO, Urban RM. Metal-ion release from titanium based prosthetic segmental replacements of long bones in baboon: a long term study. J Orthop Res 1984;1(4):421–430.

87. Williams DF. The properties and clinical use of cobalt-based alloys. In: Williams DF, ed. CRC biocompatibility of clinical implant materials. 1981: 99–124. vol 1.

88. Hughes AV, Sherlock DA, Hamblen DL, Reid R. Sarcoma at the site of a single hip screw. J Bone Joint Surg 1987;69-B:470.

89. Rostlund T. On the development of a new arthroplasty. With special emphasis on the gliding elements in the knee. Goteborg University, Sweden, 1990.

90. Crowninshield R. An overview of prosthetic materials for fixation. Clin Orthop 1988;235:166.

91. Feith R. Side effects of acrylic cement implanted into bone. Acta Orthop Scand 1975;46(suppl 161).

92. Mjoberg B, Pettersson H, Rosenquist R, Rydholm A. Bone cement, thermal injury and the radiolucent zone. Acta Orthop Scand 1984;55:597–600.

93. Huiskes R. Some fundamental aspects of human joint replacement. Acta Orthop Scand 1980;51(suppl 185).

94. Barth E, Sullivan T, Berg EW. Particulate size versus chemical composition of biomaterials as determining factors in macrophage activation. Trans 37th Annual ORS 1991;16.

95. Horowitz SM, Glautsch TL, Frondoza CG, Riley L. Macrophage exposure to methylmethacrylate leads to mediator release and injury. J Orthop Res 1991;9:406–413.

96. Maguire JK, Coscia MF, Lynch MH. Foreign body reaction to polymeric debris following total hip arthroplasty. Clin Orthop 1987;216:213–223.

97. Quinn J, Joyner C, Triffitt JT, Athanasou NA. Polymethylmethacrylate-induced inflammatory macrophages resorb bone. J Bone Joint Surg 1992;74-B:652–658.

98. Knutsson K, Tjornstrand B, Lidgren L. Survival of knee arthroplasty for rheumatoid arthritis. Acta Orthop Scand 1985;56:422–425.

99. Toksvig-Larsen S, Ryd L. Temperature elevation during knee arthroplasty. Acta Orthop Scand 1989;60:439–442.

100. Toksvig-Larsen S, Ryd L, Lindstrand A. An internally cooled sawblade. Acta Orthop Scand 1990;61(4):321–323.

101. Toksvig-Larsen S, Ryd L, Lindstrand A. On the problem of heat generation in different bone cutting. Studies on the effect of liquid cooling. J Bone Joint Surg 1991;73-B:13–15.

102. Toksvig-Larsen S. On bone cutting. Lund University, 1992.

103. Carlsson L, Rostlund T, Albrektsson B, Albrektsson T. Implant fixation improved by close fit. Cylindrical implant-bone interface studied in rabbits. Acta Orthop Scand 1988;59:272–275.

104. Toksvik-Larsen S, Ryd L. Surface flatness after bone cutting. Acta Orthop Scand 1991;62(1):15–18.

105. Burke DW, Bragdon CR, O'Connor DO, Jasty M, Haire T, Harris WH. Dynamic measurements of interface mechanics in vivo and the effect of micromotion on bone ingrowth into a porous coated surface device under controlled loads in vivo. Trans 37th Annual ORS 1991;16:103.

106. Pilliar RM, Lee JM, Maniatopoulos C. Observation on the effect of movement on bone ingrowth into porous surfaced implants. Clin Orthop 1986;208:108–113.

107. Little RB, Weavers HW, Siu D, Cooke TDV. A three-dimensional finite element analysis of the upper tibia. J Biomech Eng 1986;108:111–119.

108. Ochoa NA, Heck DA, Brandt KD, Hillberry BM. The effect of intratrabecular fluid on femoral head mechanics. J Rheumatol 1991;18(4):580–584.

109. Ivarsson I, Gillquist J. The strain distribution in the upper tibia after insertion of two different unicompartmental prostheses. Clin Orthop 1992;279:194–200.

110. Natarjan R, Andriacchi TP. The influence of displacement incompatibilities on bone ingrowth into porous tibial components. Trans 34th Annual ORS 1988;13:331.

111. Hvid I. Trabecular bone strength at the knee. Clin Orthop 1988;227:210–221.

112. Manley MT, Stulberg BN, Stern LS, Watson JT, Stulberg SD. Direct observation of micromotion at the implant-bone interface with cemented and non-cemented tibial components. Trans 33rd Annual ORS 1987;12:436.

113. Stulberg BN, Watson JT, Stulberg SD, Bauer TW, Manley MT. A new model to assess tibial fixation: II concurrent histologic and biomechanical observations. Clin Orthop 1991;263:303–309.

114. Kenna RV, Hungerford DS. Design rational for the Porous Coated Anatomic total knee system. In: Hungerford DS, Krackow KA, Kenna RV, eds. Total knee arthroplasty. A comprehensive approach. Baltimore: William & Wilkins, 1984:71–88.

115. Weinans H, Huiskes R, Grootenboer HJ. Trends of mechanical consequences and modeling of a fibrous membrane around femoral hip prostheses. J Biomech 1990;23:991–1000.

116. Rubin CT, Lanyon LE. Osteoregulatory nature of mechanical stimuli: function as a determinant for adaptive remodeling in bone. J Orthop Res 1987;5:300–310.

117. Huiskes R, Nunamaker D. Local stress and bone adaptation around orthopedic implants. Calcif Tissue Int 1984;36:S110-S117.

118. Aspenberg P, Goodman SB, Toksvig-Larsen S, Ryd L, Albrektsson T. Intermittent micromotion inhibits bone ingrowth: titanium implants in rabbits. Acta Orthop Scand 1992;63(2):1.

119. Cameron HU, Pilliar RM, MacNab I. The effect of movement on the bonding of porous metal to bone. J Biomech 1973;7:301–311.

120. Goldstein SA, Ku JL, Hollister S, Kayner DC, Matthews LS. The effect of applied stress on experimentally controlled remodeling in trabecular bone. Trans 36th Annual ORS 1986;11:432.

121. Draenert K. Histomorphology of the bone-to-cement interface: remodeling of the cortex and revascularization of the medullary canal in animal experiments. In: The hip. Proceedings of the 9th open scientific meeting of the Hip Society. St. Louis: CV Mosby, 1981:71–110.

122. Linder L, Carlsson AS. The bone-cement interface in hip arthroplasty. A histologic and enzyme study of stable components. Acta Orthop Scand 1986;57:495–500.

123. Dawson JM, Bartel DL. Consequences of an interface fit on the fixation of Porous-Coated tibial components in Total Knee replacement. J Bone Joint Surg 1992;74-A:233–238.

124. Mayor MB, Collier JP, Surprenant VA, Surprenent HP, Dauphinais LA. The success of pegs, stems, and screws as adjuvant means of fixation of tibial prostheses as measured by radiographic and histologic examination. In: Annual meeting of the AAOS. New Orleans: 1990:124.

125. Sumner DR, Jacobs JJ, Turner TM, Urban RM, Galante JO. The amount and distribution of bone ingrowth in tibial components retrieved from human patients. Trans 35th Annual ORS 1989;15:375.

126. Levack B, Revell PA, Freeman MAR. Presence of macrophages at the bone-cement interface of stable hip arthroplasty components. Acta Orthop Scand 1987;58:384–387.

127. Maloney WJ, Jasty M, Harris WH, Galante JO, Callaghan JJ. Endosteal erosions in association with stable uncemented femoral components. J Bone Joint Surg 1990;72-A:1025–1034.

128. Maloney WJ, Jasty M, Rosenberg A, Harris WH. Bone lysis in well-fixed cemented femoral components. J Bone Joint Surg 1990;72-B(6):966–970.

129. Goodman SB, Fornasier VL, Kei J. The effects of bulk versus particulate ultra high molecular weight polyethylene on bone. J Arthroplasty 1988;3(suppl):41–46.

130. Nolan JF, Bucknill TM. Aggressive granulomatosis from polyethylene failure in an uncemented knee replacement. J Bone Joint Surg 1992;74-B:23–24.

131. Murray DW, Rushton N. Macrophages stimulate bone resorption when they phagocytose particles. J Bone Joint Surg 1990;72-B(6):988–992.

132. Howie DW, Vernon-Roberts B, Oakeshott R, Manthey B. A rat model of resorption of bone at the cement-bone interface in the presence of polyethylene wear particles. J Bone Joint Surg 1988;70-A:257–263.

133. Schmalzried TP, Jasty M, Harris WH. Periprosthetic bone loss in total hip arthroplasty. J Bone Joint Surg 1992;74-A:849–863.

134. Heinegard D. Personal communication, 1992.

135. Nilsson KG, Karrholm J. Micromotion of the femoral component in Miller-Galante knee arthroplasty. Trans 38th Annual ORS 1992;17(2):378.

136. Mjoberg B, Franzen H, Selvik G. Early detection of prosthetic-hip loosening. Acta Orthop Scand 1990;61(3):273–274.

137. Snorrason F, Karrholm J. Primary stability of a threaded cementless acetabular prosthesis. J Bone Joint Surg 1990;72-B(4):647–652.

138. Snorrason F, Karrholm J. Early loosening of revision hip arthroplasty. A roentgen stereophotogrammetric analysis. J Arthroplasty 1990;5(3):217–229.

139. Nilsson KG, Broback LG, Karrholm J. Does a stem on the tibial component improve fixation of the uncemented Freeman-Samuelson prosthesis? Acta Orthop Scand 1989;60(suppl 231):34.

72

Cementless Total Knee Arthroplasty

Aaron G. Rosenberg and Jorge O. Galante

Ten years have passed since the introduction of total knee arthroplasty components designed to be fixed by bone ingrowth, and it is not yet clear what their appropriate place is in the management of the arthritic knee. Thus, many experienced knee surgeons appear to rely on this fixation method almost exclusively, while others use it rarely if at all. The initial design of cementless components was based on concerns regarding loosening of cemented devices in younger, heavier and more functionally demanding patients.

While the etiology of prosthetic loosening in total knee arthroplasty (TKA) is complex (involving issues of technique, alignment, and prosthetic design), the agent utilized to fix the prosthetic device, methylmethacrylate, has been considered a major factor. Bone cement is brittle, prone to fatigue failure, and a poor transmitter of tensile and sheer stress (1). Bone cement is capable of producing massive osteolysis, and, even when stable, an increased load, combined with the cement's finite fatigue life, may render it a potentially weak link in the chain of requirements for prosthetic survival (2, 3).

However, recent long-term follow-up as well as survival studies of well aligned, cemented total knee arthroplasties have revealed excellent function and prosthetic survival at between 10 and 15 years (4–6). Indeed, a favorable comparison has been made with cemented total hip arthroplasty, where bone-cement interface analysis appears to demonstrate that the well-cemented and well-aligned total knee arthroplasty will probably have superior survival when compared to cemented total hip arthroplasty (7). Thus, at the knee, there may be little need for alternate forms of fixation.

Nonetheless, cementless knee arthroplasty remains popular and is becoming increasingly better understood physiologically. The premises underlying the use of bone ingrowth fixation in total knee arthroplasty are: 1) that the theoretical disadvantages of cement will be eliminated, 2) fixation comparable to cement will be achieved, with similar clinical results obtained, and 3)

the result will be more durable. The purpose of this chapter is to evaluate these premises. An initial discussion of ingrowth process biology is followed by a review of the application of these principles to the design requirements of contemporary total knee arthroplasty. Specific clinical applications of this technology are reviewed, including both current indications and reported results.

Ingrowth Biology

For the purposes of this discussion, biologic ingrowth is defined as the fixation of an underlying substrate to bone by the ingrowth of bone into a porous structured coating. While both thorough and limited reviews of bone ingrowth biology have recently been published (8–12), a brief overview will help orient the reader to the application of biologic ingrowth requirements to total knee design. Many of the issues discussed with reference to this process may bear on other uncemented fixation techniques (such as press-fit implantations or fixation by polyethylene pegs), but these are beyond the scope of this discussion.

Bone ingrowth is known to occur if an appropriate porous structure is intimately applied to a living bone surface (and held in place for sufficient time) with a minimum of motion between porous surface and bone. Thus the prerequisites of ingrowth (loosely described) are the following: (*a*) appropriate porous structure, (*b*) intimate contact, (*c*) lack of relative motion.

While the majority of work done on bone ingrowth has taken place in animal models, recent widespread human implantation has led to sufficient histologic retrieval to indicate that the physiologic phenomenon observed in the laboratory is similar to that which occurs in humans.

Many of the histologic features of ingrowth resemble bone repair in the healing of cortical defects (13, 14). The void spaces in the porous structure fill with hematoma and inflammatory cells following the trauma of implantation. In the canine model, the inflammatory cellular infiltrate (pleuripotential mesenchymal cells) is replaced directly by bone approximately 2 weeks after implantation. Remaining fibrous and cellular components in the void spaces are replaced by this woven bone over the next 4 weeks with lamellar bone remodeling soon following (Fig. 72.1). This bone, which is now part of the local skeletal structure, fully interdigitates with the porous structure and accounts for the strength of fixation.

Thus, in the ideal environment of intimate contact and in the absence of substrate-bone interface motion, no cartilaginous precursor to bone is formed. However, if bone ingrowth does not occur, it is likely that a fibrous connective tissue (which may be highly organized and provide some degree of fixation, again, dependent on the physical environment) will invade the pore spaces. This type of ingrowth in which fibrocartilaginous or mineralized cartilage tissue is present appears to be related to excessive interface motion or gaps between bone and porous surface (15).

An important and unanswered question is whether any "non-bone" yet ingrown tissue may be replaced by bone at a time period after the fibrous tissue has matured and fills the void spaces. The similarities between bone ingrowth and primary fracture healing as well as between fibrous ingrowth and fibrous nonunion of fractures is intriguing. The possibility that the fibrous ingrowth "nonunion" might be converted to a bone ingrowth or a healed fracture situation by appropriate stimulation is an appealing theoretical possibility.

Remodeling

Long-term remodeling of bone in the implant setting is most likely controlled by factors related to Wolff's Law and governed by the load transmission from implant to bone. Lack of load transfer has been demonstrated to produce poor quality ingrowth (12). Thus, the ingrowth process requires a balance: sufficient loading of the interface to promote bone accretion, but not so much as to cause sufficient interface motion to prevent ingrowth. Studies of bone remodeling about porous-coated implants have tended to confirm that stress fields in bone surrounding porous-coated implants can be radically changed from normal and are dependent on prosthetic design and placement of ingrowth surfaces (16, 17). In a study designed to evaluate such parameters, the amount and pattern of bone ingrowth in a porous-coated canine femoral hip stem was seen to change over time (17). With porous surfaces along the entire length of the prosthesis, retrieval at 1 month showed uniform ingrowth along the entire surface, while at 6 months, proximal and distal ingrowth was greatly increased in comparison to midstem. This pattern was considered to reflect interface stresses as affected by the stem's material properties, geometry, and location of ingrowth surface. Other investigators have noted a similar relationship (18), and these parameters remain of primary concern in the design of "ingrowth" implants.

Ingrowth Histology

Both quantitative as well as qualitative information regarding the efficacy of this type of fixation may be provided by histologic evaluation. Retrieved specimens are cut, ground, and surface-stained with toluidine blue and basic fuchsin after embedding in methylmethacrylate. Microscopic evaluation for cellular infiltrates, inflammatory response, the architecture, pattern, and location of fibrous and bone tissue, as well as the occurrence of and response to wear debris may be carried out.

Bone ingrowth may be quantitatively assessed by point counting. Measurements of interest include the volume fraction and extent of ingrowth. Volume fraction is determined using a test point grid that allows characterization of the tissue or material at each point. The volume fraction of bone ingrowth is calculated by dividing the number of grid intersections where bone is found by the difference between the total number of grid intersections and the number of intersections where metal is encountered. The measurement of this quantity has been automated with the use of backscatter scanning electron microscopy coupled with digital image analysis (19).

Extent of ingrowth is determined by examining microscopic fields encompassing the entire depth of the porous coating. Topographical maps of the entire retrieved specimen may be constructed demonstrating areas and patterns of ingrowth (Fig. 72.2). Any bone penetrating the porous surface by an arbitrary amount (for these criteria, we have used the measurement of ½ of a metal fiber diameter) may be considered as ingrowth. Extent of ingrowth is then represented by evaluating multiple fields for the presence of bone and dividing the number of fields with bone by the total number of fields. This quantity can also be measured with backscatter scanning electron microscopy (19).

Fixation Strength

An important parameter for measuring fixation quality is the difficulty of dislodging an implanted structure. This represents the ultimate success or failure of the purported purpose of ingrowth-fixation of the device. Measurement of these forces may be affected by testing design, and testing design must be considered when comparisons of strength of fixation studies are attempted.

In general, initial strength of fixation is dependent on mechanical implant parameters such as the "tightness" of a press fit or the use of adjunct fixation. While initially less than the immediate strength achieved with bone cement, several studies of nonloaded ingrowth implants placed in cancellous bone have shown strength of fixation to increase rapidly and then plateau at 2 weeks (1.4 to 2.6 MPa)(13, 14). This is in the range of the trabecular bone strength (20). Interfacial shear strength of implants placed in cortical bone more closely reflects the strength of cortical bone (approximately 15 MPa), although peak strength values in cortical bone are not reached until about 8 weeks. Strength of fixation may be useful in evaluating parameters in-

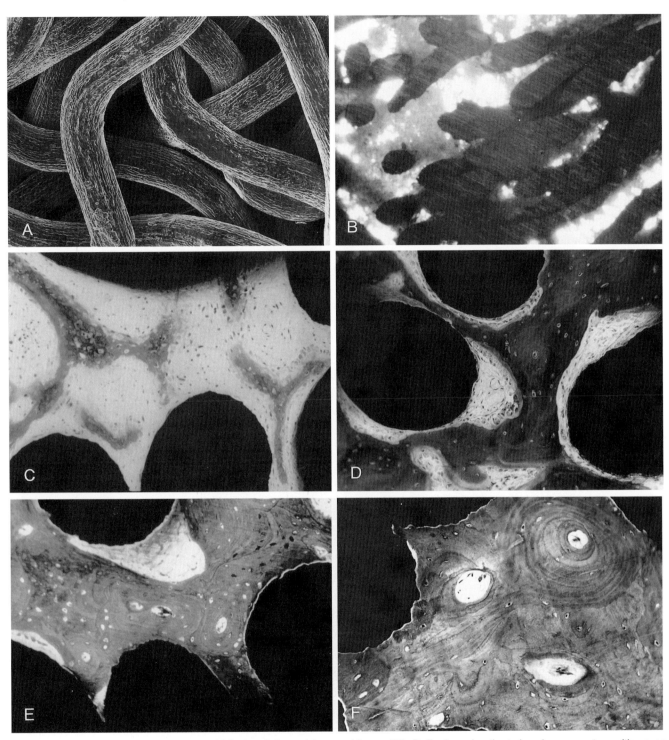

Figure 72.1.   A, Porous ingrowth substrate, kinked and sintered titanium fiber at 250 × magnification. Note three dimensional interconnecting porosity. **B,** Similar ingrowth substrate–histomicrograph at mag × 250. Approximately 48 hours after implantation. Darker segments represent cross sections of titanium wire. Interspersed in the porous layer is a hematoma resulting from the trauma of implantation. Canine model. **C,** By 2 weeks, a cellular infiltrate has replaced the hematoma. This pleuripotential mesenchymal tissue fills the porous space and is already forming strands of woven bone. Note rimming osteoblasts surrounding young trabeculae. Canine model.

Mag. × 400. **D,** By 6 weeks, the trabeculae are mature with woven bone remodelling to lamellar systems. A fibrous cellular layer remains interposed between bone and metal substrate. Note presence of osteoblasts and osteoclasts in this actively remodeling bone. Canine model. Mag × 400. **E,** At 6 months, the bone demonstrates mature osteonal systems and in many places no fibrous layer is interposed between fiber wire and bone. Canine model. Mag × 400. **F,** 10-year retrieval from primate implantation. Mag × 400. Note lack of fibrous layer. Mature osteonal bone predominates.

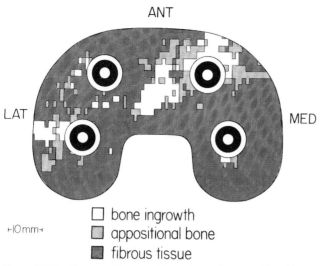

Figure 72.2. Topographic map of bone ingrowth, appositional bone, and fibrous tissue from a titanium fiber metal tibial tray retrieved at revision surgery. These maps may yield valuable information on bone ingrowth patterns and the effects of various design parameters (Used with permission from Sumner DR, Galante JO. Bone Ingrowth. In: Evarts, CM, ed. Surgery of the musculoskeletal system. New York: Churchill Livingstone, 1992).

hibiting or enhancing ingrowth and are a useful mechanical adjunct to histologic studies.

Pore Size Requirements

The effect of pore size on ingrowth was first studied using ceramics where pore size was easily controlled. Bobyn has demonstrated ingrowth of mineralized bone into pores of 50 micrometers (μm) (21). Osteonal remodeling is seen as the pore size rises above 100 μm (13, 14), and, between 50 and 100 μm, the strength of fixation increases with increasing pore size (22, 23). Most studies have confirmed that strength of fixation is not affected by pore size between 150 μm to 400 μm (21, 24, 25) and that strength of fixation is lowered between 400 μm to 800 μm (21), presumably due to smaller amounts of the void space being occupied by bone.

Other important variables in the design of a porous surface for ingrowth are particle interconnectivity and volume fraction of porosity, parameters that may affect the material strength of the substrate and the "openness" of the pores.

Apposition to Bone

Gaps at the interface between porous substrate and bone are known to decrease ingrowth and hence the strength of fixation. While gaps of up to 2 millimeters (mm) may be bridged by bone in an unloaded setting (26), they may take up to 12 weeks to fill in (27). In our laboratory, unloaded specimens were studied in a model that demonstrated bone ingrowth across 3 mm gaps. However, the ingrowth was only occasionally present and was decreased when compared to historic controls (28). The ability of the ingrowth phenomena to bridge gaps bears directly both on implant design and on the

fashioning of bone surfaces in knee replacement and is discussed in detail below.

Interface Motion

Interface motion has been demonstrated to inhibit the quality and quantity of ingrowth bone at a porous surface. As mentioned, bone ingrowth has been noted in mechanically stable implants and fibrous ingrowth in less stable implants (10). While the requirements for ingrowth are multifactorial and while both the degree of contact and micromotion are most likely to interact in a complex manner, achieving initial mechanical stability and thus minimizing micromotion is a prime consideration in the design of total knee arthroplasty components that will be expected to achieve bone ingrowth (29). Relative displacements of 28 μm have been found to be consistent with bone ingrowth with fibrous fixation at 150 μm of motion (30). Bone ingrowth has been noted in canine femoral hip stems at initial micromovement of 56 μm (31). Toksvig-Larsen, et al. (32) have reported on a micromotion chamber, which can be manipulated to achieve 250 μm or 500 μm motion. Manipulation at 500 μm 20 times (over a 30 second interval) daily, effectively inhibited bone ingrowth in 7 of 8 chambers. Twenty cycles of 250 μm did not inhibit ingrowth (3 of 3 ingrown). Even 500 μm of motion once daily was compatible with ingrowth (3 of 6 chambers ingrown). Clearly, the parameters of time, motion, and displacement interact in a complex fashion. Further interaction with the multiple factors influencing ingrowth renders this subject complex and clearly requiring further research.

Ingrowth Enhancement

In the setting where the ideal parameters for ingrowth cannot be achieved, enhancement methods may be useful. These methods may be important in situations where implant stability is not ideal or where extensive gaps are present, such as in a primary TKA with imperfect bone cuts or where there is a lack of initial mechanical stability due to poor adjunctive fixation. This may also be represented in a revision setting.

Studies evaluating a multitude of potential enhancing agents have been reported with the most commonly studied agents being autogenous (5, 28, 33–38) and allogeneic (35, 39) bone graft, calcium phosphate preparations including coatings and granules (25, 40–45), electrical stimulation (46, 47, 48–51), and other bone induction agents (52, 53).

In both nonloaded gap models (28, 34, 35), canine TKA revision models (36, 38), and loaded, nongap human retrieval models, autograft has been shown to enhance ingrowth. However, in comparison to a tight press-fit model, without loading, supplemental autograft demonstrated no enhancement in both a gap (54) or press-fit model (37). A weight-bearing gap study reported less ingrowth with autograft than with a control (33). A concern with all settings where graft or other potential "enhancement" agents are placed between live bone and the ingrowth surface is that these agents will block the pores and hence act as an ingrowth deterrent.

Fresh frozen allograft has demonstrated enhancement in nonweight-bearing gap models (35, 39) and in revision THA models (36), where freeze dried allograft has been less effective (28, 34). Calcium phosphate coatings have demonstrated the ability to "orient" initial bone ingrowth so that strength of fixation is enhanced at early time periods when compared with controls (25, 40). In a typical study, a calcium phosphate coating (applied by plasma flame spraying) was compared to an untreated titanium fiber metal unloaded implant (55). Untreated implants had lower strength of fixation at 4 weeks (24%) but was similar at 1, 2, and 6 weeks. In the untreated group, the bone was randomly distributed in the voids, while, in the coated implants, most of the bone within the void spaces was in direct contact with the calcium-phosphate-coated metal fibers. While similar findings have been noted in various implant models (43, 56–60), other studies have shown a negative or variable effect from similar coatings (25, 37, 41, 44, 61, 62). These contrary findings may be due to the transient nature of the benefit noted with these coatings, or to solubility characteristics of the coating, or to multiple other variables that differ in the various experimental models reported.

Granular calcium phosphate materials appear to enhance gap defect healing but appear ineffective when a tight press-fit model is employed (33, 35, 39, 63). In general, the bulk of experimental evidence points to a significant difference between enhancement with and without gaps present. In nongap, tight press-fit models, the presence of substances between the pores and the live bone may inhibit ingrowth by "blocking" pores. In such a setting, the use of calcium phosphate coatings may orient early ingrowth bone and enhance early strength of fixation only. In models where gaps are present, autograft bone proves more successful than allogeneic in most studies (64), and allogeneic bone is occasionally matched in efficacy by calcium phosphate granular preparations.

For a more detailed discussion of ingrowth enhancement, the reader is referred to a recent review of this subject (12).

Ingrowth Inhibition

In addition to interface gaps and excessive motion inhibiting ingrowth, other chemical and physical modalities may produce the same effect (12). These include: warfarin (Coumadin) (65), indomethacin and other nonsteroidal antiinflammatory agents (66, 67), chemotherapeutic agents (65), and ionizing radiation (68, 69). In general, anything known to have a deleterious effect on bone healing may be considered to have a similar effect on the ingrowth process.

Total Knee Arthroplasty Design Criteria

Understanding of ingrowth biology applied to the problem of providing lasting fixation of total knee arthroplasty components has centered on two primary conditions: attaining sufficient component stability in the immediate postoperative period (preventing micromo-tion and allowing for ingrowth to occur) and minimizing stress alterations in bone (which accompany prosthetic implantation), so that severe stress shielding and adverse bone remodeling is avoided.

Ingrowth surfaces have been provided on several types of condylar prostheses (meniscal bearing, rotating platform, cruciate sparing, cruciate sacrificing). However, the purpose here is not to compare prosthetic designs in terms of articulation function, but rather to evaluate the mechanisms by which these devices are designed to allow ingrowth fixation to occur.

Surface Material

Much of the initial research on porous ingrowth physiology utilized ceramics and polymers, but these have been deemed unsuitable (by most) for prosthetic fixation purposes due to their inadequate material properties. Commercially available devices consist almost exclusively of porous metallic coatings. These surfaces meet the ingrowth requirements for porosity while providing requisite mechanical properties, such as strength and fatigue resistance. Both titanium and cobalt-chrome-molybdenum alloys have been used. While claims have been made that there is a small carcinogenic risk in cobalt-chrome alloy implantation (70), titanium has been shown to be a poor bearing surface unless properly treated (71). The relative merits of each material are beyond the scope of this chapter. Two basic types of true porous surfaces are currently used: beaded and meshed.

It should also be mentioned that finned polyethylene pegs have been utilized with and without supplementary ingrowth surfaces to provide both temporary and permanent fixation (72–76). Of historical interest is Ring's arthroplasty, utilizing titanium "fins" with macro porous holes to achieve fixation (77).

Ingrowth surfaces in contemporary clinical use include cobalt chrome beads on a cobalt chrome substrate found in the Porous-Coated Anatomic (PCA) knee (Howmedica; Rutherford, NJ); titanium beads on titanium substrate in the Microloc knee (Johnson & Johnson Orthopedics; New Brunswick, NJ); a beaded system with cobalt chrome femoral and titanium tibial component (Press-Fit condylar; Johnson & Johnson; New Brunswick, NJ); and a titanium mesh system on a nitrided titanium alloy substrate (MGII; Zimmer; Warsaw, IN). Neither clinical nor experimental data on ingrowth into these varied surfaces would appear to recommend one surface over another in terms of ingrowth potential.

Interface failure may be a prelude to clinical failure in a cemented total knee, with prostheses-cement or cement-bone failure leading to increased motion at the interface with resultant increased peak stresses, further loosening, and clinical symptoms. Failure of the porous surface at its junction with the prosthetic substrate may be an additional complicating factor in the ingrowth setting. Failure at the porous-coating substrate level may be expected to be more prevalent in situations where the prosthesis bone interface is not secured by excellent ingrowth and where increased micromotion is present. This problem has been reported extensively and almost exclusively at the knee with beaded surfaces.

Gross, et al. reported 40 PCA implants with loose beads noted in 23 knees (11 femoral, 16 tibial, and 1 patellar component), correlating loose beads with radiolucent lines and progressive bead shedding with radiolucent line progression (78). Similar progressive ingrowth surface deterioration with prosthetic loosening has been reported by Knahr, et al. (79). The possibility of intraarticular migration of these metallic fragments and subsequent development of accelerated wear and prosthetic failure has been documented by Cooke, et al.(80). Ryd demonstrated PCA bead shedding in 12 of 13 uncemented tibial components (81) and Rosenqvist, et al. found over half of cemented and uncemented PCA beaded components to have bead shedding (82). In the majority, shedding was associated with radiolucency and occurred after 3 months implantation. Novacheck, et al. reported similar findings in uncemented PCA components (83) but noted a lower incidence of shedding in cemented components (44% versus 10%). Here again, radiolucent lines were significantly correlated with bead loosening. These problems may be reduced with improved contemporary manufacturing techniques.

While these reports of bead loosening are noted in only one prosthetic type (PCA), it must be noted that this phenomenon is not likely found only in this prosthesis. Haynes and Freedman (84) have demonstrated that individual beads or bead aggregates of less than 300 μm are not resolvable and are, hence, invisible using standard radiograph techniques. The PCA prosthesis associated with the reports of bead shedding used larger beads (700 to 750 μm) than is utilized with other devices (Low Contact Stress or LCS; Depuy, Warsaw, IN). All such beaded surfaces may undergo this type of shedding with smaller particles being radiographically undetectable. Mesh surfaces may be less susceptible to individual fiber shedding due to multiple welds along small segments of the surface and the overall integrity of the ingrowth substrate, which is a single, formed material. However, catastrophic separation of this substrate from the underlying prosthetic component has been noted in total hip components fixed with early sintering techniques (85).

Motion and Fixation

Both an appropriate porous ingrowth surface and viable bone are required for fixation by ingrowth. In addition, the two surfaces must be in intimate contact and maintained without excessive motion until the ingrowth process has occurred.

In general, prosthetic design allows the uniform presentation of flat prosthetic surfaces to the underlying bone. Initial intimate contact is achieved through a combination of prosthetic design and surgical technique. As the bone surfaces must be cut to mate with the prosthetic surface, accurate cutting of the bone is essential in providing initial intimate contact with the prosthesis. To this end, most prosthetic devices designed for ingrowth capability have instrumentation designed to minimize errors in the cutting of flat bone surfaces. An excellent review of technical factors in the cutting of bone surfaces is available (86). Even in the ideal setting

of the laboratory, so-called "flat" cut tibial surfaces have been shown to present irregularities on a microscopic level (87), where the surface actually appears as a series of irregular peaks and valleys. Hence, the rigid tibial component may only have multiple areas of point contact with the cut bone surface.

The porous surface-bone interface must remain in sufficient apposition following implantation to allow ingrowth to occur, and each component (femoral, tibial, and patellar) has unique design features which must be taken into account when considering the potential for interfacial motion following implantation. Excessive motion (as described in the previous section) will lead to the ingrowth of fibrous tissue and fibrocartilage at the interface. Two types of motion must be taken into account: rigid body motion—the tendency of the component to move in a direction the bone is not (subsidence, liftoff, tilt, shear), and tangential displacements—caused by a difference in elastic modulus of the porous coating and the bone.

The femoral component, by its box-like configuration, appears to provide adequate intrinsic resistance to rigid body motion by virtue of shape alone. The more precise the press fit of the anterior and posterior condylar surfaces, the greater the increase in frictional forces tending to immobilize this component. The anterior and posterior surfaces tend to resist anterior-posterior translation, flexion-extension tilt, and rotation. Metaphyseal lugs or pegs distally tend to prevent medial-lateral tilt, medial lateral translation, and rotation.

The patellar component presents unique problems to ingrowth applications, with forces at the bone-prosthetic interface highly dependent on the patello-femoral junction design. The most common porous interface is a flat surface with pegs and, while seemingly more effective in resisting compression, rotation, and shear, this configuration depends on peg interference fit with resulting interfacial frictional forces resisting tilting and lift-off. While insetting the patellar component in bone may help in resisting such forces, all noncompressive forces (shear, tilt) must be borne by the peg-plate junction until ingrowth has occurred. Consequently, patellar-component failure was a common feature of early metal backed patellar design. Additional difficulties with patellar fixation include the unique configuration of the bone itself. The cut surface may result in bone with varied bone quality available at the ingrowth surface. Additionally, problems of patellar tilting and subluxation may substantially increase those forces tending to dislodge the component. For a more complete review, the reader is referred to reports documenting this problem (88–90).

From a design standpoint, fixation on the tibial side has been considered the most problematic; thus, most of the research and modifications of cemented design to cementless design have involved this component. The magnitude of micro-motion at the tibial prosthetic bone interface has been evaluated both in vivo (91–97) and by finite element methods (98).

Observations in hemiarthroplasty and total arthroplasty cementless tibial trays fixed with simple interference fit peg fixation under eccentric physiologic loads has revealed micromotion sufficient to prevent ingrowth (150 to 300 μm)(99). While pure compressive loads are relatively easily resisted simply by compression of the underlying bone, such loads are not a realistic modeling of in vivo forces that may lead to tilting or liftoff and include both shear and eccentric compressive loading.

In a comparison of various stems and pegs in preventing torque and shear displacements, the addition of cruciate-shaped blades to a central stem inhibited both motions more than a simple stem alone (97). In this study, four pegs provided similar motion reduction to the blade plus stem configuration and was better than two pegs.

Whitesides evaluated stemmed tibial components with the addition of screws to fix the tibial component and/or a sleeve added to the stem (92). Under all loading conditions, the screws provided the greatest reduction in micromotion. These finding were also noted in our laboratory where micromotion reduction was enhanced by a placement of four screws and further improved with additional screws (95). Other investigators (100) have demonstrated the enhanced fixation capabilities of larger screws (6.5mm versus 3.8mm) in tibial components.

Direct comparisons of the mechanical stability of various commercially available tibial components have been reported. Voltz, et al. (96) found the Anatomic Medullary Knee (AMK) (Depuy; Warsaw, IN) component with four 6.5mm screws to achieve slightly greater mechanical stability than either the Whitesides' OrthoLoc I (Dow-Corning; Arlington, TN) utilizing a stem or the Miller-Galante I (Zimmer; Warsaw, IN) components that utilized four smaller screws and pegs. All showed much greater stability than the PCA (Howmedica; Rutherford, New Jersey) components with two pegs and only one screw.

Shimagaki, et al. (94) compared the PCA, Whitesides' Ortholoc I and Tricon (Richards Medical; Memphis, Tennessee) tibial components. (The Tricon has initial stability imparted by 29mm diameter polyethylene posts, each with eight polyethylene flanges.) In this study, the only component with screw fixation (PCA) was least stable to medial-lateral liftoff, and its stability was similar with or without placement of the single screw.

The Tricon demonstrated good liftoff stability but demonstrated considerable sinking under load. This may represent the flanged pegs preventing full initial seating of the component. The Whitesides component with large central stem and sleeve appeared to be most stable. Cameron demonstrated that the addition of a large central stem to the Tricon M (polyethylene finned peg) component reduced tibial component subsidence and improved the clinical result (101).

Thus, a central stem, blades affixed cruciate fashion to a stem, and, most importantly, screws have been shown to reduce micromotion of tibial components. As far as screws are concerned, larger, more peripherally placed, and a greater number of screws, all appear to enhance fixation. The addition of a stem to a tibial component that is also fixed by screws appears to decrease micromotion only in the setting of "poor quality" proximal tibial bone (102, 103).

When two different materials are compressed along their interface, variation of the elastic modulus between the two materials will lead to differences in the relative tangential strain (displacement) of the opposing surfaces when loaded. This is called tangential displacement, and represents an additional type of displacement that must be considered. Cancellous proximal tibial bone has an elastic modulus more than an order of magnitude less than most metallic porous materials (9, 10, 20, 104–106). Finite element analysis of a tibial tray rigidly fixed to cancellous bone predicts that such modulus mismatch would cause displacements of up to 150 microns at the tibial periphery (107). Active in-vitro displacements of this nature have been measured (107) with the greatest displacements noted at the periphery (100 to 200 μm) and lower displacements noted centrally (Fig. 72.3).

Lower displacements are also seen in the vicinity of peripheral pegs, which may inhibit such motion.

In addition to the agreement between the mathematical model and the mechanical test specimens, these displacement patterns appear to correlate with patterns of ingrowth noted in retrieved specimens from both human implantation and animal experimentation (15). Implanted titanium-beaded tibial components retrieved from canines 2 years after implantation revealed bone ingrowth approaching 100% at the pegs and 60% at the tibial plateau. This finding was consistent in all retrieved specimens (108).

In a similar study (15) of cementless canine total knee arthroplasty utilizing three pegs in a titanium mesh ingrowth surface tibial tray, we found consistent ingrowth into and in the immediate vicinity of the pegs (1 to 3mm radius). More variable plate ingrowth ranged from 12.0% to 81.1% with a mean of 34.6%. Ingrowth was noted most frequently in the central region of the component in the area between the pegs and over the medial aspects of the component.

Furthermore, tibial plate material properties may influence component stability. Whitesides compared CoCr and Ti6A14V tibial trays under various loading conditions and found significantly less displacement in the titanium trays under a variety of loading conditions with both hard and soft bone (109).

Bone Remodeling

Investigators remain concerned about extensive bone remodeling around porous-coated implants (110). In experimental models, stress shielding effects have been noted in extensively coated porous femoral total hip and surface hip stems (9, 13, 17). While animal studies of a porous-coated, stemmed femoral component have shown distal bone resorption with adverse remodeling changes, 5-year follow-up of porous ingrowth stemmed PCA tibial components showed no radiographically apparent adverse remodeling effects (111).

Finite element analysis used to predict bone remodeling around a flat tibial ingrowth tray with two in-

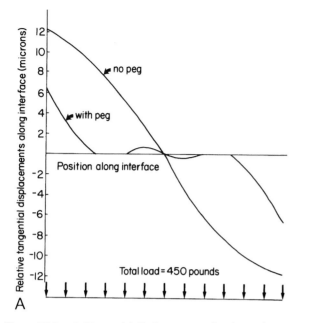

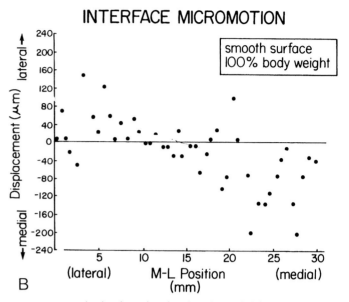

Figure 72.3. **A,** Tangential displacements take place when two materials of differing elastic modulus are compressed. Relative motion perpendicular to the applied force is different for the two materials with resultant displacement between the opposing surfaces. This finite element analysis represents position along a tibial component interface on the X axis and ranges from one edge of the plate to the opposite edge. The Y axis represents relative tangential displacements in microns. The two plots represent the interface with and with-out pegs projecting from the plate into the underlying bone. Note the relative lack of displacement centrally in both settings. Note how without pegs the displacements increase relatively rapidly out from the center. Note how pegs modulate this effect (Courtesy R. Natarajan). **B,** Canine in-vivo experimental measurement of interface micromotion due to tangential displacements. Note maximal displacements at smooth plate periphery (Courtesy R. Natarajan).

growth pegs found bone density should increase about the pegs and decrease in the plateau periphery (16). However, bone mineral density studies of the tibial plateau beneath 14 uncemented PCA tibial components implanted an average of 3.5 years showed no adverse remodeling (112).

Loading characteristics of porous-coated femoral and tibial components with long smooth pegs on the femoral and a large smooth stem on the tibial component were evaluated by Whitesides (113). Strain gauge studies demonstrated high strains in the tibial metaphyseal cortex 3 cm and 6 cm from the cut proximal tibial surface. One hundred ten similar cementless tibial components evaluated radiographically showed central proximal cancellous bone hypertrophy under the tibial plate at 3 months with 13% showing more diffuse proximal hypertrophy. By 1 year, the hypertrophic bone appeared to extend in a band to the cortical metaphysis 3 to 6 cm from the proximal tibia and was associated with peripheral proximal atrophy consistent with the strain gauge studies. Distal femoral hypertrophy was noted where the distal bone surface component contact was intimate, with atrophy noted where gaps were present.

While the possibility of adverse bone remodeling must be taken into account in the design of cementless total knee components, no significant clinical problems have been noted with current clinical designs.

Summary of Cementless TKA Design Considerations

While the above discussion reviews many of the requirements necessary to achieve ingrowth of a porous surfaced knee arthroplasty, it may be useful to briefly summarize those features of design and implantation needed to achieve a successful result.

The primary requirements of ingrowth are intimate contact and minimization of interface motion. At surgery, intimate contact must be achieved by the use of precise surgical technique with attention paid to component fit on bone surfaces. Gaps between bone and porous surface will likely diminish ingrowth across these gaps. Convex surfaces will provide for a "teeter-totter" effect. Concave surfaces are more stable but will still cause extensive gapping. Strictly flat surfaces are the ideal.

Initial stability must be enhanced by various means to allow for ingrowth to occur over a biologic time frame. The box-like configuration of the femoral component does not appear to require more than a tight press (frictional) fit (with the addition of smooth metaphyseal pegs). The tibial component should employ screws or may employ press-fit stems or broad keels in addition to pegs to provide enhanced immediate stability. Fully coated long stems may result in significant stress shielding with adverse bone remodeling and should be avoided.

Interaction of femoral and tibial components should avoid constraint to prevent the transmission of "stabilizing" reaction forces to the interface of prosthesis and bone. Although several knees with ingrowth potential have a posterior stabilized mechanism, the majority of ingrowth and press-fit knees are constrained only by virtue of retained ligaments, with conformation of distal femoral and polyethylene tibial surfaces providing only minimal restraint.

Finally, the alignment of the limb and ligamentous stability of the articulating surfaces must minimize eccentric loading of the components. Most modern instrumentations systems are designed to produce a mechanically neutral axis to the limb to minimize eccentric loading of the components. While eccentric loading due to malalignment or instability may reduce the long-term survival of cemented components, it may preclude ingrowth and jeopardize even the early result of cementless components.

Clinical Results of Cementless Systems

What follows is a review of reported results with several established cementless systems.

Whitesides' Ortholoc I and II

Whitesides has presented data on a large personal series of arthroplasties using his own prosthetic design, the Ortholoc I and its modified successor, the Ortholoc II (Fig. 72.4). The femoral component has two smooth metaphyseal pegs and avoids porous surfaces on the anterior and posterior flanges. The initial tibial component utilized smooth pegs and a smooth central stem with the newer components using additional screws for enhanced initial stability (114). This series represents consecutive cases with cementless fixation without exclusion of patients based on age, diagnosis, or bone quality. Over a 2½-year period, 304 Ortholoc I knees were implanted, with 60 knees lost to follow-up. Follow-up ranged from 24 to 67 months and averaged 38, with age averaging 65 (18 to 86). Of the 304 implants, 94% were osteoarthritic and 4% rheumatoid. Using a Hospital for Special Surgery (HSS) scoring system, 80% were excellent, 13% good, 6% fair, and 1% poor.

In a comparison of results between the Ortholoc I and II at 1-year follow-up, a statistically significant lowering of pain scores at 1 year with the use of screws in the tibial component was noted. In a more recent review of 1100 knees (481 Ortholoc I and 629 Ortholoc II) (115), approximately 10% were lost to follow-up. In the first series, only one case of component loosening was noted, and none occurred in the second series. Pain relief at 1 year was greater in the components fixed with screws but was comparable at 2 years. In the group utilizing screws, no difference in pain scores was noted for sex or age (above or below 65) at either 1-year or 2-year follow-up. In a separate review of rheumatoid patients (average age 62 years) at 1 to 7 years follow-up, the average Knee Society knee scores improved 56 points to a mean of 88. Two revisions (4%) were required but neither for component loosening, and only one patient had moderate pain.

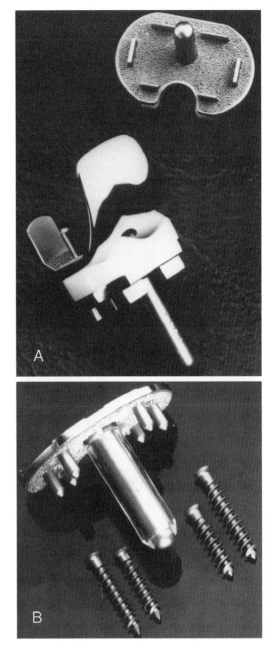

Figure 72.4. **A,** OrthoLoc I— Note small pegs and moderately long stem (Courtesy Dow-Corning, Arlington, TN). **B,** OrthoLoc II—Updated version incorporated new peg design and has added screws to improve initial fixation (Courtesy Dow-Corning, Arlington, TN).

Polyethylene Pegs

Use of the flanged polyethylene peg for definitive and adjunctive fixation has been reported. Albrektsson and Herberts (72) reported 108 ICLH knees implanted consecutively for 2 to 8 years. The tibial component was not metal backed and has no porous ingrowth surface. Fixation was only by polyethylene flanged pegs. Eleven arthroplasties failed by aseptic loosening. Utilizing a

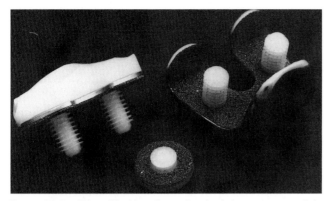

Figure 72.5. Tricon-M—Note flanged polyethylene pegs used for initial fixation. Note beaded, porous ingrowth surface (Courtesy Richards, Memphis, TN).

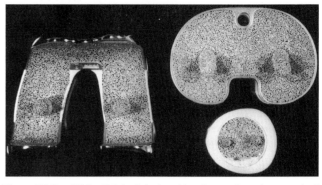

Figure 72.6. PCA—Original design. Note ingrowth surfaces on both femoral and tibial pegs and single screw design for tibial component (Courtesy Howmedica, Rutherford, NJ).

similar tibial component, Samuelson (116) followed 221 TKAs at 5 to 9 years. Of the 221 TKAs, 22 (10%) were revised for subsidence and symptoms, while an additional 21 patients had minimally symptomatic subsidence or progressive radiolucency. Laskin (76) reported on the Tricon-M knee, which used similar pegs as adjunctive fixation in a tibial component with a beaded porous undersurface (Fig. 72.5). A minimum 2-year follow-up of 96 patients (42 with osteoarthritis and 54 with rheumatoid arthritis) revealed comparable postoperative results in the two groups with mean HSS scores of 81 and 83. Three patients required revision for aseptic loosening. Cement was used when the tibial bone was soft or cysts prevented fixation of the pegs. When compared to the cementless group, the cemented patients took less time on the average to achieve a pain-free result.

Low Contact Stress (LCS) Meniscal Bearing Implant

Buechel has reported on a meniscal bearing implant (the LCS) with several varieties of bearing surfaces. (In this system, ingrowth stems and pegs are utilized for fixation of the tibial component). In a 12-year follow-up for cemented knees and 6-year follow-up for cementless, comparable survival rates were noted (117). Of primary cementless knees, 98% had good to excellent results at 2- to 7-year follow-up (118). In this series, no specific criteria for the use of cement or cementless fixation was noted.

Porous-Coated Anatomic (PCA) Prosthesis

Among the earliest knee arthroplasties designed for use without cement is the Porous-Coated Anatomic (PCA) prosthesis (Fig. 72.6). It achieves fixation with a microporous beaded surface of cobalt chrome, and the tibial component utilizes two small, posteriorly directed pegs and a single anterior screw. There are multiple reports published by the developers concerning results (1, 119, 120). Recently they reviewed results of cementless implantation of the prosthesis in their patients 50 years of age or younger (121), a group that should represent the highest stress levels for tests of the stability of the cementless system.

A total of 52 knees were implanted with 4 lost to follow-up. Follow-up time averaged 51 months (28 to 90 months). The average age at surgery was quite young, 40 for patients with osteoarthritis, 36 for rheumatoid, and 35 for osteonecrosis. Using a 100 point rating scale (which assigns 50 points for absence of pain and 50 points for normal examination and muscle strength), the average score at follow-up was 90 points. One tibial base plate placed on an autografted plateau defect subsided and required revision. Only one other tibia had complete radiolucency and was asymptomatic. No other signs or symptoms of tibial loosening were noted. Three patellar components were revised and no femoral components were revised. Fluoroscopically assisted roentgenograms were taken at follow-up with 65% of tibial components showing no lucency and the remainder showing small, scattered non-progressive lucencies.

Similar results with cementless fixations have been seen in other reports from this group. In a study of rheumatoid patients, those fixed with cementless technique had better knee scores than those that were cemented (91% good to excellent versus 81%) (122). In another study (123), comparing 18 patients at an average 5-year follow-up, each of whom had a cemented PCA on one side and cementless on the other, no differences in knee score, pain score, or range of motion were seen. No preference for one type of fixation over the other was apparent.

However, other investigators have noted less success with a cementless versus cemented comparison using this prosthesis. Rorabeck and Bourne (124) compared 110 cemented Kinematic II knees with 50 cementless PCA knees. The average age of the cemented knees was 70 (52 to 88) and 59 for cementless knees (22 to 82), with all knees followed 2 to 3 years. A similar mix of osteo- and rheumatoid arthritis was noted in each group. The patients were rated using a modified HSS score at final follow-up. Cemented knees averaged 9 points higher (88 versus 79) than the cementless and were also noted to have a greater range of motion (the average arc was 1 to 106 degrees versus 5 to 97 degrees).

Kilgus and Moreland (125) reported on 38 cementless PCA knees and compared them with 90 cemented PCA knees (including 7 revisions). The cementless patients were on the average 15 years younger (65 versus 50). Cemented knee patients were pain-free in 46% of the cases compared to 30% of cementless knees. Of cementless patients under the age of 40, 25% had more than occasional and slight pain while none of the cemented knees had these complaints. A complete radiolucency under the tibial plateau was noted in 25% of cementless knees. Minimal subsidence and tilting were seen in 54% of the lateral tibial radiographs and in 28% of the anteroposterior radiographs. Only 3% of cemented components demonstrated similar changes.

Rand, et al. (126) noted a similar discrepancy in knee scores when comparing cemented to uncemented PCA arthroplasty with 97% of the cemented group experiencing good to excellent results versus 83% in the cementless group. Similarly, a longer follow-up by Moran, et al. (127) revealed an 84% 5-year survival rate and 77% 6-year survival rate in a cohort of 108 PCA knees implanted without cement. The authors of the study did not recommend use of the prosthesis without cement. In a similar vein, Eskola, et al. (128) reported that at 2- to 4-year follow-ups (average 3.2 years) only 71 of 92 implantations performed without cement showed no clinically evident loosening. These conflicting results from multiple investigators most likely represent technical difficulties with implantation but, alternatively, may be manifestations of inherent prosthetic design features.

Anatomic Graduated Component (AGC) Total Knee

In an early report on the Anatomical Graduated Component (the AGC) total knee (Biomet, Inc.; Warsaw, Indiana) Ritter, Faris, and Keating (129) compared 192 cemented versus 54 uncemented implantations, with the cementless patients averaging 11 years younger (60 versus 71). At 2 years, a large difference in survival was noted: 97.4% for cemented and 76.5% for cementless knees. Of the surviving knees, 98.4% of the cemented were good to excellent versus 85.2% of the cementless. The authors cautioned against cementless implantation of this prosthesis. The same authors reported (in the same year) a comparison of 331 cemented and 78 cementless AGC arthroplasties. At 5 years, the survival rate was 98% for the cemented group and only 81% in the cementless population (130). Interestingly, in a report two years later, the authors reported survival data on 331 cemented and 72 cementless knees with survivorship of 99% versus 88% (131). This is similar to the reported findings of Nielsen, et al. (132), who reported on 103 unselected cases utilizing uncemented AGC components. Nielsen reported on 94 knees at 36 months follow-up with 2 cases of loose tibial components revised, 2 radiographically loose but asymptomatic components, 1 septic loosening and 4 patients with nonprogressive tibial lucencies. Overall survival was 87.1% with a success rate (no radiographic signs of loosening) of 90.7%.

Miller-Galante

Our experience with cementless fixation of total knee components has been with the Miller-Galante arthroplasty (Fig. 72.7). A full description of the arthroplasty components and implantation technique is available elsewhere (133). The knee is a condylar type with posterior cruciate retention and utilizes titanium fiber mesh as the ingrowth substrate. Four short ingrowth pegs with central holes and 4 screws are utilized to enhance initial fixation stability. Between February 1984 and February 1987, 283 TKAs were performed in 251 patients (134). The series was prospective, but the choice of fixation method was not randomized. The decision between cemented versus cementless fixation was based on patient age, the subjective quality of bone stock, prosthetic fit, and the ability of the patient to comply with initial weight-bearing restrictions.

Of the 145 cemented TKAs performed in 123 patients, five (3%) were lost to follow-up and one patient was bedridden because of a stroke, leaving 139 cemented knees in 117 patients (96%).

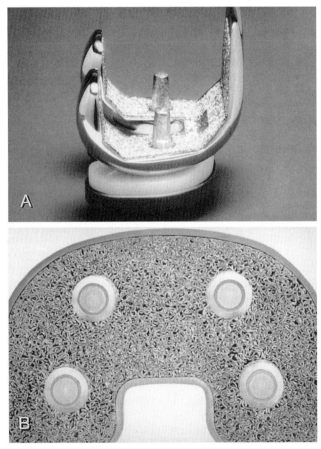

Figure 72.7. **A,** Miller-Galante I—Note smooth femoral pegs and ingrowth surface on the remainder of the femoral component (Courtesy Zimmer, Warsaw, IN). **B,** Miller-Galante I—This close-up of the tibial component reveals porous undersurface, porous-coated pegs and provisions for four screw initial fixation (Courtesy Zimmer, Warsaw, IN).

Of the 138 cementless TKAs performed, three (2%) were lost to follow-up study and three (2%) were unable to return for examination, leaving 132 knees in 122 patients (96%). The average follow-up time was 43 months in the cemented group and 44 months in the cementless group.

Of the 139 cemented TKAs done in 117 patients, 82 (70%) were in women and 35 (30%) were in men. The average age of the patient was 70 years (with a range of 31 to 97 years). Nineteen (17%) were excluded from the study: Eleven patients (15 knees) died during the three year interval after surgery. Eight knees failed and required revision of all components, leaving 98 patients with 116 cemented knees for clinical follow-up study.

Of the 132 cementless knees in 122 patients, 77 (57%) were in women and 55 (43%) were in men. The average age in the cementless group was 59 years (with a range of 19 to 76 years). Of the 132 cementless TKAs performed, 123 knees in 113 patients were clinically followed for over 3 years. Three patients (3 knees) died before completion of the 3-year follow-up study, and 6 knees (5%) failed, requiring revision.

For purposes of evaluating results and comparing pain, limp, and support scores, patients with TKA failure requiring component removal were separated from patients whose prostheses remained in place. Patients who required reoperation or patellar component revision were included in all analyses.

Diagnoses were similar in both groups; approximately 80% of the patients had osteoarthrosis and 15% had rheumatoid arthritis, with 5% having other diagnoses. Preoperative knee scores were slightly but significantly different. The cemented knees averaged 48 points (with a range of 13 to 78), and cementless knees averaged 52 points (with a range of 23 to 78) (p<0.05).

The average postoperative knee score was 89 points (with a range of 57 to 100) in the cemented group and 93 points (with a range of 57 to 100) in the cementless group. This difference was significant (p<0.05). A larger percentage of patients with cementless fixation had an excellent result (85%). Correspondingly, the cemented group had more good results (23%). Fair results were seen in 3% of the cementless knees and 4% of the cemented, and poor results were seen in one of the cementless and one of the cemented groups. Five (4%) of the cementless and seven (6%) of the cemented group required revision and were considered failures.

A comparison of pain, limp, and need for support showed no difference between groups. Preoperative range of motion (ROM) was similar in both groups. The cemented group averaged 101 degrees (range 15 to 140 degrees) and the cementless group averaged 103 degrees (range 15 to 145 degrees). The postoperative average ROM was also similar: 105 degrees (range 45 to 140 degrees) in the cemented group and 109 degrees (range 70 to 132 degrees) in the cementless group. A larger percentage of cementless knees achieved over 100 degrees of active flexion (66% versus 52%).

Failures requiring revision or removal of the prosthesis were seen in 8 of the cemented knees (6%). In this group, 3 patients had revision for chronic pain of unde-

termined etiology; no evidence of sepsis or loosening was noted. Two revisions were for postoperative skin slough, 2 for instability, and 1 for late hematogenous sepsis.

In the cementless group, there were 6 failures requiring revision (5%). One patient had a two-stage revision for a hematogenously acquired infection, 2 patients had loose tibial components requiring exchange to a cemented component, 1 patient had chronic pain of undetermined etiology, 1 patient suffered a full-thickness skin slough secondary to severe vasculitis and required revision to an arthrodesis, while 1 patient had material failure of a femoral component.

Reoperation was required in 10 patients (9%) with cement fixation: 5 for patellar realignment, 1 for repair of a late traumatic quadriceps rupture, 1 for below-knee amputation for postoperative vascular insufficiency, and 3 for revision of a failed patellar component.

Reoperation was required in 14 patients (11%) with cementless knees: 1 patient had exploratory surgery of the prosthesis when a saphenous neuroma was discovered, but the components were well fixed and the articular surface of the tibia component was exchanged to explore the tibial component; 13 cementless patellar components required reoperation for component failure. Of these 13, 11 were revised to cemented components and 2 were treated by component removal.

Radiolucent lines about the cementless femoral component were rare with no more than 3% of patients showing partial nonprogressive lucency. Partial nonprogressive tibial plate lucencies were common, but complete tibial plate lucencies were seen in three asymptomatic cases (Fig. 72.8). Radiolucent lines about pegs or screws were noted in 4%. Only one tibial component was noted to subside.

Similar results were noted with this prosthesis fixed without cement by Joseph and Kaufman (135). They followed 43 Miller-Galante knees fixed without cement. Patients were followed from 2 to 4.5 years (for an average of 3.6 years). Using a modified HSS rating scale, the average postoperation score was 93 with excellent results in 80%, good in 11%, and fair in 9%. There were no femoral or tibial component failures.

Further follow-up of 6 to 8 years in our own series (unpublished data) revealed no cementless components demonstrating evidence of progressive radiolucency, loosening, or late subsidence. Of interest, however, is the presence at between 6 to 8 years of subtle osteolytic lucencies about individual tibial screws. This phenomenon (see below) is manifested as 1 mm lucencies about a single screw in 4 cases. It may presage more extensive changes in the future, as has already come to the attention of the orthopedic community.

Osteolysis

Osteolysis, as a response to unstable metallic implants and failed cemented total hip arthroplasties (136), is not a new phenomenon in orthopedics. However, long-term follow-ups of cemented total knee arthroplasties have not cited osteolysis as a complication or noted it other

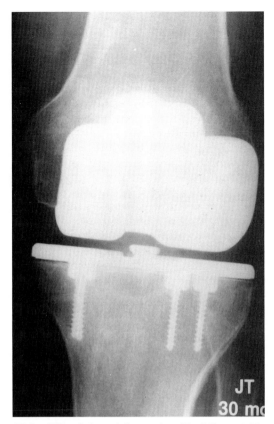

Figure 72.8. Miller-Galante I Cementless Total Knee at 30 months follow-up. Note complete radiolucent line under tibial plate. Despite this evidence of failure of ingrowth into the plate, the patient has no pain and functions at a high level.

than as a byproduct of an unstable migrating component (4, 5, 6). More recently, it has been associated with well-fixed, bone-ingrown cementless total hip components (137) as well as a failure mechanism in total knee components (138). The best documented report cites experience with the Synatomic and the Arizona Knee (Depuy, Warsaw, Indiana) (138). In this study, Engh and associates carefully demonstrate design problems with: (*a*) excessively thin modular polyethylene tibial components, (*b*) medial tibial eminence prominence with subsequent abrasive wear, (*c*) secondary wear and impingement of the tibial locking pin, and (*d*) decreased tibiofemoral congruency, as all contributing to excessive polyethylene and metal particulate wear and resulting in massive osteolysis in both loose and well-fixed total knee arthroplasties. In a series of 174 consecutive prostheses, 16% were associated with osteolysis, with over 50% of these requiring revision.

This knee design is not alone in demonstrating this problem. Both Mintz, et al. (139) and Kilgus, et al. (140) have noted similar phenomenon with the PCA knee, both reporting approximately 10% of cases demonstrating significant polyethylene thinning, catastrophic polyethylene failure, or massive osteolysis. Problems of excessive or even normal wear may surface in various designs at later time intervals and must be rigorously sought by investigators evaluating these devices. Recent

reports of catastrophic polyethylene failure due to manufacturing processes must lead to caution on the part of manufacturers and surgeons alike when contemplating design changes as well as implantation of these devices. It may well be that, over the long term, ingrowth surfaces will not be able to prevent the accumulation of wear debris at the prosthesis bone interface as well as cement has apparently done in the past.

Retrieval Studies

Analysis of retrieved specimens is essential in determining the physiologic response to prosthetic implantation. Mayor and Collier (141) examined 40 retrieved total knee specimens. While the reasons for implant removal were not available, they felt these cases were "short term only and derive from the worst cases." Femoral components appeared to be uniformly well fixed by bone. Patellar components were evenly divided with 50% showing some ingrowth and 50% showing none. Tibial components showed essentially no bony ingrowth with only a single large porous tibial stem showing any sign of ingrowth. However, fibrous ingrowth was uniformly noted at the tibial plate and appeared, by its orientation, to subserve a mechanical anchorage function.

Cook, et al. (142) reviewed 26 femoral, 34 tibial, and 25 patellar ingrowth components retrieved for malposition, instability, unexplained pain, late infection, postmortem, amputation, or after trauma. All components appeared to be well fixed to host bone, and specimens demonstrating clear evidence of subsidence or demarcation were excluded. In contrast to the previous study, 50% of the femoral components showed no ingrowth, and 34% showed only 2% or less of the surface ingrown, and that mainly on ingrowth pegs. Tibial components fared worse (although better than in the previously noted study) with 61% showing no ingrowth, 21% had 2% ingrowth or less, 15% had 2% to 5% ingrowth, and only one component (3%) had more than 5% surface ingrowth. Peg ingrowth in the tibia was only partial and spotty with occasional peripheral (cortical rim) ingrowth being the only other ingrowth seen.

At odds with these reports (which do not clarify the specific clinical reasons for removal) are the findings from our laboratory (143). Eighteen retrieved Miller Galante I tibial components were studied; 10 were removed for unexplained pain, 3 for ligamentous instability, 1 for aseptic loosening, and 4 for infection. Of the 13 components in the first 2 groups, the average extent of bone ingrowth was 27% (standard deviation 17%) with an average volume fraction of bone ingrowth of 10.4% (s.d. 8%). Ingrowth was more common in the pegs than in the plate at almost a 2 to 1 ratio and was most common in the central, not the peripheral part of the plate. A statistical correlation was noted between diminished amount of ingrowth and depth of tibial resection. Patients in the aseptically loose and infected groups had much less ingrowth. The loose component had only 1.5% tibial surface ingrowth and the infected trays averaged only 11.1%.

Attempts to correlate radiographs obtained with retrieval specimens is hampered by evidence that radiographs obtained without fluoroscopic guidance fail to reveal the vast majority of radiolucent lines below flat tibial tray surfaces (144).

Indications and Conclusions

As discussed in the opening paragraphs of the chapter, the utilization of porous ingrowth fixation of total knee components remains controversial, with experienced knee surgeons spanning the spectrum from those who utilize cementless fixation in all cases (unless a specific contraindication exists) to those who do not use it at all. Clearly, the data supporting the utilization of ingrowth fixation are not yet sufficient either in length of follow-up or in experience outside that of the developers of individual devices to warrant wholesale acceptance or rejection of the premises governing the use of ingrowth total knee devices. Ingrowth fixation is a biologic and time-dependent phenomenon with relatively narrow environmental parameters for success. Clinical results over the short term are thus more likely to be highly dependent on implantation technique and prosthetic alignment than are results that may be achieved with cement. At the current time, there is no compelling evidence that revision of loose cementless components is easier or will result in a higher quality revision results than comparable surgery to revise cemented components. Consequently, a clear clinical role for ingrowth fixation of total knee components has not yet emerged. As a confounding factor, some investigators have found that well designed press-fit components without ingrowth potential fare well over 2 to 3 year follow-up (145), while other investigators report failure rates of 10% (146) and 20% (147), raising the question of whether or not "fixation" of components is necessary to provide good clinical function. In light of the controversy, and in light of the excellent track record of cemented components, our own policy has been selective. Of concern is the patient who will load the knee in such a way as to fatigue the cement bond to failure either through weight and/or activity level or simply by duration. For these reasons, the relative indications for cementless application have been in the physiologically younger, heavier, and more active patient. In general, we would expect a cemented implant to do well over the patient's lifetime when the patient is above the age of 70. For patients below the age of 60 and otherwise healthy and active with no other limiting factors or contraindications, we have tended to use cementless implants. Thus, as the patient's potential activity level or longevity increases, we tend to use cementless implants, and, with the decreasing potential of these factors, we tend to use cemented implants. The patient's weight, per se, has rarely entered into preoperative planning in this regard although it may be a reasonable factor to consider. In addition, the knee must be replaceable with a minimally constrained device and the majority of the components supported by viable bleeding bone. The components must achieve sufficient initial stability to warrant ce-

mentless surgery; and the underlying bone must be sufficiently strong to support the prosthesis under weight-bearing loads.

While most of these criteria are subjective, evidence has been presented that cementless fixation works as well in the elderly (148) or in the rheumatoid patient (149, 150) (patients who presumably have compromised bone stock). Clearly, indications must be based on long-term results of cementless as well as cemented implants in the populations under discussion.

In our minds, relative contraindications would include the converse of indications for cementless implants, that is, elderly, inactive, and osteopenic patients (even though successful cementless implantation has been reported in these patients) (149, 150). Certainly, the inability to obtain excellent initial living bone-porous surface congruency and component stability would call for the use of methylmethacrylate.

Hybrid arthroplasty with cemented tibial and patellar components and cementless femoral components appear to offer little advantage over classical cemented techniques where femoral component problems are relatively rare. Indeed, the use of cementless components has been shown to be associated with increased blood loss (151, 152).

Further long-term clinical, animal, and retrieval studies will be necessary to clarify the utility of this ingrowth fixation method. Until such time, we believe the patient should be fully informed about the experimental nature of this fixation technique, and the individual surgeon must carefully define the indications for the technique in the performance of total knee arthroplasty.

References

1. Hungerford DS, Kenna RV. Preliminary experience with a porous-coated total knee replacement used without cement. Clin Orthop 1983;176:93–107.
2. Freeman MAR, Bradley GW, Revell PA. Observations upon the interface between bone and polymethylmethacrylate cement. J Bone Joint Surg, 1982;64–B:489–496.
3. Jones LC. Hungerford DS. Cement disease. Clin Orthop 1987;225:192–203.
4. Ranawat CS, Boachie-Adjei O. Survivorship analysis and results of total condylar knee arthroplasty: Eight-to-eleven year follow-up period. Clin Orthop 1988;226:6–13.
5. Vince KG, Insall SN, Kelly MA. The total condylar prosthesis, ten-to-twelve year results with a cemented knee replacement. J Bone Joint Surg 1989;71-B:793–797.
6. Volatile TB, Ewald FC, Friedman RS, et al. Ten year results of 139 duocondylar total knee replacements. Orthop Trans 1986;10:491.
7. Ewald FC, Hsu HP, Walker PS. Is kinematic total knee replacement better than total hip replacement. Orthop Clin N Amer 1989;20:79–88.
8. Haddad RJ, Cook SD, Thomas KA. Current concepts review-biological fixation of porous coated implants. J Bone Joint Surg 1987;59-A:1459–1566.
9. Pilliar RM. Porous-surfaced metallic implants for orthopedic applications. J Biomed Mater Res 1987;21(A1):1–33.
10. Spector M. Bone ingrowth into porous metals. In: Williams, D.F. (ed) Biocompatibility of Orthopedic Implants. Vol II. Boca Raton, FL: CRC Press, 1982:89–128.
11. Spector M. Historical review of porous-coated implants. J Arthroplasty 1987;2:163–177.
12. Sumner DR, Galante JO. Bone ingrowth. In: Evarts CM, ed. Surgery of the Musculoskeletal System. 2nd Ed. New York: Churchill Livingstone, 1990:131–176.
13. Galante JO, Rostoker W. Fiber metal composites in fixation of skeletal prostheses. J Biomed Mater Res (Symp) 1973;4:42–61.

14. Lembert E, Galante JO, Rostoker W. Fixation of skeletal replacement by fiber metal composites. Clin Orthop Rel Res 1972;87:303–310.
15. Cameron HU, Pilliar RM, McNab I. The rate of bone ingrowth into porous metals. J Biomed Mater Res 1976;10:295–302.
16. Orr TE, Beaupre GS, Carter DR, Schurman DJ. Computer predictions of bone remodeling around porous coated implants. J Arthroplasty 1990;5:191–200.
17. Turner TM, Sumner DR, Urban RM, Rivero DP, Galante JO. A comparative study of porous coatings in a weight bearing total hip arthroplasty model. J Bone Joint Surg 1986;68-A:1396–1409.
18. Heldley AK, Clarke IC, Kozinn SC, et al. Porous ingrowth fixation of the femoral component in a canine surface replacement of the hip. Clin Orthop 1982;163:300–309.
19. Sumner DR, Bryan JM, Urban RM, Kuszak JR. Measuring the volume fraction of bone ingrowth: A comparison of three techniques. J Orthop Res 1990;8:448–452.
20. Galante JO, Rostoker W. Physical properties of trabecular bone. Calcif Tis Res 1970;5:236–246.
21. Bobyn JD, Pilliar RM, Cameron HU, and Weatherly GC. The optimum pore size for the fixation of porous-surface metal implants by the ingrowth of bone. Clin Orthop Rel Res 1980;150:263–270.
22. Robertson DM, St.Pierre L, Chakal R. Preliminary observations of bone ingrowth into porous materials. J Biomed Mater Res 1976;10:335–344.
23. Welsh R, Pilliar RM, McNab I. The role of surface porosity in fixation to bone and acrylic. J Bone Joint Surg 1971;53-A:963–977.
24. Cook SD, Walsh KA, Haddad RJ. Interface mechanics and bone growth into porous materials. J Biomed Mater Res 1985;193:271–280.
25. Berry JL, Geiger JM, Moran JM, Skraba JS, Greenwald AS. Use of tricalcium phosphate or electrical stimulation to enhance the bone-porous implant interface. J Biomed Mater Res 1986;20:65–77.
26. Bobyn JD, Pilliar RM, Cameron HU, Weatherly GC. Osteogenic phenomena across endosteal bone-implant spaces with porous surfaced intramedullary implants. Acta Orthop Scand 1981;52:154–153.
27. Cameron HU, Pilliar RM, McNab I. The rate of bone ingrowth into porous metals. J Biomed Mater Res 1976;10:295–302.
28. Kienapfel H, Sumner DR, Turner T, Urban R, Skipor AK, Yang A, Galante JO. Time response of implant fixation of porous-coated implants to treatment with autograft and freeze-dried allograft in the presence of interface gaps. Trans Soc Biomat 1990;13.
29. Sumner DR, Turner TM. Enhancement of biological fixation in cementless total knee arthroplasty. In: V. Goldberg, ed. Controversies in Total Knee Arthroplasty. New York: Raven Press, 1991.
30. Pilliar RM, Lee JM, Maniatopolous C. Observations on the effect of movement on bone ingrowth into porous-surfaced implants. Clin Orthop 1986;208:108–113.
31. Zalenski E, Jasty M, O'Connor DO, Page A, Krushell R, Gragdon C, Russotti G, Harris WH. Micromotion of porous-surfaced, cementless prostheses following six months of in vivo bone ingrowth in a canine model. Trans Orthop Res Soc 1987;12:293.
32. Toksvig-Larsen S. Aspenberg P, Ryd L, Albrektsson T, Thorngren KG. The micromotion chamber. Trans Orthop Res Soc 1991;16:497.
33. Kang JD, McKernan DJ, Kruger M, Mutschler T, Thompson WH, Rubash HE. Defect filling and bone ingrowth: A comparative study in a canine fiber metal total hip model. Trans Orthop Res Soc 1989;14:552.
34. Kienapfel H, Sumner DR, Turner T, Urban R, McLeon B, Yang A, Galante JO. Efficacy of autograft, freeze dried allograft and fibrin glue to enhance fixation of porous coated implants in the presence of interface gaps. Trans Orthop Res Soc 1990;15:432.
35. Lewis GC, Jones LC, Connor KM, Lennox DW, Hungerford DS. An evaluation of grafting materials in cementless arthroplasty. Trans Orthop Res Soc 1987;12.319.
36. McDonald DJ, Fitzgerald RH, Chao EYS. Comparison of autograft and allograft in the enhancement of biological fixation of a canine porous femoral component. Trans Orthop Res Soc 1987;12:483.
37. Rivero DP, Fox J, Skipor AK, Urban RM, Galante JO. Calcium phosphate-coated porous titanium implants for enhanced skeletal fixation. J Biomed Mater Res 1988;22:191–201.
38. Turner TM, Urban RM, Sumner DR, Galante JO. Bone ingrowth in cementless revision of an aseptically loosened canine THA mode. Trans Orthop Res Soc 1989;14:551.
39. Soballe K, Hansen ES, Rasmussen HB, Pedersen CM, Buenger C. Early fixation of allogeneic bone graft in titanium and hydroxyapatite coated implants. Trans Orthop Res Soc 1989;14:385.
40. Beight J, Radin S, Cuckler J, Ducheyne P. Effect of solubility of calcium phosphate coatings on mechanical fixation of porous ingrowth implants. Trans Orthop Res Soc 1989;14:334.
41. Cook SD, Thomas KA, Kay JF, Jarcho M. Hydroxyapatite-coated porous titanium for use as an orthopedic biologic attachment system. Clin Orthop 1988;230:303–312.
42. Ducheyne P, Hench LL, Ragan A, Martens W, Bursens A, Mulier JC. Effect of hydroxyapatite impregnation on skeletal bonding of porous coated implants. J Biomed Mater Res 1980;14:225–237.
43. Jasty M. Rubash HE, Paiement C, Bragdon C, Parr J, Harrigan TP, Harris WH. Stimulation of bone ingrowth into porous surfaced total joint prosthesis by applying a thin coating of tricalcium phosphate-hydroxyapatite. Trans Orthop Res Soc 1987;12:318.
44. Mayor MB, Collier JP, Hanes CK. Enhanced early fixation of porous-coated implants using tricalcium phosphate. Trans Orthop Res Soc 1986;11:348.
45. Soballe K, Hansen ES, Rasmussen HB, Juhl GI, Pedersen CM, Knudsen V, Hvid I, Buenger C. Enhancement of osteopenic and normal bone ingrowth into porous-coated implants by hydroxyapatite coating. Trans Orthop Res Soc 1989;14:554.
46. Colella SM, Miller AG, Stang RH, Stoebe TG, Spengler DM. Fixation of porous titanium implants in cortical bone enhanced by electrical stimulation. J Biomed Mater Res 1981;15:37–46.
47. Dallant P, Meunier A, Christel P, Guillemin G, Sedel L. Quantitation of bone ingrowth into porous implants submitted to pulsed electromagnetic fields, In: Lemons, J.E., ed. Quantitative Characterization and Performance of Porous Implants for Hard Tissue Applications. Philadelphia: ASTM Special Technical Publication 1987;953.286–293.
48. Park JB, Salman NN, Kenner GH, Von Recum AF. Preliminary studies on the effects of direct current on the bone/porous implants interface. Ann Biomed Eng 1980;8:93–101.
49. Shimizu T, Zerwekh JE, Videman T, Holmes RE, Mooney V. The effect of pulsing electromagnetic field on bone ingrowth into porous calcium ceramics. Trans Orthop Res Soc 1987;12:234.
50. Weinstein AM, Klawitter JJ, Cleveland TW, Amoss DC. Electrical stimulation of bone growth into porous A1.MDSD/20.MDSD/3. J Biomed Mater Res 1976;10:231–247.
51. Rivero DP, Landon GC, Skipor AK, Urban RM, Galante JO. Effect of pulsing electromagnetic fields on bone ingrowth in a porous material. Trans Orthop Res Soc 1986;11:492.
52. Alberts LR. Effects of periosteal activation agent on bone repair and bone ingrowth. J Biomed Mater Res 1987;21:429–442.
53. Longo JA, Weinstein AM, Hedley AK. The effects of collagen on tissue growth into a porous polyethylene ingrowth model. In: Christel P, Menuier A, Lee AJC, eds. Biological and biomechanical performances of biomaterials. Amsterdam: Elsevier Science Publishers, 1986:483.
54. Wang GJ, Shen WJ, Chung KC, Balian G, McLaughlin RE. Demineralized bone matrix in revision arthroplasty. Trans Orthop Res Soc 1989;14:336.
55. Rivero DP, Fox J, Skipor AK, Urban RM, Galante JO, Rostoker W. Effects of calcium phosphates and bone grafting materials on bone ingrowth in titanium fiber metal. Trans Orthop Res Soc 1985;10:191.
56. Jones LC, Kay JF, Freeburger A, Opishinski DJ, Hungerford DS. Effect of hydroxylapatite coating on osteogenesis across an interface gap. Trans Orthop Res Soc 1991;16:549.
57. Cook SD, Thomas KA, Dalton JE, Volkman T, Kay JF. Enhancement of bone ingrowth and fixation strength by hydroxylapatite coating porous implants. Trans Orthop Res Soc 1991;16:550.
58. Stevenson S, Tisdel CL, Parr JA, Bensuras J, Goldberg VM. Site of implantation and HA/TCP coating affect bone ingrowth into titanium fiber metal implants. Trans Orthop Res Soc 1991;16:544.
59. Soballe K, Hansen ES, Rasmussen HB, Bünger C. Hydroxyapatite implant coating modifies membrane formation during unstable mechanical conditions. Trans Orthop Res Soc 1991;16:35.
60. Soballe K, Hansen ES, Rasmussen HB, Jorgenson PH, Bünger C. Tissue ingrowth into titanium and hydroxyapatite-coated implants during stable and unstable mechanical conditions. J Orthop Res 1992;10:285–299.
61. Moron A, Caja VL, Egger EL, Gottsauner-Wolf F, Rollo G. Interface strength and histomorphometric quantification of hydroxyapatite-coated and uncoated porous titanium implants. Trans Orthop Res Soc 1992;17:365.
62. Corlsson L, Regnoer L, Johansson C, Gottlander M, Herberts P. Histomorphometric comparison of titanium and hydroxyapatite-coated implants in the human arthritic knee. Trans Orthop Res Soc 1992;17:267.
63. Russotti GM, Okada Y, Fitzgerald RH, Chao EYS, Gorshi JP. Efficacy of using a bone graft substitute to enhance biological fixation of a porous metal femoral component. In Brand RA, ed. The Hip. St. Louis: CV Mosby Co, 1987.
64. Kienapfel H, Sumner DR, Turner TM, Urban RM, Galante JO. Efficacy of autograft and freeze-dried allograft to enhance fixation of porous coated implants in the presence of interface gaps. J Orthop Res 1992;10:423–433.
65. Lisecki EJ, Cook SD, Dalton JE, Callahan BC, Wolff JD, Banks RE. Attachment of HA coated and uncoated porous implants is influenced by methotrexate and Coumadin. Trans Orthop Res Soc 1992;17:368.
66. Longo JA, Magee FP. Perioperative indomethacin and its effects on porous ingrowth and screw fixation. Trans Orthop Res Soc 1991;16:524.
67. Thomas KA, Cook SD, Dalton JE, Baffes GC, Brown TD, Halvorson TL. The effects of postoperative indomethacin therapies upon biological ingrowth fixation. Trans Orthop Res Soc 1991;16:31.

68. Wise MW, Robertson ID, Lackiewicz PF, Thrall DE, Metcalf M. The effect of radiation therapy on the fixation strength of an experimental porous coated implant in dogs. Clin Orthop 1990;261:276–280.

69. Sumner DR, Turner TM, Pierson RH, Kienapfel H, Urban RM, Liebner EJ, Galante JO. Effects of radiation on fixation of noncemented porous-coated implants in a canine model. J Bone Joint Surg 1990;72-A, 1527–1533.

70. Black J. Metallic ion release and its relationship to oncogenesis. In: Fitzgerald RH, ed. The hip-proceedings of the thirteenth open scientific meeting of the hip society. St. Louis: CV Mosby, 1985:199–213.

71. Agins HJ. Alcock NW, Barsal M, et al. Metallic wear in failed titanium alloy total hip replacements: A histological and quantitative analysis. J Bone Joint Surg 1989;70A:347–359.

72. Albrektsson BEJ, Herberts PH. ICLH knee arthroplasty. A consecutive study of 108 knees with uncemented tibial component fixation. J Arthroplasty 1988;3:145–156.

73. Freeman MAR, Blaha JD, Bradley GW, Insler HP. Cementless fixation of ICLH tibial component. Orthop Clin N Amer, 1982;13:141–154.

74. Freeman MAR, McLeod HC, Leval JP. Cementless fixation of prosthetic components in total arthroplasty of the knee and hip. Clin Orthop 1983;176:88–94.

75. Freeman MAR, Samuelson KM, Bertin KC. Freeman-Samuelson total arthroplasty of the knee. Clin Orthop 1985:192:46–58.

76. Laskin RS. Tricon-M uncemented total knee arthroplasty. A review of 96 knees followed longer than 2 years. J Arthroplasty 1988;3:27–38.

77. Ring PA. Uncemented surface replacement of the knee joint. Clin Orthop 1980;148:106–111.

78. Cheng CL, Gross AE. Loosening of the porous coating in total knee replacement. J Bone Joint Surg 1988;70-B:377–381.

79. Knahr K, Salzer M, Schmidt W. A radiological analysis of uncemented PCA tibial implants with a follow-up period of 4–7 years. J Arthroplasty 1990;5:131–141.

80. Cooke TDV, Collins A, Wevers HW. Failure of a knee prosthesis accelerated by shedding of beads from the porous metal surface. Clin Orthop 1990;258:204–208.

81. Ryd L. Micromotion in knee arthroplasty [Thesis]. Lund, Sweden: Department of Orthopaedic Surgery,University Hospital, 1985.

82. Rosenqvist R, Bylander B, Knutson K, Rydholm V, Rooser B, Egund N, Lidyren L. Loosening of the porous coating of bicompartmental prosthesis in patients with rheumatoid arthritis. J Bone Joint Surg 1986;68-A:538–542.

83. Novacheck I, Buchanan JR, Gause TM, Greer RB. Significance of bead loosening in the porous coated anatomic total knee arthroplasty. Orthop Trans 1988;12(3):546.

84. Haynes DW, Freedman EL. The radiographic resolution of beads from porous coated joint prostheses. J Arthroplasty 1990;5:117–122.

85. Rosenberg AG. Cementless total hip arthroplasty: Femoral remodeling and clinical experience. Orthopedics 1989;12:1223–1238.

86. Krackow KA. The technique of total knee arthroplasty. St Louis: CV Mosby, 1990:378–382.

87. Toksvig-Larsen S, Ryd L. Surface flatness in orthopedic bone cutting. Trans Orthop Res Soc. 1991;16:564.

88. Bayley JC. Scott RD. Further observations on metal backed patellar component failure. Clin Orthop 1988;236:82–87.

89. Rosenberg AG, Andriacchi TP, Barden R. Patellar component failure in cementless total knee arthroplasty. Clin Orthop 1988;236:106–114.

90. Stulberg JD, Stulberg BN, Humati Y, Tsao A. Failure mechanisms of metal backed patellar components. Clin Orthop Rel Res 1988;236:88–105.

91. Branson PS, Steege JW, Wixson RL, Lewis J, Stulberg SD. Rigidity of initial fixation with uncemented tibial knee implants. J Arthroplasty 1989;4:21–25.

92. Miura H, Whitesides LA, Easley JC, Amador DD. Effects of screw and sleeve on initial fixation of uncemented total knee tibial components. Trans Orthop Res Soc 1988;13:474.

93. Sherazi-Adl A, Ahmed AM. Micromotions at the bone/prosthesis interface in porous surface metal tibial implants—An axisymmetric finite element study. Trans Orthop Res Soc 1986;11:262.

94. Shimagaki H, Bechtold JE, Sherman RE, Gustilo RB. Stability of initial fixation of the tibial component in cementless total knee arthroplasty. J Orthop Res 1990;8:64–71.

95. Strickland AB, Chan KH, Andriacchi TP, Miller J. The initial fixation of porous coated tibial components evaluated by the study of rigid body motion under static load. Trans Orthop Res Soc 1988;13:476.

96. Volz RG, Nisbet JK, Lee RW, McMurtry MG. The mechanical stability of various noncemented tibial components. Clin Orthop 1988;226:38–42.

97. Walker PS, Hsu HP, Zimmerman RA. A comparative study of uncemented tibial components. J Arthroplasty 1990;5:245–253.

98. Tissakht M, Ahmed AM, Mulas G. Experimental validation of a finite element method for the prediction of bone-prosthesis interface relative displacement. Trans Orthop Res Soc 1990;15:471.

99. Watson JT, Stulberg BN, Bauer TW, Manley MT. Bone ingrowth fixation in metaphyseal bone: A canine model of knee arthroplasty. Orthop Trans 1986;10:582.

100. Finlay JB, Harada I, Bourne RB, Rorabeck CH, Hardie R, Scott MA. Analysis of the pull-out strength of screws and pegs used to secure tibial components following total knee arthroplasty. Clin Orthop 1989;247:220–231.

101. Cameron HV. Noncemented tibial components: Does a stem help? Contemp Orthop 1992;24:326–330.

102. Lee RW, Volz RG, Sheridan DC. The role of fixation and bone quality on the mechanical stability of tibial knee components. Clin Orthop 1991;273:177–183.

103. Miura H, Whitesides LA, Easley JC, Amador DD. Effect of screws and a sleeve on initial fixation in uncemented total knee tibial components. Clin Orthop 1990;259:160–168.

104. Finlay JB, Bourne RB, Kreamer WS, Moroz T, Rorabeck CH. Stiffness of bone underlying the tibial plateaus of osteoarthritic and normal knees. Clin Orthop 1989;247:193–201.

105. Hvid I, Moller JJ. Tibial plateau strength patterns in experimental modular knee replacements. Arch Orthop Trauma Surg 1985;104:57–61.

106. Williams JL, Lewis JL. Properties of an anisotropic model of cancellous bone from the proximal tibial epiphysis. J Biomech Eng 1982;104:50–56.

107. Natarajan R, Andriacchi TP. The influence of displacement incompatibilities on bone growth in porous tibial components. Trans Orthop Res Soc 1988;13:331.

108. Manley MT, Stulberg BN, Stern LS, Watson JT. Direct observation of micromotion at the implant-bone interface with cemented and non-cemented tibial components. Trans Orthop Res Soc 1987;12:436.

109. Yoshii I, Whitesides LA, White SE. The effect of material properties of the tibial tray on micromovement—CoCr vs. Ti6A14V. Trans Orthop Res Soc 1991;16:167.

110. Bobyn JD, Cameron HV, Abdulla D, Pilliar RM, Weatherly GC. Biologic fixation and bone modeling with an unconstrained canine total knee prosthesis. Clin Orthop 1982;166:301–316.

111. Kim YH. Knee arthroplasty using a cementless PCA prosthesis with a porous coated central tibial stem. Clinical and radiographic review at five years. J Bone Joint Surg 1990;72-B:412–417.

112. Bohr HH, Lund B. Bone mineral density of the proximal tibia following uncemented arthroplasty. J Arthroplasty 1989;2:309.

113. Whitesides LA, Pafford J. Load transfer characteristics of a noncemented total knee arthroplasty. Clin Orthop 1989;239:168–177.

114. Whitesides LA. Clinical results of Whitesides' Ortholoc total knee replacement. Orthop Clin N Am 1989;20(1):113–124.

115. Whitesides LA. The effect of patient age, gender and tibial component fixation on pain relief after cementless total knee replacement. Clin Orthop 1991;271:21–27.

116. Samuelson K, Nelson L. An all-polyethylene cementless tibial component. A five-to-nine year follow-up study. Clin Orthop 1990;260:93–97.

117. Buechel FF, Pappas MJ. Long term survivorship analysis of cruciate-sparing versus cruciate-sacrificing knee prostheses using meniscal bearings. Clin Orthop 1990;260:162–169.

118. Buechel FF, Pappas MJ. New Jersey low contact stress knee replacement system. Orthop Clin North Am, 20(2):147–177. 1989.

119. Hungerford DS, Krackow KA, Kenna RV. Two-to-five year experience with a cementless porous coated total knee prosthesis. In: Rand JA, Dorr LD, eds. Total arthroplasty of the knee. Proceedings of the Knee Society, 1985, 1986. Rockville, MD: Aspen Publishers, 1986;215–235.

120. Kenna RV, Hungerford DS. Design rationale for the porous coated anatomic total knee system. In: Total Knee Arthroplasty: A Comprehensive Approach. Baltimore: Williams & Wilkins, 1984:71–88.

121. Hungerford DS, Krackow KA, Kenna RV. Cementless total knee replacement in patients 50 years old and under. Orthop Clin N Am 1989;20(1):131–145.

122. Ebert FR, Krackow KA, Lennox DW, Hungerford DS. Minimum 4 year follow-up of PCA total knee arthroplasty in rheumatoid patients. J Arthroplasty 1992;7:101–108.

123. Dodd CAF, Hungerford DS, Krackow KA. Total knee arthroplasty fixation. Comparison of the early results of paired cemented versus uncemented porous coated anatomic knee prostheses. Clin Orthop 1990;260:66–70.

124. Rorabeck CH, Bourne RB, Nott L. The cemented kinematic II and the non-cemented porous coated anatomic prostheses for total knee replacement. J Bone Joint Surg 1988;70-A:483–490.

125. Kilgus DJ, Moreland JR, Mesna DP, Graver JD. The PCA knee: The two-to-five year UCLA experience. Orthop Trans 1988;12(3):705.

126. Rand JA, Bryan RS, Chao EYS, Ilstrup DM. A comparison of cemented versus cementless porous coated anatomic total knee arthroplasty. In: Rand JA, Dorr LD, eds. Proceedings of the Knee Society, 1985–1986. Rockville, MD: Aspen Publishers, 1986.

127. Moran CG, Pinder IM, Lees TA, Midwinter MS. Survivorship analysis of the uncemented porous-coated anatomic knee replacement. J Bone Joint Surg 1991;73-A:848–857.

128. Eskola A, Vahvanen V, Santavirta S, Honkanen V, Slotis P. Porous-coated anatomic (PCA) knee arthroplasty. Three year results. J Arthroplasty 1992;7:223–228.

129. Ritter MA, Campbell E, Faris PM, Keating EM. The AGC 2000 total knee arthroplasty with and without cement. Am J Knee Surg 1989;2(4):160–163.

130. Ritter MA, Keating EM, Faris PM. Design features and clinical results of the anatomic graduated components (AGC) total knee replacement. Contemp Orthop 1989;19:641–647.

131. Kavolus CH, Ritter MA, Keating ME, Faris PM. Survivorship of cementless total knee arthroplasty without tibial screw fixation. Clin Orthop 1991;273:170–176.

132. Nielsen PT, Hansen EB, Rechangel K. Cementless total knee arthroplasty in unselected cases of osteoarthritis and rheumatoid arthritis. A 3 year follow-up study of 103 cases. J Arthroplasty 1992;7:137–143.

133. Rosenberg AG, Barden RM, Galante JO. A comparison of cemented and cementless fixation with the Miller-Galante total knee arthroplasty. Orthop Clin N Am 1989;20(1):97–111.

134. Rosenberg AG, Barden RM, Galante JO. Cemented and ingrowth fixation of the Miller-Galante Prosthesis. Clinical and roentgenographic comparison after three to six year follow-up studies. Clin Orthop 1990;260:71–79.

135. Joseph J, Kaufman EE. Preliminary results of Miller-Galante uncemented total knee arthroplasty. Orthopedics 1990;13(5):511–516.

136. Harris WH, Schiller AL, Scholler J-M; Freiberg RA, Scott R. Extensive localized bone resorption in the femur following total hip replacement. J Bone Joint Surg 1976;58-A:612–618.

137. Maloney WS, Jasty M, Harris WH, Galante JO, Callahan JJ. Endosteal erosion in association with stable uncemented femoral components. J Bone Joint Surg 1990;72-A:1025–1034.

138. Peters PC, Engh GA, Dwyer KA, Vinh TN. Osteolysis after total knee arthroplasty without cement. J Bone Joint Surg 1992;74-A:864k–876.

139. Mintz L. Tsao AK, McCrae CR, Stulberg SD, Wright T. The arthroscopic evaluation and characteristics of severe polyethylene wear in total knee arthroplasty. Clin Orthop 1991;273:215–224.

140. Kilgus DJ, Moreland JR, Finerman GA, Funahashi TT, Tipton JS. Cata-strophic wear of tibial polyethylene inserts. Clin Orthop 1991;273:225–231.

141. Mayor MB, Collier JP. The histology of porous coated knee prostheses. Ortho Trans 1986;10(3):441.

142. Cook SD, Barrack RL, Thomas KA, Haddad RJ. Quantitative histologic analysis of tissue growth into porous total knee components. J Arthroplasty 1989;(suppl):533–543.

143. Kienapfel H, Sumner DR, Jacobs JJ, Turner TM, Urban RM, Galante JO. Quantitative topographic evaluation of bone ingrowth in tibial components removed from human patients. In Clinical Implant Materials. G. Heimke, U. Slotesa, A.G.C. Lee (eds.), Amsterdam, Elsevier, 415–420, 1990.

144. Mintz AD, Pilkington CAJ, Howie DW. A comparison of plain and fluoroscopically guided radiographs in the assessment of arthroplasty of the knee. J Bone Joint Surg 1989;71-A.1343–1347.

145. Rackemann S, Mintzer CM, Walker PS, Ewald FC. Uncemented press-fit total knee arthroplasty. J Arthroplasty 1990;5:307–314.

146. Allan DG, Butuk D, Gross A. Nonporous press-fit tibial components in total knee arthroplasty. Orthopaedic Transactions, pg. 74, J Bone Joint Surg, Fall 1991.

147. Nafel A, Nielsen S, Kristensen O, Hvid I. The press-fit Kinemax knee arthroplasty. High failure rate of non-cemented implants. J Bone Joint Surg 1992;74-B:243–246.

148. Hoffman AA, Beck SW, Wyatt RB. Cementless total knee arthroplasty in patients over 65 years old. Orthop Trans 1989;13(1):74.

149. Armstrong RA, Whitesides LA. Results of cementless total knee arthroplasty in an older rheumatoid arthritis population. J Arthroplasty 1991;6:357–362.

150. Stuchin SA, Ruoff M, Matanese W. Cementless total knee arthroplasty in patients with inflammatory arthritis and compromised bone. Clin Orthop 1991;273:42–51.

151. Kelman GL, Laskin RS. The effect of cement on postoperative bleeding following total knee replacement. Complic Orthop 1987;2:100–112.

152. Mylod AG, France MP, Muser DE, Parsons JR. Perioperative blood loss associated with total knee arthroplasty. A comparison of procedures performed with and without cementing. J Bone Joint Surg 1990;72-A:1010–1012.

73

Soft Tissue Balancing and Total Knee Arthroplasty

Philip M. Faris

Introduction

Total knee arthroplasty is generally a very satisfactory and enduring method of relieving pain and improving function for the many persons who suffer various arthritic afflictions of the knee. The technology of total knee arthroplasty, especially prosthetic designs and instrumentation modification, has evolved rapidly since the procedure's inception. Prostheses have been designed and redesigned in attempts to simulate normal human anatomy and kinematics. As prosthetic design has evolved, more precise instrumentation has also been designed to place these implants in correct anatomical positions, angles, and centers of rotation. However, despite their best efforts, designers and manufacturers have been unable to match the infinite number of human anatomic variables, angles, radii of curvatures, or static and dynamic soft tissue constraints that dictate the fluid motions of the human knee.

At best, current techniques in total knee arthroplasty are an effort to adapt soft tissue tensions, bony anatomy, and kinematics to an implanted prosthetic device that will function relatively normally and endure for an extended period of time. Soft tissue balancing remains the most subjective and, therefore, most artistic of these techniques.

In this chapter, I will try to describe the techniques for soft tissue balancing, particularly when related to intramedullary femoral instrumentation. Techniques of soft tissue balancing with intramedullary instrumentation are similar to those employed during extramedullary instrumentation. However, because of the current widespread use of intramedullary instrumentation, the extent of soft tissue balancing has decreased. Without the use of tensor devices, soft tissue balancing has become a more subjective accompaniment to total knee replacement than when tensor devices were used to aid in determining soft tissue tensions. Soft tissue balancing, when using intramedullary devices, is as-sessed and performed prior to and after bony cuts, as well as after placement of the trial and final prostheses. Prior to the bone cuts, soft tissue releases to balance the knee are done in anticipation of their eventual necessity. Usually these are done in those knees with rather marked varus or valgus deformities. During the course of the procedure, soft tissue tensions can be judged by assessing the flexion and extension gaps after the femoral and tibial cuts with finger tensioning. Tension can also be gauged after placement of the components by palpation of the ligamentous structures and by observation of the knee during passive range of motion testing.

Medial Side

The medial side of the knee is the side most commonly balanced during soft tissue release. Some release of the medial side of the knee is performed in nearly all total knee replacements due to the fact that exposure of the proximal tibia requires release of the medial soft tissue envelope, which includes the medial meniscotibial ligaments. In addition to this, the majority of total knee instrumentation systems dictate transection of the tibia at a 90 degree angle to the longitudinal axis of the tibia in the coronal plane. When this is coupled with the instruments that dictate cutting the distal femur based on the anatomy of the femoral condyles, a relative tightness of the medial side is created in both extension and flexion.

Soft tissue release on the medial side of a knee with valgus deformity should extend only midway around the medial aspect of the proximal tibia, to preserve as much of the medial stabilizing structures as possible.

The exposure of a varus knee should extend around the posterior medial aspect of the tibia nearly to the posterior cruciate ligament. This release, when combined with section of the patellofemoral ligaments and resection of the anterior cruciate ligament, allows lateral retraction of the patellar mechanism and disloca-

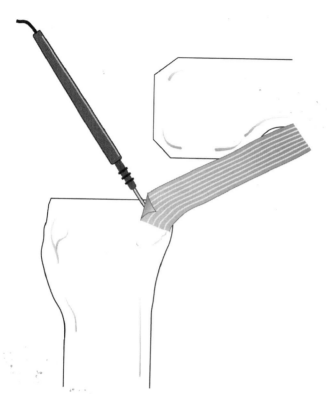

Figure 73.1.   Further exposure of medial tibia with release of the semimembranosus muscle.

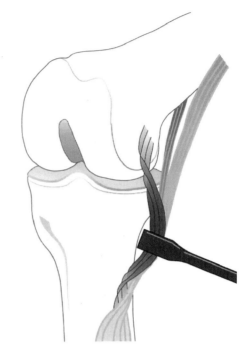

Figure 73.2.   Elevation of medial structures with elevator deep to the superficial medial collateral ligament.

tion of the tibia anteriorly from under the distal femur. This amount of exposure, when combined with occasional partial release of the semimembranosus muscle (Fig. 73.1), allows correction of most varus deformities without further release of the superficial medial collateral ligament. To allow subperiosteal elevation of the medial envelope, a periosteal elevator is placed beneath the superficial medial collateral ligament to retract and protect these soft tissues during the exposure (Fig. 73.2). If further release of the medial soft tissue envelope is necessary, then a periosteal elevator is passed along the medial proximal tibia beneath the superficial medial collateral ligament elevating it along with the entire soft tissue envelope on the medial side of the knee. The insertion of the pes anserine tendons is preserved if possible. In severe deformities, this release may be accompanied by a palpable sliding sensation on the medial side of the knee with valgus stress. Accompanying the soft tissue release, osteophytes underlying the medial collateral ligament on the medial femoral condyle should be removed by using an osteotome or rongeur.

Valgus Deformity

As described earlier, when exposing the valgus knee for total knee replacement, the medial capsular envelope should be exposed only to the midportion of the medial tibial plateau. This retains as much medial envelope stability as possible while still allowing extensive exposure on the lateral side. The patellar tendon is retracted ante-

riorly. The lateral meniscus should be transected and the proximal lateral tibial plateau should be exposed around to the midportion of Gurdy's tubercle. This allows exposure of nearly the entire anterior aspect of the proximal tibia prior to patellar mechanism dislocation.

With the knee flexed and the patella dislocated, the patellofemoral ligaments should be released to allow further relaxation of tension on the quadriceps mechanism. The initial lateral release, appropriate for all valgus knees, may be accomplished by subperiosteally releasing the iliotibial band from its insertion into Gurdy's tubercle (Fig. 73.3). This is done with either a curved osteotome or a sharp periosteal elevator. A complete iliotibial band release, including all of the anterior insertion of the tendinous portions of the iliotibial band is a necessity. The extent of this release can be discerned by extending the knee and palpating the iliotibial band to make sure that no fibers remain attached to Gurdy's tubercle. In approximately 70% of cases, particularly in valgus deformities of less than 15 degrees and in those with a competent medial collateral ligament, this release will be adequate for deformity correction. Further releases are then performed as necessary beginning with the posterior lateral capsule of the knee.

Further releases will be necessary in more severe cases. Several methods have been described. The choice of technique can be made based on the type of prosthesis chosen by the surgeon, the age of the patient, and the competency of the medial collateral ligament. When using a posterior-cruciate-sparing prosthesis with relatively unconstrained femoral and tibial articulations, rotational stability is important. In this configuration, we prefer to release the popliteus tendon and fibular

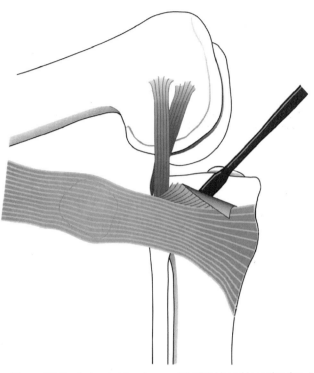

Figure 73.3. Lateral side release of iliotibial band insertion for proximal tibia.

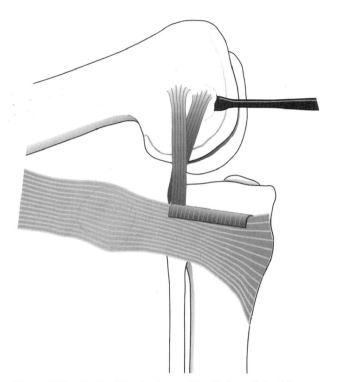

Figure 73.4. Further lateral release of the fibular collateral ligament and popliteus tendon.

collateral ligament from the lateral condyle of the femur along with their bony insertions by passing an osteotome subperiosteally beneath them (Fig. 73.4). This leaves these structures attached by their overlying soft tissue sleeve and helps to maintain rotational stability. In a younger, more active population with an incompetent medial collateral ligament, these releases may be combined with medial collateral ligament tightening as described by Krackow, et al. (1, 2). I have no experience with this tightening technique and refer the reader to Dr. Krackow's description in this volume.

When posterior cruciate substituting devices are used, then considerably more constraint in rotation is imparted by the prosthetic design. This constraint allows more extensive release of the lateral soft tissues on the femur and can include transection of the popliteus and fibular collateral ligament as well as release of the lateral and posterior capsule off of the femur as described by Insall (2). During this release, careful coagulation of the lateral geniculate artery complex must be performed to prevent hematoma formation.

In severe valgus deformities in the elderly patient, in which the medial collateral is lax, with distraction of the medial compartment, it may be prudent to proceed with a constrained type of total knee replacement such as the Insall-Burstein constrained condylar design, which substitutes for the medial collateral ligament (3–7). However, this design does not preclude the necessity for lateral soft tissue release. If adequate lateral release is not performed, excessive stress will be transferred to the central cam mechanism resulting in cold

flow deformation or cam dislocation. Using these techniques, nearly all valgus deformities may be corrected.

Another technique for release of the lateral side of the knee for valgus deformity is that described by Keblish, which includes a lateral surgical approach to the knee (9–13).

Peroneal nerve palsy occurs more frequently in valgus deformities with fixed flexion contractures. Patients should be informed of this complication preoperatively. We do not expose the peroneal nerve, but leave it undisturbed in its vascularized sheath.

Flexion Contractures

Flexion contractures occur in conjunction with both varus and valgus deformities. Flexion contractures of up to 15 to 20 degrees are usually corrected by simple resection of osteophytes in the posterior compartment and collateral ligament balancing techniques. However, flexion contractures that are fixed and greater than 20 degrees may require posterior release and/or an increase in the amount of distal femoral bone resected. All attempts should be made to correct flexion contractures without resection of significant amounts of distal femoral bone. Flexion contracture is generally corrected by release of the posterior capsule off the posterior distal femur. After all bony cuts have been performed and osteophytes have been removed from the posterior aspect of the femur using curved osteotomes and curettes, the trial components are placed, and tibial extension is tested. If flexion contracture remains, it

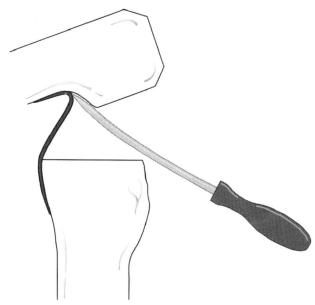

Figure 73.5. Stripping of posterior capsule from the femur using a curved elevator or osteotome.

must be corrected prior to placement of the final components. This is done by placing a posterior force on the tibia with the knee flexed to 120 degrees and transposing it proximal in relationship to the femur. The femur is then elevated anteriorly by an assistant, thus allowing exposure of the posterior aspect of the femur. Using a periosteal elevator or scalpel, the posterior capsule is elevated off the posterior femur up to and including the origins of the gastrocnemius muscle (Fig. 73.5). The release is performed incrementally with intermittent rechecks using the trial components. Gastrocnemius muscle release should be the last release performed in this sequence, and it should also be incremental, based on sequential rechecks of extension. In nearly all flexion contractures, this type of release will allow full extension of the knee.

Further release may be performed by releasing and excising the posterior cruciate ligament, in which case a posterior cruciate substituting type of knee replacement will be required. This extensive release, however, increases the flexion gap relative to the extension gap. If this extensive soft tissue release allows complete extension with minimal resection of the distal femur, then some distal femur should be resected. However, if the resulting flexion contracture would require resection beyond the origins of the collateral ligaments, then transverse posterior capsular release and/or hamstring release may be performed. Transverse capsular release, as described by Insall (14), is performed by placing curved hemostats, using blunt dissection, along the posterior aspect of the posterior capsule (10). The capsule is then sharply incised. This technique is hazardous because of the proximate placement of the popliteal artery and vein. Great care must be taken to avoid injury to these vessels. If injury occurs, then repair of the vessels should not be delayed.

Posterior Cruciate Ligament

In our experience, one of the more common causes of lack of knee flexion and posterior knee pain post arthroplasty is tightness of the posterior cruciate ligament. Because of the inability of current instrumentation to duplicate normal translations during range of motion, the posterior cruciate ligament may not be appropriately tensioned after placement of the arthroplasty components. Excess tightness of the posterior cruciate ligament inhibits knee flexion. When the posterior cruciate ligament is too tight, two things may occur. The ligament may remain intact and prevent knee flexion, or the ligament may rupture, which will allow the prosthesis to function but with posterior tibial sagging.

During surgery, posterior cruciate ligament tension should be assessed by observing passive flexion with a flat trial tibial component. If, during knee flexion, the posterior cruciate ligament is too tight, the tibial component will tilt upward, which indicates that the femoral component is rolling back too far on the tibial component (Fig. 73.6A). This increases the posterior compressive load, and causes the anterior tibial component to lift off. Other means of posterior cruciate tension assessment include direct palpation during flexion to see if the ligament is tight and impinging across the back of the tibial component. Either of these findings indicate the necessity of balancing the posterior cruciate ligament.

Our technique for releasing the posterior cruciate ligament is subperiosteal dissection of the ligament from the posterior aspect of the tibia. In this technique, the tibia is dislocated anteriorly, a periosteal elevator is used to retract the substance of the posterior cruciate ligament posteriorly, and electrocautery is used to incrementally release the ligament off the back of the tibia (Fig. 73.6B). After every 2 to 3 mm increment of release, the components are replaced, and the knee is put through a full range of motion. When the tibial component does not lift off anteriorly, the ligament is under the proper tension and will allow satisfactory flexion of the knee (Fig. 73.6C).

We have found this technique to be quite helpful in allowing total knee replacements to flex well after surgery. In our series, we found no dislocations and no apparent incidence of posterior sagging.

Discussion

The object of soft tissue release around total knee replacement is to correct acquired malalignments, and at the same time, allow prosthetic reconstruction of a compromised knee that will move smoothly through an arc of motion. The arthroplasty must provide enough stability and normal kinematics to allow a normal gait, relieve pain, and, hopefully, to impart the ability to climb steps and continue with normal life functions. When properly performed soft tissue releases are combined with well-conceived bone cuts and adequate prosthetic design, an arthroplasty that functions smoothly, competently, and dependably results.

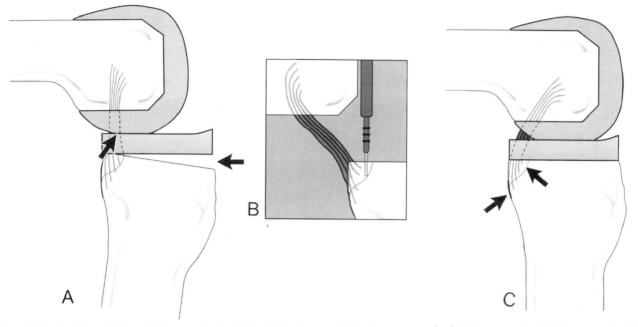

Figure 73.6.   A, Upward tilting of the anterior lip of the tibial trial component during knee flexion indicates tight posterior cruciate ligament. **B,** Release of posterior cruciate ligament from tibial insertion, using electrocautery. **C,** Satisfactory, smooth flexion arc after ligament release.

References

1. Krackow KA, Jones MM, Teeny SM, Hungerford DS. Primary total knee arthroplasty in patients with fixed valgus deformity. Clin Orthop 1991; 273:9.
2. Insall JN. Surgery of the Knee, New York: Churchill Livingstone, 1984:642.
3. Sculco TP. Total condylar III prosthesis in ligament instability. Orthop Clin North Am 1989; 20:(2).
4. Stern SH, Moeckel BH, Insall JN. Total knee arthroplasty in valgus knees. Clin Orthop 1991;(273).
5. Hohl WM, Crawfurd E, Zelicof SB, Ewald FC. The total condylar III prosthesis in complex knee reconstruction. Clin Orthop 1991; (273).
6. Rand JA. Revision total knee arthroplasty using the total condylar III prosthesis. J Arthroplasty 1991; 6(3).
7. Shaw JA, Balcom W, Greer RB. Total knee arthroplasty using the kinematic rotating hinge prosthesis. Orthopaedics 1989;12:(5).
8. Kavolus CH, Faris PM, Ritter MA, Keating EM. The total condylar III knee prosthesis in elderly patients. J Arthroplasty 1991;6:(1).
9. Keblish PA. Valgus deformity in TKR: The lateral retinacular approach. Proceedings American Academy of Orthopaedic Surgeons 53rd Annual Meeting, New Orleans, Louisiana, Feb. 20–25, 1986.
10. Keblish PA. Valgus deformity in TKR: The lateral retinacular approach. Proceedings American Academy of Orthopaedic Surgeons 53rd Annual Meeting, New Orleans, Louisiana, Feb. 20–25, 1986.
11. Keblish PA. The lateral approach in valgus TKR. Proceedings American Academy of Orthopaedic Surgeons 54th Annual Meeting, San Francisco, California, Jan. 22, 1987.
12. Keblish PA. The lateral approach to the valgus knee: Surgical technique and analysis of 53 cases with over two-year follow-up evaluation. Clin Orthop 1991; (271).
13. Buechel FF. A sequential three-step lateral release for correcting fixed valgus knee deformities during total knee arthroplasty. Clin Orthop 1990; (260).
14. Insall JN. Surgery of the Knee. New York: Churchill Livingstone publishers, 1984:643.

74

Fixed Flexion Contracture

Clifford W. Colwell, Jr.

Introduction

Flexion contracture of the knee represents one of the most complex and disabling deformities within total knee replacement surgery. The deformity may be created by soft tissue or bone, or both. Most patients with a fixed flexion deformity have an inflammatory arthritis with associated synovitis and marked pain. They often position their knee in moderate flexion to assist in pain control, with subsequent exaggeration of the deformity (Figs. 74.1–74.3). To constitute a true fixed flexion contracture, the deformity must persist despite local or general anesthetic that alleviates the pain. Flexion deformities in inflammatory arthritis of the knee range from severe (90 degrees of flexion) in wheelchair-bound patients to mild (less than 10 degrees of flexion) in ambulatory patients; however, even relatively mild, persistent flexion contractures cause a significant ambulatory deficit. These patients are unable to obtain full extension for adequate relaxation of the quadriceps mechanism, known as the "screw home" phenomenon in the normal knee, with a significant decrease in overall endurance. Therefore, the correction of the flexion deformity is a tremendous advantage during any total knee arthroplasty.

Surgical Procedure

For a fixed deformity to pose a significant surgical challenge, the deformity must usually exceed 30 degrees. This is in contrast to most patients with degenerative arthritis of the knee who have some degree of flexion contracture that can be quite easily managed by the routine surgical technique of total knee replacement. As the knee assumes a more flexed attitude in more severe flexion deformities, the anatomic description is as follows: the collateral ligaments begin to pass posterior to the midline of the tibia and femur in the sagittal plane, where they shorten, resulting in a fixed soft tissue deformity. In the most severe types of flexion deformities, there is an associated bone defect of the posterior condyles of the femur and in the posterior one-third of the tibial plateau. The "routine" fixed flexion deformity associated with inflammatory arthritis usually is an associated varus or valgus component, bone loss, and soft tissue contractures of both the cruciate and collateral ligaments involved.

The challenge of knee replacement surgery is to accomplish multiple goals efficiently and safely with the best possible outcome. In the case of fixed flexion deformities, one of the important goals is improved effective range of motion. As has been indicated in previous articles in the literature, the most significant common denominator of postoperative range of motion in total knee arthroplasty is the patient's preoperative range of motion. Therefore, although the surgical goal of repairing a fixed flexion contracture would be to increase the extension arc, it is important to realize that, if at all possible, the surgeon does not want to lose an equal arc of flexion, thereby causing a different type of disability. Therefore, approaching a fixed flexion deformity surgically requires a systematic approach toward soft tissue and bone deformities. This requires initial soft tissue releases, followed by appropriate bone resection and then fine balancing of soft tissue prior to the completion of the procedure.

Soft Tissue Approach

The skin incision for fixed flexion contraction surgery is usually the same as the skin incision for other total knee replacements; it should be straight, with the distal extension just beyond the tibial tubercle, ending proximally 10 cm above the patella. Although a "subvastus" approach can be used with a mild flexion contracture, a median parapatellar rectus-splitting incision offers more adequate exposure for the contracted knee. There is general elongation of the quadriceps mechanism with this deformity, and, therefore, the patella can generally

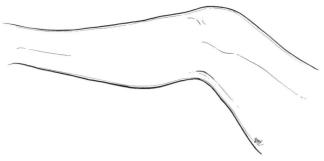

Figure 74.1. Flexion contracture under anesthesia.

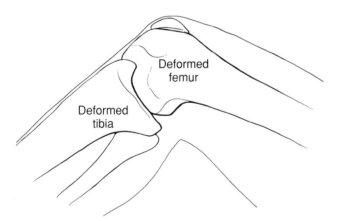

Figure 74.2. Photograph showing flexion contracture under anesthesia.

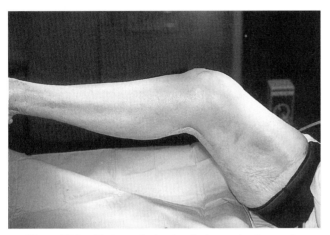

Figure 74.3. Bony deformity with longstanding flexion contracture.

be everted without difficulty. If not, a lateral retinacular release should be done early in the surgical procedure to allow adequate eversion of the patella.

The medial collateral ligament is approached as in any primary total knee replacement. Distally, the superficial fibers of the medial collateral ligament can be elevated from the bony surface of the tibia quite easily (Fig. 74.4). The deep fibers of the medial collateral lig-

ament can then be elevated from the proximal tibia with a scalpel, cutting Sharpey's fibers and maintaining the entire medial collateral ligament as a soft tissue sleeve. The medial meniscus, with its intimate attachment to the medial collateral ligament through its coronary ligament, can then be sharply dissected, leaving a few of the fibers of the medial meniscus attached to the medial collateral ligament. Any osteophytes on the medial border of the tibial plateau and femoral condyle should be removed by means of rongeurs so that, in an extended position postoperatively, the medial collateral ligament will not be "tented" over the osteophytes in the mid-sagittal plane. The medial collateral ligament dissection has to be carried posteriorly as far as the semimembranosus attachment on the posterior tibia (Fig. 74.5). This maneuver, and the excision of the anterior cruciate ligament (if still present), will allow for translocation of the tibia anteriorly.

Bony Approach

Usually one can approach the femur for bony excision following the adequate elevation of the medial collateral ligament, the excision of the anterior cruciate ligament, and adequate translation of the tibia anteriorly. If not, then one must excise the posterior cruciate ligament, which almost always remains intact but contracted.

If there is tightness on the lateral portion of the knee secondary to associated flexion and valgus deformity, release of the lateral structures has to be carried out prior to the bone resection of the distal femur. In fact, lateral tightness may be approached in the same way as medial tightness. The lateral collateral ligament must be elevated from the femoral side rather than the tibial side as in the medial collateral ligament. The femoral attachments of the lateral collateral ligament and popliteus tendon are very closely associated. They may be elevated as a sleeve, starting distally and moving proximally along the lateral femoral condyle (Fig. 74.6). Again, any osteophytes on the lateral femoral condyle or lateral proximal tibial plateau can now be removed with rongeurs to provide relief for the lateral collateral ligament.

With respect to the bony resection, the distal femur is best approached following intramedullary instrumentation. The femur is easily instrumented and the femoral cuts are generally more accurate when done in this manner. The distal femoral cut initially requires no more removal of bone than that of a standard total knee replacement without a fixed flexion contracture. The ultimate limit of resection is the soft tissue attachment of the posterior cruciate and collateral ligaments, although, in most cases of severe deformity, the posterior cruciate ligament will need to be sacrificed. Excessive femoral resection will also move the joint line proximally, negatively affecting extension stability and patellofemoral forces (Fig. 74.7).

Following distal femoral excision, conventional anterior and posterior femoral cuts are made with the anterior cortex of the femur as the guide for resection in order to avoid femoral notching. It is important to externally rotate the femoral component in order to better

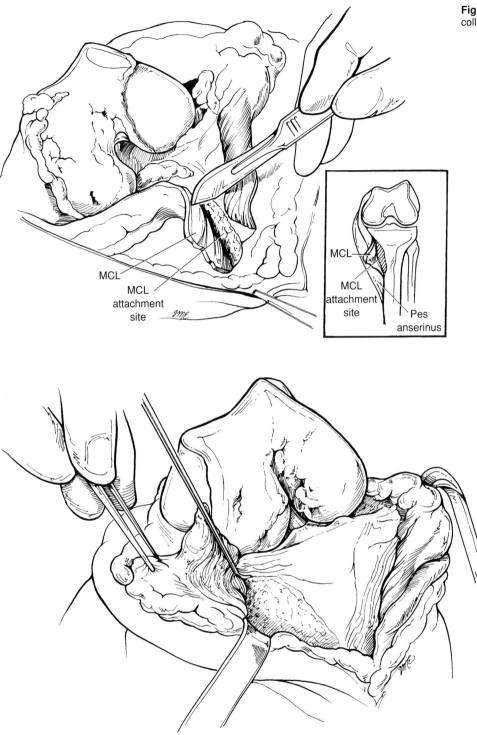

Figure 74.4. Surgical dissection of medial collateral ligament.

MCL

MCL attachment site

MCL

MCL attachment site

Pes anserinus

Figure 74.5. Completed elevation of medial collateral ligament.

equalize the flexion gaps and to better center the patella within the trochlea. Chamfer cuts can then be made for five-sided fixation of the femoral component.

Following adequate femoral resection, the proximal tibia can then be approached. It is also important not to excise excessive tibial bone because of two separate factors (Fig. 74.8): first, flexion stability is lost with ex-cessive tibial loss, and, second, tibial bone stock be-comes worse due to the inverted "cone" effect of the proximal tibia in metaphyseal bone. If, indeed, both ex-cessive tibia and femur are resected, the patient will suffer an extensor lag. The tibia may be cut perpendicu-lar to the long axis of the tibia in the coronal plane and in the sagittal plane, or it may be cut with a posterior

Figure 74.6. Elevation of lateral complex from femur.

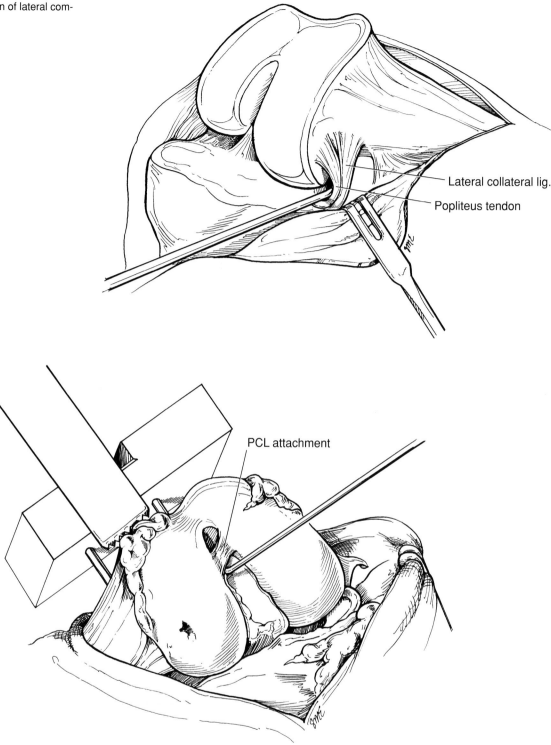

Lateral collateral lig.

Popliteus tendon

PCL attachment

Figure 74.7. Minimal distal femoral cut.

slope in the sagittal plane to more closely approximate the normal tibial slope.

Following the tibial resection, there will now be adequate space to approach the posterior structures that are the major deforming force in fixed flexion contracture. In almost all cases, the posterior cruciate ligament requires sacrifice because of its shortening during the prolonged flexed position. This can be most easily accomplished in the area of the intercondylar notch proximally on the femur, giving additional access to the posterior soft tissue structures of the femur (Fig. 74.9). The posterior portion of the femur is most easily visualized

Figure 74.8.   Minimal tibial cut.

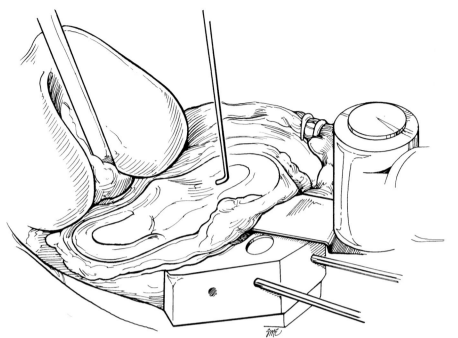

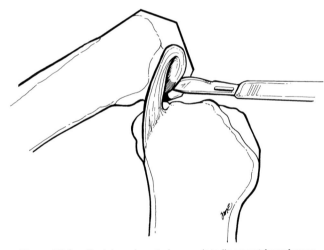

Figure 74.9.   Excision of posterior cruciate ligament from femur.

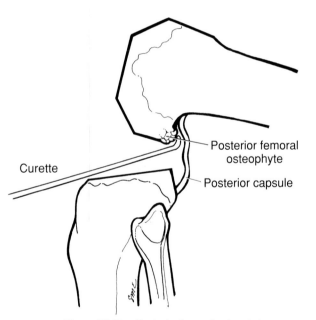

Posterior femoral osteophyte

Posterior capsule

Curette

Figure 74.10.   Posterior femoral osteophyte.

in a 90 degree flexed knee position with an intramedullary rod in the femur helping with the elevation and providing better access to the posterior aspect of the femur. All posterior osteophytes and loose bodies can be removed from the posterior condyles of the femur with a right angle curette as well as any remaining portions of medial or lateral femoral osteophyte formation (Fig. 74.10). On removing the osteophytes, the posterior capsule attachment on the femur can be well visualized; now, from both medial and lateral approaches, it can be stripped in the coronal plane in 90

degrees of flexion to protect the posterior vessels (Fig. 74.11).

There is no necessity for an incision through the posterior capsule, which may jeopardize the posterior neurovascular structures. If it is still not possible to obtain full extension after stripping the posterior capsule from the femur, the proximal heads of the gastrocnemius complex on the femur can also be stripped far proximally on the femur (Fig. 74.12). With ready access to the posterior tibia, it is also possible to elevate the posterior structures from the tibia; the structures accessible to elevation in-

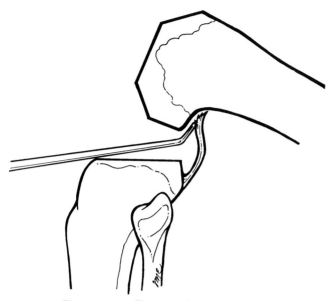

Figure 74.11. Elevation of posterior capsule.

Figure 74.12. Elevation of gastrocnemius.

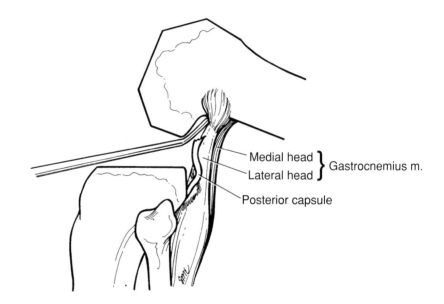

clude the distal attachment of the posterior cruciate ligament, if necessary, and the medial and lateral hamstring attachments. If it is necessary to release the entire pes anserinus, this release can be most easily accomplished from the anterior and medial aspect of the tibia.

In earlier descriptions of flexion contracture in the literature, it was recommended that the peroneal nerve be explored, particularly in cases where the flexion contracture is associated with a valgus deformity. This is unnecessary and may compromise the nerve blood supply. Unless there is a congenital shortening, this exploration is not recommended.

During prolonged flexion contracture of the knee, the tissues of the lateral retinaculum almost universally become tightened; therefore, a lateral patellar retinacular release is uniformly required, both for better tracking of the patellar mechanism and to decrease the overall load on the patella femoral joint. This can be accomplished routinely through an inside-out approach 1 inch from the lateral border of the patella after stripping of the synovium. Both superficial and deep fibers of the lateral retinaculum should be released as far distally as Gerdy's tubercle, along with release of the tensor fascia lata. The patella should track in the trochlea with a "no-thumb" technique. Most often the superior lateral genicular vessels can be dissected free, but, if they contribute to lateral subluxation, they may require division by electrocoagulation.

Implant Type

All components are now inserted, and the stability of the knee joint is checked. In most cases a minimally constrained prosthesis may be used in either a cruciate-sparing design if the posterior cruciate was left intact or cruciate-substituting design if the posterior cruciate ligament was sacrificed. Depending on the degree of bony and soft tissue releases, the knee may require a more fully constrained prosthesis such as are available from various manufacturers. There are essentially no indications for a hinged-type prosthesis.

Postoperative Rehabilitation

Following the surgical procedure, the knee should be able to be fully extended with the implant in place (Figs. 74.13 and 74.14); if the knee cannot be extended at the time of surgery, it is unlikely to extend fully in the postoperative period. The knee should then be splinted in full extension. Although the patient is ambulatory on the first postoperative day, it is recommended that the knee be kept in full extension for 2 to 3 days before starting active flexion exercises. In severe flexion contractures, there is often a prolonged extensor lag that recovers slowly. Every contracted knee requires splinting in an extended position during part of both day and night activities for approximately 6 weeks in order to prevent reformation of the flexion contracture. Active

flexion exercises are required to maintain an adequate flexion arc and to maintain extension. The full range of the extension arc will be gained after approximately 6 months, although flexion range may continue to improve over a 3-year period.

Expected Result

Patients with severe flexion contractures have a higher manipulation rate than do noncontracted patients. If the patient is to be manipulated, the manipulation should be carried out within the first 3 weeks following the surgical procedure. Manipulation is less likely to improve extension than it is to improve flexion.

Suggested Readings

Insall JN. *Surgery of the knee.* New York: Churchill Livingstone, 1984: 587–695.
Daniel DM, Akeson WH, O'Connor JJ, eds. New York: Raven Press, 1990.
Krackow KA. *The technique of total knee arthroplasty.* St. Louis: CV Mosby 1990:249–372.
Rand JA ed. *Total knee arthroplasty.* New York: Raven Press, 1993:115–153.

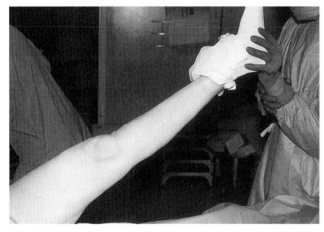

Figure 74.13.   Photograph showing postoperative full extension.

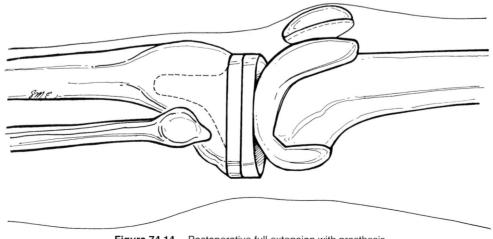

Figure 74.14.   Postoperative full extension with prosthesis.

75

Bone Defects in Total Knee Arthroplasty

Richard S. Laskin and Stephen C. Saddler

Introduction

The long-term results of total knee replacement have been excellent with clinical and radiographic survivorship of over 75% in rheumatoid patients and 90% in osteoarthritic patients at 10 years after the arthroplasty. The most common cause of failure in the remaining patients has been mechanical loosening of one or more of the components. Although the cause of this loosening has been multifactorial, the requirements that the components initially be seated on a proper flat base has been paramount. Unfortunately, in many cases bone loss from the tibia or femur occurs in advanced arthritis leading to an incomplete base for the prosthetic component. This chapter addresses the problem of this bone loss, its etiologies, and its treatment.

Etiology

There are several major etiologies of periarticular bone loss in the patient with advanced arthritis. These etiologies are stress overload collapse, subarticular cysts, prior trauma, developmental abnormalities, and tumors. In the patient undergoing revision total knee arthroplasty, there may also be bone loss resulting from numerous causes.

Statistically, the most common cause of bone loss is stress overload on the concave side of an angular deformity (i.e., the medial side of a varus knee) (Fig. 75.1). The initial response to stress overload is subarticular hypertrophy in response to Wolf's Law. With time, however, the overload can lead to microfractures that can coalesce and collapse. Microfractures are often associated with the presence of subchondral cysts, the latter possibly the result of "pressure injection" of synovial fluid through the Haversian channels of the cartilage-denuded articular surface. Such cysts have been described both in osteoarthritis and in rheumatoid arthritis and are often lined with a layer of synovium. Erosive cysts secondary to pigmented villonodular synovitis can often give a similar radiographic picture, although the clinical history of recurrent bloody effusions usually helps make this latter diagnosis evident.

Bone loss on a traumatic basis most often occurs in the patient with a prior tibial plateau fracture. Distal femoral fractures usually result not in bone loss but rather in angular deformities at the diaphyseal metaphyseal junction. Bone loss can be seen in several developmental disorders, including Blount's disease and agenesis of the lateral femoral condyle. Finally, periarticular tumors, such as chondroblastoma or giant cell tumor can lead to large cavities in the tibial metaphysis.

The largest bone defects are usually encountered at revision surgery with removal of previous total knee implants. Osteolysis secondary to particulate debris (mainly polyethylene), osteomyelitic bone erosion, and bone that is avulsed at the time that the components are removed are the most common etiologies in these cases. The last etiology can be a particular problem in those implants with porous coated stems or pegs into which there has been ingrowth of host bone.

Classification

Dorr (1) has described a simplified classification of bone deficiency, based on the type of surgery and the location of the defect.

Primary surgery
Peripheral defect
Central defect
Revision surgery
Peripheral defect
Central defect

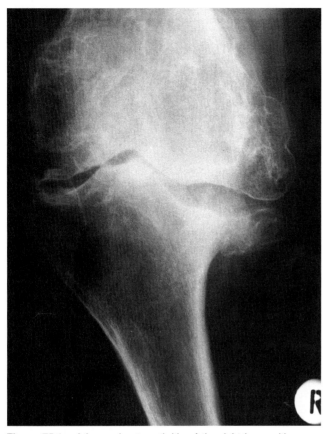

Figure 75.1. Advanced osteoarthritis of the right knee with a progressive varus deformity in a 72-year-old male. There is a segmental defect of the medial tibial plateau.

Rand (2) described four types of defects. His classification was based both on the amount of condylar involvement and on the depth of the defect.

Percentage of Condylar Involvement		Depth (mm)
Minimal	< 50%	< 5 mm
Moderate	50–70 %	5–10 mm
Extensive	70–90 %	> 10 mm
Cavitary	> 90 %	
Intact peripheral rim		
Deficient peripheral rim		

Bargar and Gross (3) have proposed a comprehensive evaluation of bone defects that enables investigators to directly compare treatment and outcome modalities by the type of defect. For both the femur and tibia, four types of defects are described. These are as follows:

1. Segmental: Lack of both cortical and cancellous bone at the level of the joint surface (called peripheral defects or uncontained defects in other systems);
2. Cavitary: Lack of cancellous bone at the level of the joint surface with an intact peripheral rim (also known as a contained defect);

3. Intercalary: Defect in the center of the bone, usually below the joint surface, with intact bone proximally and distally (as with a cyst in the low metaphyseal area);
4. Discontinuity: Fracture or segmental absence of bone.

For the patella there are three similar categories:

1. Segmental: Loss of patellar bulk or thickness;
2. Cavitary: Lack of cancellous bone with an intact peripheral rim or shell;
3. Discontinuity: fracture.

The depth of the defect is noted for both the femur and tibia in three zones. For the femur, the initial reference point is at the level of the epicondyles of the additional reference lines 1 and 2 cm distally. For the tibia, the reference point is the top of the tibial tubercle with two supplemental reference lines, one at the tip of the fibular head and another 1 cm proximal to this. Three femoral and three tibial grades are thus described (Fig. 75.2).

The volume of the defects are made from preoperative x-rays, or, more accurately, from measurements made at surgery. Finally, in an attempt to allow comparison among investigators, the authors assign a point score to each type of defect based on the severity and on the relative difficulty of management. These points are added together to provide a score for a particular patient.

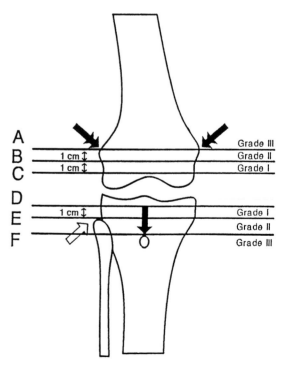

Figure 75.2. A grading system for bone defects about the knee, devised by Bargar.

Surgical Options for Bone Defects

The basic goal in treating bone defects during total knee arthroplasty is to completely support the implant. There are numerous ways to achieve this goal. Included among them are ignoring the defect; resecting bone to the bottom of the defect; filling the defect with cement; filling the defect with bone graft, either autologous or heterologous; filling the defect with prosthetic wedges and using custom components.

Prior to any decision about how to treat the defect, the surgeon should first perform a "standard" resection. Often defects that appear quite large either on preoperative x-rays or at the time of arthrotomy, shrink markedly in size after the proximal tibia has been removed.

The following sections concentrate primarily on bone defects in the proximal tibia since these are the most common defects seen in primary knee replacement. The indications, contraindications, advantages, and disadvantages apply as well to bone loss in the distal femur. Finally, bone loss in the patella presents certain specialized problems that are discussed separately.

Ignoring the Defect

This method is rarely used and is applicable only for very small defects, either segmental or cavitary, that encompass less than 5% of the resected surface. Even for these small defects, filling with bone or cement is more appropriate in the overwhelming majority of cases.

Windsor, Insall, and Sculco (4) discussed the surgical technique of shifting the position of the tibial component away from the defect. This technique, however, required a downsizing of the tibial component and had the potential to alter the force transmission across the implant to the host bone with the chance of early loosening (2). Such downsizing is especially problematic if the component is to be inserted cement-free. We have shown that lack of coverage out to the cortical rims of the tibia led to a statistical increase in the rate of subsidence of an uncemented tibial component (5).

Lotke (6) published his 3- to 8-year results using this method of downsizing to avoid a tibial defect. He found no long-term failures in patients with defects up to 20 mm treated by shifting the component. In his group of patients with defects greater than 20 mm and less than 50% surface of the hemiplateau, he shifted the component and used a cement wedge. He noted no mechanical failures in this group.

Ignoring the defect and shifting the component is not normally a method that is applicable to femoral bone loss. Downsizing in the medial to lateral plane on the femur usually requires a downsizing in the anteroposterior plane, and this can lead to either notching of the femoral cortex or laxity of the flexion space.

Resecting Bone to the Bottom of the Defect

In theory, this is the easiest, fastest, and most cost efficient method of treating bone defects during total knee replacement. The problem, of course, is that the greatest strength and quantity of bone is usually found adjacent to the joint surface, and overzealous resection can result in an implant seated on a shell of cortical bone with little cancellous support. Furthermore, the strength of trabecular bone, especially on the tibia, decreases with distance from the articular surface (7, 8). Finally, too low a resection of the tibia results in the necessity for a very thick tibial component, and this can lead to impingement of the implant and the patella.

Hvid (9) and Sneppen (10) generated strength profiles of the proximal tibia in cadaver bones using an osteopenetrometer and showed that the highest areas of strength of the medial condyle were located centrally and anteriorly. They showed that the lateral tibial condyle had a more restricted area of high strength and that this area was located in the posterior region of the condyle. Trabecular bone strength decreased with increasing distance from the subchondral resection surface. This diminution was most pronounced in the areas of high strength. In a related study, Hvid (11) evaluated 150 consecutive total knee arthroplasties at the time of surgery. They demonstrated that the distribution of bone strength between the condyles was dependent on knee alignment, being greatest medially in the varus knees while being diffusely distributed in the valgus knees. Harada (12) demonstrated that the ultimate compressive strength of the proximal tibia was greater in men than in women and, in addition, the distribution of the areas of maximum strength shifted location with increasing depths of resection.

Andrews and Barmada (13) performed a study in which they resected paired cadaver tibial specimens just below the articular surface and compared them to tibiae resected at 6 mm and at 12 mm below the joint line. In each case, a stemmed tibial component was cemented on the resected surface and the composite evaluated with a superincumbant load. They determined that the implant was best supported if the resection was within the first 1 to 2 mm below the articular surface. They then found a slight drop-off in strength, which extended all the way down to 12 mm below the articular surface.

In theory, therefore, it would appear that resection of the tibia immediately below the articular surface should yield the strongest support for the implant. Unfortunately, this resection results in elevation of the prosthetic joint line since the overwhelming majority of the extension space must be created by removal of bone from the distal femur. Such joint line elevation, especially in those knees in which the posterior cruciate ligament is retained, leads to an increased tension in the periarticular capsular ligaments with a diminution in potential knee flexion (14).

In order to retain the joint line at its normal level and to minimize the resection required in the proximal tibia, we have evolved the following surgical technique (15). The distal femur is resected, removing an amount of bone equal in thickness to the distal thickness of the femoral component being used. Next, the knee is fully extended and the collateral ligaments tensed with laminar spreaders. Soft tissue contractures are released in a standard way. A block, equal in thickness to the combined thickness of the femoral component and the thinnest tibial component for the total joint prosthesis being used, is then placed at the level of the femoral cut. Its distal portion is marked.

Using this method, we found that the amount of tibia that was resected varied from 2 mm or 9 mm with a mean of 5 mm. The large scatter was the result of the variation in the compliance of the collateral ligamentous tissues. It is this variation in compliance that prevents choosing any one arbitrary thickness of bone to remove in each and every knee.

Dorr (16) reported an increase of tibial radiolucencies when greater than 5 mm of bone was removed. We have not seen this in our series.

Lowering the resection line for the femur (actually elevating the resection line) leads to an abnormal elevation of the joint line. Proximal elevation likewise diminishes the amount of posterior condylar bone available to support the implant, and, as such, this technique should not be used for more than 3 to 4 mm in extent.

Filling the Defect with Cement

Biomechanical studies of the proximal tibia have shown that cement is a poor mechanical supporting material when used unsupported (17). The method of failure may include cement shrinkage and the development of laminations leading to fragmentation. Although cement can be used to fill small contained defects, it should not be used for peripheral defects.

There are conflicting reports as to whether reinforcement of the cement with screw or wire mesh increases its strength. Freeman (18) reported satisfactory results in total knee arthroplasties in which he employed screws to reinforce cement for proximal tibial defects. His follow-up, however, averaged only 32 months. Although there were tibial radiolucencies present in all of these knees, none were progressive.

Ritter (19) reported on 57 total knee arthroplasties, followed up to 7 years, using the technique of screws in cement. He found nonprogressive radiolucencies in 165 knees; however, no radiolucencies were present around the screw threads or the stems. He theorized that these radiolucencies were caused by poor penetration of the cement at the time of initial surgery. He had no cement failures. He then followed a subsequent group in which he extensively exposed the cancellous bed of the tibial defect to allow better cement penetration; he found no cement bone radiolucencies in 11 knees that he followed for over 2 years.

Most femoral defects are contained with intact peripheral rims that are capped by the implant. As such, they can usually be safely filled with cement and the implant adequately stabilized.

Bone Grafting Using Autologous Bone

From a purely philosophical viewpoint, the ideal material to fill a bone defect encountered during total knee arthroplasty would be bone itself. Cancellous bone is both osteoconductive and osteoinductive, is readily available, and is easy to trim to conform with any defect. Dorr and Ranwat (20) have suggested that bone grafting is the ideal treatment when there is greater than

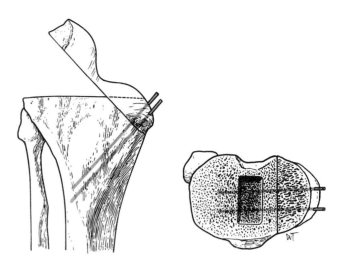

Figure 75.3.   The Sculco technique of filling a defect in the tibia with bone taken from the distal femur.

50% loss of the hemiplateau and when the defect is greater than 5 mm below the resection line.

Sources for the autogenous bone include the distal femoral condyles, the posterior femoral condyles, the intercondylar area of the femur, or iliac crest. Several techniques for using such bone have evolved.

Sculco (8) suggested using bone taken from the distal femoral resection. After performing his standard tibial resection, he removed the sclerotic base from the defect. Graft was temporarily affixed using Steinman pins and then was trimmed. To prevent intrusion of cement between the host bone and graft, a small batch of doughy polymethyl methacrylate (PMMA) was used initially as a sealant prior to cementing the permanent tibial component (Fig. 75.3)

Windsor, Insall, and Sculco (4) described a self-locking dowel technique in which the defect that was present after his standard tibial resection was reshaped into a trapezoid. The sclerotic underlying bone was removed with a high speed drill. The bone graft was shaped into a matching trapezoid and wedged into position in the defect. Although K-wires were used to hold the graft during cementing of the component, they were then removed. The results using this and the Sculco technique were excellent, with many cases developing no radiolucencies or collapse when followed for over 5 to 7 years.

Dorr (20) and his coworkers described a 3 to 6 year follow-up of 24 total knee arthroplasties with proximal tibial defects treated by bone grafting using autogenous bone. There was union in 22 of the 24 cases. Incorporation of the graft was documented by tomograms, bone scans, and bone biopsy. There was collapse of only 1 graft; this was attributed to residual varus alignment post operatively.

Scuderi et al. (21) reported similar results. They reviewed the 3-year follow-up of 26 total knee arthroplasties performed using bone graft. All grafts were found to have become incorporated within 1 year. They reported excellent results in 85%, good results in 12%, and fair results in only 4%. There were 2 knees with nonprogressive radiolucencies. One radiolucency was secondary to collapse of the graft. Similar good results have been reported by Altchek (22) and Aglietti et al. (23).

Poorer results were seen in a series we reported in 1989 (24). Four knees demonstrated collapse and dissolution within the first year. In 4 additional knees, there were radiolucencies between the graft and the proximal tibia. Nine of the knees were biopsied at over 1 year after the arthroplasty, and only 4 of these showed live osteocytes in lacunae in the bone graft. The overall success rate was only 67%. The bone used for the grafting was harvested from the posterior femoral condyle. In retrospect, this choice may have been inappropriate since it was primarily cortical and subchondral rather than cancellous, and this may have led to the failures seen.

Springorum and DeNicola (25) described a method of bone grafting that they called the basket-plasty technique (Fig. 75.4). They affixed titanium mesh as a cup or basket surrounding peripheral tibial bone defects and filled the mesh with crushed cancellous autogenous bone. Their results at 3 years were excellent with no evidence of subsidence of the prostheses or apparent fragmentation of the graft material.

Ultimately, the following factors have been essential for bone grafting to be effective: adequate surface preparation; graft fixation either by screw, pins, or the dowel technique; complete graft coverage by the tibial

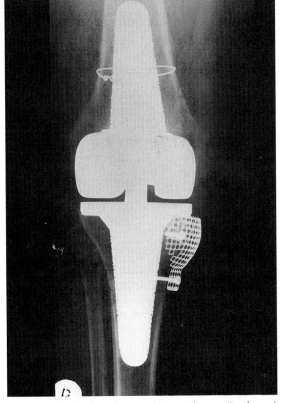

Figure 75.4. The basket-plasty technique of correcting for a defect by filling a mesh with cancellous bone.

component; proper limb alignment; and the use of a stemmed component (8, 26) in an attempt to unload some of the stresses on the graft surface. There is no uniform agreement, however, about how long or how thick the stem should be and whether it should be cemented or press-fit. Brooks, Walker, and Scott (17) determined that a 70 mm long intramedullary tibial stem could shield the proximal cancellous bone by 30%. The study by Bourne and his associates (26) further demonstrated that one could have significant stress shielding with the use of very long intramedullary stems. Bourne presently uses press fit, noningrowth, 70 mm stems and, in the short term, has not noted stress shielding of the proximal tibia. All of the authors who have described good results have used cancellous bone for the graft and have avoided large cortical fragment structural constructs.

There have been no long term studies on the use of bone graft to fill defects on the femoral side. Again, since most defects can be capped by the femoral component, bone grafting is a useful procedure. On occasion, for patients with extreme erosion of one condyle (usually the lateral condyle in a valgus knee), the bone removed from the medial side may be affixed to the lateral side with several K-wires or small screws. Posterior femoral bone loss is more difficult to treat by bone grafting because of the technical problems associated with proper placement and fixation of the graft.

Bone Grafting Using Allograft Bone

Allograft bone has been used primarily for filling defects during revision total knee arthroplasty. The experience of using large fragment allografts comes primarily from the work in tumor surgery. In a review of 600 massive cadaveric allograft transplants, Mankin (27) reported an overall success rate of 80%. Failures were secondary to fracture, nonunion and infection with the majority of the failures occurring within the first year after surgery.

In a review of 20 revision total knee arthroplasties, Whiteside (28) reported the results of using allograft cancellous bone chips. There was apparent incorporation in all cases with no evidence of loosening of the tibial components.

Mnaymneh (29) reviewed the results of 10 revision arthroplasties using massive allografts. There was union in 86% of the cases, although 2 of the allografts fractured. A similar review of a small series of massive allografts by Wilde (30) likewise revealed radiographic incorporation of the allograft in most cases.

The technique of a "bone within a bone" allograft has been described by Hedley. The senior author has personally used this technique in 5 cases. In a short follow-up, there has been good stability of the tibial component with no evidence of subsidence.

Modular Wedges and Custom Implants

Brooks, Walker, and Scott (17) reported on a study of wedge-shaped defects that such defects formed in the medial plateau of cadaveric tibiae. The defects were filled using a variety of materials; the constructs were then placed under an axial and a varus load. The least deflection of the tibial tray was seen when a custom tibial component was used. Metal wedge spacers provided almost equivalent support. Cement, either alone or with screws, gave poor results; leaving the tray unsupported was the least effective.

Clinical results with modular metal wedges have been excellent. Brand et al. (31) reviewed the 3-year follow-up results of 20 TKAs performed using modular wedges. There were no failures and the incidence of nonprogressive radiolucencies was only 27%. In a study by Rand (2), 28 TKAs were performed using modular metal wedges. The Hospital for Special Surgery (HSS) knee scores at 2 years were excellent in 79% and good in 21%. There were no failures of either the wedges or the tibial components.

Rand has reported primarily on the use of small segment tibial wedges, while use of larger hemiplateau and full plateau wedges have been described by Windsor (4). It is generally accepted that, if these larger types of wedges are to be used, there should be a tibial stem on the prosthesis as well (Fig. 75.5).

Augments have great applicability in the treatment of bone loss in the femur. Both posterior femoral and distal femoral augments are available in a variety of sizes. When both posterior and distal augments are used, we normally use a press-fit centralizing femoral stem as well. Unfortunately, augments are usually not available for anterior femoral bone loss.

The metal wedges are affixed to the components either by cement or by screws. Although both methods of fixation have yielded good short-term results, concerns remain about whether the cement will fragment, and whether there will be fretting corrosion between the screws and the wedges.

The major objection to custom devices relates to their expense and to the time required for their fabrication. Moreover, although the size and shape of these devices are determined through preoperative x-ray films and/or through tomography, often the defects found at the time of surgery do not exactly match the implant, thus rendering it relatively useless. The ability, therefore, to customize the prosthesis, "on the table," using a variety of wedges and stems has proven to be a substantial benefit for those patients with large defects.

Bone Loss from the Patella

Bone loss from the patella is usually seen in three clinical situations: in a patient with a prior fracture or partial patellectomy, in a patient with severe inflammatory erosive arthritis, and in the patient undergoing total knee arthroplasty revision. Bone grafting is usually not applicable nor is filling a large area with cement. One method of filling defects is to use a biconvex patellar implant. This surgical technique retains the peripheral cortical bone of the patella for support of the implant and restores the quadriceps moment arm (32).

Summary

In summary, it is crucial that the base that supports the femoral or tibial component be flat in order to avoid

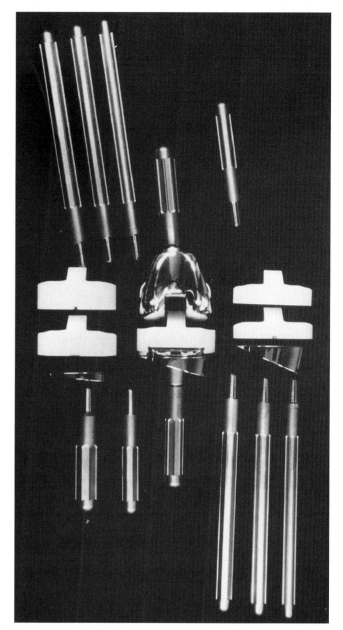

Figure 75.5. A system of metal wedges and intramedullary stems used for knees with severe bone loss and instability.

toggling or rocking the implant. Defects in the underlying bone, therefore, must be addressed by one of the techniques described above. There is still no general agreement on whether wedges or bone grafts are more applicable, although there is some thought that due to their ability to become incorporated into host bone, grafts may be preferable to wedges in younger patients, with the reverse being the case in older patients.

References

1. Dorr LD. Bone grafts for bone loss with total knee replacement. Orthop Clin North Am (US) 1989; 20 (2):179–187.

2. Rand J. Bone deficiency in total knee arthroplasty. Use of metal wedge augmentation. Clin Orthop 1991; 271:63–71.
3. Bargar WL, Gross TP. A classification of bone defects in total knee arthroplasty (Personal communication).
4. Windsor RE, Insall JN, Sculco TP. Bone grafting of tibial defects in primary and revision total knee arthroplasty. Clin Orthop 1986; 205:132–137.
5. Laskin RS. Tricon-M Uncemented Total Knee Arthroplasty. J Arthroplasty 1988;3:27–38.
6. Lotke PA, Womg R, Ecker M. The management of large tibial defects in primary total knee replacement. Orthop Trans 1985; 9:425.
7. Bargren JH, Day WH, Freeman MAR, Swanson SAV. Mechanical tests on the tibial components of nonhinged knee prosthesis. J Bone Joint Surg [Br.] 1978; 60:256–261.
8. Goldstein W, Sonstegard M. Conference report. The 26th Annual Meeting of the Orthopaedic Research Society. Engineering Medicine 1980; 9:227–231.
9. Hvid I, Hansen SL. Trabecular bone strength patterns at the proximal tibial epiphysis. J Orthop Res 1985; 3:464–472.
10. Sneppen D, Christensen P, Larsen H, Vang PS. Mechanical testing of trabecular bone in total knee replacement. Development of an osteopenetrometer. Int Orthop (SICOT) 1981; 5:251–256.
11. Hvid I. Trabecular bone strength at the knee. Clin Orthop 1988; 227:210–221.
12. Harada Y, Wevers HW, Ir I, Cooke TDV. Distribution of bone strength in the proximal tibia. J Arthroplasty 1988; 3(2):167–175.
13. Andrews SA, Marbada R. Tibial resection in total knee arthroplasty. A Scientific Exhibit at the 59th Annual Meeting of the American Academy of Orthopaedic Surgeons, Washington DC, 1992.
14. Laskin RS, Matson F: The influence of joint position during total knee replacement. Orthop Trans 1987; 11–3:535.
15. Laskin RS. The spacer block technique for determining the level of tibial plateau resection in total knee replacement. Am J Knee Surg S 1992; 5(4):184–189.
16. Dorr LD, Conaty JP, Schreiber R, Mehne DK, Hull D. Technical factors that influence mechanical loosening of total knee arthroplasty. In: Dorr LD.
17. Brooks PJ, Walker PS, Scott RD. Tibial component fixation in deficient tibial bone stock. Clin Orthop (US) 1984; 184:302–308.
18. Freeman MAR, Bradley GW, Revell PA. Observations upon the interface between bone and polymethylmethacrylate cement. J Bone Joint Surg 1982; 64B(4):489–493.
19. Ritter M. Screw and cement fixation of large defects in total knee arthroplasty. J Arthroplasty 1886; 1(2):125–129.
20. Dorr LD, Ranawat CS, Sculco TA, McKaskill B, Oriesek BS. Bone grafting for tibial defects in total knee arthroplasty. Clin Orthop 1986; 205:153–165.
21. Scuderi GR, Insall JH, Haas SB, Becker-Fluegel NW, Windsor RE. Inlay autogenic bone grafting of tibial defects in primary total knee arthroplasty. Clin Orthop 1989; 248:93–97.
22. Altchek D, Sculco TP, Rawlins B. Autogenous bone grafting for severe angular deformity in total knee arthroplasty. J Arthroplasty 1989;4(2):151–155.
23. Aglietti P, Buzzi R, Scrobe F. Autologous bone grafting for medial defects in total knee arthroplasty. J Arthroplasty 1991; 6(4):287–294.
24. Laskin RS. Total knee arthroplasty in the presence of large bony defects of the tibia and marked knee instability. Clin Orthop
25. Springorum HW, De Nicola WL. A new technique of defect filling in cementless total knee arthroplasty. In: Total knee replacement. Laskin, RS, ed. New York: Springer-Verlag, 1991; 232–234.
26. Bourne RB, Finlay JB. The influence of tibial component intramedullary stems and intramedullary stems and implant-cortex contact on the strain distribution of the proximal tibia following total knee arthroplasty. An in vitro study. Clin Orthop (US) 1986; 208.95.
27. Mankin HJ, Springfeld DS, Gebhardt MC, Tomford WW. Current status of allografting for bone tumors. Orthopedics 1992; 15(10):1147–1157.
28. Whiteside LA. Cementless reconstruction of massive tibial bone loss in revision total knee arthroplasty. Clin Orthop (US) 1989; 248:80–86.
29. Mnaymneh W, Emerson RH, Borja F, Head WC, Malinin TI. Massive allografts in salvage revisions of failed total knee replacements. Clin Orthop (US) 1990; 260:144–150.
30. Wilde AH, Schickendantz MS, Stulberg BN, Go RT. The incorporation of tibial allografts in total knee arthroplasty. J Bone Joint Surg (US) 1990; 72-A(6):815–824.
31. Brand MG, Daley RJ, Ewald FC, Scott RD. Tibial tray augmentation with modular metal wedges for tibial bone stock deficiency. Clin Orthop 1989; 248:71–79.
32. Gomes LSM, Bechtold JE, Gustilo RB. Patellar prosthesis positioning in total knee arthroplasty: A roentgenographic study. Clin Orthop. 1988; 236:72–80.

Postoperative Care for Disorders of Articular Cartilage

76

Rehabilitation Following Total Knee Arthroplasty

Raymond P. Robinson, Peter T. Simonian, and Kathleen J. McCann

Rehabilitation following total knee arthroplasty involves the manipulation of physical, emotional, and financial factors in an effort to help the patient achieve four goals: to relieve pain; to achieve normal knee and overall function; to achieve physical and emotional independence; and to accomplish this at minimal cost. When considering these goals, one must remember that patients recovering from total knee replacement surgery are also recovering from their preoperative states. Rarely do patients come to knee replacement surgery without first going through a prolonged period of knee pain and weakening. Additionally one must realize that patients are not the only individuals requiring attention. Patients may have family and friends playing important supportive roles at home.

The following is a review of rehabilitation approaches after total knee arthroplasty. The literature on controversial topics is presented first, then my opinion is described, based on my 12-year experience with cemented prostheses. During this time more than 1100 Total Condylar, Insall Burstein Posterior stabilized I (Zimmer Inc., Warsaw, Indiana, Johnson & Johnson, Raynham, Massachusetts), and Insall Burstein Posterior Stabilized II (Zimmer Inc., Warsaw, Indiana) implants have been implanted on our total joint replacement service.

Patient Expectations and Patient Education

Ideally, rehabilitation for total knee replacement surgery begins long before the patient is admitted to the hospital. Patients, their families, and friends are often understandably uninformed about the surgery and postoperative recovery. They may have unrealistic expectations regarding (*a*) the length of the hospital stay, (*b*) the patient's condition on arriving at home, (*c*) the length of recovery, and (*d*) the long-term limitations advisable for a patient with a total knee replacement. All of these issues should be covered repeatedly before surgery, in words the patient and support group can understand. A brochure that reiterates the information is also helpful. Such a brochure acts as a reference and allows the patient to share the details of surgery and recovery with family and friends. The written material must be consistent not only with the verbal description provided but also with the routines of your own institution.

Length of Hospital Stay

The preoperative office visit provides an excellent opportunity to help patients and their support groups to begin thinking about discharge from the hospital. The patient and family must be prepared for the possibility of a very brief stay in the hospital. Controlling the length of hospital stay has become one of the important factors in controlling the overall cost of the patient's care. The reasons for being in the hospital must be clear to patients and their support groups. A social worker is invaluable in facilitating discharge plans before hospitalization.

In our experience, there is not a "usual" length of hospital stay for a patient recovering from total knee replacement surgery. Discharge from our orthopaedic ward after unilateral total knee replacement has, on average, occurred on the seventh postoperative day. Twenty percent of the unilateral total knee replacement patients are discharged from the orthopaedic ward to an in-house rehabilitation service within the medical center. For bilateral total knee replacements, discharge has, on average, occurred on the sixth postoperative day. Sixty-three percent of the bilateral knee patients are discharged to the rehabilitation ward.

For most patients the day of discharge is determined by their ability to achieve 6 goals. They must (*a*) be able to get in and out of bed independently; (*b*) be able to use the bathroom facilities; (*c*) be able to walk the distances required in their home environment, using a walker or crutches for balance; (*d*) be able to negotiate stairs safely; (*e*) be able to adequately control pain through oral medications; and (*f*) be able to flex and extend the operated knee sufficiently to be confident that motion will progress uneventfully. We agree with those who consider 70 to 75 degrees of knee flexion an adequate goal for hospital discharge (1–3). Dorr suggests that unilateral knees reach 65 to 70 degrees of active flexion and bilateral knee patients achieve 80 to 90 degrees of flexion before hospital discharge (4).

Patient Condition on Arrival Home

By the time most patients have been discharged from the hospital or rehabilitation ward, they should be able to act independently in the home environment. Patients will be able to walk from room to room in their homes, get to the bathroom and back, get in and out of bed, and go up and down stairs. They will not, however, be able to do activities that require stamina, such as going shopping, doing housework, or preparing a major meal. These types of activities would be inappropriate because they tend to require endurance that the patient does not have. Postoperative fatigue that limits these activities can be overwhelming.

Therapy directed by a therapist is usually not necessary after hospital or rehabilitation unit discharge. Nevertheless, the patient should not consider discharge from the hospital and departure from the therapist as the end of aggressive rehabilitation. Most patients go home very capable of continuing on their own the rehabilitation program they learned in the hospital. When outpatient rehabilitation is required, a therapist near home can be recommended, or in special cases, the patient can be kept close to the medical center. We have found that a nearby hotel or inn is valuable for patients who need to be near the medical center for outpatient rehabilitation but live a long distance away. Frequent sessions with a physical therapist, use of a constant passive motion machine, and even knee manipulations can all be done on an outpatient basis when necessary.

Length of Recovery

The term *recovered* means different things to different patients. Some patients feel they are recovered when they regain their personal independence. This personal independence is usually achieved by the time they are discharged from the hospital. Others consider themselves recovered when they return to driving a car at 6 to 8 weeks (5). Yet most patients do not really feel recovered until 3 months after surgery, when they sense that their stamina has returned. The return of stamina allows the patient to resume a more active life-style. That does not mean, however, that 3 months marks the end of improvement. Motion will continue to improve up to 1 year after surgery (2). Strength may continue to improve for an even longer period of time (4). If recovery to the patient means the end of improvement then recovery can take 1 to 2 years.

Limitations after Recovery

The patient should be informed that limitations are advisable, even after full recovery. This is true although the knee may feel like a natural knee. Phrases such as "the day the prosthesis is implanted is the day it starts to wear out" help the patient appreciate the long-term concerns regarding polyethylene wear and mechanical loosening (6). Knee joint reaction forces of 2 to 5 times body weight during normal ambulatory activities and up to 24 times body weight during more vigorous activities have led us to advise our patients to keep their body weight under control (7). In addition, patients should avoid lifting and carrying heavy loads and avoid vigorous activities, especially those involving high impact. Activities such as walking, swimming, low-resistance bicycling, gentle cross-country skiing on level surfaces, golf, and rowing are suggested as proper methods for achieving and maintaining good conditioning. Dorr suggests that golf may not be advisable because of the rotational component of the swing (4). We have been allowing our patients to play golf and have not seen any mechanical loosening of components as a result over the last 12 years.

Patients with multiple joint involvement or multiple systems disease may pose unique situations for rehabilitation. The usual goals for discharge should be altered to fit each patient. Patients with limited goals may require more or even less time in the hospital.

Efforts to first reach the six goals required for discharge from the hospital and ultimately the four final goals of the entire rehabilitation effort can be uneventful for many individuals. However, factors such as pain, knee swelling, knee stiffness, postoperative recumbency, weakness, and emotional difficulties can make the rehabilitation of other patients a challenge.

Control of Postoperative Pain

Pain following total knee replacement surgery can be severe and can interfere with rehabilitation efforts. Coutts, in his initial report on the use of constant passive motion after total knee replacement surgery, comments that intermittent passive motion of the knee by therapists has proven unsatisfactory because of pain (8). Pain should be controlled to allow appropriate early rehabilitation. Woolfe suggests that as pain develops, substance P is released. Once substance P is released, sustained changes occur in the dorsal horn, resulting in prolonged and exaggerated transmission of pain (9). This may explain why pain is more difficult to control after it begins. Thus, the most effective way to control postoperative pain is to attempt to prevent it from occurring.

Postoperative pain after total knee replacement is best controlled by coordinating the choice of intraoperative anesthesia with the selection of appropriate postoperative analgesia. General anesthesia does not provide postoperative pain control. Therefore, strong and immediate postoperative analgesia is essential. Loading doses of narcotic or nonnarcotic analgesics can be combined with patient-controlled analgesia (PCA) to provide effective pain relief (10, 11). The patient using the PCA, however, must be alert enough to cooperate. Adequate loading doses of analgesics are necessary to establish good pain control that can then be maintained by the patient.

The concept of a PCA unit allowing the patient to control the administration of analgesic medications was introduced by Sechzer in 1965 (12). Today numerous commercial PCA units exist that combine a drug reservoir, an accurate infusion pump, a variable-demand dose element, a button for the patient to trigger the drug-delivery system, and a lockout mechanism to prevent a second dose of analgesic medication before the patient has experienced the effect of the first dose (10). PCA units have a high patient satisfaction rate, equivalent or superior pain relief at lower overall doses, reduced or unchanged sedation levels, and minimal delay between pain and relief, compared with conventional narcotic therapy (13). Scalley et al. reported a trend toward shorter hospitalization times after total knee and total hip replacement surgery using PCA (14).

Spinal or epidural anesthesia with bupivacaine or tetracaine can provide 3 to 4 hours of intraoperative anesthesia and postoperative analgesia (15). Longer anesthesia and analgesia can be provided with continuous spinal or epidural techniques. One must anticipate when they become ineffective and be prepared with narcotic or nonnarcotic analgesics. The PCA again is an effective technique to use in this situation.

Intrathecal morphine was reported to be an effective analgesic in animals by Yaksh and Rudy in 1977 and in humans by Wang et al. in 1979 (16, 17). Reports of respiratory depression, however, dampened the enthusiasm for intrathecal opioid in the early 1980s. Kalso reported in 1983 that prolonged analgesia without respiratory depression could be achieved using bupivacaine and much smaller doses of intrathecal morphine than were used earlier (18). Spinal anesthesia combining bupivacaine and a preservative-free form of morphine (Duramorph) generally results in 3 to 4 hours of operative anesthesia and 18 to 24 hours of postoperative analgesia (19). Although doses of 0.3 to 0.4 mg of intrathecal Duramorph have not been associated with the respiratory depression seen with larger doses, patients should still be observed and monitored for several hours postoperatively. Additional narcotics should be avoided, and naloxone should be available at the bedside (19). When the patient begins to experience pain, intramuscular nonnarcotic analgesics such as ketorolac tromethamine can be administered without concern about additional narcotic sedation. If pain is not adequately controlled with nonsteroidal antiinflammatory medications, parenteral or oral narcotics should be given. Pain generally returns gradually as the effect of the Duramorph subsides.

Brown et al. reported that ketorolac tromethamine, a nonsteroidal analgesic given intravenously or intramuscularly, is an effective nonnarcotic medication for controlling postoperative pain (20, 21). The pain relief resulting from 30 mg of intramuscular ketorolac was comparable to that from 12 mg of morphine when both were administered every 2 hours as needed. A maximum of 20 doses or 5 days of both medications were used. Ketorolac-treated patients had fewer adverse events than those treated with morphine. In our prac-

tice, intramuscular ketorolac has been used effectively combined with patient-controlled analgesia to control postoperative pain after the effect of the operative anesthetic and intrathecal Duramorph have worn off. The pain relief obtained allows early rehabilitation efforts to progress. Nausea, gastrointestinal bleeding, and reduced renal function are potential complications to be aware of when prescribing ketorolac.

Continuous epidural anesthesia or continuous epidural narcotics can also be used to provide extended periods of pain relief postoperatively. Mahoney et al. compared three groups of patients following total knee replacement surgery done under general anesthesia (22). One group received parenteral meperidine hydrochloride or morphine for analgesia. A second group of patients received periodic epidural injections of morphine. A third group received continuous epidural infusions of a very dilute concentration of bupivacaine hydrochloride and Duramorph. All of the patients receiving epidural catheters had them inserted at surgery. Good to excellent pain relief was reported in 86% of the epidural morphine group and 88% of the epidural bupivacaine and Duramorph group, compared with 61% of the parenteral meperidine or morphine group (22). Mahoney et al. noted that the epidural groups obtained greater knee range of motion during the first 72 hours and required a shorter hospital stay. This beneficial effect on rehabilitation was thought to result from reduced postoperative pain. The administration of the epidural analgesia in addition to the intraoperative general anesthetic increased the cost and duration of surgery (22).

Techniques that do not involve medications have also been advocated to control postoperative pain and enhance rehabilitation efforts. Walker et al. evaluated the effectiveness of constant passive motion machines, continuous cooling pads, and transcutaneous electrical nerve stimulation (TENS) in controlling pain after total knee replacement surgery (23). They found that the total hospital pain medication consumption was significantly lower in patients using the continuous passive motion machine than in the control group. Neither TENS units nor continuous cooling pads had a significant effect on total hospital pain medication consumption (23). Dorr also reported that the use of TENS units did not result in less postoperative pain in the routine postoperative total knee patient but did seem to help in patients with low pain tolerance and those who were depressed (4). Cohn et al. reported that the use of continuous cooling pads reduced the use of injectable and oral pain medication after arthroscopically assisted anterior cruciate ligament reconstruction (24). They also found that the use of continuous cooling pads reduced oral pain medication consumption.

The patient should be told to expect postoperative pain after total knee replacement surgery. Pain may be most intense immediately after surgery, with initial mobilization, and with knee range of motion exercises. Patients who are not informed of these pain patterns in advance may become unnecessarily anxious and fear that something has gone wrong.

Control of Swelling

Swelling after total knee replacement surgery can interfere with rehabilitation. It is often an acute problem and at times can be a chronic problem. Swelling can interfere with efforts to regain motion and can contribute to the patient's pain. Historically, efforts to control swelling have included elevation of the limb and application of compression dressings. Brodell et al. reviewed the historical evolution of the Robert Jones Bandage and monitored intramuscular compartment pressures under the dressing after total knee replacement surgery (25). They found that the dressing increased compartment pressures and helped reduce bleeding, tissue edema, and the size of effusions and hemarthroses. Less bulky compression dressings became necessary when CPM machines were used for immediate motion postoperatively. (8, 26). Some surgeons splint the knee after surgery for 2 to 3 days in a bulky compression dressing with splints to control pain and swelling and maintain extension, changing to a less bulky dressing to begin range of motion (1, 27).

Efforts to control swelling have also included the use of elastic compression stockings, sequential pneumatic compression stockings, continuous cooling pads, and constant passive motion machines. Properly fitting thigh-high elastic compression stockings have been shown to control swelling by providing a gradually decreasing compression of the lower extremity from the ankle to the groin (28, 29). Sequential intermittent compression stockings carry the concept of compression further, actively pumping fluid from the extremity (30). These techniques can be used to reduce swelling after knee replacement surgery.

For many years, application of cold to a swollen limb has been routine for controlling pain and swelling after acute injuries. Continuous cooling pads have been designed to apply the same principle after knee surgery. Hecht et al. reported that application of cold did decrease postoperative swelling after total knee replacement surgery (31). Cohn et al. found that the application of continuous cooling pads in anterior cruciate reconstruction patients resulted in less use of injectable Demerol, an easier conversion to oral medication, decreased use of oral pain medications, and greater ease in range of motion efforts (24). The use of continuous cooling pads did not, however, reduce the length of hospital stay or the amount of blood loss or improve postoperative range of motion (23, 24).

The use of a constant passive motion machine following total knee replacement surgery results in a significant reduction in knee swelling (1, 4, 8, 32). Coutts et al. reported a near absence of wound edema and effusion when using the CPM. They postulated that the passive motion of the limb assisted venous and lymphatic flow and prevented back-diffusion of fluids into the extracellular spaces, resulting in less edema (8). The CPM unit is also an effective way of elevating the limb.

Chronic swelling and venous stasis can occur following total knee replacement surgery, as a result of proximal deep vein thrombosis. Even if recanalization of the proximal vein occurs following treatment, patients may still develop ambulatory venous hypertension and chronic leg swelling (33). Efforts to reduce the incidence of proximal deep vein thrombosis in total knee arthroplasty patients not only would be expected to reduce the risk of pulmonary embolism but also would be expected to decrease the occurrence of chronic postoperative swelling and venous stasis changes.

Other patients have chronic swelling in the leg preoperatively. These patients may have venous or lymphatic insufficiency, or they may have fluid retention from systemic causes. Patients with preoperative chronic swelling should be thoroughly evaluated. The patient should be informed that swelling may be greater postoperatively and that the swelling may consequently impede acquiring knee motion and comfort. Patients with chronic preoperative swelling pose a special problem and should be considered for elevation of the extremity, use of a constant passive motion machine, sequential intermittent compression stockings, and long-term use of elastic support stockings.

Sympathetic dystrophy can occur after total knee replacement and can cause chronic knee swelling, pain, and stiffness (6, 34). Katz and Hungerford reviewed 36 patients with reflex sympathetic dystrophy affecting the knee. Five of these knees developed sympathetic dystrophy following total knee arthroplasty (34). Sympathetic dystrophy is considered rare in the knee and is manifested by four features: (a) intense and prolonged pain, (b) vasomotor disturbances, (c) delayed functional recovery, and (d) trophic changes (35). Patients tend to complain of pain out of proportion with the severity of the operation. They may have knee stiffness, although stiffness may only be mild (34). The diagnosis of reflex sympathetic dystrophy should be suspected when the patient has the aforementioned symptoms. The most important diagnostic tool still remains the patient's response to a lumbar sympathetic block (34).

Treatment of reflex sympathetic dystrophy consists of combining the disruption of lumbar sympathetic function by either pharmacologic agents or sympathectomy, along with physical therapy (34–36). Treatment is most successful when begun less then 6 months after the onset of symptoms (37). Cooper reported 11 of 14 patients diagnosed with reflex sympathetic dystrophy of the knee who experienced complete resolution of symptoms when treated with a continuous epidural anesthetic, continuous passive motion, manipulation as necessary, muscle stimulation, and alternating hot and cold soaks (35).

Author's Preferred Approach

Our postoperative routine to control swelling consists of the use of postoperative drains, the application of a compressive dressing, and elevation of the postoperative extremity with pillows or a folded blanket under the calf. The gatch of the bed can be lifted to increase elevation if necessary. The patient's heels are kept off the bed to prevent pressure necrosis. Specifically, the dressing consists of a nonstick layer and sterile gauze on the wound, a double layer of cotton wrapping from the ankle to the groin, an elastic wrap, a thigh-high sequential intermittent compression stocking, and a Velcro strap knee immobilizer splint. On the second postoperative day, the drains are removed, the immobilizer is unstrapped, and limited active or active-assisted knee range of motion is begun. On the third postoperative day, the compression dressing is removed. If the wound is healthy, knee range of motion exercises are advanced. The same sequential intermittent compression stocking and knee immobilizer are used as necessary throughout the patient's stay in the hospital. A CPM machine is used when knees are either unusually swollen or are expected to have unusual postoperative swelling. As the patient becomes more active, periods of leg elevation during nonambulatory moments in addition to the use of elastic support stockings are recommended to continue to reduce swelling.

Patient Mobilization

General Principles of Rehabilitation

The orthopaedic surgeon should be aware of all aspects of patient rehabilitation and should take an active role in patient recovery. Three general principles attributed to Otto Aufranc by Chandler are important guidelines to consider when one begins efforts to mobilize the patient after total knee replacement surgery (27). The first principle is to teach patients how to do their own exercises and not do them for them. Chandler emphasizes that passive stretching exercises are not appropriate. Active or active-assisted exercises lead to better success (27). Chandler also stresses that patients must take responsibility for their own recovery.

The second principle states that all exercises should be done in or near the patient's room, not in a special therapy area (27). Therapy sessions after the patient is brought to a separate therapy area tend to be too lengthy and result in patient fatigue. Frequent shorter sessions are endured better by the patient, such as three to four 10- to 15-minute visits by the therapist at the bedside. Ideally, the same therapist should see the patient each day for rehabilitation. Patients should not consider therapy as something that is done only with the therapist, but rather, they should consider therapy as their own responsibility to be done in any location, including their own home. "Homework assignments" can be given to the patient to continue rehabilitation efforts when the therapist is not present.

The third principle is that exercises should not be painful. Short periods of discomfort or aching caused by demands on tissues are appropriate, but activities or exercises that result in persistent pain should be avoided.

Author's Preferred Approach

Mobilization of the total knee patient begins as soon as the patient is awake and hemodynamically stable. This may occur in the afternoon of the day of surgery, if the procedure is done in the morning. An overhead trapeze is attached to the bed, allowing patients to independently adjust their position in bed. Ankle plantar flexion and dorsiflexion exercises; isometric quadriceps,

gluteal, and hamstring tightening exercises; well-leg strengthening exercises; and upper extremity strengthening exercises can begin as soon as the patient can cooperate. Adequate postoperative analgesia is critical during such early rehabilitation efforts.

Postoperative Day 1. Most patients can get out of bed on the first postoperative day. Patients may notice that they do not have the control of their leg to which they are accustomed. The degree of lack of control may vary with the surgical exposure used. The subvastus exposure, for example, can allow active straight leg raising by the first postoperative day (38, 39). A longitudinal exposure through the extensor mechanism usually results in more prolonged extensor mechanism weakness. Active straight leg raising in knees exposed through an extensor splitting exposure is more commonly achieved by the second or third postoperative day (1). Patients may comment that their leg "feels like it belongs to someone else" or that their leg "won't move when I tell it to." Reassure the patient that these observations are normal and temporary. The patient is encouraged to sit on the edge of the bed and, after a moment, stand by the bedside and transfer to a bedside chair, even if assistance is needed. A walker or crutches are used for balance. Weight bearing on the operative leg is allowed as comfort permits. The knee immobilizer is worn while standing or walking, to prevent unexpected knee flexion. The immobilizer can be discontinued for walking when the patient can do a straight leg raise independently.

Postoperative Days 2 and 3. On the second and third postoperative days, patients are encouraged to walk the farthest distance that they can retrace to the bed. By postoperative day 3, this distance may be approximately 20 meters. Each day patients are encouraged to walk farther and sit in the chair longer. Patients are also encouraged to get dressed in ordinary clothes, such as athletic shorts or sweat pants, rather than remaining in a hospital gown. As strength improves, the patient can transfer and walk independently, using a walker or crutches for balance.

Stairs

An important part of patient mobilization is teaching patients the proper techniques for ascending and descending stairs. They are advised to think about how many stair steps they will need to negotiate at home. Going up stairs with crutches is best done by placing the unoperated leg on the first step, followed by the operative leg, and then the crutches. The patient may also use a stairwell handrail with one hand and place both crutches under the other arm. One of the crutches may be turned horizontally and grasped with the hand supported by the crutch (Fig. 76.1, A). If the patient is using a walker, the walker is turned sideways, so that the patient is standing inside the open area. The legs of the walker facing the step are placed on the first step. One hand grasps the up-tilted handgrip of the walker while the other grasps the stair handrail (Fig. 76.2, A). The patient steps up with the unoperated leg and follows with the operated leg. The walker is then pulled up to the next step.

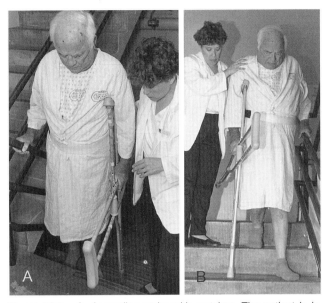

Figure 76.1. **A,** Ascending stairs with crutches. The patient is instructed to lead with the unoperated leg. **B,** Descending stairs with crutches, the patient leads with the operated leg.

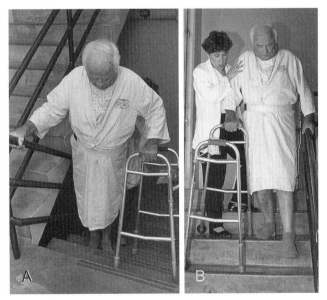

Figure 76.2. **A,** Ascending stairs with the walker, the patient grasps the upper grip of the walker and leads with the unoperated leg. **B,** Descending stairs with the walker, the patient leads with the operated leg.

When going down stairs, the patient is instructed to step close to the first step. A crutch is placed on the first step with one hand holding the other crutch horizontally, while grabbing the stair handrail with the other. Descending, the patient leads with the operated leg and follows with the unoperated leg (Fig. 76.1, *B*). Going down stairs with a walker requires the same technique as going up. The walker is placed sideways, and the two legs are tilted down on the first step. The patient grasps

the uppermost handgrip while the other hand grips the stair handrail; then steps down with the operated leg and follows with the unoperated leg (Fig. 76.2, *B*).

The walker is used differently when the patient has to negotiate a one-step entryway. To reach the top of the single step, the patient comes close to the step and places the entire walker on the stair. The patient then steps up with the unoperated leg and follows with the operated leg. Going down, the entire walker is placed down, off the step, and the patient steps down with the operated leg first.

It is acceptable for the patient to go up stairs backward; this may be easier if the patient's arms are too weak to help lift the body up forward. The patient should still be instructed to go down stairs forward.

Aids to Assist Function

Another element in the mobilization process is occupational therapy (OT). Occupational therapy helps some total knee patients anticipate the functional limitations they may experience when they arrive home after surgery. Routine occupational therapy assessment is not required for the typical patient recovering from a unilateral total knee replacement operation. Patients who have limited upper extremity function, limited back mobility, visual deficits, or limited motion or function of the opposite lower extremity often benefit from occupational therapy assessment. For example, bilateral total knee replacement patients may require an elevated toilet seat and a variety of reaching aids to assist in activities of daily living (Fig. 76.3, *A–D*).

Regaining Knee Motion

Motion Requirements

One of the most challenging goals following total knee arthroplasty surgery is regaining knee motion. Knee flexion and extension after recovery should be sufficient to enable the patient to return to normal activities. Gait analysis, performed on a group of normal patients similar in age to those undergoing total knee arthroplasty, helps one appreciate knee motion requirements during activities of daily living. Level walking results in an average 54 degrees of knee flexion (95% confidence limits: 42 to 67 degrees) (40). One hundred four degrees of knee flexion is necessary for climbing stairs (95% confidence limits: 99 to 108 degrees), 97 degrees for descending stairs (95% confidence limits: 94 to 100 degrees) (40), and 105 degrees of knee flexion is reported to be necessary to rise from a chair (41, 42). These motions vary, depending on the length of the patient's legs, the height of the step, and the height of the chair. In my practice, patients generally require at least 105 degrees of active or active-assisted knee flexion, measured in the office, before they report being able to rise comfortably from a chair and ascend and descend stairs in a normal manner. Other activities, such as squatting or getting up from a seated position on the floor or bathtub, require even more knee flexion. We expect patients to reach at least 120 degrees of knee flexion after routine total knee arthroplasty.

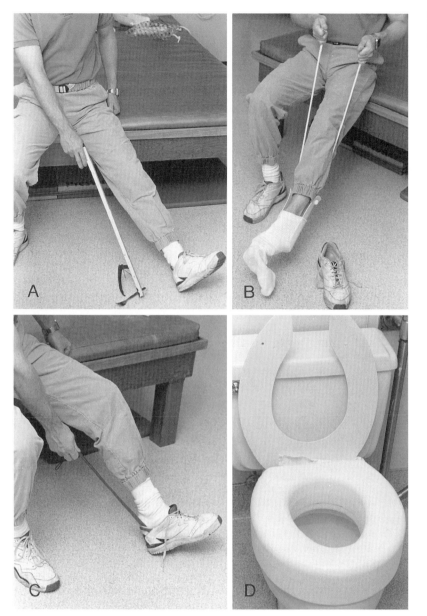

Figure 76.3. A, A reaching aid for picking up objects. **B,** A reaching aid to put on a sock. **C,** A long-handled shoe horn. **D,** Elevated toilet seat.

During level walking, the knee, on average, reaches 2 degrees of knee flexion (95% confidence limits: −4 to 8 degrees) (40). Clinically, we have observed that total knee arthroplasty patients report functional limitations when they have more than 10 degrees of flexion contracture.

Predicting Postoperative Knee Motion

Flexion

A statistically significant correlation has been described between preoperative and postoperative knee motion (6, 27, 43). Poor motion after total knee arthroplasty can be anticipated, particularly when the preoperative knee flexion is less than 75 degrees (43). The diagnosis also influences postoperative motion (42). Fox and Poss reported that patients with rheumatoid arthritis permitting less than 95 degrees of knee flexion preoperatively achieved less than 95 degrees of flexion postoperatively. Rheumatoid patients who had more than 105 degrees of flexion preoperatively tended to have more than 105 degrees of knee flexion postoperatively. The length of time that knee motion is limited preoperatively may also be an important factor in predicting postoperative motion (42). Additionally, the design of the prosthesis influences postoperative knee motion (6, 42). By considering one family of implants, the effect of design can be clearly demonstrated. The original Total Condylar design, introduced in 1974, allowed an average 90 degrees of knee flexion (44). The Insall Burstein Posterior Stabilized I (Zimmer Inc., Warsaw, IN; Johnson & Johnson, Raynham, MA) total condylar prosthesis introduced in 1978 included a cam function and other design features that increased knee flexion by enhancing posterior femoral rollback during knee flexion (45). The average flexion reported in knees receiving this newer design was 115 degrees (45). In 1988, the Insall Burstein Posterior Stabilized II (Zimmer Inc., Warsaw, Indiana) total condylar implant was introduced. It was designed to allow even more knee flexion (46).

Surgical technique can also influence postoperative knee motion (6, 42). A tight patellar retinaculum that is not released can limit knee flexion. Patients who have had a lateral retinacular release have an easier time with postoperative knee motion (6). In my own practice, a lateral retinacular release is performed in 74% of total knee arthroplasty procedures. If implant surfaces are not positioned properly, in posterior cruciate-retaining designs, flexion can be limited as the posterior cruciate tightens (6). With any implant design, discrepancy between the kinematics imposed on the knee by the implant and those imposed by soft tissue constraints can result in plowing of prosthetic joint surfaces (47). This can limit knee motion. Insall has used the term *kinematic conflict* to describe this situation (6). Knees with previous growth or traumatic disturbances that have altered the positions of ligamentous structures are particularly vulnerable to kinematic conflict when prostheses are inserted without regard to these soft tissue abnormalities. Knee deformities such as these pose particularly challenging problems for the total knee surgeon. At times, osteotomies are necessary to correct deformity before implantation of the knee prosthesis.

Finally, patient motivation, body habitus, range of motion of the opposite knee, and extent of physical therapy have been other factors believed to be related to postoperative knee flexion after total knee arthroplasty (6, 42).

Extension

As with flexion, limited extension after total knee arthroplasty may be influenced by prosthesis design and surgical techniques. Schurman et al., reporting on a series of total condylar knee replacements, found that virtually all improvement in knee extension occurred at the time of surgery (2). They believed that efforts to achieve maximum extension during surgery were imperative. No significant improvement in extension was observed after discharge from the hospital (2). Tanzer and Miller, on the other hand, studied 35 knee replacements using the Miller-Galante prostheses. They concluded that significant improvement in knee flexion contracture can occur postoperatively and that complete correction of flexion deformities at the time of surgery by resecting more bone is not necessary (48). We prefer to make every effort to achieve less than a 10 degree flexion contracture by the end of surgery and by the time of hospital discharge. In our experience, further knee extension does occur over the first 6 months after surgery.

Acquiring Knee Motion

Therapy techniques designed to increase knee range of motion after total knee replacement surgery vary from institution to institution and among individual therapists. It is best to give patients a consistent program for achieving knee motion, so that they may acquire independence with the program sooner. To this end, it is preferable that the same therapist work with the patient each day or at least that the same routine be taught to the patient throughout the recovery. For some patients, even subtle differences in a therapy program can result in confusion. The orthopaedic surgeon, therapists, and nurses need to consider a variety of techniques, some of which may work better for one patient than others. Remember the three principles of Otto Aufranc, as a rehabilitation program develops for each patient (27): (a) the exercises should be appropriate for patients to do on their own; (b) the exercises should not involve special equipment or need to be done in special locations; and (c) the program should not result in persistent pain. Below are a series of passive, active, and active-assisted techniques to help the patient advance knee range of motion.

Flexion

Knee Flexion over a Folded Pillow. The knee immobilizer is removed while the patient remains in bed in the supine position. A folded pillow is placed under the operative knee. The patient is instructed to relax and allow the knee to flex over the pillow. If knee flexion is too painful, have the patient press the heel down into the therapist's hand. The therapist gently lowers this hand while pressure is being applied.

Passive Knee Flexion over the Side of the Bed. Chandler and Krackow both describe a passive knee flexion exercise on the side of the bed (27, 49). The patient is instructed to sit on the bed, with the feet over the side edge. By slowly moving the body toward the edge of the bed, the ankle, calf, and knee lose support, resulting in gradual increases in knee flexion. This is done until the patient reaches a position of maximum comfortable flexion. Chandler points out that this technique is only effective up to 90 degrees of flexion (27).

Polishing the Floor. The patient is instructed to sit in a solid chair with armrests. A towel is positioned under the foot, on a smooth floor. The patient is instructed to "polish the floor" by moving the foot forward and backward several times. This is not a side-to-side motion (Fig. 76.4, A and B). The knee is then actively extended to achieve a self-facilitated contraction relaxation mechanism. The patient is encouraged to pull the foot farther back each time. After 5 to 10 repetitions, the patient brings the foot back as far as possible in the polishing routine. In this position of maximal flexion, the therapist's foot is placed in front of the patient's foot to prevent slippage; the therapist must not push with this foot. The patient is then instructed to scoot as close as possible to the front edge of the chair (Fig. 76.5). This is done three to five times. The knee flexion is measured on the last effort.

Flexion Sitting in a Chair. The patient sits in a chair with the knee maximally flexed. The foot is firmly planted on the ground. The patient is then instructed to move the thigh forward while contracting the hamstrings to bend the knee farther than is comfortable (27, 49). The maximum flexed position is held for 10 seconds. The patient is instructed to do the exercise 10 times a session.

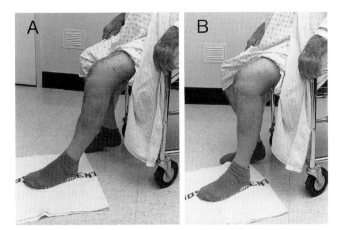

Figure 76.4. **A,** Active knee flexion exercise in the sitting position. **B,** The patient is instructed to actively bring the foot back as if polishing the floor.

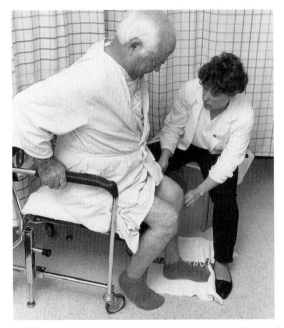

Figure 76.5. The patient is instructed to scoot to the front edge of the chair and actively flex the knee. This is done while the therapist holds a foot on the floor, preventing the operated knee from extending. Maximum knee flexion is measured with a goniometer.

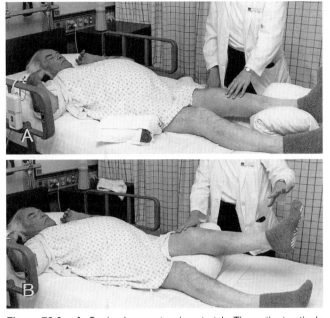

Figure 76.6. **A,** Supine knee extension stretch. The patient actively pushes the knee toward the bed. **B,** Terminal knee extension with the distal thigh supported on a pillow.

Flexion in a Standing Position. The patient is instructed to walk up to an elevated step or stool with crutches or walker. By placing the foot on progressively higher steps, more knee flexion is accomplished (27, 49). Moving the thigh forward and contracting the hamstrings as in the chair technique will result in further flexion.

Hands and Knees Flexion. A patient who can comfortably kneel on a soft surface can be instructed to get into a hands-and-knees position on the bed. Knee flexion can be increased by having the patient move the buttocks posteriorly toward the heels by pushing with the hands while contracting the hamstrings (27).

Stationary Bicycle. The stationary bicycle is a valuable aid in acquiring knee flexion (6, 27). The patient is instructed to begin with the seat high to limit the knee flexion required to peddle. As comfort permits, the seat can be lowered to increase knee flexion.

Extension

Supine Knee Extension Stretch. Place a folded pillow or blanket under the ankle of the operative leg. Instruct the patient to allow the leg to relax. After a few moments have the patient contract the quadriceps to press the knee down toward the bed (Fig. 76.6, *A*). Hold the extension for 10 seconds. Measure the extension accomplished.

Terminal Knee Extension. A folded pillow is placed under the knee. Alternatively, a sling supported from an overhead frame can be used to support the knee. The patient is instructed to extend the knee actively and hold for 10 seconds (Fig. 76.6, *B*). If one needs to facilitate quadriceps contraction, the therapist can lift the heel, bring the knee into extension, and ask the patient to maintain the extension and then to slowly lower the foot back to the bed.

Prone Knee Extension. The patient is asked to move into the prone position. The knee rests in extension on the bed. By contracting the quadriceps and balancing the lower extremity on the toes, further knee extension is achieved (27).

Knee Extension Standing. The patient is instructed to stand with the crutches or walker and extend the knee fully in a heel-strike position. The heel is placed on the floor slightly in front. The heel is then dragged backward along the floor, contracting the quadriceps and hip extensors and extending the knee

(27). The patient is instructed to repeat this same maneuver during each step in ambulation.

Knee Extension While Walking. Patients with limited knee extension will tend to lift the heel off the floor too early at the end of stance phase. The patient should be instructed to keep the knee extended and keep the heel down at the end of stance phase. A shorter stride often helps the patient accomplish this (27).

Constant Passive Motion Machines

In recent years, the use of constant passive motion (CPM) has been advocated as a routine in postoperative total knee rehabilitation. (8, 26, 32, 50). The earliest reported clinical use of continuous passive motion in the knee was by Nickel in 1960, following a synovectomy in a patient with rheumatoid arthritis (8, 51). In 1975, Salter reported his studies on the biological effect of CPM on healing articular cartilage defects (52). He later reported the beneficial effects of CPM on intraarticular fracture healing, cartilage preservation in septic joints, and tendon healing (53–55). This work led to the reduction of postoperative immobilization time in knee surgery as well as in surgery on many other joints. The concept of early motion, and the concept that such motion could be used to orient collagen fibers in an advantageous way, led Coutts to develop a constant passive motion machine to be used after total knee replacement surgery (8).

As one reviews the many reports regarding CPM machines and total knee replacement surgery, it is important to remember that early knee range of motion is not achieved with a machine exclusively. Physical therapy routines influenced by the same early motion studies began including early ambulation and knee mobilization techniques. Of equal importance is that during the early enthusiasm for passive motion using machines, prosthetic designs were changing to provide more motion, surgical techniques such as the subvastus exposure were being introduced to reduce early postoperative quadriceps weakness, postoperative analgesia options were being improved, and criteria for hospital discharge were changing (11, 17, 37, 44–46). All of these changes have affected the rehabilitation of the total knee arthroplasty patient. Any decision today regarding the routine use of the CPM must take all of these changes into account.

The initial report on the use of CPM following total knee arthroplasty compared a group of patients who were placed on CPM machines immediately after surgery with a group of patients immobilized for 3 days and then begun on conventional physical therapy (8). The patients treated with CPM (*a*) acquired knee flexion faster, (*b*) achieved superior knee flexion at 1 year, (*c*) were more comfortable, (*d*) had less knee edema and effusion, (*e*) had a shorter hospital stay, (*f*) demonstrated increased venous flow (might be expected to reduce the incidence of thrombophlebitis), and (*g*) avoided the need for later manipulation of the knee under anesthesia (8). Retrospective studies that followed this report confirmed that knees treated with CPM progressed more rapidly with early knee flexion than knees that were first immobilized and then treated with conventional physical therapy (51, 56). If 90 degrees of knee flexion remained a criterion for hospital discharge, then patients treated with CPM could be discharged from the hospital earlier (51). Not only could the discharge occur earlier, but there was less need for knee manipulation (56). However, these studies did not find a statistically significant improvement in ultimate knee motion using CPM (51, 56).

Five prospective randomized studies have compared total knee arthroplasty patients with knees treated with CPM with those treated with immobilization followed by conventional physical therapy. These studies have extended the observations in the earlier reports. Goll et al. found no statistically significant decrease in the incidence of thrombophlebitis or pulmonary embolism using CPM (57). They did, however, report a reduced incidence of wound complications, a faster recovery, and a shorter hospital stay in the CPM group. The CPM patients averaged 16 days in the hospital (57).

Vince et al. reported a prospective randomized study in which a group of patients begun on CPM in the recovery room achieved 90 degrees of knee flexion faster than a control group. Ultimate range of motion was not determined by whether one used a CPM machine, but rather by the implant design and surgical techniques (58). They found a 30% reduction in thrombophlebitis distal to the knee but concluded that no direct evidence equated CPM machine use with a decreased risk of pulmonary emboli. They resorted to knee manipulation less frequently in the CPM group. Vince et al. suggested that the use of CPM would enable patients who were unwilling or unable to participate aggressively in postoperative rehabilitation to achieve flexion more easily after total knee replacement surgery and would also help them avoid manipulation (58).

Ritter et al. reported a consecutive series of bilateral simultaneous total knee replacement patients who had one knee randomly selected to begin use of a CPM machine on the first postoperative day (1). The Anatomically Graduated Component (AGC) 2000 (Biomet, Warsaw, Indiana) posterior cruciate retaining condylar implant was used on all knees. Both knees were dressed in bulky compressive dressings for the first 24 hours. During this time, patients were instructed in bilateral isometric quadriceps exercises, gluteal sets, ankle dorsiflexion and plantar flexion exercises, assisted straight leg raises, and ambulation with a walker, weight bearing as tolerated. On the second postoperative day, both bulky dressings were removed and conventional physical therapy techniques begun to regain knee motion and strength. The control side was kept in a knee immobilizer between therapy sessions until the ability to do an active straight leg raise was achieved. This was usually accomplished on the second or third postoperative day. A knee immobilizer was still worn on the control side at night to prevent knee flexion contracture. The other leg was placed in a CPM unit for 20 hours a day. Patients were allowed out of the machine for physical therapy, meals, bathing, toilet needs, and ambulation. Seventy degrees of flexion was considered to be appropriate for discharge from the hospital. Ritter et al. reported no statistically significant difference in range of motion at the average 8-day discharge time. No difference in knee motion was observed between the two groups 2 months, 6 months, or 1 year after surgery. There was, however, a significant decrease in knee swelling with the CPM machine. The CPM-treated knee appeared to be generally weaker, as reflected by a greater extension lag and more flexor tightness. Initial adjustments of the machine and later efforts to maintain correct alignment were tedious, time consuming, and painful to the patient. Use of a CPM machine increased expenses because of the cost of the equipment and the increased staff time needed to set up and use it. Ritter et al. concluded that compared with their non-CPM rehabilitation routine, the CPM machine was neither cost-effective nor beneficial.

McInnes et al. conducted a randomized prospective study to evaluate the efficacy of CPM in total knee arthroplasty patients (32). They reported that compared with patients treated with a more conventional physical therapy program, CPM patients had less knee swelling and a reduced risk of requiring knee manipulation under anesthesia. They concluded that avoiding knee manipulation would lower the cost of treatment of a group of total knee arthroplasty patients if one used CPM routinely. The study reported that there was little or no difference in patient pain, quadriceps strength, active knee flexion, active knee extension, or length of hospital stay.

Johnson reported a prospective randomized controlled study comparing total knee replacement patients treated postoperatively with immobilization in a splint for 7 days and patients treated immediately postoperatively with CPM (59). Not surprisingly, the CPM group achieved flexion earlier and were discharged from the hospital sooner than the group immobilized for such an extended time. In this carefully selected group of patients, the CPM was not associated with an increased incidence of superficial infection or wound-healing problems, as had been observed earlier by Maloney et al. (51). Transcutaneous oxygen tension measurements were used to assess viability of the tissues around the wound during knee range of motion. Findings revealed that knee flexion above 40 degrees during CPM progressively reduced the oxygenation of the wound, particularly during the first 3 postoperative days. This was especially true in the lateral wound flap (59).

My interpretation of present physical therapy knee mobilization techniques, our own experience with CPM, and the present literature regarding CPM, is as follows: (a) early use and motion of the knee after total knee replacement surgery is advisable unless extensor mechanism disruption, wound drainage, or wound-healing complications prevent it; (b) motion past 40 degrees during the first 3 postoperative days may be dangerous in some patients because of reduced blood flow to the wound edges (59); (c) early knee motion can be safely accomplished by the use of a CPM machine, but it can also be safely accomplished by early patient mobiliza-

tion and active-assisted knee motion exercises (1, 8, 32, 59); (d) the CPM machine is helpful in controlling swelling (1, 8, 32); (e) the use of the CPM machine involves additional cost (1, 23); (f) the use of CPM reduces the frequency of later knee manipulation under anesthesia and therefore eliminates the cost for such a procedure; (g) early physical therapy knee mobilization techniques must be accompanied by adequate analgesia.

Each institution must decide whether the CPM technique of acquiring early motion is cost-effective. In our medical center, the CPM machine has been discontinued for *routine* use after total knee arthroplasty because it did not prove to be cost-effective. The CPM is, however, invaluable to those patients who (a) are unwilling or unable to participate aggressively in postoperative rehabilitation; (b) are anticipated to have unusual problems with postoperative swelling; (c) are not demonstrating satisfactory progress in knee motion after surgery; or (d) are expected to have poor range of motion postoperatively because they had poor motion preoperatively. Using these criteria, the CPM machine was used on 22% of the senior author's total knee procedures. The CPM machine used in this way has reduced the incidence of knee manipulation from 20% to 6%.

Author's Preferred Program to Regain Knee Motion

At the end of surgery, the knee is splinted in maximum extension. When the patient is in bed, the knee immobilizer splint continues to support the knee in an extended position. Later, when the knee is out of the immobilizer, the leg is supported with a pillow under the distal calf to encourage knee extension. The tendency for the patient and the inexperienced staff to place a pillow under the knee should be discouraged. Although resting with the knee in a position of mild flexion is more comfortable, it can cause a flexion contracture that can be difficult to eliminate.

On the first postoperative day, the patient sits on the edge of the bed with the immobilizer in place. After a moment's rest, the patient stands, bearing weight on the operative extremity as tolerated with assistance from the therapist. If comfort permits, the patient is allowed to transfer for a short time to a chair next to the bed. No formal knee motion exercises are attempted. Some slight knee motion does occur in the brace as the patient sits and stands.

Knee flexion and extension exercises are begun on the second postoperative day. Appropriate analgesia is important at this stage to allow motion to begin. The physical therapist instructs the patient in supine knee extension, stretching, and terminal knee extension exercises with the compressive dressing in place. The knee immobilizer is removed for the exercises (Fig. 76.6, *A* and *B*).

On the third postoperative day, the patient's compressive dressing is removed. If the wound is benign and deep drainage is absent, knee motion exercises are advanced. The patient continues the supine knee stretching and terminal knee extension exercises and begins knee motion in the sitting position by "polishing the

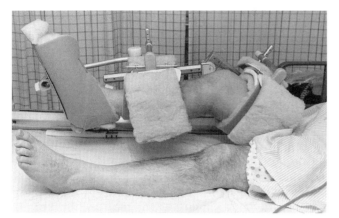

Figure 76.7. The constant passive motion (CPM) machine. Sutter 7000 Litelift with permission (Sutter Corporation, San Diego, CA).

floor." The flexion and extension achieved are written in large numbers on a board in the room so the patient and the professional staff can see the accomplishments. Patients who are not progressing satisfactorily with knee flexion, patients in whom we expect unusual swelling, or patients who are unwilling or unable to participate in knee motion therapy are begun on a CPM machine (Fig. 76.7).

When the patient can do an active straight leg raise and has less than a 15-degree extension lag, the knee immobilizer is removed during ambulation. The immobilizer is still recommended at night for patients who have a flexion contracture greater than 10 degrees. Knee extension exercises while standing and walking are begun at this time. Patients are expected to achieve at least 70 degrees of knee flexion with a flexion contracture of 10 degrees or less before discharge from the hospital.

Knee motion goals do not necessarily determine the time of discharge from the hospital. A patient may reach 70 degrees of knee flexion but not yet be able to walk distances or negotiate stair climbing well enough for discharge. Other patients may be discharged without reaching 70 degrees of knee flexion. A number of factors may change the usual knee motion goals. Patients demonstrating proficiency in knee motion exercises can be discharged as soon as they are independent. Such patients can be followed carefully as outpatients. Limited preoperative range of motion may alter postoperative knee motion expectations. These patients may be discharged earlier than usual, anticipating a more prolonged outpatient therapy program. As an outpatient, CPM therapy or even knee manipulation under anesthesia can be considered. Wound necrosis or wound drainage may require complete cessation of knee motion efforts. Dorr stressed the importance of stopping knee motion if wound drainage occurred. He found that the infection rate in knees with drainage was 5% (4). Knees with wound drainage, deep necrosis, or wounds that are of concern should be immobilized until the concern is over. In some cases, this immobilization may continue for months. Hospitalization during this time is usually unnecessary. Surgical exposures such as the

Coonse and Adams patellar turn down approach and the tibial tubercle release are necessary at times to enhance exposure (60, 61). These approaches can result in 4 to 6 weeks of immobilization.

After discharge from the hospital, patients are encouraged to continue the knee motion exercises learned in the hospital and to incorporate other activities to enhance knee motion and strength. Activities of daily living become excellent knee exercises. Walking, sitting down and rising from the toilet or chair, and negotiating stairs are examples of beneficial knee exercise. The use of a stationary bicycle is also strongly recommended.

Results

To provide information for this chapter, we recalled prospectively accumulated data on a series of 205 primary Insall Burstein Posterior Stabilized II total knee replacements completed by the senior author. One hundred seventy-seven knees had degenerative joint disease, 7 had rheumatoid arthritis, 13 had posttraumatic arthritis, 3 had avascular necrosis, and 5 had other diagnoses. Using the rehabilitation techniques described and the discharge goals outlined, unilateral knee replacement patients in this series were discharged from the hospital on postoperative day 7 ($\pm$2), ranging from 3 to 16 days. Twenty percent of these patients were transferred from the orthopaedic ward to a rehabilitation unit for an average 9 ($\pm$3) days, ranging from 1 to 15 days. Bilateral simultaneous total knee replacement patients were discharged on postoperative day 6 ($\pm$2), ranging from 4 to 16 days. Sixty-three percent of these patients were transferred to the rehabilitation ward for an average 8 ($\pm$3) days, ranging from 2 to 14 days. At discharge from the hospital or rehabilitation ward, knee range of motion in this series averaged an 8 ($\pm$4; 0 to 20) degree flexion contracture and 78 ($\pm$10; 52 to 120) degrees of flexion. At 6 weeks, the flexion contracture averaged 5 ($\pm$4; 0 to 25) degrees and flexion averaged 97 ($\pm$15; 55 to 128) degrees. By 3 months, the flexion contracture averaged 4 ($\pm$4; 0 to 12) degrees and flexion averaged 107 ($\pm$13; 55 to 135) degrees. At 6 months, the flexion contracture averaged 2 ($\pm$3; 0 to 19) degrees and flexion averaged 113 ($\pm$13; 65 to 135) degrees. At the 1-year office visit, the flexion contracture averaged 2 ($\pm$2; $-$5 to 12) degrees and flexion averaged 115 ($\pm$14; 60 to 140) degrees. Over the past 6 months, hospital stays for unilateral total knee patients have been reduced on average to 6 days.

Knee Manipulation

The use of either CPM or non-CPM techniques during early knee range of motion efforts may, in some patients, still fail to achieve the expected knee motion. In these situations, whether the patient is still in the hospital or is an outpatient, knee manipulation under anesthesia can be considered. Ranawat, reporting on a series of duocondylar knees, found that the manipulated knees did not have better flexion than those that were not manipulated. Fox et al. reviewed a series of primarily Duo-Patella (Cintor Division, Johnson & Johnson, Raynham, Massachusetts) knee replacements in 70%

rheumatoid patients (42). Patients who failed to achieve 90 degrees of flexion by the end of 2 weeks were manipulated. They found that knee range of motion was improved only temporarily. This temporary improvement in motion helped facilitate rehabilitation efforts. However, at 1 year there was no difference in knee range of motion between the knees that were manipulated and those that were not manipulated. Fox et al. concluded that routine manipulation after total knee replacement surgery was not justified for the purpose of improving ultimate knee flexion. Nevertheless, it was appropriate to facilitate rehabilitation in patients with poor motion at the 2-week period (42). Insall found knee manipulation after total knee replacement to be an indispensable aid to physical therapy, but not a substitute for therapy (62). He believed that knee manipulation prevented permanent restriction of knee range of motion in certain patients who are difficult to identify until it is too late for manipulation to be helpful (62). He recommended manipulating the knee when necessary, 2 to 3 weeks postoperatively. Insall further stated that in rare cases, success with manipulation occurred as late as 2 years after surgery. In general, manipulation later than 3 months was felt to be difficult. Knee manipulation was less common, in Insall's experience, when lateral retinacular releases were performed. Knee manipulation combined with a lateral retinacular release and open release of adhesions is occasionally necessary in particularly difficult cases (62).

Chandler suggested that knee manipulation was seldom necessary (27). If knee motion plateaued at 60 to 70 degrees of flexion by 10 to 14 days after surgery, knee manipulation should be considered. He added that in 5 years using the CPM machine, only one patient needed manipulation. CPM has reduced the need for manipulation of knees under anesthesia in total knee arthroplasty surgery (27, 32).

To our knowledge, a prospective randomized study of patients, all thought to be candidates for knee manipulation, with knees that are manipulated and knees that are not manipulated, has not been reported. Studies regarding manipulation tend to compare patients believed to need manipulation with patients who are not (49). Whether the patient who is left alone with poor early postoperative motion will eventually achieve as much knee motion as the patient with poor early postoperative motion treated with CPM and knee manipulation is still not clear.

The aforementioned reports regarding knee manipulation are difficult to compare because they deal with a variety of implants and different postoperative rehabilitation programs. As implant designs improved to allow greater knee flexion and as rehabilitation programs stressed earlier range of motion, the necessity for knee manipulation under anesthesia has decreased. In my own practice in the last 2 years, 6% of the knees have been manipulated under anesthesia in an effort to help the patients progress in their rehabilitation. Using the CPM machine for patients having difficulty with knee motion has helped our rehabilitation program, reducing the necessity for manipulation.

Several investigators have looked for factors that might predict the necessity for manipulation of the knee after total knee arthroplasty. In a series of Insall Burstein Posterior Stabilized I knee replacements, Figgie et al. reported that joint line elevation positively correlated with an increased incidence of manipulation (63). Fox and Poss, reporting on primarily rheumatoid patients, found that patients over 70 years of age required manipulation more often (42). Daluga et al., reporting on a series of posterior-stabilized knee arthroplasties, found that a 12% increase in the AP dimension of the natural femoral condyles, caused by placement of the prosthetic femoral component, significantly predisposed patients to manipulation (41). Factors such as knee alignment, joint line elevation, AP placement of the tibial component, patellar height, obesity, patient age, preoperative flexion, and single versus bilateral knee implants did not correlate positively with the occurrence of knee manipulation (41).

When manipulation is performed, it should be done under appropriate anesthesia. This can be either general or regional anesthesia. Regardless of the type of anesthesia used, complete muscle relaxation is critically important. Manipulation is done slowly. The surgeon's hand or ear is placed on the knee to detect the popping sensations resulting from rupturing adhesions. The flexion force is applied in the midtibial area and not at the ankle, to avoid a long moment arm. Load can be applied with either the hand or the axilla of the manipulator, but the force must be applied gradually and steadily (Fig. 76.8). As the popping sensations are felt and the knee sags into further flexion, the motion achieved can be measured, and further force should not be applied.

While manipulation of total knee replacements may become necessary in certain cases, complications can arise. Examples of complications under anesthesia are anesthetic risks, supracondylar fractures, wound dehiscence, patellar ligament avulsion, and hemarthrosis

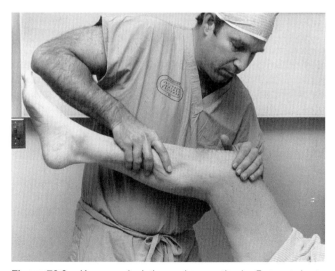

Figure 76.8. Knee manipulation under anesthesia. Pressure is applied firmly and steadily. A hand or ear on the knee allows sensation of adhesions rupturing.

(41–43). Daluga et al. believed that quadriceps adhesions were a factor leading to manipulation and that rupture of these adhesions led to heterotopic bone formation. The consequences of such heterotopic bone are not clear (41). Manipulation under anesthesia is also expensive, which has an impact on the overall cost of patient care (32).

Recovering Strength and Stamina

Two aspects of strength recovery should be considered: the return of muscle strength and the return of overall body strength and stamina. Return of muscle strength is critical to achieving a comfortable and optimally functional result (4, 64). The time it takes to recover muscle strength is often underestimated by both the patient and the surgeon. Postoperative weakness results from both the surgery and the deconditioned state of the patient before surgery. Dorr found that by 6 months after surgery, the total knee patient had only recovered 50% of normal muscle strength (4). By 1 year, the patient had recovered 80% of normal strength. As a result of weakness, the patient may notice a tight or band-like feeling around the knee as well as aching pain from the patellofemoral mechanism up to 6 months after surgery (4).

Muscle strengthening should begin early but gently. Townley even begins exercises a few weeks before surgery (3). Insall cautions not to stress strengthening exercises for the first 5 days after surgery, because of concern about damaging the capsular repair (6). He reports encountering cases of patellar dislocation during early physical therapy with weights. Early efforts at strengthening should be gentle and should not aggravate pain.

Ankle pumps can be started as soon as the patient is awake after surgery. Periodic dorsiflexion and plantar flexion of the ankle and moving the foot around in a circle tend to be tolerated well. Isometric exercises, including tightening the quadriceps, gluteal muscles, and hamstrings, can begin with the patient in the knee splint while lying supine in bed on the first day after surgery. Straight leg raising exercises can be initiated when comfortable. Some patients can begin doing straight leg raises on the first postoperative day. More often, the patient cannot accomplish a straight leg raise until the second or third postoperative day. At times, the patient may take even longer.

After the knee has become more comfortable and the patient has progressed with knee motion, isometric strengthening exercises in a variety of positions can begin. Sitting in a chair, isometric exercises can be done by placing the foot under any immovable object (27). Hamstring isometric exercises can be performed by placing the heel of the operative leg against the front leg of a chair while sitting or against the toes of the opposite foot. Gastrocnemius isometric exercises can be done by standing on tiptoes and holding the position for 10 seconds (27). Such isometric exercises can be done in sets of 10, 10 times a day.

Muscle atrophy following knee surgery has been attributed to a reflex response of muscles to the trauma of surgery and the resulting inhibition of muscle usage (64, 65). Efforts to avoid such atrophy, using electrical muscle stimulation, have been proposed (64). Coutts et al. combined the use of CPM and electrical muscle stimulation after total knee replacement surgery. Their results suggested a positive effect on muscle strength, but the advantages were not clear (64).

Exercises remain the cornerstone of treatment to regain muscle strength after total knee surgery. As strength and function return, more generalized exercises are recommended. These exercises include walking, swimming, and low-resistance bicycling. Ideally, these exercises should correspond to the interests and life-style of each patient.

Besides the loss of muscle strength, the patient will find that stamina is dramatically reduced after surgery. The feeling of fatigue can be overwhelming. In general, the patient is dominated by this feeling and finds that it takes about 3 months to resolve. We have discovered nothing to reduce this period of fatigue. Patients should be repeatedly reminded that such fatigue is normal after a total knee replacement operation and that it will soon disappear.

Emotions

It is not possible to describe a single pattern of patient emotional responses resulting from total knee arthroplasty. Some patients remain optimistic and positive throughout the entire experience, while others develop varying degrees of postoperative depression. Muller has recognized that the best results after knee surgery tend to occur when the patient approaches rehabilitation with a positive and active attitude (66). Depression can interfere with efforts to foster such a positive outlook. Understanding the anxiety, confidence, fear, hope, disappointment, and pride felt by the patient is important in assisting the patient maintain a positive attitude.

Preoperatively, many patients experience a period of anxiety and fear. It is quite natural for anyone to be anxious before having an operation, but sometimes a patient experiences additional anxiety caused by factors that can be addressed by the physician. Patients, for example, may be concerned about their families during and after their surgery; they may fear that they will wake up during the operation or that their leg will not be straight after surgery. The surgeon cannot alleviate the patient's natural anxiety related to having an operation, but by taking the time to discuss some of the patient's concerns, unnecessary anxiety can sometimes be reduced.

After the surgery, patients are often relieved and pleased that everything has gone well. This might be called the period of elation. Patients who have received intrathecal Duramorph or continuous epidural anesthesia may be particularly elated because they are not only past the surgery but they may also be free of pain. If the patient conveys a feeling of relief, it is appropriate to share the experience with them. Nevertheless, it is also important to remind the patient and the family that there is a long recovery ahead, which will be difficult at times and will require their cooperation. I tend to say, "Remember, it takes 3 months to recover from this operation."

As the patients are mobilized and as they begin the difficult task of recovering knee motion and strength, they feel the full impact of rehabilitation. The combination of postoperative fatigue, loss of independence, pain, and the realization of the length and difficulty of rehabilitation can result in depression. Patients, at this point, can get lost in the moment-to-moment fluctuations of their recovery and not be aware of their progress. Asking them to observe their improvement by remembering what they were like a week ago or 2 weeks ago is an effective motivational device. Patients often need encouragement and reassurance. It is helpful to explain that other patients experience the same problems. In elderly patients, postoperative confusion can exaggerate the depression. Psychiatric consultation can at times be advisable. However, reassuring patients that their feelings are normal and temporary is usually sufficient.

Three months after surgery, most patients feel that the period of fatigue is over. Optimism returns. They should be encouraged to get on with their lives and begin doing the activities that interest them. They should also be advised that although they have improved dramatically during the 3 months after surgery, they will continue to improve more gradually as they regain further motion and strength.

Cost

The cost of rehabilitation after total knee arthroplasty is a relatively new concern that has not been addressed in previous textbooks. One of the major factors affecting cost of patient care after surgery is the duration of hospital stay. Efforts to reduce the length of hospital stay have resulted in progressively shorter periods of rehabilitation in the hospital. In the past, reducing the intensity of physical therapy occurring at the time of hospital discharge was equated with slowing or even ultimately thwarting the patient's ability to achieve the desired result (49). It was believed that one could be more confident of the patient's achieving full knee range of motion if they were kept in the hospital until they reached 90 or 95 degrees of flexion (49). If third-party payers insisted on discharge sooner, one could expect patients to lose ground rather than make further motion progress (49). In the interest of maximizing the quality of outcome "and maintaining at least a modicum of humanity and practicality," the patient should be kept in the hospital until formal physical therapy sessions are no longer productive (49). Such an approach has resulted in excellent outcomes after total knee arthroplasty (26, 49). However, the long hospital stay results in considerable cost.

Others have had equally excellent outcomes with dramatically different rehabilitation routines. Townley, for example, has reported that with proficient surgical technique using his prosthesis, a prolonged regimen of physical therapy in the hospital is not necessary (3). Patients can be started on a program of self-motivated exercises at home 2 weeks before surgery. Postoperatively, patients can continue the same exercise program that they learned before surgery, under the guidance of a therapist. Patients can be discharged from the hospital when they are ambulating safely and have 70 degrees of knee flexion. Patients are assessed as outpatients at 6 weeks to determine whether more aggressive therapy or knee manipulation is necessary (3).

These two rehabilitation approaches are dramatically different. The former describes aggressive, in-house therapy under the watchful eyes of the surgeon and physical therapist, while the latter emphasizes confidence in the patient's ability to learn the appropriate exercises and progress independently. Problems that arise from the latter approach are addressed later on an outpatient basis. The more watchful approach costs more because of longer hospital stays and charges for repeated formal physical therapy sessions. If both rehabilitation philosophies result in the same excellent clinical outcome, then we must look closely at the less costly approach. On the other hand, we must be careful to avoid reducing the quality of outcome by drawing simplistic conclusions about these two different rehabilitation approaches. Factors that may not be obvious, such as the surgeon's patient education skills, surgical technique, and prosthetic choices may be making the less aggressive therapy approach successful. Prospective randomized studies will be critical in determining how further reductions in hospital stay and further reliance on self-motivated exercises affect clinical outcomes after total knee arthroplasty.

Other observations have suggested that outcomes after routine total knee arthroplasty may not be dramatically affected by reductions in physical therapy. In our experience, knees that are immobilized in extension because of skin necrosis or wound drainage still acquire excellent knee flexion when knee motion exercises are delayed for 4 or 6 weeks. Clinical outcomes of total hip and total knee replacement patients receiving dramatically different amounts of physical therapy do not differ (67). The opportunity to study such a situation resulted from fiscal pressures that forced a reduction in the amount and quality of physical therapy available at one institution. Despite the reduction in formal physical therapy from one group to the other, Liang et al. were unable to demonstrate any major differences in length of hospital stay, functional status at discharge, or numbers of surgical complications between the two groups (67). Observations such as these require further study. Third-party payers, however, must realize that regardless of what studies reveal for the routine cases, some patients will still require prolonged physical therapy and hospitalization after total knee arthroplasty.

Devices such as the constant passive motion machine, continuous cooling pads, and patient-controlled analgesia machines have all been introduced to advance the ease of recovery and the quality of outcome after total knee arthroplasty (8, 13, 24, 32). Some devices have been developed to reduce the cost of patient care by reducing the length of time the patient is hospitalized or by preventing further costly procedures (8, 13, 32).

Unfortunately, these devices themselves add additional cost, not only from the expense of the equipment but also the expense of personnel to set up and use the equipment properly (1). The effect on outcome and the cost for each new device introduced must be determined by careful prospective randomized studies. These studies must also be repeated whenever other features of the patient's rehabilitation change. The use of the CPM machine, for example, when compared with rehabilitation techniques avoiding early knee and patient mobilization, was a cost-effective approach (8). As non-CPM rehabilitation routines, surgical techniques, and implant designs changed, the routine use of the CPM machine was no longer cost-effective (1). Rehabilitation of our patients must be constantly monitored to assure the highest quality outcomes and the most cost-effective techniques.

Acknowledgments

The authors would like to thank Glenn Harvey PA-C for his excellent care of patients, Thomas Lorig, R.N., for accumulating and assessing data, and Rebecca Lee for her help in preparing this manuscript.

References

1. Ritter MA, Gandolf VS, Holston KS. Continuous passive motion versus physical therapy in total knee arthroplasty. Clin Orthop 1989;244:239–243.
2. Schurman DJ, Parker JN, Ornstein D. Total condylar knee replacement: a study of factors influencing range of motion as late as two years after arthroplasty. J Bone Joint Surg 1985;67-A:1006–1014.
3. Townley CO. The anatomic total knee resurfacing arthroplasty. Clin Orthop 1985;192:82–96.
4. Dorr LD, Leffers D. Rehabilitation and assessment of knee function after total knee arthroplasty. In: Ranawat CS, ed. Total condylar knee arthroplasty. New York: Springer-Verlag, 1985:105–115.
5. Warren M, Owen JW. The effect of total hip replacement on driving reactions. J Bone Joint Surg 1988:70-B:202–205.
6. Insall JN. Total knee replacement. In: Insall JN, ed. Surgery of the knee. New York: Churchill Livingstone, 1984:587–695.
7. Burstein AH. Biomechanics of the knee. In: Insall JN, ed. Surgery of the knee. New York: Churchill Livingstone, 1984:21–39.
8. Coutts RD, Toth C, Kaita JH: The role of continuous passive motion in the rehabilitation of the total knee patient. In: Hungerford DS, Krackow KA, Kenna RV, eds. Total knee arthroplasty: a comprehensive approach. Baltimore: Williams & Wilkins, 1983:126–132.
9. Woolf CJ. Recent advances in the pathophysiology of acute pain. Br J Anaesth 1989;63:139–146.
10. Owen H, White PF. Patient controlled analgesia: an overview. In: Sinatra RS, ed. Acute pain: mechanisms and management. St. Louis: Mosby Year Book, 1992:151–164.
11. Albert TJ, Cohn JC, Rothman JS, Springstead J, Rothman RH, Booth RE. Patient-controled analgesia in a postoperative total joint arthroplasty population. J Arthroplasty 1991;6(suppl):S23-S28.
12. Sechzer PN. Patient-controled analgesia (PCA): a retrospective. Anesthesiology 1990;72:735–736.
13. Angel JM, McKay WR. PCA and post surgical outcome: influence on morbidity and length of hospital stay. In: Sinatra RS, ed. Acute pain: mechanisms and management. St. Louis: Mosby Year Book, 1992:201–204.
14. Scalley RD, Berquist K, Cochran RS. Patient-controled analgesia in orthopedic procedures. Orthop Rev 1988;17(11):1106–1113.
15. Moore DC. Spinal anesthesia: bupivacaine compared with tetracaine. Anesth Analg 1980;59:743–750.
16. Yaksh TL, Rudy TY. Studies on the direct spinal action of narcotics in the production of analgesia in the rat. J Pharmacol Exp Ther 1977;202:411–428.
17. Wang JK, Nauss LA, Thomas JE. Pain relief by intrathecally applied morphine in man. Anesthesiology 1979;50:149–151.
18. Kalso E. Effects of intrathecal morphine injected with bupivacaine on pain after orthopaedic surgery. Br J Anaesth 1983;415–422.
19. Gwirtz KH. Single-dose intrathecal opioid in the management of acute postoperative pain. In: Sinatra RS, ed. Acute pain: mechanisms and management. St. Louis: Mosby Year Book, 1992:253–268.
20. Brown CR, Moodie JE, Wild VM, Bynum LJ. Comparison of intravenous ketorolac tromethamine and morphine sulfate with treatment of postoperative pain. Pharmacotherapy Suppl 1990;10(6):116S-121S.
21. Brown CR, Mazzulla JP, Mok MS, Nussdorf RT, Rubin PD, Schwesinger WH. Comparison of repeat doses of intramuscular ketorolac tromethamine and morphine sulfate for analgesia after major surgery. Pharmacotherapy 1990;10(6):45S-50S.
22. Mahoney OM, Noble PC, Davidson J, Tullos HS. The effect of continuous epidural analgesia on postoperative pain, rehabilitation, and duration of hospitalization in total knee arthroplasty. Clin Orthop 1990;260:30–37.
23. Walker RH, Morris BA, Angulo DL, Schneider J, Colwell CW. Postoperative use of continuous passive motion, transcutaneous electrical nerve stimulation, and continuous cooling pad following total knee arthroplasty. J Arthroplasty 1991;6,2:151–156.
24. Cohn BT, Drageger RI, Jackson DW. The effect of cold therapy in the postoperative management of Pain in patients undergoing anterior cruciate ligament reconstruction. Am J Sports Med 1989;17:344–349.
25. Brodell JD, Axon DL, Evarts CM. The Robert Jones dressing. J Bone Joint Surg 1986;68B:776–779.
26. Hungerford DS, Krackow KA. Total joint arthroplasty of the knee. Clin Orthop 1985;192:23–33.
27. Chandler HP: Postoperative management and follow-up evaluation. In: Hungerford DS, Krackow KA, Kenna RV, eds. Total knee arthroplasty: a comprehensive approach. Baltimore: Williams & Wilkins, 1983:110–125.
28. Lewis CE Jr, Antoine J, Mueller C, Talbot WA, Swaroop R, Edwards WS. Elastic compression in the prevention of venous stasis: a critical reevaluation. Am J Surg 1976;132:739–743.
29. Sigel B, Edelstein AL, Savitch L, Hasty JH, Felix WR. Type of compression for reducing venous stasis: a study of lower extremities during inactive recumbency. Arch Surg 1975;110:171–175.
30. Nicolaides AN, Fernandes e Fernandes J, Pollock AV. Intermittent sequential pneumatic compression of the legs in the prevention of venous stasis and postoperative deep venous thrombosis. Surgery 1980;87:69–76.
31. Hecht PJ, Bachmann S, Booth RE Jr, Rothman RH. Effects of thermal therapy on rehabilitation after total knee arthroplasty: a prospective randomized study. Clin Orthop 1983;178:199–201.
32. McInnes J, Larson MG, Daltroy LH, Brown T, Fossel AH, et al. A controlled evaluation of continuous passive motion in patients undergoing total knee arthroplasty. JAMA 1992;268(11):1423–1426.
33. Rutherford RB. The role of thrombectomy in the management of iliofemoral venous thrombosis. In: Rutherford RB, ed. Vascular surgery. Philadelphia: WB Saunders, 1989:1569–1574.
34. Katz MM, Hungerford DS. Reflex sympathetic dystrophy affecting the knee. J Bone Joint Surg 1987;69-B:797–803.
35. Cooper DE, DeLee JC, Ramamurthy S. Reflex sympathetic dystrophy of the knee: treatment using continuous epidural anesthesia. J Bone Joint Surg 1989;71-A:365–369.
36. Schutzer SF, Gossling HR. Current concepts review: the treatment of reflex sympathetic dystrophy syndrome. J Bone Joint Surg 1984;66-A:625–629.
37. Ogilvie-Harris DJ, Roscoe M. Reflex sympathetic dystrophy of the knee. J Bone Joint Surg 1987;69-B:804–806.
38. Hofmann AA, Plaster RL, Murdock LE. Subvastus (southern) approach for primary total knee arthroplasty. Clin Orthop 1991;269:70–77.
39. Peters PC Jr, Knezevich S, Engh GA, Dwyer KA, Preidis FE. Comparison of the subvastus quadriceps-sparing and standard anterior quadriceps-splitting approaches in total and unicompartmental knee arthroplasty. AAOS meeting, Washington, D.C., 1992:44.
40. Otis JC. Department of Biomechanics, The Hospital for Special Surgery, New York, New York, Nov 3, 1992. Personal communication.
41. Daluga D, Lombardi AV, Mallory TH, Vaughn BK. Knee manipulation following total knee arthroplasty: analysis of prognostic variables. J Arthroplasty 1991;6,2:119–128.
42. Fox JL, Poss R. The role of manipulation following total knee replacement. J Bone Joint Surg 1981;63-A:357–362.
43. Ritter MA, Stringer EA. Predictive range of motion after total knee replacement. Clin Orthop 1979;143:115–119.
44. Insall JN, Scott WN, Ranawatt CS. The total condylar knee prosthesis: a report of two hundred and twenty cases. J Bone Joint Surg 1979;61-A:173–180.
45. Insall JN, Lachiewicz PF, Burstein AH. The posterior stabilized condylar prosthesis: a modification of the total condylar design. J Bone Joint Surg 1982;64-A:1317–1323.
46. Striplin DB, Robinson RP. Posterior dislocation of the Insall Burstein II

posterior stabilized total knee prosthesis. Am J Knee Surg 1992; 5, 2:79–83.

47. Frankel VM, Burstein AH, Brooks DB. Biomechanics of internal derangement of the knee: pathomechanics as determined by analysis of the instant center of motion. J Bone Joint Surg 1971;53-A:945–962.

48. Tanzier M, Miller J. The natural history of flexion contracture in total knee arthroplasty: a prospective study. Clin Orthop 1989;248:130–134.

49. Krackow KA. Postoperative period. In: Krackow KA. The technique of total knee arthroplasty. St. Louis: C. V. Mosby Company, 1990:385–424.

50. Freeman MAR, Samuelson KM, Bertin KC. Freeman-Samuelson total arthroplasty of the knee. Clin Orthop 1985;192:46–58.

51. Maloney WJ, Schurman DJ, Hangen D, Goodman SB, Edworthy S, Bloch DA. The influence of continuous passive motion on outcome in total knee arthroplasty. Clin Orthop 1990;256:162–168.

52. Salter RB, Simmonds DF, Malcolm BW, Rumble EJ, Macmichael D, Clements ND. The biological effect of continuous passive motion on the healing of full-thickness defects in articular cartilage. J Bone Joint Surg 1980;62-A:1332–1251.

53. Salter RB, Harris D. The healing of intraarticular fractures with continuous passive motion. AAOS Lecture Series 1979;28:102.

54. Salter RB, Bell RS, Keeley FW. The protective effects of continuous passive motion on living articular cartilage in acute septic arthritis: an experimental investigation in the rabbit. Clin Orthop 1981; 159:223–247.

55. Salter RS, Bell RS. The effect of continuous passive motion on the healing of partial thickness lacerations of the patellar tendon of the rabbit. Presented at the 27th Annual ORS, Las Vegas, Nev., Feb 1981:82.

56. Romness DW, Rand JA. The role of continuous passive motion following total knee arthroplasty. Clin Orthop 1988;226:34–37.

57. Goll SR, Lotke PA, Ecker ML. Failure of continuous passive motion as prophylaxis against deep venous thrombosis after total knee arthroplasty. In: Ranawat CS, ed. Total condylar knee arthroplasty. New York: Springer-Verlag, 1985:299–305.

58. Vince KG, Kelly MA, Beck J, Insall JN. Continuous passive motion after total knee arthroplasty. J Arthroplasty 1987;2,4:281–284.

59. Johnson DP. The effect of continuous passive motion on wound-healing and joint mobility after knee arthroplasty. J Bone Joint Surg 1990;72-A:421–426.

60. Coonse K, Adams JD. A new operative approach to the knee joint. Surg Gynecol Obstet 1943;77:344–347.

61. Masini MA, Stulberg SD. A new surgical technique for tibial tubercle transfer in total knee arthroplasty. J Arthroplasty 1992;7(1):81–86.

62. Insall JN. Miscellaneous items: arthrodesis, the stiff knee, synovectomy, and popliteal cyst. In: Insall JN, ed. Surgery of the knee. New York: Churchill Livingstone, 1984:729–741.

63. Figgie HE III, Goldberg VM, Heiple KG, Heiple KG, Moller HS, Gordon NH. The influencew of tibial-patellofemoral location on function of the knee in patients with the posterior stabilized condylar knee prosthesis. J Bone Joint Surg 1986;68-A:1035–1040.

64. Coutts RD, Rosenstein A, Stewart WT, Martin TP, Akeson WH. The effect of muscle stimulation in the rehabilitation of patients following total knee replacement. In: Ranawat CS. ed. Total-condylar knee arthroplasty: technique, results, and complications. New York: Springer-Verlag, 1985:306–316.

65. Smillie S. Injuries of the knee joint. Edinburgh: E & S Livingstone, 1962.

66. Muller W. Postoperative rehabilitation. In: Muller W. The knee: form, function, and ligament reconstruction. Berlin: Springer-Verlag, 1983:266–307.

67. Liang MH, Cullen KE, Larson MG, Schwartz JA, Robb-Nicholson, Fossel AH, Roberge N, Poss R. Effects of reducing physical therapy services on outcomes in total joint arthroplasty. Med Care 1987;25(4):276–285.

SECTION

XIV

Patellofemoral Complications in Disorders of Articular Cartilage

77

Biomechanics of the Patellofemoral Articulation Relevant to Total Knee Replacement

Abdul M. Ahmed

Introduction

Since the introduction of total knee replacement (TKR) surgery in the late 1960s, the design of the replacement components has evolved considerably. Among the many factors stimulating this process are two complex interacting demands: replication of motion and stability and increased durability of the components and their fixation. Until recently, attention has been focused on tibial component design and those features of the femoral component that pertain to the tibiofemoral articulation.

Initial TKR designs did not provide for patellar resurfacing. The high incidence of patellofemoral symptoms, however, motivated introduction of all-polyethylene patellar components in the early 1970s, particularly for patients with rheumatoid arthritis. Since then, patellar resurfacing has become increasingly common. Although complications related to the early designs of patellar components were often reported (1, 2), they were overshadowed by the inadequacies of fixation of the tibial component and of the design of the tibiofemoral articulation. In the early 1980s, a new generation of TKR components was introduced with near-anatomic shapes for the tibial and femoral articulating surfaces, to allow greater motion, and with metal backing for the tibial and patellar components, to allow for more even stress distribution at the fixation interfaces. The metal surfaces later provided the potential for porous ingrowth fixation. With these new designs, patellar complications became more frequent. The complications involved instability and maltracking of the patella, mechanical failure of the prosthesis, excessive wear, patellar fracture, failure of fixation, and soft-tissue impingement (3–18). In the early 1990s, the second most frequent reason for the failure of knee arthroplasty, after deep sepsis, was considered to be related to the patellofemoral articulation (19).

It is then not surprising that many surgeons advocate the abandonment of current designs of the patellar com-

ponent pending further research (4, 5, 14), while others suggest avoidance of the routine use of the patellar prosthesis altogether (20). As a consequence, reports are increasing from surgeons electing to leave the patella unresurfaced (21–23). While this might be the right option for some patients regardless of the performance of the patellar component, many patellas do require resurfacing. From this perspective, improvements are necessary in the design of the patellofemoral components when the patella needs to be resurfaced and in the design of the trochlear groove of the femoral component for cases when the patella is best left unresurfaced. It is expected that, similar to the evolution of the design of the tibiofemoral components, rigorous biomechanical criteria will be used for the design of the next generation of patellofemoral components. In this light, it would be appropriate to review the biomechanics of the patellofemoral articulation in order to identify the particular features of this articulation that are likely to be relevant in the formulation of the necessary design criteria for the *articular surfaces* of the components. Such a review is the objective of this chapter.

First, the general biomechanical functions and the gross biomechanical features of the patellofemoral articulation are briefly summarized. This is followed by a more detailed review of three aspects of the biomechanics of the articulation:

1. The relationship between the forces acting on the patella
2. The characteristics of the patellofemoral contact
3. The patellar tracking pattern

The chapter ends with an overview of the above three aspects of the patellofemoral biomechanics and their implications for the improvement of the components.

This chapter is based primarily on results from our laboratory, where the biomechanics of the patellofemoral articulation are investigated in vitro using different combinations of three knee simulations. However, some features of the basic simulations are different among the various experiments. To avoid unnecessary duplication within the chapter text, the features of the simulations are summarized in Appendix I in a unified manner.

Biomechanical Function

The patella serves three biomechanical functions:

1. It increases the moment-arm of the extensor mechanism of the knee and thus reduces the quadriceps tension necessary to extend the knee against a given flexion moment. This function is illustrated by a simplified case of the forces acting on the lower leg corresponding to a phase of a "static" functional activity as shown in Figure 77.1, *A*. The foot-floor reaction force, *F*, assumed to be vertical (i.e., the frictional force component of the reaction is assumed to be negligible), tends to flex the knee with a flexion moment equal to the product of $|F|$ (i.e., the magnitude of *F*) and the moment-arm *a*. If there are no other flexion moments present (such as those caused by the flexor muscles), then this moment needs to be balanced by an extensor moment caused by the patellar tendon and equal to the product of the magnitude of the tension in the tendon, $|T_P|$, and its moment-arm *b*, such that

$$|T_P| \cdot b = |F| \cdot a \qquad \text{(Eq. 77.1)}$$

In the absence of the patella, when the quadriceps tendon slides directly on the femoral trochlear surface, the extensor moment-arm *b* would be shorter, shown as *b'* in Figure 77.1, *B*. This decrease in the

length of *b* requires a proportionate increase in $|T_P|$ to balance the same flexion moment ($|F| \cdot a$). From an analysis of the geometry of the patellofemoral articulation, it is estimated that, in general, the presence of the patella reduces the patellar tendon tension requirement (and, hence, approximately, the quadriceps tension requirement) by 20% to 30%.

2. The patella facilitates realignment of the diversely oriented tension vectors of the individual muscle components of the quadriceps groups to an appropriate "central" vector to transmit the tension to the patellar tendon. It has been suggested that this function of the patella decreases the possibility of dislocation of the extensor mechanism (24).

3. The patella converts what would have otherwise been contact between the quadriceps tendon and the articular cartilage of the trochlear surface of the femur to contact between the articular cartilage of the retropatellar surface and the articular cartilage of the trochlear surface. The latter type of contact allows relatively friction-free sliding and also avoids compressive stresses on the tendon.

Biomechanical Features

The patellofemoral articulation is characterized by three gross biomechanical features. Understanding these features is important for the interpretation of the more detailed characteristics of the articulation and is discussed below.

Magnitude of forces. The magnitude of the forces acting on the patella will, of course, depend on the type of activity and the knee flexion angle. Nevertheless, it is worth noting that even during certain routine activities, the magnitudes can be relatively large. This feature is illustrated by referring to the simplified case of the forces acting on the lower leg as shown in Figure 77.1, *A* and by rewriting Equation 77.1 in the following form:

$$|T_P| = (a / b) \cdot |F| \qquad \text{(Eq. 77.2)}$$

In functional activities involving deep flexion, the ratio of the moment-arms (*a* / *b*) can be greater than 3 and the foot-floor reaction ($|F|$) greater than 1 body weight. In such cases, the patellar tendon tension ($|T_P|$) can exceed 3 times body weight. Although the exact relation between $|T_P|$ and the magnitudes of the other two forces acting on the patella (i.e., the patellofemoral joint reaction and the quadriceps tension) is the subject of a subsequent section, nevertheless, it will suffice to mention here that the magnitudes of all three forces are of the same order. It is worth noting that more detailed analyses of the forces acting on the lower leg indicate that the patellofemoral joint reaction can be greater than 3 times body weight while rising from a chair (25) and stair walking (26, 27), and greater than 5 times body weight while standing on the balls of the feet with the knee flexed at 80° (28).

Direction of forces. Although the directions of the muscular and tendon forces acting on the patella are such that their resultant vector is oriented mainly to-

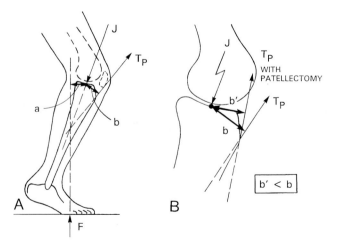

Figure 77.1. A, Simplified representation of the forces acting on the lower leg (tibia-foot unit). *F*, foot-floor reaction; *J*, tibiofemoral joint reaction; *T*$_P$, patellar tendon tension; *a*, moment-arm of *F*; *b*, moment-arm of *T*$_P$. Note that the three forces, *F*, *J* and *T*$_P$ are concurrent. **B,** Schematic drawing illustrating the decrease in the length of the moment-arm *b*, when the quadriceps tendon slides directly on the trochlear surface (as would be the case after patellectomy).

wards the posterior direction, there is, nevertheless, a significant component pointing toward the lateral direction. As shown in Figure 77.2, the frontal plane projections of the quadriceps tension vector (T_Q) are angulated with respect to the patellar tendon tension vector (T_P) by the Q angle. The vector sum of the two forces, therefore, has a component directed towards the lateral side (the valgus component) that tends to subluxate the patella. This effect is pronounced near knee extension where the Q angle is maximum, and it is counterbalanced partly by the medial retinaculum and partly by the patellofemoral contact force. Their respective contributions depends on the flexion angle. Although precise measurements of Q angle as a function of knee flexion are not available, the valgus component can be estimated at approximately 21%–26% of T_P (or T_Q) if the Q angle is assumed to be in the range 12° to 15°. The magnitude of the force, however, will be affected by a variation of the Q angle that results from passive axial rotation of the tibia, increasing with external rotation and decreasing with internal rotation.

Relative motion. The relative motion at the patellofemoral articulation occurs entirely through sliding action. This is unlike, say, the case in the tibiofemoral articulation where a significant fraction of the relative motion is due to rolling. With increasing flexion and while the patella slides distally and posteriorly on the trochlear surface, the contact area on the retropatellar surface gradually shifts proximally from the lower pole to the upper border of the surface. In the knee flexion range of 0° to 120° (for an average sized specimen), the net patellar motion is around 7 to 8 cm. During this motion, the contact area slides by about 4.5 to 5.5 cm on the trochlear surface and 2 to 2.5 cm on the retropatellar surface.

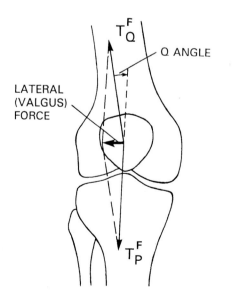

Figure 77.2. Schematic drawing illustrating the lateral (valgus) force caused by the Q angle. $T_Q{}^F$ and $T_P{}^F$ are the frontal-plane projections of the T_Q and T_P vectors and the lateral force is the vector sum of $T_Q{}^F$ and $T_P{}^F$.

Forces Acting on the Patella

The general objective of this section is to identify the particular geometric features of the patellofemoral articulation that govern the relationship between the patellar tendon tension (T_P) and the other forces acting on the patella. It might be assumed that the magnitude of T_P is known a priori, obtained by an analysis of the forces acting on the lower leg as illustrated by the simplified example of the previous section or as derived by more detailed analysis by previous authors (25–28). Once the particular features of the articulation relating the forces are established, it would be possible to evaluate how the design of the patellofemoral components might influence the characteristics of the patellofemoral joint reaction and the quadriceps force.

Force Analysis

For the purpose of the present analysis, it will be adequate to consider a simplified two-dimensional (i.e., planar) representation of the joint as shown in Figure 77.3. In this representation, the tensions in each part of the quadriceps muscle group and the contact forces between the facets of the patella and the femur are represented by their respective resultant forces, the quadriceps tension (T_Q) and the patellofemoral joint reaction (*PFJR*). These two forces, along with the tension in the ligamentum patellae (T_P) are the three forces that act on the patella. As these three forces are not parallel (for equilibrium), they must be concurrent and must act in one plane. However, the location of that plane varies with the knee flexion angle because of the dependence of the directions of the T_P and T_Q vectors on the flexion angle. Even at a given flexion angle, the location of that plane relative to the anatomic planes is difficult to define because none of the vectors are parallel to any of the anatomic planes. While, for the *flexed* knee, the plane is roughly parallel to the sagittal plane (approximately as shown in Fig. 77.3) near *extension*, it rotates about a vertical axis to be angulated closer to the frontal plane, (approximately as shown in Fig. 77.2). For the purpose of our analysis, it would be adequate to assume that this plane is the general plane of motion of the patella relative to the femur.

Early methods to relate the magnitudes of the three forces assumed that the patella acted as a section of a "frictionless pulley" (24, 29–34). In this assumption (Figure 77.3, *A*), the patella is considered to "rotate" relative to the trochlear surface about a point coinciding with the approximate center of the trochlear arc. Thus, regardless of the flexion angle, the magnitudes of T_Q and T_P will be identical and the line of action of the *PFJR* will be the bisector of the angle between the lines of action of T_Q and T_P. Using the elementary law of sines, the equations relating the magnitudes of the forces are:

$$|T_Q|/|T_P| = 1 \qquad \text{(Eq. 77.3)}$$

$$|PFJR|/|T_P| = [\sin(180° - 2\beta)]/[\sin\beta] \quad \text{(Eq. 77.4)}$$

where 2β is the angle between the lines of action of T_Q and T_P and is termed the patellar mechanism angle.

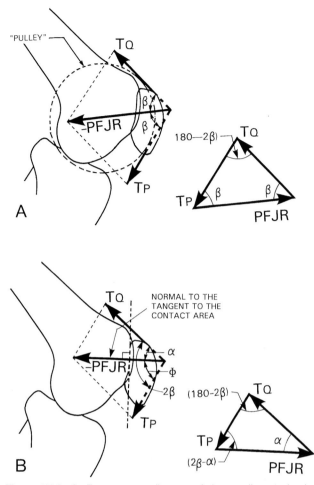

Figure 77.3. A, Force vector diagram of the patellar mechanism based on the "frictionless pulley" assumption. T_Q, quadriceps tension (resultant); T_P, patellar tendon tension; *PFJR*, patellofemoral joint reaction (resultant); β, half of patellar mechanism angle. **B,** Force vector diagram of the patellar mechanism based on the assumption that patellofemoral contact is frictionless, i.e., *PFJR* is normal to the tangent to the contact area, where α is the angle between T_Q and *PFJR*.

From the above two equations, it is noted that, if the patella is assumed to act as a "frictionless pulley," then the magnitudes of the three forces are related by only *one* geometrical parameter of the patellofemoral articulation, that is the patellar mechanism angle 2β. In accordance with Equation 77.4 for a given $|T_P|$, $|PFJR|$ will decrease with an increase in the angle 2β, i.e., with greater knee extension.

Several investigators have determined, however, that the "frictionless pulley" representation fails to reflect the basic mechanics of the patellofemoral articulation (34–39). A principle of contact mechanics dictates that, in the absence of friction, the lines of action of *PFJR* must be normal to the common tangent to the contacting surfaces at the point (or line) of contact. In this case, if the profile of the trochlear surface in the plane of patellar motion is reasonably close to a circular arc, only then would the "frictionless pulley" representation be appropriate. Otherwise, the relationship between the

magnitudes of the three forces must take into account the condition that the line of action of *PFJR* is constrained to be normal to the common tangent. Referring to Figure 77.3, *B* and again using the law of sines, the relations between the force magnitudes are rederived as:

$$|T_Q|/|T_P| = [\sin(2\beta - \alpha)]/(\sin \alpha) \quad \text{(Eq. 77.5)}$$

$$|PFJR|/|T_P| = [\sin(180 - 2\beta)]/(\sin \alpha) \quad \text{(Eq. 77.6)}$$

where 2β remains as the patellar mechanism angle and α, the new angle, is the angle between the lines of action of T_Q and *PFJR*. (The equations could have been equally derived using the angle between the lines of action of T_P and *PFJR*, i.e., the angle β = 2β − α).

From the above two relations, it is noted that the magnitudes of the three forces are now related by *two* geometrical parameters of the patellofemoral articulation: the patellar mechanism angle 2β, and the angle between the lines of action of *PFJR* (constrained to be normal to the common tangent) and T_Q, i.e., α. The latter angle is a property of the geometry of the motion-plane profile of the trochlear surface. It is noted that, if this profile were a circular arc, then α (or φ) would have been equal to β and Equations 77. 5 and 77.6 would have reduced to Equations 77.3 and 77.4, respectively. According to Equation 77.6, for a given $|T_P|$ and 2β, the $|PFJR|$ will increase with an increase in the angle α, and for a given $|T_P|$ and α, the $|PFJR|$ will decrease with an increase in the angle 2β.

Experimental Validation

The foregoing analysis of the patellar force system has been investigated in detail (41), and the salient findings are summarized briefly. Figure 77.4 shows the results of measurement of the angles β and α as a function of knee flexion angle η. The measurements were made from lateral radiographs of 42 fresh-frozen specimens taken while the specimens were subjected to a $|T_Q|$ of 50 N. The data indicate that apart from a small range of flexion angle around 45°, at other flexion angles, the angle α departs significantly from β. When these values of the two angles are used to predict the ratio ($|T_Q|$ / $|T_P|$), using Equations 77.3 and 77.5, the results obtained are shown in Figure 77.5, *A* and are compared to measurements. These measurements were made on 10 fresh-frozen specimens subjected to two loading conditions: the first simulating the static lifting maneuver (Simulation 1, Appendix I), and the other simulating the "leg-raising" exercise (Simulation 2, Appendix I). In both cases, $|T_P|$ was measured directly using a buckle transducer. The results of Figure 77.5, *A* indicate that the variation of the ratio ($|T_Q|/|T_P|$) with flexion angle is complex, first decreasing with flexion (up to η ~30°), then increasing (up to η ~ 90°), and finally decreasing again with further flexion. Equation 77.5 appears to predict not only the characteristic variation of the ratio with knee flexion, but also its magnitude with reasonable accuracy. When it is recognized that Equation 77.3 predicts a ratio of 1 at all flexion angles, it becomes evi-

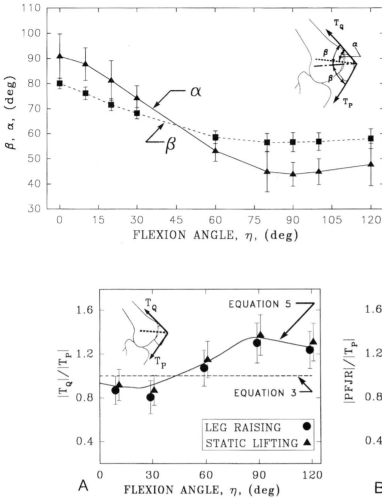

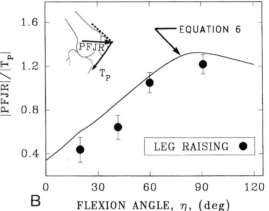

Figure 77.4. Effect of knee flexion angle η on the geometric parameters, β and α, which govern the relationship between the patellar forces (Fig. 77.3B). The vertical bars represent ±1 standard deviation of the measurements. (Adapted with permission from Ahmed AM, Burke DL, Hyder A. Force analysis of the patellar mechanism. J Orthop Res 1987;5:69–85.)

Figure 77.5. A, Comparison of the predicted (Equations 77.3 and 5) and the measured ratios of the magnitudes of the quadriceps tension ($|T_Q|$) and the patellar tendon tension ($|T_P|$). **B,** Comparison of the predicted (Equation 77.6) and the measured ratios of the magnitudes of the patellofemoral joint reaction ($|PFJR|$) and the patellar tendon tension ($|T_P|$). The vertical bars represent ±1 standard deviation of the measurements. (Adapted with permission from Ahmed AM, Burke DL, Hyder A. Force analysis of the patellar mechanism. J Orthop Res 1987;5:69–85.)

dent that the pulley representation of the patella is an oversimplification of the actual mechanics of the patellofemoral articulation.

Figure 77.5, B compares the variation of the ratio ($|PFJR|/|TP|$) with knee flexion angle η, predicted using Equation 77.6, with those interpreted from the retropatellar pressure distribution measurements reported in an earlier study (35). In that study, measurements were made in 24 fresh-frozen specimens subjected to a loading condition simulating the "leg-raising" exercise (Simulation 2, Appendix I), and the pressure distribution was measured using a custom-made plastic microindentation transducer. The results of Figure 77.5B indicate that, although differences exist between the measured and the predicted values of the ratio, nevertheless, the measured values are in general agreement with the trend predicted by the analysis, assuming the line of action of *PFJR* to be constrained to be normal to the contact surface. Equation 77.6 predicts that for a

given value of $|T_P|$, $|PFJR|$ will increase with flexion angle up to around η = 60°, where the two magnitudes become nearly identical and remain so up to around η = 100°. For knee flexion beyond this angle, prediction will be only approximate because of the onset of direct contact between the quadriceps tendon and the trochlear surface. Although the angles β and α (Fig. 77.4) used in Equation 77.6 were measured by taking into account the effect of the tendofemoral contact on the line of action of T_Q, nevertheless, Equation 77.6 itself is derived by excluding the possibility of force transmission across this contact. Therefore, the equation will overestimate $|PFJR|$ at flexion angles greater than 100°.

Finally, the results of a recent study (42) involving direct measurement of $|PFJR|$ in *prosthetic* joints under loading conditions simulating level walking (Simulation 3, Appendix I) are shown in Figure 77.6. The measurements were made in 7 fresh-frozen specimens using a 5-mm thick custom-made force-plate transducer im-

Figure 77.6. Comparison of the predicted (intact articulation) and measured (prosthetic articulation) magnitudes of the patellofemoral joint reaction ($|PFJR|$) as a function of percent gait cycle corresponding to level walking. The prediction is based on Equation 77.6 and the data of Figure 77.4.

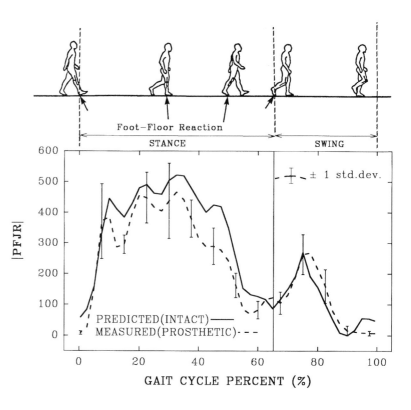

planted at the interface of the patellar prosthesis and the patellar bone. The knee prosthesis used was the Miller-Galante II (Zimmer, Warsaw, IN). The design of this prosthesis and its placement were such that the moment-arm b of the patellar tendon tension T_P was identical to that in the intact joint in the flexion range 30° to 80°. Outside this range, the moment-arm was increased, but by less than 10%. In Figure 77.6, the measured $|PFJR|$ is compared to that predicted for the *intact* joint using Equation 77.6 and the values of β and α as shown in Figure 77.4. (In the prediction, $|T_P|$ was first calculated from the flexing/extending moment component of the foot-floor reaction, inertial and gravitational forces, applied in the loading simulation.) Although exact agreement between the predicted and the measured $|PFJR|$ cannot be expected because of the differences between the two cases in the location of the patellofemoral contact areas and the contact surface profiles (both affecting the angle α), nevertheless, the analysis appears to predict, with reasonable accuracy, the complex variation of $|PFJR|$, as it corresponds to level walking.

Design Implications

Having identified the features of the patellofemoral articulation that govern the forces acting on the patella, it is possible to discuss how component design might affect the magnitude of the patellofemoral joint reaction force. In general, the design might affect two gross features. The first is the location of the patella relative to the femur in the anterior-posterior direction, say, by the choice of the thicknesses of the patellar component and the anterior flange of the femoral component, or by the

choice of the placement of the femoral component relative to the femoral axis. The second is the geometry of the motion-plane profile of the trochlear surface as designed to conform with the anatomic or domed shapes of the design of the patellar surface. The first effect will influence the patellofemoral joint reaction in two ways: by altering the moment-arm b of the patellar tendon tension T_P and, by altering the patellar mechanism angle 2β. If, for example, the patella is displaced anteriorly from its normal anatomic position, the length of the moment-arm b will be increased, so that to balance the same flexion moment, the $|T_P|$ (and hence $|T_Q|$) required will be proportionately decreased (Equation 77.1). At the same time, however, the angle 2β will be decreased, which means that for a given $|T_P|$, $|PFJR|$ will be increased (Equation 77.6). The exact magnitudes of these two opposing influences will depend on the knee flexion angle. For example, at a flexion angle of 60°, it can be estimated that an anterior displacement of the patella by 5 mm from its normal position would increase the moment-arm b by around 10% and decrease the angle 2β by 3%. The net effect would be a reduction of $|PFJR|$ by 8% for an identical flexion moment.

The second effect involving the geometry of the motion-plane profile of the trochlear surface will influence the patellofemoral joint reaction by altering the angle α. If for example, the design of the femoral component is such that the motion-plane profile is a circular arc representing the average size and relative location of the trochlear profile, then α will be decreased in the knee flexion range 0° to around 45° but increased for flexion angles beyond this range. Consequently, for a given $|T_P|$, $|PFJR|$ will be decreased in the low flexion and increased in the high flexion range. It can be estimated that, although the decrease would be marginal (<3%), the increase could be as high as 10 to 15% at a flexion angle of 90°.

Contact Characteristics

This section reviews the features of patellofemoral contact pertinent to knee arthroplasty. When the patella is resurfaced, then the one relevant feature is the *location* of the contact area relative to the contacting surfaces. Any alteration to this location, either by the design of the patellar component, or by placement of the component relative to the patella, will affect the line of action of *PFJR* and hence the angle α (Fig. 77.3, *B*). Consequently, in accord with Equations 77.5 and 77.6, for a given $|T_P|$, both $|T_Q|$ and $|PFJR|$ will differ from their normal magnitudes. On the other hand, if the patella is left unresurfaced, a practice that is becoming increasingly common as noted earlier, then a knowledge also of the *magnitude* of the contact area, indicative of the average contact pressure, and of the contact *pressure distribution* on the retropatellar surface becomes equally important. This is because the geometry of the patellar articulation on the femoral component should be such that contact between this surface and the retropatellar cartilage does not generate pressures that are detrimental to cartilage.

Location of Contact

The features of the patellofemoral contact area have been investigated by many authors (24, 26, 29, 30, 43–47). In terms of the location of this area at various knee flexion angles, there is general agreement among the available results (24, 26, 35, 43). This is because, owing to the stiffness of the patellar tendon, the location of the patella on the femoral trochlear surface is relatively insensitive to the forces acting on the patella and, in general, on the knee joint. Typical results obtained when an unconstrained fresh-frozen knee specimen is subjected to loads simulating the static lifting maneuver (Simulation 1, Appendix I) are shown in Figure 77.7. At full extension, the location of the patella is such that its lower pole is either above the osteochondral ridge or makes only marginal contact with the ridge. At around 15° of flexion, the lower pole of the patella first makes firm contact with the trochlear surface. With increasing flexion, the contact area appears as a well-defined transverse band extending to both sides of the ridge separating the medial and lateral facets of the retropatellar surface. Up to a flexion angle of around 100°, the contact band, while shifting progressively distally on the trochlear surface, shifts towards the superior border of the patella on the retropatellar surface. Beyond this flexion angle, the patella enters the intercondylar notch area of the femur with a gradual decrease in contact in the central area of the retropatellar surface and a corresponding increase in the areas in apposition to the inner flanks of the condyles. At around 130° of flexion, the center of the retropatellar surface loses contact, with contact occurring only at two iso-

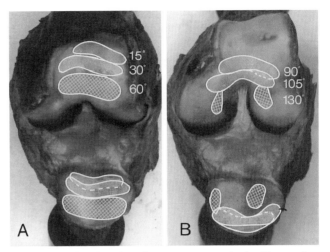

Figure 77.7. The location of contact area on the trochlear surface and the retropatellar surface of various knee flexion angles. Note that the specimen is from a left limb. **A,** flexion angles 15°, 30°, 60°. **B,** flexion angles 90°, 105°, 130°.

lated areas of the medial and lateral edges of the surface. Although, the above describes the general pattern of variation in the location of the contact area with knee flexion angle, it must be understood that considerable differences exist between specimens. For example, in specimens with high-riding patella, the sequence of variation in the location of the contact area, will occur at correspondingly lower knee flexion angles, while the opposite will be true for specimens with low-riding patella.

Contact Area

Unlike the location of the contact area, the magnitude of the contact area is very sensitive to the characteristics of the forces acting on the patella, particularly to $|PFJR|$ and to the line of action of T_P, the latter influencing the flexion of the patella at high knee flexion angles. Moreover, it is now known that the accuracy of measurement is particularly susceptible to the technique employed (48). Therefore, it is understandable that considerable difference exists among the results of different investigators (24, 26, 35, 43, 46). Nevertheless, the general trends can be illustrated adequately using the results of two studies that employ different patellofemoral loading conditions and different measurement techniques (Fig. 77.8). In the first study (35), the simulated loading condition corresponded to the "leg-raising" exercise (Simulation 2, Appendix I) and measurements were made in 24 fresh-frozen specimens using the plastic microindentation transducer. In the second study (23), the loading condition simulated was the static lifting maneuver (Simulation 1, Appendix I), and measurements were made in 6 fresh-frozen specimens using the commercially available Fuji Prescale pressure sensitive film. The results of both sets of measurement (Fig. 77.8) show that with increasing flexion, the contact area gradually increases up to $\eta = 60°$, where it occupies between 30%–40% of the total retropatellar surface

Figure 77.8. The average ratio of contact area to the retropatellar surface area as a function of knee flexion angle as measured under two different knee loading conditions. The vertical bars represent ±1 standard deviation of the measurements.

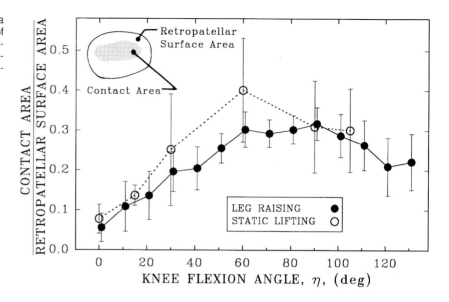

area (12–13 cm^2). With a further increase in flexion, the results of the first study (leg raising simulation) show the area to remain nearly constant up to $\eta = 90°$ and then to decrease up to $\eta = 120°$. In contrast, the results of the second study (static lifting simulation) indicate a significant decrease in contact area with increasing flexion directly from $\eta = 60°$ onward. The differences between the two sets of results are fairly typical of the differences among the results of different investigators (24, 26, 35, 43, 46).

Average Contact Stress

The average contact stress or pressure can now be easily determined by dividing the applied contact force ($|PFJR|$) with the measured contact area. This parameter is a fair global indicator of the stress-state of the contacting cartilages. Since the contact area does not increase in direct proportion to the contact force, the average contact stress itself is a function of the contact force. This function, although over a limited range of contact force, has been measured in an earlier study (35). In Figure 77.9, variations of the average contact stress with the contact force for the patellofemoral articulation are compared to those for the tibiofemoral articulation for representative knee flexion angles. For the tibiofemoral articulation, the contact force is the axial component of the tibiofemoral joint reaction J of Figure 77.1, *A*. In Figure 77.9, regions corresponding to the maximum contact force and the flexion angle associated with a number of dynamic functional activities have been indicated as shaded areas. Predictions of Matthews, et al. (26) for the patellofemoral articulation and of Morrison (31, 32) for the tibiofemoral articulation were used to identify these areas. The results indicate that for identical walking or climbing activity, the maximum average contact stress on the patellofemoral articulation is always higher than in the tibiofemoral articulation. The difference is relatively less (< 40%) during level walking and walking up-ramp. During walking down-ramp and climbing upstairs or downstairs, how-

ever, the patellofemoral articulation can be expected to experience contact stresses that are more than twice those in the tibiofemoral articulation.

Contact Pressure Distribution

The contact pressure distribution, even more than the magnitude of the contact area, is sensitive to the characteristics of the forces acting on the patella (35). In addition, the pattern of pressure distribution varies considerably among specimens (35) and is also affected by the quality of the contacting cartilages (45). As such, selection of a general pattern for the purpose of illustration is difficult. Nevertheless, the characteristics of the contact pressure distribution might be discerned by comparing the distribution in the intact articulation with an unresurfaced patella against the femoral component of different knee replacement designs. The results of an on-going study (23) that has been undertaken to investigate the causes of residual anterior knee pain in some patients after TKR without patellar resurfacing are reviewed below.

In this study, pressure distribution is measured using the Fuji Prescale pressure sensitive film, while fresh-frozen knee specimens are subjected to loads corresponding to the static lifting maneuver (Simulation 1, Appendix I). Following measurements in the intact joint, measurements are repeated with the following prostheses: MGII (Zimmer, Warsaw, IN), AMK (DePuy, Warsaw, IN), Whitesides Ortholoc (Dow Corning Wright, Arlington, TN), PFC (Johnson & Johnson, New Brunswick, NJ), and IBII (Zimmer, Warsaw, IN). During implantation of the prosthesis, care is taken to maintain a constant joint line and equal flexion and extension gaps. Capsular soft tissue releases are performed as required.

Contact pressure distributions in the intact articulation and the distributions when the unresurfaced patella articulates with the various designs of the femoral component, are qualitatively compared in Figure 77.10, using the results obtained from one specimen. Results

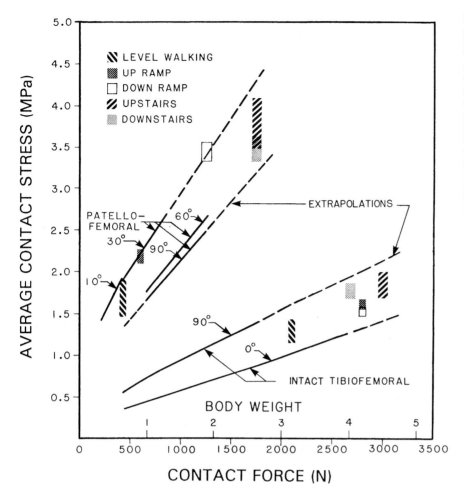

Figure 77.9. Average contact stress (or pressure) as a function of contact force for the patellofemoral and tibiofemoral articulations. The contact force for the patellofemoral articulation is $|PFJR|$ (Fig. 77.3), and for the tibiofemoral articulation, it is the compressive component of J (Fig. 77.1A). The various knee flexion angles corresponding to the individual curves have been indicated in the figure. The regions corresponding to the maximum contact force and knee flexion angle for some walking activities are shown as shaded areas. (Adapted with permission from Ahmed AM, Burke DL, Yu A. In-vitro measurement of static pressure distribution in synovial joints. Part II: Retropatellar surface. J Biomech Eng 1983; 105:226–236.)

of quantitative analysis of the measurements from 6 specimens, in terms of the magnitude of the contact area subjected to different levels of pressure, are shown in Figure 77.11.

Although the contact area appears as a continuous transverse band (in the flexion range of 0° to 105°) for the intact articulation, the highest pressures tend to occur at two separate locations, one near the central ridge but generally biased towards the medial facet and the other at the lateral facet (Fig. 77.10). Also, the pressure distributions tend to be fairly nonuniform, particularly at higher flexion angles, which in this case also corresponds to a higher $|PFJR|$. For example, the results of Figure 77.11 for the 90° flexion angle show that, although approximately 2.5 cm^2 of the total contact area is subjected to pressures below 3 MPa (megapascals), areas of 0.8 cm^2, 0.5 cm^2 and 0.3 cm^2 are subjected to pressures in the ranges 3–4 MPa, 4–5 MPa, and greater than 5 MPa respectively. However, as noted earlier, the exact pattern of pressure distribution is known to be particularly sensitive to differences in the patellar loading condition.

The findings of the study in terms of the alteration of the contact characteristics when an unresurfaced patella articulates with the femoral components of different designs, are summarized as follows:

1. Location of contact: In knee flexion from 0° to 60°, the contact area remains approximately stationary relative to the retropatellar surface, and it is located at the center of the surface. With flexion beyond 60°, the pressure in the midzone of the contact area progressively decreases until the area appears as two isolated zones, one on the medial facet and the other on the lateral facet. The location of these zones relative to the retropatellar surface, however, is generally different from those of the high-pressure zones in the intact articulation. In femoral components designed with the central notch extending more into the anterior flange, the apex of the central ridge of the retropatellar surface tends to impinge in the notch. This effect is seen as an abrupt change in the shape of the contact area to one that conforms with the outline of the notch (e.g., the PFC prosthesis at 90° and the AMK at 105° in Fig. 77.10).

2. Magnitude of contact area: Although the magnitude of the contact area remains relatively unaltered in the knee flexion range 0° to 30°, it decreases by 15% to 35% at higher flexion angles, depending on the type of the femoral component. Consequently, the average contact stress on the retropatellar surface is increased in direct proportion. In this context, it is worth noting that for identical functional activities,

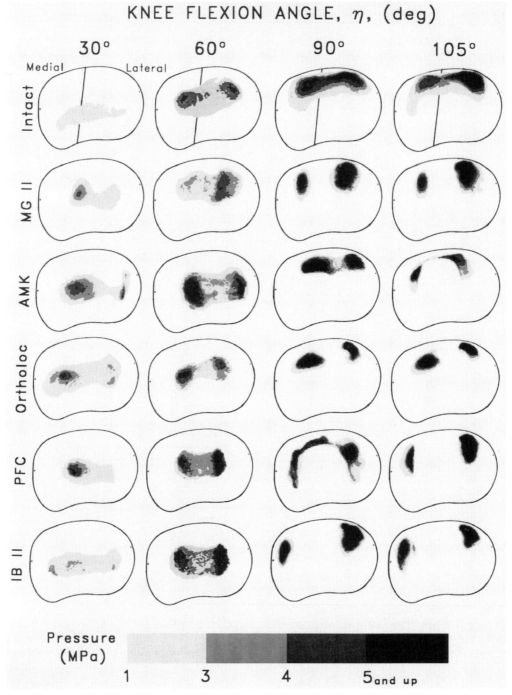

Figure 77.10. Comparison of the contact pressure distributions measured in the intact articulation *(first row)* with those measured when the intact patella articulates with the femoral components of different designs of TKR components.

the average contact stress on this surface is already very high compared to those on the tibial or femoral surfaces in the tibiofemoral articulation (Fig. 77.9).

3. Pressure distribution: With knee flexion beyond 30°, the proportion of contact area subjected to higher pressures increases significantly in comparison to the intact articulation. For example, the results of Figure 77.11 for a 90° flexion angle, show that the area of contact subjected to pressures above 5 MPa

increases from around 0.3 cm^2 to 0.7–1.1 cm^2 depending on the type of femoral component.

Design Implications

Considering contact characteristics, the design of the patellofemoral components must first ensure that the magnitude of the contact area, and hence contact stress, is compatible with the particular wear and degradation properties of the materials of the component.

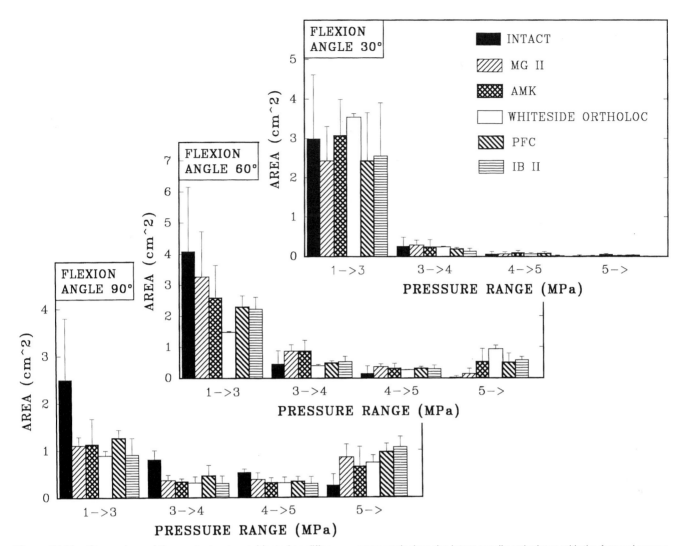

Figure 77.11. Comparison of the contact areas subjected to different pressure levels measured in the intact articulation with those measured when the intact patella articulates with the femoral components of different designs of TKR components.

Therefore, exact duplication of the contact characteristics of the intact articulation is irrelevant, as long as the location of the contact area relative to the retropatellar surface geometry (affecting the angle α, Fig. 77.3, *B*) can be maintained close to its normal location throughout the flexion range. In the intact articulation, with increasing flexion, the location shifts progressively from the lower pole to the upper border of the retropatellar surface. For patellar components with "dome" or "button" shaped articular surfaces, the contact area tends to localize at the transverse midline of the component (42). Thus, it can be estimated that for a given $|T_P|$, at a flexion angle of 30°, $|PFJR|$ will increase by around 9%, and at an angle of 90°, it will be decreased by 19%.

If the patella is left unresurfaced, then the design of the patellar surface of the femoral component must ensure that the retropatellar cartilage is not subject to adverse average or maximum contact pressures. The results presented in this section indicate that such adverse condition may result when an unresurfaced patella articulates with a femoral trochlea that has been designed for a nonanatomic patellar resurfacing. Therefore, for articulation with the unresurfaced patella, the patellar surface of the femoral component must be designed specifically to conform more with the normal trochlear topography than in the present designs.

Tracking Characteristics

The objective of this section is to review the characteristics of patellar tracking and to identify the features of the patellofemoral articulation that govern them. This is necessary in order to establish specific design criteria so that the patellofemoral components can avoid problems of maltracking. The design must allow knee flexion up to the desired limit, while maintaining retinacular balance throughout the flexion range and providing adequate patellar stability near knee extension.

Patellar tracking consists of relatively high displacements in the plane of patellar motion (in-plane displacements), as well as small but significant displacements in the other planes (out-of-plane displacements). Since maltracking essentially consists of aberrations in the out-of-plane displacements, control of these displacements is of primary concern in the design of the patellofemoral components. Considerable disagreement exists among the published results (49–53) over the characteristics of these displacements. This is due partly to inadequacies in the definition of the displacement measurement coordinate system and partly to inaccuracies in the method of measurement. A recent study (52), provides the results of very accurate measurements, but only for 4 specimens. Even from these results, the general characteristics are difficult to establish because of the wide differences in the results between the 4 specimens. Therefore, the review of this section has been based on results of two recently completed studies in our laboratory. The first study (54) involved measurements in 22 fresh-frozen specimens that were subjected to the loading conditions simulating the static lifting maneuver (Simulation 1, Appendix I), and the second study (55) involved measurements in 8 fresh-frozen specimens subjected to load-histories corresponding to level walking (Simulation 3, Appendix I). In both studies, patellar displacements relative to the femur were measured using a 6-degrees-of-freedom electromechanical goniometer with inaccuracy limits of ±0.5 mm for translations and ±0.5 for rotations. In the following sections, patellar translations are presented as translations of the *centroid* of the patella relative to the fixed femur (based on the direction of the *femoral-shaft axis*) and the patellar rotations are expressed as rotations about its own anatomically defined axes. In addition, the patellar translations are normalized with respect to the width of the specimen to allow comparison of the translations measured in specimens of different size.

In-Plane Displacements

The measured in-plane displacements are shown in Figure 77.12, where the patellar flexion has been plotted as a function of knee flexion angle η, (Fig. 77.12, A), and

the patellar anterior-posterior and proximal-distal translations for various values of η have been cross-plotted to illustrate directly the patellar in-plane track (Fig. 77.12, B). The results of Figure 77.12, A show that the patellar flexion increases in unison with that of the knee, although at a lesser rate; the net patellar rotation is around 85° in the η range of 0° to 120°. In Figure 77.12, B, the superposition of the radiographic outline of an average-sized specimen on the measured in-plane tracks indicates that the tracks correspond reasonably well with the trochlear topography. In general, the characteristics of all three in-plane displacements are fairly consistent between specimens and relatively insensitive to the loading condition.

Out-of-Plane Displacements

The measured out-of-plane displacements as functions of knee flexion angle, η, are shown in Figure 77.13. Unlike the in-plane displacements (Fig. 77.12), these displacements are found to differ markedly between specimens, as indicated by the large standard deviations, and they are also sensitive to the patellar loading conditions, as indicated by the differences in the results obtained for the two simulations. Nevertheless, the general features of these displacements can be ascertained from the results of the static lifting simulation covering the η range of 0° to 120°. Since the displacement varies in a complex manner with η, it would be convenient to divide the range of η into three segments: 0° to 30°, 30° to 90°, and 90° to 120°. In the initial range, with increasing flexion, the patella undergoes a medial translation, a medial tilt, and a lateral rotation in the coronal plane (the lower pole turning towards the head of the fibula). In the midrange of η, the direction of the translation and the senses of the tilt and rotation are all opposite to those in the initial range. In the final range of η, the patellar tilt undergoes a second reversal of sense, while the translation and the rotation continue as in the midrange. On an average, in the η range of 0° to 120°, the patella undergoes a lateral translation of 11 mm, a

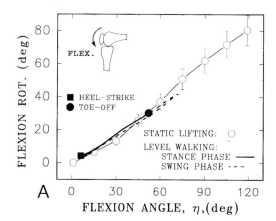

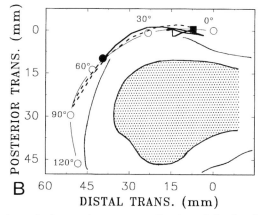

Figure 77.12. **A,** Patellar flexion as a function of the knee flexion angle. **B,** The average in-plane tracking pattern of the patella superimposed on the tracing of the lateral x-ray of an average-size specimen. Note that for the results from the level walking simulation, the

knee flexion angles corresponding to patellar locations along the track have not been indicated (for clarity) and are not necessarily identical to those from the static lifting simulation. The maximum flexion angle in the former case is 70°.

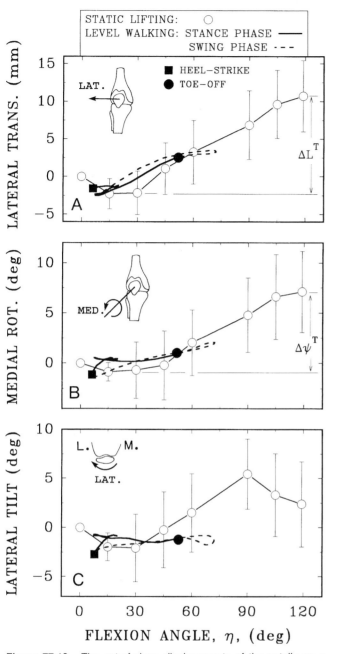

Figure 77.13. The out-of-plane displacements of the patella as a function of knee flexion angle; **A**, medial-lateral translation, **B**, rotation in the coronal plane (rotation), **B**, rotation in the transverse plane (tilt). The vertical bars represent ±1 standard deviation of the measurements.

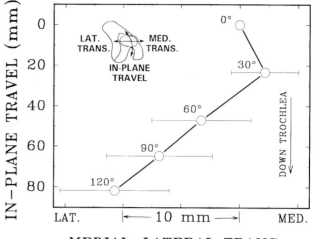

MEDIAL–LATERAL TRANS.

Figure 77.14. The average out-of-plane tracking pattern of the patella, i.e., patellar medial-lateral translation as a function of its in-plane travel. Note that the direction of the medial-lateral translation as shown in the figure corresponds to that for the right knee. Note also, that for the in-plane travel (vertical axis) a different scale has been used than for the medial-lateral translation (horizontal axis). Therefore, this track is not a pictorial representation of the actual track, unlike the case for the in-plane track shown in Figure 77.12, B.

lateral tilt of 8° and a medial rotation of 7°. The patellar out-of-plane track, i.e., its medial-lateral translation as a function of its in-plane travel or track-length, is shown in Figure 77.14. It must be emphasized that the patellar medial-lateral translation in this figure is measured with respect to the axis of the femoral-shaft. If, for example, the measurements were made with respect to the mechanical axis of the leg, then the track would indicate much less medial-lateral translation compared to that shown in the figure. The figure illustrates the character-

istic pattern of the patellar out-of-plane track with knee flexion: an initial sharp medial shift as the patella enters the trochlea, followed by a reversal in the direction of the shift and a progressive increase in the lateral shift as it travels down the trochlea.

Although the foregoing provides the general features of the out-of-plane tracking pattern, an understanding of the pattern remains incomplete in the absence of an explanation of the causes of the wide differences in the results between specimens. In general, the differences are of two types. The first type involves the transition flexion angle between the initial and the midrange where all three displacements reverse their direction or sense. On average, this transition flexion angle is around 30°, but the range of variation is as large as 0° to 45°. Although as yet not confirmed by measurements, it is expected that this variation is due to differences in the relative location of the patella in the sagittal plane. For high-riding patellae, the transition flexion angle will be smaller, while the opposite will be true for low-riding patellae. The second type of difference between specimens involves the magnitude of the displacements. This difference can only be explained on the basis of the governing mechanics of the out-of-plane tracking pattern. An attempt toward such an explanation is provided in the following section.

Mechanics of Patellar Tracking

The patellar tracking pattern can be expected to be governed by the variation with knee flexion of the mechanical balance between the external force system imposed on the patella (T_Q and T_P) and the restraining force generated by the geometric interaction of the articular surfaces (*PFJR*). In general, it is expected that near knee extension, when the patella is only partly inside or even outside the trochlea, the directions of the T_Q and T_P vectors will dominate the tracking pattern. On the other hand, for knee flexion angles above 30°, when the patella articulates fully with the trochlear surface, the trochlear topography, which governs the direction of *PFJR*, will dominate the tracking pattern. The trochlea is in the form of a shallow "S" curve whose long-axis is inclined medially towards the osteochondral ridge and is approximately parallel to the femoral mechanical axis. The inclination of the curve-axis might be expected to impart the medial-lateral translation while the curve itself might be expected to impart the rotation of the patella in the coronal plane. Also, the prominence of the lateral femoral condyle relative to the medial condyle is likely to control the tilt of the patella.

In order to establish quantitative correlation between features of the trochlear topography and the tracking pattern, the trochlear topography was mapped in detail in 8 fresh-frozen specimens, subsequent to patellar displacement measurements. From this map, the trochlear curve was determined as the locus of the deepest points of the trochlea as shown in Figure 77.15, *A*. Relative to this curve, contour lines of equal height were established. A two-dimensional representation of these contour lines is shown in Figure 77.15, *B*. Figure 77.15, *B* also shows the two indices used to characterize the trochlear curve: (*a*) the lateral offset *X* and, (*b*) the change in inclination *Y*. Since the objective is to correlate the patellar tracking pattern with the trochlear topography, only the patellar displacements in the knee flexion range where they are expected to be influenced by the topography are correlated with these indices. These displacements are those associated with knee flexion from around 30°. More precisely, for the patellar

medial-lateral translation, it is the lateral translation from its most medial location, i.e., the maximum lateral translation (ΔL^T, Fig. 77.13, *A*), and for the patellar rotation, it is the medial rotation from its most laterally rotated position, i.e., the maximum medial rotation ($\Delta = \Psi^T$, Fig. 77.13, *B*). In Figure 77.16, *A*, the individual maximum lateral translations, as defined above, measured in the 8 specimens are plotted as a function of the lateral offset *X* measured in the corresponding specimens. The slope of 1.0 for the regression line (r = .95) suggests the dominant influence of the trochlear inclination on this translation. The regression line for the maximum medial rotation in the coronal plane with the change in inclination θ, however, shows a slope of only 0.31 (Fig. 77.16, *B*). This suggests that, although the sense of rotation is certainly controlled by θ, the magnitude of the rotation is only partly influenced by θ even in the flexed knee. The direction of the T_Q vector can then be expected to equally influence this rotation.

The influence of the direction of T_Q on the patellar tracking pattern is yet to be measured in detail. Nevertheless, the extent of the influence can be assessed from the results of two different tests, both involving measurement of patellar medial-lateral translation as a function of the Q angle, the latter controlling the direction of T_Q. In the first test (55), measurements were made in 8 fresh-frozen specimens subjected to loading conditions simulating level walking (Simulation 3, Appendix I), and in the second test (57), 5 fresh-frozen specimens were subjected to loads corresponding to the "leg-raising" exercise (Simulation 2, Appendix I). The results of the first test are shown in Figure 77.17, *A* where the patellar out-of-plane track, measured with a normal Q angle, is compared to that measured when the Q angle was increased by 7.5°. It is noted that during the swing phase of level walking, the out-of-plane track with an increased Q

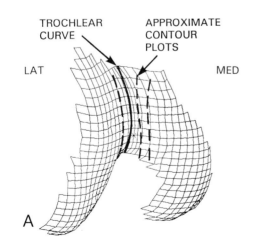

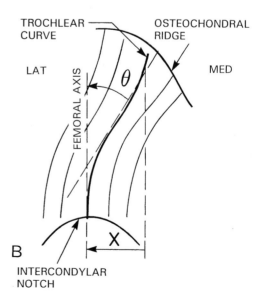

Figure 77.15. **A,** A representative surface topography of the femoral trochlea, illustrating the trochlear curve and contour lines. **B,** Contour plot of the developed surface of the trochlea and definition of the two indices: lateral offset *X,* and change in inclination θ, for the characterization of the trochlear topography.

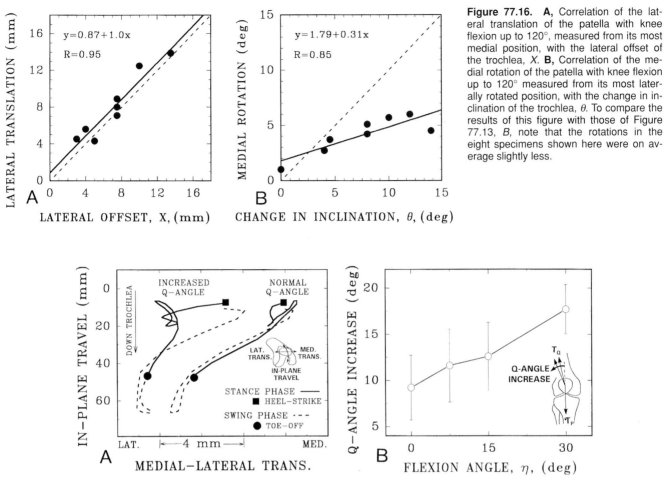

Figure 77.16. **A,** Correlation of the lateral translation of the patella with knee flexion up to 120°, measured from its most medial position, with the lateral offset of the trochlea, *X*. **B,** Correlation of the medial rotation of the patella with knee flexion up to 120° measured from its most laterally rotated position, with the change in inclination of the trochlea, *θ*. To compare the results of this figure with those of Figure 77.13, *B*, note that the rotations in the eight specimens shown here were on average slightly less.

Figure 77.17. **A,** Comparison of the out-of-plane track measured with a normal Q angle with that measured with an increase in Q angle by 7.5°, corresponding to knee loading conditions simulating level walking. To compare the results of this figure with those of Fig- ure 77.14, note that in the simulated level walking, the maximum knee flexion angle is only 70°. **B,** The maximum increase in Q angle prior to patellar dislocation as a function of knee flexion angle.

angle, although offset laterally by around 2 mm, follows closely the pattern of the normal track. On the other hand, during the stance phase, when $|T_Q|$ is relatively high, the track with an increased Q angle deviates markedly towards the lateral direction, particularly near full extension. The fact that the influence of Q angle is more pronounced near extension is supported by the results of the second test shown in Figure 77.17, *B*. In the figure, the maximum increase in Q angle prior to patellar dislocation is plotted as a function of the knee flexion angle, η. Patellar dislocation is defined as the condition of an abrupt increase in the patellar lateral translation with increasing Q angle. On average, the increase in Q angle necessary for dislocation is around 8° at $\eta = 0°$ and 16° at $\eta = 30°$.

On the basis of the foregoing results, it is possible to establish the governing mechanics of the patellar tracking pattern with the schematic of Figure 77.18. For this explanation, it will be convenient to follow the track with knee extension rather than flexion, i.e., in a direction opposite to that considered so far. At high flexion angles, say at $\eta = 90°$, the patella can be considered to

be stably located in the depth of the trochlea. With knee extension up to around $\eta = 30°$, the patella slides along the trochlea, its location dictated by the trochlear inclination with respect to the axis of the femoral shaft (Fig. 77.18, *A*). As noted earlier, the trochlea is inclined approximately along the mechanical axis of the femur. Thus, the patellar in-plane track is approximately in the plane of the tibial flexion/extension rotation. During this part of the patellar travel, an increase or decrease in the lateral component of T_Q will tend only to offset the track in the medial-lateral direction, without affecting its general pattern (for example, Fig. 77.17, *A*). Although the inclination of the trochlea controls the location of the patella, the curve associated with the inclination is excessive in order to impart a corresponding rotation of the patella in the coronal plane against the opposing influence of the direction of T_Q. The gradual shift of location of the patellar contact area toward the lower pole with knee extension allows the patella to pivot more readily to orient itself along the T_Q vector while maintaining its location within the trochlea (Fig. 77.18, *A*). Thus, up to $\eta = 30°$, although the *location* of the patella

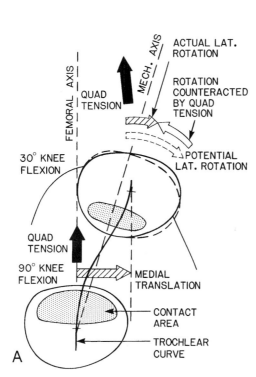

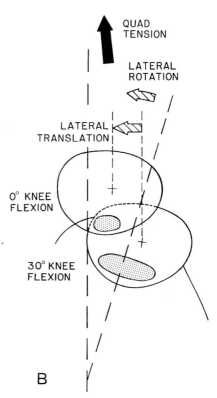

Figure 77.18. Schematic representation of the governing mechanics of the patellar out-of-plane translation and coronal-plane rotation. Note that the displacements are exaggerated for the purpose of illustration. **A,** Knee extension from 90° to around 30°. **B,** Knee extension from around 30° to full extension.

is dictated by the trochlear topography, its *orientation* is influenced equally by the direction of T_Q.

With knee extension beyond $\eta = 30°$, the patella progressively exits from the trochlea with a gradual decrease in the influence of the trochlear topography and a corresponding increase in the influence of the direction of T_Q (and of T_P) on its location and orientation (Fig. 77.18, *B*). This causes the reversal in the direction of the medial-lateral translation and the sense of the coronal-plane rotation of the patella at η around 30°. The lateral translation of the patella with extension from $\eta = 30°$ effectively reduces the *potential* increase in Q angle with knee extension. Nevertheless, the resultant Q angle remains sufficiently high for the patella to be more vulnerable to dislocation because of any additional increase in this angle near knee extension. Thus, for $\eta < 30°$, the tracking pattern appears to be governed by a subtle balance between the characteristics of the quadriceps force and the trochlear topography.

Design Implications

From the point of view of tracking characteristics, the design of the patellofemoral components needs to ensure, (*a*) knee flexion to the desired limit, (*b*) retinacular balance throughout the range of flexion, and, (*c*) patellar stability. To allow knee flexion in the desired range, the *length* of the track of the resurfaced patella (i.e., the net translation of the centroid of the construct) must not exceed the corresponding length in the intact articulation. Ideally, the *location* of the track relative to

the femoral geometry, the *shape* of the track, and the patellar *rotations* associated with tracking, all need to be replicated to maintain retinacular balance. Although the out-of-plane tracking pattern is complex, nevertheless, for knee flexion angles greater than 30° ($\eta > 30°$), the pattern has been found to be dictated primarily by the trochlear topography. Thus, for articulation in the range $\eta > 30°$, if the patellar surface of the femoral component is designed to conform with the anatomic trochlear topography, and its placement during surgery is made accordingly, then both the retinacular balance and the range of flexion will be maintained. Because the Q angle is reduced for $\eta > 30°$, the normal depth of the trochlea, if replicated in the patellar surface of the femoral component, can be expected to provide, adequate stability simultaneously.

For articulation near extension, i.e., $\eta < 30°$, the design features necessary to provide both adequate tracking and stability characteristics are not as clear. One option would be to design the surface of the proximal part of the anterior flange of the femoral component to conform with the trochlear topography such that the shape and the relative location of the proximal edge of the flange replicate the osteochondral ridge. In this case, the resurfaced patella would undergo the normal lateral translation with knee extension (Fig. 77.18, *B*), as it gradually slides out of the femoral component with a consequent reduction of the *potential* Q angle. However, with knee flexion/extension, the potential abrading and impingement of the patellar component with the proximal edge of the femoral component are likely to aggravate problems of wear and degradation of the component materials. Therefore, a better option would be to extend the anterior flange proximally to ensure continuous and smooth travel of the contact area in this range of knee motion. This, of course, is the option used in the current designs of the femoral component. However, in such designs, the surface features of the anterior flange should be such as not to aggravate the vulnerability of the patella to dislocation by preventing it from its normal lateral translation with knee extension for $\eta < 30°$. Two approaches to the design can be envisaged. In one, an appropriate lateral bend can be incorporated in the groove of the patellar surface to allow normal tracking. In this case, however, the depth of the groove needs to be sufficient to prevent dislocation under aberrant loading conditions such as those associated with an increased Q angle. In the second approach, the patellar surface can be made relatively flat to allow free medial-lateral translation of the patella corresponding not only to that in normal tracking but also to aberrant conditions. In the latter case, under conditions of dislocation in the intact articulation, the patella would merely translate more laterally rather than suffer dislocation.

Overview

From a biomechanical point of view, the design of TKR components for the patellofemoral articulation ought to be simpler than for the tibiofemoral articulation. This is because, firstly, the former is not subjected to the variety of complex *external* load conditions that are experienced by the latter, whether in habitual activities or accidentally. Secondly, patellar resurfacing does not involve removal of load-bearing soft-tissue structures, such as the menisci and the anterior or both cruciates, as in the resurfacing of the tibiofemoral articulation. In the latter case, the design of the articular surfaces of the components needs also to incorporate the biomechanical stabilizing functions of the removed structures, while maintaining the normal functions of the remaining structures. Design of the patellofemoral components is spared from such complex demands and can be viewed as an application of the concept of pure resurfacing of the articular surfaces. Nevertheless, the biomechanics of the patellofemoral articulation are not so simple that they can be ignored in the design of the components and their placement during surgery.

The various design implications of the patellofemoral biomechanics discussed in the individual sections of this chapter can now be subjected to an overview, not only to illustrate the interrelationship between them, but also to develop the necessary design criteria based on biomechanical performance requirements. The following is an attempt in this direction.

1. **Range of knee flexion and retinacular balance**. To ensure knee flexion in the desired range, the design of the patellofemoral components should be such that the *length* of the patellar track (i.e., the net translation of the patella) in this range does not exceed the length in the intact articulation. This can be assured if the tracking patterns, in-plane (Fig. 77.12, *B*) and out-of-plane (Fig. 77.14), are replicated by shaping the patellar surface of the femoral component to conform with the trochlear topography. In this case, the patellar *rotations* (Figs. 77.12, *A*, 77.13, *B* and *C*) will also be close to their normal values, which along with the replication of the normal translations, will automatically ensure maintenance of the retinacular balance throughout the flexion range. This, of course, will be true only if the original balance in the intact articulation was normal.

2. **Quadriceps function and patellofemoral joint reaction**. To ensure that for a given loading condition (i.e., $|T_P|$), the magnitudes of the quadriceps force ($|T_Q|$) and the patellofemoral joint reaction ($|PFJR|$) are maintained identical to that in the intact articulation, the design of the components should be such that the moment-arm b of the patellar tendon tension T_P (Fig. 77.1), the patellar mechanism angle 2β (Fig. 77.3), and the angle α (Fig. 77.3, *B*) are not altered from their corresponding values in the intact articulation. If the in-plane tracking pattern (Fig. 77.12, *B*) is reproduced as found desirable in the paragraph above, then the magnitude and variation with flexion angle of the moment-arm b and of the angle 2β (Fig. 77.4) will be automatically reproduced. In this case, for a given $|T_P|$, $|T_Q|$ and $PFJR$ will be close to those in the intact articulation. In addition, if the variation of the relative location of the patellofemoral contact area with flexion angle (Fig. 77.7) is reproduced by design, then the magnitude and variation of the angle α (Fig. 77.4) will also be replicated, ensuring that the magnitudes of both forces are identical to those in the intact articulation at all flexion angles.

3. **Patellar stability**. To ensure patellar stability, the design of the patellofemoral components should be such as to maintain the out-of-plane tracking pattern (Fig. 77.14) in the presence of medial-lateral forces, such as the lateral or valgus force due to the Q angle (Fig. 77.2). In the *flexed* knee, if the out-of-plane tracking pattern is reproduced by shaping the patellar surface of the femoral component to conform with the trochlear topography, as required in the paragraph on Range of Knee Flexion above, then adequate stability can be expected for any reasonable design of the patellar component. On the other hand, for articulation near knee *extension*, where the Q angle is the highest, it has been argued that the replication of the trochlear topography is not advisable. The anterior flange of the femoral component must then incorporate special features in order to, (*a*) reproduce the normal out-of-plane tracking pattern (Fig. 77.14), which reduces the *potential* increase in the Q angle with extension, and, (*b*) provide additional stability to counter the increased vulnerability of the patella to dislocation, because of, say, an increase in Q angle (Fig. 77.17, *B*).

4. **Contact stress**. For the minimization of wear and degradation of the component materials, the design

of the components should be such as to minimize the contact stress by maximizing the contact area. This is particularly true for contact at high flexion angles where $|PFJR|$ is high (Fig. 77.5, *B*). If the patellar surface of the femoral component is designed to conform with the trochlear topography as found desirable above (in the paragraph on the Range of Knee Flexion), then the surface profile of the patellar component needs to be optimized to achieve maximum contact area in this range of flexion. It is worth noting that recent results suggest that in current designs of patellofemoral components, the patellofemoral contact area is approximately 21% of that in the intact articulation (58), and that the corresponding contact pressure exceeds the compressive yield strength of the polyethylene (UHMWPE) used for patellar components in TKR (59).

5. **Contact pressure distribution (unresurfaced patella).** To avoid adverse contact conditions on the retropatellar cartilage, the average and the maximum contact stresses must not exceed their respective normal magnitudes. As in the previous paragraph, this is critical for articulation at high flexion angles where $|PFJR|$ is high. In the current designs of TKR components, this condition does not appear to be met (Figs. 77.10 and 77.11). If, again, the patellar surface of the femoral component is designed to conform with the trochlear topography, this requirement will be automatically satisfied. In addition, the intercondylar notch in the femoral component should be located and shaped so as to ensure smooth sliding of the unresurfaced patella at high flexion angles. Results accrued so far suggest that this condition can be satisfied by avoiding extension of the intercondylar notch of the femoral component too far into the anterior flange (Fig. 77.10).

The criteria for the design of the *articular surfaces* of the patellofemoral components identified in the above discussion are summarized below and also highlighted schematically in Figure 77.19. The criteria are as follows:

1. Reproduction of the in-plane and out-of-plane tracking patterns for knee flexion angles greater than 30°.
2. Maintenance of retinacular balance and enhancement of patellar stability for articulation near knee extension.
3. Maximization of component contact area, particularly for articulation in the flexed knee.
4. For TKR without patellar resurfacing, provision of compatible contact stress conditions, with particular emphasis on contact stress conditions for articulation in the flexed knee.
5. For TKR without patellar resurfacing, provision of conditions for smooth sliding of the patella for articulation near the intercondylar notch area of the femoral component.

It has been shown that Criteria 1 and 4 are satisfied by shaping the patellar surface of the femoral component to conform to the trochlear topography. Also, it appears that Criterion 5 can be met by limiting the extension of the intercondylar notch into the anterior flange. However, the exact design features for optimum satisfaction of Criteria 2 and 3 require further basic research.

Apart from the foregoing, the design of the patellofemoral components must also consider anatomic variations, fixation stresses, requirements of the tibiofemoral component design, and surgical techniques. These factors often conflict with those based purely on patellofemoral biomechanics. The challenge remains to de-

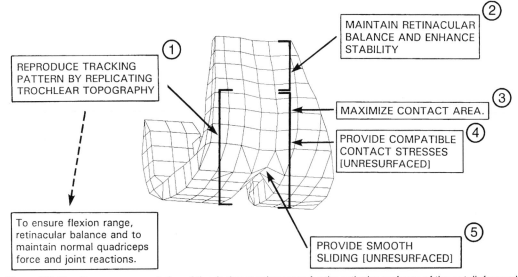

Figure 77.19. Summary presentation of the design requirements for the articular surfaces of the patellofemoral components formulated on the basis of patellofemoral biomechanics.

velop a design, which, while satisfying the biomechanical criteria, also satisfies these other, equally important demands of the arthroplasty.

Future Perspective

The increasing concern stemming from the inadequacies of the current designs of the patellofemoral components is certain to stimulate improvement. Basic research on the biomechanics of the articulation of the knee will refine the design criteria. In addition, innovative concepts are expected to be applied to satisfy these design specifications. However, the evolution of component design is likely to be inhibited, if it is not accompanied by a parallel evolution in surgical technique. This important point is illustrated as follows.

In current surgical practice, patellar component placement is accomplished without the aid of instrumentation. Since under this condition, accurate placement of the component is difficult, the preferred shape of the component has remained limited to those which are relatively insensitive to the precision of placement in terms of general tracking characteristics (e.g., dome- or button-shaped components). It is understood that a more anatomic design, if placed inaccurately during surgery, would predispose the component to maltracking. Since satisfactory fulfillment of the criteria, such as those formulated in this chapter, cannot be envisaged by a design whose performance would remain unaffected by inaccuracies in placement, acceptance of modification in surgical technique must accompany an improved design. Such modification is expected to include, similar to the current standard practice for the placement of the tibiofemoral components, the accurate assessment of patellar alignment prior to surgery and the use of instrumentation for the placement of the patellar component during surgery. In the author's opinion, in the absence of such a change in TKR surgical concept, it will be fruitless to rely only on design improvements to achieve satisfactory long-term performance of the patellofemoral components.

Acknowledgment

I am greatly indebted to my associates C. McLean and N.A. Duncan, who were responsible for the collection, analysis, and interpretation of all of the more recent results presented in this chapter; without their enthusiastic contribution, the preparation of the manuscript would not have been possible. The author is also grateful to his colleague, Dr. M. Tanzer, who initiated the research on the contact characteristics of the unresurfaced patella in TKR that is reported here; he supplied many valuable suggestions from the surgical perspective. Grateful acknowledgment is made to J. Casey for his dedicated assistance on the many aspects of preparation of the chapter and to A. Cianci for her meticulous production of the manuscript. Finally, the author is indebted to the Medical Research Council of Canada for continual support of the research reported in the chapter.

References

1. Clayton ML, Thirupathi R. Patella complications after total condylar arthroplasty. Clin Orthop Rel Res 1982;170:152–155.
2. Scott RD, Turoff N, Ewald FC. Stress fracture of the patella following duopatellar total knee arthroplasty with patellar resurfacing. Clin Orthop Rel Res 1982;170:147–151.
3. Aglietti P, Buzzi R, Gaudenzi A. Patellofemoral functional results and complications with the posterior stabilized total condylar knee prosthesis. J Arthroplasty 1988;3:17–23.
4. Bayley JC, Scott RD. Further observations on metal-backed patellar component failure. Clin Orthop Rel Res 1988;236:82–87.
5. Bayley JC, Scott RD, Ewald FC, Holmes GB. Failure of the metal-backed patellar component after total knee replacement. J Bone Joint Surg 1988;70A:668–674.
6. Briard JL, Hungerford DS. Patellofemoral instability in total knee arthroplasty. J Arthroplasty 1989;S87–S97.
7. Figgie HE, Goldberg VM, Figgie MP, Inglis AE, Kelly M, Sobel M. The effect of alignment of the implant on fractures of the patella after condylar total knee arthroplasty. J Bone Joint Surg 1989;71A:1031–1039.
8. Goldberg VM, Figgie HE, Inglis AE, et al. Patellar fracture type and prognosis in condylar total knee arthroplasty. Clin Orthop Rel Res 1988;236:115–122.
9. Grace JN, Rand JA. Patellar instability after total knee arthroplasty. Clin Orthop Rel Res 1988;237:184–189.
10. Hozack WJ, Goll SR, Lotke PA, Rothman RH, Booth RE. The treatment of patellar fractures after total knee arthroplasty. Clin Orthop Rel Res 1988;236:123–127.
11. Kirk P, Rorabeck CH, Bourne RB, Burkart B, Nott L. Management of recurrent dislocation of the patella following total knee arthroplasty. J Arthroplasty 1992;7:229–233.
12. Lombardi AV, Engh GA, Volz RG, Albrigo JL, Brainard BJ. Fracture/dislocation of the polyethylene in metal-backed patellar components in total knee arthroplasty. J Bone Joint Surg 1988;70A:675–679.
13. Rosenberg AG, Andriacchi TP, Galante JO. Patellar component failure in cementless total knee arthroplasty. Clin Orthop Rel Res 1988;236:106–114.
14. Stulberg SD, Stulberg BN, Hamati Y, Tsao A. Failure mechanisms of metal-backed patellar components. Clin Orthop Res Rel 1988;236:88–105.
15. Thorpe CD, Bocell JR, Tullos HS. Intra-articular fibrous bands: Patellar complications after total knee replacement. J Bone Joint Surg 1990;72A:811–814.
16. Vernace JV, Rothman RH, Booth RE, Balderston RA. Arthroscopic management of the patellar chunk syndrome following posterior stabilized total knee arthroscopy. J Arthroplasty 1989;4:179–182.
17. Wasilewski SA, Frankl U. Fracture of polyethylene of patellar component in total knee arthroplasty, diagnosed by arthroplasty. J Arthroplasty 1989;S19–S22.
18. Windsor RE, Scuderi GR, Insall JN. Patellar fractures in total knee arthroplasty. J Arthroplasty 1989;(suppl)S63–S67.
19. Rand JA. Patellar resurfacing in total knee arthroplasty. Clin Orthop Rel Res 1990;260:110–117.
20. Abraham W, Buchanan JR, Daubert H, Greer RB, Keefer J. Should the patella be resurfaced in total knee arthroplasty? Efficacy of patellar resurfacing. Clin Orthop Rel Res 1988;236:128–134.
21. Smith SR, Stuart P, Pinder IM. Non-resurfaced patella in total knee arthroplasty. J Arthroplasty 1989;S81–S86.
22. Enis JE, Gardner R, Robledo MA, Latta L, Smith R. Comparison of patellar resurfacing versus non-resurfacing in bilateral total knee arthroplasty. Clin Orthop Rel Res 1990;260:38–42.
23. McLean CA, Tanzer M, Laxer E, Casey J, Ahmed AM. The effect of femoral component designs on the contact and tracking characteristics of the unresurfaced patella in TKA. Transactions, 40th Annual Meeting, Orthop Res Soc 1994;19(2):821.
24. Ficat RP, Hungerford DS. Disorders of the patello-femoral joint. Baltimore: Williams & Wilkins, 1977:1–249.
25. Ellis MI, Seedhom BB, Amis AA, Dowson D, Wright V. Forces in the knee joint whilst rising from normal and motorized chairs. Eng Med 1979;8:33–40.
26. Matthews LS, Stonstegard DA, Henke JA. Load bearing characteristics of the patellofemoral joint. Acta Orthop Scand 1977;48:511–516.
27. Reilly DT, Martens M. Experimental analysis of the quadriceps muscle force and patellofemoral joint reaction force for various activities. Acta Orthop Scand 1972;43:126–137.

28. Bishop RED, On the mechanics of the human knee, Eng Med 1977;6:46–54.
29. Bandi W. Chrondromalacia patellae und femoro-patellare arthrose. Atiologie, klinik and therapie. Helv Chir Acta 1972;119(suppl):3–70.
30. Goymann V, Muller HG: New calculation of the biomechanics of the patellofemoral joint and its clinical significance. In: Ingwersen OS, et al. ed. The Knee Joint. Amsterdam: Excerpta Medica, 1974:16–21.
31. Morrison JB. Function of the knee joint in various activities. Biomed Eng 1969;4:573–580.
32. Morrison JB. The mechanics of the knee joint in relation to normal walking. J Biomechanics 1970;3:51–61.
33. Perry J, Antonelli D, Ford W. Analysis of knee joint forces during flexed-knee stance. J Bone Joint Surg 1975;57A:961–967.
34. Schmidt GL: Biomechanical analysis of knee flexion and extension. J Biomech 1973;6:79–92.
35. Ahmed AM, Burke DL, Yu A. In-vitro measurement of static pressure distribution in synovial joints. Part II: Retropatellar surface. J Biomech Eng 1983;105:226–236.
36. Bishop RED, Denham RA. A note on the ratio between tensions in the quadriceps tendon and infra-patellar ligament. Eng Med 1977;6:53–54.
37. Buff HV, Jones LC, Hungerford DS. Experimental determination of forces transmitted through the patellofemoral joint. J Biomech 1988;21:17–24.
38. Ellis MI, Seedhom BB, Wright V, Dowson D. An evaluation of the ratio between the tensions along the quadriceps tendon and the patellar ligament. Eng Med 1980;9:189–194.
39. Huberti HH, Hayes WC, Stone JL, Shybut GT. Force ratios in the quadriceps tendon and ligamentum patellae. J Orthop Res 1984;2:49–54.
40. Maquet PGJ. Biomechanics of the knee. Berlin: Springer-Verlag, 1976:134–136.
41. Ahmed AM, Burke DL, Hyder A. Force analysis of the patellar mechanism. J Orthop Res 1987;5:69–85.
42. McLean CA, Ahmed AM: Direct measurement of the prosthesis/bone interface loads in the patellar prosthesis during simulated static and dynamic activities. Transactions, 38th Annual Meeting, Orthop Res Soc 1992;17(1):269.
43. Aglietti P, Insall JN, Walker PS, Trent P. A new patella prosthesis. Clin Orthop Rel Res 1975;17:175–187.
44. Goodfellow J, Hungerford DS, Zindel M. Patellofemoral joint mechanics and pathology, 1. Functional anatomy of the patellofemoral joint. J Bone Joint Surg 1976;58:287–290.
45. Huberti HH, Hayes WC. Patellofemoral contact pressures. The influence of Q angle and tendofemoral contact. J Bone Joint Surg 1984;66A:715–724.
46. Seedhom BB, Tsubuku M. A technique for the study of contact between visco-elastic bodies with special reference to the patellofemoral joint. J Biomech 1977;10:253–260.
47. Ferguson AB, Brown TD, Fu FH, Rutkowski R. Relief of patellofemoral contact stress by anterior displacement of the tibial tubercle. J Bone Joint Surg. 1979;61A:159–166.
48. Ateshian GA, Kwak SD, Soslowsky LJ, Grelszmer RP, Mow VC. Contact area measurements in diarthrodial joints: A comparison with a new stereophotogrammetry method. Transactions, 39th Annual Meeting, Orthop Res Soc 1993;18(2):347.
49. Fujikawa K, Seedhom BB, Wright V. Biomechanics of the patellofemoral joint. Part I: A study of the contact and congruity of the patellofemoral compartment and movement of the patella. Eng Med 1983;12:3–11.
50. Reider B, Marshall JL, Ring B. Patellar tracking. Clin Orthop Rel Res 1981;157:143–143.
51. Sikorski JM, Peters J, Watt I. The importance of femoral rotation in chondromalacia patellae as shown by serial radiography. J Bone Joint Surg 1979;61B:435–442.
52 van Kampen A, Huiskes R. The three-dimensional tracking pattern of the human patella. J Orthop Res 1990;8:372–382.
53. Veress SA, Lippert FG, How MCY, Takamoto T. Patellar tracking pattern measurement by analytical x-ray photogrammetry. J Biomech 1979;12:639–650.
54. Ahmed AM, Duncan NA, Chan KH. The three-dimensional tracking characteristics of the patella in simulated functional activities. Submitted: J Biomech, 1993.
55. McLean CA, Ahmed AM. The effect of dynamic loading and Q- angle on the patellar tracking pattern. Transactions, 40th Annual Meeting, Orthop Res Soc 1994;19(2):666.
56. Ahmed AM, Duncan NA, Tanzer M. The medial-lateral shift and spin of the patella are correlated with the geometric features of the femoral trochlea. Transactions, 40th Annual Meeting, Orthop Res Soc 1994;19(2):666.
57. McLean CA, Ahmed AM. Biomechanics Laboratory, Mechanical Engineering Department, McGill University. Unpublished data.
58. Kim W, Chao EYS, Rand JA. Comparative evaluation of patellofemoral contact area in different total knee designs. Transactions, 38th Annual Meeting, Orthop Res Soc 1992;17(2):326.
59. Hayes WC, Lathi VK, Takeuchi TY, Hipp JA, Myers ER, Dennis DA. Patellofemoral contact pressures exceed the compressive yield strength of UHMWPE in total knee replacements. Transactions, 39th Annual Meeting, Orthopaedic Research Society, 1993;17(2):421.

Appendix I

The results of the measurements presented in this chapter were carried out on fresh-frozen knee specimens subjected to loads simulating three functional activities. The simulation method and conditions for each of them are briefly summarized below.

1. Static lifting maneuvre. For this simulation, a quadriceps simulation apparatus detailed in an earlier paper (1) and shown in Figure 77.A.1 was used. The femur of the specimen was fixed to the loading platform of the apparatus (a) while the tibia was allowed to swing freely. At first, a foot-floor reaction (F, Fig. 77.1A) of 334 N was applied to an extension of a tibial intramedullary rod (b), ensuring that the line of action of this reaction, with respect to the knee joint geometry, was such as to reproduce the knee force and torque corresponding to a specified flexion angle during static lifting. The torque was then balanced by a simulated quadriceps tension. Two methods were used for the application of this tension. In one, a toggle clamp (not shown in Fig. 77.A.1) was attached to the common tendon of the rectus femoris and the vastus intermedius, and tension was applied to the clamp by a hydraulic actuator (c) and wire-pulley assembly (d), ensuring that its line-of-action corresponded to that of the rectus tension.

A force transducer (e) incorporated in the tension wire was used to measure the applied quadriceps tension. The results shown in Figure 77.5A were measured under this condition. In the second method, a close fitting cap was bolted firmly to the patella (f). Three tension bands (g), simulating three muscle groups of the quadriceps were attached to the cap and tensioned by three independent hydraulic actuators through three wire-pulley assemblies. The pulleys simulated the points of origin of the muscle groups. Three muscle groups were selected: (a) vastus lateralis; (b) vastus intermedius, rectus femoris combined with the vastus medialis longus, and (c) vastus medialis oblique. The tension distribution among the groups was set according to their cross-sectional areas as reported in (2). The results shown in Figures 77.7, 77.8, 77.10 to 77.14, and 77.16 were measured under the above conditions. It is worth mentioning that, with a foot-floor reaction of 334 N, the net quadriceps tension varies from around 250 N at 10° flexion to 1000 N at around 90° flexion.

2. Leg raising exercise. The apparatus used for this simulation was very similar to that used in the foregoing simulation and has been described in detail elsewhere (2). In this case, at first, the simulated quadriceps force was applied to the specimen. To prevent knee extension from the desired flexion angle, the tibial intramedullary rod was held in a bracket (not shown in Fig. 77.A.1) such that the rod was free to rotate axially

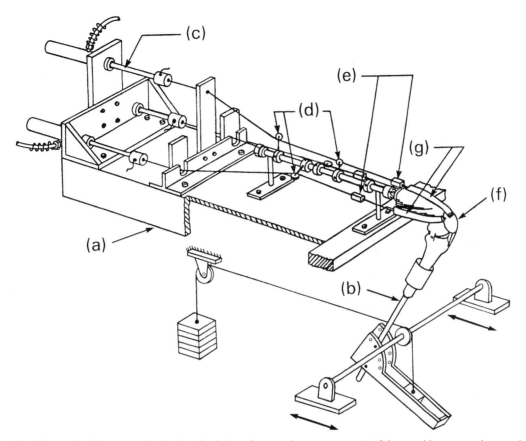

Figure 77.A.1. Quadriceps simulation appartus for the simulation of the static lifting maneuver; *a,* loading platform; *b,* tibial intramedullary rod; *c,* hydraulic actuator for application of tension; *d,* tension wire-pulley assemblies (the pulleys simulating the point of origin of the various components of the quadriceps muscle group); *e,* force transducer; *f,* patellar cap; *g,* bands used to simulate tension in the components of the quadriceps.

and slide laterally. Measurements were made with two values of the net quadriceps tension, 734 N and 668 N. The results of Figure 77.5*B* were obtained with the former value, while all other results measured using this simulation reported in the chapter corresponded to the latter value. Similar to the case described in the "Static lifting maneuver" above, three methods were used to simulate the quadriceps tension. In one, tension was applied by a clamp attached to the common tendon of the rectus and the intermedius (results of Fig. 77.5*A* and 77.17*B*). In the second case, tension was applied to the patellar cap (*F* in Fig. 77.A.1) using *five* tension bands, simulating individually all 5 quadriceps muscle components (results of Figs. 77.5*B*, 77.8 and 77.9).

3. Level walking. For this simulation, a novel unconstrained dynamic knee simulator detailed in Appendix Reference 3 and shown schematically in Figure 77.A.2 was used. In the simulator, the controlled parameters are the time-histories of the flexion angle and of the two main components of the foot-to-floor reaction: the flexing/extending moment and the tibial axial force. Two flexible cables, acted upon by stepping motors,

replicate the lumped actions of the extensor and flexor muscle groups by controlling the flexion angle time-history of the joint (Fig. 77.A.2, *A*). The extensor cable is inserted at the patella, thus including the patellofemoral joint mechanics. Concurrently and independently, two linear electrohydraulic actuators are used to apply the time-histories of the foot-to-floor reaction components. The tibial axial actuating force is applied through a cable/pulley mechanism to the tibia (Fig. 77.A.2, *B*). The individual controllers of the motors and the actuators are synchronized by a microcomputer. The simulator has been programmed to replicate the controlled parameters corresponding to level walking that are available in the literature. Independent measurement of the parameters has shown satisfactory replication.

References

1. Ahmed AM, Burke DL, Hyder A. Force analysis of the patellar mechanism. J Orthop Res 1987;5:69–85.
2. Ahmed AM, Burke DL, Yu A. In-vitro measurement of static pressure distribution in synovial joints. Part II: Retropatellar surface. ASME J Biomech Eng 1983;105:226–236.
3. McLean CA, Ahmed AM. Design and development of an unconstrained dynamic knee simulator. ASME J Biomech Eng 1993;115:144–148.

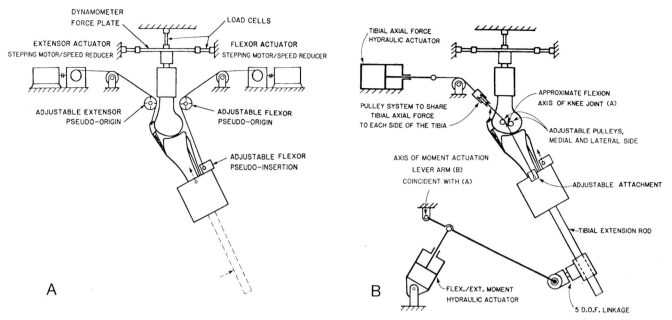

Figure 77.A.2. Schematic representation of the actuation system of the dynamic knee simulator; **A,** muscle actuation; **B,** foot-floor reaction actuation. Please note that for clarity, the moment actuation lever arm axis *A* has been shown displaced. In the simulator, it is coincident with the approximate knee joint flexion axis *B*. (Reproduced with permission from McLean CA, Ahmed AM. Design and development of an unconstrained dynamic knee simulator. ASME J Biomech Eng 1993;115:144–148).

78

Design of the Patellofemoral Joint in Total Knee Arthroplasty

Timothy M. Wright

Routine resurfacing of the patella as part of knee arthroplasty remains controversial (1), although functional performance is enhanced with total replacement of the patellofemoral joint (2–4). The controversy persists mainly because the complication rates caused by pain and instability, for example, are comparable whether or not the patella is resurfaced. In fact, patellar complications account for about half of all complications noted in total knee replacement. While some complications caused by resurfacing of the patellofemoral joint are related to implant design, most are certainly more influenced by surgical technique and the bone and soft tissue anatomy of the knee (5, 6). Therefore, the importance of patellar and femoral component design on the clinical results of knee arthroplasty is limited, compared with the importance of reconstructing appropriate anatomy.

As with any total joint prosthesis, the design of implants to replace the patellofemoral joint requires consideration of three important factors: range of motion, kinematics, and long-term performance. Adequate functional performance of the knee requires a large range of motion in flexion-extension, exceeding at least 100 degrees. The role of the natural patella in providing an adequate lever arm and appropriate protection to the quadriceps tendon as it traverses the knee joint must be maintained after resurfacing, to assure proper functional motion between the femur and the tibia. The implant design must also provide long-term stable fixation, adequate mechanical strength, and wear resistance.

Range of Motion and Kinematics

Normal Knee

The patellofemoral joint experiences large contact forces as it acts to change the direction of the quadriceps muscle force while the muscle force passes around the knee during flexion and extension. Contact forces approach one and one-half times body weight for level walking and exceed three times body weight for strenuous activities (7, 8).

For the natural patella, the lateral and medial facets maintain an adequate contact area with the femur throughout the range of motion of the knee. Contact areas are in the range of 2½ to 4 cm^2, resulting in contact pressures as high as 12 MPa under a maximal applied moment (8). In general, contact pressures increase with flexion angle and increase as the quadriceps angle (Q angle) deviates from normal. With increased flexion angle, the radius of curvature of the femoral anatomy decreases significantly as the patella begins to contact the femoral condyles rather than the patellar groove. The decreased radius causes a decrease in contact area and an increase in contact pressure between the patella and the femur. Deviation in Q angle will substantially unload one of the facets, decreasing contact area on the facet, with a concomitant increase in pressure on the opposite facet.

The kinematics of the natural patella are complex and are controlled by the position of the femur and tibia relative to one another and relative to the patella, as well as by the muscle and ligamentous forces applied to the patella. The bony anatomy of the patella and the patellar groove of the femur provides some constraint to the patellofemoral joint. The anatomy of the contacting surfaces is not symmetrical in that the patellar groove is tilted laterally a few degrees. During flexion, the anatomic constraints and the soft tissue forces cause the patella to both rotate and tilt with respect to the femur and to shift medially as much as 5 mm (9–11).

Knee Replacement

Both range of motion and kinematics are important in patellofemoral implant design. Range of motion of a total knee design is generally controlled by the shape and kinematics of the femorotibial articulation. The need for a large range of motion together with the requirement for bicondylar femorotibial surfaces leads to the same dilemma as in the natural patella: changing articulating geometries with decreased contact areas as flexion and contact forces increase.

The need for appropriate kinematics presents an even greater problem in that patellar component design alone cannot be expected to provide the necessary constraint for all patients. Moreover, as with the natural knee joint, the stability of the patellofemoral joint in total knee replacement depends on the constraint (or stability) of the femorotibial joint. For example, patellar instability was a more common complication of knee joint designs with constrained, hinged femorotibial joints than with less constrained designs (Grace). The hinged designs eliminated both internal-external and varus-valgus rotation, greatly altering the kinematics of the remaining natural patella.

Three general solutions to range of motion and kinematics problems for the patellofemoral joint exist in contemporary total knee implant designs. One common solution uses anatomic shapes for both the patellar component and the patellar groove on the femoral component. Examples include the Howmedica Kinemax and the Richards RMC Anatomic designs. The design goals for such components are to provide a more conforming patellar track (i.e., a more anatomic track) than in less constrained alternative designs and to maximize contact area, thereby minimizing contact pressures (12).

An advantage of closely imitating normal anatomy in the patellar groove of the femoral component is that the surgeon can choose not to resurface the patella. Disadvantages with anatomically shaped patellar and femoral components include the surgical skill required to achieve both appropriate alignment between the three joint components and adequate soft tissue balance throughout the range of motion. Kinematics are difficult to assess passively at surgery, since kinematics will depend on the action of muscle forces and soft tissue constraints. Another disadvantage of anatomic designs is that a larger inventory is required to include both right and left femoral components.

A second solution is to replace the anatomy of the natural patellofemoral joint with a spherical, dome-shaped patellar component contacting a single radius of curvature patellar groove on the femoral component. An example is the Insall/Burstein design. The first widely accepted design type used to resurface the patella, the primary advantage of the dome design is that it eliminates the importance of rotatory alignment between the patellar and femoral components, because the spherically shaped contacting surfaces are free to rotate. The symmetrical shape of the femoral component has the added advantage of reducing inventory by eliminating the need for right and left femoral components.

The third patellofemoral design solution is the introduction of an additional articulation within the patellar component itself. This solution includes a polyethylene insert that can rotate with respect to a metal backing fixed to the remaining bony patella. The insert can have an anatomic articulating geometry. An example is the LCS design. The added rotational degree of freedom between the insert and the backing is intended to have the same advantage as the dome design, in that rotational alignment of the patellar component with respect to the femoral component is not critical. The rotational degree of freedom provided at the polyethylene–metal backing interface allows an anatomic shape at the patellofemoral joint. An added advantage is that the joint contact forces, which might be expected to rotate the entire patella during functional activities and thus increase stress at articulating and fixation interfaces, instead cause rotation about the additional articulation. The disadvantage is that the additional polyethylene-metal interface provides another source of wear. Though clinical results have been generally favorable (13), this design approach has also been criticized in that the minimal amount of patellar rotation may not require an additional degree of freedom (14).

No well-controlled clinical studies exist that allow conclusions about the effect of design on clinical outcome, and few experimental studies have directly assessed the effect of patellofemoral design on kinematics. In a clinical study comparing a dome design with a more congruent design, Bindeglass et al. (6) found that design type did not affect the kinematics of the patellofemoral joint. Patellar alignment seemed more dependent on the preoperative alignment of the natural patella than on design or surgical soft tissue reconstruction.

Experimental studies are significantly limited because the functional forces and the active soft tissue constraints are difficult to recreate in vitro. Nonetheless, such studies have been used to provide general indications of design effects. For example, Cepulo and colleagues (15) measured the medial-lateral stability of seven different patellar implant designs, including both anatomic and dome-shaped designs. Shear load was applied across the patellofemoral joint with the knee positioned in 15, 30, and 110 degrees of flexion. The results showed that the design of the patellar component alone did not necessarily influence stability. For the designs tested, the resistance to lateral displacement of the patellar component depended more on the design of the patellar groove than on the femoral component. For example, the design that exhibited the greatest stability was a dome design with a deep patellar groove.

In other experimental studies (10, 11), three-dimensional motion of the patella was measured in cadaver knees with and without total joint components implanted. Flexion of the knee was created by pulling on the quadriceps. In contrast to the study in which pure shear loads were applied to the patellofemoral joint (15), the study of more natural motion of the knee joint concluded that a high lateral ridge on the patellar groove of the femoral component was effective in preventing patellar dislocation (10). The dome design with its vertical femoral groove was found to create a patellar tracking pattern quite different from that of the natural patella (10, 11), with significantly different medial-lateral displacement and rotational variations throughout the range of motion.

Long-Term Survival

Fixation

As with most total joint implant components, fixation of patellar components was first accomplished with acrylic bone cement, and this mode of fixation remains the "gold standard." Early designs included supplemental fixation in two forms. A central peg was provided on the anterior surface of the component. The peg protruded into a hole cut into the cancellous bone of the patella. A small undercut around the periphery of the component was also provided to act as a cement dam. These supplemental features provided resistance to torsional and shear loads across the bone-implant interface and have remained important features of many contemporary designs.

Most early designs of patellar components were fabricated from polyethylene to provide a low-friction articulation with the polished surface of the cobalt alloy femoral component. In the early 1980s, however, two concepts were introduced that led to alterations in patellar design. One concept dealt with the effect of stiffening surface replacement components, such as total knee tibial plateaus and total hip acetabular cups, which require direct load transfer through the component to the underlying cancellous bone. Theoretical analyses (16, 17) showed that stiffening an all polyethylene component by adding a metal backing, joint contact loads were distributed over a larger area of the cancellous bone, thus reducing the chances of bone failure and subsequent component loosening. The same effect was assumed to be important for the patellar component.

The second concept dealt with the ability to achieve biologic fixation of implant components by the ingrowth of tissue into porous layers on the component surface. The possibility of fixation without cement was attractive, both because such fixation might be permanent and because cement fixation was believed to be primarily responsible for creating particulate debris that could cause a biologic reaction in the surrounding tissues, which, in turn, could lead to loosening (18). Introduced for the femoral and acetabular components of total hip replacements (19), bone ingrowth was shown to occur into porous metallic coatings.

The development of these two concepts led to the introduction of metal-backed and porous-coated patellar components as well. Most of these designs have not, however, achieved clinical success. The reasons stem from both design and biologic considerations. The clinical justification for stiffening the patellar component by adding a metal backing was lacking. Loosening of patellar components was not a major complication and was not caused by cancellous bone failure, as had been clearly demonstrated for other types of surface replacements. Successful biologic fixation is often difficult to achieve. For example, Vigorita and colleagues (20) recently examined postmortem knee specimens containing porous-coated knee implants that had been functioning successfully. They found that although the patellar components showed more bone ingrowth than the femoral and tibial components, only 29% of the porous layer was filled with bone (Fig. 78.1). Furthermore, cement debris was not the only culprit invoking a detrimental biologic reaction. Polyethylene debris is now recognized as just as deleterious as cement debris in causing osteolysis of the surrounding bone (21–23).

An important requirement of bone ingrowth into a porous implant is initial rigid fixation. In metal-backed, porous-coated patellar designs, initial fixation is usually obtained through the use of multiple metal pegs, sometimes porous-coated as well. Clinical experience has shown that fatigue fracture of these pegs can occur. Failures have occurred primarily in components with porous coatings on the pegs. Bone ingrowth occurred predominately into the pegs and not into the rest of the metal backing, so that a considerable amount of the joint loads was transferred through the pegs to the ingrown bone (24). Eccentric joint loads across the patellofemoral articulating surface created large shear

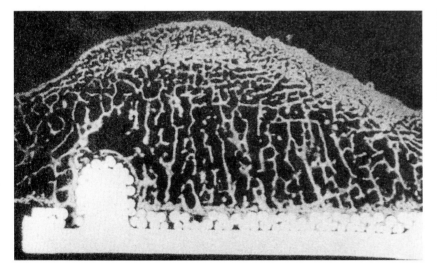

Figure 78.1. Cross-sectional microradiograph of a porous-coated patellar implant retrieved at autopsy, showing bone ingrowth. (From Vigorita VJ, Minkowitz B, Dichira JF, Higham PA. A histomorphometric and histologic analysis of the implant interface in five successful, autopsy-retrieved, noncemented porous-coated knee arthroplasties. Clin Orthop 1993;293:211–218.)

stresses at the junction between the peg and the metal backing, leading to fatigue failure of the pegs (25, 26).

Wear

The large contact forces applied across the patellofemoral joint during normal activities and the large range of motion through which the joint passes make wear of the articulating surfaces unavoidable. As with the natural patella, contact between the patellar and femoral components is generally conforming only near full extension, regardless of design. Through much of the rest of the range of motion, the component surfaces become less conforming, as the patellar component contacts the femoral condyles. The resulting decrease in contact area and the higher joint loads that accompany activities requiring considerable knee flexion combine to increase contact pressure and, therefore, increase the stresses occurring on and within the polyethylene. Since wear mechanisms in polyethylene will be more severe the higher the contact stresses, the shapes of the articulating surfaces of the femoral and patellar components and the resulting contact areas are important design considerations.

Experimental Studies of Contact

Initial contact areas between the patellar and femoral components have been measured experimentally for a number of different design types. These measurements were performed by applying a physiologic load across the joint and measuring the resulting contact area, using a technique such as pressure-sensitive film interposed between the surfaces. The film creates a color patch corresponding to those areas in which the contact pressure exceeded some minimal level. In general, the experimental results showed that the contact areas of contemporary designs are only a fraction of those measured for the natural patella. For example, Cepulo and colleagues (15), in their study of seven different commercially available designs, measured contact areas

of less than 0.2 cm^2 at full flexion for all the designs. Near full extension, the measured contact areas were typically 1 to 1.5 cm^2

In a similar study, Kim and colleagues (27) also measured contact areas for a number of contemporary designs, including all three of the general design solutions (anatomic, dome, and rotating). The patellofemoral joints were loaded in a number of different positions, including medial-lateral tilt of the patella by ±15 degrees and ±10 degrees of medial-lateral rotation and anteroposterior tilt. The contact areas were averaged for all positions tested and reported as a percentage of the contact area measured on the natural patella (Fig. 78.2). As with the results from Cepulo et al. (15), the measured contact areas were less than half those measured in the natural patella, even for components designed to have anatomically shaped articulating surfaces. These results reflect not only the difficulty of designing a conforming patellofemoral geometry throughout the range of motion but also the higher elastic moduli of polyethylene and metal compared with cartilage.

The combination of small contact areas and large physiologic loads creates large contact pressures and, therefore, large stresses in the polyethylene. For example, the pressure-sensitive film used by Cepulo and colleagues (15) in their contact area measurements recorded contact pressures that exceeded 25 MPa for all designs when the knee was tested in 30 and 110 degrees of flexion. In contrast, the yield stress for polyethylene is only 19 MPa (28), so that material in the region of contact could be expected to plastically deform.

Recently, Hsu and Walker (29) investigated the wear behavior of a number of different patellofemoral designs, using a knee joint simulator. The simulator went through a flexion angle from 55 to 100 degrees at 32 cycles of flexion per second. The applied load was 1500 newtons for most of the tests. Distilled water was used as a lubricant. Though this study could be criticized from a number of experimental considerations, the results

Figure 78.2. Contact area (as a percentage of the contact area on the natural patella) for a number of different types of patellofemoral joint designs (27). The axisymmetric designs were of the anatomic type, and the one- and two-plane symmetric designs were of the dome type.

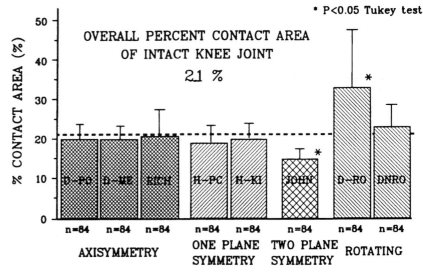

	Test		Base	Load (Newtons)	Number of cycles	Result of test
1	Metal-backed dome	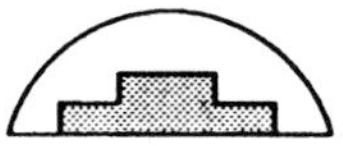	Pedilen	750	192,000	metal penetrated
2	All-plastic dome	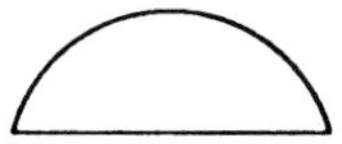	Pedilen	1,500	1,652	Pedilen crushed under load points
3	All-plastic dome	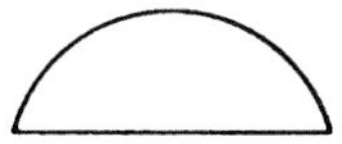	bone	1,500	3,000	bone crushed under load points
4	Metal-backed dome	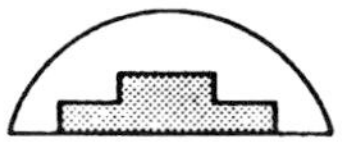	Pedilen	1,500	5,352	metal penetrated
5	All-plastic conforming	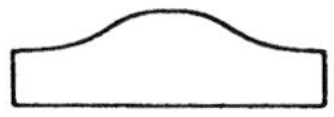	bone	1,500	70,000	some plastic deformation
6	Metal-backed conforming	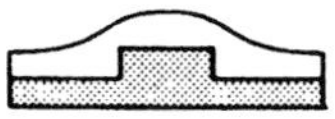	bone	1,500	600,000	partial wear through
7	Metal-backed conforming	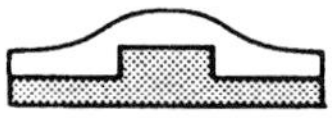	bone	1,500	600,000	partial wear through

Figure 78.3. A review of the experimental results from Hsu and Walker (29), obtained by cyclically loading patellofemoral joint replacements on a knee simulator apparatus.

generated wear-damage modes consistent with those observed in retrieved components, particularly in terms of the contrast in failure modes between all polyethylene and metal-backed component designs (Fig. 78.3).

Observations from Retrieved Components

Evidence of both wear and gross plastic deformation can be found on patellar components retrieved at revision or removal surgery (30–32). Dome-shaped components, for example, experienced considerable damage to the articulating surfaces. The amount of damage was shown to positively correlate with patient weight, patient age, the length of time the component had been implanted, and the range of motion achieved by the patient postoperatively (30, 31). Damage was more severe in components retrieved from male patients than in those retrieved from female patients. All of these clinical factors would be expected to increase either the loads across the patellofemoral joint, the number of load cycles that the joint had to withstand, or both.

Design factors also affected the damage. In particular, a femoral component design with a smaller radius of curvature on the inner edge of the femoral condyles (the original Insall/Burstein Posterior Stabilized design) generated significantly more damage than a design with a larger radius of curvature (the original Total Condylar) (30). These condylar edges contact the patellar component through much of the range of motion. The smaller radius of curvature decreases the contact area between the apposing metal and polyethylene surfaces, leading to increased contact stresses and increased stresses within the polyethylene.

The primary wear-damage modes observed on patellar surfaces are scratching, deformation, and burnishing. These modes, usually associated with abrasive wear mechanisms, dominate because the contact area on the patellar component does not change position appreciably as the knee goes through the range of motion. Points on the polyethylene surface do not, therefore, experience large fluctuations in stresses as the contact area sweeps across them, as has been postulated for tibial components (33, 34). In tibial components, the rollback of the femoral component causes the contact area to sweep across the plateau, so that points on the surface see stresses that alternate between compression and tension. These alternating, cyclic stresses are responsible for pitting and delamination, damage modes associated with fatigue failure mechanisms.

Gross deformation of polyethylene patellar components was also evident in retrieved components (Fig. 78.4). The amount of gross deformation was inversely related to the amount of wear damage observed on the articulating surface (30), though no explanation for this correlation currently exists. The deformation was considerable, and originally circular components often permanently deformed into elliptical shapes in which the major and minor axes differed by more than 5%. Polyethylene deformation occurred in metal-backed patellar components as well. Most metal-backed designs rely on a mechanical interference or dovetail connection to keep the polyethylene and metal portions bonded to one another. The attachment point between the two portions often is designed near the periphery of the component, close to the contact area where large poly-

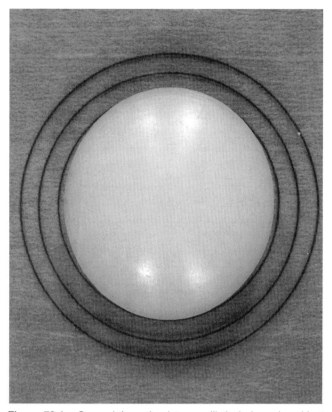

Figure 78.4. Gross deformation into an elliptical shape is evident on this retrieved dome-shaped component that was circular before implantation.

ethylene stresses would be expected. When the polyethylene undergoes large permanent deformation, however, the attachment is compromised, and the polyethylene dissociates from the metallic portion of the component (35–39). The dissociation has often been associated with significant wear and fracture of the polyethylene.

Analytical Studies of Patellofemoral Component Contact

Few analytical studies have examined the stresses occurring on and within patellar components. As with experimental studies, analytical studies can be limited by assumptions about the applied loads and boundary conditions affecting the structure being considered. But such studies do provide an economical means for investigating the effect of parametric changes in important design variables. For example, Bartel et al. (33) used analytical finite element techniques to investigate the effects of component geometry and material properties on the stresses occurring in polyethylene tibial and acetabular components. Their results showed the importance of polyethylene thickness, conformity of the articulating surfaces, and the elastic modulus of the polyethylene in controlling stresses associated with wear damage. In general, stresses increased as component thickness decreased, as the articulating surfaces became less conforming, and as the elastic modulus of

the polyethylene increased. The latter circumstance could occur from intentional alterations in the polyethylene material at the time of fabrication (e.g., the addition of reinforcing carbon fibers) or from chemical degradation of the polyethylene.

The influence of thickness on polyethylene stresses is certainly important to the performance of patellar total knee components. The thickness of patellar implants is usually on the order of only a few millimeters in the regions of contact with the femoral component, so the stresses would be expected to be quite high. This conclusion is consistent with the experimental measurements of contact stresses, which showed stress values well in excess of the yield stress of polyethylene. Furthermore, when a metal backing is included on the component, it is often added at the expense of decreasing the thickness of the remaining polyethylene to maintain the overall thickness of the component. The decreased thickness would be expected to increase stresses even further, as would the addition of a generally unbonded metallic backing (40). Polyethylene thickness is, therefore, one of the major factors explaining the poor mechanical performance of metal-backed patellar components.

Recently, Elbert and colleagues extended the investigation of polyethylene stresses to include patellar components with convex articulating surfaces (41, 42). The goals of the study were to determine the magnitude and distribution of stresses on and within the patellar component and to examine the effect on the stresses of assuming the patellar surface had experienced wear and deformation through use. Three-dimensional finite element models of a dome-design patellar component were constructed. Two different geometries were used to model the articulating surface of the component. In one model, the geometry of the surface was that of a newly manufactured component. In the second model, the surface geometry was that of a retrieved patellar component with two worn and deformed contact areas. The component had been implanted in an active male patient for 15 months before being removed as part of revision surgery for a loosened tibial component. The worn contact areas resulted from articulation with the femoral condyles while the component had been implanted. Within the contact areas, the articulating surface was no longer convex, but rather had worn and deformed into a concave geometry.

Both models included a metal backing to which the polyethylene was assumed to be rigidly fixed. The contact load was 750 newtons and was obtained from a force analysis of the patella for a 76-kg individual during normal gait. Several types of stresses were examined: the range of maximum principal stress and the maximum shear stress (both of which have been implicated in wear-damage mechanisms involving fatigue fracture of polyethylene (33, 34)) and the von Mises stress (which can be used as a yield criterion for material failure through permanent deformation).

The results of the analyses showed that the range of maximum principal stress and the maximum shear stress were more severe when the surface geometry

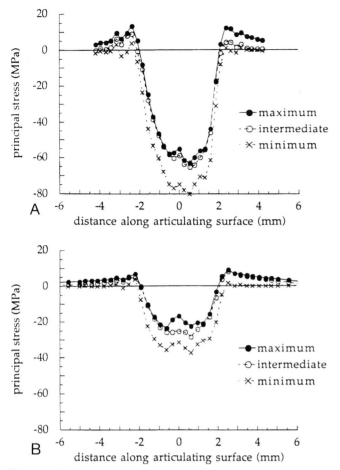

Figure 78.5. Principal stresses plotted against the distance along the articulating surface for the analytical models of Elbert and colleagues (41, 42). **A,** Results from the model in which the patellar component had the geometry of a newly manufactured dome-shaped patellar component. **B,** Results from the model with the geometry of a retrieved component.

was convex (as in a newly manufactured component) than when the surface geometry matched that of a retrieved component. The range of maximum principal stress was about 70 MPa for the new-component geometry (Fig. 78.5A). The range decreased by more than half when the surface geometry was that of the retrieved component (Fig. 78.5B). For either geometry, the principal stresses were compressive in the contact area and were tensile at the articulating surface at the edge of the contact area.

The largest maximum shear stress was found about 1 to 2 mm below the surface, similar to the situation in concave polyethylene tibial components in total knee replacements (33). As with the range of maximum principal stress, the maximum shear stress was much larger in the geometry of a newly manufactured component than in the retrieved patellar geometry. The maximum shear stress for the newly manufactured geometry was also greater than had been previously reported for tibial components (33), while the maximum shear stress for the retrieved patellar component geometry was similar to that found for tibial components.

For both component geometries, the von Mises stress was at or near the yield stress for polyethylene within the contact area. The von Mises stress reached 40 MPa for the new component geometry and 20 MPa for the retrieved geometry. The magnitudes of these stresses are consistent with the gross deformation often observed in retrieved patellar components and suggest that permanent deformation would have continued in the retrieved component had it remained implanted beyond 15 months.

Summary

Patellar resurfacing in total knee arthroplasty has proven effective at relieving pain and restoring function. Patellar complications remain a serious problem, but are more affected by anatomy and surgical technique than by component design. As with other total joint implants, however, there are design factors that are important to the mechanical performance of the device. The orthopaedic surgeon can make a rational choice based on consideration of these factors.

References

1. Abraham W, Buchanan JR, Daubert H, et al. Should the patella be resurfaced in total knee arthroplasty? Efficacy of patellar resurfacing. Clin Orthop 1988;236:128–134.
2. Cameron HU. The patella in total knee arthroplasty. In: Laskin RS, ed. Total knee replacement. London: Springer-Verlag, 1991:199–210.
3. Soudry M, Mestriner LA, Binazzi R, Insall JN. Total knee arthroplasty without patellar resurfacing. Clin Orthop 1986;205:166–170.
4. Picetti GD, McGann WA, Welch RB. The patellofemoral joint after total knee arthroplasty without patellar resurfacing, J Bone Joint Surg 1990;72A:1379–1382.
5. Grace J, Rand JA. Patellar instability after total knee arthroplasty. Clin Orthop 1988;237:184–189.
6. Bindeglass DF, Cohen JL, Dorr LD. Patellar tilt and subluxation in total knee arthroplasty. Relationship to pain, fixation, and design. Clin Orthop 1993;286:103–109.
7. Reilly DT, Martens M. Experimental analysis of the quadriceps muscle force and patello-femoral joint reaction force for various activities. Acta Orthop Scand 1972;43:126–137.
8. Huberti HH, Hayes WC. Patellofemoral contact pressures. The influence of Q-angle and tendofemoral contact. J Bone Joint Surg 1984;66A:715–724.
9. Van Kampen A, Huiskes R, Blankevoort L, Van Rens ThJG. The three-dimensional tracking pattern of the patella in the human knee joint. Trans Orthop Res Soc 1986;11:386.
10. Rhoads DD, Noble PC, Reuben JD, et al. The effect of femoral component position on patellar tracking after total knee arthroplasty. Clin Orthop 1990;260:43–51.
11. Kaltwasser P, Uematsu O, Walker PS. The patello-femoral joint in total knee replacement. Trans Orthop Res Soc 1987;12:292.
12. Hungerford DS, Kenna RV. Preliminary experience with a total knee prosthesis with porous coating used without cement. Clin Orthop 1983;176:95–107.
13. Buechel FF, Rosa RA, Pappas MJ. A metal-backed rotating-bearing patellar prosthesis to lower contact stress. An 11-year clinical study. Clin Orthop 1989;248:34–49.
14. Freeman MAR, Samuelson KM, Elias SG, et al. The patellofemoral joint in total knee prostheses. Design considerations. J Arthroplasty 1989;(suppl):S69-S74.
15. Cepulo AJ, Stahurski TM, Moran JM, et al. Mechanical characteristics of patello-femoral replacements. Trans Orthop Res Soc 1983;8:41.
16. Bartel DL, Burstein AH, Santavicca EA, Insall JN. Performance of the tibial component in total knee replacement. J Bone Joint Surg 1982;64A:1026–1033.
17. Pedersen DR, Crowninshield RD, Brand RA, Johnston RC. An axisymmetric model of acetabular components in total hip arthroplasty. J Biomech 1982;15:305–315.
18. Willert H-G, Semlitsch M. Reactions of the articular capsule to wear

products of artificial joint prostheses. J Biomed Mater Res 1977;11:157–164.

19. Engh CA, Bobyn JD. Biologic fixation in total hip arthroplasty. Thorofare, N.J.: Slack, 1985.

20. Vigorita VJ, Minkowitz B, Dichira JF, Higham PA. A histomorphometric and histologic analysis of the implant interface in five successful, autopsy-retrieved, noncemented porous-coated knee arthroplasties. Clin Orthop 1993;293:211–218.

21. Schmalzried TP, Kwong LM, Jasty M, et al. The mechanism of loosening of cemented acetabular components in total hip arthroplasty: analysis of specimens retrieved at autopsy. Clin Orthop 1992;274:60–78.

22. Tsao A, Mintz L, McCrae CR, et al. Severe polyethylene wear in failed PCA total knee arthroplasties. J Bone Joint Surg 1993;75A:19–26.

23. Engh GA, Dwyer KA, Hanes CK. Polyethylene wear of metal-backed tibial components in total and unicompartmental knee prostheses. J Bone Joint Surg 1992;74B:9–17.

24. Dawson JM, Bartel DL. Consequences of an interference fit on the fixation of porous-coated tibial components in total knee replacement. J Bone Joint Surg 1992;74A:233–238.

25. Rosenberg AG, Andriacchi TP, Barden R, Galante JO. Patellar component failure in cementless total knee arthroplasty. Clin Orthop 1988;236:106–114.

26. Cheal EJ, Gerhart TN, Hayes WC. Failure analysis of a porous coated patellar component. In: Lewis JL, ed. Computational methods in bioengineering. New York: American Soc Mech Eng, 1989:211–221.

27. Kim W, Chao EYS, Rand JA. Comparative evaluation of patellofemoral contact area in different total knee designs. Trans Orthop Res Soc 1992;17:326.

28. Wright TM, Rimnac CM. Ultra-high-molecular-weight polyethylene. In: Morrey BF, ed. Joint replacement arthroplasty. New York: Churchill Livingstone, 1991:37–45.

29. Hsu H-P, Walker PS. Wear and deformation of patellar components in total knee arthroplasty. Clin Orthop 1989;246:260–265.

30. Figgie MP, Wright TM, Santner T, Fisher D, Forbes A. Performance of dome-shaped patellar components in total knee arthroplasty. Trans Orthop Res Soc 1989;14:531.

31. deSwart RJ, Stulberg BN, Gaisser DM, Reger SI. Wear characteristics of all polyethylene patellar components: a retrieval analysis. Trans Orthop Res Soc 1989;14:367.

32. Hood RW, Wright TM, Fukubayashi T, Burstein AH. Retrieval analysis of total knee prostheses. A method and its application to 48 total condylar prostheses. J Biomed Mater Res 1983;17:829–842.

33. Bartel DL, Bicknell VL, Wright TM. The effect of conformity, thickness, and material on stresses in UHMWPE components for total joint replacement. J Bone Joint Surg 1986;68A:1041–1051.

34. Bartel DL, Rimnac CM, Wright TM. Evaluation and design of the articular surface. In: Goldberg V, ed. Controversies of total knee arthroplasty. New York: Raven Press, 1991:61–74.

35. Rosenberg AG, Andriacchi TP, Barden R, Galante JO. Patellar component failure in cementless total knee arthroplasty. Clin Orthop 1988;236:106–114.

36. Bayley JC, Scott RD, Ewald FC, Holmes GB Jr. Metal backed patellar component failure following total knee replacement. J Bone Joint Surg 1988;70A:668–674.

37. Lombardi AV Jr, Engh GA, Volz RG, Albrigo JL, Brainard BJ. Fracture/dissociation of the polyethylene in metal-backed patellar components in total knee arthroplasty. J Bone Joint Surg 1988;70A:675-679.

38. Stulberg SD, Stulberg BN, Hamati Y, Tsao A. Failure mechanisms of metal-backed patellar components. Clin Orthop 1988;236:88–105.

39. Sutherland CJ. Patellar component dissociation in total knee arthroplasty: a report of two cases. Clin Orthop 1988;228:178–181.

40. Bartel DL, Wright TM, Edwards D. The effect of metal backing on stresses in polyethylene. In: Hungerford DS, ed. The hip. St. Louis: CV Mosby, 1983:229–239.

41. Elbert K, Bartel D, Wright T. The effect of conformity on stresses in dome shaped polyethylene patellar components. J Orthop Res, submitted.

42. Elbert K. Analysis of polyethylene in total joint replacement [Dissertation]. Ithaca, N. Y.: Cornell University, 1991.

79

Patellar Complications Related to Tracking

William J. Hozack

Soft Tissue Impingement
Instability
    Pathogenesis and Prevention
    Lateral Retinacular Release
    Treatment
    Conclusions

Dealing properly with the patellofemoral joint during total knee arthroplasty presents a major challenge to the reconstructive orthopaedic surgeon. Failure to meet this challenge can lead to a variety of problems including fracture, wear, instability, and soft tissue impingement (9, 17, 18, 24, 28). Directly or indirectly, each of these individual problems can usually be traced to an underlying problem with patellar tracking. This chapter reviews the scope of patellar complications related to tracking, including etiology, pathogenesis, prevention, and treatment. Since fracture and wear complications are discussed elsewhere, this chapter concentrates on the problems of soft tissue impingement and instability.

Soft Tissue Impingement

Soft tissue impingement encompasses a spectrum of problems related to fibrous tissue formation around the patella (Fig. 79.1). This fibrous tissue probably represents a response to abnormal pressure and contact of the patella and its component against the other components in the total knee replacement, although Cameron (8) feels that some fibrous tissue formation with associated crepitation would occur in all total knee replacements. While annoying, this "meniscus" of fibrous tissue might actually protect the underlying patellar button from wear. For the most part, however, aggressive fibrous tissue formation leads to symptoms such as pain, limitation of motion, or persistent and annoying crepitus necessitating operative intervention.

Three variations of the syndrome of soft tissue impingement have been described. Pettine and Bryan (30) described a phenomenon of dense fibrous hypertrophy. Their five patients developed enlarged painful infrapatellar masses that led to reduced motion. This enlarged fibrotic infrapatellar fat pad responded well to excision, but excision of the fat pad at the original surgery did not seem to protect against this complication. No pathogenetic mechanism was identified.

Another variation of this syndrome has been described by Thorpe et al. (40). In 11 of 635 total knee arthroplasties, painful crepitus and maltracking of the patella was attributed to intraarticular fibrous bands (Fig. 79.2). Symptoms occurred as the knee was brought from the flexed position into extension, but range of motion was not decreased. The pathogenesis of the symptoms was tethering of the patella by fibrous bands, either superiorly and transversely (type I), laterally (type II), or inferiorly (type III). The pathogenesis of the fibrous bands was not clear as no specific abnormality of patellofemoral or femorotibial mechanics could be identified. Arthroscopic treatment appeared to successfully eradicate symptoms.

Possibly the most common presentation of the soft tissue impingement syndrome is the patellar clunk syndrome (19) (Fig. 79.3). It consists of patellar pain with a normal range of motion. A catch or clunk of the patella is noted upon knee extension. While the pathology is a prominent fibrous nodule at the proximal pole of the patella (akin to the type I lesion described by Thorpe et al. (40)), the pathogenesis is not clear (Fig. 79.4). It is most likely related to changes in the mechanics about the patellofemoral joint after total knee replacement, as first outlined by Figgie et al. (10). In their review of 116 total knee arthroplasties, they found a significant increase in the development of symptoms secondary to fibrous tissue formation with a failure to maintain a normal joint line location after surgical reconstruction of the degenerated knee. This finding was echoed by Aglietti et al. (1, 2).

Another potential source of this syndrome may be related to component design. As noted by several authors (1, 2, 19), the early posterior-stabilized total condylar knee design with a sharp femoral component anterior notch may have served as a source of irritation, resulting in fibrous tissue formation. Hirsh et al. (16) also implicated impingement against components as a cause, although they believed that the tibial eminence might be

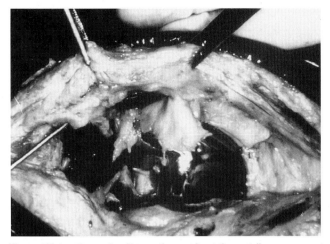

Figure 79.1. Excessive fibrous tissue about the patellar component in this patient required surgical excision. Femoral component to the *right,* tibial component to the *left,* patellar component in *center.*

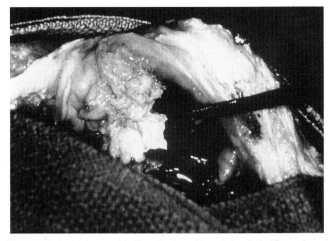

Figure 79.3 Hypertrophic fibrous tissue at proximal patellar pole resulting in "patellar clunk" syndrome. Side view, *left* is proximal, femoral component is at the *bottom,* forceps point to partially inverted patellar button, and fibrous nodule is in the *center.* (Reproduced with permission from Hozack WJ, Booth RE. Patellar complications in total knee arthroplasty. Complications in Orthopaedics 1991;March/April:57–73.)

Figure 79.2. **A,** Type I fibrous band. Fibrous band prevents the patella from seating well into the sulcus of the femoral component. This type of fibrous band may cause symptoms similar to those of the "patellar clunk syndrome." **B,** Type II fibrous band. This type of fibrous band tethers the patella laterally as the knee bends and extends. **C,** Type III fibrous band. This fibrous band extends from the distal pole of the patella to the intercondylar notch, tethering the patella inferiorly. (Reproduced with permission from Thorpe CD, Bocell JR, Tullos HS. Intra-articular fibrous bands: patellar complications after total knee replacement. J Bone Joint Surg 1990;72A:811–814.

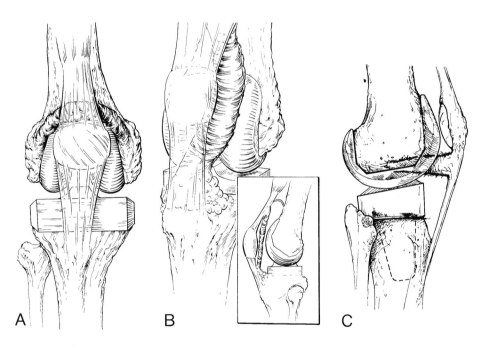

A B C

the source of impingement. Probably, the combination of patella baja and component design leads to the patella clunk phenomenon—my recent experience with a modified femoral component design has seen a reduction, but not complete elimination, of patellar clunk symptoms. The key in avoiding this problem is to try to maintain an anatomic joint line during surgery, to avoid patella baja, and to avoid femoral components with sharp intercondylar notch outlines.

Treatment alternatives for soft tissue impingement problems include conservative modalities, operative excision with or without component revision, and arthroscopic intervention. Case reports in the literature as-

cribe success to each of these choices (1, 2, 4, 16, 19, 40, 41). In an attempt to provide a rationale for treatment, a review of 1484 posterior-stabilized total knee arthroplasties was undertaken at my institution (3). Twenty patellar clunks in 19 patients (6 men and 13 women, with an average age of 69 years at arthroplasty) were identified. The clunks developed at an average 10.6 months (range 2 to 34 months) post–prosthetic implantation. All patients exhibited an audible or palpable clunk, and eight experienced pain when extending the knee from flexed position. Only 4 of the 20 clunks resolved with nonoperative measures, which included quadriceps-strengthening exercises and cortisone injec-

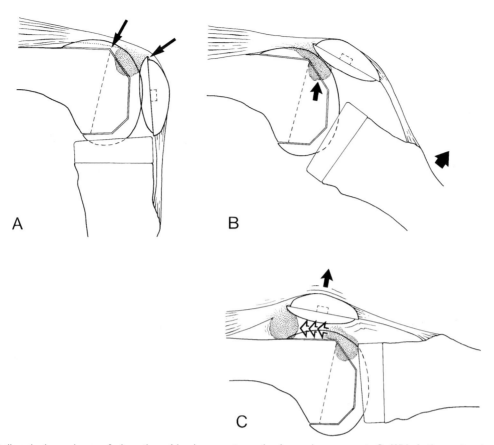

Figure 79.4.   Patellar clunk syndrome. **A,** Location of impingement (*arrows*). Most common area is at anterosuperior intercondylar notch area of femoral component. Secondarily, an overhanging patellar component may impinge as shown. **B,** As knee is brought toward extension, fibrous nodule is locked into the intercondylar notch area of the femoral component. **C,** With further extension, the nodule suddenly pops and comes to lie proximally. The patient experiences clunking sensation at this point. (Reproduced with permission from Hozack WJ, Booth RE. Patellar complications in total knee arthroplasty. Complication in Orthopaedics 1991;March/April:57–73.)

tions. Fourteen surgical procedures—11 arthroscopic debridements and 3 arthrotomies with patellar button revision—were performed in 10 patients. Although the clunk resolved after nodular excision in all patients, four clunks recurred after arthroscopic debridement. No recurrences were seen following arthrotomy, nodule extirpation, and button revision. Six clunks persist. Of these six patients, four have refused surgical intervention, and two developed recurrences after arthroscopic debridement but have refused additional operative intervention.

Based on my experience and that of others, the following treatment guidelines are recommended. Conservative measures (quadriceps exercises and injections) are unlikely to eliminate symptoms. However, in some instances, this initial conservative approach can alleviate symptoms sufficiently to avoid surgical intervention. If the conservative approach fails, arthroscopic debridement is indicated (Fig. 79.5). However, in up to one third of patients, symptoms may recur. Arthrotomy should be reserved for those patients with recurrences after arthroscopic debridement and those with either a loose or malpositioned patellar component.

Instability

Patellar instability is the most frequent extensor mechanism complication. Most often manifested as subluxation or dislocation, it is likely that many instances of patellar component wear or patellar fracture can be traced to a derangement of patellar tracking (Figs. 79.6 and 79.7) (13, 23, 39). Dislocation of the patella is rare but usually quite dramatic (11). Subluxation of the patella can be much more subtle. However, both dislocation and subluxation are caused by the same underlying pathogenetic mechanisms: limb malalignment, component malalignment, improper component design, improper patellar preparation, muscle imbalance, and trauma. Remember that each of these mechanisms continues to operate, even if the patella is not resurfaced (38).

Pathogenesis and Prevention

Limb malalignment in the form of excessive valgus of the anatomic femorotibial axis causes patellar instability by creating an abnormal Q angle, thereby altering the pull of the quadriceps muscle (Fig. 79.8). The overall limb alignment may be still normal, yet component

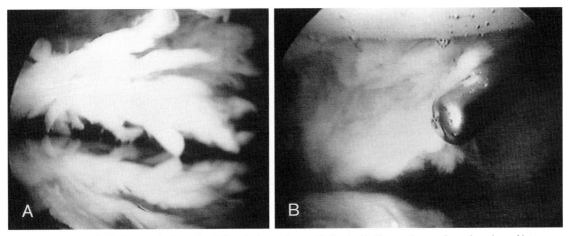

Figure 79.5. **A,** Arthroscopic view of patellar clunk syndrome. Patient with fibrous tissue obscuring view of knee joint. **B,** Postarthroscopic resection. The patellar component is visible at the *top*.

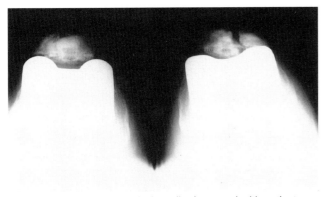

Figure 79.6. Bilateral vertical patellar fractures in this patient are most likely related to abnormal patellar tracking.

malalignment may be severe enough to cause patellar instability (Fig. 79.9). While much of the attention in patellofemoral instability has focused upon the patella, subtle abnormalities with femoral or tibial position and alignment are probably the most common sources of this problem.

Placing the femoral component in more than 7 degrees of valgus with respect to the axis of the femur may create a situation in which the resultant force of the quadriceps tends to cause the patella to subluxate laterally. This is most common in the degenerative valgus knee in which the distal lateral femoral condyle has significantly eroded (Fig. 79.10). In this situation, intramedullary instrumentation of the femur for the distal femoral cut can avoid improper femoral component alignment.

Medial-lateral position of the femoral component also affects patellar stability (Fig. 79.11). In a cadaveric study, Rhoads et al. (33) found that 5 mm of medial displacement of the femoral condyle increased medial patellar tilt during the initial 60 degrees of flexion. The femoral component in this study included a high lateral flange constraining the patellar component so that no increase in dislocation or subluxation was seen.

Rather, increased pressure was created within the patellofemoral joint—this could translate in the clinical situation to eccentric wear, component fracture, or component dissociation. Without the flange to prevent patellar instability, dislocation or subluxation is likely. More lateral placement of the femoral component seems to reduce this problem.

Rotational abnormalities of femoral component position also predispose to instability of the patellar component. With internal rotation, a medial shift of the patellar groove occurs with a resultant increase in tension on the lateral retinacular structures (33). This internal rotation is usually caused by the use of instrumentation that references the posterior femoral condyles for femoral component position (5). Unrecognized deficiencies of the posterior lateral femoral condyle obligate an internal rotation to the femoral component (Fig. 79.12).

Clinically, there are two reliable techniques to avoid this problem. If a proper tibial cut has already been made, the femoral anteroposterior cutting guide can be externally rotated to balance the flexion gap (Fig. 79.12). That is, the surgeon converts the flexion gap from a trapezoid to a rectangle. Alternatively, the surgeon can rotate the cutting guide externally just to the point where anterior femoral notching would occur. As of now, there are no data to suggest that external rotation of the femoral component to this extent (usually less than 5 degrees) will adversely affect knee mechanics (33).

Tibial component alignment errors can also influence patellofemoral functional results (27). These errors are more important as femorotibial component congruence increases. Nagamine et al. (29) evaluated patellar shift with various degrees of internal and external rotation of partially constrained tibial components in cadaveric specimens. Externally rotating the partially constrained tibial tray caused the tibia to rotate internally with flexion and significantly shifted the patella medially. While internally rotating the tibial tray did not cause subluxation, the tibia itself did externally rotate with flexion, thus causing

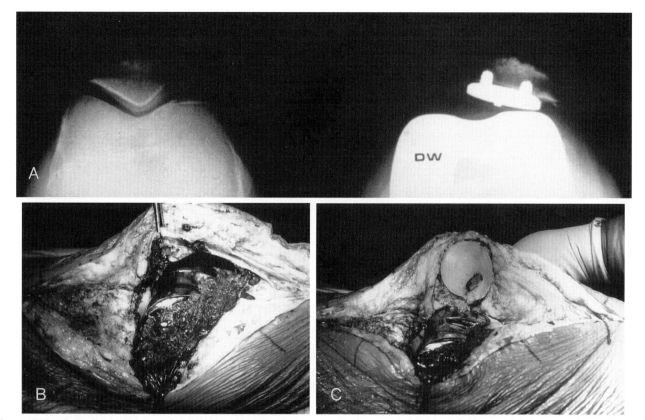

Figure 79.7.   A, Radiographic view of metal-backed patellar component with instability and polyethylene wear. **B,** Intraoperative picture of extensive black synovitis created by metal-on-metal contact. **C,** After removal of black synovitic material, the area of excessive polyethylene wear on the patellar component is easily visible.

an increase in the Q angle. The authors believed that while subluxation was prevented by the expanded lateral flange on the femoral component, internal rotation of the tibial component could lead to wear, fracture, or dissociation. Without the constraint of the lateral femoral flange, patellofemoral instability would result. As suggested by Merkow et al. (27), "correct rotational positioning of the tibial component is best achieved by aligning the intracondylar eminence of the tibial component with the tibial crest in the sagittal plane" (Fig. 79.13).

However, overemphasis on placing the tibial component in the external rotation is unwise. Exaggerated external rotation of the tibial plateau leads to a mismatch of the arc of motion of the knee determined by the ligaments and that imposed by the femorotibial congruency. This can lead to abnormally high contract stresses between the femoral component and the tibial plateau, thus promoting excessive polyethylene wear (Fig. 79.14). The best compromise is to perform component trial reductions before selecting tibial rotational alignment. Using a pegless tibial trial, the knee should be taken through a full range of motion several times. In doing so, the tibial component trial will generally seek its correct rotational alignment, based on the femoral component alignment and the overall ligament tension.

The actual femoral component design plays an important role in patellofemoral stability. Several authors suggest that merely deepening the anterior femoral groove can be beneficial. Freeman (12) suggests a 5-mm deepening. Yoshii et al. (42) demonstrated an increase in patellofemoral stability by deepening the femoral groove 1 mm from an initial 3 mm. This study also demonstrated the added benefit of a raised lateral femoral flange. However, a high femoral flange may prevent patellofemoral instability but at the cost of abnormal wear, increased patellar fracture, and increased incidence of patellar component dissociation (Fig. 79.15). This is also true of anatomically designed patellar components. Slight malrotation of these components can have serious consequences (11). Therefore, a dome-shaped patella is recommended. Remember, design modifications of the femoral and patellar components alone will be insufficient if other factors potentiating patellar instability are ignored.

Errors in preparation of the patella are easy to make but difficult to appreciate intraoperatively. Ideally, the patella should be cut to create a symmetrical remnant onto which the patella component is placed. Furthermore, the overall height of the patella should be maintained. Increases in patellar height increase the stresses on the lateral retinacular structures and can lead directly to dislocation or subluxation (Fig. 79.16). Proximal or distal asymmetry of the cut can have the same effect. An asymmetric cut with selective overthickening of the lateral side of the patella again increases lateral

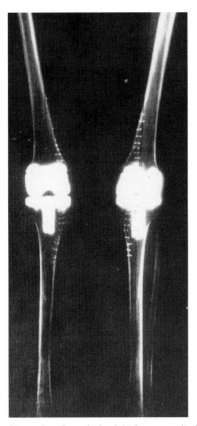

Figure 79.8. Excessive Q-angle in right knee results in patellar instability. The patellar component is just visible over the superolateral edge of the femoral component.

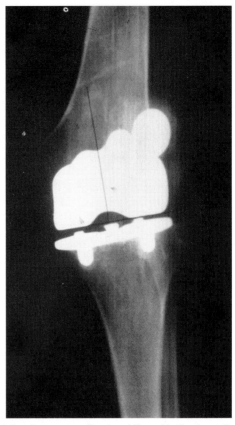

Figure 79.9. Severe patellar instability with fixed patellar dislocation. Aside from soft tissue imbalance, component alignment was a critical etiologic factor. Tibial component is in 7 degrees of varus and femoral component is in 12 degrees of valgus. Three-component revision was necessary to correct this problem. (Reproduced with permission from Hozack WJ, Booth RE. Patellar complications in total knee arthroplasty. Complications in Orthopaedics 1991;March/April:57–73.)

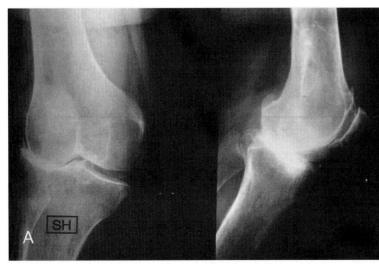

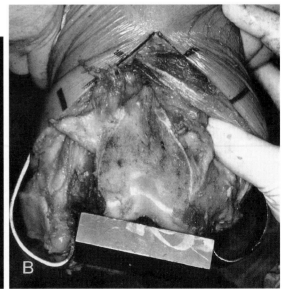

Figure 79.10. **A,** Radiographic view of valgus knee with deficiency of distal-lateral femoral condyle. **B,** Intraoperative view of the same knee with block on distal femur after anterior cut was made. A distal cut made parallel to the distal femur would result in a femoral component being placed in excessive valgus with respect to the long axis of the femur. In this situation, intramedullary instrumentation would avoid an incorrect distal femoral cut and, therefore, improper femoral component alignment.

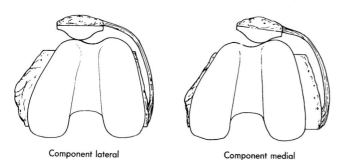

Component lateral   Component medial

Figure 79.11. Illustration of how medial placement of the femoral component increases the tension on the lateral retinacular structures and predisposes to patellar instability or abnormal patellar plastic wear. (Reproduced with permission from Krackow KA. The technique of total knee arthroplasty. St. Louis, CV Mosby, 1990.)

retinacular tightness, thus leading to subluxation (Fig. 79.17).

Accurate patellar resection requires proper exposure. All osteophytes must be removed. The goal is to cut the patella parallel to its anterior surface. Caliper measurement before and after cutting aids in proper resection technique (32). Direct palpation of the patella is critical. Bimanual palpation of the patella, using the thumb and forefinger of each hand, allows the surgeon to better assess the three-dimensional shape of the patella after the initial cut—evaluating the symmetry or lack thereof in both the proximal-distal and medial-lateral direction. Secondary cuts should be made until the patella surface is deemed proper.

After bony resection, the patellar surface is rarely circular—rather it is oblong from medial to lateral (Fig. 79.18). As discussed by Briard (5) and evaluated by Yoshii (42) in cadaveric specimens, medial placement of a symmetrical dome-shaped patellar component allows proper patellar component tracking without excess tightening of the lateral retinacular structures (Fig. 79.19). An alternative, an eccentrically domed patellar component, achieves the same results with more complete coverage of the patellar bone (5).

Trauma or poor suturing technique can also lead to rupture of the medical retinacular structures and thus patellar femoral instability. While uncommon, these complications demand immediate surgical correction.

Lateral Retinacular Release

Assessing the lateral retinacular structures is an important surgical step in total knee replacement. Failure to perform a lateral retinacular release when indicated can lead to patellofemoral instability. However, performing a lateral retinacular release cannot by itself restore patellofemoral stability if the previously mentioned pathogenic mechanisms—limb malalignment, component malalignment, and patellar preparation errors—are not corrected first.

Assuming that these pathogenic mechanisms are not in play, there are times when the patellofemoral joint is not "balanced" after placement of components. The motion of the patella with respect to the femur must be ob-

served directly. In addition, the "no-thumb technique" must be used (i.e., no external pressure should be exerted by the surgeon or the assistant onto the patella during the stability evaluation (37)). Any subluxation or even tilting of the patellar component is best treated via lateral release. Rae et al. (31) recommended a "one stitch" test. A single suture placed adjacent to the patella to close the capsule should not cut out during flexion. If it does, a lateral retinacular release is needed.

The exact technique of lateral retinacular release varies from surgeon to surgeon. However, before undertaking a lateral retinacular release, several bands of tissue stretching from the femur to the patella (patellofemoral capsular ligaments) should be incised (Fig. 79.20). Only if patellofemoral subluxation persists after this simple step, should formal retinacular release be undertaken. In general, a lateral release is best done from an intracapsular approach, to minimize soft tissue dissection superficial to the patella. Significant decrements in transcutaneous oxygen tension and increases in wound discoloration and superficial wound infection have been demonstrated after a lateral retinacular release (20). An intracapsular approach with preservation of the superolateral genicular vessels minimizes the serious consequences of delayed wound healing. The lateral retinaculum is incised approximately 1.5 to 2 cm lateral to the lateral patellar edge, placing it between the fibers of the iliotibial band and the patella (27). As demonstrated by Kayler and Lyttle (21), lateral retinacular releases within 1.5 cm of the patella seriously compromise lateral parapatellar circulation and intraosseous blood flow. Occasionally, a partial lateral retinacular release may be sufficient for patellofemoral stabilization. If not, this incision is carried proximally past the superior lateral genicular vessels traversing horizontally 1 to 2 cm below the inferior border of the vastus lateralis muscle (Brick, 1988) and then preserved if possible (Fig. 79.21).

Much attention has been focused upon the advisability and consequences of a lateral retinacular release. Scuderi et al. (36) did a clinical and scintigraphic evaluation of 36 total knee arthroplasty patients. Technetium bone scans revealed a higher incidence of vascular compromise (56% versus 15%) in knees with a lateral release than in those without. This effect upon the circulation was confirmed in a later scintigraphic study by McMahon et al. (26). In these two studies, no attempt was made to preserve the superior lateral genicular artery system. These reports and that by Brick and Scott (6) suggest that lateral retinacular release leads to avascular necrosis of the patella, thus predisposing to patellar fracture. In contrast, Ritter et al. (1989) studied 48 total knee arthroplasty patients who underwent bilateral replacements in which only one side underwent lateral retinacular release, and found no clinical or radiographic differences. Furthermore, scintigraphic evaluation revealed no evidence of patellar avascular necrosis. Another study by Ritter and Campbell (34) found a statistically significant higher incidence of fracture in patients who did not undergo lateral retinacular release (1.5% of 471 total knee arthroplasties) as compared to

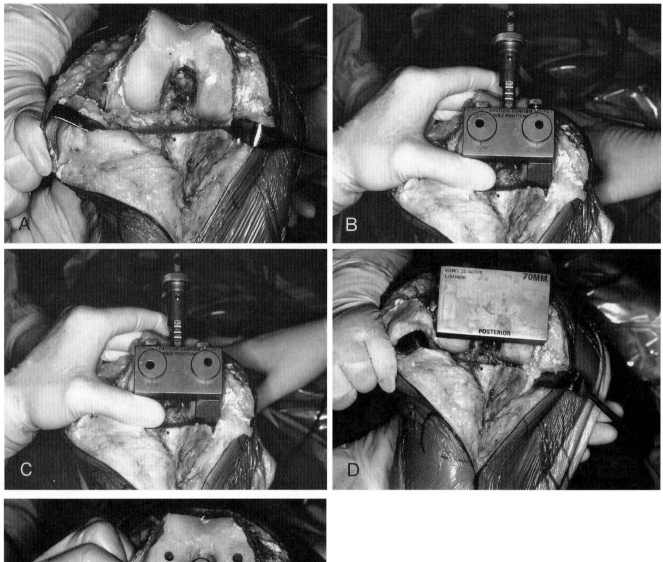

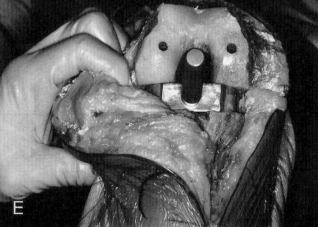

Figure 79.12. **A,** Anatomic positioning of the femoral component referencing the posterior femoral condyles will result in internal rotation of the femoral component. This will lead to increased patellofemoral instability. **B,** A femoral component cutting guide referencing the posterior femoral condyle is placed. The drill holes are placed in the anatomic position. **C,** By rotating the left drill hole guide, the femoral component is externally rotated in the femur. **D,** Placement of the anterior-posterior femoral cutting guide showing external rotation of the guide on the distal femur. Notice the asymmetric cut of the posterior femoral condyles, with less being cut from the posterior lateral femoral condyle. In addition, the flexion gap is now equal both medially and laterally. **E,** External rotation of the femoral component results in improved patellofemoral stability and equality of the flexion gap and, therefore, improved femorotibial stability in flexion.

Rotational malalignment = patellar dislocation

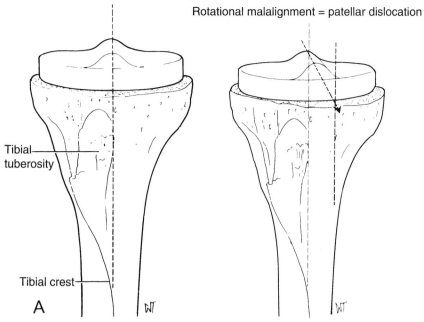

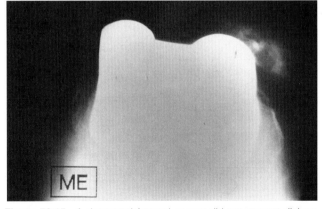

Figure 79.13.   A, Rotational malalignment of the tibial component as shown results in patellar dislocation. As the knee moves through the range of motion, the tibia is forced into external rotation by the congruency of the femoral and tibial components. This exaggerates the Q-angle and potentiates patellar instability. Correct alignment of the tibial component with the medial border of the tibial tuberosity will

minimize this problem. (Reproduced with permission from Merkow RL, Soundry M, Insall JN. Patellar dislocation following total knee replacement. J Bone Joint Surg 1985;67A:1321–1327.) **B,** Intraoperatively, this position is easily identified and marked to avoid inadvertent internal rotation of the tibial component during the surgery.

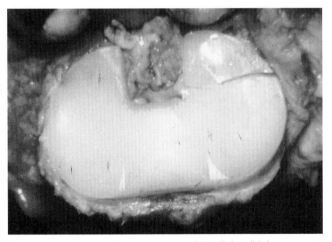

Figure 79.14.   Excessive external rotation of the tibial component can result in a mismatch of the arch of motion of the knee determined by the ligaments and the arc of motion imposed by the femoral-tibial congruency. The result is exaggerated and premature polyethylene wear.

Figure 79.15   A deepened femoral groove did not prevent dislocation in this patient. The surgeon cannot rely solely on component design to ensure patellofemoral stability.

those who received a lateral retinacular release (3.6% of 84 total knee arthroplasties). The likely explanation is that patellar fracture is more closely related to the abnormal stresses of instability than to avascular necrosis. As Merkow (27) observed, although there is a recognized risk of vascular damage to the patella with lateral retinacular release, the problems of patellar instability are overriding, and therefore adequate lateral retinacu-

lar release takes precedence over considerations of patellar vascularity.

Treatment

Considering the complexity of the pathogenesis of patellofemoral impingement, it is unwise to presume that treatment will be straightforward or simple. I am increasingly convinced that attempts at soft tissue re-

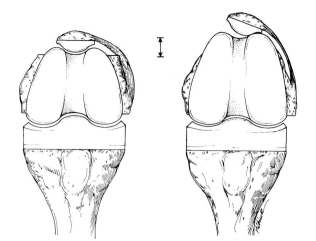

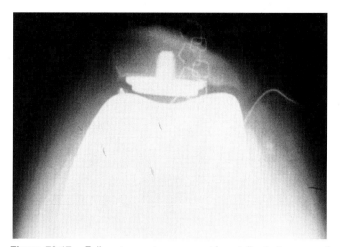

Figure 79.16. Increasing patellar height through either increased thickness of the reconstructed patella or increased thickness of reconstructed femur results in increased tension on the lateral retinacular structures and, therefore, a tendency to either patellar instability or premature patellar wear or fracture. (Reproduced with permission from Krackow KA. The technique of total knee arthroplasty. St. Louis: CV Mosby, 1990.)

Figure 79.17. Failure to create a symmetric patellar in the coronal plane contributed to instability in this patient. Patella revision, proximal quadriceps realignment, and tibial tuberosity transfer were required to correct the problem. (Reproduced with premission from Hozack WJ, Booth RE. Patellar complications in total knee arthroplasty. Complications in Orthopaedics 1991;March/April:57–73.)

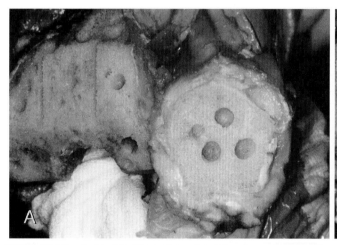

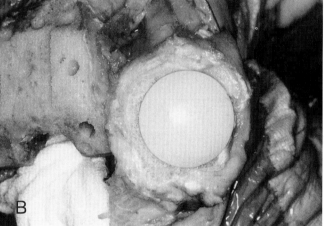

Figure 79.18. **A,** Asymmetric surface of patella after resection cut and preparation for patellar component placement. **B,** Placement of the patellar component trial emphasizes the asymmetry of the resid-

ual patellar bone. The patellar component should be placed as medially as possible, to insure proper component tracking.

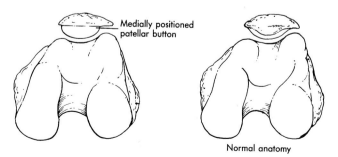

Figure 79.19. Diagrammatic representation of medially positioned patellar button which allows patellar component tracking in a more normal configuration without excess tightening of the lateral retinacular structures. (Reproduced with permission from Krackow KA. The technique of total knee arthroplasty. St. Louis: CV Mosby, 1990.)

alignment should be sublimated to attempts to correct the real source of the problem. That is, since the problem of patellofemoral instability is most commonly related to a component position error, component revision should be considered before soft tissue realignment as a means of correcting patellofemoral instability.

Soft tissue realignment can be performed proximal or distal to the patella. Although each of these procedures incorporates a lateral retinacular release into the procedure, lateral release alone rarely corrects the problem. However, Bocell et al. (4) successfully treated two patients with patellar subluxation using arthroscopic lateral retinacular releases. Merkow et al. (27)

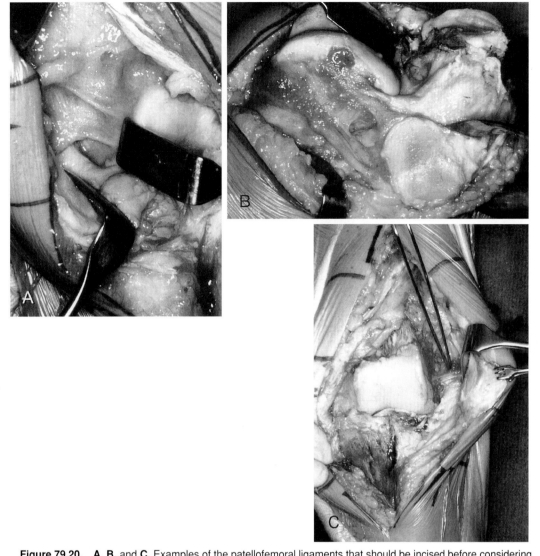

Figure 79.20.   A, B, and **C,** Examples of the patellofemoral ligaments that should be incised before considering a lateral retinacular release.

described the technique of proximal realignment with satisfactory results in 12 of 12 cases. Grace and Rand (15) also advocated proximal realignment. This technique involves a lateral retinacular release with imbrication and overlap of the medial quadriceps (Fig. 79.22). Early mobilization and motion were encouraged.

However, most authors emphasize distal realignment procedures (5, 21, 25, 28). The advantage of distal realignment is an improvement in the Q angle; the main disadvantage is patellar tendon rupture. A variety of new techniques have been advocated to minimize this significant complication, and the specifics of each author's technique are contained in the original articles (Figs. 79.23 and 79.24). In common they include the following points of technique:

1. A lateral retinacular release;
2. Thick and long medial and lateral soft tissue flaps to

avoid skin slough and to provide adequate soft tissue coverage;
3. Osteotomy of the tibial eminence and crest, extending at least 6 cm in length, 1 cm in width, and 4 to 5 mm in depth;
4. Preservation of distal attachments of the bony segment;
5. Preparation of the bed for the osteotomized segment with a bur, thus creating a cancellous surface;
6. Medial rotation of the osteotomized segment without anterior translation;
7. Secure fixation with screws, staples, or wire;
8. Immobilization in a cast or splint for 6 weeks.

In addition, both Masini and Stulberg (25) and Kirk (21) warn about compartment syndrome and recommend considering anterior compartment fasciotomy as a prophylactic measure.

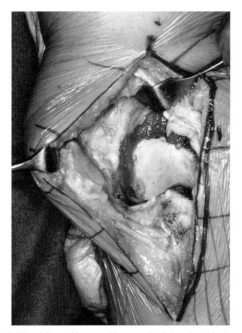

Figure 79.21. View of knee with superior lateral genicular vessels exposed halfway between the two retractors.

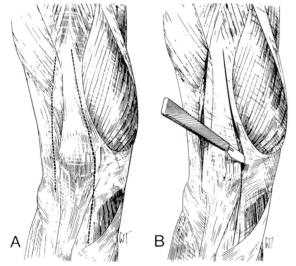
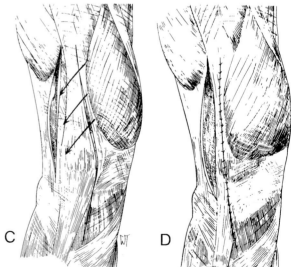

Figure 79.22. **A,** Two deep incisions are made into the quadriceps mechanism. The first enters the knee joint by a capsular incision that extends along the muscular tendinous extension of the vastus medialis and then distally across the medial corner of the anterior surface of the patella and along the medial margin of the patellar tendon. The second deep incision is a lateral release that extends proximally cutting the fibers of the vastus lateralis. **B,** To preserve the continuity of the medial flap, the quadriceps expansion overlying the medial part of the patella must be carefully preserved and separated from the underlying bone by sharp dissection. **C,** Realignment is accomplished by advancing the medial flap containing the vastus medialis laterally and distally and aligned with fibers of the oblique portion of the vastus medialis (*arrows*) over the anterior surface of the patella. **D,** After suturing the edge of the advanced medial flap in place near the lateral margin of the patella, the suture line is straight along the front of the patella, and the lateral release should be opened widely. (Reproduced with permission from Merkow RL, Soundry M, Insall JN. Patellar dislocation following total knee replacement. J Bone Joint Surg 1985;67A:1321–1327.)

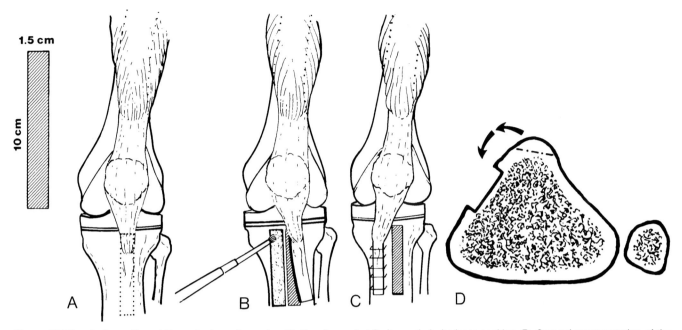

Figure 79.23. **A,** An outline of the osteotomy is made with the dimensions as shown. A lateral retinacular release is performed before osteotomy. **B,** A bur is used to create a cancellous bed with the dimensions of the graft and corresponding to the thickness of the graft. **C,** The graft is transferred medially, and power staples or other secure fixation is used. Note that the staples do not perforate the graft but fix it snugly in its inset position. **D,** Coronal representation of the transfer. Note that the transferred bone is inset into the tibia. (Reproduced with permission from Masini MA, Stulberg SD. A new surgical technique for tibial tubercle transfer in total knee arthroplasty. J Arthroplasty 1992;7:81–86.)

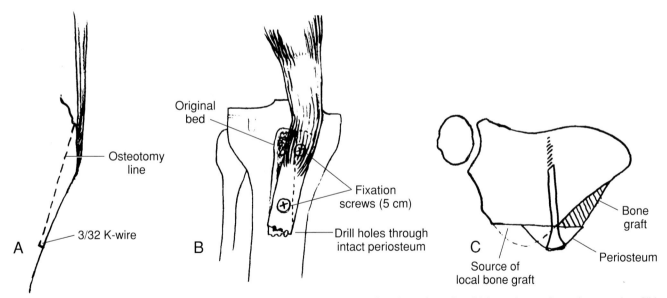

Figure 79.24. **A,** The osteotomy of the tibial tuberosity extends from behind the patellar tendon to a drill hole 5 to 6 cm distally. **B,** The tubercle is rotated medially, leaving the distal periosteum intact, and fixed with one or two screws. **C,** Medial rotation uncovers the cancellous bone laterally, which can be used as a bone graft to fill in the medial overhang. (Reproduced with permission from Briard JR, Hungerford DS. Patellofemoral instability in total knee arthroplasty. J Arthroplasty 1989;(suppl):87–97.)

Conclusions

In the current operative setting, with our relatively crude surgical techniques, perfect patellofemoral tracking after total knee replacement is rarely achieved. Subtle instabilities generally remain but usually do not lead to a serious problem. However, a greater understanding of the pathogenesis of the various problems related to patellar tracking can certainly minimize these occurrences, if not entirely eliminate them. With a greater awareness of abnormal patellar tracking problems, the surgeon should anticipate better clinical results for the patient.

References

1. Aglietti P, Buzzi R. Posteriorly stabilized total condylar knee replacement. J Bone Joint Surg 1988;70B:211–216.
2. Aglietti P, Buzzi R, Gaudenzi A. Patellofemoral functional results and complications with the posterior stabilized total condylar knee prosthesis. J Arthroplasty 1988;3:17–25.
3. Beight J, Booth RE, Hearn S, Hozack WJ. Patellar clunk syndrome following posterior stabilized total knee arthroplasty: results of treatment. Presented at the Knee Society, San Francisco, Calif., 1993.
4. Bocell JR, Curtis CD, Tullos HS. Arthroscopic treatment of symptomatic total knee arthroplasty. Clin Orthop 1991;271:125–134.
5. Briard JL, Hungerford DS. Patellofemoral instability in total knee arthroplasty. J Arthroplasty 1989;(suppl):87–97.
6. Brick GW, Scott RD. Blood supply to the patella—significance in total knee arthroplasty. J Arthroplasty 1989;(suppl):75–79.
7. Brick GW, Scott RD. The patellofemoral component of total knee arthroplasty. Clin Orthop 1988;231:136–178.
8. Cameron HU, Cameron GM. The patellar meniscus in total knee replacement. Orthop Rev 1987;16:75–79.
9. Clayton ML, Thirupathi R. Patellar complications after total condylar arthroplasty. Clin Orthop 1982;170:152–155.
10. Figgie HE, Goldberg VM, Heiple KG, Moller HS, Gordon NH. The influence of tibial-patellofemoral location on function of the knee in patients with the posterior stabilized condylar knee prosthesis. J Bone Joint Surg 1986;68A:1035–1040.
11. Flandry F, Harding AF, Kesler MA, Cook SD, Haddad RJ. A chronically dislocating prosthetic patella. Orthopaedics 1968;11:457–460.
12. Freeman MAR, Samuelson KM, Elias Marrorenzi LJ, Gokcay EI, Tuke M. The patellofemoral joint in total knee prosthesis—design considerations. J Arthroplasty 1989;(suppl):69–74.
13. Goldberg VM, Figgie HE, Inglis AE, et al. Patellar fracture type and prognosis in condylar total knee arthroplasty. Clin Orthop 1988;236:115–121.
14. Gomes LSM, Bechtold JE, Gustilo RB. Patellar prosthesis positioning in total knee arthroplasty. Clin Orthop 1988;236:72–81.
15. Grace JN, Rand JA. Patellar instability after total knee arthroplasty. Clin Orthop 1988;237:184–189.
16. Hirsh DM, Sallis JG. Pain after total knee arthroplasty caused by soft tissue impingement. J Bone Joint Surg 1989;71B:591–592.
17. Hozack, WJ. Extensor mechanism complications of total knee arthroplasty. Semin Arthroplasty 1991;2:40–45.
18. Hozack WJ, Booth RE. Patellar complications in total knee arthroplasty. Complications in Orthopaedics 1991;March/April:57–73.
19. Hozack WJ, Rothman RH, Booth RE, Balderston RA. The patellar clunk syndrome: a complication of posterior stabilized total knee arthroplasty. Clin Orthop 1989;241:203–208.
20. Johnson DP, Eastwood DM. Lateral patellar release in knee Arthroplasty: effect on wound healing. J Arthroplasty 1992;7:427–431.
21. Kayler DE, Lyttle D. Surgical interruption of patellar blood supply by total knee arthroplasty. Clin Orthop 1988;229:221–227.
22. Kirk P, Rorabeck CM, Bourne RB, Burkart B, Nott L. Management of recurrent dislocation of the patella following total knee arthroplasty. J Arthroplasty 1992;7:229–233.
23. Lombardi AV, Engh GA, Volz RG, Albrigo JL, Brainard BJ. Fracture/dissociation of the polyethylene in metal-backed patellar components in total knee arthroplasty. J Bone Joint Surg 1988;70A:675–679.
24. Lynch AF, Rorabeck CH, Bourne RB. Extensor mechanism complications following total knee arthroplasty. J Arthroplasty 1987;2:135–140.
25. Masini MA, Stulberg SD. A new surgical technique for tibial tubercle transfer in total knee arthroplasty. J Arthroplasty 1992;7:81–86.
26. McMahon MS, Scuderi GR, Glashow JL, Scharf SC, Meltzer LP, Scott WN. Scintigraphic determination of patellar viability after excision of infrapatellar fat pad and/or lateral retinacular release in total knee arthroplasty. Clin Orthop 1990;260:10–16.
27. Merkow RL, Soudry M, Insall JN. Patellar dislocation following total knee replacement. J Bone Joint Surg 1985;67A:1321–1327.
28. Mochizuki RM, Schurman DJ. Patellar complications following total knee arthroplasty. J Bone Joint Surg 1979;61A:879–883.
29. Nagamine R, Whiteside LA. The effect of tibial tray malrotation on patellar tracking in total knee arthroplasty. Trans Orthop Res Soc 1992;38:271.
30. Pettine KA, Bryan RS. A previously unreported cause of pain after total knee arthroplasty. J Arthroplasty 1986;1:29–33.
31. Rae PJ, Noble J, Hodgkinson JP. Patellar resurfacing in total condylar knee arthroplasty: technique and results. J Arthroplasty 1990;5:259–265.
32. Rand JA. Patellar resurfacing in total knee arthroplasty. Clin Orthop 1990;260:110–117.
33. Rhoads DD, Noble PC, Reuben JD, Mahoney OM, Tullos HS. The effect of femoral component position on patellar tracking after total knee arthroplasty. Clin Orthop 1990;260:43–51.
34. Ritter MA, Campbell ED. Postoperative patellar complications with or without lateral release during total knee arthroplasty. Clin Orthop 1987;219:163–168.
35. Ritter MA, Keating EM, Faris PM. Clinical roentgenographic and scintigraphic results after interruption of the superior lateral genicular artery during total knee arthroplasty. Clin Orthop 1989;248:145–151.
36. Scuderi G, Scharf SC, Meltzer LP, Scott WN. The relationship of lateral releases to patella viability in total knee arthroplasty. J Arthroplasty 1987;2:209–214.
37. Scott RD. Prosthesis replacement of the patellofemoral joint. Orthop Clin North Am 1979;10:129.
38. Smith SR, Stuart P, Pinder IM. Nonresurfaced patella in total knee arthroplasty. J Arthroplasty 1989;(suppl):81–86.
39. Stulberg SD, Stulberg BN, Hamati Y, Tsao A. Failure mechanisms of metal-backed patellar components. Clin Orthop 1988;236:88–104.
40. Thorpe CD, Bocell JR, Tullos HS. Intra-articular fibrous bands: patellar complications after total knee replacement. J Bone Joint Surg 1990;72A:811–814.
41. Vernace JV, Rothman RH, Booth RE, Balderston RA. Arthroscopic management of the patellar clunk syndrome following posterior stabilized total knee replacement. J Arthroplasty 1989;4:179–182.
42. Yoshii I, Whiteside LA, Anouchi YS. The effect of patellar button placement and femoral component design on patellar tracking in total knee arthroplasty. Clin Orthop 1992;275:211–219.

80

Patellar Fracture and Breakage

Matthew J. Kraay and Victor M. Goldberg

Incidence

The incidence of patellar fracture following total knee arthroplasty has varied widely. Cameron and Fedorkow (1) reported an incidence of patellar fracture of 21.4% with the ICLH prosthesis. They attributed these fractures to extensive resection of the posterior two-thirds of the patella and breaching of the anterior cortex during preparation for the central fixation peg.

Grace and Sim (2) reported an incidence of patellar fracture of 0.15% in 8249 total knee arthroplasties. The incidence in primary total knee arthroplasties was 0.12%, and the incidence in revision total knee arthroplasties was 0.61%. There was no statistically significant difference in the incidence of patellar fracture in patients with rheumatoid arthritis versus those with osteoarthritis. The fat pad was excised in all patients, and a lateral release was performed in only 3 of 12 knees complicated by patellar fracture.

Etiology

Several clinical reviews have implicated avascular necrosis of the patella in patellar fracture following total knee arthroplasty (1, 3–7). Total knee arthroplasty performed using a medial parapatellar approach invariably sacrifices the superior-medial genicular and the inferior-medial genicular arteries to the patella. Several other technical considerations including lateral retinacular release, excision of the patellar fat pad, and anterolateral capsular release from the tibia also potentially compromise patellar vascularity. Until recently, the significance of these aspects of the surgical technique of total knee arthroplasty was not well understood.

The extra- and intraosseous vascular anatomy of the patella has been described by Scapinelli (8). The extraosseous blood supply to the patella consists of an anastomotic vascular ring that surrounds the patella and lies in the thin layer of loose connective tissue covering the dense fibrous expansion of the quadriceps mechanism. The major vessels contributing to this anastomotic circle are the supreme genicular, medial superior genicular, medial inferior genicular, lateral superior genicular, and lateral inferior genicular arteries and the anterior tibial recurrent arteries (Fig. 80.1). The lateral superior genicular and the medial superior genicular arteries converge and anastomose with the supreme genicular artery at the level of the superior pole of the patella, just anterior to the insertion of the quadriceps tendon. Before reaching the margins of the patella ligament, the lateral inferior and the medial inferior genicular arteries each divide into three branches: the ascending parapatellar artery, the oblique prepatellar artery, and the transverse infrapatellar artery. The ascending parapatellar arteries branch upward along the margins of the patella to anastomose with the descending branches of the superior genicular arteries. The oblique prepatellar branches converge centrally toward the anterior surface of the patella along with other smaller branches from the vascular anastomotic ring. The transverse infrapatellar branches anastomose behind the patellar ligament and give off polar vessels that course between the ligament and the patellar fat pad and enter the patella behind the origin of the patellar ligament. The delicate network of arteries in the front of the patella provides nutrient vessels entering the anterior surface of the patella.

The intraosseous vascular anatomy of the patella has been grouped into two main systems by Scapinelli. The midpatellar vessels that enter the vascular foramina located in the middle third of the anterior surface of the patella course obliquely upward and ramify within the cancellous bone right up to the chondro-osseous junction (Fig. 80.2). The second interosseous vascular system arises from the polar vessels that originate from the infrapatellar anastomosis behind the patellar ligament. These vessels course upward, supply the inferior third of the patella, and communicate with branches of the

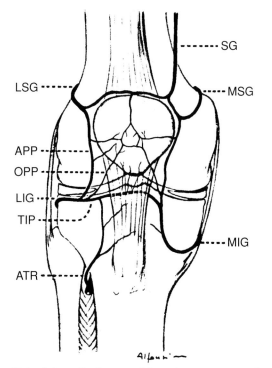

Figure 80.1 Schematic diagram of the extraosseous vascular supply to the patella as determined by Scapinelli. *LSG,* lateral superior genicular artery; *APP,* ascending parapatellar artery; *OPP,* oblique prepatellar artery; *LIG,* lateral inferior genicular artery; *TIP,* transverse infrapatellar artery; *ATR,* anterior tibial recurrent artery; *SG,* supreme genicular artery; *MSG,* medial inferior genicular artery. (Reproduced with permission from Scapinelli R. Blood supply of the human patella. J Bone Joint Surg (Br) 1967;49B:564.)

midpatellar system within the cancellous bone of the patella.

Contrary to the findings of Scapinelli, Bjorkstrom and Goldie (9) have demonstrated an intratendinous vascular supply to the superior pole of the patella from within the quadriceps tendon. Small arterial branches originating from deep peripatellar arteries penetrate the medial and lateral borders of the patella. This additional vascular supply is independent of the extraosseous anastomotic ring described by Scapinelli and appears to be age-dependent.

Several studies have suggested an association between lateral retinacular release and avascular necrosis of the patella following total knee arthroplasty. Wetzner et al. (6) performed pre- and perioperative radionucleotide bone scans on 37 consecutive patients undergoing 41 total knee arthroplasties. They noted a significant association between lateral retinacular release and diminished patellar radionucleotide uptake on postoperative bone scans. Progressive increase in patellar radionucleotide uptake was noted on follow-up bone scans at 2 and 3 months postoperatively in patients who had avascular changes in the patella perioperatively. Scuderi et al. (10) evaluated 36 knees with radionucleotide bone scanning following total knee arthroplasty. Sixteen knees had a lateral release that consisted of incision of the lateral capsule and lateral retinacu-

lum, which presumably interrupted the anterior tibial recurrent and superior and inferior lateral geniculate arteries. The incidence of a "cold" bone scan in knees requiring a lateral release was 56%. Similar findings were noted in only 15% of knees not requiring a lateral release. Follow-up bone scans of knees with apparent avascularity of the patella showed progressive increase in patellar radionucleotide uptake between 3 and 10 months postoperatively. McMahon et al. (11) studied the effect of lateral release and excision of the patellar fat pad in 70 total knee arthroplasties evaluated by radionucleotide scanning. The technique of lateral release included sacrifice of the superior lateral geniculate artery and release of the anterolateral capsule, with presumed disruption of the lateral inferior geniculate artery. As noted by Scuderi et al., there was a significantly increased incidence of "cold" bone scans in patients requiring a lateral release compared with those who did not require a lateral release. There was no significant difference in the incidence of a cold postoperative bone scan between those patients who had or did not have the excision of the infrapatellar fat pad.

Ritter et al. (12) evaluated 48 patients undergoing simultaneous bilateral total knee arthroplasty with lateral retinacular release of one knee only. The lateral superior genicular artery was sacrificed in those patients with a lateral release. The infrapatellar fat pad was not excised, and lateral dissection of the tibia was limited to minimize compromise of the lateral inferior genicular artery and the anterior tibial recurrent artery. Clinical and radiographic results showed no difference between the knees with or without lateral release. Postoperative bone scans done between 1 and 12 years postoperatively failed to demonstrate any difference in patellar vascularity between knees with or without lateral release. Based on their results, the authors concluded that adequate blood supply to the patella can be maintained despite transection of the medial superior and lateral superior genicular arteries if the circumpatellar anastomotic ring and arterial contributions from the infrapatellar fat pad and quadriceps tendon are undisturbed. These authors' previous report of a significantly decreased incidence of patellar stress fractures and other patellar complications in patients with lateral release compared with patients without lateral release following total knee arthroplasty further supports their conclusions (13).

Kayler and Lyttle (14) investigated the effects of several aspects of the surgical procedure on patellar blood supply, using an injection technique. Their results suggested that if the anastomotic ring around the patella is maintained by even a single supplying artery, arterial blood flow may still reach the substance of the patella. Procedures that disrupt the vascular ring close to the periphery of the patella reduced intraosseous blood flow. A medial arthrotomy too close to the patella, radical excision of the patellar fat pad, lateral retinacular release performed too close to the patella, and cauterization of the prepatellar vessels resulted in absence of vascular filling. Based on their results, the authors recommended avoiding cauterization of the prepatellar

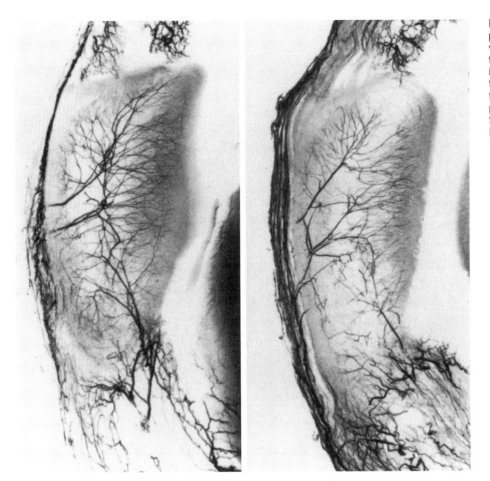

Figure 80.2. Photograph of sectioned patellae, demonstrating the intraosseous vascular anatomy using an injection technique. Note major vascularity entering through foramina on the anterior surface of the patella and the inferior pole of the patella posterior to the ligamentum patellae. (Reproduced with permission from Scapinelli R. Blood supply of the human patella. J Bone Joint Surg (Br) 1967;49B:565).

vessels on the anterior surface of the patella, avoiding close dissection around the periphery of the patella before patellar osteotomy, and avoiding damage to the anastomotic ring by a deep saw cut of the patellar articular surface, which might damage the infrapatellar blood supply.

In summary, certain variations in the surgical technique can have a significant effect on patellar vascularity following resurfacing. Despite concerns about patellar vascularity, lateral retinacular release and centralization of the extensor mechanism is mandatory if there is a tendency for patellar subluxation or dislocation.

Avascularity may be minimized by performing the lateral release away from the lateral patella and by maintaining the lateral superior genicular artery. The latter may not always be possible, and the contribution of the lateral superior genicular artery after lateral release may be questionable. Dissection around the anterior lateral corner of the proximal tibia may disrupt the lateral inferior genicular artery and should be minimized. Extensive debridement of the patellar fat pad may compromise the patellar blood supply. However, patellar revascularization seems to occur promptly and reliably after surgery. Without malalignment or instability, the significance of patellar avascularity is minimal (10–12).

Several mechanical factors probably play a role in fracture of the resurfaced patella. Obviously, excessive resection leaving a thin patella predisposes to fracture. In general, we attempt to restore the normal patellar height by measuring the thickness of the patella before resection and then resecting at a level that restores this thickness with the component. This typically leaves a patella at least 14 mm thick. We avoid resecting to less than 14 mm because of concerns about weakening the underlying bony patella. Reuben et al. (15) measured patellar strains after patellar resurfacing using a knee joint simulator. Patellae thinner than 15 mm suffered increased strain.

Patellar components with large central fixation pegs may weaken the patella. Patellar components with multiple smaller pegs may reduce the risks of fracture. Violation of the anterior cortex of the patella should be avoided.

Basic patellofemoral mechanics help explain the etiology of patellar fractures. Patellofemoral joint reaction forces have been estimated to exceed seven times body weight for activities involving marked knee flexion (16). The normal patellofemoral contact moves from distal to proximal as knee flexion increases. Deep knee flexion consequently results in significant eccentric loading and shear stresses across the patellofemoral joint, which

Figure 80.3.   A, Effect of tibial component rotation on extensor mechanism alignment. The diagram on the *left* depicts proper rotational positioning of the tibial component. With internal rotation of the tibial component as seen on the *right,* the effective quadriceps angle increases, predisposing to patellar malalignment and eccentric loading. (Reproduced with permission from Merkow et al. Patellar dislocation following total knee replacement. J Bone Joint Surg 1985;67A:132.) **B,** Rotational malalignment of the femoral component can also contribute to patellar malalignment and eccentric loading of the implant. With internal rotation of the femoral component, the effective quadriceps angle is increased, with the potential for eccentric loading of the prosthesis and instability. (Reproduced with permission from Figgie, et al. The effect of alignment of the implant on fractures of the patella after condylar total knee arthroplasty. J Bone Joint Surg 1989;71A:1031–1039.)

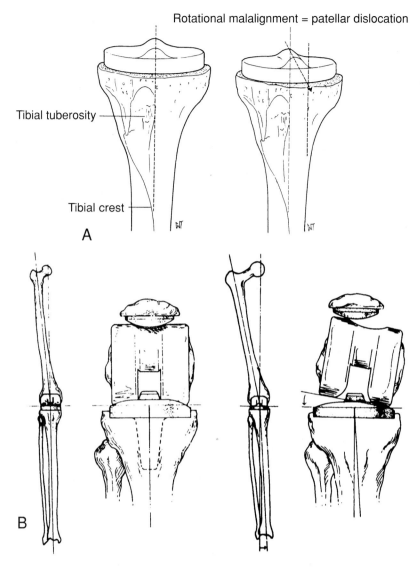

may lead to bone or implant failure. Improvements in total knee prosthesis design and kinematics, which have resulted in reproducibly better flexion may contribute to patellar fracture by this mechanism.

Several other aspects of surgical technique can produce patellofemoral malalignment and eccentric loading of the patella in the coronal plane. Patellofemoral malalignment is often the result of soft tissue imbalance between the medial and lateral peripatellar restraints and may often be prevented by a lateral retinacular release and secure medial retinacular repair. More severe malalignment is frequently caused by tibial and femoral component malpositioning. Careful intraoperative assessment of limb alignment and component positioning is essential when the patella tracks abnormally. Excessive limb valgus (more than 9 degrees) or femoral component positioning of more than 12 degrees valgus may produce abnormal patellar tracking and eccentric patellar loading. Excessive internal rotation of the tibial or femoral component (Fig. 80.3, *A* and *B*) increases the Q angle and contributes to abnormal patellar tracking and

eccentric loading. Proximal joint line position resulting from excessive distal femoral resection, anterior positioning of the femoral component, or a femoral component that is undersized in the anteroposterior dimension produces similar problems (Fig. 80.4).

Thermal necrosis from polymerization of polymethylmethacrylate has been suggested as another potential cause of patellar fracture. The extent to which this occurs is unknown.

Classification of Patellar Fractures

Several different classification schemes have been described for treatment of patellar fractures following total knee arthroplasty. Windsor et al. (7) established two general classifications: traumatic fractures and fatigue, or stress, fractures. Traumatic fractures result from significant injury and usually result in significant displacement of the fracture fragments. Fatigue fractures occur spontaneously, without any significant trauma, are generally asymptomatic, and are often

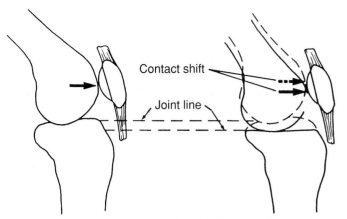

Figure 80.4. Change in position of the joint line may also contribute to eccentricity of patellar loading in a proximal-to-distal fashion. (Reproduced with permission from Rosenberg et al. Patellar component failure in cementless total knee arthroplasty. Clin Orthop 1988;236:112–113.)

Table 80.1. Patellar Fracture Type

Type 1	No involvement of implant-cement composite or quadriceps mechanism
Type 2	Involvement of implant-cement composite and/or quadriceps mechanism
Type 3a	Inferior pole fracture with patellar ligament disruption
Type 3b	Inferior pole fracture without patellar ligament disruption
Type 4	Fracture-dislocation of patella

found incidentally on routine follow-up radiographs. Windsor et al. further classify fractures into vertical, transverse, comminuted, and avulsion types, which may be either displaced or nondisplaced.

Our classification system based on treatment of patellar fractures complicating total knee arthroplasty has proved useful for prognosis and treatment (17, 18) (Table 80.1). Type 1 fractures do not involve the implant-cement composite or quadriceps mechanism. Type 2 fractures involve the implant-cement composite and/or quadriceps mechanism. Type 3a consists of inferior pole fractures with patellar ligament rupture, while type 3b consists of inferior pole fractures without patellar ligament rupture. Type 4 fractures are fracture-dislocations of the patella.

Treatment and Clinical Results

Extensor mechanism disruption, manifested by separation of the patellar fragments and an extensor lag, has been an important determinant of surgical versus nonoperative treatment. Loosening of the patellar prosthesis as a result of the patellar fracture must be considered. The patellar prosthesis and polymethylmethacrylate limit internal fixation options.

Roffman et al. (4) reported a good result in one patient with a minimally displaced transverse fracture of the patella, with an extensor lag of only 10 degrees, who was treated with closed immobilization. A poor clinical result was obtained in another patient with a proximal pole fracture with 2 cm of displacement and a 60-degree extensor lag who was treated surgically with cerclage suture fixation of the patella and suture of the extensor retinaculum. Clayton and Thirupathi (3) reported disappointing results in five of six patellar fractures treated with a variety of surgical techniques including patellectomy, fragment excision, and extensor mechanism repair.

Scott et al. (5) reported satisfactory results in three patients with patellar stress fractures with fragment displacement of less than 13 mm who were treated nonoperatively. In two of these cases, no treatment was rendered because the patients were asymptomatic, and the fractures were noted as incidental findings on follow-up radiographs. One patient treated with a patellectomy and one patient treated with excision of a distal pole fragment and recementing of a patellar prosthesis had satisfactory results. One patient with initial fragment displacement of 48 mm had multiple attempts at internal fixation and eventually required a patellectomy. Scott and associates recommended initial splinting in extension for 4 weeks. Surgical treatment was recommended only if pain or significant extensor lag persisted. They also suggested that patellectomy provided a good result if the fracture could not be surgically repaired.

Several large, recent clinical series have further defined the role of operative versus nonoperative treatment. Grace and Sim (2) reviewed 12 patellar fractures following 8249 total knee arthroplasties performed at the Mayo Clinic. Treatment was based on fracture displacement, extent of comminution, and fixation of the patellar component. Four fractures with minimal displacement (less than 5 mm), with little or no comminution, and with an intact patellar prosthesis were treated nonoperatively with 6 weeks of immobilization. Three of the four patients treated nonoperatively had a satisfactory result with minimal complications. Fractures with displacement exceeding 5 mm, extensive comminution, or a loose patellar implant were treated surgically. Four of these knees were treated by total patellectomy, two by partial patellectomy, one with tension-band wiring, and one with cerclage wiring. Three had significant postoperative complications: a quadriceps tendon rupture, a recurrent fatigue fracture, and a deep infection. Four of five patients treated with patellectomy or partial patellectomy regained prefracture functional status; no patient with internal fixation regained prefracture functional status. Satisfactory results were obtained in five of eight patients treated surgically.

Hozack et al. (19) reviewed 21 patellar fractures following total knee arthroplasty after a variety of arthroplasty or fracture treatment techniques. Seven were nondisplaced (less than 2 mm). Satisfactory results were obtained with closed treatment in both knees with minimally displaced fractures without comminution. Patellectomy provided satisfactory results in four of five minimally displaced, comminuted patellar fractures. Although none of the conservatively treated patients developed an extensor lag, four of the five patients with patellectomy had a decrease in quadriceps strength. Treatment results in patients with displaced (greater than 2 mm) patellar fractures varied widely. Operative treatment was satisfactory in two patients with displaced pole fractures. Fragment excision and quadriceps repair were satisfactory in two patients and unsatisfactory in two patients with displaced pole fractures. Patellectomy resulted in a satisfactory outcome in only two of six patients with displaced fractures. Clinical results correlate with an extensor lag at the time of initial presentation. Satisfactory results of nonoperative or operative treatment were obtained in 78% of patients without an extensor lag, compared with satisfactory results in only 31% of patients with an extensor lag at the initial evaluation. Hozack and colleagues recommended nonoperative treatment in all patients with nondisplaced patellar fractures, regardless of their physical findings. Persistent pain or extensor mechanism dysfunction can be treated with patellectomy, with the expectation of a satisfactory result. Patients with displaced fractures but without an extensor lag can also be treated nonoperatively with frequent satisfactory results. Results with open reduction and internal fixation were generally poor. Fragment excision and patellar tendon reattachment provided satisfactory results in displaced distal pole fractures.

Using their classification, Windsor et al. (7) have suggested the following guidelines for management of patellar fractures complicating total knee arthroplasty. Treatment recommendations for comminuted or vertical-type fractures, regardless of displacement, consist of 6 weeks of immobilization in a cylinder cast. In these authors' experience, comminuted fractures frequently consolidate and require no further treatment after discontinuation of immobilization. In their experience, vertical fractures usually heal without further displacement or disruption in the fixation of the patellar component. They recommend open reduction and internal fixation of transverse patellar fractures with more than 2 cm of displacement that are associated with a significant extensor lag and quadriceps weakness. Cerclage wiring of the patella and repair of the extensor retinaculum with cylinder cast immobilization is recommended as an alternative to standard internal fixation techniques, which are difficult in the resurfaced patella fixed with polymethylmethacrylate. Nondisplaced transverse fractures are in general treated with immobilization in a cylinder cast. A loose patellar component should be removed. A new patellar prosthesis may often be reimplanted, but removal of the loose component alone generally relieves pain. With severely comminuted patellar fractures associated with an extensor lag, removal of the patellar component, partial patellectomy, and repair of the extensor retinaculum may be necessary. Windsor and colleagues also recommended immobilization for small proximal or distal avulsion fractures of the patella. They

have performed arthroscopic patellar debridement after partial patellectomy and patella component removal when pain and patellofemoral crepitation has continued despite a thorough trial of physical therapy and antiinflammatory medications.

Our experience with the treatment of 36 patellar fractures following total knee arthroplasty has been reported (17, 18). Fourteen fractures were through the superior pole or body of the patella but did not disrupt either the implant bone interface or the quadriceps mechanism (type 1 fractures). All had good or excellent results following treatment. Similarly, two type 3b fractures, which by definition did not disrupt the bone cement interface or extensor mechanism, obtained an excellent result following treatment.

Fracture of the inferior pole of the patella with rupture of the patellar ligament (type 3a fractures) occurred in eight knees. Surgical treatment consisted of repair of the ruptured patellar ligament in seven knees and was recommended in the other. Despite surgical treatment, the average postoperative knee score was 63 points, and five knees were considered poor results using the University Hospitals of Cleveland quantitative knee scoring system.

Six knees had a type 4 fracture-dislocation. All were treated operatively. The average postoperative knee score after fracture dislocations was 67 points, with four knees considered unsatisfactory.

All six knees with patellar component loosening (type 2 fracture) required surgical treatment. Extensor mechanism repair was also necessary in two of these cases. The average postoperative knee score for these knees was 75 points; however, four were unsatisfactory.

We have observed an association between patellofemoral malalignment and the occurrence, severity, and prognosis of patellar fractures following total knee arthroplasty. Careful preoperative radiographic and intraoperative assessment of both limb and component alignment and positioning is essential to identify any factors predisposing to patellar fracture. Component revision is frequently necessary to correct any malalignment contributing to patellar failure.

Detailed radiographic analysis of the knees complicated by patellar fracture was performed using previously defined alignment criteria (18) (Table 80.2, Fig. 80.5–80.10). None of the 36 knees met all of the criteria for neutral alignment. Sixteen knees had minor malalignment, and 20 had major malalignment. Only one knee with minor malalignment resulted in a fracture with implant loosening or extensor mechanism disruption. In the remaining 15 knees with minor malalignment and without patellar loosening or extensor disruption, nonoperative treatment produced good or excellent results in all cases. Of the 20 knees with major malalignment, surgery was performed in 18 knees. In 15, this was limited to extensor mechanism reconstruction only. Four of these knees had an excellent or good result, three had a fair result, and eight had a poor result. The average knee score for this group of surgically treated patients was 60 points. Three-component revision was performed in three knees, with a patellectomy

Table 80.2. Neutral Alignment Range

1. Change in joint line (JL′–JL) ≤8 mm
2. A-P position of tibial component:
   C_L prosthesis posterior to C_L tibia
3. Patellar height (P) between 10 and 30 mm
4. Tibial component centralized in medial-lateral plane:
   E–F = 0 – 4 mm
5. Restoration of medial femoral condyle height:
   W–W′ ≤ 4 mm
   Z–Z′ ≤ 2 mm
   (W + Z) – (W′ + Z′) ≤ 5 mm
6. Angle between axis of femoral component and anatomic axis of femur = 5 ± 4°
   Angle between posterior surface of anterior flange of femoral component and immediately adjacent femoral cortex = 0 – +4°
7. Angle between tibial component and anatomic axis of tibia = 90 ± 2° on AP and lateral radiograph
8. Restoration of limb mechanical axis to 0 ± 4°
   Malrotation of tibial or femoral component of ≤ 5°
9. Patellar coverage > 90%
10. Patellar resection (Q) ≤ 40%

Failure to meet criteria 1–8 constitutes MAJOR malalignment with the exception of the following, which are considered MINOR malalignment:

   W–W < 7 mm
   JL–JL′ > 8 < 13 mm

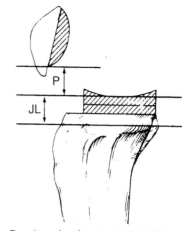

Figure 80.6 Drawing showing measurements on a lateral radiograph after a total knee replacement. *P* is the patellar height, measured from the joint line of the tibial prosthesis to the distal pole of the patellar prosthesis. *JL′* is the postoperative distance from the tibial tubercle to the distal surface of the tibial component. (Reproduced with permission from Figgie, et al. The effect of alignment of the implant on fractures of the patella after condylar total knee arthroplasty. J Bone Joint Surg 1989;71A:1031–1039.)

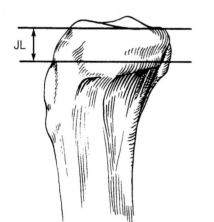

Figure 80.5. Lateral view of the proximal part of the tibia. This drawing shows the measurement of *JL* (the distance from the tibial tubercle to the tibial plateau) on a preoperative lateral radiograph of the knee. (Reproduced with permission from Figgie, et al. The effect of alignment of the implant on fractures of the patella after condylar total knee arthroplasty. J Bone Joint Surg 1989;71A:1031–1039.)

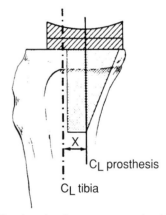

Figure 80.7. Drawing showing measurements of the tibial plateau on a postoperative lateral radiograph of the knee. C_L *tibia* is the anatomic axis of the tibia; C_L *prosthesis* is the midline of the prosthesis; *X* is the posterior distance that the prosthesis was set from the anatomic axis of the tibia. (Reproduced with permission from Figgie, et al. The effect of alignment of the implant on fractures of the patella after condylar total knee arthroplasty. J Bone Joint Surg 1989;71A:1031–1039).

performed in two of these cases. In two of the three knees, satisfactory alignment was restored, with an excellent result in both.

This study suggests that patellar fractures not associated with loosening of the patellar component, disruption of the extensor mechanism (type 1 or 3b fractures), and without major malalignment may be treated satisfactorily without surgery. Nonoperative treatment generally consists of immobilization with a knee immobilizer, partial weight bearing with crutches, and use of

antiinflammatory medications until the acute symptoms subside. Physical therapy is generally initiated after 4 to 6 weeks of immobilization and consists of active motion and quadriceps-strengthening exercises.

Despite surgery, types 2, 3a, and 4 fractures were frequently associated with an unsatisfactory outcome. Thirteen of 18 arthroplasties with major malalignment that persisted following treatment resulted in unsatisfactory outcomes. Three knees had complete revision knee arthroplasty. Two were revised to within the neu-

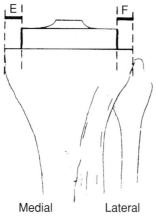

Figure 80.8. Anterior view of the tibial plateau. Distance *E* represents the offset of the implant from the medial border of the medial tibial plateau, and distance *F* represents the offset of the lateral border of the implant from the lateral aspect of the lateral tibial plateau. (Reproduced with permission from Figgie, et al. The effect of alignment of the implant on fractures of the patella after condylar total knee arthroplasty. J Bone Joint Surg 1989;71A:1031–1039).

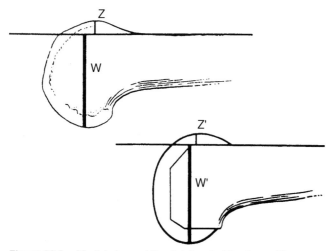

Figure 80.9. Medial views of the distal part of the femur. The *upper figure* shows the medial femoral condyle before the operation and the lower figure, after the operation. Distance *W* is the maximum height of the posterior part of the medial femoral condyle, measured from the articular surface of the condyle to a line tangent to the anterior surface of the femur. Distance *Z* represents a similar measurement for the anterior part of the condyle. Distances *Z'* and *W'* represent these measurements on the postoperative radiographs. (Reproduced with permission from Figgie, et al. The effect of alignment of the implant on fractures of the patella after condylar total knee arthroplasty. J Bone Joint Surg 1989;71A:1031–1039.)

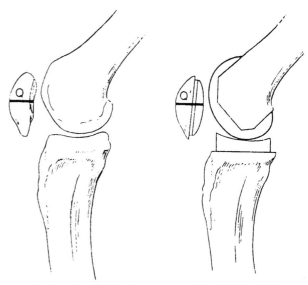

Figure 80.10. Lateral views of the knee preoperatively *(left)* and postoperatively *(right)*. Distance *Q* is the maximum thickness of the anatomical patella, and *Q'* is the maximum thickness of the prosthetic reconstruction. (Reproduced with permission from Figgie, et al. The effect of alignment of the implant on fractures of the patella after condylar total knee arthroplasty. J Bone Joint Surg 1989;71A:1031–1039.)

tral range and resulted in an excellent result. Fifteen of 16 knees with minor malalignment that was still present following treatment had a satisfactory outcome. Several previously defined alignment criteria may influence the rate, severity, and prognosis of patella fractures complicating total knee arthroplasty. While minor implant malalignment usually is associated with fractures that do well with nonoperative treatment, major malalignment is often associated with extensor disruption and component loosening that require surgery. Patellar fracture type and outcome were not related to the degree of coverage of the patella, the amount of bone resected at the time of the initial arthroplasty, or the final thickness of the patella.

Metal-backed Patellar Component Failure

Failure of metal-backed porous-coated patellar components has been well documented (20–26) and is related to both implant design and mode of fixation. While there may be some theoretical advantage to metal backing of patellar components (27), clinical failures with a wide variety of metal-backed patellar components raise serious questions as to whether these design objectives can be successfully met.

As previously mentioned, estimates of patellofemoral joint reaction forces exceed seven times body weight for some activities involving marked knee flexion (16). Study of normal patellofemoral kinematics has shown that the location of patellofemoral contact changes in a distal-to-proximal fashion as knee flexion increases. Activities involving knee flexion consequently result in eccentric loading of the patella. As the eccentricity of loading increases, an increasing component of the patellofemoral joint reaction force resolves as shear force on a dome-shaped patellar prosthesis (Fig. 80.11). Problems with patellar tracking secondary to limb or component malalignment or soft tissue balance exacerbate this problem. Patellar tilt caused by asymmetric resection or changes in the joint line position can have similar effects. Patient factors such as body weight, activity level, and postoperative knee motion have been associated with metal-backed patellar component failures, presumably because of shear component overloading.

The effect of eccentric loading on a domed-shaped patellar component is responsible for many of the observed problems with metal-backed patellar components. Three general mechanisms of uncemented patellar component failure have been identified (24) (Fig. 80.12). When bone has grown into the pegs, but not the metal baseplate, the fixation pegs may fail at their junction with the component as a result of the shear loads transmitted from the shear across the interface. Delamination or dissociation of the polyethylene from the underlying metal base can be caused by these shear forces. Failure can also result from local wear over a point of stress concentration or minimal material thickness associated with the underlying metal backing.

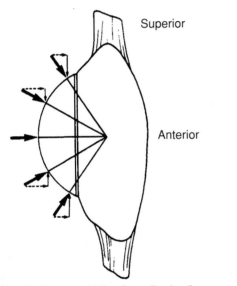

Figure 80.11. As the eccentricity of patellar loading on a dome-shaped patella increases, an increasing component of the patellofemoral joint reaction force resolves as a shear force. (Reproduced with permission from Rosenberg, et al. Patellar component failure in cementless total knee arthroplasty. Clin Orthop 1988;236:112,113.

A definite relationship between polyethylene wear, polyethylene thickness, and articular congruence has been demonstrated, and a minimal polyethylene thickness of 8 mm has been recommended for low conformity articulations such as the tibial component (28). This may be even more important considering the high loads and small contact areas of the patellofemoral joint (26). The limitations imposed by patellar implant size versus bony patella size and compromise of patellar polyethylene thickness by the underlying metal backing make the development of a reliable metal-backed patellar component uncertain. Modified dome components with improved patellofemoral congruity may normalize patellofemoral loads, minimize shear forces on the implant, and make metal backing feasible (29). Considering the severity and increasing frequency of complications associated with both cemented and uncemented metal-backed patellar components, we do not recommend their continued use at this time.

Diagnosis and Treatment of Metal-backed Patellar Component Failure

While patellar component loosening can usually be determined by plain radiography, the diagnosis of polyethylene wear or patellar component failure can be difficult. The clinical presentation of metal-backed patellar component failure is variable (21, 22, 26). Often times the patient may relate an acute onset of audible, grating patellofemoral crepitation after a specific episode involving significant knee flexion and stressing of the patellofemoral joint. This is usually associated with acute or delayed anterior knee pain and later development of an effusion. This scenario indicates catastrophic patellar component failure with metal-on-metal articulation of the failed patellar and femoral components. In other patients, the clinical presentation is insidious, with gradual development of peripatellar pain and an effusion. We have observed asymptomatic patellar component failure at the fixation peg junction in the presence of a well-developed patellar meniscus.

Regardless of symptoms, patients with metal-backed patellar components warrant a high index of suspicion in view of the increasing frequency of problems with these designs. Prompt diagnosis may prevent damage to

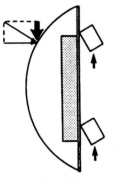

Peg failure

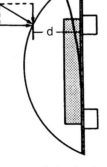

Delamination

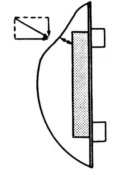

Wear

Figure 80.12. Three general mechanisms of patellar component failure as a result of the shear forces generated by eccentric loads on a dome-shaped patella. (Reproduced with permission from Rosenberg, et al. Patellar component failure in cementless total knee arthroplasty. Clin Orthop 1988;236:112,113).

the femoral component and metallosis. Examination often shows patellofemoral crepitation, boggy synovitis, and a massive effusion, which makes the diagnosis rather certain. Physical findings in patients presenting early can be subtle and consist only of mild peripatellar pain or a minor effusion.

Plain radiography may demonstrate peg failure at the junction with the metal base, or occasionally a lucency in the suprapatellar pouch from the dissociated polyethylene surface. The Merchant or other tangential views of the patellofemoral articulation may demonstrate loss of interposed polyethylene between the femoral and patellar component metal backing or patellar malalignment. Radiographs should be carefully evaluated for limb or component malalignment, which frequently contributes to patellar subluxation and patellar component failure. Aspiration may reveal discolored synovial fluid in association with metallosis or even polyethylene wear debris. Frequently, the diagnosis is uncertain and can only be confirmed by arthroscopy or arthrotomy. When metal-backed patellar failure is suspected and arthroscopy or exploration is contemplated, the knee should be immobilized, and the diagnosis confirmed without delay.

Revision of the failed metal-backed patellar component can be complicated by several factors. Damage to the femoral component frequently makes revision of this component necessary. Uncomplicated removal of the uncemented femoral component often allows exchange with a new cemented prosthesis. Posterior cruciate ligament competence may be compromised by removal of a well-fixed femoral component or by the extensive synovectomy necessary if associated metallosis is present. A posterior cruciate ligament–substituting prosthesis should be considered in this situation.

Component positioning and axial and rotational alignment should be carefully evaluated intraoperatively because of the association of malalignment with patellar component failure. Component malalignment may warrant tibial or femoral component revision to ensure adequate extensor mechanism alignment. The metal-backed patellar component should be carefully removed to minimize bone stock loss. Usually, the failed patellar component can be successfully revised with a cemented, all-polyethylene component. Rarely, patellar bone stock will be insufficient for resurfacing, and a patelloplasty will be required.

References

1. Cameron HU, Fedorkow DM. The patella in total knee arthroplasty. Clin Orthop 1982;165:197–199.
2. Grace JN, Sim FH. Fracture of the patella after total knee arthroplasty. Clin Orthop 1988;230:168–175.
3. Clayton ML, Thirupathi R. Patellar complications after total condylar arthroplasty. Clin Orthop 1982;170:152–155.
4. Roffman M, Hirsh DM, Mendes DG. Fracture of the resurfaced patella in total knee arthroplasty. Clin Orthop 1980;148:112–116.
5. Scott RD, Turoff N, Ewald FC. Stress fractures of the patella following duopatellar total knee arthroplasty with patellar resurfacing. Clin Orthop 1982;170:147–151.
6. Wetzner SM, Bezreh JS, Scott RD, Bierbaum BE, Newberg AH. Bone scanning in the assessment of patellar viability following knee replacement. Clin Orthop 1985;199:215–219.
7. Windsor RE, Scuderi GR, Insall JN. Patellar fractures in total knee arthroplasty. J Arthroplasty 1989;(suppl)S63–67.
8. Scapinelli R. Blood supply of the human patella. J Bone Joint Surg (Br) 1967;49B:563–570.
9. Bjorkstrom S, Goldie IF. A study of the arterial supply of the patella in the normal state, in chondromalacia patellae and in osteoarthrosis. Acta Orthop Scand 1980;51:63–70.
10. Scuderi G, Scharf SC, Meltzer LP, Scott WN. The relationship of lateral releases to patellar viability in total knee arthroplasty. J Arthroplasty 1987;2:209–214.
11. McMahon MS, Scuderi GR, Glashow JL, Scharf SC, Meltzer LP, Scott WN. Scintigraphic determination of patellar viability after excision of infrapatellar fat pad and/or lateral retinacular release in total knee arthroplasty. Clin Orthop 1990;260:10–16.
12. Ritter MA, Keating EM, Faris PM. Clinical roentgenographic, and scintigraphic results after interruption of the superior lateral genicular artery during total knee arthroplasty. Clin Orthop 1989;248:145–151.
13. Ritter MA, Campbell ED. Postoperative patellar complications with or without lateral release during total knee arthroplasty. Clin Orthop 1987;219:163–168.
14. Kayler DE, Lyttle D. Surgical interruption of patellar blood supply by total knee arthroplasty. Clin Orthop 1988;229:221–227.
15. Reuben JD, McDonald CL, Woodard PL, Hennington LJ. Effect of patellar thickness on patellar strain following total knee arthroplasty. J Arthroplasty 1991;6:251–258.
16. Reilly DT, Martens M. Experimental analysis of the quadriceps muscle force and patellofemoral joint reaction force for various activities. Acta Orthop Scand 1972;43:126–137.
17. Goldberg VM, Figgie HE, Inglis AE, Figgie MP, Sobel M, Kelly M, Kraay M. Patellar fracture type and prognosis in condylar total knee arthroplasty. Clin Orthop 1988;236:115–122.
18. Figgie HE, Goldberg VM, Figgie MP, Inglis AE, Kelly M, Sobel M. The effect of alignment of the implant on fractures of the patella after condylar total knee arthroplasty. J Bone Joint Surg 1989;71A:1031–1039.
19. Hozack WJ, Goll SR, Lotke PA, Rothman RH, Booth RE. The treatment of patellar fractures after total knee arthroplasty. Clin Orthop 1988;236:123–127.
20. Bayley JC, Scott RD. Further observations on metal-backed patellar component failure. Clin Orthop 1988;236:82–87.
21. Bayley JC, Scott RD, Ewald FC, Holmes GB. Failure of the metal-backed patellar component after total knee replacement. J Bone Joint Surg 1988;70A:668–674.
22. Lombardi AV, Engh GA, Volz RG, et al. Fracture/dissociation of the polyethylene in metal-backed patellar components in total knee arthroplasty. J Bone Joint Surg 1988;70A:675–679.
23. Rand JA. Cement or cementless fixation in total knee arthroplasty. Clin Orthop 1991;273:52–62.
24. Rosenberg AG, Andriacchi TP, Barden R, Galante JO. Patellar component failure in cementless total knee arthroplasty. Clin Orthop 1988;236:106–114.
25. Rosenberg AG, Barden RM, Galante JO. Cemented and ingrowth fixation of the Miller Galante prosthesis. Clin Orthop 1990;260:71–79.
26. Stulberg SD, Stulberg BN, Hamati Y, Tsao A. Failure mechanisms of metal-backed patellar components. Clin Orthop 1988;236:88–105.
27. Goldstein SA, Coale E, Weiss AC, et al. Patellar surface strain. J Orthop Res 1986;4:372–377.
28. Bartel DL, Bicknell VL, Wright TM. The effect of conformity, thickness and material on stresses in ultra-high molecular weight components for total joint replacement. J Bone Joint Surg 1986;68A:1041–1051.
29. Hsu H, Walker PS. Wear and deformation of patellar components in total knee arthroplasty. Clin Orthop 1989;246:260–265.

81

Extensor Mechanism Rupture

Roger H. Emerson, Jr.

Introduction

The extensor mechanism of the knee consists of the quadriceps muscle and tendon, patella, and patellar retinaculum, patellar tendon, and tibial tubercle. This mechanism provides for active extension of the knee with the patella acting as a fulcrum over the trochlea of the femur. The patellar tendon links the patella to the tibia, and the quadriceps tendon links the patella to the quadriceps muscle. Extensor mechanism rupture commonly refers to rupture of the major soft tissue portions of the extensor mechanism, that is, the quadriceps tendon and patellar tendon. Patellar fracture, tibial tubercle fracture, and patellar instability are separate but related problems.

The most common pathological conditions of this mechanism are disorders of patellar tracking (8, 11) and fractures of the patella itself (18). Extensor mechanism ruptures are comparatively rare, but clinically significant, since the resulting loss of quadriceps function produces such a profound disability for the knee; with rare exception, this problem requires surgical intervention to restore function. The best reconstructive techniques for these ruptures remain controversial because of inconsistent outcomes in some clinical settings after treatment. Surprisingly, despite the profound functional consequences of extensor rupture, Siwek and Rao found that 38% were initially misdiagnosed (30).

Extensor mechanism rupture is seen in three clinical settings:

1. Chronically ill patients, usually spontaneous, as, for example, in dialysis patients (17);
2. Very active patients, usually posttraumatic (30);
3. After knee surgery, both anterior cruciate ligament reconstruction (14) and total knee replacement (18).

Extensor mechanism rupture after total knee replacement has been especially problematic, and is, therefore, discussed in more detail.

Biomechanical Factors Affecting the Extensor Mechanism

The force of body weight produces a flexion force across the knee that is balanced by the force of the quadriceps muscle acting through the quadriceps tendon and patella tendon. The joint reaction force acting across the patellofemoral joint is the result of these two force vectors. The patella serves as the fulcrum directing the forces. As knee flexion increases, the quadriceps force must, of necessity, increase to balance the increased body weight produced by the longer moment arm of the femur (20). Therefore, while the patella and extensor mechanism functions as a pulley, it is not a pure pulley mechanism because the amount of force transferred from the quadriceps muscle to the patellar ligament depends on the angle of knee flexion (which in turn determines such factors as the tibial-femoral contact and the angle of the patellar ligament). This extension torque is maximum at around 25 degrees of knee flexion (1).

Femoral rollback, the anterior to posterior translation of the tibiofemoral contact point with knee flexion, is a function of the four-bar linkage of the anterior and posterior cruciate ligaments (9). It also influences the mechanical efficiency of the quadriceps muscle and the resulting strain in the extensor mechanism. Sledge and Walker have calculated that, in the absence of physiologic rollback, the quadriceps force must be more than doubled to maintain balance between the weight-bearing force and the quadriceps force (31). Andriacchi, et al. have found that in the absence of this rollback the reduction of quadriceps mechanical efficiency is greatest at 60 degrees of flexion (1).

The effect of total knee implant design on extensor mechanism strain has been studied with variable findings. Reuben, et al. found no difference in anterior patellar strain between posterior cruciate ligament retaining and substituting designs (26). McLain, et al.

found, as predicted, that anterior patellar strain is higher in the Total Condylar design (Zimmer, Warsaw, IN) that sacrifices the posterior cruciate ligament compared to the Robert Brigham design that preserves the posterior cruciate ligament and to the Insall-Burstein prosthesis that has a cam mechanism substituting for the posterior cruciate ligament. However, sectioning of the posterior cruciate ligament in the Robert Brigham design did not result in an increase in patellar strain, indicating that other design features also play a role in patellar strain (20). Neither of these studies, however, assessed any difference in rollback between the various study designs.

Patellar strain is also determined by the thickness of the patella. Reuben, et al. have shown that, when performing a total knee replacement at the time of patellar resurfacing, anterior patellar strain increases with the amount of bone resected and is highest when the boney patellar remnant is less than 1.5 cm thick (26).

Incidence and Pathomechanics

Extensor mechanism rupture is not a very common problem. In the nonimplant population, Siwek and Rao found only 67 cases accumulated over a 10-year period from 4 different hospitals. (30) Murzac, et al. found only 45 cases at a major medical center over a twelve-year period (22). Commonly, those patients with a quadriceps tendon rupture are older than those with a patellar tendon rupture (15, 22, 30); for example, the median age for quadriceps ruptures was 63 years compared to 45 years for patellar injuries in Larsen and Lund's series (15).

Siwek and Rao found that most of the extensor mechanism ruptures in their series occurred after "acute trauma." Certain diseases seemed to predispose to rupture, e.g., gouty arthritis, psoriatic arthritis, long standing diabetes mellitus, and rheumatoid arthritis. The only bilateral rupture (in this case, patellar tendons) occurred in a patient with rheumatoid arthritis treated with both systemic steroids and intraarticular steroids (30). Murzac, et al. found that 79% (19 of 24) of the patellar tendon ruptures in their series were due to "indirect trauma," typically a rapid loading of the tendon, such as jumping, and that 16 of the 19 ruptures occurred at the inferior pole of the patella. Similarly, most of the quadriceps ruptures (20 out of 21) were found to follow indirect injury, usually a stumble or slip. Only 1 of the quadriceps ruptures occurred while playing a sport, whereas 12 patellar tendon ruptures occurred during sports (22).

In the total knee implant population, the overall incidence of extensor mechanism complications following surgery can be high, from 4.9 to 16% (4, 18, 19). For example, Lynch, et al. reported a 10% incidence in a series of 281 total knee arthroplasties followed for an average 42 months. They noted 3 quadriceps tendon ruptures, 4 patellar tendon ruptures, along with 5 patellar fractures, 11 recurring patellar subluxations, 4 anterior pain problems attributed to the patella, and 1 malpositioned patella (18).

Quadriceps tendon rupture after total knee replacement is unusual and appears to be less common than patellar tendon rupture, despite the older average age of the typical knee implant patient. Very little information is available in the orthopedic literature about this problem. Kirgis has reported 1 rheumatoid patient with a spontaneous quadriceps rupture attributed to repeated steroid injections (13). Gustilo and Thompson have reported 1 quadriceps tendon rupture attributed to impingement of the patellar prosthesis, which was positioned slightly off the bone at the location of the rupture and was presumed to have abraded the tendon (10). Doolittle and Turner have reported a quadriceps tendon rupture in an implant patient following a Roux-Goldthwaite procedure for recurrent dislocations (in a knee that had had several previous operations for patellar dislocations) (4). Lynch, et al. have reported 3 quadriceps ruptures, all having had a lateral retinacular release (18).

Patellar tendon rupture after total knee replacement has been studied better than quadriceps tendon rupture. The incidence of patellar tendon rupture in the total knee implant population is small, reported by Rand and his coauthors as a complication in 0.17% of total knee surgeries at the Mayo Clinic between 1973 and 1985 (24). Cadambi and Engh have reported an incidence of 0.55% patellar tendon ruptures, (5 out of 915 knee arthroplasties) from the Anderson Clinic (2).

The cause of patellar and quadriceps tendon ruptures after total knee surgery is multifactoral, involving mechanical, vascular, and surgical technique factors. Emerson, Head, and Malinin found that most patellar tendon ruptures after total knee arthroplasty developed atraumatically with a progressive extensor lag (5). Gustilo and Thompson have also reported that most patellar tendon ruptures occur late, suggesting to these authors that impingement of part of the prosthesis on the patellar tendon, or removal of too much bone from the patella at the time of resurfacing with weakening of the extensor tissues, or a devascularization process from the surgical exposure is the likely cause of most patellar tendon ruptures in this clinical setting (10). Acute patellar tendon avulsion at the time of surgery is less common but can certainly occur. It occurs more commonly in patients with rheumatoid arthritis (33), in more complicated knee replacement surgeries (19), and especially, in those patients with motion restricted to less than 70 degrees, as reported by Rand, et al. (24). Cadambi and Engh found that 6 of the 8 patellar tendon ruptures in their series occurred acutely, 3 at surgery and 3 soon afterwards. They stressed the importance of proximal release of the quadriceps mechanism in the stiff knee to protect the tibial tubercle tendon insertion. Others have also emphasized the importance of protecting the patella tendon as much as possible during the actual surgery (24).

The role played by the vascular supply in the various pathologic conditions of the extensor mechanism has been of intense interest recently. The arterial blood supply to the extensor mechanism has been studied. Three vessels contribute to the medial side: the superior genicular, the medial superior genicular, and the medial inferior genicular. Only two vessels contribute to the lateral side: the lateral inferior genicular, and lateral superior genicular (27). DePalma has reported that surgery on a fractured patella will increase the incidence of avascular necrosis, especially of the upper pole fragment (3). Scapinelli reported 37 cases of avascular necrosis out of 41 patellas with a transverse fracture pattern following a circumferential suturing technique, which, he theorized, disrupts the radial anastomosis surrounding the patella. He noted, however, that there was no adverse clinical consequence of the necrosis (27). Insall, W. Scott, and Ranawat noted more patellar fractures in total knee replacements that had undergone a lateral release. Avascular necrosis was found in 1 retrieval specimen (12). After a lateral release, Scuderi, et al. have reported 9 of 16 knees, or 56%, demonstrating cold bone scans of the patella compared to 3 of 20 knees, 15%, with no lateral release. The abnormal scans had returned to normal by 3 months. There was 1 patellar fracture associated with a lateral release in this series, successfully treated nonoperatively (28). However, Ritter, et al., looking at 48 knees undergoing bilateral simultaneous total knee arthroplasty (with only 1 knee having had a lateral release) found no difference in the rate of patellar fractures between those with lateral releases and those without lateral releases (25). In addition, Figgie, et al. studied a series of patella fractures after total knee arthroplasty and found that, out of 36 patella fractures, only 6 had a lateral release. They concluded that lateral release played no causative role in most patellar fractures (7).

As for patellar tendon ruptures, Gustilo and Thompson speculate that devascularizing incisions about the patellar tendon can lead to tendon rupture (10). Similarly, Lynch, et al. found that lateral release seemed to predispose to quadriceps rupture; they recommended careful protection of the blood supply of the quadriceps and patellar tendon at the time of surgery. They specifically recommended avoiding bringing the lateral release too high proximally and too close to the quadriceps tendon; they also recommended preservation of the fat pad about the patellar tendon (18). Laskin reported one patellar tendon rupture (out of three in his series) where he performed a complete excision of the fat pad and a simultaneous lateral release adjacent to the patellar tendon. He indicated, however, that, in over 500 cases of fat pad excision alone, he saw no patellar tendon ruptures (16).

Rand, et al. reported 4 patients who had a failed proximal realignment for patellar dislocation (lateral release and vastus medialis advancement) who subsequently underwent distal alignment by tibial tubercle transfer with resulting patellar tendon rupture (24). Therefore, vascular insults to the extensor mechanism are common, but, fortunately, they do not usually result in adverse clinical consequences. They must, however, be considered a risk factor for extensor mechanism rupture. Similarly, the literature does not suggest a strong relationship between component design or alignment and extensor mechanism rupture. Nevertheless, certain

design features predispose to patellofemoral problems. Older hinged knee prostheses have a higher incidence of patella wear and dislocations, as reported by Mochizuki, et al. (21), who nonetheless, had no patellar fractures or patellar tendon disruptions in their series of 86 patients. Rand, et al. reported that 50% of the patellar tendon ruptures in their series were in fixed-hinge designs, although this series was from the era when hinged knee arthroplasties were more commonly used (24). MacCollum, et al. have reported a series of 87 knees with 5 patellar fractures (6%) and 2 patellar tendon ruptures (2.4%), with an overall 16% patellofemoral complication rate, when using a design with a conforming femoral trochlea and eccentrically shaped patella, i.e., the Porous-Coated Anatomic (PCA) (Howmedica) knee. Of the 5 patella fractures in this report, 2 had persisting lateral patellar subluxation, despite a 39% rate of lateral patellar retinacular release. They attributed the high rate of these patellofemoral problems to the higher forces on the extensor mechanism in this design setting, especially with imperfect patellar tracking. However, the two patellar tendon ruptures occurred at the time of surgery, one in a revision case and the other in a conversion of a high tibial osteotomy, implicating the complexity of the surgery rather than the design of the components in the tendon ruptures (19). Lynch, et al., however, found no difference in overall extensor mechanism complications between the PCA and the Kinematic (less constrained) designs, ("Kinematic Condylar," Howmedica) (18).

Figgie and coworkers (7) found that femoral and tibial component alignment correlated with patellar fractures. They distinguished between major and minor component malalignments, described in an earlier study (8), in which they hypothesized that the resulting component mismatch, the joint line shift or "flexor/extensor imbalance," causes a fatigue fracture of the patella. The type and severity of fractures correlated with minor or major malalignment categories. No mention of soft tissue rupture was made in this study, but it follows that alignment problems that predispose to fatigue fracture of the patella might also risk patellar and quadriceps tendon rupture.

Treatment and Clinical Results

Rupture of the extensor mechanism requires surgical repair under ordinary clinical circumstances. Extensor mechanism repair has typically been divided into acute repairs (usually within the first 2 weeks) and delayed repairs. The results of acute repair are generally better than those of late repair, when soft tissue contractures, joint stiffness, and extensor lag have developed.

In the nonimplant patient, early repair of quadriceps tendon ruptures with end-to-end sutures has been consistently satisfactory, whereas several authors have recommended supplemental fixation for early repair of patellar tendon ruptures (15, 30, 32). Murzic, et al. have reported 83% good to excellent results with direct patellar tendon repair alone. All early repairs were performed with nonabsorbable suture and eight other repairs used reinforcing techniques, either a cerclage wire or free fascia lata graft woven through the patellar and the tendon (22).

Clinical results following extensor mechanism repair in the nonimplant population have varied. Using only strength and motion criteria, Siwek and Rao found that patients with early quadriceps repairs do very well, achieving either excellent or good status. The results of late repair were less favorable. Half of the patients (3 of 6) suffered weakness, loss of motion, and were graded as unsatisfactory. With early patellar tendon repair, 24 of 25 patients had good to excellent results; surprisingly, most of the delayed repairs, 5 of 6, also were graded good or excellent. The only reruptures in this series were two immediate patellar tendon repairs, occurring with subsequent sports activities. Usually no clinical symptoms accompanied the measurable quadriceps atrophy of most patients in this series, regardless of the timing of the repair (30).

Murzac, et al., with pain as an additional follow-up parameter, reported 2 patellar tendon repairs and 1 quadriceps repair with only fair results, due to patellofemoral pain. They report 1 rerupture in both the patellar tendon and quadriceps tendon groups. Isokinetic testing showed that 7 of the 11 tested after patellar tendon repair achieved 80% of the contralateral quadriceps power, whereas only 3 of 8 patients tested after quadriceps repair achieved 80% of the contralateral side (22).

Larsen and Lund analyzed the painful knees in their series and found that all demonstrated maltracking of the patellofemoral joint on tangential x-ray views. They also point out that not all patients with maltracking had pain. Patellar tendon repair patients were more likely to have pain than quadriceps repair patients, a finding which the authors attributed to the higher relative loss of tissue elasticity with patellar tendon surgery (as compared to quadriceps tendon surgery), a loss leading to high patellofemoral compressive forces in the patellar tendon group (15).

The total knee replacement patient with rupture of the extensor mechanism represents a small subgroup of patients with extensor mechanism rupture, but one which has presented exceptional challenges. While the incidence of rupture is low, the functional outcome after treatment has been consistently inferior to results in the nonimplant population, with permanent bracing a frequent outcome (4, 10, 19).

Very little has been published about quadriceps tendon repair after total knee replacement. Anecdotal reports indicate that end-to-end repair can be successful, but with frequent complications and diminished functional results. The tendon repair should be protected for several months (10, 18). Lynch, et al. have reported 3 quadriceps repairs, 1 that ruptured at 6 weeks postrepair, and the other 2 that had diminished knee flexion (70 degrees) and extensor lags of 12 and 19 degrees (18).

No single quadriceps repair technique has been reported in a substantial patient series, but, assuming that rupture of the quadriceps tendon after total knee arthroplasty occurs in the setting of a structurally compromised tendon with rerupture common, reinforcement

techniques or tissue augmentation techniques make the most sense. Free fascia lata grafts and quadriceps turndown flaps have been used for this purpose (22, 29).

Treatment of patellar tendon rupture following total knee replacement has proved to be as problematic as quadriceps tendon rupture. Again, no one technique universally has been shown to be successful. Of the 18 knees in the Mayo Clinic series, reported by Rand, et al., 16 knees underwent repair, mostly by primary resuture, with only 4/16, or 25%, achieving a healed repair. The most successful technique in this series was staple fixation with 6 weeks of immobilization (24). Lynch, et al. performed primary repairs in 4 patellar tendon ruptures resulting in 3 healed repairs, although with persisting extensor lags, and 1 rerupture treated with a brace (18). Gustilo and Thompson have reported 2 patellar tendon repairs, both with primary suture and with autograft tendon augmentation (1 semitendinosis tendon and 1 iliotibial band) with figure-of-eight wire support (Fig. 81.1). One of these two repairs ruptured (10).

These results again suggest that there is often insufficient autogenous tissue remaining to effect a durable repair. Unfortunately, in the author's experience, this lack of autogenous tissue is the most common clinical situation when patellar tendon rupture accompanies total joint replacement; this observation probably explains the clinical difference between patellar tendon reconstruction in the implant and nonimplant groups. Most patellar tendon ruptures after total knee arthroplasty develop insidiously through a combination of vascular and mechanical factors (discussed above) that lead to an attritional failure of the tendon. At surgery, there is often little recognizable patellar tendon tissue remaining. Despite this, primary patellar tendon repair has a role in treatment of the acute rupture and when there is sufficient remaining tendonous tissue. Typically, this occurs when the patellar tendon ruptures at surgery, usually avulsed from the tibial tubercle. There must be enough tendon substance to make the repair; simultaneous autogenous tissue augmentation and wire reinforcement, as depicted in Figure 81.1, seem sensible, given the experience with unreinforced primary repair (24, 30). The literature supports a long period of bracing and protection from extremes of motion, i.e., from 6 to 18 weeks (2, 24). Reruptures are likely to occur.

When primary repair does not seem feasible, the surgical reconstruction must restore autogenous or allograft tissue to the knee. Recently, Cadambi and Engh have reported 7 patients who underwent successful reconstruction of the patellar tendon using doubled semitendinosis tendon and an 18-week period of cast and brace protection. If the semitendinosis was very small, the reconstruction was further augmented with the gracilis muscle, in 2 cases (Fig. 81.2) (2). No preoperative traction was used. The ligament graft was placed through a drill hole in the inferior pole of the patella or was weaved through the quadriceps tendon if the bone remnant was insufficient. The authors avoided joint motion for 6 weeks, followed by 3 additional months during which time flexion was limited to 60 degrees. They based their technique on the work of Noyes, et al. who

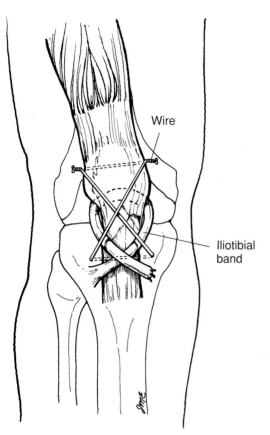

Figure 81.1. Primary resuture technique augmented with the iliotibial band and figure-of-eight tension band wire. The semitendinosis could also be used. This technique could be used for either an implant or nonimplant patient.

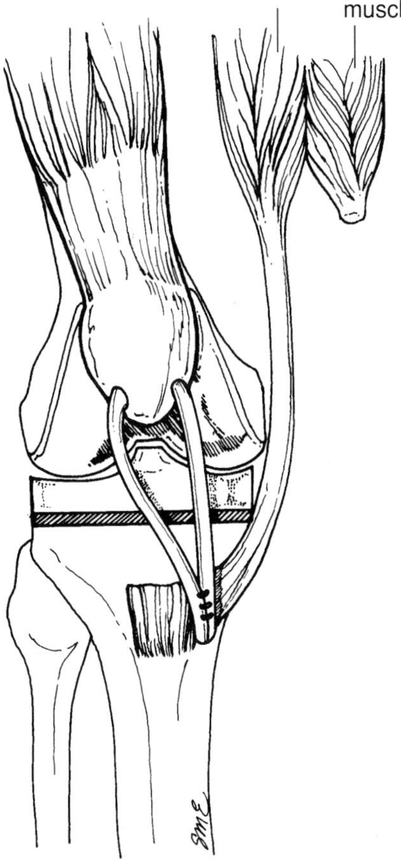

Gracilis m.   Semitendinosis muscle belly

Figure 81.2. Reconstruction of the patellar tendon using a doubled semitendinosis tendon. This technique requires a very long length of tendon, best obtained by harvesting the tendon through a separate incision.

showed that the semitendinosis tendon has about 50% of the strength of the patellar tendon (23).

When primary repair was not deemed feasible after patellar tendon rupture following total knee arthroplasty, I have resorted to an allograft of the extensor mechanism, consisting of tibial tubercle, patellar tendon, patella, and quadriceps tendon, an allograft described by Emerson, Head, and Malinin (5). The underlying rationale is to return structurally sound tissue to patients in cases where a severe deficiency occurs. It follows logically that no autogenous tissue should be removed from the patient if the goal is to add tissue, not diminish it. In addition, the patient's patellar remnant and scarred patellar ligament are retained to provide coverage of the graft by as much host tissue as possible. Another advantage of the allograft is that the graft can be anatomically situated over the knee joint; frequently, the patient's own patella cannot be brought to an anatomic position. Preoperative traction, as advocated by some, is best avoided because of the adjacent prosthetic joint.

Both freeze-dried and fresh frozen grafts have been used with equal success in our experience to date. The allograft patella has been resurfaced, although this may not be necessary. The bone resection should be conservative (Fig. 81.3 and 81.4). The entire surface of the bony patella remnant should be covered by the component to avoid concentrated stress. The graft should be handled carefully, avoiding placement of any piercing or crushing clamps on the allograft that could permanently damage the graft and predispose to failure. This technical point cannot be overemphasized.

The allograft tibial tubercle is keyed into an appropriately sized slot cut from the proximal tibia (Fig. 81.5), attempting to medialize the location slightly to minimize the "Q" angle and enhance tracking. The patella should articulate with the femoral flange in full extension. The allograft tubercle should be anatomically positioned in terms of tubercle elevation. Depressing the tubercle will increase patellar strain, a circumstance which is undesirable. Elevating the tubercle would be theoretically advantageous, making for a "Maquet osteotomy" effect, but the skin in this area of the knee is invariably thin with little subcutaneous tissue covering the graft. Wound closure with skin tension would compromise healing. The tubercle is rigidly fixed with bone screws and further supported with cerclage wire.

The quadriceps mechanism is sutured to the graft to maintain a horizontal inclination of the graft with

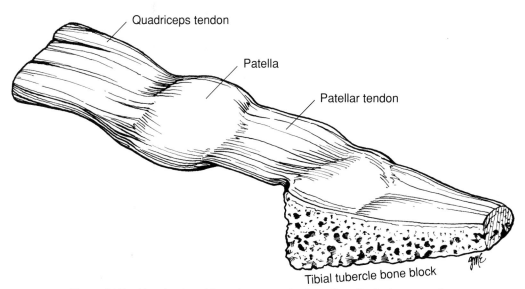

Figure 81.3. Line drawing of the extensor mechanism allograft prior to preparation.

smooth tracking in the trochlea (Fig. 81.6). The allograft should be placed under the host quadriceps muscle as much as possible, to provide a healthy vascularized bed for graft healing and to protect the graft from a superficial wound healing problem. In the few patients who retained their own normal patella, the prosthesis has been removed but the bony remnant has been left in situ, helping to anchor the quadriceps portion of the graft and serving as protection of the proximal allograft from the adjacent wound, as discussed above. Usually, the autogenous patella has been retracted proximally for a long time and cannot be brought down to the correct position on the femoral component. Ideally, the entire graft would be covered by host muscle or joint capsule. This is not anatomically feasible, and the allograft patellar tendon and tubercle remain subcutaneous.

Postoperatively, the knee is placed in a hinged knee brace. The patient is allowed 60 degrees of motion for the first 6 weeks. The brace is continued with a 90 flex-

ion degree stop for the next 6 weeks, allowing the patient to gradually increase range of motion as comfort allows. The patient is encouraged to use walking aids until the gait is smooth. The grafted leg should not be used to push up from a chair. Stair climbing should be one step at a time to protect the grafted knee.

The author is following 15 patellar tendon allografts at this time, with 8 patients more than 3 years after reconstruction. Except for one young patient, age 36, the remainder have been elderly at the time of their surgery, with their average age 74 years. There have been no tibial tubercle nonunions. There was 1 postoperative quadriceps junction failure early in the series and 1 graft rupture at 6 months. The latter was attributed to surgical damage to the graft at the time of surgery. Based on this experience of graft damage, no crushing or piercing instruments should be applied to the graft. Recently, one patellar component has come loose, but the graft remained intact and has continued to function after removal of the loose patellar button. Using the technique

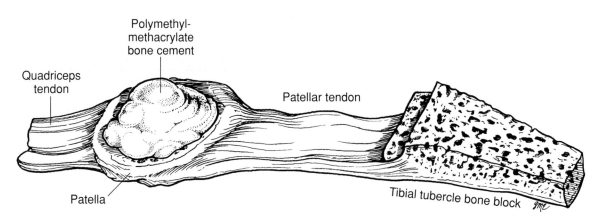

Figure 81.4. Patella facets have been resected and polymethylmethacrylate cement placed on the bony surface prior to insertion of the component.

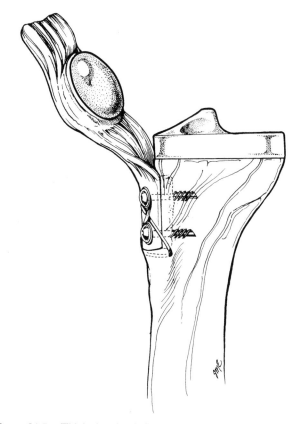

Figure 81.5. Tibial tubercle of allograft mechanism is keyed into the proximal tibia and held with screws and a tension-band wire.

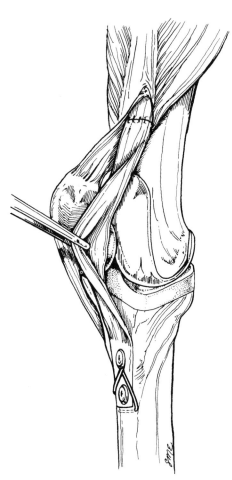

Figure 81.6. The quadriceps tendon on the allograft is sutured to the host quadriceps tendon, maintaining moderated tension on the extensor mechanism. The patella should articulate with the patellar flange of the femoral component. The host soft tissue sleeve should ideally cover as much of the allograft as possible.

as described, all patients have been able to regain functional extensor function.

The most difficult task with this technique is soft tissue tension and balance. Several patients, early in the series, had persisting extensor lags and tilting patellar grafts due to insufficient tensioning of the reconstruction. No grafts have dislocated. With improved surgical technique, the more recent extensor allograft patients have achieved full, active extension with better tracking of the grafts in the trochlea of the femur.

With a chronic extensor rupture, the quadriceps muscle shortens. At the time of surgery, the graft, therefore, must be under tension, even at full knee extension. Sixty degrees of passive motion on the operating room table is all that is sought. With time, as the contracted quadriceps stretches to its more normal functional length, knee motion improves. All knees in our series have gained at least 90 degrees of motion. As a group, prosthetic knees with a patellar tendon rupture have good motion before tendon reconstruction because the flexion is unopposed by the tethering, and flex without the tethering effect of the quadriceps. No vigorous attempt was made to return motion to the patient, for fear of disrupting the graft-host junction.

While the short-term success of this technique appears to be satisfactory, the long-term durability is as yet unproven.

References

1. Andriacchi TP, Stanwyck TC, Galante JO. Knee biomechanics and total knee replacement. J Arthroplasty 1986; 1:211–219.
2. Cadambi A, Engh GA. Use of a semitendinosis autogenous graft for rupture of the patellar ligament after total knee arthroplasty. J Bone Joint Surg 1992; 74A:974–979.
3. DePalma AF. Diseases of the knee. Philadelphia: JB Lippincott, 1954:218.
4. Doolittle KH, Turner RH. Patellofemoral problems following total knee arthroplasty. Orthop Rev 1988; 17:696–702.
5. Emerson RH, Head WC, Malinin TI. Reconstruction of patellar tendon rupture after total knee arthroplasty with an extensor mechanism allograft. Clin Orthop 1991; 260:154–161.
6. Figgie HE III, Goldberg VM, Heiple KG, Holler HS, Godgon NH. The influence of tibial-patellofemoral location on function of the knee in patients with the posterior stabilized condylar knee prosthesis. J Bone Joint Surg 1986; 68A:1035–1040.
7. Figgie HE III, Goldberg VM, Figgie MP, Inglis AE, Kelly M, Sobel M. The effect of alignment of the implant in fractures of the patella after condylar total knee arthroplasty. J Bone Joint Surg 1989; 71A:1031–1039.
8. Fulkerson JP, Shea KP. Current Concepts Review: Disorders of the patellofemoral alignment. J Bone Joint Surg 1990; 72A:1424–1429.
9. Goodfellow J, O'Connor J. The mechanics of the knee and prosthesis design. J Bone Joint Surg 1978; 60B:358–369.

10. Gustillo RB, Thompson R. Quadriceps and patellar tendon ruptures following total knee arthroplasty. In: Rand JA, Dorr LD, eds. Total arthroplasty of the knee. Rockville, Maryland: Aspen, 1987:45.

11. Inoue M, Konsei S, Hitoshi H, Horibe S, Ono K. Subluxation of the patella. J Bone Joint Surg 1988; 70A:1331–1337.

12. Insall JN, Scott WN, Ranawat CS. The total condylar knee prosthesis. J Bone Joint Surg 1979; 61:173–180.

13. Kirgis A. Spontaneous ruptures of the extensor mechanism of the knee following joint replacement in patients with rheumatoid arthritis. (Ger) Zeitschrift Für Orthopadie Und Ihre Grenzgebiete 1988; 126:519–525.

14. Langan P, Fontanetta AP. Rupture of the patellar tendon after use of its central third. Orthop Rev 1987; 16:317–321.

15. Larsen E, Lund PM. Ruptures of the extensor mechanism of the knee joint. Clin Orthop 1986; 213:150–153.

16. Laskin RS: Total condylar total knee replacement in rheumatoid arthritis. J Bone Joint Surg 1981; 63A:29–35.

17. Lauerman WC, Smith BG, Kenmore PI. Spontaneous bilateral rupture of the extensor mechanism of the knee in two patients on chronic ambulatory peritoneal dialysis. Orthopedics 1987; 10:589–591.

18. Lynch AF, Rorabeck CH, Bourne RB. Extensor mechanism complications following total knee arthroplasty. J Arthroplasty 1987; 2:135–140.

19. MacCollum MS, Karpman RR. Complications of the PCA anatomic patella. Orthopedics 1989; 12:1423–1428.

20. McLain RF, Bargar WF. The effect of total knee design on patellar strain. J Arthroplasty 1986; 1:91–98.

21. Mochizuki RM, Schurman DJ. Patellar complications following total knee arthroplasty. J Bone Joint Surg 1979; 61A:879–886.

22. Murzic WJ, Hardaker WT, Goldner JL. Surgical repair of extensor mechanism ruptures of the knee. Complic Orthop 1992; 7:276–279.

23. Noyes FR, Butler DL, Grood ES, Zernicke RE, Hefzy MS. Biomechanical analysis of human ligament grafts used in knee-ligament repairs and reconstructions. J Bone Joint Surg 1984; 66A:344–352.

24. Rand JA, Morrey BF, Bryan RS. Patellar tendon ruptures after total knee arthroplasty. Clin Orthop 1989; 224:233–238.

25. Ritter MA, Keating EM, Faris PM. Clinical, roentgenographic, and scintigraphic results after interruption of the superior lateral genicular artery during total knee arthroplasty. Clin Orthop 1989; 248:145–151.

26. Reuben JD, McDonald CL, Woodward PL, Hennington LJ. Effect of patella thickness on patella strain following total knee arthroplasty. J Arthroplasty 1991; 6:251–258.

27. Scapinelli R. Blood supply of the human patella. Its relation to ischemic necrosis after fracture. J Bone Joint Surg 1967; 49B:563–570.

28. Scuderi G, Scharf SC, Meltzer LP, Scott WN. The relationship of lateral releases to patella viability in total knee arthroplasty. J Arthroplasty 1987; 2:209–214.

29. Scuderi, C. Ruptures of the quadriceps tendon. Am J Surg 1958; 95:626–634.

30. Siwek CW, Rao JO. Ruptures of the extensor mechanism of the knee joint. J Bone Joint Surg 1981; 63A:932–937.

31. Sledge CB, Walker PS. Total knee arthroplasty in rheumatoid arthritis. Clin Orthop 1984; 182:127–136.

32. Walker LG, Glick H. Bilateral spontaneous quadriceps tendon ruptures. Orthop Rev 1989; 18:867–871.

33. Wolfe AM, Hungerford DS, Krackow KA. Jacobs MA. Osteotomy of the tibial tubercle during total knee replacement. J Bone Joint Surg 1989; 71A:848–852.

SECTION

XV

General Complications in Disorders of Articular Cartilage

82

Thromboembolic Disease

Phillip J. Mosca and Steven B. Haas

Introduction

Thromboembolic disease continues to pose a major threat to patients undergoing major knee surgery. Patients having surgical procedures such as total knee replacement (TKR) and high tibial osteotomy without prophylaxis have been shown to have deep vein thrombosis rates of 50 to 80% (1, 2, 3). While the majority of these clots occur in the calf veins and resolve without symptoms, many may propagate to the proximal veins, leading symptomatic deep vein thrombosis and pulmonary emboli.

Surgeons may find it easy to ignore thromboembolic disease, since the occurrence of clinically significant pulmonary embolism is relatively uncommon and the symptoms are often confused with other cardiac and pulmonary conditions found in an older population. The true incidence of symptomatic and fatal pulmonary embolism is probably underestimated since many pulmonary emboli do not occur until several weeks or months following surgery.

Prevention appears to be the best solution to the thromboembolic disease problem. This is especially true if one considers the risks involved with treatment of early proximal deep vein thrombosis and pulmonary embolism. One study from our institution showed that heparin therapy used within the first 5 days following total joint replacement surgery was associated with a 51% complication rate (4). Untreated patients with symptomatic pulmonary embolism have also been shown to suffer a high mortality rate (5). Clearly the answer is prevention.

While there is no ideal prophylactic regimen, several modalities have been shown to be both safe and effective in lowering the incidence of pulmonary embolism. When choosing the appropriate prophylactic regimen for the knee surgery patient, one must remember that the pathogenesis and epidemiology of thromboembolic disease in hip and knee surgery are different. For example, total hip replacement patients more commonly develop isolated proximal thrombi while TKR patients generally form calf thrombi. Additionally, warfarin has been shown to prevent the occurrence of deep vein thrombosis after total hip replacement while its efficacy in preventing deep vein thrombosis after TKR is less clear.

The surgeon should therefore choose an appropriate prophylactic regimen for knee surgery patients. This regimen can then be adjusted to meet the individual patient's need.

This chapter begins with a review of the pathogenesis and pathophysiology of thromboembolic disease. The clinical presentation and diagnostic tests are described; followed by a review of the best studied prophylactic and treatment modalities. The chapter concludes with a summary and recommendations for routine prophylaxis and treatment.

Pathogenesis

The development of a deep venous thrombosis is a multifactorial process (6). Virchow's triad, hypothesized in 1856 (7), has been the basis of our understanding of the pathogenesis of deep venous thrombosis. Studies have shown that changes in the constituents of the blood resulting in hypercoagulability, changes in the lining of the vessel wall, and changes in blood flow are primary mechanisms in the development of deep venous thrombosis.

Anatomy and Physiology

The venous drainage of the lower extremity varies anatomically. Blood travels back to the heart through the deep veins, the muscular veins, and the superficial veins. The deep and superficial systems are connected by communicating or perforating veins. Although there are four systems of veins, only blood clots in the deep system are considered "deep vein thrombosis" (8). The deep veins of the lower extremity consist of the deep plantar veins of the foot; the three paired veins of the leg named by the artery they surround (the posterior tibial veins, the anterior tibial veins, and the peroneal veins), the popliteal vein; and the superficial and deep femoral veins.

The veins in the soles of the feet and the plantar arch drain into the posterior tibial veins. The veins of the dorsum of the foot drain into the anterior tibial veins. The posterior tibial veins, the anterior tibial veins, and the peroneal veins form the popliteal vein. The popliteal vein continues proximally and becomes the superficial femoral vein. About 9 cm inferior to the inguinal ligament, the superficial femoral vein receives the deep femoral vein. This confluence forms the common femoral vein that, slightly more proximal, receives the saphenous vein. After it passes posterior to the inguinal ligament, the common femoral vein becomes the external iliac vein. The external iliac vein, upon joining with the internal iliac vein becomes the common iliac vein that, in joining with its counterpart, forms the vena cava.

Physiologically, most of the circulating volume of blood is contained in the venous system that, for the most part, acts as a capacitor. Of the three major types of veins, cutaneous, splanchnic and skeletal muscular veins, the skeletal muscular veins have little or no innervation by the sympathetic nervous system. Vasoconstriction of these vessels is limited, and, therefore, blood must be aided on its course back to the heart by the muscle pumps and the valves within the veins. The muscle pump results from muscular activity of the lower extremity that squeezes the veins and thereby increases their intraluminal pressure. The valves prevent distal reflux of blood in the deep veins and prevent reflux of blood from the deep to the superficial system. The valves also indirectly decrease the venous hydrostatic pressure by dividing the long column of blood, which would be present without the valves, into small columns of blood that exert smaller hydrostatic pressures (6).

On a cellular level, abnormal thrombogenesis is avoided because intact venous endothelium is nonthrombotic secondary to the attached glycosaminoglycans. Endothelial cells also produce prostacyclin, which is an antiplatelet aggregation agent, and plasminogen activators, which lyse intravascular fibrin (9).

Etiology

As mentioned earlier, Virchow's triad is the basis for our understanding of the etiology of deep vein thrombosis. Many authors believe that stasis is probably the most important factor in the development of deep vein thrombosis (10). Others feel that stasis works in concert with hypercoagulability and/or vessel wall damage (9, 11, 12). Many experiments and studies suggest that hypercoagulability is an essential factor in the initiation of deep venous thrombosis (9, 11, 13).

Changes in Blood Flow

Changes in the flow of blood are factors to consider in the pathogenesis of deep vein thrombosis. As blood courses the valve cusps, eddy currents form that increase platelet deposition at the base of the valve cusps (14, 15). With decreased blood flow, red and white blood cells as well as platelets can "silt" in a valve pocket where they can become bound and anchored by fibrin. This acts as a nidus for the thrombus that will continue to grow with successive layers of cells and fibrin.

A decrease in blood flow, stasis, can increase viscosity and decrease the clearance of activated clotting factors by the liver and reticuloendothelial system. With stasis, there may be an inability for blood components to mix properly, i.e., esterases mixing with their inhibitors (16). Clinically, we know that stasis of the blood in the veins of the lower extremity is associated with deep vein thrombosis formation (17). As early as 1793, Baillie reported that inferior vena cava obstruction decreased blood flow and led to deep vein thrombosis (18). Studies of patients with paralyzed lower extremities secondary to stroke (19, 20) or spinal cord injury (21–25) revealed a high incidence of deep vein thrombosis in the affected limb. When examining unilateral paralysis, the incidence of deep vein thrombosis was higher in the paralyzed leg when compared to the nonparalyzed leg (25).

Changes in the Lining of the Vessel Wall

Endothelial cell damage with exposure of subendothelial structures, especially collagen, induces platelet aggregation and activation. It also initiates the blood coagulation cascade via the extrinsic route. Investigators believe that there must be injury to the vein wall for thrombus to form (10). Clinically, there is a high incidence of deep vein thrombosis in patients who have major orthopaedic surgery that requires soft tissue manipulation and damage, i.e., total hip replacements, total knee replacements or hip fracture-procedures (1–3, 26–34).

Using electron microscopy, investigators were able to show that stasis and trauma allow white blood cells to adhere to the vessel wall. These white blood cells would then translocate to the basement membrane where they caused a patchy endothelial desquamatization, exposing subendothelial collagen that can induce thrombus formation (12).

The functioning of the endothelial cell is very important for homeostasis. As mentioned earlier, endothelial cells produce tissue plasminogen activator and prostacyclin. When the cell malfunctions causing a decrease in the production and/or release of tissue plasminogen activator or decrease in the prostacyclin activity, recurrent deep vein thrombi have been shown to occur (35–42). Other factors such as antithrombin III (43, 44), Factor VIII (45–47) and glycosaminoglycans (48–50) especially, heparin sulfate, have been found in endothelial cells. Their contributions to the pathogenesis of deep vein thrombosis, as well as that from tissue plasminogen activator and prostacyclin, have yet to be determined fully.

Changes in Blood Constituents

Changes in the coagulation factors following orthopaedic (16, 51–54) and nonorthopaedic surgery (55–58) have been reported. The level of fibrinogen and coagulation factors II, V, VII, and XII have all been shown to increase after surgery; but there have been no studies that show these factors cause deep vein thrombosis (51). Antithrombin III has been studied extensively and its deficiency is accepted as a cause of deep vein thrombosis (9, 17, 54, 59, 60). Antithrombin III is an alpha-2 globulin in the blood that inactivates thrombin (factor IIa), factor Xa and factor IXa (61). Antithrombin III is an important heparin cofactor, and when bound to heparin, antithrombin III has a higher rate of inactivation than the above mentioned coagulation factors. Levels of antithrombin III decrease after orthopaedic surgery (62, 63). Recent studies using antithrombin III in combination with subcutaneous heparin as a prophylactic agent after total hip and total knee replacement support this etiology by showing a decrease in the incidence of deep vein thrombosis as compared to a control group (60, 61, 64, 65). Protein-C deficiency, protein-S deficiency and hereditary heparin cofactor II deficiency have also been studied; their deficiencies increased the risk of recurrent deep vein thrombosis in certain families (66–72).

It is well known that platelets play a major role in arterial thrombosis, but few data support their role in the development of venous thrombosis (73, 74). Early studies incorporating aspirin as prophylaxis in patients who receive total hip replacements showed its effectiveness, but these studies have been disputed (33, 75–78). Following surgery, the number and the activity of platelets increase (57–59, 79–81). Recently, it was reported that there was no correlation between platelet activation and the occurrence of deep vein thrombosis after total hip arthroplasty (82). All this contradicting data leaves the role of platelets in the development of deep venous thrombosis unknown.

Macroscopically, it is felt that deep vein thrombosis formation in the surgical patient starts intraoperatively, or in the early postoperative period, and frequently originates in the deep veins of the calf. Several studies have shown that it is unusual for an orthopaedic patient to have a deep vein thrombosis prior to surgery (28, 83). Doing serial venography, Maynard, et al. (83) showed that 86% of the thrombi that were identified in patients in the postoperative period were found "post-op day number one".

Once thrombi have formed, they may spontaneously lyse, become organized, or extend in either an antegrade or retrograde manner. If obstruction occurs, the thrombus will grow in a retrograde manner (9). Extension of a calf clot occurs in 5 to 30% of all patients with calf clots (84). Clots that are smaller than 5 cm in length are less likely to propagate (26, 85). Extension of calf thrombi often proceeds to embolization (53).

The frequency of pulmonary embolism following a calf thrombosis has not been extensively studied. The risk of a silent pulmonary embolism has been estimated to be 8 to 18%. The risk of symptomatic pulmonary embolism appears to be 2 to 4%, while the risk of fatal pulmonary embolism is not known but appears to be less than the risk noted in total hip replacement, that is, 1 to 3% (84). In a study at our institution, patients who were identified as having calf thrombi had a 6.9% incidence of positive lung scans and 1.7% incidence of symptomatic pulmonary embolism (86).

Clots in the proximal deep venous system are more dangerous than distal clots because of the fact that proximal clots tend to be large and have a much greater risk of embolization.

Risk Factors

There have been many risk factors identified that may potentiate deep venous thrombosis in the general population (87). Although these factors may signal which patients develop deep venous thrombosis, we feel that major knee surgery has such a great impact on the development of deep vein thrombosis that the usual risk factors have less effect. In total knee replacement surgery, two factors, identified as having a positive correlation with deep vein thrombosis formation, include old age and hypertension (3, 26).

Clinical Presentation

The clinical presentation of deep vein thrombosis is highly varied. Most of the time, the patient has no signs or symptoms. Other times, symptoms are generalized and include calf pain, which may be dull and achy and aggravated by standing or walking; swelling; pyrexia of unknown origin; and discoloration of the skin of the leg (88). Because of the varied clinical presentation and the fact that postoperative knee surgery patients have swollen and painful calves anyway, one can gather that the clinical diagnosis of deep vein thrombosis after knee surgery is unreliable and nonspecific. The clinical diagnosis of deep vein thrombosis in the hospital population has been reported to be 50% accurate (89), although a more recent report showed a 14% accuracy rate (2).

Diagnostic testing, although not 100% accurate, does aid in diagnosing deep vein thrombosis. One needs to correlate the signs and symptoms with the diagnostic test results to determine the appropriate treatment protocol.

Diagnostic Tests for Deep Vein Thrombosis

Diagnostic tests that are used to evaluate the postoperative orthopaedic patient include venography and sonography. Iodine-125-labeled fibrinogen scans and impedance plethysmography are nonspecific tests that have little use in this patient population.

Venography

Contrast venography is often referred to as the gold standard for diagnosing deep vein thrombosis. It has been used extensively for the past 20 years. The basic technique is to inject contrast into the veins of the foot and then x-ray the leg. At our facility, we use the technique described by Rabinov and Paulin (8), but with the addition of tourniquets at the lower leg to favor venous blood flow through the deep veins. Fifty to 100 cc of Conray 43 (iothalamate meglumine) is used. The test is done under continuous fluoroscopic monitoring. The advantages of this test include:

1. Direct visualization of the thrombi
2. Sensitivity to both proximal and distal deep vein thrombosis
3. Confirmation or exclusion of the diagnosis is usually achieved in one session.

The disadvantages include the need for *(a)* specialized staff members and *(b)* venous access, anaphylactoid reaction to the contrast, risk of extravasation, inability to visualize the deep femoral vein or the internal iliac vein, and postvenography syndrome. The venographic dye, Isopaque (meglumine metrizoate), has been reported to precipitate thrombosis in 7% of patients (90), although we have seen a much lower complication rate at our institution (83). Contraindications for this test relate to the contrast material and include patients with acute renal failure, patients with chronic renal failure and a serum creatinine greater than 3 mg/100 ml, and patients with idiosyncratic reactions. A newer nonionic contrast material is available for patients who are allergic to the ionic contrast material or who cannot tolerate a large fluid load.

Sonography

The use of sonography to detect thrombi of the lower extremity is a diagnostic test that has been gaining popularity over the last few years. With technologic improvements and expert technicians, sonography can be of great benefit.

The current technique for assessing thrombi with ultrasound is B-mode ultrasound. Ultrasound, originally described in 1976 (91), has evolved many clinical applications. B-mode ultrasound uses high frequency sound waves to produce a two-dimensional image. When a thrombus is present, the B-mode ultrasound may visually show it, may reveal a noncompressible vein, or it may show a certain percentage of change in the vein diameter during a Valsalva maneuver. Studies have shown that compressibility is the best criterion for detecting deep vein thrombosis (92–96). Clinically, the test results are reliable in detecting a proximal deep vein thrombosis in symptomatic patients and postoperative patients (92, 93, 97). In symptomatic patients, the sensitivity of this test ranges from 83 to 100%; the specificity ranges from 86 to 100% (97). Although a number of studies has shown that B-mode ultrasound is highly sensitive, there was one report of low sensitivity in asymptomatic patients (98). The advantages of this test include the fact that it is painless, noninvasive, quick, and does not expose the patient to x-ray irradiation. There are no absolute contraindications to the test. A main disadvantage is that ultrasound testing is extremely operator-dependent. In one report, a learning curve was documented over a 2-year period with the sensitivity improving from 67 to 83% and specificity improving from 99 to 100% (93). Other disadvantages include the expense of the equipment and the inability to image middle and distal calf veins and iliofemoral veins. Detecting isolated calf thrombi with B-mode ultrasonography has been reported to be 36% sensitive (92). Proponents of this test contend that calf deep vein thrombi are not clinically significant, but that when they become clinically significant, i.e., by propagation to proximal deep vein thrombi, they will be detected by B-mode ultrasound.

Iodine-125-Labeled Fibrinogen Leg Scanning

In the past, this test has been used extensively in general surgery patients. The basis for this test is the fact that radioactive-labeled fibrinogen is incorporated into a clot as it forms. The reported sensitivity is 95% in symptomatic general surgery patients with recent onset of deep vein thrombosis (99, 100). The results in the orthopaedic patient have not been as encouraging. It is nonspecific because of accumulation of fibrin in areas where no deep vein thrombosis is present, the wound and the operative site (101). We do not recommend this test as a screening test in the postoperative knee surgery patient.

Impedance Plethysmography

Impedance plethysmography is also a poor test to detect deep vein thrombosis in the postoperative orthopaedic patient. In asymptomatic patients, it has an overall accuracy of 60 to 70% (102). Two large studies comparing impedance plethysmography with venography (103) and impedance plethysmography with [125I]fibrinogen and venography (104) in patients who underwent hip surgery revealed a sensitivity of 12% and 29%, respectively, and a specificity of 99% and 98%, respectively. These tests are noninvasive and have a low chance of morbidity and mortality. However, because of their inaccuracy, we do not recommend their use in the postoperative knee surgery patient.

Pulmonary Embolism

Pulmonary embolism is one of the most feared complications of total knee arthroplasty. The incidence of asymptomatic pulmonary embolism detected by $\dot{V}/\dot{Q}$ lung scans has been reported in up to 17% of cases (26). There are 600,000 cases of symptomatic pulmonary embolism in the United States per year, and 200,000 patients die of pulmonary embolism per year in the United States (105). Most pulmonary emboli are asymptomatic and may occur unnoticed. In healthy individuals, hemodynamic changes are not evident until more than half of the pulmonary arterial tree is involved (106). But, in patients with a compromised respiratory system, small pulmonary emboli may cause severe symptoms and death. The signs and symptoms of pulmonary embolism are nonspecific and the results of $\dot{V}/\dot{Q}$ scans can be inconclusive (107). Therefore, one must have a high index of suspicion when diagnosing pulmonary embolism.

Most pulmonary emboli originate from thrombi formed in the veins of the lower extremity. Therefore, the pathogenesis and the risk factors for pulmonary embolism are similar to those of deep vein thrombosis. Knee surgery is a risk factor in thromboembolic disease. Total knee arthroplasty has such a strong correlation with deep vein thrombosis and pulmonary embolism that most studies have not shown a correlation with other risk factors, such as obesity, diabetes, malignancy, or infection. The size and location of the thrombus are other important determinants of pulmonary embolism risk. Thrombi that are greater than 5 to 6 cm in length or those proximal to the calf have an increased chance of embolizing to the lung.

Clinical Presentation

As stated previously, the signs and symptoms of pulmonary embolism vary and are nonspecific. Symptomatic patients may present with dyspnea; pleuritic pain, if the periphery of the lung is involved, tachypnea; tachycardia; and fever. On physical examination, the neck veins may be distended, changes in heart sound may be auscultated, and symptoms of deep venous thrombosis may be elicited. Patients suspected of having a pulmonary embolism should always be examined for signs and symptoms of deep vein thrombosis.

Diagnostic Tests for Pulmonary Embolism

As with deep vein thrombosis, clinical diagnosis of pulmonary embolism is unreliable. One needs to combine clinical signs and symptoms with objective testing to diagnose PE. The gold standard in diagnosis of pulmonary embolism is angiography but its invasiveness and unavailability at all centers make it a test that is used infrequently.

Arterial Blood Gases

Arterial blood gas results may reveal a low arterial PO_2 with an increase in the A-a gradient. A low arterial Pco_2 may also be noted secondarily to the transient tachypnea.

Electrocardiogram

Changes on electrocardiograms (ECGs) are seen in massive pulmonary embolisms. The changes are related to right ventricular function and to the increased pulmonary pressure that accompanies pulmonary embolism. The classic finding is described as a prominent S wave in lead I, a Q wave in lead III and T-wave inversions in lead III (S-1, Q-3, T-3). Other findings may include T-wave inversions in leads V1, V2, V3, and possibly V4 and the presence of a right bundle branch block pattern. New onset atrial fibrillation may also present as a first sign of pulmonary embolism.

Chest X-ray

Findings on chest x-ray are nonspecific and usually not helpful alone but may be needed for comparison with a ventilation-perfusion scan (108). Chest x-ray findings that suggest a pulmonary embolism include:

1. Infarct shadows, usually wedge shaped
2. Linear atelectasis
3. Loss of lung volume
4. A small pleural effusion (109).

Ventilation-Perfusion Scintigraphy

Ventilation-perfusion scintigraphy or V̇/Q̇ scanning is a noninvasive technique that can be of significant assistance in the detection of pulmonary embolism.

Perfusion scintigraphy is a very sensitive test for detecting pulmonary embolism, but the technique is not specific for pulmonary embolism (110). A normal perfusion scan has a very high negative predictive value for detecting pulmonary embolism (111). An abnormal perfusion scan may not necessarily mean a pulmonary embolism is present (low positive predictive value).

The test is performed by injecting radioactive isotopes into a peripheral vein and then imaging the lung in eight views: anterior, posterior, right lateral, left lateral, right anterior oblique, left anterior oblique, right posterior oblique, and left posterior oblique (108). Technetium-99m-labeled albumin microspheres and technetium-99m-labeled macroaggregated albumin are two commonly used agents. They are pure gamma emitters having a short half-life (6 hours) and expose the body to a low dose of radiation (108). A perfusion defect when imaging signifies a decrease or occlusion of blood flow. Besides an embolus, other causes of perfusion defects must be ruled out, i.e., obstructive airway disease, infection, and neoplastic disease (108).

Although perfusion scanning can be performed alone to detect pulmonary embolism, the specificity of the test is significantly increased with the addition of ventilation scanning. Ventilation scans are performed by having the patient inhale radioactive agents that do not diffuse into the circulation. The four most commonly used ventilation agents are xenon-133, xenon-127, krypton-81m, and technetium-99m-DTPA (diethylene triamine pentraacetate) aerosols (108). Theoretically, this test should be performed before perfusion scanning. In collecting the data, views similar to the perfusion scan are obtained.

The scans are assessed using the criteria shown in Table 82.1. Many studies have been conducted to assess the accuracy of V̇/Q̇ lung scans. The results of the scans are varied, and, because of this, a classification has been established (108, 112). Accordingly, using these classifications, the probability that a patient has a pulmonary embolism is 0% for a normal scan result; 0% to 5% for a very low scan result; less than 10% for a low scan result; 10% to 85% for an intermediate scan result; and greater than 85% for a high scan result.

Pulmonary Arteriography

Pulmonary arteriography is probably the most definitive and accurate procedure for diagnosing pulmonary embolism (108). The test may be indicated to confirm or exclude a diagnosis. It should be performed in 24 to 48 hours after the onset of symptoms because clot lysis can lead to nonspecific vascular defects. A catheter is usually passed over a wire that initially is inserted into the femoral vein. If clots are suspected in the femoral

Table 82.1. Ventilation-Perfusion Lung Scan Criteria

Probability	Classification
High Probability	≥ 2 Large (> 75% of a segment) segmental perfusion defects without corresponding ventilation or roentgenographic abnormalities or substantially larger than either matching ventilation or chest roentgenogram abnormalities.
	-or-
	≥ 2 Moderate segmental (≥ 25% and ≤75% of a segment) perfusion defects without matching ventilation or chest roentgenogram abnormalities and 1 large mismatched segmental defect
	-or-
	≥ 4 Moderate segmental perfusion defects without ventilation or chest roentgenogram abnormalities
Intermediate Probability	Not falling into normal, very-low-, low-, or high-probability categories
	-or-
(Indeterminate)	Borderline high or borderline low
	-or-
	Difficult to categorize as low or high
Low Probability	Nonsegmental perfusion defects (eg, very small effusion causing blunting of the costophrenic angle, cardiomegaly, enlarged aorta, hila, mediastinum, and elevated diaphragm)
	-or-
	Single moderate mismatched segmental perfusion defect with normal chest roentgenogram
	-or-
	Any perfusion defect with a substantially larger chest roentgenogram abnormally
	-or-
	Large or moderate segmental perfusion defects involving no more than 3 segments in 1 lung region with matching ventilation defects either equal to or larger in size and chest roentgenogram either normal or with abnormalities substantially smaller than perfusion defects
Very-low Probability	> 3 Small segmental perfusion defects (<25% of a segment) with a normal chest roentgenogram
	-or-
	≥ 3 Small segmental perfusion defects with a normal chest roentgenogram
Normal	No perfusion defects present
	-or-
	Perfusion outlines exactly the shape of the lungs as seen on the chest roentgenogram (hilar and aortic impressions may be seen, chest roentgenogram and/or ventilation study may be abnormal)

veins or above, the catheter may be passed through the antecubital vein or through the jugular vein. After the catheter reaches the heart, it is advanced through the tricuspid valve and the pulmonary valve. Once in the pulmonary artery, dye is injected to detect any large emboli that may be present. If not, the catheter is advanced into specific branches with the injection of dye and continuous fluoroscopic monitoring.

The advantage of this test is its accuracy. Disadvantages include its invasiveness, risk of complications, the need for qualified personnel, and the need for a catheterization laboratory. Absolute contraindications include a recent myocardial infarction and uncontrolled left ventricular failure. Relative contraindications are related to the contrast material and include renal failure and a serum creatinine of more than 3 mg/dl.

Complications of pulmonary arteriography include adverse reaction to the contrast material, renal failure, cardiac arrhythmias, endocardial or myocardial injury, cardiac arrest, dislodgment of venous, cardiac or pulmonary artery emboli, and death. Because of the 3.5% morbidity rate and the 0.2% mortality rate, this test should obviously not be used for screening (113).

Postphlebitic Syndrome

Besides pulmonary embolism, another sequela of deep vein thrombosis is postphlebitic syndrome. Postphlebitic syndrome is generally considered a complication of proximal vein thrombosis, although postphlebitic syndrome has been seen in patients with distal deep vein thrombosis. The syndrome presents months to years after deep vein thrombosis. The etiology is thought to be due to the high intravenous pressure that can result from outflow obstruction, by valve destruction, or by narrow veins secondary to recanalization of the thrombosed veins. The high pressure is thought to eventually cause the valves of the perforating vein to malfunction, resulting in blood flow from the deep system into the superficial system. The high pressure in the superficial system leads to the symptoms of swelling, edema, pigmentation, and induration around the ankle and lower leg, and, possibly, ulcerations of the leg, especially around the medial malleolus (10, 114, 115).

Studies reveal that postphlebitic syndrome following isolated calf deep vein thrombosis is uncommon. However, patients with calf thrombi have shown persistent flow changes which were subclinical (116). The incidence of postphlebitic syndrome following proximal deep vein thrombosis is higher. In patients with untreated proximal deep vein thrombosis who were followed for more than 10 years, the frequency of leg edema and skin changes was over 90% (117). Despite anticoagulation therapy and, in some cases, thrombolytic therapy, patients with proximal thrombi can still develop postphlebitic syndrome, emphasizing prophylaxis as the best form of treatment (118–120).

Prophylaxis

The incidence of venographically defined deep vein thrombosis in patients who have had total knee arthroplasty without prophylaxis has ranged from 70 to 84% (1–3). The incidence of asymptomatic pulmonary embolism following TKA has been reported to be between 7 and 17%; the incidence of symptomatic pulmonary embolism has been reported to be between 1 and 10% (2, 3), and the incidence of fatal pulmonary embolism is currently unknown, but appears to be less than the 1 to

3% rate reported after total hip replacement (2, 3, 121). Understanding the increased risk that knee surgery, especially total knee replacement, has on the development of deep vein thrombosis and pulmonary embolism, one must consider prophylaxis for all patients who will have major knee surgery. In contrast, young patients undergoing arthroscopic knee surgery have not been shown to have an increased risk of development of deep vein thrombosis; a deep vein thrombosis rate of 4% has been reported (29).

In evaluating the literature on deep vein thrombosis prophylaxis, one must not only compare the rates of deep vein thrombosis that have been reported, but also the diagnostic means of assessing for deep vein thrombosis. As mentioned earlier, the clinical diagnosis of deep vein thrombosis is extremely difficult in this patient population. At this time, the gold standard for assessing thrombosis in clinical studies is ascending venography.

Prophylactic agents that have been studied in patients who undergo major knee surgery include pharmacologic agents such as aspirin, warfarin, dextran, heparin, low molecular weight heparin, and mechanical agents, such as pneumatic compression boots.

Pharmacologic Agents

Aspirin

Aspirin (acetylsalicylic acid) is a nonsteroidal antiinflammatory agent that irreversibly inhibits the cyclooxygenase of platelets, thereby inhibiting the synthesis of thromboxane A2. Thromboxane A2 causes platelet aggregation and vasoconstriction (73). Aspirin has been reported to be an effective antithrombotic agent in patients with ischemic heart disease and cerebrovascular disease (73). It gained popularity as a prophylactic modality in orthopaedic patients after early reports of success. Follow-up reports and further evaluations revealed that it is not effective in preventing deep vein thrombosis in patients who have total knee and hip replacements. We do not recommend its use as a single prophylactic agent in major knee surgery.

The incidence of deep vein thrombosis when aspirin was used prophylactically in knee surgery patients ranged from 41 to 78% (2, 3, 30, 33, 122–124). There has been only one small study that showed a deep vein thrombosis rate of 8% (122). Risks of using aspirin include gastric mucosa erythema, gastric erosions, and gastric ulcers (73). These side effects appear to be dose related. Most regimens employ aspirin by mouth, 325 mg to 650 mg BID.

Although aspirin has little effect in preventing deep vein thrombosis after TKA, if aspirin is combined with routine venographic screening and treatment of detected thrombi, it appears to be associated with a low rate of symptomatic and fatal pulmonary emboli (86).

Warfarin

Warfarin is becoming an increasingly popular form of prophylaxis following knee surgery because of its encouraging results following total hip replacement.

Warfarin is an oral anticoagulant that inhibits the blood coagulation cascade by affecting the synthesis of active vitamin K-dependent coagulation factors (factors II, VII, IX, and X) as well as protein C. Since warfarin inhibits synthesis of active coagulation factors, it has no effect on the existing circulating coagulation factors. Therapeutic anticoagulation is reached from 24 to 36 hours after the initial dose of warfarin. There have been two protocols described in the literature for using warfarin in the prophylaxis of orthopaedic patients. The low-dose protocol entails dosing of 10 mg on the night of surgery or the night prior to surgery and then dosing to keep the prothrombin time between 1.2 to 1.5 times the control prothrombin time. Rates of deep vein thrombosis using this method range from 35 to 59% with one study reporting a deep vein thrombosis rate of 25% (3, 30, 125–128). The two-step protocol begins 10 to 14 days preoperatively and maintains a prothrombin time of 1.5 to 3 seconds above the control prothrombin time. Postoperatively, the prothrombin time is maintained at 1.5 times the control prothrombin time. A deep vein thrombosis rate of 21% was reported (129).

Risks when using this medication include bleeding, and, although rare, warfarin-induced skin necrosis. Another pitfall associated with warfarin is the need to monitor the prothrombin time. The advantages of warfarin prophylaxis are twofold: a) warfarin can be continued as treatment if a thrombus is detected and b) the oral route of administration.

Although warfarin appears to be an effective agent in reducing the deep vein thrombosis rate after hip replacement surgery, its efficacy in total knee replacement is not clear. Warfarin may limit propagation and embolization of a thrombus, but it has not clearly been shown to decrease the occurrence of deep vein thrombosis.

Dextran

Dextran is a neutral polysaccharide molecule that is a product of bacterial metabolism. Dextran 40 and dextran 70 are two commercially available preparations. Initially used as plasma expanders, they also exhibited antithrombotic properties. Dextrans seem to increase blood flow by decreasing blood viscosity. They also decrease platelet adhesiveness, decrease clotting factor VIII, and cause the fibrin network that forms in thrombi to be defective and to lyse more easily. They also enhance fibrinolysis and protect plasmin from inhibitory effects. These effects are still not adequately understood (130). The dosage varies among studies but usually includes a loading dose of dextran administered intravenously and followed by a continuous IV drip for 3 to 5 days. Clinical trials have shown deep vein thrombosis rates of 50 and 100% (60, 65, 128, 129). Side effects include bleeding, possible allergic reaction, and volume overload that can lead to pulmonary edema. Intravenous access must be maintained during the treatment. Although dextran has been shown to be effective in prophylaxis after hip surgery (131–133), it has not been effective in preventing deep vein thrombosis after major knee surgery.

Heparin

Heparin is a mixture of very large molecules of mucopolysaccharide-glycosaminoglycans. The molecular weight ranges from 5000 to 30,000 daltons. It has been shown to be an effective anticoagulant. The mechanism of action, mediated through antithrombin III and heparin cofactor II, is by inhibition of the blood coagulation cascade. Subcutaneous heparin has been commonly used in general surgery patients and is also popular in Europe; however, fixed dose subcutaneous heparin does not appear to be effective in decreasing the rate of deep vein thrombosis after total knee replacement. Heparin has been used in a few prophylactic protocols. When low-dose heparin prophylaxis was employed (heparin 5000 units subcutaneously, BID), deep vein thrombosis rates of 50 and 53% were recorded (3). A deep vein thrombosis rate of 34% was reported when adjusted-dose heparin was used (129). In this study, heparin was given subcutaneously, and the partial thromboplastin time (PTT) was kept between 31.5 to 36 seconds. Low-dose heparin has been combined with antithrombin III, dihydroergotamine, sulfinpyrazone, and intermittent pneumatic compression devices. The action of low-dose heparin and antithrombin III has been studied in knee surgery, revealing deep vein thrombosis rates of 25 and 28% (60, 65).

Risks with the use of heparin include bleeding and thrombocytopenia. Because antithrombin III is a blood product, there is a risk of transmitting blood-borne disease.

Adjusted dose heparin probably has beneficial effects, but further investigation is needed to confirm its effectiveness in patients undergoing knee surgery. Low-dose heparin is felt to be ineffective. Low-dose heparin and antithrombin III appear to be effective but this combination is still in the experimental stage.

Low Molecular Weight Heparin

Low molecular weight heparin is a relatively new prophylactic modality that has been popular in Europe and is being tested extensively in the United States. Low molecular weight heparin was developed in the 1970s and was shown to have very good antithrombotic activity, and, when compared to standard heparin, to have less bleeding per unit of equivalent antithrombotic activity. Low molecular weight heparin is the fractionated form of heparin with a molecular weight ranging from 4000 to 6000 daltons. Numerous forms of low molecular weight heparin are available. Dalteparin and Flaxiparin are formed by nitrous acid depolimerization; Logiparin by heparinase depolimerization; RD 1185 by peroxide degradation; and Enoxaparin by beta-elimination. All low molecular weight heparin contains the specific pentasaccharide that binds antithrombin III. Because of its smaller size, the low molecular weight heparin can bind antithrombin III and this complex can inactivate coagulation factor Xa to a greater extent than factor IIa. Its size also inhibits it from binding to heparin cofactor II, a mediator that inactivates factor IIa, specifically. Low molecular weight heparins have high bioavailability at low doses because, unlike standard heparin, they only bind to one circulating protein. Studies have shown that once or twice per day dosing is effective in decreasing the rate of deep vein thrombosis without the need to monitor the partial thromboplastin time (61). There have been many studies in patients who have had total hip replacement and have shown deep vein thrombosis rates of 8 to 30% (134–138). Two studies employing low molecular weight heparin in patients undergoing total knee replacement revealed deep vein thrombosis rates of 17 and 26% (139, 140).

As with heparin, bleeding and thrombocytopenia are risks that need to be considered when using low molecular weight heparin.

One type of low molecular weight heparin, enoxaparin (Lovenox, Rhone-Poulenc Rorer), has recently been approved by the FDA for deep vein thrombosis prophylaxis in patients who have total hip replacement. Although these drugs are not FDA approved for patient who have total knee replacement, the results are promising. More research in patients having major knee surgery is warranted.

Mechanical Devices

Mechanical devices and physical agents have been used as deep vein thrombosis prophylaxis in a variety of surgical procedures. Early mobilization, constant passive motion machines, and graded compression stockings are all advocated, but are insufficient alone in preventing deep vein thrombosis in patient undergoing TKA. A number of intermittent pneumatic compression devices are available; they include calf- and thigh-length boots. Both appear to be effective in preventing deep vein thrombosis following knee surgery.

Intermittent Pneumatic Compression Devices

Intermittent pneumatic compression devices include polyvinyl boots or leggings, stockings with inflatable bladders and multicompartment vinyl leggings (141). Generally, the pressures reach between 35 to 55 mm Hg and inflate in cycles of 60 to 90 seconds (normal venous refilling takes 60 to 90 seconds). The devices are thought to decrease stasis, understandable as the result of periodically raising intraluminal venous pressure, but it is also felt that intermittent compression increases the activity of the fibrinolytic system. Knight, et al. (142) theorized that occlusion of the veins and direct compression of the vein walls release fibrinolytic activators.

Usually, a boot is applied to the nonoperated leg preoperatively and the other boot is applied to the operated leg postoperatively. The boots are continued until the patient is ambulating independently.

The incidence of deep vein thrombosis has been reported to be 7.5 to 33% (30, 33, 125, 127, 128, 143, 144) after unilateral total knee replacement. One study examined thrombi according to size and found that intermittent pneumatic compression boots reduced the rate of large thrombi to 6%, while patients on aspirin had a rate of large thrombi of 31% (33). Patients undergoing simultaneous bilateral total knee replacement are at increased risk for the development of deep vein thrombosis and were found to have a 48% incidence of deep vein thrombosis despite the use of compression boots (33). There is minimal morbidity associated with the use of this device. We recommend that dressings not be excessively bulky. Its use is contraindicated in patients with peripheral arterial disease. It is effective in reducing the incidence of deep vein thrombosis after unilateral TKA and especially effective in preventing the formation of large thrombi.

Combination of Prophylactic Agents

Few studies have looked at combination prophylaxis. This is difficult to study because a large number of patients are required to prove a statistically significant incremental benefit. Pharmacologic agents combined with intermittent pneumatic compression devices (IPCD) have been used in arthroplasty patients. The combination of dextran and thigh-high IPCD, aspirin and thigh-high IPCD, and warfarin and thigh-high IPCD have been studied in patients undergoing total hip replacement. Harris, et al. (145) found that the combination of dextran and IPCD, when compared to 1.2 grams of aspirin daily and 0.3 grams of aspirin daily showed a significant reduction in the rate of deep vein thrombosis. But when combinations of IPCD with aspirin or with warfarin were compared to IPCD alone, no significant differences in proximal deep vein thrombosis formation were noted (146). The combination of IPCD and warfarin was compared to IPCD alone in patients undergoing TKA. There was no statistically significant difference between the two groups (30).

Combined modalities may have a beneficial effect on decreasing the incidence of deep vein thrombosis, which has, as yet, not been shown.

Treatment

Treatment of deep vein thrombosis in the postoperative knee patient is not without complications. The goal of treatment must be defined. Preventing embolization of the clot is a main concern because of the possibility of fatal pulmonary embolism. Morbidity from postphlebitic syndrome and pulmonary hypertension are other concerns. In deciding on the treatment, numerous considerations must be assessed. The location of the thrombi is important with respect to the risk of embolization. The symptomatology of the patient may determine what action, if any, is taken. The age and medical status of the patient are also considered. Finally, the time from surgery until the detection of the thrombi is important to assess the risks of bleeding complications if anticoagulation therapy is considered.

Besides bedrest and elevation of the affected leg, treatment regimens include anticoagulants and vena cava interruption devices. There is little indication for thrombolytics and surgical intervention in the postoperation knee surgery patient.

Anticoagulants

The most commonly used anticoagulants are heparin and warfarin. In the treatment of deep vein thrombosis,

the classic dosing of anticoagulants with the administration of intravenous heparin for 10 days and warfarin therapy starting 5 days after the start of heparin therapy has been questioned. Administration of IV heparin for a total of 5 days with warfarin dosing starting on the first day of heparin therapy was as effective as the standard dosing (147). The warfarin is continued for 6 weeks to 3 months. Studies have shown that a moderately intense regimen of warfarin, keeping the international normalized ratio (INR) between 2.0 to 2.3 (prothrombin time at 1.3 to 1.5 times normal), has been both effective and yielded less bleeding complications than a more intense, standard regimen (148). A recent report in the *New England Journal of Medicine* found that treatment of symptomatic deep vein thrombosis in medical patients with acenocoumarol, a warfarin-like drug, was less effective than treatment with heparin initially, followed by acenocoumarol (149). Warfarin alone may, however, be an acceptable form of treatment for asymptomatic, isolated calf thrombi detected in the postoperative TKA patient.

Anticoagulants inhibit the coagulation cascade and, therefore, have no effect on clot lysis. The lysis of clot is secondary to the body's own fibrinolytic cascade.

Complications with heparin in the postoperative total joint patient have been studied. They include bleeding from the operative site, gastrointestinal bleeding, thrombocytopenia, venous thrombosis, and arterial thrombosis (4). Bleeding was related to the day the heparin therapy was started. If heparin was administered within the first 5 days after surgery, bleeding from the wound occurred in about 50% of the patients. The occurrence of wound bleeding dropped to 15% when heparin was started more than 1 week after surgery. Thrombocytopenia occurred in about 4% of the patients studied. Overall, heparin therapy had to be discontinued in 35% of the patients because of local or systemic complications related to heparin. The main complication with warfarin use in the treatment of deep vein thrombosis is bleeding. The rate of bleeding is related to the intensity of the therapy. Hull, et al. (148) reported a decrease in bleeding complications from 22.4 to 4.3% when a moderately intense regimen of warfarin was used.

Early studies showed that low molecular weight heparin is as effective as continuous IV heparin in the treatment of proximal vein thrombosis (150). Low molecular weight heparins are newer drugs that are still under study. Although not FDA-approved for the treatment of deep vein thrombosis, they may prove to be a simpler and safer way to treat thrombi.

Vena Cava Filters

The Greenfield filter is the most widely used vena cava filter in the United States. The filter is placed percutaneously in the infrarenal vena cava and stops the migration of emboli to the lungs. It has been shown to be very effective in reducing pulmonary embolism while still maintaining blood flow. A long-term follow-up study revealed a recurrent embolism rate of 4% and a patency rate of 98% (151). The classic indications for

Table 82.2.   Deep Vein Thrombosis (DVT) Rates in Patients Who Had Total Knee Arthroplasty (TKA)

Study	Type of Prophylaxis	Number of Patients	Calf DVT Rate %[a]	Proximal DVT Rate %[a]	All DVT Rate %[a]
Aspirin					
Haas (33) unilateral TKA	650 mg BID	36	47	0	47
bilateral TKA	650 mg BID	22	64	4	68
Lynch (123)	650 mg BID	150	36	5	41
Lotke (26)	650 mg BID	175	40	31	72
Stulberg (3)	650 mg BID	450	46	10	56
Lotke (124)	325 mg BID	166[b]	47	10	57
McKenna (122)	325 mg TID	9	c	c	78
	1300 mg TID	12	c	c	8
Warfarin					
Stulberg (3)	Low-dose warfarin	17	41	12	53
Lotke (124)	Low-dose warfarin	146[d]	42	11	53
Graor (128)	Low-dose warfarin	c	c	c	59
Friedman (140)	Low-dose warfarin	147	c	10.2	43
Hodge (125)	Low-dose warfarin	48	29	6	35
Lynch (30)	Low-dose warfarin	282	c	c	40
Kaempffe (127)	Low-dose warfarin	24	17	8	25
Francis (129)	Two-step warfarin	14	c	c	21
Dextran					
Francis (65)	10 ml/kg	38	63	11	74
Graor (128)	over 12 hrs	c	c	c	50
Stulberg (60)	then	22	64	18	82
Francis (129)	7ml/kg/24 hrs	8	c	c	100
Heparin					
Stulberg (3)	Low-dose heparin	64	42	11	53
	Low-dose heparin starting preoperation	24	38	12	50
Graor (128)	Adjusted-dose heparin	c	c	c	34
Francis (65)	AT III & heparin	39	15	13	28
Stulberg (60)	AT III & heparin	20	15	10	25
Leclerc (139)	LMWH (Enoxaparin)	65[e]	17	0	17
Friedman (140)	RDH[e]	150	c	6	26
	RDH[e]	149	c	4.7	29
Intermittent Pneumatic Compression Devices					
Haas (33) unilateral TKA	Thigh-length IPCD[g]	36	22	0	22
bilateral TKA	Thigh-length IPCD	25	40	8	48
Graor (128)	Calf-length IPCD	c	c	c	33
Hodge (123)	Calf-length IPCD	81	27	6	33
Lynch (30)	Calf-length IPCD	307	c	c	11
Kaempffe (127)	Thigh-length IPCD	26	12	23	35
Hood (143)	Calf-length IPCD	25	8	0	8
Hull (144)	Calf-length IPCD	32[e]	6.3	0	6.3

[a] =all thrombi were venographically detected
[b] = 104 patients had total knee replacement, & 62 patients had total hip replacement
[c] = data not specified
[d] =76 patients had total knee replacement; 70 patients had total hip replacement
[e] =participants had various types of knee surgery.
[f] = reconstituted depolimerized heparin
[g] = intermittent pneumatic compression devices

Greenfield filter placement include recurrent embolism, despite anticoagulation, or deep venous thrombosis with a contraindication to, or complication of, anticoagulant therapy. Insertion of a Greenfield filter has recently been advocated as prophylaxis in the high-risk patient undergoing total hip or total knee replacement as well as part of the treatment of deep vein thrombosis in patients in which anticoagulation therapy is contraindicated or anticoagulant therapy has failed (152).

The filters have no effect on the dissolution of thrombi and, therefore, no effect on the risk of postphlebitic syndrome. Complications are unusual but can occur. At insertion, there is a risk from local anesthesia injection, a risk of filter misplacement (2.6%), and risk of bleeding at the insertion site. Over the long run, migration of the filter or bleeding secondary to puncture of the aorta or puncture of the surrounding structures can occur, although rarely.

Table 82.3. Suggested Thromboembolic Prophylactic and Treatment Regimens in Total Knee Arthroplasty (TKA)

	Unilateral TKA	One-Stage Bilateral TKA
Prophylaxis	Pneumatic compression boots	Pneumatic compression boots and low dose warfarin that is continued for a 6-week course
	Routine DVT screening performed prior to discharge	
Treatment of Calf Thrombi	Low dose warfarin therapy for 6 weeks -or- Follow-up duplex ultrasound	
Treatment of Large Proximal Thrombi	Greenfield Filter -or- Anticoagulation with heparin/warfarin for 6 weeks to 3 months	
Treatment of Symptomatic Pulmonary Emboli	Greenfield Filter -or- Anticoagulation with heparin/warfarin for 3 to 6 months	

Thrombolytics

Thrombolytics, such as streptokinase and urokinase, lyse thrombi and are used mainly for massive pulmonary emboli. Complete clot lysis occurs in 30 to 40% of patients medicated with this regimen. Due to the exceedingly high risk of bleeding, there are virtually no indications for thrombolytics in postoperative patients who develop deep venous thrombosis.

Surgical Intervention

Surgical intervention, i.e., venous thrombectomy or pulmonary embolectomy, is performed only in desperate cases. These cases include venous obstruction that leads to cerulea dolens and limits the viability of the leg and cases in which patients with massive pulmonary embolization do not respond to thrombolytics and vasopressors (153).

Recommendations for Deep Vein Thrombosis Prophylaxis

Patients undergoing major knee surgery, such as total knee replacement should receive an effective primary prophylactic agent to prevent thromboembolic disease. The ideal medication would inhibit all thrombus formation, yet allow healing of the surgical site without bleeding or other complications. Of course, there is no such medication. Intermittent pneumatic compression boots appear to be the best modality for prevention of thrombus formation after TKA (33, 143, 154). Another acceptable prophylactic regimen is low-dose warfarin. Low molecular weight heparins may prove to be an effective prophylactic agent in patients who undergo TKA; however, studies are not completed, and the drug is not FDA approved for use in TKA (Tables 82.2 and 82.3).

Despite primary prophylaxis, some patients will develop deep vein thrombi that are mostly limited to the distal calf veins. Prior to discharge, patients should undergo routine screening with either duplex ultrasonography or venography. Since duplex ultrasound scanning is not sensitive for detection of calf thrombi, a follow-up duplex study may be beneficial for detecting distal thrombi which may propagate.

An alternative to prophylaxis and screening is low-dose warfarin either alone or preferably with pneumatic compression boots. The compression boots, if used, may be removed once the patient is ambulating. The warfarin is continued for a 6-week period postoperatively.

Recommendations for Deep Vein Thrombosis Treatment

Most physicians agree that large proximal thrombi and symptomatic pulmonary emboli should be treated aggressively with anticoagulation or with the use of a vena cava filter. Controversy exists whether to treat calf thrombi in postoperative patients. We have previously shown that, although not catastrophic, calf thrombi do subject the patient to an increased risk of pulmonary embolism (86). We recommend that patients who are identified postoperatively as having calf thrombi should be started on low-dose warfarin therapy and should be continued for 6 weeks after surgery. If no anticoagulation is started, it would be prudent to have a follow-up duplex ultrasound to detect any proximal propagation. We do not feel that calf thrombi detected in the early postoperative period should be routinely treated with heparin because of the risk of complication with anticoagulation therapy in the early postoperative period (2, 4).

Patients who develop large proximal thrombi or symptomatic pulmonary embolism in the early postoperative period require more aggressive therapy. In addition to medical treatment (i.e., IV fluids, oxygen, possible ventilation support, etc.), these patients require a Greenfield filter or anticoagulation with heparin followed by long-term warfarin therapy. The choice of whether to use a Greenfield filter or anticoagulation must be individualized. If heparin is chosen in the early postoperation period, one must be cautious not to give large boluses of heparin that may transiently raise the partial thromboplastin time to greater than 100 seconds. The warfarin must be continued for 3 to 6 months. In this early postoperation period, we have chosen to use a Greenfield filter to avoid the possibility of bleeding complications.

References

1. McKenna R, Bachmann F, Kullshal SP, Galante JO. Thromboembolic disease in patients undergoing total knee replacement. J Bone Joint Surg 1976; 58A(7):928–932.
2. Lotke PA, Ecker ML, Alavi A, Berkowitz H. Indications for the treatment of deep venous thrombosis following total knee replacement. J Bone Joint Surg 1984; 66A(2):202–208.
3. Stulberg BN, Insall JN, Williams GW, Ghelman B. Deep vein thrombosis following total knee replacement. J Bone Joint Surg 1984; 66A(2):194–201.
4. Patterson BM, Marchand R, Ranawat C. Complications of heparin therapy after total joint arthroplasty. J Bone Joint Surg 1989; 71A(8):1130–1134.
5. Barritt DW, Jordan SC, Brist MB. Anticoagulant drugs in the treatment of pulmonary embolism: A controlled trial. Lancet 1960; 18:1309–1312.
6. Kraritz E, Karino T. Pathophysiology of deep vein thrombosis. In: Leclerc JR. Venous thromboembolic disorders. Philadelphia: Lea and Febiger, 1991:54–64.
7. Virchow R. Neuer Fall von tödlicher Emboli der Kungerarterien. Arch Path Anat 1856; 10:225.
8. Rabinov K and Paulin S. Roentgen diagnosis of venous thrombosis in the leg. Arch Surg 1972; 104:134–144.
9. Lowe LW. Venous thrombosis and embolism. J Bone Joint Surg 1981; 63B(2):155–167.
10. Nadrowski LF. Deep venous thrombosis: Recent advances in pathogenesis and treatment. Surg Annu 1991; 23:147–173.
11. Wessler S, Yin ET. Experimental hypercoagulable state induced by factor X: Comparison of the non-activated and activated forms. J Lab Clin Med 1968; 72:256.
12. Stewart GJ. The role of the vessel wall in deep venous thrombosis. In: Nicolaides AN, ed. Thromboembolism, aetiology, advances in prevention and management. Lancaster: MTP, 1975.
13. Browse NL, Burnard KG, Thomas ML. Diseases of the veins: Pathology, diagnosis and treatment. Baltimore: Edward Arnold, 1988:454.
14. McLachlin AD, et al. Venous stasis in the lower extremity. Ann Surg 1960; 152:678–683.
15. Cotton LT, Clark C. Anatomical localization of venous thrombosis. Ann R Coll Surg Engl 1965; 36:214–224.
16. Leclerc JR. Venous thromboembolic disorders. Philadelphia: Lea and Febiger, 1991:55.
17. Sevitt S, Gallagher N. Venous thrombosis and pulmonary embolism: A clinico-pathological study in injured and burned patients. Br J Surg 1961; 48:475–489.
18. Browse NL, Burnand KG, Thomas ML. Diseases of the veins: pathology, diagnosis and treatment. Baltimore: Edward Arnold, 1988:9.
19. Gibberd FB, Gould SR, Marks P. Incidence of deep vein thrombosis and leg oedema in patients with strokes. J Neurol Neurosurg Psych 1976; 39:1222–1225.
20. Warlow C, Ogston D, Douglas AS. Deep venous thrombosis of the legs after strokes: Part I Incidence and predisposing factors. Br Med J 1976; 1:1178–1182.
21. Green D, Lee MY, Ito VY, et al. Fixed vs. adjusted-dose heparin in the prophylaxis of thromboembolism in spinal cord injury. JAMA 1988; 260(9):1255–1258.
22. Chu DA, Ahn J, Ragnarsson K, et al. Deep venous thrombosis: Diagnosis in spinal cord injured patients. Arch Phys Med Rehabil 1985; 66:365–369.
23. Perkash A. Experience with the management of thromboembolism in patients with spinal cord injury: Part I Incidence, diagnosis and role of some risk factors. Paraplegia 1978–1979; 16:322–331.
24. Todd JW, Frisbie JH, Rossier AB, et al. Deep vein thrombosis in acute spinal cord injury: A comparison of 125-I-fibrinogen leg scanning, impedance plethysmography and venography. Paraplegia 1976; 14:50–57.
25. Cope C, Rayes T, Skversky N. Phlebographic analysis of the incidence of thrombosis in hemiplegia. Radiology 1973; 109:581–584.
26. Lotke PA, Wong RY, Ecker ML. Asymptomatic pulmonary embolism after total knee replacement. Orthop Trans 1986; 10(3):490.
27. Morrey BF, Adams RA, Ilstrup DM, Bryan RS. Complications and mortality associated with bilateral or unilateral total knee arthroplasty. J Bone Joint Surg 1987; 69A(4):484–488.
28. Cohen SH, Ehrlich GE, Kauffman MS, Cope C. Thrombophlebitis following knee surgery. J Bone Joint Surg 1973; 55A(1):106–112.
29. Stringer MD, Steadman CA, Hedges AR, Thomas EM, Morley TR, Kakkar VV. Deep vein thrombosis after elective knee surgery. J Bone Joint Surg 1989; 71B(3):492–497.
30. Lynch JA, Baker PL, Polly RE, et al. Mechanical measures in the propylaxis of post-operative thromboembolism in total knee arthroplasty. Clin Orthop 1990; 260:24–29.
31. Harris WH, Salzman EW, Desanctis RW. The prevention of thromboembolic disease by prophylactic anticoagulation. J Bone Joint Surg 1967; 49A(1):81–89.
32. Haake DA, Borkman SA. Venous thromboembolic disease after hip surgery. Clin Orthop 1989; 242:212–231.
33. Haas SB, Insall JM, Scuderi GR, Windsor RE, Ghelman B. Pneumatic sequential compression boots compared with aspirin prophylaxis of deep vein thrombosis after total knee arthroplasty. J Bone Joint Surg 1990; 72A(1):27–31.
34. Hull RD, Raskob GE. Prophylaxis of venous thromboembolic disease following hip and knee surgery. J Bone Joint 1986; 68A(1):146–150.
35. Isacson S, Nilsson IM. Defective fibrinolysis in blood vein walls in recurrent "idiopathic" venous thrombosis. Acta Chir Scand 1972; 138:313–319.
36. Johansson L, Hedner U, Nilsson IM. A family with thromboembolic disease associated with deficient fibrinolytic activity in vessel walls. Act Med Scand 1978; 203:477–480.
37. Jorgensen M, Mortensen JZ, Madsin AG, Thorsen S, Jacobsen B. A family with reduced plasminogen activator activity in blood associated with recurrent venous thrombosis. Scand J Haematol 1982; 29:217–223.
38. Ljungner H, Berqvist D, Isacson S. Plasminogen activator activity of superficial veins in acute deep venous thrombosis. Vasa 1982; 11:174–177.
39. Stead NW, Bauer KA, Kinney TR, et al. Venous thrombosis in a family with defective release of vascular plasminogen activator and elevated plasma factor VIII, von Willebrand's factor. Am J Med 1983; 74:33–39.
40. Stormorken H, Lund M, Holmsen I. Vessel wall activator (tPA) as evaluated by poststasis euglobulin lysis time (PELT) in recurrent deep venous thrombosis. In: Jespersen, Kluff C, and Korsgaand O, eds. Clinical aspects of fibrinolysis and thrombolysis. Esbjerg: South Jutland University Press, 1983.
41. Sundqvist S-B, Hedner U, Kullenberg HKE, Bergentz S-E. Deep venous thrombosis of the arm: A study of coagulation and fibrinolysis. Br Med J 1981; 283:265–267.
42. Lanham JG, Levin M, Brown Z, Gharavi AE, Thomas PA, Hanson GC. Prostacyclin deficiency in a young woman with recurrent thrombosis. Br Med J 1986; 292:435–436.
43. Awbrey BJ, Hoak JC, Orwen WG. Binding of human thrombin to cultured human endothelial cells. J Biol Chem 1979; 254:4092–4095.
44. Chan V, Chan TK. Antithrombin III in fresh and cultured human endothelial cells: A natural anticoagulant from the vascular endothelium. Thromb Res 1979; 15:209–213.
45. Bloom AL, Giddings JC, Willes CJ. Factor VIII on the vascular intima: Possible importance in haemostasis and thrombosis. Nature 1973; 241:217–219.
46. Holmberg L, Mannucci BM, Turesson I, Ruggeri ZM, Nilsson IM. Factor VIII antigen in the vessel wall in von Willebrand's disease and hemophilia A. Scand J Haematol 1974; 13:33–38.
47. Jaffe EA, Hoyer LW, Nachman RL. Synthesis of antihemophilic factor antigen by cultured human endothelial cells. J Clin Invest 1973; 52:2757–2764.
48. Gore I, Larkey BJ. Functional activity of aortic mucopolysaccharides. J Lab Clin Med 1960; 56:839–846.
49. Izuka K, Murata K. Inhibitory effects of human aortic and venous acid glycosaminoglycans on thrombus formation. Atherosclerosis 1972; 16:217–224.
50. Nakazawa K, Murata K. Acidic glycosaminoglycans in three layers of human aorta: Their different constitution and anticoagulant function. Paroi Asterielle 1975; 2:203–208.
51. Paramo JA, Rocha E. Changes in coagulation and fibrinolysis after total hip replacement and their relations with deep vein thrombosis. Haemostasis 1985; 15:345–352.
52. Gray DH, Mackie CEJ. The effects of blood transfusion on the incidence of deep vein thrombosis. Aust N Z J Surg 1983; 53:439–443.
53. Philbrick JT, Becker DM. Calf deep venous thrombosis: A wolf in sheep's clothing? Arch Int Med 1988; 148:2131–2138.
54. Houghton GR, Papadakis EG, Rizza CR. Changes in blood coagulation during total hip replacement. Lancet 1978; 1:1336–1338.
55. Foster DP, Whipple CH. Blood fibrin studies: Fibrin influenced by cell injury, inflammation, intoxication, liver injury and the Eck fistula: Notes connecting the origin of fibrin in the body. Am J Physiol 1922; 58:407–411.

56. Egeberg O. Changes in the coagulation system following major surgical operations. Acta Med Scand 1963; 171:679–684.

57. Godal HC. Quantitative and qualitative changes in fibrinogen following major surgical operations. Acta Med Scand 1962; 171:687–694.

58. Ygge J. Studies on blood coagulation and fibrinolysis in conditions associated with an increased incidence of thrombosis: Methodological and clinical investigations. Scand J Haematol Suppl 1970; 11:1–45.

59. Browse NL, Burnard KG, Thomas ML. Disease of the veins: Pathology, diagnosis and treatment. Baltimore: Edward Arnold, 1988:445–446.

60. Stulberg BN, Francis CW, Pellegrini VD, et al. Antithrombin III/low dose heparin in the prevention of deep vein thrombosis after total knee arthroplasty. Clin Orthop 1989; 248:152–157.

61. Hirsh J, Levine MN. Low molecular weight heparin. Blood 1992; 79(1):1–17.

62. Fredin H, Nilsson B, Rosberg B, Tengborn L. Pre- and post-operative levels of antithrombin III with special reference to thromboembolism after total hip replacement. Thromb Haemost 1983; 49(3):158–161.

63. Gitel SN, Salvati EA, Wessler S, Robinson HJ, Worth MH. The effects of total hip replacement and general surgery on antithrombin III in relation to venous thrombosis. J Bone Joint Surg 1979; 61A:653–656.

64. Francis CW, Pellegrini VD, Marder VJ, et al. Prevention of venous thrombosis after total hip arthroplasty: Antithrombin III and low dose heparin compared with dextran 40. J Bone Joint Surg 1989; 71A(3):327–335.

65. Francis CW, Pellegrini VD, Stulberg BN, Miller ML, Totterman S, Marder VJ. Prevention of venous thrombosis after total knee arthroplasty: Comparison of antithrombin III and low dose heparin with dextran. J Bone Joint Surg 1990; 72A(7):976–982.

66. Bertina RM, Broekmans AW, Van Der Linden IK, Mortens K. Protein C deficiency in a Dutch family with thrombotic disease. Thromb Haemost 1982; 48:1–5.

67. Broekmans AW, Veltkamp JJ, Bertina RM. Congenital protein C deficiency and venous thromboembolism: A study of three Dutch families. N Engl J Med 1983; 309:340–344.

68. Griffin JH, Evatt B, Zimmerman TS, Kleiss AJ, Wideman C. Deficiency of protein C in congenital thrombotic disease. J Clin Invest 1981; 68:1370–1373.

69. Horellow MH, Conrad J, Bertina RM, Samama M. Congenital protein C deficiency and thrombotic disease in nine French families. Br Med J 1984; 289:1285–1287.

70. Marlar RA, Endres-Brooks J. Recurrent thromboembolic disease due to heterozygous protein C deficiency. Thromb Haemost 1983; 50:331–334.

71. Pabinger-Fasching I, Bertina RM, Lechner K, Niessner H, Koriniger CH. Protein C deficiency in two Austrian families. Thromb Haemost 1983; 50:810–813.

72. Tran TH, Marbet GA, Duckert F. Association of hereditary heparin cofactor II deficiency with thrombosis. Lancet 1985; 2:413–414.

73. Hirsh J, Salzman EW, Harker L, et al. Aspirin and other platelet active drugs: Relationship among dose, effectiveness and side effects. Chest 1989; 95(suppl 2):12s–16s.

74. Salzman EW, Harris WH, De Sanctis RW. Reduction in thromboembolism by agents affecting platelet function. N Engl J Med 1971; 284:1287–1292.

75. Harris WH, Salzman EW, Athanasoulis CA, Waltman AC, De Sanctis RW. Aspirin prophylaxis of venous thromboembolism after total hip replacement. N Engl J Med 1977; 297:1246–1249.

76. DeLee JC, Rockwood CA. The use of aspirin in thromboembolic disease. J Bone Joint Surg 1980; 62A(1):149–152.

77. Butterfield WJH, Hicks BH, Ambler AR, et al. Effects of aspirin on postoperative venous thrombosis. Lancet 1972; 2:441–444.

78. Stamatakis JD, Kakkar VV, Lawrence D, Bentley PG, Nairn D, Ward V. Failure of aspirin to prevent post operative deep vein thrombosis in patients undergoing total hip replacement. Br Med J 1978; 1:1031.

79. Emmons PR, Mitchell JRA. Post operative changes in platelet-clumping activity. Lancet 1965; 1:71–75.

80. Warren R, Lauridsen J. Belko J. Alterations in numbers of circulating platelets following surgical operation and administration of adrenocorticotrophic hormone. Circulation 1953; 7:481–486.

81. Wright H, Payling. Changes in the adhesiveness of blood platelets following parturition and surgical operations. J Pathol Bacteriol 1942; 54:461–468.

82. Paramo JA, Rocha E. Deep vein thrombosis and related platelet changes after total hip replacement. Haemostasis 1985; 15:389–394.

83. Maynard MJ, Sculco TP, Ghelman B. Progression and regression of deep vein thrombosis after total knee arthroplasty. Clin Orthop 1991; 273:125–130.

84. Leclerc JR. Natural history of venous thromboembolism In: Leclerc JR. Venous thromboembolic disorders. Philadelphia: Lea and Febiger, 1991:166–175.

85. Kakkar VV, Howe CT, Flanc C, Clarke MB. Natural history of postoperative deep-vein thrombosis. Lancet 1969; August 2:230–233.

86. Haas SB, Tribus CB, Insall JN, Becker MW, Windsor RE. The significance of calf thrombi after total knee arthroplasty. J Bone Joint Surg 1992; 74B:799–802.

87. Browse NL, Burnard KG, Thomas ML. Diseases of the veins: Pathology, diagnosis and treatment. Baltimore: Edward Arnold, 1988:456–459.

88. Browse NL, Burnard KG, Thomas ML. Disease of the veins: Pathology, diagnosis and treatment. Baltimore: Edward Arnold, 1988:475–477.

89. Cranley JJ, Canos A, Sull WJ. The diagnosis of deep venous thrombosis: Fallibility of clinical symptoms and signs. Arch Surg 1976; 111:34–36.

90. Albrechtsson U, Olsson CG. Thrombotic side-effects of lower-limb phlebography. Lancet 1976; 2:723–724.

91. Day TK, Fish PJ, Kakkar VV. Detection of deep vein thrombosis by Doppler angiography. Br Med J 1976; 1:618–620.

92. Lensing AWA, Prandoni P, Brandjes D, et al. Detection of deep vein thrombosis by real-time B-mode ultrasonography. N Engl J Med 1989; 320:342–345.

93. Woolson ST, Pottorff G. Venous ultrasonography in the detection of proximal vein thrombosis after total knee arthroplasty. Clin Orthop 1991; 273:131–135.

94. Froehlich JA, Dorfman GS, Conan JJ, Urbanek PJ, Herndon JH, Aaron RK. Compression ultrasound for the detection of deep venous thrombosis in patients who have a fracture of the hip. J Bone Joint Surg 1989; 71A(2):249–256.

95. Tremaine MD, Choroszy CJ, Gorden GH, Menking SA. Diagnosis of deep venous thrombosis by compression ultrasound in knee arthroplasty patients. J Arthroplasty 1992; 7(2):187–192.

96. Ginsberg JS, Caco CC, Brill-Edwards PA, et al. Venous thrombosis in patients who have undergone major hip or knee surgery: Detection with compression US and impedance plethysmography. Radiology 1991; 181:651–654.

97. Leclerc JR. Venous thromboembolic disorders. Philadelphia: Lea and Febiger, 1991:215–216.

98. Davidson BL, Elliott CG, Lensing WA. Low accuracy of color doppler ultrasound in the detection of proximal leg vein thrombosis in asymptomatic high-risk patients. Ann Intern Med 1992; 117:735–738.

99. Hull R, et al. Combined use of leg scanning and impedance plethysmography in suspected venous thrombosis: An alternative to venography. N Engl J Med 1977; 296:1497–1500.

100. Kakkar VV, et al. 125-I-labled fibrinogen test adapted for routine screening for deep vein thrombosis. Lancet 1970; 1:540–542.

101. Harris WH, Salzman EW, Athanasoulis C, Waltman AC, Baum S, DeSanctis RW. Comparison of warfarin, low-molecular-weight dextran, aspirin, and subcutaneous heparin in prevention of venous thromboembolism following total hip replacement. J Bone Joint Surg 1974; 56A(8):1552–1562.

102. Leclerc JR, Illescas F, Jarzem P. Diagnosis of deep vein thrombosis. In: Leclerc JR. Venous thromboembolic disorders. Philadelphia: Lea and Febiger, 1991:196–204.

103. Paiement G, et al. Surveillance of deep vein thrombosis in asymptomatic total hip replacement patients: Impedance phlebography and fibrinogen scanning vs. roentgenographic phlebography. Am J Surg 1988; 155:400–404.

104. Cruickshank MK, et al. An evaluation of impedance plethysmography and 125-I-fibrinogen leg scanning in patients following hip surgery. Thromb Haemost 1989; 62:830–834.

105. Dalen JE, Alpert JS. Natural history of pulmonary embolism. Prog Cardiovasc Dis 1975; 17:259–270.

106. Browse NL, Burnard KG, Thomas ML. Diseases of the veins: Pathology, diagnosis and treatment. Baltimore: Edward Arnold, 1988:559.

107. Leclerc JR. Venous thromboembolic disorders. Philadelphia: Lea and Febiger, 1991:229.

108. Smith R and Alderson PO. Ventilation-Perfusion scintigraphy in pulmonary embolism. In: Loken MK, ed. Pulmonary nuclear medicine. East Norwalk, CT: Appleton and Lange, 1987:51–79.

109. Fraser RG, Pare JAP. Pulmonary thromboembolism. In Fraser RG, Pare JAP, Editors: Diagnosis of diseases of the chest. Philadelphia: Saunders, 1978; 2 ed:1143–1160.

110. Anderson PO, et al. Ventilation-perfusion lung imaging and selective pulmonary angiography in dogs with experimental pulmonary embolism. J Nucl Med 1978; 19:164–171.

111. Kipper MS, Moser KM, Kortman KE, Ashbum WL. Long-term follow-up of patients with suspected pulmonary embolism and a normal lung scan: Perfusion scans in embolic suspects. Chest 1982; 82:411–415.

112. PIOPED Investigators. Value of the ventilation/perfusion scan in acute pulmonary embolism: Results of the prospective investigation of pulmonary embolism diagnosis. JAMA 1990; 263(20):2753–2759.

113. Mills SR, et al. The incidence, etiologies and avoidance of complications of pulmonary angiography in a large series. Radiology 1980; 136:295–299.

114. Dalen JE, Paraskos JA, Ockene IS, Alpert JS, Hirsch J. Venous thromboembolism: Scope of the problem. Chest 1986; 89(suppl 5):370s–373s.

115. Hirsch J, Hull RD. Natural history and clinical features of venous thrombosis. In: Colman RW, et al. ed. Hemostasis and Thrombosis. New York: JB Lippincott Co., 1987; 2nd ed.:1209–1210.
116. Browse NL, Burnard KG, Thomas ML. Diseases of the veins. Pathology, diagnosis and treatment. Baltimore: Edward Arnold, 1988:307–310.
117. Bauer G. A roentgenological and clinical study of the sequels of thrombosis. Acta Chir Scand 1942; 86:1–126.
118. Arnesen H, Heilo A, Jakobsin E, Ly B, Skaga E. A prospective study of streptokinase and heparin in the treatment of deep vein thrombosis. Acta Med Scand 1978; 203:457–463.
119. Elliot MS, Immelman EF, Jeffery P, et al. A comparative randomized trial of heparin versus streptokinase in the treatment of acute proximal venous thrombosis: An interim report of a prospective trial. Br J Surg 1979; 66:838–843.
120. Schulman S, Lockner D, Granqvist S, et al. A comparative randomized trial of low-dose versus high-dose streptokinase in deep vein thrombosis of the thigh. Thromb Haemost 1984; 51:261–265.
121. Consensus Development Panel. Prevention of venous thrombosis and pulmonary embolism. JAMA 1986; 256:744–749.
122. Mckenna R, Galante J, Bachmann F, Wallace DL, Kaushal SP, Meredith P. Prevention of venous thromboembolism after total knee replacement by high-dose aspirin or intermittent calf and thigh compression. Br Med J 1980; 280:514–517.
123. Lynch AF, Bourne RB, Rorabeck CH, Rankin RN, Donald A. Deep-vein thrombosis and continuous passive motion after total knee arthroplasty. J Bone Joint Surg 1988; 70A:11–14.
124. Lotke PA, Palevsky H, Keenan A, Meranze S, Steinberg ME, Ecker ML, in press, 1991.
125. Hodge WA. Warfarin and sequential calf compression in the prevention of deep vein thrombi following total knee replacement. Presented at the Knee Society, Las Vegas, February, 1989.
126. Hodge WA. Prevention of deep vein thrombosis after total knee arthroplasty. Clin Orthop 1991; 271:101–105.
127. Kaempffe FA, Lifeso RM, Meinding C. Intermittent pneumatic compression versus coumadin: Prevention of deep vein thrombosis in lower-extremity total joint arthroplasty. Clin Orthop 1991; 269:89–79.
128. Graor RA, Davis AW, Borden LS, Young J. Comparative evaluation of deep vein thrombosis prophylaxis in total joint replacement patients. Presented at American Association of Orthopaedic Surgeons, Las Vegas, February, 1989.
129. Francis CW, Marder VJ, Evarts CM, Yaukoolbodi S. Two-step warfarin therapy. Prevention of postoperative venous thrombosis without excessive bleeding. JAMA 1983; 249:374–378.
130. Salemark L, Wieslander JB, Dougan P, Arnljots B. Studies of the antithrombotic effects of dextran 40 following microarterial trauma. Br J Plastic Surg 1991; 44:15–22.
131. Ahlberg A, Nylander G, Robertson B, et al. Dextran in prophylaxis of thrombosis in fractures of the hip. Acta Chir Scand 1968; 387(suppl):83–85.
132. Johnsson SR, Bygdeman S, Eliasson R. Effect of dextran on postoperative thrombosis. Acta Chir Scand 1968; 387(suppl):80.
133. Evarts CM, Feils EJ. Prevention of thromboembolic disease after elective surgery of the hip. J Bone Joint Surg 1971; 53A:1271–1280.
134. Eriksson B, et al. Thrombosis prophylaxis with low molecular weight heparin in total hip replacement. Br J Surg 1988; 75:1053–1057.
135. Eriksson B, Kalebo P, Anthmyr BA, Wadenvik H, Tengborn L, Risberg B. Prevention of deep vein thrombosis and pulmonary embolism after total hip replacement. Comparison of a low molecular weight heparin and unfractionated heparin. J Bone Joint Surg 1991; 73A:484–493.
136. Planes A, Vochelle N, Mazas F, et al. Prevention of postoperative venous thrombosis: A randomized trial comparing unfractionated heparin with low molecular weight heparin in patients undergoing total hip replacement. Thromb Haemost 1988; 60:407–410.
137. The Danish Enoxaparin Study Group. Low-molecular-weight heparin (Enoxaparin) vs dextran 70: The prevention of postoperative deep vein thrombosis after total hip replacement. Arch Intern Med 1991; 151:1621–1624.
138. Planes A, Vochelle N, Fagola M, et al. Once-daily dosing of Enoxaparin (a low molecular weight heparin) in prevention of deep vein thrombosis after total hip replacement. Acta Chir Scand Suppl 1990; 556:108–115.
139. Leclerc JR, Geerts WH, Desjardins L, et al. Prevention of deep vein thrombosis after major knee surgery: A randomized, double-blind trial comparing a low molecular weight heparin fragment (Enoxaparin) to placebo. Thromb Haemost 1992; 67:417–423.
140. Friedman RJ, Lotke PA, Hofmann AA, Groth HE, Drennan DB, Chenault CS, et al. Reconstituted depolymerized heparin versus warfarin in the prevention of deep vein thrombosis following total hip and knee arthroplasty. Orthop Trans 1993; 16(3):712.
141. Tarnay TJ, Rohr PR, Davidson AG, Stevenson MM, Byars EF, Hopkins GR. Pneumatic calf compression, fibrinolysis, and the prevention of deep venous thrombosis. Surgery 1980; 88:489–496.
142. Knight MTN, Dawson R. Effect of intermittent compression of the arms on deep venous thrombosis in the legs. Lancet 1976; 2:1265–1267.
143. Hood RW, Flawn LB, Insall JN. The use of pulsatile compression stockings in total knee replacement for prevention of venous thromboembolism: A prospective study. Presented at the Orthopaedic Research Society, New Orleans, January, 1982.
144. Hull R, Delmore TJ, Hirsh J, et al. Effectiveness of intermittent pulsatile elastic stockings for the prevention of calf and thigh vein thrombosis in patients undergoing elective knee surgery. Thromb Resear 1979; 16:37–45.
145. Harris WH, Athanasoulis CA, Waltman AC, Salzman EW. Prophylaxis of deep-vein thrombosis after total hip replacement. Dextran and external pneumatic compression compared with 1.2 or 0.3 gram of aspirin daily. J Bone Joint Surg 1985; 67A:57–62.
146. Woolson ST, Watt JM. Intermittent pneumatic compression to prevent proximal deep venous thrombosis during and after total hip replacement: A prospective, randomized study of compression alone, compression and aspirin, and compression and low-dose warfarin. J Bone Joint Surg 1991; 73A:507–512.
147. Hull RD, Raskob GE, Rosenbloom D, et al. Heparin for 5 days as compared with 10 days in the initial treatment of proximal vein thrombosis. N Engl J Med 1990; 322:1260–1264.
148. Hull R, Hirsh J, Jay R, et al. Different intensities of oral anticoagulant therapy in the treatment of proximal-vein thrombosis. N Engl J Med 1982; 307:1676–1681.
149. Brandjes DPM, Heijboer H, Buller HR, De Rijk M, Jagt H, Wouter Ten Cate J. Acenocoumarol and heparin compared with acenocoumarol alone in the initial treatment of proximal-vein thrombosis N Engl J Med 1992; 327(21):1485–1489.
150. Hull RD, Raskob GE, Pineo GF, et al. Subcutaneous low-molecular-weight heparin compared with continuous intravenous heparin in the treatment of proximal-vein thrombosis. N Engl J Med 1992; 326:975–982.
151. Greenfield LJ, Michna BA. Twelve year clinical experience with the Greenfield vena caval filter. Surgery 1988; 104:706–712.
152. Emerson RH, Cross R, Head WC. Prophylaxtic and early therapeutic use of the Greenfield filter in hip and knee joint arthroplasty. J Arthroplasty 1991; 6:129–135.
153. Miller GA, Hall RJC, Paneth M. Pulmonary embolectomy, heparin, and streptokinase: Their place in the treatment of acute massive pulmonary embolism. Am Heart J 1977; 93:568–574.
154. Salzman EW, Hirsh J. Prevention of venous thromboembolism. In: Colman RW, Hirsh J, Marder VJ, and Salzman EW, eds. Hemostasis and thrombosis: Basic principles and clinical practice. New York: J.B. Lippincott Co., 1987:1262.

83

Mechanical Failure: Implant Breakage and Loosening

Gerard A. Engh and Kimberly A. Dwyer

Implant Breakage

Introduction

Breakage is a rare cause of total knee implant failure and is not usually listed as a reason for revision in most long-term follow-up clinical reports. Fracture of the original all-polyethylene tibial components occurred infrequently. Ultra high molecular weight polyethylene (UHMWPE), with a relatively low modulus of elasticity compared to subchondral bone, will suffer coldflow and will deform while in service, but it does not usually fracture. The introduction of metal-backing for patellar and tibial components was perceived as a way of (*a*) curbing the coldflow and deformation observed with all-polyethylene tibiae; (*b*) distributing stresses to the underlying subchondral bone more evenly to reduce the potential for subsidence and loosening; and (*c*) providing a surface for biologic fixation. Conservative tibial bone resections have generally been advocated in order to preserve the better quality subchondral bone for tibial tray fixation; however, for a given flexion-extension gap, this limits the available space for the tibial component. The combination of metal-backing and conservative bone resections has inadvertently led to widespread use of thin metal trays and thin polyethylene inserts that have been prone to failure by wear and fracture (1–4).

Thin tibial and patellar metal-backed implants have demonstrated acceptable performance in a low demand environment with ideal extremity and implant alignment. This situation does not always exist. Most reports of implant breakage have identified an adverse environment as a major contributor to fatigue failure of the components. Specifically, excess patient weight (5–7), malalignment (8–9), instability, and/or poor quality bone (7, 10) have been associated with fracture (1, 11). Breakage is more likely to occur in younger, heavier, and more active individuals, particularly if correct axial alignment has not been restored with the arthroplasty.

It has been estimated in a static knee model that 5 degrees of malalignment doubles the compressive load on one side of the tibial component, creating tensile loads in the opposite compartment (12). Static radiographic analysis is a useful approximation of stresses within the joint, relative to angular relationships at the knee, but the analysis does not take into consideration the muscle forces and alterations in gait pattern that come with changes in extremity alignment. Weight-bearing activities place high stresses on all three components of a prosthetic knee replacement even under ideal conditions. Peak loads in normal gait have been estimated at 1.5× to 5× body weight with stair climbing or strenuous activity. Clearly, excess body weight, malalignment, and high activity level may lead to implant failure.

Mandatory Reporting of Implant Failures

The Food and Drug Administration (FDA) has required mandatory reporting of failure and breakage of prosthetic devices since December 1984. Four hundred forty knee implant fractures have been reported from December 1984 to July 1992 (13). The actual incidence of failures almost certainly exceeds this number because of incomplete reporting. Effective November, 1991, "User Facilities" were mandated by federal law to report the removal of any prosthetic device regardless of the reason for failure. Compliance with these regulations should improve with time and should provide useful information for the medical community.

The cursory information that has been provided to the FDA is summarized in Table 83.1. Information concerning implants under investigation as part of a federally supervised Investigational Device Exemption (IDE) or a premarket notification (510 (k)) is complete, but only for the relatively short-term time interval of these studies. Implants that are not part of a government study, but that frequently fail are occasionally reported. The surgeon is more likely to notify the manufacturer of repeat occurrences. The failure rate by fracture of any

Table 83.1. Knee Arthroplasty: Device Fractures/Breakages Reported to the F.D.A. (Dec. 1984-July 1992)

Component	Number of Cases
Femoral	82
Tibial[a]	162
Patellar[a]	140
Femoral or tibial stems	14
Pins, clips, axles	6
Unidentified component[b]	37
Total	441

[a]Note: Tibial Components include tibial tray and/or bearing fractures; Patellar Components include backing, polyethylene and/or peg fracture.
[b]Note: Reported data does not always provide complete information.

specific prosthesis is unknown. The FDA does not know the number of implants at risk for any given design or the true number of failures. The FDA data permit only generalizations about components that have failed.

In general, metal-backed tibial and patellar components have fractured more frequently than femoral components. The polyethylene tibial inserts and the polyethylene portion of metal-backed patellae can wear and fracture or dissociate from their metal backing. The base metal tray can fracture and the pegs or stems that help anchor a component can shear or fracture from the component. This chapter discusses the information that has been reported relating to cases of tibial insert fracture, tibial tray fracture, femoral component fracture, and breakage of the metal-backed patellar components.

Tibial Polyethylene Insert Fracture

Clinical Presentation

The patient with a fractured polyethylene bearing usually presents with recent pain and an effusion. These symptoms are secondary to a hypertrophic synovitis associated with wear particles of polymethylmethacrylate, polyethylene, and/or metal. Mechanical symptoms may develop with large fragments of polyethylene acting as loose bodies within the knee. Weight-bearing radiographs demonstrate loss of the space between the metal tibial baseplate and the femoral component that is usually occupied by the polyethylene insert (Fig. 83.1, A and B). The likelihood of this complication increasing with time in situ underscores the importance of annual clinical and radiographic examinations. The fluid from a knee with a broken or severely worn component is usually serosanguineous. Polarized light microscopic analysis may demonstrate small and large particulate material from the damaged surfaces.

Technical Aspects

Polyethylene breakage is primarily a complication of the thin tibial inserts that were introduced in conjunction with metal-backing of the tibial components. Metal-backing requires that the polyethylene thickness is less for any given level of bone resection. The minimally acceptable thickness of the metal baseplate to avoid

breakage is on the order of 2 to 4 mm (14). Metal-backing, combined with the philosophy of conservative bone resections to preserve the highest quality bone for implant fixation, has compelled surgeons to routinely use thin polyethylene inserts with an actual thickness of less than 8mm. In fact, communication with implant manufacturers has revealed that over 50% of the total knees performed in the United States in the past decade have used polyethylene inserts of less than 8mm thick, which puts many devices at risk for failure. In vitro studies (15) have substantiated that thin polyethylene (less than 8mm thick) is at risk for more rapid wear because of higher Von Mises stresses within the polyethylene. Retrieved implants in our laboratory have always demonstrated significant wear prior to implant fracture, suggesting that, because of its susceptibility to wear, polyethylene less than a few millimeters thick, is at particular risk for breakage (Fig. 83.2).

Polyethylene fractures only if the yield strength is exceeded. UHMWPE has a yield strength of 10–14 MPa. Contemporary posterior cruciate ligament sparing designs, by necessity, must reduce articular conformity to permit tri-planar motion. As the conformity is decreased, the contact area between the femoral and tibial components is reduced, leading to higher stresses, since the same load is being applied to a smaller area. Malalignment and instability can exacerbate these high stresses, particularly with flat-on-flat designs that are prone to point contact and edge-loading.

Of the 209 fractured tibial components reported to the FDA, 64 were the tibial bearings. Information regarding the thickness of the bearings and the clinical environment in which they were used is unavailable. The majority of the polyethylene insert fractures were cruciate sparing, minimally congruent designs.

Our impression, from analysis of our own retrievals, is that gradual polyethylene wear contributes to joint laxity. This wear decreases the very limited translational stability of the tibiofemoral interface and leads to edge loading. The asymmetric wear of the central eminence in our retrieved polyethylene inserts confirms this hypothesis. The tibial surface fractures when the sharp corner of the femoral component overloads the polyethylene (Fig. 83.3). This usually occurs at the medial border of the tibial polyethylene due to a varus thrust in normal gait and to the normal concentration of loads through the medial compartment of the knee.

The mobile polyethylene bearings in the Low Contact Stress knee (LCS, DePuy, Warsaw, IN) have fractured when the bearings translate to a position where they are unsupported by the metal baseplate. The movements of these UHMWPE bearings require that proper ligament balance and joint line level be established by the surgeon at the time of arthroplasty. A similar process can occur with the UHMWPE patellar component of this design. The bearings fracture if they translate to a position in which adequate support from the metal baseplate is lost. Fracture of the UHMWPE bearings of the Mobile Bearing knee were not part of the original 510(k) clinical investigation and so were not reported to the FDA. In the FDA Summary of Safety and Effectiveness of the

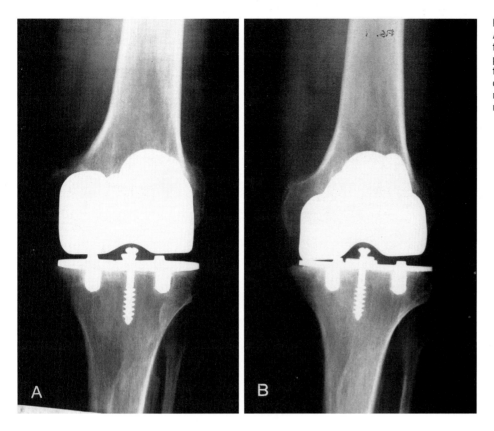

Figure 83.1. **A,** A 2-year postoperative AP radiograph of a cementless PCA total knee arthroplasty. **B,** The 4-year postoperative AP radiograph shows full thickness polyethylene wear and metal-on-metal contact in the medial compartment. (Figure 83.1*B*, reprinted with permission from J Bone Joint Surg-(Am))

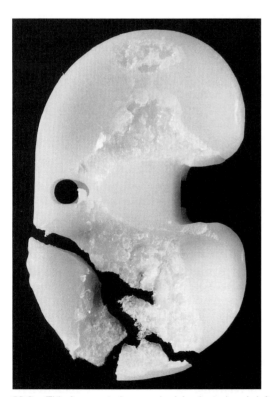

Figure 83.2. This fragmented, severely delaminated and deformed polyethylene insert was retrieved after 89 months in situ from a 200 pound 52-year-old man. The heat-pressed polyethylene of this 7mm metal-backed tibial component failed secondary to catastrophic polyethylene wear. (Figure 83.2 reprinted with permission from J Bone Joint Surg (Br))

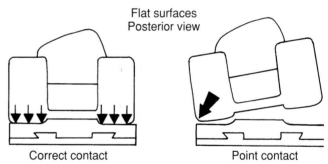

Flat surfaces
Posterior view

Correct contact   Point contact

Figure 83.3. A flat-on-flat articulation is not well tolerated and when associated with malalignment or instability can create point contact loading and accelerated polyethylene damage.

LCS Meniscal Bearing Knee, with follow-up between 3 and 5 years and a revision rate of 3.7%, bearing fracture was not listed as a complication. Meniscal extrusion occurred in two cases (0.6%), but was not included in cases requiring revision.

An independent clinical study of 557 primary meniscal bearing knees listed bearing fracture in 4 cases and meniscal extrusion in an additional 5 knees (Lou Jordan, M.D., unpublished data, 1992). Of these knees, 329 had been followed for 2 or more years. The earliest fracture of a bearing occurred at 33 months; trauma was implicated in each case of fracture. Breakage of a bearing was associated with the sudden onset of pain, an effusion, and increased varus-valgus laxity. The diagnosis is confirmed by displacement of the bearing marker from the dovetail groove of the tibial baseplate, usually anteriorly and beneath the patella. Replacement with thicker bearings has been the treatment for this complication. The mechanism of LCS failures relates primarily to inadequate ligament balance or to implant malposition at the time of surgery.

Posterior stabilized tibial components substitute for posterior cruciate ligament function with a polyethylene post that articulates with the cam of the femoral component. Stresses on the post depend on the location of contact between the cam and post. The location of contact moves up the post as the knee flexes: the greater this distance, the higher the shear stress at the base of the post. Contact location varies with different posterior stabilized configurations. Implants need to be thoroughly tested for fatigue strength of the post. At the Hospital for Special Surgery, none of the original Insall-Burstein designs have failed in this location; however, various other designs have failed by this mechanism (Steve Li, Ph.D., HSS, NY, personal communication).

Constrained condylar implants, that provide varus-valgus as well as anteroposterior stability, carry even higher loads through the post of the tibial component. A reinforcing bar has been added to augment the strength of many such designs.

Tibial Tray Fracture

Clinical Presentation

The diagnosis of a broken metal tibial tray is frequently not made until the component is inspected at revision surgery. Preoperative radiographs usually do not demonstrate the broken piece. A fractured prosthesis, therefore, must be included in the differential diagnosis of a patient that develops late onset of pain following total knee arthroplasty, particularly with components that have been known to fail because of materials or design weaknesses. Progressive subsidence of a component and the resulting malalignment create an environment that contributes to this complication.

Design Factors and Case Reports

Several designs of metal-backed tibial components have fractured (1, 7, 10, 16). Specific clinical factors associated with failure were active and heavy individuals, implant malalignment (either initially or after implant subsidence following fixation failure), tibial bone defects, or poor quality bone beneath the metal tibial platform. Design deficiencies were also implicated in these failures. The 5 major factors influencing success or failure of a design are the following: (1) tray thickness, (2) tray material, (3) manufacturing techniques, (4) in situ loading, and (5) design/shape. These 5 factors are discussed in detail below. It should, however, be noted that the surgeon must share the responsibility for implant success or failure through proper patient selection consistent with long-term durability of the arthroplasty.

1. Implant manufacturers (Table 83.2) have minimized the thickness of metal to permit thicker polyethylene for any given level of bone resection. The conserva-

Table 83.2. Commercially Available Metal Tibial Trays: Materials and Thicknesses

Device	Material	Thickness (MM)
Whitesides I	CoCr	4.2
Whitesides II	CoCr	2.1
PCA	CoCr	1.8
AMK textured edition	Ti-6A1-4V	4.0
AMK	Ti-6A1-4V	3.1
Natural Knee	Ti-6A1-4V	2.8
Miller Galante	Ti-6A1-4V	2.7
PFC	Ti-6A1-4V	1.4

*Adapted by permission from D. Kelman.

tive bone resections preferred by many surgeons create a limited flexion-extension space for adequate combined metal and polyethylene thickness of at least 10 to 12 mm. The thickness of commercially available metal tibial trays varies from 1.5 mm to almost 5 mm (14). A thicker tray possesses greater strength at the expense of thinner polyethylene.

2. The two alloys available for contemporary tibial trays are Ti-6Al-4V and CoCrMo. Titanium alloys are much "easier" to manufacture than CoCr. Also, Ti-6Al-4V has a higher yield strength and a lower modulus of elasticity than CoCr, which makes it appear better suited for orthopaedic applications. However, titanium alloy is extremely notch sensitive, meaning that irregularities or notches in the surface structure are more likely to propagate into fractures. This lowers fatigue strength to much less than cobalt-chrome and may affect the performance of Ti-6Al-4V in situ.

3. The heat treatment required to apply a porous coating on a titanium alloy or a CoCr alloy alters the microstructure of the metal and reduces its fatigue strength (16). Applying a porous coating on titanium further increases its notch sensitivity and reduces the fatigue strength of the base metal. A post-sintering heat treatment improves titanium's fatigue strength by 15% (17), but has no effect on notch sensitivity. Thus, the manufacturing processes required to produce a porous-coated titanium implant may adversely alter its mechanical properties.

The Press-Fit Condylar knee (PFC, Johnson and Johnson, Raynham, Mass.) is an example of a design incorporating the above three potentially detrimental design choices: thin (approximately 1.5mm), Ti-6Al-4V alloy with porous coating on the tibial tray. Cook (2) reported two PFC tibial trays that fractured after 28 and 35 months respectively. Scanning electron microscopy of the fracture surfaces revealed that fatigue was the mechanism of failure. Cantilever loading may contribute to failure in tibial components that demonstrate incomplete bone ingrowth (Fig. 83.4).

4. Metal tibial trays have relatively high stiffness compared to the supporting cancellous bone. Micromo-

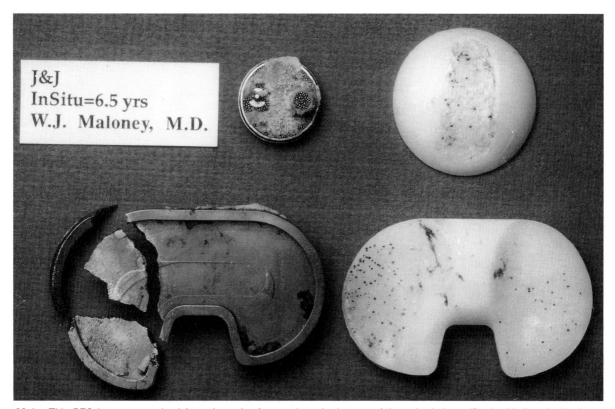

Figure 83.4. This PFC knee was revised for pain and a fractured tibial baseplate after 6.5 yrs in situ.. Also note the extensive bead shedding that has damaged the metal base plate and created third body wear of the polyethylene. (Device kindly submitted to our laboratory by W. Maloney, M.D.)

tion between the tray and bone occurs with each loading cycle because of this modulus mismatch, and it is pronounced if a layer of fibrous tissue is present. A three-dimensional finite element analysis of a commercially available 3mm thick CoCr tibial tray with a central stem subjected to peak loads of normal gait determined that the endurance limit of the tray was exceeded when it was supported by a 1mm fibrous membrane (18, 19). This analysis predicted early failure (10^4 cycles) of the original Porous Condylar Anatomic (PCA, Howmedica, Rutherford, NJ) knee. Fracture occurred through slots in the metal tibial tray that were designed to provide access to the bone-cement interface adjacent to the stem if removal were necessary (10). Although the slots were deleted, fatigue failure has remained a problem (1). Two additional fractured PCA trays have been submitted to our lab. Their CoCrMo baseplates were less than 2 mm thick. The sintering involved in the application of a porous surface may have weakened the substrate metal (16) (Fig. 83.5).

5. Additional design features that increase the risk for failure include: sharp corners, edges, prominences on the component, and screw holes or slots in the metal baseplate. A rigidly fixed central stem transfers cantilever bending stresses to the tray itself. Design features such as sharp corners, edges, prominences on the component, and screw holes and slots in the metal baseplate are stress risers that further increase

the risk of tray fracture. An in vitro test that compared commercially available tibial trays identified fracture initiation and propagation in such areas (14). Clinical confirmation was reported with the Kinematic tibial tray: the relatively sharp corner of the tibial baseplate, created as a recess for preserving the posterior cruciate ligament, was implicated in clinically observed failures. Tibial component fractures in 2 heavy, active patients occurred at this corner of the baseplate, which acted as a stress riser (7).

A patient from the Anderson Clinic sustained a tibial plateau fracture 1 year after total knee replacement with a Kinematic total knee. This fracture healed with residual tibia vara and an abnormal mechanical axis of the lower extremity. The metal tray subsequently fractured through the medial plateau. Cantilever bending secondary to a rigidly fixed, cemented central stem was implicated in these tibial component failures.

Surgeons must thoughtfully evaluate the implants that he or she plans to use in primary and revision total knee surgery. The tibial baseplate should have a cross-sectional thickness of at least 3mm, particularly if it is manufactured from titanium. The design may compensate for material weakness, if, for example, there are struts underneath or rails into which the articular polyethylene slides, which also function as "I" beams. Porous-coated tibial components of CoCrMo will have less notch sensitivity than the same component of tita-

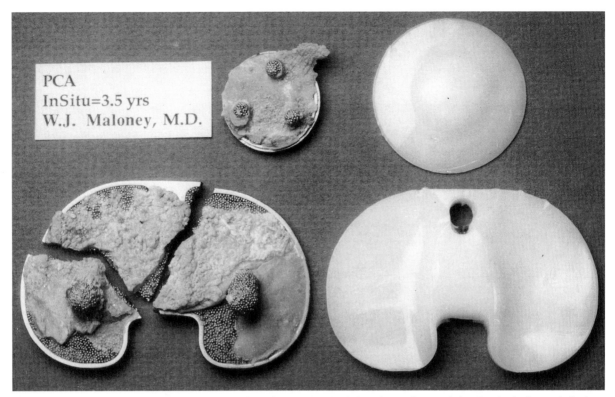

Figure 83.5. This PCA tibial baseplate fractured into three large pieces and several smaller pieces after 41 months in situ. Radiographs demonstrated loosening and subsidence. Note that the tibial polyethylene is not fractured despite the broken cobalt chrome tray. (Device kindly submitted to our laboratory by W. Maloney, M.D.)

nium. Corners, edges, and prominences should be contoured gently. The locking mechanism for modular tibial inserts should not weaken the metal tray. Screw holes must be kept away from the periphery of the tray. The juncture of stem to baseplate should be tapered to the baseplate and should be of sufficient strength and should not fracture when support beneath the plateau portion of the implant is deficient.

Patellar Component Fracture

Clinical Presentation

Fracture of all polyethylene patellar components of total knee arthroplasties appears to be infrequent. Metal-backed patellar components have not, however, shared the same low failure rates. Three series have described the clinical presentation of failed metal-backed patellae (20–22). Fractures of metal-backed patellae rarely occur within the first year of implantation. The patient may relate an acute event at which time the polyethylene either fractured or dissociated from its metal backing or the onset may be insidious with nothing more than low grade pain, an effusion, and a "noisy, squeaky" knee. The patient may describe this as a "grating" noise occurring with activities that load the patellofemoral joint, such as climbing stairs. In several of the failed metal-backed patellae at the Anderson Clinic, the patient did not present to the doctor for 6 months to a year from onset of these symptoms.

Examination of the knee in which the patellar component has broken confirms an effusion, which, if aspirated, is characteristically serosanguineous. A rough grating and audible scraping is present clinically with extension of the knee. The separated polyethylene can become a loose body that leaves the uncovered metal backing to articulate with the femoral component. Radiographs are frequently negative, but may show the soft tissue outline of the loose polyethylene.

A complete synovectomy is needed at revision surgery to remove this tissue, laden with particulate metallic debris. The articulating surface of the femoral component may be damaged from contact with the metal-backing and may require revision, particularly if it is a titanium implant. A more difficult decision must be made when slight burnishing and mild scratching on a well-fixed CoCr femoral component is identified. The potential for accelerated polyethylene damage of the revised patellar component and the tibial articulation from the unrevised femoral component must be considered.

Technical Aspects

The problems of thin polyethylene are present with metal-backed patellae. Many failed designs of metal-backed patellae have been reported: the domed PCA, PFC, Synatomic, Miller Galante, and Microloc designs. The thin polyethylene of these designs led to accelerated wear until fracture occurred and the polyethylene disassociated from its metal backing. Stress risers were created by sharp metal corners or edges for locking the polyethylene to the metal-backing in some designs (20, 23).

Metal-backed patellae have failed at the junction of fixation posts to the implant (2). Forty-one of the 142 patellar component failures reported to the FDA were patellar peg fractures (13). Twelve fiber-mesh titanium Miller-Galante (Zimmer, Warsaw, Indiana) patellar components from a reported series of 122 cementless total knee arthroplasties experienced fatigue fracture at the peg-plate juncture (24). Preferential bone ingrowth into the pegs concentrated stresses at the base of the pegs (Fig. 83.6). The application of titanium fiber mesh to the substrate may have contributed to fracture. Retrievals of implants at the Anderson Clinic include 1 case in which a fixation peg sheared from the back of a PFC metal-backed patella and 2 cases of failure of all 4 fixation pins of a Synatomic (DePuy, Warsaw, Indiana) patella. The PFC patella was porous-coated titanium and the root diameter of the CoCr Synatomic pins was less than 2mm.

Femoral Component Fracture

Condylar femoral component designs, except for the Whitesides II Ortholoc knee (Dow Corning Wright, Arlington, TN), are rarly broken. Of the 82 fractured

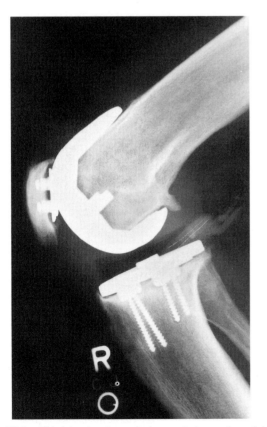

Figure 83.6. This lateral radiograph demonstrates preferential bone ingrowth into the porous-coated titanium mesh pegs. A wide radiolucency exists along the metal-bone interface where bone resorption has occurred.

femoral components reported to the FDA, 39 were the Whitesides Ortholoc design. This CoCrMo femoral component had a substrate metal thickness at the junction of the posterior chamfer of less than 2 mm, which predisposed to fracture. Whitesides has independently reported this complication (25), and the implant has been modified. Cook reported 1 fatigue failure of an Ortholoc femoral component: the device fractured at the posteromedial condyle after 20 months (2). Implants fabricated in titanium may also be subject to failure at this same juncture, a type of failure that points up once again the notch sensitivity of this material.

Revision Component Fracture

Deficient bone stock in revision surgery often requires intramedullary canal support with long-stemmed implants. Revision implants must maintain their integrity under adverse loading conditions at the junction of the stem and the prosthesis, since bone support is usually deficient. Sixteen failures reported to the FDA were of stem fracture, with 12 of these being tibial stems. A 6% breakage rate of the Kinematic Rotating Hinge prosthesis (Howmedica, Rutherford, N.J.) at the junction of the stem and the tibial baseplate was reported from a series of 50 total knee arthroplasties (26). In the 1-to-3 year follow-up of the uniaxial, Vitallium GUEPAR hinge (developed in 1970) 2 of 108 arthroplasties had fractured femoral stems (27). The porous-coated stem of the revision PCA femoral component was welded to the implant. One patient, at the Anderson Clinic with bilateral revision PCA knees, fractured at the stem-implant weld of both femoral components. This failure of the prosthesis was identified on preoperative radiographs by a change in the angle between the component and its stem (Fig. 83.7, *A*, *B* and *C*). Since high stress is imparted at the stem-component junction, a stem attachment that is located away from this area of stress concentration may be preferable. The stem-implant junction should be capable of bearing full loads despite complete loss of bone support beneath the condyles or plateau of the component.

The thin metal-backing of a primary knee system may be too weak for a revision case with compromised bone support. Revision implants should be robust. The metal of both the femoral and tibial components can be augmented, since in most revision cases ample room is present for a thicker component.

Fixation Failure/Implant Loosening

Historical Perspective

The most common reason for total knee arthroplasty failure over the history of this procedure has been loosening of the implant. Factors that have been associated with loosening include: infection, implant constraint, failure to achieve neutral mechanical alignment, instability, and cement technique. The clinical presentation of the patient with a loose component is the same regardless of the cause: pain that is frequently associated with angular deformity of the knee. The radiographic features include a widening radiolucent zone between

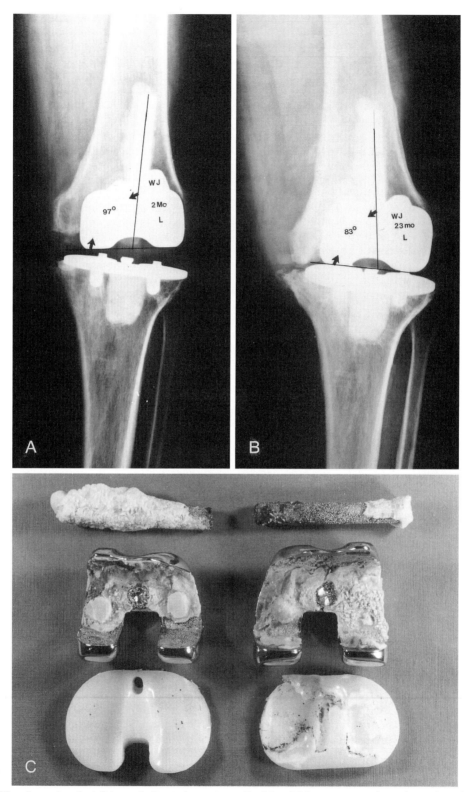

Figure 83.7. Two AP radiographs of a left knee: **A,** 2 months postoperatively and **B**, 23 months postoperatively of a cemented revision PCA knee. During this time frame the porous-coated stem, which was welded to the femoral component, fractured at the weld. The femoral component subsided medially as evidenced by the 14 degree change in the stem-component angular relationship. A similar scenario developed on the contralateral side. **C,** The retrieved cemented

Revision PCA components from the patient described in **A** and **B**. The left knee was revised after 31 months in situ and the right after 67 months. Both porous-coated CoCr stems failed at the stem-component weld. Significant polyethylene wear, including delamination and third-body wear secondary to bead shedding was observed bilaterally.

the implant and the adjacent bone and subsidence of the implant.

Infection must never be overlooked as a cause of implant loosening. Infection can occur early or late and can present with or without signs of systemic toxicity. The symptoms are frequently the same as those seen with aseptic loosening. A progressive radiolucency between a prosthesis and its adjacent bone must always be considered an infection until proven otherwise. Negative aspirates from the knee, normal sedimentation rates and C-reactive protein, and negative Gallium and Indium scans do not rule out infection of a prosthetic device. The patient should be advised that even in the presence of normal tests, infection may be discovered intraoperatively and require the removal of the prosthetic devise.

Evolution of Implant Designs

The earliest implants that replaced the tibiofemoral joint were metal-on-metal hinged designs, such as the Walldius, Stanmore, and GUEPAR prostheses, that permitted motion about a single axis. The loosening rates for these linked devices in early studies is inaccurately reported because the tibial and femoral components were implanted without the use of cement. The lack of rigid implant fixation was not considered to be a significant source of pain with these early press-fit, hinged components. Infection necessitated revision in approximately 10% of the cases (28–31).

Subsequent studies, in which cement was used and follow-up was less than 5 years, reported loosenings that required revision in 10 to 25% of cases (31, 32). The rate of loosening was much higher for osteoarthritic knees in active individuals. Radiographic criteria for loosening had not been established and, therefore, were not reported. Deep infection remained a problem in 10% of cases (33, 34)

Single axis hinge designs were followed by implants that permitted biplanar motion. The Attenborough, the Kinematic rotating hinge, and the Noiles prostheses all provided rotation through the tibial bearing. These linked implants used polyethylene bearings to reduce friction and were fixed to bone with cemented stems on both the tibial and femoral side. The major mechanism of failure was aseptic loosening, although deep infection continued to be a problem in most reports. The Attenborough prosthesis had a reported loosening rate of 20 to 30% (35, 36) with follow-up less than 6 years. In one series, the Noiles prosthesis demonstrated radiographic subsidence in 94% of the cases at 5 years (37). Loosening of the implant was associated with pain and widening radiolucencies, but angular deformity was prevented by the long intramedullary stems.

The high failure rates of constrained knee prostheses used in the 1960s clearly was a problem of constraint. Hinged devices, even with rotating bearings, did not permit triplanar motion of the knee, essential for normal ambulatory activities. Stems enhanced the initial fixation stability of the implant and ensured proper alignment of the components by acting as intramedullary guides. Thus, neither malalignment nor ligament imbalance were related to implant failure in these designs. The high stresses transmitted by a constrained implant to the fixation interface exceeded the strength of the cement bond, particularly in younger, more active individuals (Fig. 83.8). Linked devices are of historical interest only in the management of knee arthritis.

High loosening rates restricted design evolution to the semiconstrained cruciate-sacrificing and to the unconstrained cruciate-sparing implants in use today. The Polycentric and Geometric implants were early nonlinked devices designed to retain the collateral and posterior cruciate ligaments for joint stability and load transfer. The Polycentric prosthesis allowed 20 degrees of axial rotation to decrease stress on the fixation interface. The Geometric knee had a single radius of curvature of the femoral component in a sagittal plane. The kinematic mismatch between implant articular geometry and ligaments led to loosening with a 10% incidence, requiring revision at 10 years, for the Polycentric knee (38), and it led to an 18% failure rate, with maximum follow-up of 8.5 years, for the Geometric implant (39).

Condylar designs were developed to permit more natural movements of the knee. The Total Condylar Knee was designed with a relatively closely matching radius of curvature between the tibial and femoral components in a coronal plane and a radius of curvature that decreased posteriorly on the femoral component. The posterior cruciate ligament was sacrificed with stability achieved by balancing the collateral ligaments in flexion and extension. The tibial component was cup-shaped in an anterior to posterior direction that did not permit femoral rollback as the knee flexed and, therefore, limited knee flexion. This degree of congruency was not associated with high loosening rates; only 2 tibias loosened in one series of 100 osteoarthritic knees with follow-up of 5 to 9 years (40); in a group of 129 Total Condylar knee replacements followed for a mean 9.1 years, 2 other tibias loosened (41). The durability of cement fixation with this implant and with other condylar designs has resulted in the widespread use of prosthetic replacement of the knee for the management of arthritis.

The Posterior Cruciate Condylar Knee, a design iteration of the Total Condylar Knee, provided a cutout in the back of the tibial component for retention of the posterior cruciate ligament. The cupped tibial component, in concert with posterior cruciate ligament retention, did not limit flexion and did not increase loosening rates. One tibial loosening was identified from a group of 88 knee arthroplasties followed for at least 5 years (42). There were incomplete radiolucencies less than 1mm in width in only 22% of cases. No revisions for tibial loosening were reported in another clinical report study of 164 Posterior Cruciate Condylar implants at 5 years (43).

The Kinematic prosthesis also retained the posterior cruciate ligament, but the tibial component was flattened posteriorly to accommodate femoral rollback with knee flexion. Loosening was not a cause for revision in a study of 192 Kinematic implants 5 to 9 years

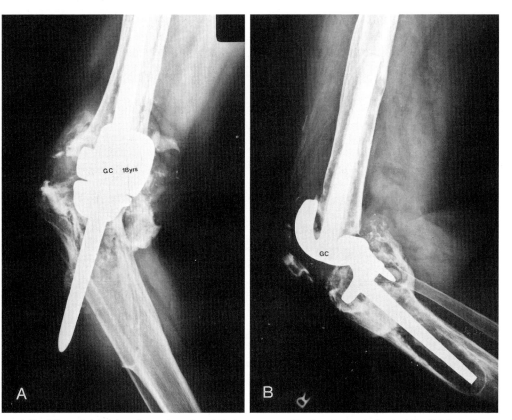

Figure 83.8. **A** and **B,** AP and lateral radiographs of a failed GUEPAR knee. The stems of the implant have loosened from their cement bed and migrated out of the tibial shaft secondary to the high constraint built into the component.

after the operation (44) This implant had a nonmodular metal-backed tibial component similar to many prosthetic knee designs in the late 1970s. Metal-backing was perceived as a way of improving the durability of tibial component fixation by reducing loads at the fixation interface (45).

The Posterior Stabilized prosthesis, introduced by Insall and Burstein, substituted for the posterior cruciate ligament and created femoral rollback through a central polyethylene post that contacted a transverse cam on the femur as the knee flexed. The post provided posterior stability to the knee. The tibial polyethylene had a posterior slope of 5 degrees and, when combined with the design of the post and cam, converted shear forces to predominantly compressive forces at the tibial fixation interface. Metal-backing was later added to the stemmed tibial component. Knee flexion was improved and excellent AP (anteroposterior) stability was maintained without increasing loosening rates (5). A survivorship report comparing results of the Posterior Stabilized knee from 289 cases performed between 1978 and 1981 with an all polyethylene tibia reported 2 loose tibial and 3 loose femoral components. A ten year success rate of 97.34% was projected (46). The same component with a metal-backed tibial component placed between 1981 and 1986 had no reported failures of metal-backed tibial components, 1 loose femoral component, and a projected 10 year survivorship of the implant of 98.75%. An independent report of 119 knees followed from 2 to 8 years identified only 2 cases of tibial loosening.

Cementless Fixation

Cementless total knee arthroplasty was developed as an alternative to conventional cement fixation to solve the problem of loosening. Many implants available today offer a porous or textured metal surface for bone ingrowth. Cementless fixation is only considered feasible with minimally congruent implants that do not transfer shear stresses to the fixation interface. Proponents of cementless fixation believe that a bone ingrown implant will be more durable because bone at the fixation interface will remodel to the demands of its environment.

Several clinical reports of cementless total knee arthroplasty have failed to demonstrate a difference in clinical scores or revision rates when compared with cement component fixation (47–49). In some studies patients were preselected for cementless fixation based primarily on the quality of bone and fit of the prosthesis obtained at the time of the arthroplasty. Preselection bias may invalidate the results of such reports. The short-term results with biologic fixation with a porous surface implant in other reports were less predictable than results with cemented devices (50–52). A comparison of 50 cemented to 41 cementless PCA knees identified lower post-operative knee scores and a higher early revision rate with the cementless group (51). The reoperation rate was higher when comparing 50 uncemented

PCA knee arthroplasties with 110 cemented kinematic knees (52) at 2 years. A survivorship analysis of 108 uncemented PCA knee replacements with an average follow-up of 64 months reported collapse of the tibial plateau in 14 cases. The cumulative rate of survival was only 77% at 6 years (53).

Implant subsidence (49, 54, 55) has been identified with cementless tibial components. Resecting the proximal tibia leaves fractured trabeculae to support the metal tray. A stereophotogrammatic method of roentgenographic analysis has demonstrated subsidence, distal migration and micromotion of tibial components (56). This motion may inhibit bone ingrowth fixation and may account for the relatively limited area and amount of bone ingrowth identified in retrieval studies (57, 58). Implant motion may also explain the higher incidence of pain seen early with the use of cementless tibial fixation (49). Hard tissue histology has confirmed that the radio-dense line beneath the tibial baseplate is new bone formation associated with interposed organized fibrous tissue (59), and does not represent bone remodeling secondary to bone ingrowth fixation. Bead shedding, another negative radiographic feature, was found in over 50% of PCA knees in 2 separate studies (60, 61). Progressive bead loss is secondary to movement of an implant, and correlates with radiolucencies on radiographs, and progressive subsidence of a component. Loose beads are occasionally seen between the articular surfaces and as such may damage the surfaces and accelerate wear.

The design of cementless tibial components continues to evolve, with modifications to the metal tray that achieve better immediate stability, and hopefully, more predictable bone ingrowth. Most cementless tibial components now include options for larger and longer modular stems, posts or cleats, and screws to enhance the mechanical interlock of the component. The Synatomic Knee, which incorporated 2 to 4 screws, demonstrated a 13.3% incidence of tibial osteolysis adjacent to the cancellous screws (62). Corrosion has been observed at the Morse tapers in total hip arthroplasty (63), which raises concern with the use of mixed-metal modular stems and wedges on both tibial and femoral components in knee surgery. The potential for debris generation from modular surfaces and fretting of screws with cementless fixation underscores the need for controlled studies before adopting changes in implant designs.

Cementless fixation is more successful with femoral than tibial components. The larger surface area for fixation of the femoral component provides better initial implant stability. Hybrid fixation, with cement stabilization of the tibial component and cementless fixation of the femoral component, has become a relatively popular alternative. Early clinical results have been favorable (64). Cementless fixation may also be possible with a posterior stabilized implant.

Long-term results with cemented condylar prostheses appear to be excellent, although the incidence of non-progressive radiolucent lines at the bone cement interface remains high (5). Uncemented fixation of any component of a total knee replacement must be thoughtfully considered until long-term results of cementless fixation have been substantiated. Radiographic assessment of cementless components is much more difficult than the radiographic evaluation of a cemented interface. The metal component blocks visualization of the fixation interface of a cementless device unless the x-ray beam is precisely perpendicular to the component. This may necessitate the use of fluoroscope controlled imaging or multiple radiographs. Different radiographic criteria are necessary when evaluating cementless components. Radiographic results should not be compared if different modes of fixation have been used.

Clinical Reports

The clinical results achieved with an implant introduced in the 1980s or 1990s cannot be compared with the results of an earlier generation of implants with a different mode of implant fixation or a different patient population. The first generation of implants came in a limited number of sizes providing incomplete coverage of the bone surfaces. Surgery was performed with relatively crude instrumentation for aligning and orienting the prosthetic components. Malalignment has been singled out as a critical factor influencing postoperative loosening and instability, and was particularly problematic in earlier knee arthroplasties. Improvements in cement technique and soft tissue balancing have evolved as greater experience has been gained with this procedure. The Total Condylar Knee was subject to deficiencies in instrumentation and implant inventory, yet maintained a relatively low loosening rate. Ninety percent survivorship at nine to eleven years with the Total Condylar Knee was achieved in a primarily rheumatoid arthritis population despite alignment between neutral and 12 degrees of valgus (5). This data should not be used to predict survivorship at longer follow-up intervals or survivorship for a younger and more active osteoarthritic patient population. It would also be incorrect to compare these results with those achieved with a later generation of implants and credit the improvement solely to a change in implant design. The improved survivorship reported with the posterior stabilized implant and with metal backing of the tibial component (46) may have been independent of these design changes and may have been the results of improved instrumentation, surgical experience including bone preparation and cement technique, and improvements in materials and manufacturing techniques. Prospective, randomized and carefully controlled trials are needed to accurately identify improvements in implant designs.

Current Concepts in Implant Loosening
Mechanical Factors

The cruciate sparing designs of today differ from the earlier condylar designs mainly by a reduction in contour between the tibial and femoral components. Most contemporary designs are flat or almost flat in the relationship of the femoral to the tibial component in both anteroposterior and medial-lateral directions and therefore provide very little constraint at the prosthetic interface. Improved knee flexibility is achieved with reduced congruency, but at the expense of higher contact stress as a result of the reduced contact area. Knee designs, in which the femoral component is flat or only slightly contoured, transmit very low shear across the component interface, thereby reducing the demand on component fixation. A contoured implant, in comparison, and particularly an AP (anterior-posterior) constrained or varus-valgus constrained device with a central articulating post, will transmit significantly more stress to the bone-implant bond. A more rigid initial fixation is required including the use of cemented and stemmed implants. Early fixation failure should be higher with the more contoured designs, but polyethylene wear should be higher with the less congruent designs because of the higher contact stresses. Likewise, range of motion theoretically should be better with a minimally constrained device, whereas knee stability should be better with more conformity between the articulating surfaces. Polyethylene wear may become a problem with increasing time in situ and may create knee instability with minimally congruent surfaces, particularly if correct alignment and ligament balance is not achieved at the time of the knee arthroplasty (Fig. 83.9, A and B).

Role of Alignment

Limb alignment has been recognized as the single most important factor influencing loosening in many designs of total knee arthroplasty (65). The mechanical axis of the limb should pass from the hip to the ankle through the center of the knee. The components should be oriented at a right angle to the mechanical axis to ensure that primarily compressive forces are transmitted to the fixation interface. Errors in limb alignment create eccentric loading of the components that can overload the fixation of the bone-implant interface. Overall varus malalignment correlates with tibial radiolucent lines and statistically greater loosening rates (66). Likewise, component malalignment is also associated with higher failure rates. Tibial components aligned in more than 4 degrees of varus had a statistically higher incidence of radiolucencies and loosening (67). Malalignment occurs because of incorrect use of the alignment system or incorrect interpretation of information that the alignment system provides. Intramedullary alignment is usually more accurate in controlling the axial alignment of the femoral component (68). Intramedullary guides require less judgment in the interpretation of the information they provide than an extramedullary guide system. Extramedullary alignment is difficult in obese patients because bony landmarks are obscured by the soft tissue; fortunately, intramedullary systems do not share this problem. Tibial alignment can be controlled with either intramedullary or extramedullary alignment devices with similar, acceptable results. The tibial shaft and ankle are easy to palpate, providing accuracy in orienting extramedullary guides. The correct rotational orien-

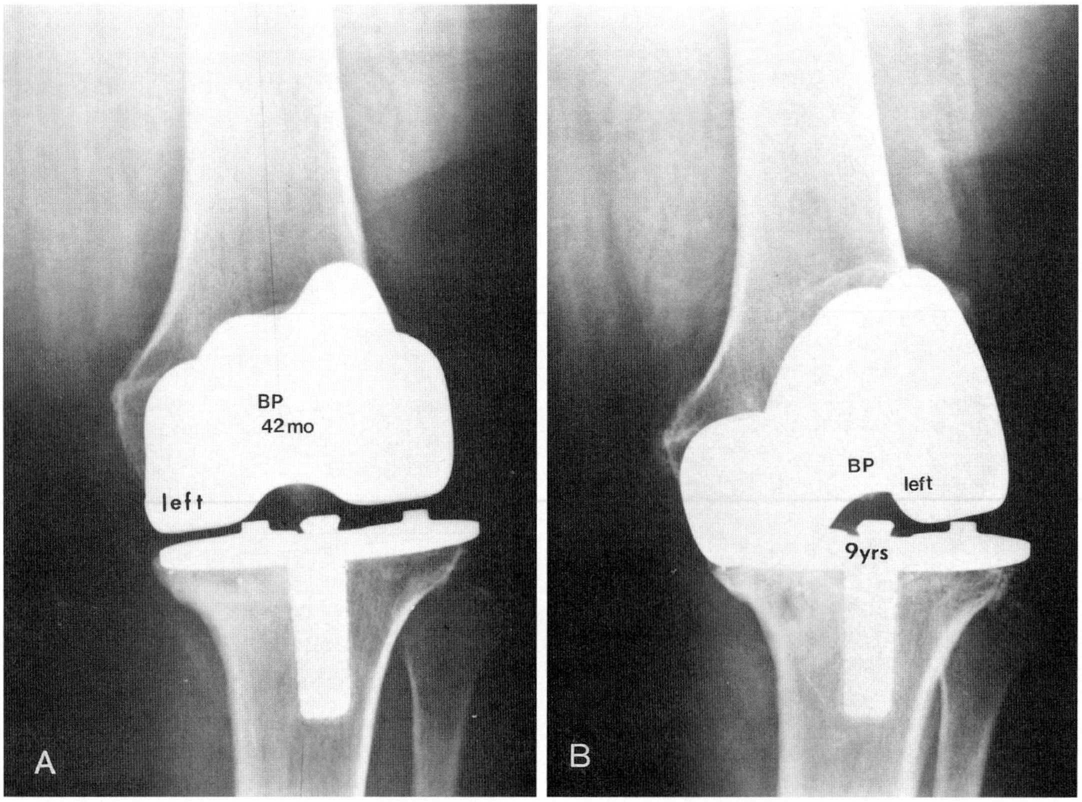

Figure 83.9. **A** and **B,** A cementless PCA knee with a non-constrained and minimally congruent articulation. The patient was pain free at 42 months but demonstrates early lateral shift of the tibia relative to the femur. The 9-year radiograph documents instability, loss of alignment, and severe polyethylene wear.

tation of the alignment device is equally important with intramedullary and extramedullary guides. Since the cutting block is oriented at an angle to the alignment device (valgus orientation of the femoral cutting block and posterior slope to most tibial cutting blocks), malrotation of the device will orient the cutting guide incorrectly for the plane of the cut. For instance, if a tibial guide with 7 degrees posterior slope is externally rotated, the posterior slope will be directed medially, creating varus with the tibial resection. This malrotation of the tibial alignment device can occur with both intramedullary and extramedullary guides.

The alignment of the entire extremity is important, and should be checked independently of the orientation of the tibial and femoral components. A few degrees of malalignment of one component may be of no consequence, but, if both components are malaligned in the same direction (i.e., varus of both components), the errors may create adverse loading conditions across the knee (Fig. 83.10). A knee that starts in varus tends to fail in varus. It is probably better to slightly overcorrect the preoperative malalignment.

Ligament Balance

Ligamentous balance goes hand-in-hand with alignment in creating a mechanically sound environment for a prosthetic device. The correct use of alignment devices will restore axial alignment of the bony structures, but will not evenly distribute loads across the knee. In most instances of deformity, if the surgeon simply corrects the static malalignment, then the ligaments will be too tight on the concave side of the preoperative deformity. The soft tissue elements must be balanced to the corrected alignment of the extremity. An incomplete release of contracted ligaments leaves inadequate space for the components on the contracted side. The surgeon has to either force components into this contracted space or use an implant that is too thin in order to bring the ligaments under proper tension on the noncontracted side. If the ligaments are incompletely released, then the compressive forces are localized to the contracted side, and tensile forces are created on the noncontracted side. Implants may subside when the support bone is insufficient. It is this author's opinion that this subsidence can even occur intraoperatively when testing a knee for stability with trial components, and it can alter component alignment as the soft bone is being compressed on the contracted side prior to final implant fixation.

Ligament imbalance can also produce an asymmetric or defective cement mantle that is apparent on immediate postoperative radiographs. A common practice is to

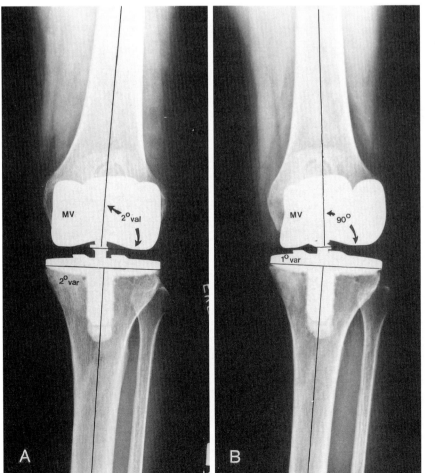

Figure 83.10. A, A nonweight-bearing radiograph obtained early post-operatively demonstrates neutral extremity alignment. Although neither component is badly aligned, the combination of inadequate valgus orientation of both components is additive. **B,** A weight-bearing radiograph demonstrates that load is concentrated in the medial compartment that may contribute to loosening.

extend the knee at the time of cement polymerization to compress the cement into cancellous bone. Contracted ligaments will compress the cement only on the tight side of the knee with this maneuver. Tension on the opposite side can create a wedged appearance or radiolucency in the cement, which has been associated with a higher loosening rate (Hardinge K, personal communication, 1992).

Ligament release should be anticipated in all knees with significant varus or valgus deformity. If preoperative examination and x-rays demonstrate the need for ligament release that are then found to be unnecessary during the operation, the bone cuts should be rechecked for correct axial alignment, and the ligaments should be inspected for inadvertent rents that may have occurred. Residual ligament imbalance may predispose the patient to early fixation failure and/or accelerated polyethylene wear (Fig. 83.11).

Posterior Cruciate Ligament

The posterior cruciate ligament (PCL) and popliteus tendon can also contribute to eccentric loads on the tibial component that may affect fixation. In a knee with a contracted PCL, the femoral condyles will roll too far posteriorly on the tibial plateau as the knee is flexed. The surgeon recognizes the posterior position of the

femoral component on the tibial plateau and a lifting up of the front of the tibial tray as the knee is flexed intraoperatively with trial components. The term "booking open" is used to describe this phenomenon. Compressive forces concentrated eccentrically at the posterior aspect of the tibial plateau must be corrected by surgically relaxing or recessing the PCL and, sometimes, the popliteus tendon. An excessively tight posterior cruciate ligament may also increase stress on the posterior aspect of the tibial component. The potential for accelerated polyethylene wear has been postulated to affect the long-term durability of the arthroplasty (69).

Mechanically Induced Loosening (Fixation Failure)

Implant loosening can occur early or late. Early implant loosening (within the first 2 years) usually represents a mechanical failure of the interlock of the implant to host bone (Fig. 83.12). This early implant loosening is more appropriately called fixation failure and is often secondary to errors in judgment at the time of surgery or to problems with the technical aspects of the surgical procedure. Extremity malalignment, soft tissue imbalance, and poor cement technique may individually, or in combination, contribute to loosening.

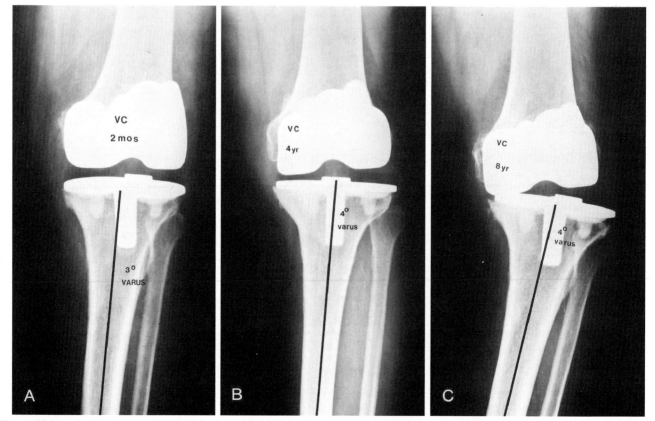

Figure 83.11. **A,** This cemented PCA implant was placed in a 78-year-old gentleman with preoperative severe varus deformity. **B,** A minimal release of contracted medial compartment ligaments is evident by asymmetric loading as seen at 4 years. **C,** By 8 years, the tibial component remains rigidly fixed to bone but the patient has developed recurrent varus malalignment, instability and severe polyethylene wear.

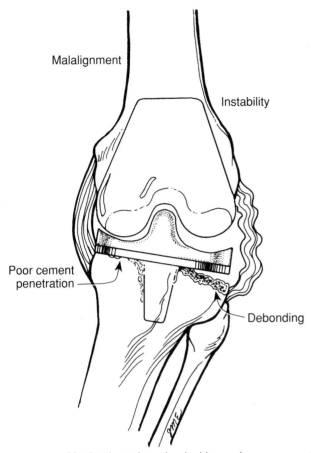

Mechanism of mechanical loosening

Figure 83.12. Factors that influence mechanical loosening include malalignment, instability, and poor initial bone preparation and bonding of cement to host bone. It is the surgeon's responsibility to create a sound mechanical environment for the prosthesis. Cementless components and more constrained implants are particularly dependent on technical aspects of the surgical procedure.

Tibial Component

The early loss of implant fixation to host bone can occur with cemented and cementless tibial components (Fig. 83.11). The tibial component is more likely to fail than the femoral component because of its smaller surface area for component fixation, the nature of the loading environment, and its less intimate fit. The density of bone of the resected proximal tibia is variable in quality. The highest quality bone of the proximal tibia is located just beneath the subchondral plate. No more than 5mm of bone should be removed from the medial tibial plateau, which equates to 8 to 10mm of bone from the lateral tibial plateau when performing a 90 degree tibial resection, because a strong correlation between radiolucencies and the depth of tibial bone resection has been identified (70). The varus knee characteristically has dense, sclerotic bone in the medial tibial plateau and osteoporotic bone on the lateral side. Resection of the proximal tibia at 90 degrees removes more bone from the lateral tibial plateau where the bone is of poorer quality in terms of compressive strength (71). Placing a

metal plate on this surface without cement, is analogous to building a house on a strong foundation built under only one end of the house. Much as the house will settle under its own weight, so will the tibial component subside into the weaker cancellous bone when it is loaded. A major advantage of cement is its provision of a composite structure in osteoporotic bone that provides strength sufficient to support a tibial component during weight-bearing activities. A stem further reduces stress on the interface. Fixation in poor quality bone is best managed with a longer stemmed implant and cement fixation.

Femoral Component

Early failure of cemented femoral components is almost nonexistent with minimally constrained components. While cementless fixation generally provides excellent short-term clinical results, these components appear to be more prone to early fixation failure, because of the greater difficulty in achieving immediate stability in the face of weight-bearing loads without cement.

Although a randomized, prospective clinical trial comparing the two methods of fixation has not been published, the only two cases of early fixation failure (of any component) with the first 600 implants of the Anatomic Modular Knee (AMK-DePuy, Warsaw, Indiana) at the Anderson Clinic were cementless femoral components (Fig. 83.13). In both cases, postoperative activity-related pain was alleviated by reinserting the femoral component with cement. The stability of the initial implant is critical if cementless fixation is selected. A false assumption is that femoral component fixation does not require an intimate fit of the component to host bone. In fact, anything less than a tight press fit should be changed to a cement bond.

Hybrid fixation of total knee implants, with cement fixation of the tibia and patella and cementless femoral fixation, has been advocated by Scott (64), based on his personal observations of an increased incidence of radiolucencies adjacent to the posterior condyles of cemented femoral components that were not present in a review of his cementless femoral implants. These radiolucencies were interpreted as bone remodeling. Scott postulated that in flexion, strong forces applied through the posterior condyles of the femoral component tend to flex the implant. Tensile forces are created secondarily in the cement mantle beneath the anterior flange that may exceed the strength of the cement bond. A cementless implant, by comparison, can remodel to loads at the bone-implant interface and can accommodate loads applied through the femoral component with the knee in flexion. This theoretical advantage of a cementless femoral component has not been substantiated by clinical results.

Patellar Component

Patellar fixation failure, reported with several designs, depends on many of the same parameters as other components. The bone must be of adequate quality to provide a stable fixation interface, particularly for cementless fixation. The implant should fully cover the

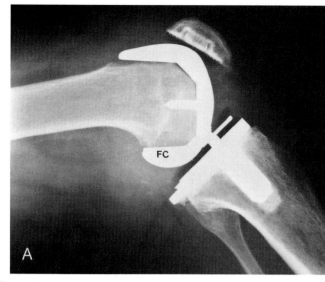

Figure 83.13. **A,** The immediate postoperative lateral radiograph of an AMK hybrid total knee replacement demonstrates a poor initial fit of the cementless femoral component. The patient complained of activity-related pain. **B,** A lateral obtained at 1 year demonstrated a circumferential radiolucency adjacent to the femoral component. Revision to a cemented femoral component relieved the patient of all his pain.

resected undersurface of the patella to maximize the area for component support. This requires an array of sizes. The patellofemoral groove must be of adequate depth and appropriate configuration to reduce the potential for subluxation, but should not be constrained to the degree that the fixation interface might be compromised as the knee flexes. The Kinematic knee prosthesis has experienced a problem with early loosening secondary to excessive constraint of a recessed patellofemoral groove (44).

Fixation posts should be of adequate size, number, and configuration to provide the necessary component stability. The original PCA patellar component had 2 relatively short porous-coated pegs that were prone to early failure. The pegs were lengthened and a third one added. The Synatomic implant provided 4 pins for initial fixation. which proved too weak to resist shear loads in 2 failed implants retrieved at the Anderson Clinic. Satisfactory results have been reported with 3 fixation posts of approximately 5mm in length (23). A fixation ring has also proved successful in achieving initial patellar stability (72).

Biological Factors

Late loosening of total knee implants is often secondary to the host biologic response to wear debris (Fig. 83.14) that weakens the mechanical bond of implant to bone established at the time of surgery (62, 73–75). Mechanical factors may contribute to late loosening, but they do not alone explain the loss of fixation of a device that has been stable for many years. The volume of particles generated from the articulation is influenced by: patient weight and activity level, duration of implantation, polyethylene thickness, and contact stresses. Wear may be accelerated by malalignment, instability, and ligament

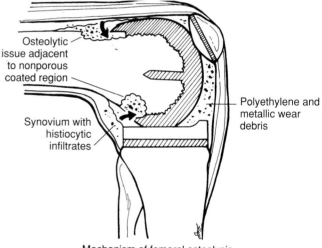

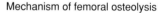
Mechanism of femoral osteolysis

Figure 83.14. Particulate wear debris gains access to the bone-implant interface in regions where the component is not rigidly bonded. Voids in the cement mantle and smooth regions of a porous-coated device provide access routes and recesses for accumulation of particulate. Osteolysis develops when the focal defense mechanism to handle foreign material is overwhelmed.

imbalance, resulting in an increased volume of particulate released into the joint.

When a total knee arthroplasty is performed, the trauma of surgery incites a fracture healing response that includes remodeling of osseous trabeculae adjacent to the implant. Bone scans demonstrate increased vascularity associated with this process. A bond is established between implant and bone that, ideally, demonstrates direct, extensive apposition of bone with metal or polymethylmethacrylate. The extent of this intimate contact varies from case to case. A cemented implant may have areas where cement is separated from bone by fibrous tissue. Bone ingrowth into a cementless implant occurs in only about 10% of the available surface area with fibrous tissue in areas not ingrown with bone. In regions of poor cement penetration, such as sclerotic bone or where smooth metal is in direct contact with bone, a fibrous tissue membrane develops. The organized fibrous tissue in such areas, adjacent to a mechanically stable cemented or cementless components, has a characteristically benign appearance without inflammatory or synovial-like cells. The radiographic appearance is also benign without widening radiolucencies or evidence of implant migration. The fibrous interface may, however, provide an avenue for incursion of particulate debris to the fixation interface, particularly at the margins of the implant (76, 77).

A total knee implant, in an engineering sense, is a wear couple of metal and polyethylene. Debris is generated by friction between the different components. The volume of particulate polyethylene particles in a total joint arthroplasty under normal conditions has been estimated at 30,000,000 particles a day. The volume of debris is influenced by a host of factors, including the size and activity of the individual, the quality (63) and thickness of the polyethylene (3, 4, 14), the surface finish of the metal counterface (78, 79), and the presence of debris within the joint that can act as an abrasive between the articulating surfaces. Most of this debris, released into the synovial confines of the knee, is phagocytosed by the synovial lining and transported through the lymphatics to regional lymph nodes. It is theorized that the synovial lining has a threshold of debris that it can tolerate. Particles that are not phagocytosed are free to migrate along the path of least resistance. A pumping action occurs with cyclic loading of the knee (77, 80, 81). Debris gains access to bone adjacent to the components wherever an intimate relationship at the fixation interface has not been established (77). A mismatch in the modulus of elasticity between metal and bone enhances this debris migration.

Metal and polymethylmethacrylate particles also may accumulate at the fixation interface. The metal-on-metal contact that occurs with failed metal-backed patellae and the use of screws to anchor cementless tibial components have been implicated as sources of metal debris with cementless total knee arthroplasty (Fig. 83.15) (62). Modular trunions of stems and wedges that are attached with screws may be additional sources of particulate debris. Titanium alloy-bearing surfaces, with wear characteristics inferior to those of CoCrMo (82–84), may yield comparatively large amounts of particulate debris.

The tissue immediately adjacent to a loose implant differs dramatically from that of a stable component (85). A dense synovial-like membrane defines the margins of this tissue. Beneath this layer are sheets of activated macrophages and giant cells in a variable stroma of fibrous tissue. Bone remodeling occurs at a rapid rate as demonstrated by a pronounced osteoclastic and os-

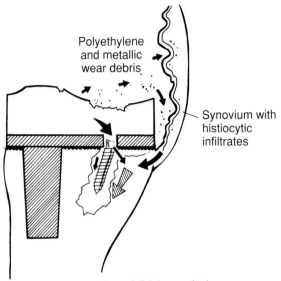

Mechanism of tibial osteolysis

Figure 83.15. Osteolysis has been demonstrated adjacent to tibial screws used with cementless component fixation. Modularity of total knee components provide additional sources of wear debris that may accelerate wear of the articulating surfaces through a third body wear mechanism.

teoblastic response in the adjacent bone. Lymphocytes are occasionally present, but polymorphonuclear leukocytes and plasma cells are generally absent, supporting the concept that infection or a cell-mediated allergic reaction is not responsible for component loosening (85).

Once implant movement begins, the tissue response at the fixation interface is altered. Motion between an implant and bone stimulates the formation of synovial-like tissue. Motion generates another source of debris as the implant moves within its cement mantle and against bone. The host defense mechanisms to an increasing volume of particulate is overwhelmed, cell damage occurs, and high levels of digestive enzymes are released from this activated membrane. An enzymatic destruction of surrounding bone leads to further loosening or periprosthetic bone loss that has been termed osteolysis (Fig. 83.16, *A* and *B*).

The role of particulate debris in prosthetic loosening was unrecognized for years because of the difficulty of identifying the presence of these microscopic particles. Chemical fixatives used in tissue preparation dissolve polymethylmethacrylate, leaving empty spaces encircled by giant cells. Sometimes, barium sulfate, used for radiographic identification of methacrylate cement, can be identified in the spaces formerly occupied by polymethylmethacrylate. Polyethylene appears clear and cannot be readily identified when viewed with transmitted light microscopy; however, polarized light is very useful for identifying polyethylene since it is birefringent. Yet, submicron particles of polyethylene remain difficult to resolve even with polarized light. Newer staining techniques, such as the modified oil red-O stain, should prove helpful in identifying debris (62, 77, 86).

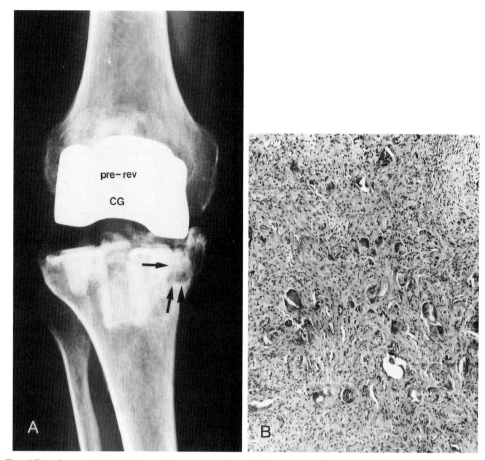

Figure 83.16. A, The AP radiograph of this Duopatellar cemented total knee implant demonstrates cavitary lesions beneath the medial tibial plateau with coldflow and subsidence of the all polyethylene tib-ial component. **B,** Tissue from the area of osteolysis demonstrates an intense giant cell and histiocytic reaction at 100X magnification in response to extensive amounts of particulate polyethylene wear debris.

The role of micron and submicron size particles remains undefined. It is becoming increasingly evident that foreign materials, including polymers and metals, that are nicely tolerated by the human body as bulk-sized components are not tolerated in microscopic amounts as particulates (87). The relationship between wear and the late loosening of a prosthetic device can be expected to stimulate new interests on the part of the vendors of prostheses in designs, materials, and manufacturing techniques that minimize wear.

The relationship between wear and contact stress is incompletely understood. Despite the differences in congruency, both highly congruent total hip replacements and minimally constrained knee implants have demonstrated evidence of polyethylene wear in radiographic and retrieval studies. Linear wear rates of 0.096mm per year have been measured in total hip replacements with 22mm femoral heads (88). Wear rates for polyethylene in knees have not been measured. Survivorship analyses and relative absence of wear in long-term clinical and radiographic studies suggest that some knee implants do not suffer from the same propensity for wear as do hip implants (5, 44) (Fig. 83.17).

Polyethylene destruction, unique to total knee replacements in the clinical literature, occurs secondary to high contact stress. This creates subsurface delamination and separation of large pieces of polyethylene (62, 75). Delamination and pitting have been reported with knee implants (particularly those sparing the posterior cruciate ligament), but are rarely seen in retrieved total hip components. Voids in the polyethylene created during fabrication may be an important factor making the material susceptible to contact stress (63). Polyethylene wear increases with duration of implantation (3), and oxidation may play a role in this phenomenon (89). The development of materials that are more resistant to oxidation and to other forms of chemical degradation as well as more stringent control of fabrication of polyethylene from powder to bulk material should improve the wear characteristics and durability of metal on polyethylene articulations.

The fixation interface may be preserved by limiting penetration and breakdown of an increasing load of particulate wear debris. Cement may block the migration of debris into cancellous bone by containing material within the synovial cavity. The fibrous tissue layer at the bone cement interface needs to be eliminated by penetration of cement into clean and dry cancellous bone at surgery. An extensively bone ingrown implant might be an equivalent seal to particulate penetration. A growing

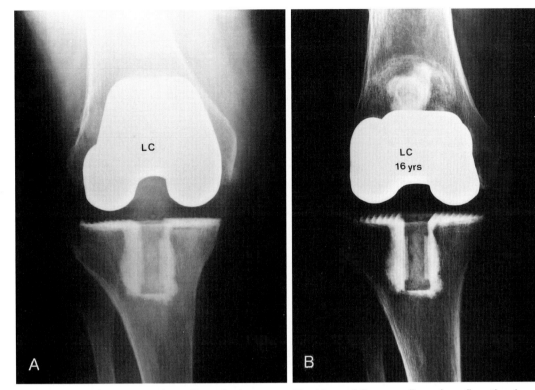

Figure 83.17.   A, The immediate postoperative radiograph of a cemented Total Condylar knee in a 60-year-old, 180-pound nurse demonstrating excellent alignment and an intact cement mantle. **B,** The 16-year follow-up radiograph confirms the absence of significant polyethylene wear in this moderately active individual.

body of evidence suggests that areas of the prosthesis not bonded to bone either by cement or bone ingrowth provide avenues for debris to follow. Either a defect in the cement mantle or a segment lacking bone ingrowth may be equally harmful in that they may provide particulate debris with access to subchondral bone.

The cause of late prosthetic loosening has gained interest because of the increasing number of patients at risk—those with total knee implants for more than 5 years. The proliferation of minimally congruent metal-backed tibial components with high contact stresses accompanied by widespread use of thin polyethylene inserts has resulted in accelerated wear of some components (3, 79). The roles of particulate debris from modular attachments and the increasing number of component parts mated with Morse tapers, threaded attachments, and screws create additional undesirable sources of metal and polyethylene wear. Since joint prostheses are mechanical bearings, there are concerns that intraarticular wear debris may create additional damage to the wear couple with longer follow-up intervals and initiate a biologic component to loosening through host tissue response to an overwhelming volume of particulate debris.

The breakdown of a stable fixation interface is often multifactorial with interaction of both mechanical and biologic factors (Fig. 83.18). Wear of polyethylene can be minimized by the orthopedic surgeon through precise surgical technique that restores correct extremity alignment, ligament balance, and an optimum fixation interface. Proper patient selection must be exercised until the science of joint replacement surgery has achieved a level of predictability and durability that can make this procedure acceptable for younger, larger, and more active individuals. In the coming decade, advances in materials science should improve the wear characteristics of polyethylene, making it less prone to chemical degradation. Designs that minimize wear debris by decreasing contact stresses at the bearing interface will be introduced, along with improved surface finishes for the metal counterpart and more stringent industry standards for all implanted devices.

References

1. Morrey BF, Chao E. Fracture of the porous-coated metal tray of a biologically fixed knee prosthesis. Clin Orthop Rel Res 1988;228:182–189.
2. Cook SD, Thomas KA. Fatigue failure of noncemented porous-coated implants. J Bone Joint Surg 1991;73-B(1):20–24.
3. Engh GA, Dwyer KA, Hanes CK. Polyethylene wear of metal-backed tibial components in total and unicompartmental knee prostheses. 1992;74-B(1):9–17.
4. Engh GA. Failure of the polyethylene bearing surface of a total knee replacement within four years: A case report. J Bone Joint Surg [Am] 1988;70-A:1093–1096.
5. Ranawat CS, Boachie-Adjei O. Survivorship analysis and results of total condylar knee arthroplasty. Eight- to 11-year follow-up period. Clin Orthop Rel Res 1988;226:6–13.
6. Rosenberg AG, Verner JJ, Galante JO. Clinical results of total condylar III prosthesis. Clin Orthop Rel Res 1991;273:83–90.

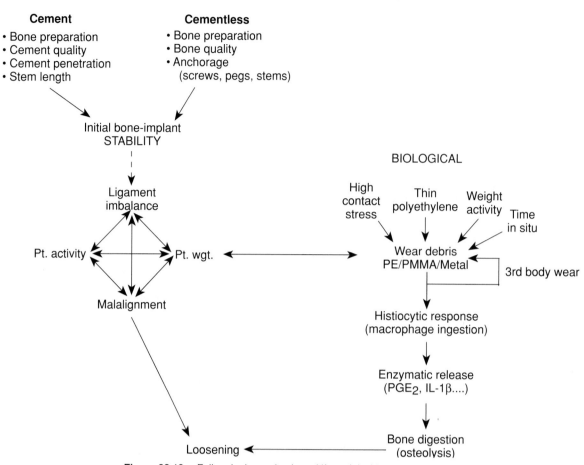

Figure 83.18. Failure by loosening is multifactorial with a combination of mechanical and biological mechanisms.

7. Scott RD, Ewald FC, Walker PS. Fracture of metallic tibial tray following total knee replacement. Report of two cases. J Bone Joint Surg 1984;66-A (5):780–782.
8. Ducheyne P, Kagan II A, Lacey JA. Failure of total knee arthroplasty due to loosening and deformation of the tibial component. J Bone Joint Surg 1978;60-A(3):384–391.
9. Cornell CN, Ranawat CS, Burstein AH. A clinical and radiographic analysis of loosening of total knee arthroplasty components using a bilateral model. J Arthroplasty 1986;1(3):157–163.
10. Gradisar IA, Hoffman ML, Askew MJ. Fracture of fenestrated metal-backing of tibial knee component. J Arthroplasty 1989;4(1):27–30.
11. Moreland JR. Mechanisms of failure in total knee arthroplasty. Clin Orthop Rel Res 1988;226:49–64.
12. Volz, RG. Basic biomechanics: lever arm, instant center of motion moment force, joint reactive force. Orthop Rev 1986;15:101.
13. MacCollum M. MDR Report. Rockville, MD: FDA. July 1992.
14. Boger J. An in-vitro test method for comparison of commercially available tibial trays. Transactions of the 39th Annual Meeting of the Orthopaedic Research Society. Orthopaedic Research Society, 1993:82.
15. Bartel DL, Bicknell VL, Wright TM. The effect of conformity, thickness and material on stress in ultra-high molecular weight components for total joint replacement. J Bone Joint Surg [Am] 1986;68A:1041–1051.
16. Cook SD, Georgette FS, Skinner HS, Haddad RJ. Fatigue properties of carbon- and porous-coated Ti-6Al-4V. J Biomed Mat Res 1984;18:497–512.
17. Cook SD, Thongpreda N, Anderson RC, Haddad Jr. RJ. The effect of post-sintering heat treatments on the fatigue properties of porous-coated Ti-6Al-4V Alloy. J Biomed Mat Res 1988;22:287–302.
18. Paganelli JV, Skinner HB, Mote Jr. CD. Prediction of fatigue failure of a total knee replacement tibial plateau using finite element analysis. Orthopedics 1988;11 (8):1161–1168.
19. Skinner HB, Mabey MF, Paganelli JV, Meagher JM. Failure analysis of

20. Lombardi AV, Engh GA, Volz RG, Albrigo JL, Brainard BJ. Fracture/dissociation of the polyethylene in metal-backed patellar components in total knee arthroplasty. J Joint Surg [Am] 1988;70-A(5):675–679.
21. Bayley JC, Scott RD, Ewald FC, Holmes GB. Failure of metal-backed patellar components after total knee arthroplasty. J Bone Joint Surg [Am] 1988;70-A(5):668–674.
22. Peters JD, Engh GA, Corpe RS. The metal-backed patella: An invitation for failure? J Arthroplasty 1991;6(3):221–228.
23. Stulberg SD, Stulberg BN, Hamati Y, et al. Failure mechanisms of metal-backed patellar components. Clin Orthop Rel Res 1988;248:152–157.
24. Rosenberg AG, Andriacchi T, Barden R, Galante JO Patellar component failure in cementless total knee arthroplasty. Clin Orthop Rel Res 1988;236:106–114.
25. Whitesides L. Fracture of the femoral component in cementless total knee arthroplasty. Trans Knee Soc 1992;1:10.
26. Rand JA, Chao YS, Stauffer RN. Kinematic rotating hinge total knee arthroplasty. J Bone Joint Surg 1987;69-A(4):489–497.
27. Jones EC, Insall JN, Inglis AE, Ranawat CS. GUEPAR Knee arthroplasty results and late complications. Clin Orthop Rel Res 1979;140:145–152.
28. Walldius B. Arthroplasty of the knee using an endoprosthesis. Acta Orthop Scand 1960;30:137.
29. Mazas FB. The GUEPAR Group: Guepar total knee prosthesis. Clin Orthop Rel Res 1973;94:211–221.
30. Jones EC, Insall JN, Inglis AE, Ranawat CS. GUEPAR knee arthroplasty results and late complications. Clin Orthop Rel Res 1979;140:145.
31. Grimer RJ, Karpinski MRK, Edwards AN. The long-term results of Stanmore total knee replacements. J Bone Joint Surg 1984;66B:55–62.

PCA revision total knee replacement tibial component. A preliminary study using finite element analysis. Orthopedics 1987;10(4):582–584.

32. Hui FC, Fitzgerald, Jr. RH. Hinged total knee arthroplasty. J Bone Joint Surg 1980;62A:513–519.
33. Bain AM. Replacement of the knee joint with the Walldius prosthesis using cement fixation. Clin Orthop Rel Res 1973;94:65–71.
34. Shiers LGP. Hinge arthroplasty of the knee(abstract). J Bone Joint Surg 1965;47B:586.
35. Kershaw CJ, Themen AEG. The Attenborough knee: A 4 to 10 year review. J Bone Joint Surg 1988;70B:89–93.
36. Simison AJM, Noble J, Hardinge K. Complications of the Attenborough knee replacement. J Bone Joint Surg 1986;68B:100–105.
37. Shindell R, Neumann F, Connolly JF, Jardon OM. Evaluation of the Noiles hinged knee prosthesis: A 5-year study of 17 knees. J Bone Joint Surg 1986;68A:579–585.
38. Gunston FH. Ten-year results of polycentric knee arthroplasty (abstract). J Bone Joint Surg 1980;62B:133.
39. Riley D, Woodyard JE. Long-term results of geometric total knee replacement. J Bone Joint Surg 1985;67B:548–550.
40. Insall JN, Hood RW, Flawn LB, Sullivan DJ. The total condylar knee prosthesis in gonarthritis: A 5- to 9-year follow-up of the first 100 consecutive replacements. J Bone Joint Surg 1983;65A:619–628.
41. Schurman JR, Borden LS, Wilde AH. Long-term results of total condylar knee prosthesis (abstract). Orthop Trans 1987;11:443.
42. Ritter MA, Gioe G, Stringer EA, Littrell D. The posterior cruciate condylar knee prosthesis: A five-year follow-up study. Clin Orthop Rel Res 1984;184:264–269.
43. Bourne MH, Rand JA, Ilstrup DM. Posterior cruciate condylar total knee arthroplasty: Five year results. Clin Orthop Rel Res 1988;234:129–136.
44. Wright J, Ewald FC, Walker PS, Thomas WH, Poss R, Sledge CB. Total knee arthroplasty with the kinematic prosthesis. J Bone Joint Surg 1990;72A:1003–1009.
45. Walker PS, Greene D, Reilly D, Thatcher J, Ben-Dov M, Ewald FC. Fixation of tibial components of knee prosthesis. J Bone Joint Surg 1981;63A:258–267.
46. Scuderi GR, Insall JN, Windsor RE, Moran MC. Survivorship of Cemented Knee Replacements. J Bone Joint Surg 1989;71-B(5):798–803.
47. Dodd CAF, Hungerford DS, Krackow KA. Total knee arthroplasty fixation. Comparison of the early results of paired cemented versus uncemented porous-coated anatomic knee prostheses. Clin Orthop Rel Res 1990;260:66–70.
48. Whitesides LA. Clinical results of Whitesides ortholoc total knee replacement. Orthop Clin North Am 1989;20(1):113–124.
49. Laskin RS. Tricon-M uncemented total knee arthroplasty. A review of 96 knees followed for longer than 2 years. J Arthroplasty 1988;3:27–38.
50. Blaha JD, Insler HP, Freeman MAR, et al. The fixation of a proximal tibial polyethylene prosthesis without cement. J Bone Joint Surg 1988;64B:326.
51. Rand JA, Bryan RS, Chao EYS, Ilstrup DM. A comparison of cemented versus cementless porous-coated anatomic total knee arthroplasty. Total arthroplasty of the knee. Proceedings of the Knee Society, 1985–1986. Rockville, MD: Aspen Pub, 1987:195–212.
52. Rorabeck CH, Bourne RB, Nott L. The cemented Kinematic-ll and the non-cemented porous-coated anatomic prosthesis for total knee replacement: A prospective evaluation. J Bone Joint Surg 1988;70-A:483–490.
53. Moran CG, Pinder IM, Lees TA, Midwinter MJ. Survivorship analysis of the uncemented porous-coated anatomic knee replacement. J Bone Joint Surg 1991;73-A(6):848–857.
54. Audell RA, Cracchiolo III A. The use of implants with polyethylene peg fixation in total knee arthroplasty. Proceedings of the Knee Society 1985–1986. Rockville, MD: Aspen Pub, 1987:179.
55. Landon GC, Galante JO, Maley MM. Non-cemented total knee arthroplasty. Clin Orthop Rel Res 1986;205:49–57.
56. Ryd L. Micromotion in knee arthroplasty. A roentgen stereophotogrammetric analysis of tibial component fixation. Acta Orthop Scand 1986(suppl)220:1–80.
57. Cook SD, Thomas KA, Haddad RJ. Histologic analysis of retrieved human porous-coated total joint components. Clin Orth Rel Res 1988;234:90–101.
58. Collier JP, Mayor MB, Surprenant VA, Surprenant HP, Jensen R. Biological ingrowth of porous-coated knee prostheses. In: Goldberg VM, ed. Controversies of Total Knee Arthroplasty. New York: Raven Press,1991:95–103.
59. Engh GA, Bobyn D. Radiographic and histologic study of porous-coated tibial component fixation in cementless total knee arthroplasty. Orthopedics 1988;11(5):725–731.
60. Rosenqvist R, et al. Loosening of the porous coating of bicompartmental prostheses in patients with rheumatoid arthritis. J Bone Joint Surg 1986;68A:538–542.
61. Cheng CL, et al. Loosening of the porous coating in total knee replacement. J Bone Joint Surg 1988;70(3):377–381.
62. Peters PC, Engh GA, Dwyer KA, Vinh TN. Osteolysis after total knee arthroplasty without cement. J Bone Joint Surg 1992;74-A (6):864–876.
63. Collier JP, Mayor MB, Surprenant HP, Dauphinais LA, Jensen RE. The biomechanical problems of polyethylene as a bearing surface. Clin Orthop Rel Res 1990;261:107–114.
64. Kobs JK, Lachiewicz PF. Hybrid total knee arthroplasty. Two- to five-year results using the Miller-Galante prosthesis. Clin Orthop Rel Res 1993;286:78–87.
65. Lotke PA, Ecker MA. Influence of positioning in total knee replacement. J Bone Joint Surg 1977;59-A:77–79
66. Ewald FC, Jacobs MA, Walker PS, et al. Accuracy of total knee replacement, component position, and relationship to bone cement interface reaction. In: Dorr LD, ed. The Knee: Papers of the First Scientific Meeting of the Knee Society. 1985:117.
67. Rand JA, Coventry MB. Ten-year evaluation of geometric total knee arthroplasty. Clin Orthop Rel Res 1988;232:168–173.
68. Engh GA, Petersen T. Comparative experience with intramedullary and extramedullary alignment in total knee arthroplasty. J Arthroplasty 1990;5(1):1–8.
69. Freeman MAR, Railton GT. Should the posterior cruciate ligament be retained or resected in condylar nonmeniscal knee arthroplasty. J Arthroplasty 1988;(suppl):S3–S12.
70. Dorr LD, Conaty JP, Schreiber R, et al. Technical factors that influence mechanical loosening of total knee arthroplasty. In: Dorr LD, ed. The Knee: Papers of the First Scientific Meeting of the Knee Society. 1985:121.
71. Harada Y, Wevers HW, Cooke TDV . Distribution of bone strength in the proximal tibia. J Arthroplasty 1988;3(2):167–175.
72. Engh GA, Dwyer KA. The anatomic modular knee (AMK)—A 2- to 4-year follow-up of the first 113 cases. Am J Knee Surg 1991;4(2):51–58.
73. Wroblewski BM. Wear of high density polyethylene on bone and cartilage. J Bone Join Surg 1979;61-B(4):498–500.
74. Dannenmaier WC, Haynes DW, Nelson CL. Granulomatous reaction and cystic bony destruction associated with high wear rate in total knee prosthesis. Clin Orthop Rel Res 1985;198:224–230.
75. Nolan JF, Bucknill TM. Aggressive granulomatosis from polyethylene failure in an uncemented knee replacement. J Bone Joint Surg 1992;74-B(1):23–24.
76. Maloney WJ, Jasty M, Harris WH, Galante JO, Callaghan. Endosteal erosion with stable uncemented femoral components. J Bone Joint Surg 1990;72-A(7):1025–1034.
77. Schmalzreid TP, Jasty M, Harris WH. Periprosthetic bone loss in total hip arthroplasty: Polyethylene wear debris and the concept of effective joint space. J Bone Joint Surg 1992;74-A (6):849–863.
78. Streicher RM, Schon R. Tribological behavior of various materials and surface against polyethylene. Transactions of the 17th Annual Meeting of the Society for Biomaterials 1991:289.
79. Dwyer KA, Topoleski LDT, Bauk DJ, Nakielny R, Engh GA. The neglected side of the wear couple: Analysis of surface morphology of retrieved femoral components. Presentation: Orthopaedic Research Society. San Francisco, CA. Feb, 1993.
80. Anthony PP, Gie GA, Howie CR, Ling RSM. Localized endosteal bone lysis in relation to the femoral components of cemented total hip arthroplasties. J Bone Joint Surg 1990;72-B(6):972–979.
81. Hendrix RW, Wixon RL, Rana NA, Rogers LE. Arthrography after total hip arthroplasty: A modified technique used in the diagnosis of pain. Radiology 1983;148:647–652.
82. Lombardi AV, Mallory TH, Vaughn BK, Drouillard P. Aseptic loosening in total hip arthroplasty secondary to osteolysis induced by wear debris from titanium alloy femoral heads. J Bone Joint Surg 1989;71-A:1337–1342.
83. Milliano T, Whitesides LA, Kaiser AD, Zwirkoski PA. Evaluation of the effect of articular surface material on a metal-backed patellar component. Transactions the 36th Annual Meeting of the Orthopaedic Research Society. Orthopaedic Research Society, 1990:279.
84. Milliano T, Whitesides LA. Articular surface material effect on metal-backed patellar components—A microscopic evaluation component. Transactions the 37th Annual Meeting of the Orthopaedic Research Society. Orthopaedic Research Society, 1991:557.
85. Goldring SR, Schiller AL, Roelke M, et al. The synovial-like membrane at the bone cement interface in loose total hip replacements and its proposed role in bone lysis. J Bone Joint Surg [Am] 1983;65-A (5):575–584.
86. Campbell PC, Schmalzried TP, Amstutz HC. Wear debris induced osteolysis as a cause of TJR failure. Transactions of the Implant Retrieval Symposium of the Society for Biomaterials. 1992:19.
87. Howie DW. Tissue response in relation to type of wear particles around failed total hip arthroplasties. J Arthroplasty 1990;5:337–348.
88. Wroblewski BM. 15–21 year results of the Charnley low-friction arthroplasty. Clin Orth Rel Res 1986;211:30.
89. Nagy EV, Li S. Analysis of retrieved knee components via Fourier transform infrared spectroscopy. The 16th Annual Meeting of the Society for Biomaterials, 1990:274.

84

Stiff Total Knee Arthroplasty

Kelly G. Vince and Edward Eissmann

Introduction

The stiff arthroplasty, whether lacking flexion, extension, or both, may be one of the most dismaying and difficult knees to revise. The problem may not be amenable to revision, and a thorough evaluation is essential prior to surgery. The stiff painful knee should be distinguished from the stiff, but pain free, arthroplasty.

Evaluation

Referred Pain

The problem may not reside in the knee itself. Pain is commonly referred to the knee from the hip and less commonly from the spine. Both areas should be evaluated prior to any knee surgery, and both areas merit close attention in the stiff, painful knee arthroplasty. If the current pain resembles that which was present prior to the primary arthroplasty, revision is unlikely to help. Whenever concurrent hip and knee problems exist, the hip should be corrected first. The painful arthritic hip definitely impairs recovery from knee arthroplasty. Flexing the knee drives the femur into the acetabulum. This is painful and precludes good motion in the knee.

Infection

The infected knee arthroplasty has many faces (2). Rarely does a patient with a septic arthroplasty suffer shaking chills and fever. More commonly, and perhaps for months, the knee may be insidiously painful and stiff. Sepsis must be considered in the painful stiff arthroplasty, and an aspiration is required. Specimens of fluid should be sent for cell count and culture. A negative aspirate from a suspicious joint should be repeated. If suspicion of sepsis persists at revision surgery despite negative aspirates, antibiotic prophylaxis may be deferred until multiple culture specimens are procured. Swabs from the interface and pieces of tissue often yield positive cultures from the infected knee when aspirates have not. No surgeon wants to unwittingly implant a prosthesis into an infected knee; and so, a revision may have to be abandoned, temporarily leaving a resection arthroplasty until final intraoperative culture results are available. Frozen sections, which are quantitatively evaluated for the number of white blood cells per high power field may help determine immediately if infection is present. Fewer than 5 cells per high power field is an unlikely finding in the presence of sepsis, and greater than 10 suggests a problem. Judgment is required when 5 to 10 cells are present.

Reflex Sympathetic Dystrophy

Reflex sympathetic dystrophy (RSD) has undergone a transformation in terminology, etiology, and pathology over the years since it was first described by Mitchell in 1862 as "causalgia" in American civil war soldiers following peripheral nerve injuries (31). Sudek, in 1900, described the "acute atrophy of bone" associated with this disorder as an entity distinct from "disuse atrophy" (46). In 1971, Lenggenhager termed the radiologic changes associated with the chronic pain and atrophic changes "Sudeck's atrophy" or "osteodystrophy" (27). Morton and Scott (1931), and later Lehman (1934), emphasized that vasospasm is involved in the pathogenesis. De Takats, in 1937, emphasized a neurovascular reflex mechanism as causative and termed the disorder "reflex dystrophy of the extremities." Evans, in 1946, stressed the importance of autonomic sympathetic input and coined the modern term "reflex sympathetic dystrophy" or RSD.

While the classic presentation of RSD, with its cardinal signs of disproportionate pain, swelling, stiffness, and discoloration, is straightforward, the multitude of variant presentations that lack the full menu of findings has led to the term "reflex sympathetic imbalance" (23) to distinguish minor forms.

The occurrence of RSD in the knee is often a diagnostic challenge. Guileful in its presentation and often chronic in its bearing, the inciting events to RSD are heterogeneous and not always obvious. In a 1986 review by Katz, et al., of 1914 recently published cases of poor results following knee arthroplasty, none were diagnosed as RSD despite 1.8% incidence of "unexplained pain" (20). An index of clinical suspicion is a necessary first step in this diagnosis. Since the same trauma that injured the knee may also trigger RSD, the establishment of another diagnosis does not rule out RSD. Three-phase bone scans, affected by the hyperemia of the condition, may be useful in establishing the diagnosis (29).

The natural history of the disorder is also varied. All studies find women at greater risk for the diagnosis (4 of 5 in Katz' 1986 study, 13 of 19 in Ogilvie-Harris 1987 study, and 25 of 36 in Katz and Hungerford' 1987 study) (20, 21, 34). The most common and distressing feature is pain. It is usually severe, persistent, and described as burning. Accompanied by edema, erythema, and warmth, it may initially be decreased by local measures, such as ice or heat, or be made worse by them. Tenderness of the joint to motion and even touch has been reported. This is the "acute" stage. Despite, and perhaps due to, the efforts of physical therapy, motion of the joint is decreased. The "dystrophic" stage is heralded by a change to cold, glossy skin. Osteoporosis is evident radiologically. If these changes persist, the insidious progression to the "atrophic" stage is entered with the knee developing contractures and atrophy of skin and muscle. Edema gives way to induration, further stiffening the knee. Sudeck's "atrophy of the bone" is evident in all three bones of the knee, but especially in the patella on axial view (1, 13).

The triggering event and subsequent development of pain is an incompletely understood phenomenon. The limited number of patients who present with this disorder prohibit statistically significant prospective double blind studies. Only crude extrapolations can be made from incomplete animal models. All contemporary authors agree that anything can be an inciting factor. Trauma, even so small as to be forgotten, can initiate the vicious cycle. Surgical interventions, physical therapy, and degenerative lesions can each be culpable in the right milieu. Generally, it can be said that partial nerve lesions cause RSD more often than complete transections, and the lower extremity is less often affected than the upper.

The incidence of RSD in the lower limb has been variously reported as 0.8% in patients after total knee replacement (TKR) (21), and as 1 in every 2000 patients after extremity trauma (36). Patman's (1973) series of 113 RSD patients found only 18 in whom the diagnosis was made by the first treating physician (35).

Various theories have been proposed linking the deranged vasomotor and autonomic signs with chronic intense pain. Livingston (1943) postulated that the initial event results in peripheral nerve irritation that contributes to an increased activity state in the internuncial neuronal pool, raising activity within the spinal cord (28). This continuously stimulates the sympathetic efferent fibers. Melzack and Wall's 1965 "gate control theory" is the most popular model (30).

A more recent hypothesis by Devor (9) suggests that injured or transected nerves have an increased accumulation of alpha adrenergic receptors on the exposed regenerating surface. The accumulation of ACH (acetylcholine) at these multiple sites leads to spontaneous depolarization, thus becoming a sort of ectopic pacemaker, bombarding and overloading the ability of the central nervous system to process sensory input. This results in paresthesias with the return of an altered sympathetic response.

While debate about the neurologic pathways continues, the sympathetic effects at the tissue level are well described. Currently, the emphasis centers around the vascular changes that occur in both soft tissue and bone. In both cases, it appears that the initial vasoconstriction is followed by regional vasodilation causing clinically apparent erythema and warmth. Det Takats and Miller (1943) used water plethysmography to demonstrate increased vascular flow in affected versus contralateral limbs in all stages of the disease (8). They postulated that dilation of the local arterial supply combined with venous constriction led to edema. In 1970, Stolte, et al. (45) described an increased oxygen content in the venous blood in RSD limbs, raising the specter of arteriovenous shunting in the precapillary network. In their 1977 book, *Disorders of the Patello-femoral Joint*, Ficat and Hungerford discuss the sympathetically induced dilation of the intraosseous vasculature, leading to increased flow and intraosseous hypertension. Ficat has demonstrated changes in the intramedullary tissues resembling avascular necrosis (AVN) using scintigraphy, biopsy, and intraosseous phlebography.

The diagnosis of reflex sympathetic dystrophy is primarily clinical. Ficat and Hungerford describe "functional exploration of the bone," using bone scan, intramedullary pressure measurements, phlebography, and biopsy. Of these, bone scan is the only one shown to have prognostic significance. Butler-Manuel, et al. (3) studied 20 patients with anterior knee pain diagnosed as atypical RSD. Sympathetic blocks were employed for treatment after bone scans were performed. Only 1 in 10 patients with a hot bone scan had a poor response to blockade, while 7 of 9 patients with a normal bone scan had a poor response. They recommend bone scan before entering into this treatment modality.

The treatment of RSD is as individual as the presentation of the disorder. Whether the reinstitution of motion promotes or relieves pain, treatments for RSD include both rest and motion. Cessation of aggressive attempts at reinstituting joint motion are necessary. Gentle active and active-assist exercises, within a comfortable arc, are appropriate. Hydrotherapy and the application of ice may be beneficial. Extreme cold may exacerbate pain. The use of transcutaneous electrical nerve stimulation (TENS) units theoretically may stimulate the inhibitory fibers, suppressing activity in the spinal cord. This would represent "closing the gate," consistent with the theories of Melzack. It has been suggested that deep friction massage releases histamine from mast cells and stimulates inhibitory fibers.

Ficat and Hungerford describe the historical compilation of medicinal agents to treat RSD (13). These have included curarizing agents, ganglionic blockers, local anesthetics, antihistamines, anabolic hormones, steroids, and others. In the lower limb, the intravenous use of ganglionic blockers via a Bier block method is not practical. Injection of local anesthetics has found little favor in and about the knee. Steroids have complications that limit their use when safer protocols are available.

Currently, the aim of most treatments is to interrupt the sympathetic flow to the extremity in an attempt to break the pain cycle. This can be attempted by pharmacologic or surgical means. Spurling, in 1930, demonstrated the validity of a cervicothoracic sympathectomy in the first documented cure of a patient with upper extremity RSD (44). Today, sympathetic blockade is diagnostic and prognostic as well as a therapeutic in RSD of the knee. So successful is pain relief, at least initially, with an accurate lumbar sympathetic block that, if there is no mitigation of the pain, the diagnosis of RSD should be questioned (40). Aggressive sympathetic blockage is now encouraged. While abandonment of this procedure has been advocated in patients who find no lasting relief after as little as 4 or 5 blocks, we have had patients develop long-term mitigation of painful symptoms after 10 to 15 blocks. Other authors (19, 24) report long-term palliation rates of 80 to 90% using this mode of therapy.

Physical therapy while the patient is under block is an important adjunct. Knee stiffness with a flexion contracture makes ambulation difficult. Even after alleviation of causalgic pain, a deformed joint may require surgical intervention to gain acceptable motion. Perioperative use of epidural Marcaine and careful attention to pain relief are essential because surgery can exacerbate the RSD (13).

While remaining a diagnostic and therapeutic challenge, patients with RSD of the knee have a variety of treatments available. The aggressive approach begins with a high index of suspicion. The sooner the diagnosis is established, the sooner treatment can begin, thus increasing chances for a successful outcome. RSD does not always present in its classic form, and covert cases abound. While most patients will respond with conservative physical therapy, the early use of sympathetic blocks must not be delayed if progress is not readily evident. The two-pronged approach consisting of interruption of sympathetic flow and reinstitution of movement has the best chance of a successful outcome. Reflex sympathetic dystrophy may be difficult to diagnose, but it creates inordinate pain and stiffness. It must be considered in all patients with painful, stiff knee arthroplasties, and revision surgery should be deferred for treatment of the neurologic disorder.

Neuromuscular Disorders

Neuromuscular disorders that increase muscle tone may limit motion or impede physical therapy. Parkinson's disease, prevalent in the age group where arthroplasty is performed, need not compromise function if the patient is ambulatory prior to arthroplasty and the Parkinson's disease is treated (50).

Disorders characterized by spasticity are most likely to result in flexion contractures that cannot easily be corrected by arthroplasty surgery. Ankylosing spondylitis, when severe, may be associated with spinal pathology and spasticity. Central nervous system disorders, such as multiple sclerosis, head trauma, and normal pressure hydrocephalus can produce disabling flexion contractures in knee arthroplasties that can be difficult, if not impossible to correct (Fig. 84.1).

Heterotopic Ossification

Heterotopic ossification can occasionally be identified in the quadriceps muscle after knee arthroplasty. It is rarely a cause of stiffness (6). Calcified tissue may appear as a periostitis and not as true heterotopic bone formation. This is shown clearly on CT scanning (Fig. 84.2). It is not clear that simple excision of heterotopic ossification followed by radiotherapy will improve motion in a stiff knee, although this may be of benefit in combination with complete revision surgery.

Surgical Technique

The appropriate surgical technique for revision of the stiff knee arthroplasty is determined by the specific causes of the stiffness and pain. The surgical planning must include a very detailed understanding of the failed knee and a plan to correct the identified problems. What aspects of the reconstruction should be manipulated to

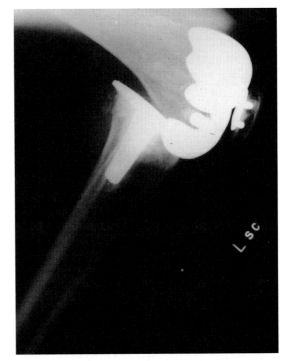

Figure 84.1. Profound flexion contracture with posterior dislocation of the knee due to spasticity resulting from normal pressure hydrocephalus. Multiple attempts at correction failed before diagnosis of spasticity was established. Agressive revision to constrained arthroplasty with limb shortening was necessary to achieve comfort in the patient who remained nonambulatory.

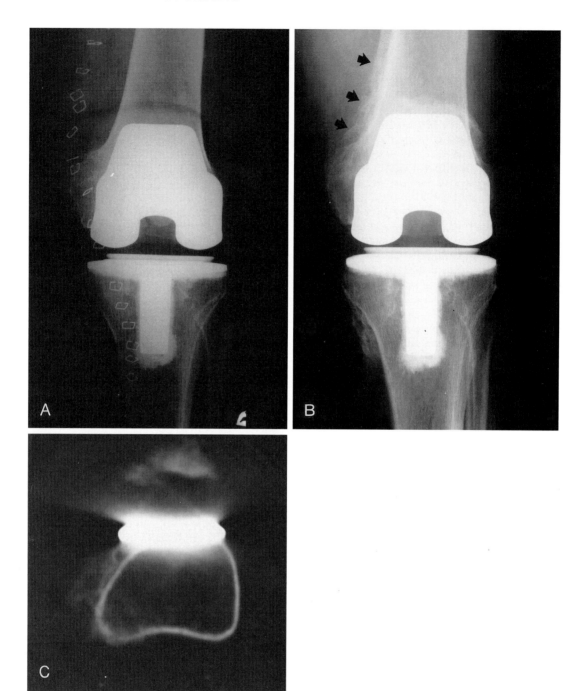

Figure 84.2. **A,** Immediate postoperative radiograph showing no heterotopic or periosteal new bone formation on medial femoral cortex. **B,** Within several weeks, calcific density appears on medial femoral cortex (*arrows*) and proximal medial tibia. Patient regained the 90 degrees of flexion that were present preoperatively. **C,** Computed tomography of the femur, at the level of the femoral flange, demonstrates that the new bone is actually periosteal in origin, where the vastus medialis was elevated for a subvastus arthrotomy.

improve or restore motion? Is a complete revision necessary or will changing the size or position of a single component suffice? What soft tissues require release or reconstruction (55)?

Manipulation

Before revision surgery is planned, manipulation under general anesthesia is often considered. While there is a place for manipulation (specifically, in the patient who has a mechanically sound reconstruction, but who has been unable or unwilling to attend to physical therapy), this procedure must be advised cautiously. Some experienced surgeons feel that manipulation is not beneficial and should be avoided (15). There is the potential for serious complications: supracondylar femur fracture, patellar fracture, and disruption of the extension mechanism.

While manipulation may not be effective, if performed, it is best performed within 6 weeks of arthroplasty. At 2 months after knee replacement, the risk of complication probably exceeds the potential for gain. The original surgeon is best equipped to perform the manipulation with the knowledge that the reconstruction inherently provides the motion that is sought by the manipulation. It is unrealistic and dangerous to expect motion from a manipulation that exceeds what was achieved in the operating room, under anesthesia, at the conclusion of the arthroplasty.

Arthroscopic Release

Arthroscopic release of intraarticular fibrosis, followed by manipulation and physical therapy, has been of modest value in some patients with stiff knee arthroplasties (5, 18, 25). This approach is predicated on the belief that the reconstruction is capable of superior motion, that the patient was unable to perform therapy, and that lysis of ensuing, secondary scar should allow motion that the patient will then maintain with an aggressive approach to therapy. Arthroscopic procedures cannot be expected to provide better motion than was present at the conclusion of the arthroplasty.

Surgical Approach for Revision

A stiff arthroplasty requires a cautious surgical exposure to spare the patellar tendon and its insertion. The quadriceps tendon should be "turned down" or the tibial tubercle elevated with an osteotomy (17, 41, 57, 59). A "femoral peel" exposure may be necessary to flex the knee (58). Extension contractures may sometimes be improved by releasing individual quadriceps tendons—the rectus for example, if it is tighter than other constituents of this muscle. Sculco and Faris (42) credited Ritter with a modification of the Thompson quadricepsplasty to increase knee flexion. Generous exposure of the proximal thigh is necessary to free the rectus femoris muscle from the vastus lateralis and intermedius muscles. Nichols and Dorr recommended closing a quadriceps turndown as a V-Y lengthening with the patella "rock solid" when the knee is flexed to 90 degrees (33). Osteotomies of the tibial tubercle provide excellent exposure of the stiff knee and avoid patellar tendon rupture (57, 59) (Fig. 84.3).

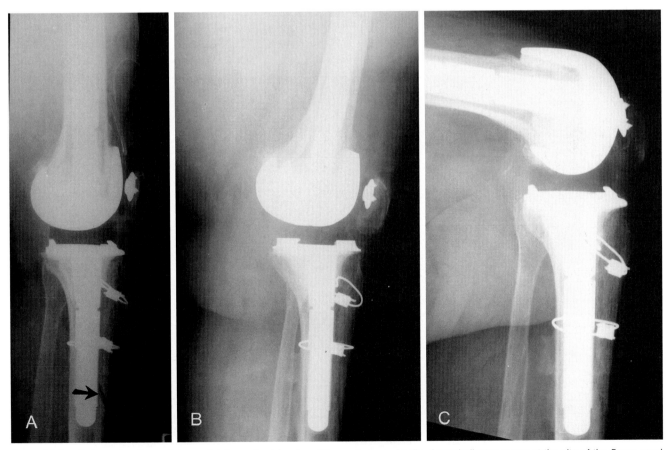

Figure 84.3.   A, Lateral radiograph immediately postrevision for stiff knee arthroplasty. The original cruciate-retaining, resurfacing arthroplasty fully extended, but flexed to only 30 degrees. The patella was low, relative to the joint line, and the tibial tubercle osteotomy was performed to provide exposure and to advance the extensor mechanism proximally. *Arrow* indicates a gap at the site of the 5 mm proximal advancement. **B,** Several months postrevision, this lateral radiograph shows healing of the osteotomy site. Recurrent patellar infera from contracture of the patellar tendon is apparent. **C,** Several months postrevision, flexion to 90 degrees has been achieved.

Primary Mechanical Impediments

Bone Blocks

Bone and osteophytes that remain on the posterior femoral condyles can limit flexion. This is a condition that merits attention at the time of primary surgery; the offending hard tissue should be removed with a curved osteotome. Adherent scar and capsule may be elevated from the condyles with benefit. This maneuver is a necessary first step in improving extension in the stiff knee (Fig. 84.4).

Gap Mismatch

The concept of balanced flexion and extension gaps was developed with the knee arthroplasties of the original total condylar vintage in the early 1970s (48, 49). The usual sequence was to create a flexion gap by resecting the proximal tibia and the posterior femoral condyles and completing soft tissue releases. The dimensions of the gap and the stability of the joint were confirmed with spacer blocks. Then, using a tensor device, the appropriate amount of distal femur was resected to create an extension gap of dimensions and tension equal to the flexion gap.

Contemporary instrument systems, usually with intramedullary guides, have foregone these steps in favor of a technique of "measured resection." This involves removal of bone that is equal in thickness to the prosthesis that will be implanted. This generally works well,

but, in cases where extensive soft tissue release is required to correct deformity, it is important to formally confirm that the flexion and extension gaps are indeed equal.

If gaps are left unequal, several situations may occur, depending on how the surgeon decides to stabilize the arthroplasty. There are 9 permutations—only one of which is desirable (Table 84.1). Two other situations feature equal gaps that have been improperly stabilized by selection of tibial inserts that are either too thick (globally tight knees) or too thin (globally unstable knees). Some of these knees may be stabilized by exchange of polyethylene tibial components. In the fortuitous situation where modular components have been implanted, this surgery may be minimal—no more than an arthrotomy. The globally stiff arthroplasty in which the thinnest available polyethylene has been used requires, at a minimum, removal of the tibial component with resection of additional tibial bone. In most cases, release of extensive secondary scarring that has occurred as the result of immobility is also necessary.

Flexion contractures (i.e., less than full extension) in the knee that flexes reasonably well, result from a relatively tight extension gap. The gap may have been left tight at the primary arthroplasty, or secondary scarring may be responsible. This type of scarring can occur in the patient who finds comfort by maintaining the knee in a flexed position during rehabilitation. This individual typically rests the flexed knee on a pillow while recum-

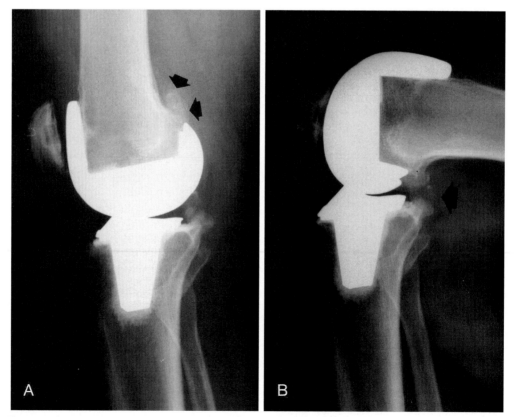

Figure 84.4.   A and **B,** Lateral radiographs in extension and flexion show how residual bone and osteophytes limit flexion, in this case at 90 degrees.

Table 84.1.

Flexion	Extension	Consequence
Stable	Stable	Balanced knee, good flexion and full extension
Stable	Tight	Flexion contracture with good flexion
Stable	Loose	Flexes well but unstable in extension with recurvatum
Tight	Stable	Extends fully but bends poorly
Tight	Tight	Globally stiff knee
Tight	Loose	Poor flexion, unstable in extension with recurvatum
Loose	Loose	Globally unstable knee
Loose	Tight	Good flexion, with potential for posterior tibial dislocation/ flexion contracture
Loose	Stable	Unstable in flexion with potential for posterior tibial dislocation/ full extension with stability

bent. As healing progresses, it becomes impossible to achieve full extension. This knee usually requires extensive release of posterior soft tissues and revision of the femoral component with resection of distal femoral bone.

Resection of additional distal femoral bone is the most efficient means of increasing the size and decreasing the tension of the extension gap. It has been observed in cadaver studies with the Total Condylar arthroplasty that every millimeter decrement in the extension gap reduces extension by about 4 degrees (43). Considering that most tibial implants are available in sizes that differ in thickness by 2 millimeters, a second best choice could create a flexion contracture approaching 10 degrees.

Resecting additional distal femur is not, however, without problems. This maneuver effectively elevates the joint line and creates a relative patella baja, albeit without a patellar tendon contracture. The posterior cruciate ligament conserving arthroplasty is particularly sensitive to proximal migration of the joint line, which tightens the ligament as the knee bends (10). Cruciate resection arthroplasty is less sensitive to proximal joint line migration (51). Resection of distal femur also shortens the limb in extension and risks an extensor lag because the quadriceps muscle remains at the original length (53). A vastus medialis advancement may diminish the lag.

There is an ineluctable relationship between stability and motion. While neither stiffness nor instability are tolerable, patients tend to function better and more comfortably with knees that are not tight. Edwards and Miller have made this point clearly (11).

The 9 permutations shown in Table 84.1 assume intact collateral ligaments. Other, more challenging problems arise in the knee with either an incompetent medial collateral ligament or in a knee with a medial to lateral imbalance in gap size. The lateral collateral liga-

ment is almost dispensable in the well-aligned knee arthroplasty. This was demonstrated by the classic techniques for correction of valgus deformities, where the recommended release at one time included transection of the lateral collateral ligament. By comparison, a stable resurfacing arthroplasty is not feasible in the absence of a structurally sound medial collateral ligament (MCL) (17).

The relationship between stability and stiffness is acute in the knee without an MCL. The uninitiated surgeon, faced with valgus instability in a knee arthroplasty may conclude (incorrectly) that a thicker tibial insert will solve the problem. This is misguided. Assuming the arthroplasty is correctly aligned in valgus, a thicker polyethylene is only effective if contractures on the lateral side (lateral collateral ligament, iliotibial band, capsule, popliteus tendon) are released so that both sides of the knee are balanced. However, if the MCL is longer and more lax than the posterior structures, then further release of the lateral side and insertion of thicker tibial components will create a flexion contracture. The knee cannot be stabilized if the MCL is completely disrupted without ligament reconstruction or recourse to a constrained prosthesis.

Component Malposition

Anterior Tibial Slope

The normal orientation of the articular surface of the proximal tibia, viewed from the side, is higher anteriorly than posteriorly. This is described as "posterior slope" and should be reestablished by the arthroplasty. Different strategies exist: the bone may either be resected at this angle or the tibial component may have the slope built into its base plate or articular surface. The arthroplasty with inadequate posterior slope or worse anterior slope, will flex poorly. Anterior slope tightens the collateral and posterior cruciate ligaments in flexion. It also impedes femoral rollback, a mechanism that facilitates flexion. Revision surgery should restore the desired posterior slope of between 3 and 7 degrees.

Flexed Femoral Component

A femoral component that has been implanted in a flexed position will not necessarily create a stiff knee. However, this orientation reduces the size of the flexion gap. If the gaps were not formally balanced during the primary arthroplasty, an imbalance may exist. This can be improved during revision surgery by restoring the femoral component position.

Oversized Components

Femoral

The anteroposterior dimension of the femoral component is the most important factor in correct component selection. If the component exceeds the size of the bone, stiffness is likely. The collateral ligaments, normally less tight in the flexed knee, become taut and limit flexion if the femoral component is oversized. The size of the femoral component in the stiff arthroplasty must be assessed carefully. Daluga, working with Lombardi,

Mallory, and Vaughn, determined that an increase in the anteroposterior dimension greater than 12% was a critical and independent predictor of poor motion and the need for a manipulation (6). Radiographs of the contralateral knee, if it does not have an arthroplasty, help determine the appropriately sized femoral component. Due to the scarring in a stiff knee arthroplasty, it may be beneficial to select a revision component that is slightly smaller than the patient's original anatomy. Stability in flexion must not, however, be compromised by a smaller femoral component and posterior stabilized-type components may be very helpful.

Tibial polyethylene

The tibial component has an equal influence on stability and motion in both flexion and extension because its entire articular surface is always in contact with the femur. Accordingly, exchanging the tibial component for a thinner insert will be appropriate for the knee that is globally tight, i.e., one that extends and flexes poorly, but that is otherwise stable and well balanced. If a flexion contracture is treated by revision to a thinner tibial insert, the knee may become unstable in flexion. Conversely, the knee that was flexing poorly (but had full extension) will develop recurvatum and instability with a thinner tibia.

Extensor Mechanism

Patella Thickness

If the polyethylene patellar dome is thicker than the amount of bone that has been resected from the articular surface, the new construct will be thicker and tighter than the original. This impedes flexion and the increased forces may lead to patellar fracture or dislocation (52). In general terms, the thickness of the resurfaced patella should not exceed 25 mm and is often much less. Clearly, there is variation between patients. Evaluation of patellofemoral radiographs of the contralateral knee may be helpful in deciding whether to revise a thick patella in a stiff knee arthroplasty.

Patella Baja

True patella baja, occurring from contracture of the patellar tendon, can cause stiffness and anterior knee pain. This differs from the patella that is low consequent to an elevated joint line, but which has a patellar tendon of normal length. The contracted patellar tendon may predate or have complicated the primary arthroplasty and is difficult to correct. Lengthening of the patellar tendon has been described but is not recommended due to the risk of disrupting the extensor mechanism (14, 22). The tibial tubercle can be advanced proximally. This cannot be expected to improve knee motion as an isolated surgical procedure, but may have some benefit during a complete revision surgery. The tip of the tubercle may avulse, leading to a disrupted extension mechanism (Fig. 84.5).

Patella baja, or a patella that is high relative to the joint line, may occur with a patellar tendon of normal length, if excessive distal femur had been resected to correct a flexion contracture, as described above. Revision surgery, with careful attention to soft tissues and to balancing flexion and extension gaps may restore patellar height.

Rotational Malposition

Rotational malposition of the femoral or tibial components, though difficult to diagnose, may be the basis for poor motion. Malrotation jams the components together painfully during flexion, causing stiffness and contributing to patellar maltracking (37, 47, 52).

Soft Tissue Problems

Posterior Cruciate Ligament Balance

Controversy persists over the role of the PCL in primary knee arthroplasty. Majority opinion supports cruciate sacrifice for revision knee surgery. It is difficult, if not impossible to consider retention of a functional PCL in the revision of a stiff TKR. This would be unwise.

The PCL may be tight despite good component position. Recession, or partial release of the PCL, is recommended in the primary arthroplasty if the femur rolls back excessively on the tibia during flexion (38). Femoral rollback, once considered desirable, if not essential, in the cruciate retaining knee arthroplasty (56) has been reevaluated (54). If rollback is associated with tightness, the knee will not flex. Marked displacement has been associated with destructive polyethylene wear of the thinner posterior surface and the see-sawing of rollback rocks the cruciate-retaining tibial component, increasing the risk of loosening (39).

Primary Soft Tissue Scarring

Poor Flexion

The quadriceps mechanism, including the 4 constituent muscles and the tendon will likely be tight and scarred in the knee that has not flexed fully because of arthritis. Once mechanical impediments, such as bone blocks and incongruent articular surfaces, have been corrected by arthroplasty, the extensor mechanism may continue to block motion. A modified quadricepsplasty may be effective, but lengthening of the extensor mechanism risks a debilitating extensor lag (41).

The collateral ligaments may be neither supple nor of normal length in the chronically arthritic knee. Limited release of both medial and lateral collateral ligaments, following classic techniques for the correction of deformity, may be necessary. The knee is at risk of instability with this approach, and some surgeons have recommended more constrained devices when revising the stiff arthroplasty.

Poor Extension

Soft tissue contractures, especially in the posterior knee, frustrate the correction of the severe flexion contracture in both primary and revision surgery. All of the techniques that have been discussed above are appropriate. The nonambulatory patient presents the greatest challenge. Profound contracture of the capsule and all

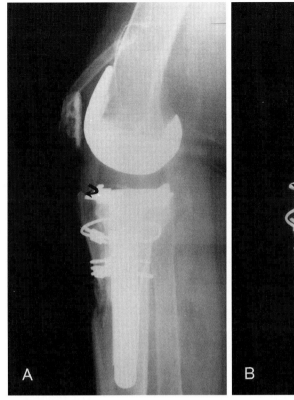

Figure 84.5. **A,** Long tibial tubercle osteotomy performed in a primary knee arthroplasty. Patient was a limited household ambulator with very stiff knees. Exposure was achieved with a long tubercle osteotomy and the tubercle was advanced proximally by 5 mm to decrease patella infera. The tip of the tubercle protrudes above the tibial base plate. (*curved arrow*). **B,** Several weeks later, the extensor mechanism has ruptured. The tip of the tubercle has broken off (*curved arrow*) and is now lying proximal to the joint line (*straight arrow*). Marked patella alta is apparent.

musculature in the back of the knee are coupled with chronic weakness of the extensor mechanism. The posterior capsule must be elevated or transected (17). The gastrocnemius muscles are frequently contracted and their origins can be released from the posterior femur. The hamstring tendons require release or lengthening that sometimes is best accomplished from separate incisions in the popliteal fossa. This may require separate procedures, although the patient can first be positioned prone for a short, percutaneous hamstring lengthening, and then repositioned for knee arthroplasty. A separate incision is safer for the peroneal nerve when releasing the biceps femoris tendon.

Secondary Scarring

Scarring may leave an otherwise sound, stable, and well-balanced arthroplasty stiff if the patient does not participate in physical therapy. Manipulation is only useful relatively soon after surgery. Revision may still be necessary to release scar tissue and symmetrically loosen the knee. The tibial component can be exchanged for a thinner insert or revised with resection of additional proximal tibia. Similarly, symmetric results can be achieved by exchanging the femoral component for a smaller size and seating it more proximally. When conforming prostheses are used, this requires revision to a smaller tibial component also.

Conversion of Arthrodesis

Conversion of a knee arthrodesis to an arthroplasty is a technically demanding procedure that is fraught with complications. While Insall lists solid, pain-free arthrodesis as a contraindication to arthroplasty (17), the conversion has been described (4, 16). Conversion without an extensor mechanism is inappropriate unless the patient understands that ambulation will only be feasible with a long leg brace. The collateral ligaments may not be functional, and a constrained device may be necessary. Only modest motion may be achievable, but even this may be greatly appreciated by the patient. The neurovascular contents of the popliteal fossa are in jeopardy, because bone cuts through the fusion mass are made with the knee extended.

Reference

1. Arlet J, Ficat P, Durroux R, et al. Histopathologie des lesions osseuses et cartilagineuses dans l'algodystrophie sympathique reflese du genou. Rev Rheum Mal Osteoartic 1981;48:315.
2. Bindelglass DF, Cohen JL and Vince KG. The infected total knee arthroplasty. Am J Knee Surg 1991;4: 94–105.
3. Butler-Manuel PA, Justins D, Heatley FW. Sympathetically mediated anterior knee pain. Acta Orthop Scan 1992;63:90–93.
4. Cameron HU. Role of total knee replacement in failed knee fusions. Can J Surg 1987;30(1):25–27.

5. Campbell ED Jr. Arthroscopy in total knee replacements. Arthroscopy 1987;3(1):31–35.

6. Daluga D, Lombardi AV, Mallory TH, Vaughn BK. Knee manipulation following total knee arthroplasty: Analysis of prognostic variables. J Arthroplasty 1991;6:119–128.

7. De Takats G. Reflex dystrophy of the extremities. Arch Surg 1937;34:939.

8. Detakas G, Miller BS. Post traumatic dystrophy of the extremities: A chronic vasodilator mechanism. Arch Surg 1943;46:469.

9. Devor M. Nerve pathophysiology and Mechanisms of Pain. J Auton Nerv Syst 1983;7:371.

10. Dorr LD, Boiardo RA. Technical considerations in total knee arthroplasty. Clin Orthop 1986;205:5.

11. Edwards E, Miller J, Chan KH. The effect of postoperative collateral ligament laxity in total knee arthroplasty. Clin Orthop 1988;236:44–51.

12. Evans JA. Reflex sympathetic dystrophy: A report on 57 cases. Ann Intern Med 1947;26:417.

13. Ficat RP, Hungerford, DS. Disorders of the patello-femoral joint. Baltimore: Williams & Wilkins, 1977

14. Figgie MP, Goldberg VM, Figgie HE, Heiple KG, Inglis AE. Salvage of the symptomatic patellofemoral joint following cruciate substituting total knee arthroplasty. Am J Knee Surg 1988;1:48–55.

15. Fox PL, Poss R. The role of manipulation following total knee replacement. J Bone Joint Surg 1981;63A:357.

16. Holden DS, Jackson DW. Considerations in total knee arthroplasty following previous knee fusion. Clin Orthop 1988;227:223–228.

17. Insall JN. Total knee arthroplasty. In: Insall JN, ed. Surgery of the Knee. New York: Churchill Livingstone, 1984.

18. Johnson DR, McGinty JB, Mason JL, et al. The role of arthroscopy in the problem total knee replacement. Arthroscopy 1990;6(1):30–32.

19. Jones D. Reflex sympathetic dystrophy of the knee. Presented at the Annual Meeting of the Western Orthopedic Society, Tuscon AZ, 1991.

20. Katz MM, Hungerford DS, Krackow KA, et al. Reflex sympathetic dystrophy as a cause of poor results after total knee arthroplasty. J Arthroplasty 1986;2:117.

21. Katz MM, Hungerford DS. Reflex sympathetic dystrophy affecting the knee. J Bone Joint Surg (Br) 1987;69-B,5:797.

22. Kaufer H, Matthews LS. Revision total knee arthroplasty: Indications and contraindications. Instructional Course Lectures. 1986;35:297–304.

23. Ladd, AL, DeHaven KE, Thanik J, et al. Reflex sympathetic imbalance: Response to epidural blockade. Am J Sports Med 1989;vol 17,5:660.

24. Lankford LL, Thompson JE. Reflex sympathetic dystrophy, upper and lower extremity: Diagnosis and management. St.Louis: CV Mosby, 1977;26:163.

25. Lee JM, DiBenedetto TD. Arthroscopic management of late fibroarthrosis following total knee replacement. Am J Knee Surgery 1989;2:42–45.

26. Lehman EJP. Traumatic vasospasm: A study of 4 cases of vasospasm in the upper extremity. Arch Surg 1934;29:92.

27. Lenggenhager K. Sudeck's osteodystrophy: Its pathogenesis, prophylaxis, and therapy. Minn Med 1971;54:967.

28. Livingston WK. Pain mechanisms. A physiologic interpretation of causalgia and its related states. New York: Macmillan 1943:212.

29. MacKinnon SE, Holder LE. The use of three-phase radio nuclide bone scanning in the diagnosis of reflex sympathetic dystrophy. J Hand Surg 1984;9:556.

30. Melzack R, Wall PD. Pain mechanisms: A new theory. Science 1965;150:971.

31. Mitchell SW. Injuries of nerves and their consequences. Philadelphia: JB Lippincott Co, 1872.

32. Morton JJ, Scott WJM. Some angiospastic syndromes in the extremities. Ann Surg 1931;94:839.

33. Nichols DW, Dorr LD. Revision surgery for stiff total knee arthroplasty. J Arthroplasty 1990;5:573–577.

34. Ogilvie-Harris DJ, Roscoe M. Reflex sympathetic dystrophy of the knee. J Bone Joint Surg (Br) 1987;69-B,5:804.

35. Patman RD, Thompson JE, Pearsson AV. Management of post-traumatic pain syndromes: Report of 113 cases. Ann Surg 1973;177:780.

36. Plewes W. Sudeck's atrophy in the hand. J Bone Joint Surg (Br) 1956;38-B:195.

37. Rhoads DD, Noble PC, Reuben JD, Mahoney OM, Tullos HS. The effect of femoral component position on patellar tracking after total knee arthroplasty. Clin Orthop Rel Research 1990;260:43–51.

38. Ritter MA, Faris PM, Keating ME. Posterior cruciate ligament balancing during total knee arthroplasty. J Arthroplasty 1988;3:323–326.

39. Ryd L, Toksvig-Larsen S. In-vivo measurements of the stability of tibial components in the postoperative phase. J Orthop Res 1992 (In press).

40. Schutzer SF, Gossling HR. Current concepts review. The treatment of reflex sympathetic dystrophy syndrome. J Bone Joint Surg 1984;4:625.

41. Scott RD, Siliski JM. The use of a modified V-Y quadricepsplasty during total knee replacement to gain exposure and improve flexion in the ankylosed knee. Orthopedics 1985;8:45.

42. Sculco TP and Faris PM. Total knee replacement in the stiff knee. Techn Orthop 1988;3:5–8.

43. Shoemaker SC, Markolf KL, Finerman GAM. In vitro stability of the implanted total condylar prosthesis. J Bone Joint Surg 1982;64A:1201–1213.

44. Spurling RG. Causalgia of the upper extremity. Treatment by dorsal sympathetic ganglionectomy. Arch Neurol Psychiat 1930;23:784.

45. Stolte BH, Stolte JB, Leyten JF. De Pathofysiologie von ist schoulderhand syndroom. Ned Tijdschr Geneeskd 1970;114:1208.

46. Sudeck, P. Über die acute entzundliche Knochenatrophie. Arch Klin Chir 1900;62:147.

47. Vince KG and Dorr LD. Revision total knee arthroplasty for aseptic failure. Techn Orthop 1987;1:83–93.

48. Vince KG and Dorr LD. Surgical technique of total knee arthroplasty: Principles and controversy. Techn Orthop 1987;1:69–82.

49. Vince KG, Insall JN. The total condylar knee prosthesis. In: Laskin R, ed. Total knee replacement. New York: Springer-Verlag, 1991.

50. Vince KG, Insall JN, Bannerman CE. Total knee arthroplasty in the patient with Parkinson's disease. J Bone Joint Surg 1989;71B:43–46.

51. Vince KG, Insall JN, Kelly M, Silva M. Long term assessment of joint line position and motion in a cruciate sacrificing knee arthroplasty. Orthop Trans 1988;12:710, 1988.

52. Vince KG and McPherson E. Patellar complications in total knee arthroplasty. Orthop Clin North Am 1993;23:675–686.

53. Vince KG. Limb length discrepancy after revision total knee arthroplasty. Techn Orthop 1988;3:35–43.

54. Vince KG. Principles of condylar knee arthroplasty: Issues evolving. Instructional Course Lectures 42. Chicago: American Academy of Orthopedic Surgery, 1993:315–324.

55. Vince KG. Revision knee arthroplasty. In: Chapman M, ed. Operative orthopedics. Philadelphia: JB Lippincott Company, 1993.

56. Walker P, Sledge C. Total knee replacement in rheumatoid arthritis. In: Insall JN, ed. Surgery of the knee. New York-Churchill: Livingstone, 1984:697–716.

57. Whitesides LA. Tibial tubercle osteotomy for exposure of the difficult total knee arthroplasty. Clin Orthop 1990;260:6–9.

58. Windsor RE and Insall JN. Exposure in revision total knee arthroplasty: The femoral peel. Techn Orthop 1988;3:1–4.

59. Wolff AM, Hungerford DS, Krackow KA, et al. Osteotomy of the tibial tubercle during total knee replacement. A report of twenty-six cases. J Bone Joint Surg 1989;71A:848–852.

85

Wound Problems in Total Knee Arthroplasty

Neil E. Klein and Christopher V. Cox

Approximately 10 to 20% of total knee replacements will have a problem with wound healing or infection, and yet these difficulties are not often addressed in today's literature (15). There are many reasons why so many wound problems occur. The knee, compared with the hip, is a relatively superficial joint, not covered by a protective layer of muscle. This superficiality makes minor wound problems serious and seems to set the stage for more wound difficulties. This chapter deals with diagnosis, treatment, and prevention of the problem wound after total knee arthroplasty (TKA).

Vascular Anatomy

The vascular anatomy of the knee has been well described (44, 59) (Fig. 85.1). The blood supply to the anterior knee forms a circular anastomotic ring around the patella, with several contributing branches. The popliteal artery gives off medial and lateral superior genicular arteries superior to the joint, which then pass anteriorly. Similarly, the medial and lateral inferior genicular arteries arise from the popliteal artery inferior to the joint line and also pass anteriorly. These four vessels are the main components of the anterior vascular anastomotic ring. The middle genicular artery also has medial and lateral branches, which course about the periphery of the menisci and then anastomose with the anterior ring.

Vessels other than the geniculars also contribute to the anterior anastomotic ring. The anterior tibial recurrent artery arises from the anterior tibial artery and joins the lateral inferior genicular. A branch of the profunda femoris anastomoses with the superior lateral genicular. The arteria genus suprema, also called the supreme genicular or descending genicular, is a branch of the superficial femoral artery. It anastomoses with the superior medial genicular as well as having direct access to the superomedial skin (9). The saphenous branch of the descending genicular anastomoses with the inferior medial genicular. This vessel augments medial skin circulation and may allow medial skin to be raised as a fasciocutaneous unit for local flap reconstruction.

Skin circulation depends on the dermal plexus, which originates directly from arterioles traveling with the subcutaneous fascia. Elevating skin flaps superficial to the fascial layer damages this circulation and may cause wound slough. Only if the superficial fascia is left attached to the subcutaneous tissue will the superficial arterial network and the circulation to the skin remain intact.

The anatomy also implies that incisions kept toward the midline will be least disruptive to the blood supply (Fig. 85.2). Quadriceps-splitting, median parapatellar incisions damage numerous branches on the medial side of the knee and contribute to decreased vascularity of deep structures. The addition of a lateral retinacular release will further damage branches to the anastomotic ring (60). Other incisions for total knee arthroplasty such as the subvastus approach seek to minimize vascular damage from dissection. A subvastus approach spares the supreme genicular on the medial side and may decrease the need for lateral retinacular release (28). The actual clinical importance of the subvastus approach with regards to wound healing and patellar vascularity has been questioned (49, 55).

Risk Factors in Wound Healing: Surgical Technique

Several specific factors can be clearly identified as detrimental to wound healing (Table 85.1). Prior skin incisions or previous procedures on the knee pose an increased risk for wound problems and deep infections (9, 25, 68). Unfortunately, it is relatively common to have other incisions on a knee that requires TKA, as these knees have often been injured or have had previous procedures. An old wound will have invariably dam-

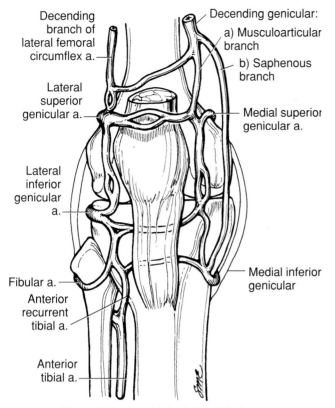

Figure 85.1. Arterial circulation of the knee.

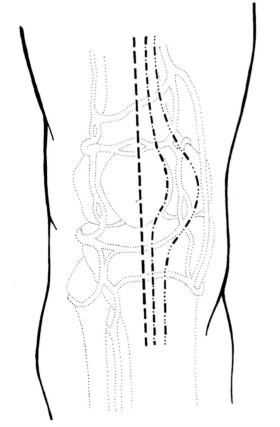

Figure 85.2. Effects of skin incisions on arteries around the knee.

Table 85.1. Risk Factors in Wound Healing

Very high risk	High risk	Low or no risk
Previous incisions	Corticosteroid use	Rheumatoid arthritis
Posttraumatic skin and scarring	Hypovolemia	Anemia
	Diabetes mellitus	NSAIDs
Cigarette smoking	Obesity	Age
	Malnutrition	Gender
	Poor surgical technique	Blood loss

aged the anastomotic network of vessels of the anterior knee. Adding a new incision can create a skin bridge with poor vascularity between the new incision and the old scar. Wide scars with thin or absent subcutaneous tissue indicate severe damage to the subdermal plexus and should serve as a red flag for potential wound problems.

The use of a medial skin incision that creates a large laterally based skin flap has been associated with poor skin viability and a higher incidence of wound problems. There seems to be a medial-side predominance in the cutaneous circulation and poorer tissue oxygenation on the lateral flap after incision. Studies comparing incisions and wound edge viability tend to confirm this asymmetry. Transcutaneous oxygen measurements have been made in TKAs that used either midline, medial parapatellar, or curved medial incisions (31, 34). There was a consistent and statistically significant lower oxygen tension on the lateral wound edge at all times and with all incisions. The more medial the incision (i.e., a larger laterally based skin flap), the lower were the lateral flap oxygen tensions. Oxygen tension returned to preoperative levels by postoperative day 8. This small study showed a clear trend of lower oxygen tension on the lateral wound edge, suggesting that incisions with larger lateral flaps could be at a higher risk for poor wound healing.

The use of lateral retinacular releases in TKA can further impair lateral circulation in the soft tissue. A standard median parapatellar approach combined with a lateral retinacular release will transect both the superior and inferior medial genicular arteries and the superior lateral genicular artery. This may potentially devitalize the patella and prepatellar skin (8, 36, 42, 60). Lateral retinacular release is associated with increased superficial wound infections and decreased lateral wound edge viability as well as decreased transcutaneous oxygen tension (33).

Other technical factors that are important for good wound healing seem obvious but merit stressing. Meticulous surgical technique and incisions of adequate length are simple but important ideas. Being gentle with retraction of skin edges, ensuring hemostasis to avoid postoperative hematomas, and closing wounds carefully are extremely important. We have observed most wound problems at the site of lateral skin retraction and patellar erosion. An incision of appropriate length obviates the need for aggressive retraction and prevents this trauma. The incision should be long enough to eliminate tension on the wound when the knee is flexed.

Correct surgical technique can reduce the risk of wound problems. When making an incision, it is best to stay toward the midline, ending the distal incision medial to the prominence of the tibial tubercle. Old incisions should be incorporated if they lie near the midline. Prior incisions that are *far* to the medial or lateral sides may be ignored if subcutaneous tissues are healthy. A preexistent transverse incision can usually be crossed at 90 degrees without worry. If curved incisions are necessary because of preexistent scars, try not to have a large laterally based skin flap. Avoid undermining large segments of skin, and always retain the superficial fascia with the subcutaneous layer.

Even the best surgical technique cannot prevent problems if the anatomy is flawed. If soft tissue coverage of the knee is poor, no incision can succeed. We have used prophylactic muscle pedicle and free flaps for soft tissue enhancement to ease exposure in this eventuality.

Impaired peripheral circulation can create the potential for wound problems. Careful examination of the patient's vascular status is essential. If suspected, preexisting arterial and/or venous problems can be diagnosed by noninvasive procedures. A limb with poor circulation will have trouble healing a surgical wound, and vascular reconstruction may be needed before knee replacement can be accomplished.

Patient Risk Factors

Corticosteroids

Beyond surgical technique, other risk factors for wound problems are less easily controlled. Patients who have been on corticosteroid medication chronically have long been presumed to be at risk for poor wound healing or infection (46, 50). Such patients are common in a joint replacement population because of the prevalence of corticosteroid therapy in people with rheumatologic diseases. Patients who have a long history of corticosteroid use have poor skin turgor and poor skin vascularity (61). Corticosteroids administered at the time of, and immediately after, surgery can influence wound healing by inhibiting fibroblast proliferation (10, 23). This slows the accumulation of collagen and thus decreases the tensile strength of the wound. McNamara and colleagues demonstrated that steroids impaired tensile strength of experimental healing wounds in rabbits and rats (41). This steroid effect abated gradually in their experiments, and they used extremely large doses of corticosteroids. What actually constitutes long-term use or risk level of corticosteroids is not known, as there is great variation in dose and duration of therapy used in the clinical population.

Collagenase, normally present in the healing wound, decreases with time. Cortisone influences collagenase activity by slowing its disappearance from wounds, thus decreasing collagen accumulation and wound strength (65, 66). The persistence of collagenase will

weaken wounds by shifting the balance between collagen production and catabolism to the collagen-breakdown side (9).

The association between the use of corticosteroids, poor wound healing, and infection, however, is not consistent. Wilson showed that when corticosteroid use was viewed independently of preoperative diagnosis, there was no increased risk of poor wound healing (68). Similarly, Garner found no relationship between the dose of corticosteroid used and the time to complete wound healing in a clinical study (17). Garner did, however, find that rheumatoid arthritics who had been on corticosteroids for more than 3 years had both longer times to complete wound healing and a higher rate of wound infections.

Current practice would indicate that there is no necessity to eliminate corticosteroid use before knee surgery, especially as such medications are usually mandatory for adequate disease control and avoiding addisonian crisis. But the long-term steroid user must be considered at greater risk for developing a wound complication.

Rheumatoid Arthritis

Rheumatoid arthritis has been proposed as a greater risk factor than osteoarthritis in wound healing and late infection (13, 25, 35, 45, 51, 54, 62, 68). Wong found a threefold increase in risk for wound problems in rheumatoid patients, as opposed to osteoarthritic patients (69). However, there is little direct evidence that the underlying disease process in rheumatoid patients affects wound healing. Garner et al. had seemingly conflicting data: the time for wound healing was the same in rheumatoid arthritic patients and in controls (17). Neither the activity of the disease nor the presence of rheumatoid factor was associated with delays in healing. But Garner et al. also found an increased incidence of wound separation and overall failure of healing in the rheumatoid patients.

Rheumatoid patients who used corticosteroids were much more likely to have a postoperative wound infection. Wilson similarly found an increased risk of infection in rheumatoid patients with total knee replacements, but again only in those who had been treated with corticosteroids (68). Most likely, the increased risk of infections or wound problems seen in rheumatoid arthritic patients is the result of long-term steroid use by these patients.

Nutrition

One might assume that malnutrition is detrimental to wound healing (15), yet even when malnourished, patients marshal proteins for wound healing (37, 52, 56). It is unlikely that severe malnutrition would be present in a candidate for total knee replacement, however, when identified, malnutrition should be corrected before surgery.

Obesity is much more common and has long been associated with poor wound healing (11, 15, 29, 46). Wong found a linear relationship between obesity and poor wound healing. Other studies on obese patients have also shown delayed healing and an increased incidence of postoperative wound drainage (68).

Obesity also creates the possibility for mechanical wound problems. In the heavier patient with a thick panniculus, the skin is less tenacious to the underlying tissues, and the shearing force of a retractor may easily tear the dermis from the subcutaneous layer. The relative paucity of circulation in fat makes this layer particularly susceptible to local trauma, and devascularization with skin necrosis or secondary infection a likely sequela.

Anemia/Hypovolemia

Anemia and more importantly hypovolemia can affect wound healing. Anemia however, unless severe, has not been shown to affect wound healing. Hypovolemia, though, has a strong effect on oxygen delivery to the wound. If normovolemia is maintained, hematocrits of 18 to 20 allow adequate wound healing (9).

Cigarette Smoking

Cigarette smoking has been shown in many studies to have a deleterious effect on wound healing (10, 43, 53). Inhalation of cigarette smoke can affect the skin microcirculation as well as healing at the cellular level. These effects have been attributed to two substances, nicotine and cotinine, which both appear in the circulation with smoke inhalation. Nicotine is a potent vasoconstrictor that increases both heart rate and blood pressure (3). This systemic vasoconstriction can also diminish blood flow to the skin and increase the risk of poor wound healing. Nicotine also increases plasma catecholamine levels, which further increase peripheral vasoconstriction (3, 43). Catecholamines impair wound epithelialization, possibly by acting as cofactors for wound hormones that inhibit epithelialization (12, 67). Nicotine, however, is rapidly metabolized, and its effects short-lived. The greater long-term problem may be from cotinine.

Cotinine is the major metabolite of nicotine in man (4). It is stored in body fat and can be released into the circulation even weeks after exposure. This effect implies that the simple cessation of smoking in the immediate perioperative period may not be sufficient to reduce the risk of smoking on wound healing. The exact biologic effects of cotinine, however, are not clear. Some have called it a potent vasoconstrictor like nicotine. Others have found it to have little or no physiologic effects (5). Cotinine has no effect on blood pressure, heart rate, and skin temperature, and in one study, has even been associated with lower blood pressure (5, 16). Regardless of cotinine's effects, restriction of cigarette smoking is one significant risk factor that can and should be eliminated as long before surgery as possible.

Diabetes

Wound problems have long been associated with diabetic patients (15, 19, 20, 40). Wong showed in a prospective study that diabetics were more likely to have a delay in wound healing, manifested by increased swelling, erythema, or wound separation (69). Why this occurs is not entirely clear, but delayed collagen synthesis and delayed wound tensile strength have been suggested (19, 20). In addition, early capillary ingrowth into wounds is retarded, and the early inflammatory response may be delayed. Also both large- and small-vessel peripheral vascular disease are common in diabetics, further inhibiting oxygen delivery to the wound. These patients are often obese and elderly and thus also have lower insulin production and higher levels of insulin resistance. All these factors confuse the issue of the true source of poor healing. In Wilson's study, in which matched controls were used, diabetes mellitus was not found to be a significant risk factor for infection in total knee replacements (68).

Insulin, in some cases, reverses the defects of capillary ingrowth and inflammation (21). Other studies though have shown insulin to have little or no effect on collagen synthesis (48, 64). Careful insulin regulation of blood sugar and control of obesity to decrease insulin resistance are desirable because these are factors over which the surgeon has control.

Continuous Passive Motion

The postoperative use of continuous passive motion (CPM) has become routine in total knee replacement, to encourage early motion. The effect of CPM on wound healing, however, is controversial. Some authors have suggested that early continuous passive motion tenses the skin, with a resultant decreased oxygenation to the skin edges (18). Johnson showed that transcutaneous oxygen tension (TcO_2) measured at the wound edges decreased with knee flexion beyond 40 degrees, especially in the first 3 postoperative days (32). Even though Johnson demonstrated no difference in wound problems between patients using CPM and those being immobilized, he proposed 40 degrees as the flexion limit in the early postoperative period. Wong, in his prospective study of 120 knees, actually found continuous passive motion helpful. He noted a reduction in wound complications from 16 to 4% when CPM was used (69). Continuous passive motion also increases the tensile strength of wounds created in mature rabbits, compared with the wounds in rabbits treated with immobilization alone (63). We use CPM routinely, following Johnson's guidelines, and have found no increase in wound problems.

Infection

Difficulty with a wound may be either mechanical, infectious, or a combination of the two. Often a "noninfected" wound will be colonized by organisms, making it difficult to determine what role the organisms are playing. A true infection may penetrate the soft tissues, contaminating the components, or may seriously involve the substance of the bone that supports them.

Treatment of a problem wound must deal with the spectrum of infectious problems as well as the mechanical ones. Management of the infected prosthesis requires an accurate bacteriologic diagnosis by aspiration cultures, and aggressive intervention with antibiotics. Debridement and flap coverage should be considered when necessary (6). Well-vascularized flaps, and particularly muscle flaps, seem to have a salutary effect on problem wounds.

Most mechanical wound problems can be corrected. Present-day flap surgery can deal with even the most distressing soft tissue difficulties. Skeletal defects, though more difficult to treat, can respond to various orthopaedic techniques and custom implants. In the presence of established deep infection, however, explantation is usually necessary.

Miscellaneous Factors

Several other factors may add risk of wound problems following TKA. These include the patient's sex and age, the amount of blood loss, and the use of nonsteroidal antiinflammatory drugs. None of these variables has ever consistently been shown to have a significant effect on wound healing (15, 39, 68, 69).

Types of Wound Problems

Wound problems fall into one of four major groups. Each is more severe and poses greater risk to the implant: (*a*) delayed healing or prolonged drainage, (*b*) minor skin necrosis and superficial infections, (*c*) tense hematomas, and (*d*) major skin necrosis with an exposed prosthesis. Any of these problems may lead to, or be a sign of, superficial or deep infection. Infection must always be considered with any wound problem. Cultures, debridements, and antibiotics should enter into the treatment as soon as infection is suspected (6). Any infection following TKA requires aggressive treatment.

Description and Treatment

As most wound problems are minor, they can usually be eliminated by timely and simple means. A common situation is the wound with prolonged serous drainage or a delay in healing (30) (Fig. 85.3). The wound usually appears otherwise benign, without erythema, tenderness, or purulence. Treatment consists of frequent dressing changes to keep the wound as clean and dry as possible, to decrease the risk of contamination. Temporarily discontinue CPM and physical therapy, and allow the limb to rest. The patient should regain the motion later. Do not use antibiotics routinely or at least not without obtaining joint aspirate for culture and sensitivity first. These wounds are usually not infected, and antibiotics may alter the flora and their sensitivities if a deep infection develops (30, 61). In addition, superficial drainage is easily contaminated and often has little relationship to the true infectious state of the knee. This type of wound problem is most commonly seen in the obese patient, the diabetic, or those on chronic corticosteroid therapy.

The second type of problem is minor skin necrosis or minor superficial infection (Fig. 85.4). Superficial wound infections range from simple suture abscesses to soft tissue infections and cellulitis superficial to the joint. Suture abscesses require only simple debridement and redressing. Superficial infections should be cultured. An aspirate of the joint for culture and cell count

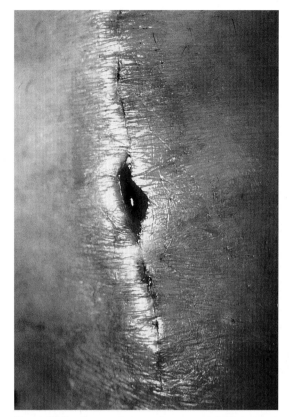

Figure 85.3. Serous drainage from an uninfected wound.

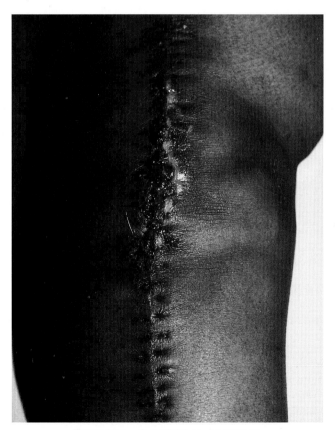

Figure 85.4. Superficial wound necrosis.

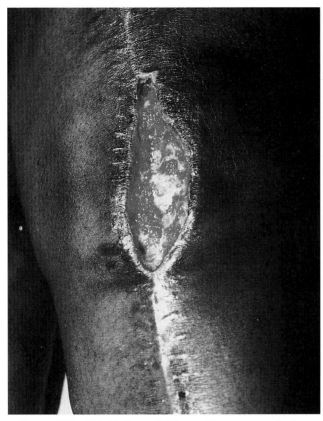

Figure 85.5. Debrided superficial wound from same patient as in Figure 85.7.

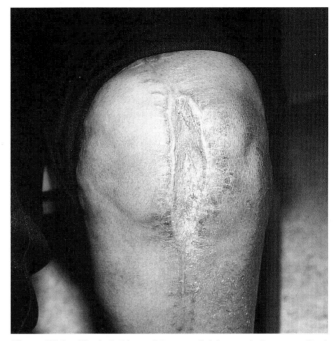

Figure 85.6. Healed skin graft to superficial wound of same patient as in Figures 85.4 and 85.5.

can be obtained if deep infection is a consideration. Antibiotics may then be started against the suspected organism and altered if necessary after the culture report is obtained. It is best to keep the limb immobilized and elevated until the drainage ceases.

Skin necrosis may lead to more serious trouble. Necrosis under 3 cm in diameter can initially be treated with immobilization and redressing (61). Debridement should suffice to remove dead tissue (Fig. 85.5). Leaving a layer of necrotic tissue to "protect the prosthesis" serves no useful function. This tissue is undoubtedly already infected and, at the very least, contaminated. Dead tissue should be completely removed. If during debridement of the wound the prosthesis is exposed or the joint is entered, the problem is obviously more serious, and closure may require a muscle flap. If the necrosis is superficial, then simple closure techniques may be adequate.

The choice of wound closure for the superficial necrosis depends on the size of the wound and the suppleness of the skin. The decision to proceed with surgical closure is based on whether the time for wound healing after a closure procedure would be shorter than the time it would take for the wound to close by secondary intention. Usually, skin grafting is the procedure of choice (Fig. 85.6). A fasciocutaneous flap, as described by Hallock, would also serve well in this instance (26).

Tense hematomas can threaten a wound from pressure and the toxic breakdown products of hemoglobin. Hematomas, if contaminated, also present a rich medium for bacterial growth. Recognition of an early postoperative hematoma can be difficult. Dressings, drainage, and postoperative swelling may all look disturbing. Copious bloody discharge into the dressing, inordinate pain, swelling, and discoloration of skin on the first postoperative day is worrisome and may indicate hematoma. Drains cannot always prevent hematoma formation, and their presence should not lull one into thinking that a hematoma is impossible.

Despite excellent hemostasis obtained before skin closure, a hematoma may still form. If a large hematoma is diagnosed, it is best to return to the operating room to reopen the wound, decompress and irrigate the joint, and obtain hemostasis (Fig. 85.7). These hematomas usually form secondary to continued bleeding from a genicular artery, but a single source may not always be found.

Major skin necrosis (Fig. 85.8) or an exposed prosthesis (Fig. 85.9) is rare, and there is no standard treatment. Treatment options for these grave conditions often involve removal of the prosthesis. However, with aggressive treatment the prosthesis may be salvaged. The first step in saving the prosthesis is exploration and debridement (Fig. 85.10). A simple secondary closure is usually not possible while still allowing a tension-free wound. More commonly, a flap reconstruction of this soft tissue deficit is required. Options for these flaps include local, random- or axial-pattern flaps, gastrocnemius muscle flaps, fasciocutaneous flaps, and free flaps (Fig. 85.11). Success with flap reconstruction in this area depends upon the viability of the flap itself as well

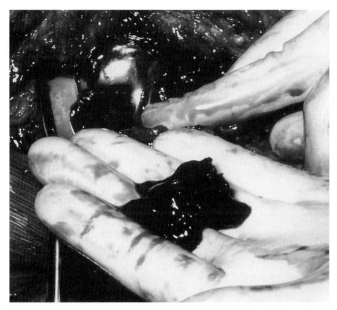

Figure 85.7.   Large hematoma at time of evacuation.

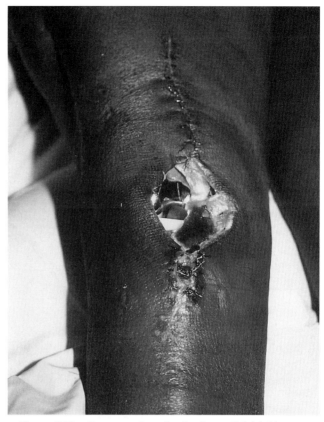

Figure 85.9.   Exposure of prosthesis after partial debridement.

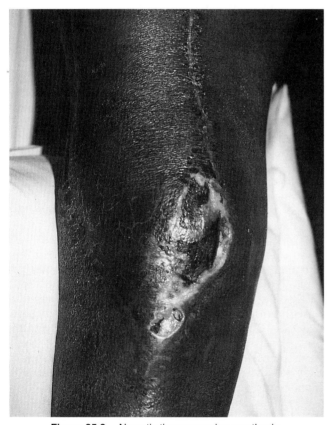

Figure 85.8.   Necrotic tissue covering prosthesis.

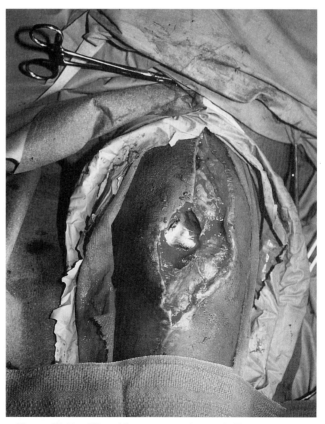

Figure 85.10.   Wound from same patient as in Figures 85.8 and 85.9 following complete debridement.

as the status of the prosthesis, if septic arthritis is causing the drainage. Even a healthy flap cannot save a prosthesis that is infected or if there is osteomyelitis. These problems must be treated concurrently with removal of the prosthesis, debridement, and antibiotics.

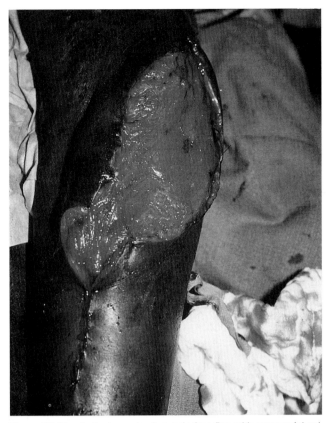

Figure 85.11. Latissimus dorsi muscle free flap with successful salvage of prosthesis in same patient as in Figures 85.8, 85.9, and 85.10.

Attempts at simple secondary closure when major skin necrosis is present have met with poor results. In a Swedish study, Bengston found that in trying to salvage 10 exposed knee prostheses, all 6 knees that had a simple secondary closure failed (2).

Cutaneous rotation flaps represent the next step in complexity for wound closure. These flaps are created by making a counterincision adjacent to the wound, moving that skin island to appose the debrided wound edges, and then skin-grafting the created defect. Lian and Cracchilo (38) reported on seven patients with major skin necrosis, of whom five had cutaneous rotation flaps and two gastrocnemius flaps for salvage. They initially irrigated and debrided the joint, followed by an average of 10 days of intravenous antibiotics. A flap procedure was then done. Four of seven healed; however, it was not specified which knees received the two gastrocnemius flaps and which had the cutaneous flaps (38).

We usually reserve skin procedures for simple superficial wounds. Muscle flaps are more reliable for wounds where prostheses are exposed. The gastrocnemius muscle flap seems well suited to salvage the severe wound (14, 27, 47, 57). It is anatomically accessible and fills empty space with vascular tissue that provokes a superior immune response (7). The medial gastrocnemius is preferable because it is longer than the lateral gastrocnemius, is more mobile, and does not endanger the peroneal nerve. The medial gastrocnemius flap eas-

ily covers the area of the patella and tibial tubercle where most wound problems seem to occur (Figs. 85.12–85.15). The lateral gastrocnemius muscle should be reserved for problems with lateral knee coverage or absent medial gastrocnemius muscle heads.

Several case reports on the use of a gastrocnemius flap with retention of the components have advanced its use in the salvage of total knee replacements. Only three studies have described more than one patient. Greenberg (24) reported on 10 patients with skin necrosis more than 1 cm in diameter. Although 8 of 10 were "salvaged," the paper did not elaborate on the two failures. In Bengston's study of 10 knees, all 4 of those covered with gastrocnemius flaps succeeded (2). Sanders (58) reported on nine exposed prostheses treated with gastrocnemius flaps. Only four of the nine healed without sequelae. The reasons for failure were not included, except that a history of deep venous thrombosis may have contributed to one flap failure.

In addition to local muscle flaps, free flaps can be used for wounds that cannot be reached or reliably covered by gastrocnemius flaps. No studies have been published regarding use of free flaps to cover exposed total knees. Latissimus dorsi and serratus anterior free flaps have successfully covered exposed endoprostheses and hardware at other sites (22). The rectus abdominis and gracilis muscles are also useful, as are some nonmuscle flaps such as the scapular and parascapular flaps.

In our series of 11 patients with infected or exposed prostheses, 2 patients were treated with latissimus dorsi muscle free flaps and 8 by covering the debrided wounds with medial gastrocnemius muscle flaps. A free flap was required in one case because of the large defect after debridement, and in the second case because of the large size and awkward lateral position of a defect that resulted from a drainage procedure done at a different hospital.

One patient with a gastrocnemius reconstruction died from a pulmonary embolus 2 weeks postoperatively. Three patients required eventual removal of the prosthesis for recurrent infection. The five other gastrocnemius salvages remain intact. Of the free flap patients, one expired from unrelated causes, 1 year after the free flap surgery, with the TKA intact. The other required removal of the prosthesis after 6 months but had a successful reimplantation under the free flap 6 months later as part of a two-stage protocol. Even if the prosthesis must be removed after a flap has been placed to attempt salvage, the success of future reimplantation is enhanced by a well-healed flap.

It remains unclear whether components that are exposed by skin and wound problems (rather than initial deep infection) represent established deep infections or "colonization." It would seem generally that removal of components and thorough debridement, followed by wound coverage and delayed reimplantation, would produce the best results. However, there seems to be some indication that if there is neither frank purulence nor necrotic debris when the wound is debrided and if the prosthetic components are stable, the prosthesis may be salvaged by flap coverage. This seems to be

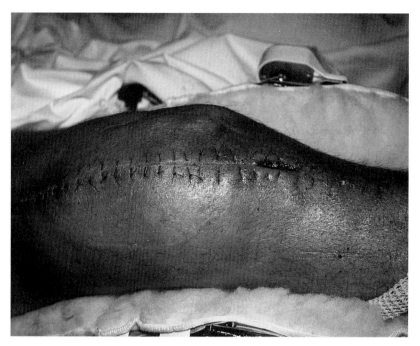

Figure 85.12. Small wound with communication to joint.

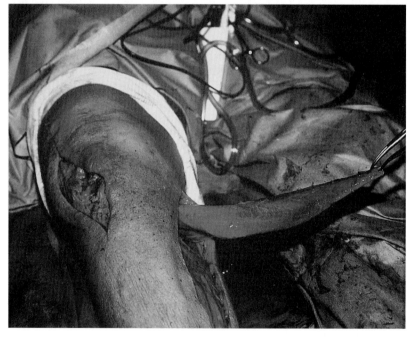

Figure 85.13. After debridement of wound from patient in Figure 85.12, with medial gastrocnemius muscle elevated.

true, especially if the wound is free from difficult organisms such as Gram-negative, anaerobic, or mixed bacteria. We were able eventually to salvage 40% of our severe wound complications.

As our one mortality indicates, these reconstructions are not without hazard. The patients are usually among the poorest of candidates for surgery. Patients with serious wound problems usually have several risk factors and additionally have been at bed rest or some degree of immobilization before the salvage flap procedure. All this must be considered before offering a muscle flap to attempt prosthesis salvage. A brief delay in surgery may

not make much difference in salvage rate of the prosthesis, but it could ensure a healthier patient who is more likely to avoid complications.

Prophylaxis

The best way to treat a wound problem is to identify it before it happens. Poor soft tissue over the knee results in a greater likelihood of postoperative wound difficulties. In our experience, a flap applied to a problem soft tissue area before the knee replacement will obviate wound problems after the knee replacement.

Figure 85.14. Debrided wound, flap passed beneath median skin bridge to soft tissue deficit.

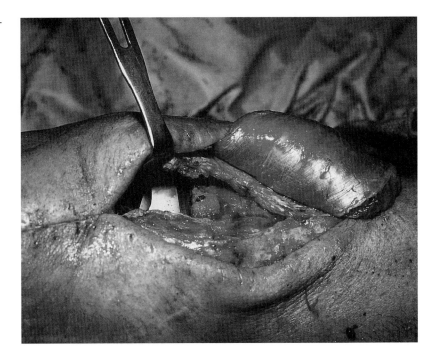

Figure 85.15. Gastrocnemius muscle flap in place over knee with split-thickness skin graft applied to exposed muscle.

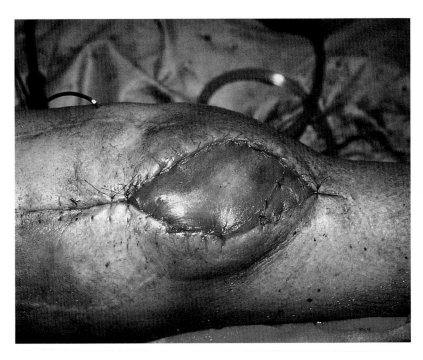

For the patient with numerous crisscrossing scars or residual atrophic skin overlying the patella or pretibial area, a gastrocnemius muscle flap or free flap can be placed preimplantation (Fig. 85.16). This allows the knee to be entered and then closed with the healthy flap that has been used to replace the unhealthy tissue (Figs. 85.17 and 85.18). The choice of flap depends on the size and location of the soft tissue deficiency. A medial gastrocnemius flap will easily cover the patella and tibial tubercle areas. The largest conceivable deficiency, extending from collateral ligament to collateral ligament,

and distal quadriceps to the tibial crest, can usually be covered with a latissimus dorsi muscle free flap. Other flaps, local or free, can be tailored to specific deficiencies by the plastic surgeon.

As with any prophylactic procedure, it is impossible to determine whether the operation would have been needed had it not been done. However, in several of our cases, total replacement would have been contraindicated because of the tremendous scarring about the knee. Of 10 patients in whom prophylactic flaps were done before total knee revision, 9 were free flaps, and 1

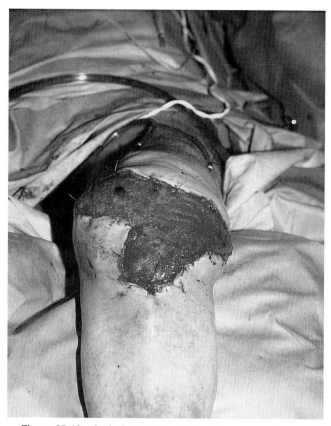

Figure 85.16. Latissimus dorsi muscle free flap to left knee in preparation for TKA to be done at a later date.

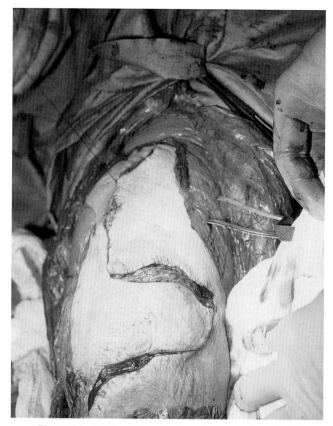

Figure 85.18. Free flap placed and wound being closed.

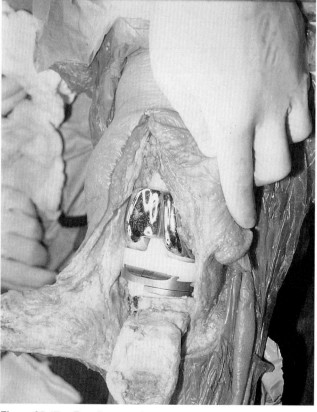

Figure 85.17. Free flap reevaluated to expose knee for revision TKA.

was a lateral gastrocnemius flap. Not one of these patients has had wound problems following eventual total knee replacement (Figs. 85.19 and 85.20). We recommend that the procedure be performed several months before the arthroplasty and that healing be complete before the subsequent surgery.

In addition to local muscle flaps and free flaps, soft tissue expansion has been used about the knee to correct tight scarring. This procedure seems to be less useful (Figs. 85.21–85.23). Combined evaluation by both orthopaedic and plastic surgeons will provide the best answer to wound problems before they occur.

Summary

Wound problems in total knee replacements are fairly common. While severe wound problems are rare, they can be catastrophic. Understanding the vascular anatomy of the knee helps explain the danger of prior incisions and supports the use of midline incisions. The surgeon must control as many of the wound healing factors as possible. Prior incisions and previous wounds are probably the greatest risk factors for severe wound complications. Treatment of prolonged drainage and minor wound breakdown is simple with use of local wound care, immobilization, and use of antibiotics where appropriate. Treatment of severe wound necrosis or the exposed prosthesis is difficult. The use of cutaneous flaps is probably insufficient, but local muscle

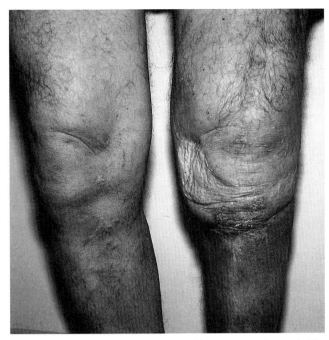

Figure 85.19. Healed free flap *(left leg)* from same patient as in Figures 85.18 and 85.20 over secondary reimplantation after 1 year.

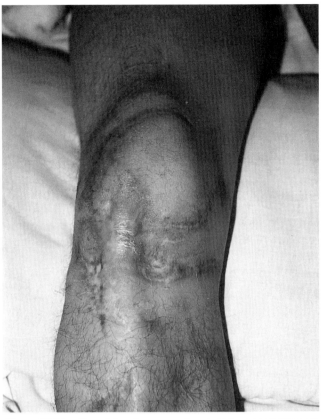

Figure 85.21. Knee injury from propeller of ski boat. Unstable scar with deficiency of soft tissue over patella and tibial crest.

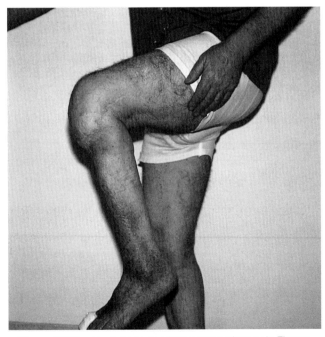

Figure 85.20. Healed free flap from same patient as in Figures 85.18 and 85.19 over secondary reimplantation after 1 year.

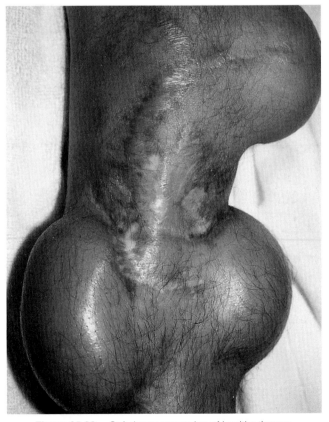

Figure 85.22. Soft tissue expansion of healthy tissues.

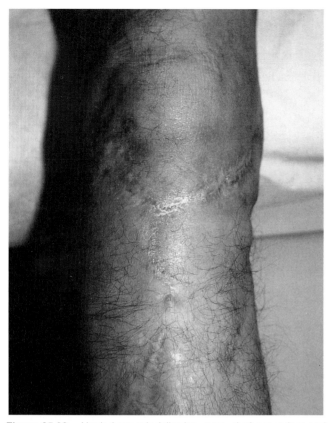

Figure 85.23. Healed wounds following removal of expanders and use of expanded local flaps to replace scarred skin over patella and tibial crest.

flaps and free flaps appear to be helpful. Prophylactic soft tissue coverage is one way to help to avoid problems in the scar-covered knee.

References

1. Alexiades M, Sands A, Craig SM, Scott WN. Management of selected problems in revision knee arthroplasty. Orthop Clin North Am 1989;20(2):211–219.
2. Bengtson S, Carlsson A, Relander M, Kuntson K, Lindgren L. Treatment of the exposed knee prosthesis. Acta Orthop Scand 1987;58:662–665.
3. Benowitz NL, Kuyt F, Jacob P III. Influence of nicotine on cardiovascular and hormonal effects or cigarette smoking. Clin Pharmacol Ther 1984;36:74–81.
4. Benowitz NL, Kuyt F, Jacob P III, Jones RT, Osman A. Cotinine deposition and effects. Clin Pharmacol Ther 1984;34(5):604–611.
5. Benowitz NL, Sharp D. Inverse relation between serum cotine concentration and blood pressure in cigarette smokers. Circulation 1989;80(5):1309–1312.
6. Bindelglass DF, Cohen JL, Vince KG. The infected total knee arthroplasty. Am J Knee Surg 1991;4:2.
7. Calderon W, Chang N, Mathes SJ. Comparison of the effects of bacterial inoculation in musculocutaneous and fasciocutaneous flaps. Plast Reconstr Surg 1986;77:785–792.
8. Clayton ML, Thiruipathi R. Patellar complications after total knee arthroplasty. Clin Orthop 1982;170:152–155.
9. Craig S. Soft tissue considerations. In: Scott WN, ed. Total knee revision arthroplasty. Orlando, FL. Grune & Stratton, 1987:99–112.
10. Craig S, Rees TD. The effects of smoking on experimental skin flaps in hamsters. Plast Reconstr Surg 1985;75(6):842–846.
11. Cruse PJ, Foord R. A prospective study of 23,649 surgical wounds. Arch Surg 1973;107:206.
12. Cryer PE, Haymond MW, Santiago JV, et al. Norepinephrine and epinephrine release and adrenergic mediation of smoking associated hemodynamic and metabolic events. N Engl J Med 1976;295:573.
13. D'Ambrosia RD, Shoji H, Heater R. Secondarily infected total joint replacements by hematogenous spread. J Bone Joint Surg 1976;58A(4):450–453.
14. Eckhardt JJ, Lesavoy MA, Dubrow TJ, Wackyum PA. Exposed endoprosthesis. Clin Orthop 1990;251:220–229.
15. Echer ML, Lotke P. Postoperative care of the total knee patient. Orthop Clin North Am 1989;20(1):55–62.
16. Freidman GD. Cigarette smoking, cotinine, blood pressure. Circulation 1989;80(5):1493–1494.
17. Garner RW, Mowat AG, Hazleman BL. Wound healing after operations on patients with rheumatoid arthritis. J Bone Joint Surg 1973;55B(1):134–144.
18. Goletz TH, Henry JH. Continuous passive motion after total knee arthroplasty. South Med J 1986;79(9):1116–1120.
19. Goodson WH III, Hunt TK. Studies of wound healing in experimental diabetes mellitus. J Surg Res 1977;22:221.
20. Goodson WH III, Hunt TK. Wound healing and the diabetic patient. Surg Gynecol Obstet 1979;149:600–608.
21. Goodson WH III, Hunt TK. Wound healing in experimental diabetes mellitus; importance of early insulin therapy. Surg Forum 1978;29:95.
22. Gordon L, Levinsohn DG. Versatility of the latissimus and serratus anterior muscle transplants in providing cover for exposed hardware and endoprostheses. Presented at Western Orthopaedic Association 1991 Annual Meeting, Tucson, AZ.
23. Green JP. Steroid therapy and wound healing in surgical patients. Br J Surg 1965;52:523–525.
24. Greenberg B, LaRossa D, Lotke P, Murphy JB, Noone RB. Salvage of jeopardized total knee prosthesis: the role of the gastrocnemius muscle flap. Plast Reconstr Surg 1989;83(1):85–89.
25. Grogan TJ, Dorey F, Rollins J, Amstutz HC. Deep sepsis following total knee arthroplasty. J Bone Joint Surg 1986;68A(2):226–234.
26. Hallock GG. Salvage of total knee arthroplasty with local fasciocutaneous flaps. J Bone Joint Surg 1990;72A(8):1236–1239.
27. Hemphill ES, Ebert FR, Muench AG. The medial gastrocnemius muscle flap in the treatment of wound complications following total knee arthroplasty. Orthopedics 1992;15(4):477–480.
28. Hoffman AA, Plaster RL, Murdock LE. Subvastus approach for total knee arthroplasty. Clin Orthop 1991;269:70–77.
29. Hood RW, Insall JN. Infected MDNM/total knee replacement arthroplasties. In: Evarts CM. ed. Surgery of the musculoskeletal system. Vol 4, chap 10. New York: Churchill Livingstone, 1983:173–188.
30. Insall JN, Scott WN, Ranawat CS. The Total Condylar Knee prosthesis: a report of two hundred and twenty cases. J Bone Joint Surg 1979;61A:173.
31. Johnson DP. Midline or parapatellar incision for knee arthroplasty. A comparative study of wound viability. J Bone Joint Surg 1988;70-B(4):656–658.
32. Johnson DP. The effects of continuous passive motion on wound healing and joint mobility after knee arthroplasty. J Bone Joint Surg 1990;72-A(3):421–426.
33. Johnson DP, Eastwood DM. Lateral patellar release in knee arthroplasty. Effect on wound healing. J Arthroplasty 1992;7(suppl):427–431.
34. Johnson DP, Houghton TA, Radford P. Anterior midline or medial parapatellar incision for arthroplasty of the knee. A comparative study. J Bone Joint Surg 1986;68-B(5):812–814.
35. Karten I. Septic arthritis complicating rheumatoid arthritis. Ann Intern Med 1969;70:1147.
36. Kayler DE, Lyttle D. Surgical interruption of patellar blood supply by total knee arthroplasty. Clin Orthop 1988;229:221–227.
37. Levenson S, Seifter E. Nutrition and wound healing. Clin Plast Surg 1977;4:375–388.
38. Lian G, Cracchiolo A, Lesavoy M. Treatment of major wound necrosis following total knee arthroplasty. J Arthroplasty 1989;(suppl):S23–32.
39. McGrath MH. The effect of prostaglandin inhibitors on wound contraction and the myofibroblast. Plast Reconstr Surg 1982;69:75.
40. McMurray JF. Wound healing in diabetes mellitus, better glucose control for better wound healing in diabetes. Surg Clin North Am 1984;64(4):769–777.
41. McNamara JJ, Lanborn PJ, Mills D, Aaby GV. Effects of short term pharmacologic doses of adrenocorticoid therapy on wound healing. Ann Surg 1969;170:199.
42. Merkow RM, Soudry M, Insall JN. Patellar dislocation following total knee replacement. J Bone Joint Surg 1985;67A:1321.
43. Mosely LH, Finseth F, Goody M. Nicotine and its effect on wound healing. Plast Reconstr Surg 1978;61(4):570–575.
44. Mueller W. The knee-form, function and ligament reconstruction. Berlin: Springer-Verlag, 1982:158–167.
45. Myers AR, Miller LM, Pinals RS. Pyarthrosis complicating rheumatoid arthritis. Lancet 1969;2:714.
46. Nelson CL. Prevention of sepsis. Clin Orthop 1987;222:66–72.
47. Peled IJ, Frankl U, Wexler MR. Salvage of exposed knee prosthesis by

gastrocnemius myocutaneous flap coverage. Orthopedics 1983;6(10):1320–1322.

48. Perlish JS, Bashley RI, Fleischmajer R. The in-vitro effect of insulin on collagen synthesis in embryonic chick tibia. Proc Soc Exp Biol Med 1973;142:1152.

49. Peters P, Knezevich S, Engh G, Dwyer K, Predis F. Comparison of the subvastus quadricep-sparing and standard anterior quadricep-splitting approaches in total and unicompartmental knee arthroplasty. Presented at American Academy of Orthopaedic Surgeons 1992 Annual Meeting, Washington D.C.

50. Petty W, Bryan RS, Coventry MB, Peterson LF. Infection after total knee arthroplasty. Orthop Clin North Am 1975;6:1005–1014.

51. Poss R, Thornhill TS, Ewald FC, Thomas WH, Batte NJ, Sledge CB. Factors influencing the incidence and outcome of infection following total joint arthroplasty. Clin Orthop 1984;182:117–126.

52. Powanda MC, Moyer ED. Plasma proteins and wound healing. Surg Gynecol Obstet 1981;153:749.

53. Rees TD, Liverett DM, Guy CL. The effect of cigarette smoking on skin-flap survival in the face lift patient. Plast Reconstr Surg 1984;73(6):911–915.

54. Rimoin DL, Wennburg JE. Acute septic arthritis complicating chronic rheumatoid arthritis. JAMA 1966;196:617.

55. Ritter MA, Campbell ED. Postoperative patellar complications with or without lateral release during total knee arthroplasty. Clin Orthop 1987;219:163–168.

56. Ruberg RL. Role of nutrition in wound healing. Surg Clin North Am 1984;64:705.

57. Salibian AH, Sanford HA. Salvage of an infected total knee prosthesis with medial and lateral gastrocnemius muscle flaps. J Bone Joint Surg 1983;65-A(5):681–684.

58. Sanders R, O'Neil T. The gastrocnemius myocutaneous flap used as a cover for the exposed knee prosthesis. J Bone Joint Surg 1981;63-B(3):383–386.

59. Scapinelli R. Studies on the vasculature of the human knee joint. Acta Anat 1968;70:305.

60. Scuderi G, Scharf SC, Meltzer LP, Scott WN. The relationship of lateral release to patella viability in total knee arthroplasty. J Arthroplasty 1987;2(3):209–214.

61. Sculco TP. Local wound complications after total knee arthroplasty. In: Ranawat CS, ed. Total-Condylar Knee arthroplasty: technique, results and complications. New York: Springer-Verlag, 1985:194–196.

62. Thomas BJ, Moreland JR, Amstutz HC. Infection after total joint arthroplasty from distal extremity sepsis. Clin Orthop 1983;181:121–125.

63. Van Royen BJ, O'Driscoll SW, Dhart WI, Salter RB. A comparison of the effects of immobilization and continuous passive motion on surgical wound healing in mature rabbits. Plast Reconstr Surg 1986;78(3):360–366.

64. Villee DB, Powers ML. Effect of glucose and insulin on collagen secretion by human skin fibroblasts in-vitro. Nature 1977;268:156.

65. Wehl LM. Hormonal regulation of macrophage collagenase activity. Biochem Biophys Res Commun 1977;74:296.

66. Werb Z. Biochemical actions of glucocorticoids on macrophages in culture. J Exp Med 1978;147:1695.

67. Westfall TC, Watts DT. Catecholamine excretion in smokers and non-smokers. J Appl Physiol 1964;19:40.

68. Wilson MG, Kelley K, Thornhill TS. Infection as a complication of total knee-replacement arthroplasty, risk factors and treatment in sixty-seven cases. J Bone Joint Surg 1990;72A(6):878–883.

69. Wong RY, Lotke PA, Ecker ML. Factors influencing wound healing after total knee arthroplasty. Orthop Trans 1986;10:497.

86

Planning and Techniques for Unconstrained Revision Total Knee Replacement

Kenneth Gustke

Introduction

A revision total knee replacement is a significantly different operative procedure from a primary total knee replacement. Usually, a revision total knee replacement requires the use of specially designed revision total knee implants. The operative procedure is more technically demanding, especially if the use of unconstrained components is the goal. The joint line position and ligamentous balancing must be perfect. Preoperative planning is necessary to assist with these intraoperative technical decisions.

Implant Considerations

Tibial Components

In general, as with any total knee replacement, the least constrained implants possible are the most desirable as long as the knee is ultimately stable (1, 2). Occasionally, very conservative bone resections can be accomplished, and, if the collateral and posterior cruciate ligaments are intact, primary total knee components can be used. This, however, is rather rare. Use of a revision system with tibia components that are asymmetrically shaped (Fig. 86.1) is even more advantageous than in primary total knee replacement. The cancellous bone in the proximal tibia in a revision situation is usually either deficient or very soft; thus, cortical bone support becomes mandatory. Because the normal tibia is wider in the anteroposterior dimension medially than laterally, asymmetrical tibial components achieve cortical contact both medially and laterally without medial undersizing or the need for lateral overhang.

Tibial bone loss secondary to erosion from a loose component or from component removal can usually be replaced with a thicker tibial liner, to reestablish the joint line. Occasionally, tibial bone loss extends distal to the proximal fibula. Most revision knee systems do not have thick enough polyethylene tibial liners to replace this amount of bone loss. Also, because the tibia becomes narrower distally, a mismatch of a required small tibial component and liner with a large femoral component can occur. A preferable solution is to use a specially designed thicker tibial revision baseplate (Fig. 86.2) that is tapered and wider proximally than distally to allow use of a wider tibial liner more compatible with the femoral component, thus producing a more normal contour to the proximal tibia.

Femoral Components

On the femoral side, distal and posterior femoral bone loss of 2 to 5 mm usually occurs after removal of a fixed cemented or uncemented component, or even more bone may be eroded by osteolysis or motion from a loose component. Accurate positioning of the femoral component is critical to proper knee balancing. If a conventional primary femoral component is used in the face of bone loss, the joint line will be displaced proximally and the anterior-posterior diameter will be narrowed. Use of revision femoral components designed with increased buildup posteriorly and distally (Fig. 86.3) is usually necessary to reestablish anatomic joint positions (1, 3).

A recent review of 91 revision total knee replacements performed by the author between January 1987 and December 1993 revealed that 36% of revised tibial components employed a primary component, whereas primary femoral components were used only 28% of the time. Use of revision femoral components is usually necessary to reestablish the correct joint line position. Primary components are used mainly in cases with minimal bone loss.

Femoral and Tibial Stems

In revision surgeries, frequently even after appropriate bone cuts, the surfaces still have cavity deficiencies, the cancellous bone is soft, and the cortices are thin. Having revision components with stems of various length and thickness to obtain endosteal cortical contact (Fig. 86.4)

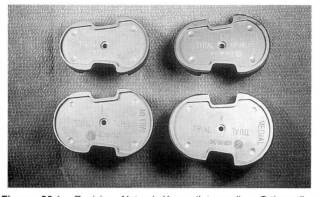

Figure 86.1. Revision Natural Knee (Intermedics Orthopedics, Austin, TX) tibial baseplate trials with asymmetrical shape. The anteroposterior diameter is wider medially.

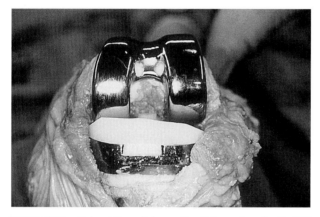

Figure 86.2. Natural Knee (Intermedics Orthopedics, Austin, TX) +14 mm revision tibial component.

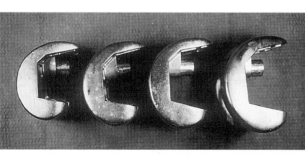

Figure 86.3. Natural Knee (Intermedics Orthopedics) revision femoral component.

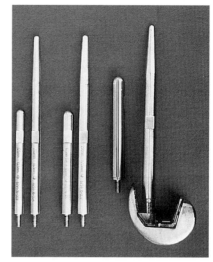

Figure 86.4. Natural Knee (Intermedics Orthopedics) revision femoral trial stems of various lengths and thicknesses.

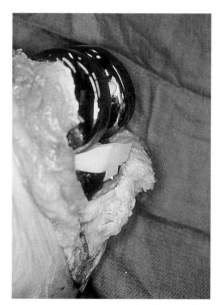

Figure 86.5. Natural Knee (Intermedics Orthopedics) ultra-congruent tibial liner with extra anterior buildup to resist posterior insufficiency.

increases implant stability (2) by redistributing some of the stresses away from the implant interface and allows for the option of uncemented fixation. The stems are usually not cemented, thereby lessening proximal stress shielding and the difficulty of later removal (4, 5).

Tibial Polyethylene Liner and Implant Constraint

If the posterior cruciate ligament is intact, a standard posterior cruciate retained tibial liner can be used. However, in the majority of knee revision surgeries, the posterior cruciate ligament is either absent or so very attenuated that it is not very functional. Even with an absent posterior cruciate ligament, a congruent or dished tibial insert will provide adequate stability if the flexion and extension spaces are tightly balanced (6). Additional posterior stability can be achieved, if needed, with an ultracongruent tibial liner, which is a dished liner with increased anterior buildup (Fig. 86.5). Another option is to use a stabilizer-type implant where the central eminence of the tibial liner is contained in a femoral housing to inhibit posterior subluxation (7). If the medial or lateral collateral ligaments are deficient, a special constrained posterior stabilizer device with a high central eminence and parallel sides congruent with the femoral housing is required, inhibiting varus-valgus motion (8–10). The author's preference is to avoid posterior stabilizer-type implants if possible because of the increased femoral bone resection required. Also, theoretically, increased stresses may be transmitted to the fixation interfaces, which can, in cases of poorer bone quality, result in early component loosening (11).

If the knee has mild lateral collateral laxity only, a congruent tibial liner combined with postoperative bracing for 3 months will usually provide ultimate stability without having to use a constrained posterior stabilizer device. Bracing alone, however, will not be successful for medial collateral insufficiency (3, 10). Fixed or rotating hinge devices are rarely necessary (12, 13). Since the Intermedics Revision Natural Knee System (Intermedics Orthopedics, Austin, TX) became available to the author in 1988, of 79 knee revisions, only one case has required the use of a posterior stabilizer implant, five cases have needed a constrained posterior stabilizer implant for medial collateral insufficiency, and two cases have required a rotating hinge implant. One of these rotating hinges was used for the revision of an extensor mechanism deficient knee, and the second was used for posterior instability associated with hamstring spasticity.

Cement Versus Cementless Fixation

The choice of cement versus cementless fixation is determined by the same criteria as in primary knee replacement; those criteria are the quality of the bone, the obtainable implant-bone stability, and the patient's age. The author has found that the bone quality in most of his patients undergoing revision total knee replacement has not been ideal for cementless fixation. A rough guide used to ascertain bone quality is whether the cancellous bone is indentable with the fingertip. Of 91 revision total knee replacements performed between January 1987 and December 1993, 14% were performed uncemented, whereas, during that same time period, cementless fixation was used in approximately 25% of the author's primary knee replacements.

Preoperative Evaluation

Reason for Revision

Preoperative evaluation is an important step in the management of the failed total knee replacement. A loose total knee replacement is fairly easy to diagnose. In the author's experience, revision knee replacement for loosening is becoming less prevalent. Of revisions performed by the author between 1987 and 1989, 88% were for loosening, but from 1990 to 1993, only 20% had the diagnosis of loosening. Most of the revisions performed by the author recently are for instability, polyethylene wear, or reimplantation after infection. With improvements in instrumentation that have provided more accurate varus-valgus alignment and with better implant design, early loosening has become less common. Instability due to ligament imbalance, component malrotation, and patellofemoral malalignment is becoming more common. These technical errors are less easily prevented by instrumentation.

Unstable Arthroplasty

In the evaluation of an unstable knee arthroplasty, it is necessary to determine why the implant is unstable. Instability can be present because the collateral ligaments are out of balance, the posterior cruciate is absent, the components are malaligned, or because the joint line is malpositioned. Physical examination and radiological examination are both necessary. Stability needs to be assessed to varus and valgus stress in 90 degrees of flexion as well as in full extension. If the knee is unstable to either varus *or* valgus stress in both flexion *and* extension, the knee probably has a loose collateral ligament or a tibial or femoral component that is malaligned. The radiograph will confirm if the instability is secondary to component malalignment. If the knee is unstable only in flexion, either to varus or valgus stress, and stable in extension, the cause is usually malrotation of the femoral component. Physical examination is the only way this condition can be diagnosed because the radiograph will appear normal. If varus as well as valgus instabilities are present in flexion *or* in extension but not in both, femoral component malposition or malsizing are likely. The flexion-extension spaces are not balanced.

If insufficient distal femur has been resected, the joint line will be brought distally. The extension space can be tensed with a thinner tibial liner or with a lower tibial bone resection, but the flexion space cannot be adequately tensed (Fig. 86.6). If too much distal femur is resected, the joint line will be more proximal. If a thicker tibial liner is used to obtain adequate tension to the extension space, the flexion space will be overstuffed, and poor flexion will result (Fig. 86.7). If a thinner tibial liner is used to allow flexion, the knee will be unstable in extension. Knowing the etiology of the instability allows appropriate corrections at the revision surgery to be made to prevent a recurrence of instability.

Joint Line Malposition

Joint line malposition is frequently observed with unstable unconstrained revision total knee replacements. Even stabilizer-type implants can be unstable with gross joint line malposition. If there is distal femoral bone loss with a primary femoral component used for replacement and if the resultant increased extension space is replaced with a thicker tibial component, stability will be present in extension. This knee will have poor flexion, however, because the narrower flexion space will not allow for that thicker tibial liner (Fig. 86.7). If posterior femoral bony deficiency is present and a smaller femoral component is used that does not adequately tense the flexion space, the knee will have good stability in extension but, again, will have flexion instability (Fig. 86.8). In the presence of posterior femoral bone loss, if an appropriately sized primary component is used and if the component is placed against the deficient bone posteriorly, allowing it to sit more anteriorly, the knee will still have flexion instability (Fig. 86.9), and the anteriorly translated femoral

Figure 86.6. Insufficient distal femoral bone resection. *Left,* The knee can be adequately tensed with a thinner tibial liner or lower tibial cut. *Right,* The flexion space remains lax with knee instability in flexion likely.

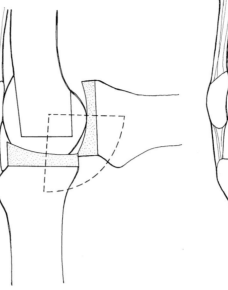
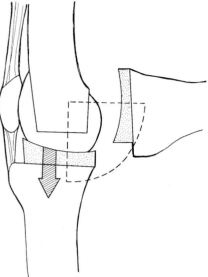

Figure 86.7. Excessive distal femoral bone resection. The knee can be adequately tensed with a thicker tibial liner, but because the flexion space will not accommodate this thickness, poor flexion will result. If a thinner tibial liner is used to allow knee flexion, the knee will be too lax in extension.

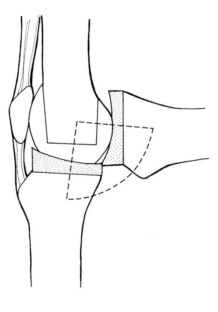
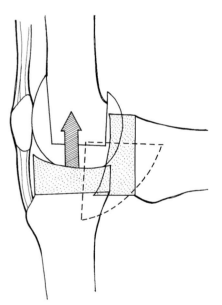

Figure 86.8. The anteroposterior diameter of the distal femur, inadequately replaced with a small femoral component, leads to laxity of the knee in flexion.

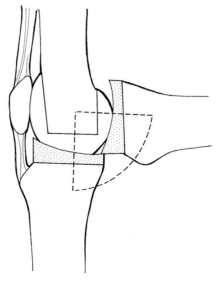
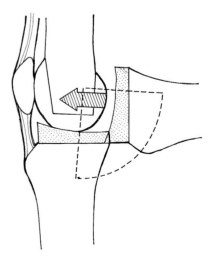

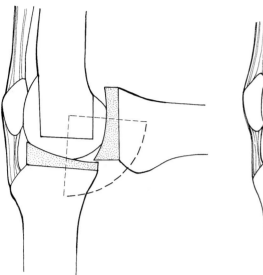 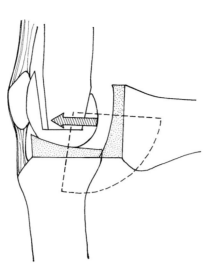

Figure 86.9. The correct size for the femoral component is shown, but is subject to anterior displacement because of posterior femoral bone loss resulting in knee laxity in flexion.

component will cause patellofemoral problems (14). The normal anteroposterior distal femoral dimension must be reestablished for proper joint mechanics.

Use of a revision femoral component with a thicker distal and posterior buildup does not negate the need to determine the correct joint line position preoperatively in order to achieve it intraoperatively. The following is an example. The postrevision total knee replacement radiograph with unconstrained implants shows what appears to be excellent component positioning (Fig. 86.10, A). However, this patient's knee subluxated posteriorly in flexion. If one were to determine the position of the normal joint line from measurements taken from the contralateral normal knee, one would be able to see that the joint line has been translated distally, thus accounting for the instability as the result of flexion laxity (Fig. 86.10, B). The second revision radiograph demonstrates correction of the joint line that has resulted in knee instability in extension and flexion (Fig. 86.10, C).

Planning Joint Line Correction

How does one go about reestablishing the joint line position correctly intraoperatively? The first and most important step is not performed intraoperatively, but preoperatively by determining where the joint line should be. Obtain the radiograph of the involved knee pre-total knee replacement. If this radiograph is not readily available, the contralateral knee can be used if it has not been operated on, or, even if it also has had a total knee replacement, it can be used as long as it is functioning well. In any case, bilateral knee radiographs should be obtained routinely in the evaluation of a problem total knee replacement in order that various measurements from anatomic points to the joint line can be taken. The case shown in Figure 86.11, A, illustrates this preoperative planning technique. Although the component alignment appears satisfactory, this patient has had instability in flexion. The first step must be to verify that the comparison knee films are the same magnification, otherwise the measurements will need to be factored by

the magnification difference. On the anteroposterior radiograph, measurements are taken from the joint line to the adductor tubercle, the lateral epicondylar ridge, and the fibular head (Fig. 86.11, B). On the lateral view, measurement is from the joint line to the junction of the posterior femoral condyle and the shaft and to the fibular head (Fig. 86.11, C). The anteroposterior diameter of the distal femur is also measured. Postoperatively, measurements should be reproduced if the posterior cruciate ligament is intact. If the posterior cruciate ligament is not intact, the femoral measurements will be the same, but the distance to the fibular head will be about 2 to 3 mm larger, owing to the need for a thicker tibial component. In the illustrated case, the joint line placement is too distal, producing the flexion instability. The templates are placed over the normal knee to determine the correct size of the femoral component by matching the anteroposterior diameter of the femur (Fig. 86.11, D). Then the correctly sized femoral template is placed over the abnormal knee, taking into consideration where the joint line should be. (Fig. 86.11, E–G). One can then determine the amount of bone resection or replacement that will be required from the femur in relation to the distal end of the existing femoral component. Similar templating is performed on the tibial side, mainly to be sure the revision system will be able to replace the bone loss present. It may not be necessary to carry out all of these measurements. The points of reference that are the most obvious on the radiograph and easiest to locate intraoperatively are the ones to use. The measurements on the postoperative radiographs should demonstrate the correct joint line position (Fig. 86.11, H and I).

Intraoperative Techniques

Implant Balancing

It is important to know the joint line position preoperatively and then to be able to determine it intraoperatively because the instrumentation cannot be relied on to determine it. The most important determination is

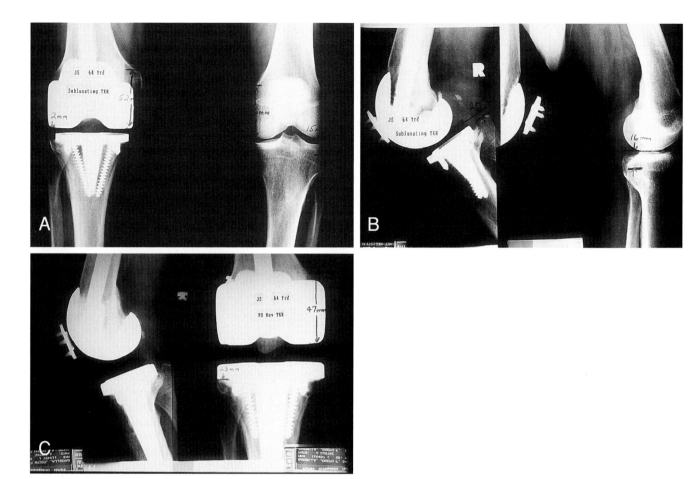

Figure 86.10. JS is a 64-year-old female; who has had a revision total knee replacement with unconstrained implants. The knee is still unstable in flexion. **A** and **B,** Comparison measurements of the joint line position to the contralateral knee demonstrates that the joint line has been distally positioned. **C,** The postrevision radiograph demonstrates appropriate joint line position, and the knee was now stable.

the position of the distal femoral cut. Obviously, the normal articular surfaces are not available as reference points as in a primary knee, from which to base a predetermined thickness of bone resection. It cannot be assumed that the correct amount of bone was resected previously. The easiest way to determine where the new distal femoral cut should be is to mark off the distance, determined from preoperative radiographs, proximal to the distal end of the existing femoral component that corresponds to the appropriate new distal femoral osteotomy site. An alternative method is to measure distal to the adductor tubercle the preoperatively determined distance to the joint line minus the thickness of the new revision component. An indirect technique using spacer blocks can also be used to determine the level of the distal femoral cut. The tibial osteotomy and the posterior femoral cuts are made first, leaving the distal and anterior femoral cuts for last. Tenser devices such as laminar spreaders are used to determine the amount of flexion space present. Then whatever amount of bone that needs to be removed from the distal end of the femur is marked to make the tensed extension space equal to the flexion space plus the difference in the distal and posterior thicknesses of the revision femoral

components. The potential problem with this technique is that it assumes a normal collateral ligament balance that may not be present.

After all the bone cuts are made, insert the trial components and always compare the varus/valgus laxity in extension and flexion. If the flexion and extension spaces are not equal, the femoral cuts need to be adjusted.

The next most difficult intraoperative determination in revision knee surgery is the femoral component rotation. Normal posterior femoral condyles are not present to use as a reference guide, as in a primary knee replacement. One may or could assume that the previous rotation was correct depending on how well the knee prior to revision is balanced in flexion to varus-valgus stress. However, a better method to determine femoral component rotation is to use a line between the medial and lateral epicondyles as a guide. But, it must be remembered that the medial epicondyle is more anterior than the lateral and that the epicondylar line forms a 6 to 8 degree angle to the posterior femoral condyles. Another preferred method to determine femoral component rotation is to use the tensor block technique with laminar spreaders. The tibial cut is made first. With the

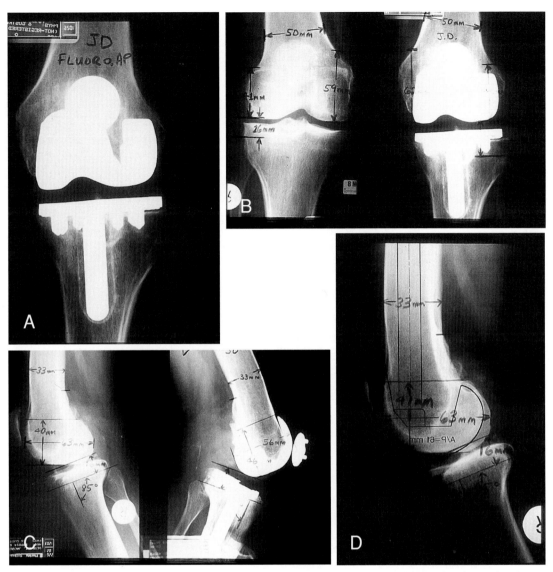

Figure 86.11.   This patient had knee instability in flexion. **A,** The radiograph demonstrates what appears to be properly positioned components. **B** and **C,** The joint line distance from the fibular head, medial and lateral femoral epicondyles, and the junction of the posterior femoral condyle and the shaft is compared on the total knee and plain knee radiographs. **D** and **E,** The appropriate size femoral component is determined from the plain radiographs. **F** and **G,** The femoral component template is placed over the abnormal knee radiograph with the joint line position predetermined. The distance of the new distal femoral osteotomy to the distal aspect of the existing femoral component is determined for later use at surgery. **H** and **I,** The postrevision radiographs demonstrate appropriate joint line position.

knee at 90 degrees of flexion, the laminar spreaders are used to tense up the medial and lateral side. The anterior and posterior femoral cuts are then made parallel to the tibial cut. It should be noted that the potential problem with this method is that it assumes that the collateral ligaments are intact and balanced.

Dealing with Bony Defects

Minimal bone loss of the distal femur can be dealt with rather easily by using a revision femoral component with increased distal and posterior femoral component thickness. Usually after making appropriate bony cuts for such a revision femoral component, there are no, or minimal, bony defects remaining. If minimal bony de-

fects are still present, they can be filled with cement or particulate bone graft, depending on whether cement or uncemented fixation is used. If initial bone loss is minimal, one can even occasionally use a primary femoral component. This situation is not common.

On the tibial side, when there is more bony erosion on one side than the other, it is very tempting to resect bone low enough to obtain good cortical bone circumferentially. This may result in such an aggressive cut that sufficient component replacement thickness is not available. The lower the cut, the poorer the bone strength (8), and the greater is the potential for ligament or patellar tendon compromise. If the tibial resection level will be close to, or below, the fibular head, it is

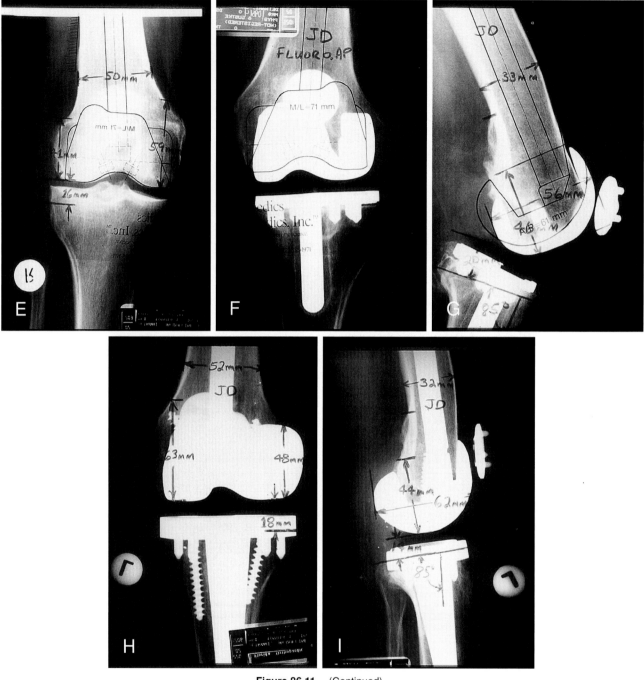

Figure 86.11. (Continued)

preferable to make a higher tibial cut as long as there is at least 50% of the cortex remaining on the deficient side. Preferably, a tibial component with an anatomic asymmetrical baseplate (wider AP diameter medially than laterally) is used to be able to contact the remaining cortex (Fig. 86.1).

Another viable option for unicondylar tibial defects is to use a metal spacer (3, 15). The author's preference is to use a flat spacer rather than a wedge because instruments can be used to make a more accurate bony cut.

Also, a flat spacer allows compression rather than shear at the interface, a preferable biomechanical loading pattern. If the defect is greater than 1 cm in height and the patient is relatively young, the author prefers to use a bulk bone graft (5, 15). Rigid graft fixation is mandatory (16). A interface perpendicular to the tibial axis is also created at the host-graft interface to lessen shear stress and to aid in better apposition. The bone graft is temporarily fixed with K-wires while the proximal tibial cut is made. The graft is permanently secured with vertical screws through the tibial baseplate, or, if the graft is very large, screws are placed obliquely through the graft into the host tibia. Use of an implant with a long wide uncemented stem will resist some of the stresses on the graft and, if uncemented, will not create stress shielding (5). If there is bicondylar tibial bone loss below the proximal end of the fibula, special tibial components such as the Intermedics +14 Revision Tibial Base Plate (Fig. 86.2) is used. With its oblique sides, this base plate provides a more natural contour, but, more importantly, allows for the use of a wider tibial liner, better matching the size of the femoral component.

Central tibial defects are less challenging (3). One can obtain circumferential cortical contact for tibial component support, and the central defects can be filled with particulate bone graft if the defects are large or if uncemented fixation is desired, or the defects can be filled with cement if they are small in size.

Collateral Ligament Balance

If the joint line is in the correct position, if the femoral and tibial component cuts are in the appropriate alignment, and if there is still varus or valgus instability in both extension and flexion, then collateral ligament imbalance is present. If there is varus or valgus instability in flexion only, the femoral component rotation should be rechecked. If there is varus and valgus laxity in flexion, but not in extension, the joint line position is incorrect.

In general, collateral ligament imbalance is addressed in a manner similar to a primary knee replacement by releasing the tight side (17). The lateral collateral ligament is released from the femur and the medial collateral ligament is released from the tibia. There may be a severe collateral ligament imbalance in revision knee arthroplasty, (greater than 1 cm). A ligament release of this degree requires the use of a thicker tibial polyethylene liner and may produce a relative patella baja with potential impingement of the patellar component against the tibial liner. In this situation, it is preferable to tighten or advance the loose collateral ligament (6). It is essential to obtain medial stability on the operating table, whereas the lateral side can be left a little loose if the knee is in the correct valgus alignment. By using a postoperative hinged brace for 3 months, the lateral side usually tightens.

Results with Unconstrained Implants for Revision Knee Arthroplasty

Between July 1988 and December 1993, revision total knee replacements were performed by the author, of which 66 used the Natural Knee (Intermedics Orthopedics, Austin, TX) system. Of these cases, 17 had primary components only. The other 49 had at least one revision component. During this period, 13 cases had implants other than Natural Knee components; of the 13 cases, 5 were partial revisions requiring compatible components, 5 were cases requiring constrained posterior stabilizer implants for medial collateral insufficiency, and the 4 other cases required rotating hinges.

In the author's series of revision total knees, the unconstrained Natural Knee System (Intermedics Orthopedics, Austin, TX) was used in 48 cases. Between January 1987 and June 1992, 39 knees with follow-up for longer than 6 months were reviewed. Utilizing a modified Hospital for Special Surgery scoring method (9), the mean score for this group was 78. There was not much difference in the knee score for the more difficult cases when revision components were used when compared with the simpler revisions where primary components were used. The mean score for the patients in which only primary Natural Knee components were utilized was 77. The mean score for the patients in which one or all Revision Natural Knee components were used was 78. Of cases in this series, 74% had a good or excellent result. These results are certainly better than reported series using constrained posterior stabilizer implants (8, 10), and they are comparable to those using a posterior stabilizer (7). Only two of the fair or poor results in this series were related to implants. One patient has fibrous ingrowth of an uncemented tibial component, but does not feel his discomfort warrants revision surgery. The other patient had persistent posterolateral instability and was stabilized by re-revision using an ultracongruent liner.

One of the main advantages of using unconstrained revision knee components is the potential for excellent knee flexion. Mean maximum flexion for the patients in the authors series with revision unconstrained components was 106 degrees, and 104 degrees for the patients with primary unconstrained components. This is approximately 15 degrees greater than the average maximum flexion for the posterior stabilized implant cases in the series described by Goldberg et al. (7).

Bulk allografts were required in 6 of the 35 patients in which Revision Natural Knee (Intermedics, Austin, TX) components were utilized. Of these cases, 4 had femoral bulk allografts only while 2 had both tibial and femoral bulk allografts. Unconstrained implants were successfully used even in these cases requiring major grafts.

Summary

In summary, the basic principles of revision knee arthroplasty include saving bone during component removal and being conservative with new bone cuts. There will often be some distal and posterior femoral bone loss, so a knee arthroplasty system with femoral components revision with increased distal and posterior buildup will usually avoid bone grafting and will allow implant-host bone contact for cementless fixation if desired. Revision components with variable length and thickness stems may be required to lessen the stresses on weak interfaces. It is important to reestablish the proper joint line position. Incorrect joint line position leading to instability is probably the most common reason for failure of revision total knee arthroplasty. If the joint line is properly reestablished, stabilizer-type devices are usually not necessary (18). Knee stability requires correct joint line position, femoral component rotation, and collateral ligament balance. In some total knee revisions, it may be preferable to advance a loose collateral ligament rather than release a tight one if significant imbalance is present. Using the techniques illustrated, successful stable knees can be achieved using unconstrained implants.

References

1. Bryan RS, Rand JA. Revision total knee arthroplasty. Clin Orthop 1982;170:116–122.
2. Rand JA, Bryan RS. Results of revision total knee arthroplasties using condylar prostheses. J Bone Joint Surg 1988; 70A:738–745.
3. Scott RD. Revision total knee arthroplasty. Clin Orthop 1988;65–77.
4. Brooks PJ, Walker PS, Scott RD. Tibial component fixation in deficient tibial bone stock. Clin Orthop 1984;184:300–302.
5. Elia EA, Lotke PA. Results of revision total knee arthroplasty associated with significant bone loss. Clin Orthop 1991; 271:114–121.
6. Jacobs MA, Hungerford DS, Krackow KA, Lennox DW. Revision total knee arthroplasty for aseptic failure. Clin Orthop 1988; 78–85.
7. Goldberg VM, Figgie MP, Figgie HE III, Sobel M. The results of revision total knee arthroplasty. Clin Orthop 1988;228:86–92.
8. Donaldson WF, Sculco TP, Insall JN, Ranawat CS. Total Condylar III knee prosthesis: Long-term follow-up study. Clin Orthop 1988;21–28.
9. Insall JN, Dethmers DA. Revision of total knee arthroplasty. Clin Orthop 1982;170:123–130.
10. Rosenberg AG, Verner JJ, Galante JO. Clinical results of total knee revision using the Total Condylar III prosthesis. Clin Orthop 1991;273:83–90.
11. Walker PS. Requirements for successful total knee replacements. Orthop Clin North AM 1989;20(1):15–29.
12. Bargar WL, Cracchiolo A III, Amstutz HC. Results with the constrained total knee prosthesis in treating severely disabled patients and patients with failed total knee replacements. J Bone Joint Surg 1980;62A:504–512.
13. Rand JA, Chao EYS, Stauffer RN. Kinematic rotating-hinge total knee arthroplasty. J Bone Joint Surg 1987;69A:489–497.
14. Figgie H E III, Goldberg VM, Heiple KG, et al. The influence of tibial-patellofemoral location on function of the knee in patients with the posterior stabilized condylar knee prosthesis. J Bone Joint Surg 1986;68A:1035–1040.
15. Rand JA. Bone deficiency in the total knee arthroplasty. Use of metal wedge augmentation. Clin Orthop 1991;271:63–71.
16. Dorr LD. Bone grafts for bone loss with total knee replacement. Orthop Clin North AM 1989;20(2):179–187.
17. Sculco TP. Total Condylar III prosthesis in ligament instability. Orthop Clin North Am 1989;20(2):221–226.
18. Cohen B, Constant CR. Subluxation of the posterior stabilized total knee arthroplasty. J Arthroplasty 1992;7(2):161–163.

87

Infected Total Knee Arthroplasty

Dean T. Tsukayama and Ramon Gustilo

Introduction

Infection of a total knee arthroplasty (TKA) is a serious complication that jeopardizes the function of the joint and occasionally threatens the life of the patient. The incidence of infection is approximately 1 to 5%. (1–3) with a higher infection rate reported with revision TKA and rheumatoid arthritis. As with all prosthetic-device-associated infections, TKA infections are characterized by persistence of the bacterial pathogen despite antibiotic therapy and often require removal of all prosthetic material to eradicate the infection. Management of these infections can also be complicated by problems with bone loss, joint instability, and necrosis of the soft tissue overlying the joint, resulting in a lower rate of successful reimplantation of an infected TKA compared to total hip arthroplasty infections (4).

The primary goals in treating the infected total knee replacement are twofold—to control the infection and to restore the prosthesis to a functional and durable state. The first consideration is to control the infection. When infection is uncontrolled, it can result in disabling pain, progressive bone loss, or even death from systemic complications. In general, therapy should be given with the intent of eradicating the infection, although in selected cases, control of infection may be limited to suppression of symptoms. For example, in cases where poor general medical condition precludes the surgery necessary to remove an infected prosthesis, a patient may be treated with an indefinite course of oral antibiotics. Our experience, however, is that suppressive antibiotic therapy is unlikely to provide satisfactory long term results (4a).

In recent years, progress has been made in determining the factors that make treating prosthetic device infections so difficult. Investigators have found that polymorphonuclear leukocyte (PMN) function is impaired in the presence of foreign bodies (5–9), and that bacteria can evade both host defense cells and antibiotics by at-taching to the prosthetic device and covering themselves with an extracellular slime known as glycocalyx (10). It also appears that bacteria become less susceptible to killing by antibiotics when associated with a foreign body (11). In most cases, removal of all prosthetic components and cement is necessary to cure the infection.

A second goal is to retain or restore optimal joint function at the completion of therapy. Ideally, one would like to complete treatment with a well-fixed, painless total knee arthroplasty in place. There is scant data to support treating the infection while retaining the original infected arthroplasty. In virtually all cases of established infection, components have to be removed, and the patient has to be entered into a two-stage protocol with delayed reimplantation after the infection has been treated (12). However, in some number of cases, the final result is less than ideal: namely, the infected prosthesis must be removed, but a replacement cannot be reimplanted, and patients are left with an arthrodesis, pseudoarthrosis, or even in rare occasions, amputation.

A key question, then, in the management of infected total knee arthroplasties from the viewpoint of eradicating infection and also preserving joint function is, "Under what circumstances should the prosthesis be removed?" In general, the answer is that an attempt at treatment while retaining the prosthesis may be made in acute infections (13–15), but clinically significant, chronic infections almost always require that the prosthesis be removed. Various classification systems, based on time of onset of infection following knee implantation and on the source of the bacteria, i.e., contamination versus hematogenous seeding, have been proposed to guide therapy. Types of infections are distinguished as early, late, and hematogenous infections. Depth of infection must also be considered (16).

At Hennepin County Medical Center, we have treated prosthetic joint infections according to a classification

1563

system based on the clinical presentation of the infection. In our experience, total knee (and hip) arthroplasty infections present in one of four clinical settings:

1. Positive intraoperative culture (PIOC);
2. Early postoperative infection (EPOI);
3. Late chronic infection (LCI);
4. Acute hematogenous infection (AHI).

In this chapter, we review the literature as it pertains to the diagnosis and management of total knee arthroplasty infections, present our management protocols based on the clinical setting, and report our results of the outcome of therapy in 46 cases.

Positive Intraoperative Culture

This is an occult infection diagnosed by multiple positive cultures obtained during revision arthroplasty (or primary arthroplasty, if the joint was previously operated on) of a knee in which infection was not suspected prior to operation. Cultures are obtained from the joint, femur, and tibia, and an infection is diagnosed if the same pathogen is recovered from two or more cultures. Cultures that are positive in the broth only are disregarded in this setting.

Occasionally, it may be difficult to distinguish clinically an insidious TKA infection from aseptic loosening. Preoperative evaluation for infection is not completely reliable, with knee aspiration yielding the pathogen in as few as 45 to 70% of cases (12, 17). In some cases, infection is not recognized until revision surgery is performed for presumed aseptic loosening (12, 18). The replacement prosthesis has already been implanted when the operative cultures become positive.

Our experience is that PIOC occurs much less frequently in total knee arthroplasties than in total hip arthroplasties. The treatment for this infection is 6 weeks of an appropriate antibiotic without any further operation. Three patients have been treated with this regimen; all remain free of infection after more than 2 years of follow-up.

Early Postoperative Infection

Early postoperative infections presumably occur as a result of contamination with bacteria introduced at the time of surgery or early in the postoperative period. The diagnosis is usually obvious with presenting symptoms of drainage, erythema, swelling, and impaired wound healing. The significance of this category of infection is that, in contrast to chronic infections, treatment with irrigation, debridement, and retention of the prosthesis may be attempted with a reasonable expectation of successful outcome. However, no consensus exists on the period of time after surgery that defines an early infection, with definition ranging from 2 weeks (13, 19, 20) to as long as 3 months (21). Successful eradication of infection and salvage of the original prosthesis with surgical debridement appears to range from 50 to 85% (13, 22).

We have defined an Early Postoperative Infection as one that occurs within 1 month after implantation of the total knee arthroplasty. In our experience, infections that are diagnosed beyond 1 month after surgery (excluding Acute Hematogenous Infection) rarely can be cured without prosthesis removal.

Treatment of this infection is surgical debridement and antibiotic therapy, while retaining the prosthesis. Surgical debridement for deep infections (those extending into the joint) includes exchange of the polyethylene liner to allow exposure posteriorly for better debridement and irrigation.

If the infection is superficial (not extending into the joint), duration of antibiotic therapy can be limited to 2 weeks. Deep infections as well as infections in which the depth of infection cannot be easily judged are treated with high-dose, intravenous antibiotics for 6 weeks. Of 16 patients with deep early postoperative infections treated with this protocol, 14 were free of infection and had retained their prostheses after at least 2 years of follow-up (for a success rate of 87%). We previously reported that 6 patients with early superficial infections were also treated successfully with debridement and 2 weeks of antibiotic therapy (16).

Late Chronic Infection

A Late Chronic Infection is a deep infection of the knee occurring later than 1 month after placement of the prosthesis, usually presenting insidiously, with gradual onset of pain and swelling. Initially, the primary consideration in the differential diagnosis is aseptic loosening of the knee. Left untreated, the infection can progress to cause wound dehiscence, draining sinuses, and bone resorption. Systemic manifestations are minimal and bacteremia is rare.

Several studies have shown that debridement alone without removal of the prosthesis is an inadequate procedure for chronic infections, with a reported success rate of 10 to 20% (19, 23). In one intriguing report, Freeman found that debridement alone was successful in 4 patients with uncemented prostheses (24). However, given the poor expected outcome with debridement, it cannot be advocated as a first procedure, because of the additional cost and morbidity of subsequent procedures that are likely to be necessary (15).

With prosthesis removal, successful eradication of infection can be achieved in 80 to 90% of cases (25–28). Although the literature reaches no consensus on this point, it is our experience that Gram-negative bacilli are no more difficult to treat than other pathogens (12). Immediate exchange arthroplasty has been reported by Goksan to be successful in 17 of 18 cases of infected TKA (25). Bengston also has reported that there was no difference in outcome of infected TKA treated with either immediate or delayed exchange arthroplasty (2). Nonetheless, delayed exchange arthroplasty has become the standard of care in the treatment of chronic TKA infections. Success in eradicating infection approaches or exceeds 90% in several reports (12, 26, 27). However, the outcome with respect to function may be somewhat less successful. Morrey found that, after an average of 8 years of follow-up, only about 53% (8 of 14) of reimplanted prostheses were still in place and only 33% were felt to be functionally successfully (17). Windsor reported good to excellent function in 63% (24 of 38) of patients with an average follow-up of 4 years (12).

There are also a number of patients with infected TKA who are not acceptable candidates for revision arthroplasty. These include patients with excessive bone loss, inadequate soft tissue, or medical contraindications to the required multiple surgical procedures. For these patients, the surgical options that remain are resection arthroplasty, arthrodesis, or amputation. Falahee has reported that resection arthroplasty eliminated infection in 89% of patients and 54% (15 of 28) could ambulate independently (29). Arthrodesis in earlier reports was found to be successful in 70 to 80% of cases (30, 31), and subsequent series have not improved upon these results (32, 33).

Our treatment of this infection begins with surgical debridement and prosthesis removal. Antibiotic-impregnated cement spacer and antibiotic beads are placed into the joint and intramedullary canal of the femur and tibia, and intravenous antibiotics are administered for 6 weeks. Upon completion of antibiotic therapy, the patient is observed for 2 weeks, and a repeat erythrocyte sedimentation rate and C-reactive protein are obtained. If no clinical signs of infection recur and if there is no laboratory evidence of ongoing inflammation, a revision

arthroplasty is done. Operative cultures are obtained, and the patient is kept on appropriate paraoperative antibiotics until all culture results are finalized. If infection persists, the patient is treated for an additional 6 weeks with high dose antibiotic therapy, but no further surgery is performed (3, 28). After a minimum of 2 years of follow-up, 14 of 17 patients (82%) treated with this protocol remain free of infection with the revision prosthesis in place.

Surgical Management for Late Chronic Infection

Delayed Exchange Arthroplasty

Radical surgery consisting of thorough debridement, total synovectomy, removal of all prosthetic components, and cement is performed (Fig 87.1 and 87.2). Intraoperative cultures and Gram stains are taken from the joint, femur, and tibia and also from the prosthetic surfaces in contact with bone and cement. Synovectomy of the suprapatellar pouch, lateral and medial recesses, and the posterior compartment is performed. The knee is copiously irrigated with a normal saline solution containing bacitracin and polymyxin. The bone cement is meticulously removed, and the adequacy of cement removal is checked by x-rays, if necessary. Tobramycin beads (90 to 120 6-mm beads) are packed into the femur and proximal tibia. The joint space is maintained by a cement spacer block impregnated with to-

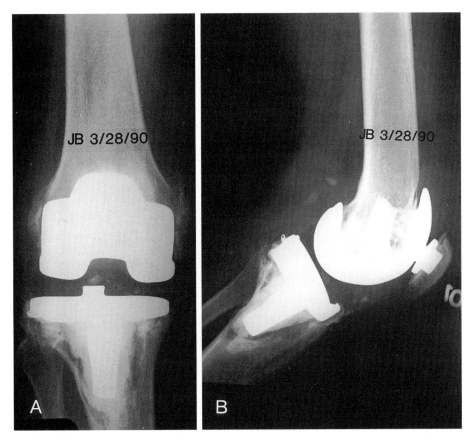

Figure 87.1. **A** and **B,** JB: Anteroposterior and lateral x-rays showed a wide and complete radiolucent line, at the cement/bone interface of the tibia component. Aspiration of the knee and culture revealed coagulase-positive staphylococci. Coagulase was positive. A previous revision surgery had been done 2 years before, prior to the onset of the present symptoms of pain and swelling. Sedimentation rate was 64mm/hr.

Figure 87.2. JB: Radical debridement was done including removal of knee components and bone cement. Antibiotic beads were used.

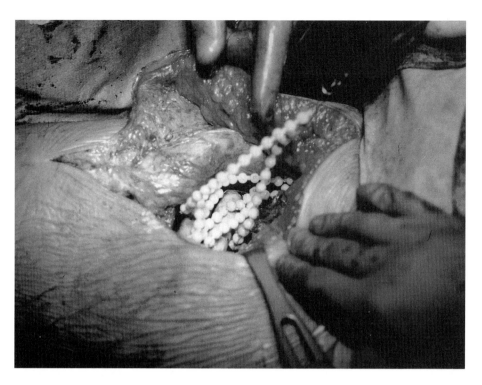

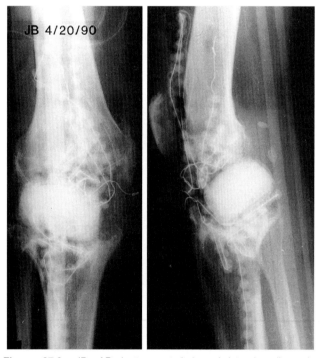

Figure 87.3. JB: AP (anteroposterior) and lateral radiographs showed the tobramycin-impregnated cement block and the tobramycin beads inserted into the joint, the distal femur, and the proximal tibia.

bramycin (2.4 g in 40 g of bone cement) (Fig. 87.3). The joint space is measured for sizing the component thickness that will be used at the time of delayed exchange. Two hemovac drains are inserted without pressure. The wound is closed in two layers in an interrupted manner.

Pressure dressings are applied with lateral and medial plaster splints with the knee in full extension. The drain is removed in 3 to 4 days when drainage is less than 25 ml in an 8-hour period. If excessive drainage persists, surgical debridement and irrigation is repeated. At 2 weeks, the sutures are removed, and the knee is placed in a knee immobilizer or a cylinder cast for 4 weeks. The patient is continued on appropriate parenteral antibiotic therapy for 6 weeks. At 6 weeks, the antibiotics are discontinued, the cast or splint is removed, and sedimentation rate and C-reactive protein are obtained. If there is suspicion of persistent infection based on laboratory data or clinical appearance, the knee is aspirated for culture and Gram stain. If there is no evidence of ongoing infection, exchange arthroplasty is done in 10 to 14 days (Fig. 87.4).

Careful preoperative planning is essential in selecting the right components and inserts, making use of a modular knee system in order to achieve optimal alignment with ligamentous stability. A posterior, stabilized module is generally used. The antibiotic cement and spacer block are removed; multiple samples are obtained for culture and Gram stain; a specimen is sent for frozen section histologic examination. The knee joint is debrided and copiously irrigated. Recutting of the distal femur and tibia is done using posterior stabilized instrumentation, and distal and posterior wedges are usually needed. The selected components are then cemented in place with antibiotics in the bone cement (1.2 to 2.4 g of tobramycin in 40 g of bone cement). The wound is closed in a regular manner with hemovac suction. Antibiotics are continued for 5 days until operative culture results are finalized. If there is no potential wound-healing problem, the knee is started on active range of motion using a continuous passive motion machine. If a

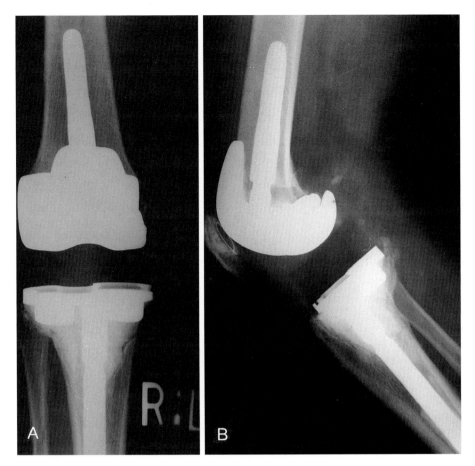

Figure 87.4. JB: AP and lateral x-rays taken 2 years after a delayed exchange to a posterior stabilized knee prosthesis revealed stable prostheses with good alignment and no recurrence of infection.

problem with wound healing is anticipated or found, the knee is placed in a knee-immobilizer cast for 2 weeks until the wound is completely healed. It is our experience that range of motion is not compromised by the short immobilization period. If the Gram stain is positive for bacteria or the frozen section shows acute inflammation during the revision surgery, the prosthesis should not be implanted, at least until culture results are known. If infection persists, the protocol for delayed exchange can be repeated. Consideration should also be given to arthrodesis as an alternative approach. Occasionally, the Gram stain and frozen section are negative and the new prosthesis is implanted, but multiple operative cultures are reported as positive in 2 to 5 days after the operation. In these cases, the antibiotic therapy (routinely given for 5 days postoperatively in all revision cases because of this possibility) is extended for 6 weeks, but no further surgery is done.

Arthrodesis

Arthrodesis has been an accepted salvage procedure for infected arthroplasty (Figs. 87.5–87.7). A variety of surgical techniques using different devices have been reported. A review of published series revealed fusion rates of 17 to 88% (30–32, 34). Failure was associated with lack of bone apposition, persistence of infection and inadequate immobilization. The indications for arthrodesis are:

1. A young patient with osteoarthritis in a single joint;
2. Poor skin envelope around the knee joint, i.e., infected skin graft or infected local flap;
3. Quadriceps or patellar tendon rupture;
4. An immunosuppressed host.

The surgical procedure consists of removal of all components and bone cement, total synovectomy, and placement of antibiotic beads. As much bone as possible is preserved. The wound is closed, and, at 2 weeks, a formal arthrodesis is carried out. The distal end of the femur and the proximal end of the tibia are recut and connected together in full extension. The three devices commonly used to achieve stability are external fixation, intramedullary nail, and double plates.

Our procedure of choice would be a long intramedullary nail inserted down to the midshaft or lower third of the tibia. The surgical technique consists of an arthrotomy of the knee and the introduction of a long guide pin from the distal femur up to and through the greater trochanter in a retrograde manner. A skin incision can be made over the trochanteric area where the pin protrudes. Then the guide pin is pushed down into the distal tibia; the femoral and tibial surfaces are aligned and opposed to each other in full extension through the knee incision, which is then closed. The intramedullary canal of the femur and tibia are reamed through the trochanteric incision to an appropriate size

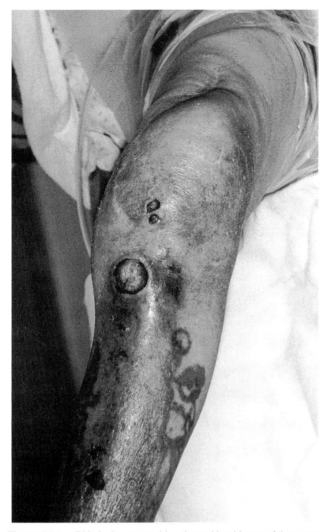

Figure 87.5. RM: A sixty-year-old patient with a history of three previous operations, including skin grafting, prolonged i.v., and oral antibiotic therapy. This resulted in failure to control infection. As shown in the photograph, knee components have been removed, revealing two draining sinuses with poor soft tissue enveloped around knee joint.

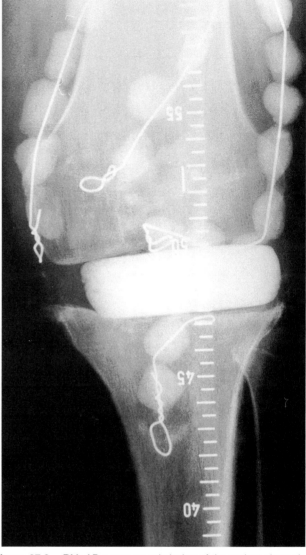

Figure 87.6. RM: AP x-rays on admission of the patient showed a cement block and antibiotic beads in place after all knee components and cement had been previously removed.

(usually not smaller than 13 mm in diameter). It is essential to know the size and length of the intramedullary nail that wil be required. This is easily determined at surgery when the infected knee components are removed. Bone grafting is usually not needed. The patient is placed in a cylinder cast for 6 weeks and allowed early weight bearing. The rate of union is very high with this technique. In the one case of nonunion we have encountered, repeat nailing with a larger nail was successful.

The main contraindication to the use of an intramedullary nail is a prosthesis or other device in the ipsilateral femur or a deformed femur or tibia. In these cases, double-plating is an alternative procedure (Fig. 87.8). Double-plating is also indicated when lengthening is needed that requires extensive bone grafting to fill the gap. External fixation is a third method for obtaining arthrodesis (Figs. 87.9 and 87.10). It requires immobilization for a minimum of 10 to 12 weeks and has been

associated with a high incidence of nonunion and pin tract infection.

The major problem with arthrodesis after removal of an infected knee prosthesis is bone loss, which results in a shortening of 1 to 3 inches after fusion. The patient must also realize that conversion of a surgically fused knee (especially fusion done for infected TKA) to a total knee replacement is not an option for the future.

Resection Arthroplasty

Resection arthroplasty (Figs. 87.11 and 87.12) should be reserved for the severely disabled patient with multiple joint disease and low functional demand.

Pain relief and control of infection are not always accomplished by this surgery (25, 30). A failed arthrodesis may result in a resection arthroplasty. Overall, patients with resection arthroplasties have inadequate pain relief and cannot stand or walk for an extended period. Often,

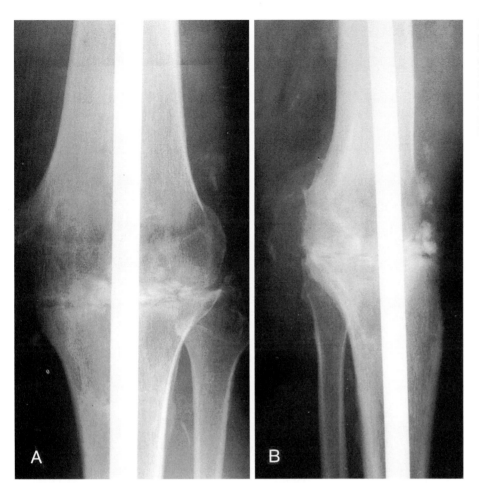

Figure 87.7. **A** and **B**, RM: Repeat surgical debridement with Intramedullary nailing of the distal femur and tibia was done; a new set of antibiotic beads and an impregnated antibiotic cement block were reinserted and 2 weeks later reamed. AP and lateral x-rays revealed progression of union at 3 months. There was no recurrence of sepsis, and patient is full weight bearing without pain.

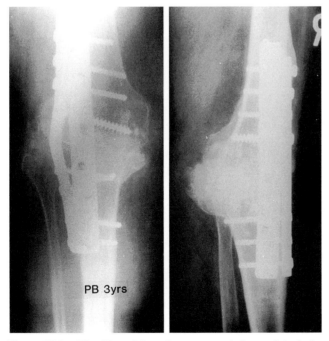

Figure 87.8. PB: AP and lateral x-ray revealed complete fusion after double-plating for an infected knee. The patient is rheumatoid and has a total hip replacement in the same extremity. There was no recurrence of sepsis.

the patient becomes wheelchair-bound, especially if there is arthritis in the contralateral leg.

Amputation

The primary indication for amputation is uncontrollable and potentially life-threatening sepsis, even after debridement and prosthesis removal. A second indication is failure to obtain wound healing after numerous surgical failures, usually in an immunocompromised patient. In an elderly patient, an above knee amputation usually results in the patient being confined to a wheelchair. It is very seldom that a patient with an amputation for an infected total knee arthroplasty, even with a good opposite leg, will choose to use an above knee prosthesis.

Acute Hematogenous Infection

As the name suggests, an Acute Hematogenous Infection presents with an acute onset of symptoms in the affected prosthetic joint and is associated with a documented or suspected bacteremia. Although this infection can occur early or late in relation to joint surgery, the typical case involves a prosthesis that has been functioning well for months or years and that suddenly becomes painful and swollen; this is associated with systemic manifestations, such as fever and chills.

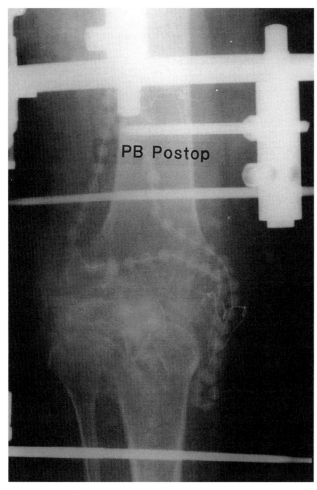

Figure 87.9. PB: AP and lateral x-rays showing external fixation for knee fusion following infected TKA. Antibiotic beads were incorporated at the initial closure and removed at 2 weeks.

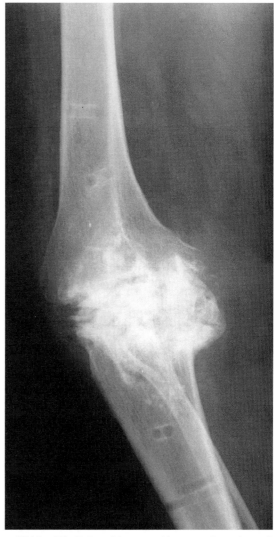

Figure 87.10. PB: Delayed bone grafting was done. Lateral x-ray revealed nonunion at 6 months. Double-plating was done to accomplish fusion.

Soft tissue infections are most frequently implicated as the source of the bacteremia (2, 35). Bengtson has reported in 2 series totaling 408 patients that 25 to 47% of all total knee arthroplasty infections were hematogenous in origin (2, 36).

An Acute Hematogenous Infection differs from a Late Chronic Infection (whose source of infection may also be hematogenous) in the length of time that the infection is present in the joint before it becomes clinically apparent.

Bliss noted that of 13 late TKA infections with acute onset of symptoms, the 4 successfully retained arthroplasties all had evidence of infection for less than 1 week prior to debridement. Borden and Gearen have advocated classification of hematogenous infections as acute if they were treated within 2 weeks of onset of symptoms. The maximum time period allowable for successful treatment with the arthroplasty in situ is unknown, but it is likely to be weeks, rather than months, with the greatest chance of success associated with the shortest duration of symptoms.

Our treatment protocol for this infection is similar to treatment for Early Postoperative Infections. Unless it

is found to be loose at surgery, the prosthesis is retained. Thorough debridement is done, including exchange of the polyethylene liner in a modular arthroplasty. Antibiotic-impregnated beads are placed for 2 weeks. Appropriate intravenous antibiotics are administered for 6 weeks. Patients are not prescribed oral antibiotics after completion of the course of intravenous therapy. Of 5 patients treated with this protocol, 3 have been cured of infection and have retained their prostheses for at least 2 years. One patient required a delayed exchange arthroplasty that was successful, and we ended with a revised arthroplasty.

Microbiology and Antimicrobial Therapy

Staphylococci are the most frequently recovered pathogens in TKA infections (37). Coagulase-positive staphylococci are often associated with a toxic presentation and purulent drainage and, in our experience, are the most frequently recovered pathogen in Early Post-

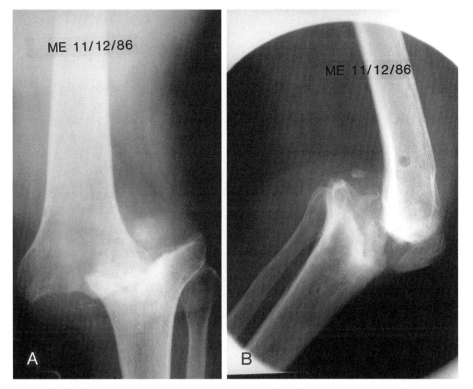

ME 11/12/86

A

ME 11/12/86

B

Figure 87.11. A and **B,** ME: A 53-year-old patient. Three years after resection and arthroplasty for infected TKA, the patient was unable to bear weight and was a very unhappy person. AP and lateral x-rays revealed unstable, displaced knee joint without components. A delayed total knee replacement was done.

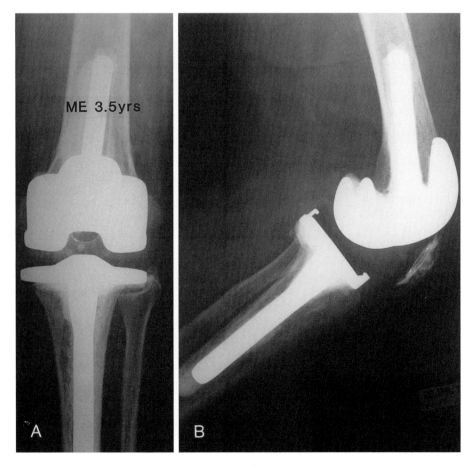

ME 3.5yrs

A

B

Figure 87.12. A and **B,** ME: Three and a half years after a delayed exchange total knee replacement, the patient is without pain and has an active range of motion from 0 to 80 degrees. AP and lateral x-rays revealed the knee components to be stable with no evidence of loosening and no recurrence of sepsis.

operative Infections and Acute Hematogenous Infections. Coagulase-negative staphylococci cause a more indolent infection, sometimes difficult to distinguish from aseptic loosening and are most often isolated in Positive Intraoperative Cultures and Late Chronic Infections. Treatment of staphylococci depends on their susceptibility to β-lactam antibiotics. If they are susceptible to oxacillin or nafcillin, these antibiotics are the agents of choice for treatment. Acceptable alternatives include first generation cephalosporins, vancomycin, and clindamycin. Staphylococci that are resistant to oxacillin, nafcillin, or methicillin (MRSA) should also be considered resistant to all other β-lactam antibiotics. For these pathogens, vancomycin is the drug of choice. For patients unable to tolerate vancomycin, treatment with trimethoprim-sulfamethoxazole or with a quinoline agent such as ciprofloxacin may be considered, depending on the results of susceptibility testing. Teicoplanin, an investigational glycopeptide, has in vitro activity against staphylococci resistant to β-lactams and may be another alternative agent if it is approved for general use. The percentage of resistant coagulase-positive staphylococci varies widely from institution to institution. The majority of coagulase-negative staphylococci are β-lactam resistant.

Penicillin is the antibiotic of choice for the treatment of streptococcal infections, but these bacteria are susceptible to many agents including other β-lactams, clindamycin, and vancomycin. Enterococci, however, can be much more difficult to treat. Ampicillin, penicillin, or vancomycin are the agents most frequently used, but enterococci resistant to each of these agents have been reported.

Gram-negative bacilli can be effectively treated with third generation cephalosporins, other extended-spectrum β-lactams, quinolones, and trimethoprim-sulfamethoxazole. Useful specific agents include ceftrixone, an intravenous agent that can be given once daily, and ciprofloxacin (and other quinolines), agents that can be given orally. Ceftazidime and imipenem are the most reliably active antibiotics against *Pseudomonas aeruginosa*.

Anaerobes, especially Gram-positive cocci such as *Peptostreptococcus*, are occasionally isolated from TKA infections. The antibiotic of choice for the treatment of anaerobic Gram-positive cocci is penicillin. Anaerobes are often found in prosthesis infections as one of several bacteria. In many of these cases, a single antibiotic with a broad spectrum of activity can be chosen to treat all significant pathogens. If this is not possible, clindamycin or metronidazole is usually added to treat the anaerobic component.

References

1. Meislin R, Zuckerman JD. Management of an infected total knee arthroplasty. Bull Hosp Jt Dis Orthop Inst 1989;49:21–36.
2. Bengtson S, Knutson K. The infected knee arthroplasty. Acta Orthop Scand 1991;62:301–311.
3. Rosenberg AG, Haas B, Barden R, et al. Salvage of infected total knee arthroplasty. Clin Orthop 1988;226:29–33.
4. Lo NN, Tsukayama DT, Wicklund B, Gustilo RB. Infected total knee replacements—Prosthesis retention or removal? Presented at the Annual Meeting of the American Academy of Orthopaedic Surgeons. New Orleans, Februrary, 1994.
4a. Tsukayama DT, Wicklund B, Gustilo RB. Suppressive antibiotic therapy in chronic prosthetic joint infections. Orthopedics 1991;14:1–4.
5. Petty W. The effect of methylmethacrylate on bacterial phagocytosis and killing by human polymorphonuclear leukocytes. J Bone Jt Surg Am 1978;60A:752–757.
6. Petty W, Caldwell JR. The effect of methylmethacrylate on complement activity. Clin Orthop 1977;128:354–359.
7. Vaudaux PE, Zulian G, Huggler E, et al. Attachment of staphylococcus aureus to polymethacrylate increases its resistance to phagocytosis in foreign body infection. 1985;50:472–577.
8. Pascual A, Tsukayama DT, Wicklund BH, et al. The effect of stainless steel, cobalt-chromium, titanium alloy, and titanium on the respiratory burst activity of human polymorphonuclear leukocytes. 1992;280:281–288.
9. Gristina A, Costerton J. Bacterial adherence to biomaterials and tissue. J Bone Joint Surg. 1985; 67A:264–273.
10. Chuard C, Lucet J-C, Rohner P, et al. Resistance of *Staphylococcus aureus*. Recovered from infected foreign body in vivo to killing by antimicrobials. J Infect Dis 1991;163:1369–1373.
11. Borden L, Gearen P. Infected total knee arthroplasty. J Arthroplasty. 1987;2:27–36.
12. Bliss DG, McBride GG. Infected total knee arthroplasties. Clin Orthop 1985;199:207–214.
13. Burger RR, Basch T, Hopson CN. Implant salvage in infected total knee arthroplasty. Clin Orthop 1991;273:105–112.
14. Rasul AT, Tsukayama DT, Gustilo RB. Effect of time of onset and depth of infection on the outcome of total knee arthroplasty infections. Clin Orthop 1991;273:98–104.
15. Morrey BF, Westhold F, Schoifet S, et al. Long-term results of various treatment options for infected total knee arthroplasty. Clin Orthop 1989;248:120–128.
16. Windsor RE, Insall JN, Urs WK, et al. Two-stage reimplantation for the salvage of total knee arthroplasty complicated by infection. J Bone Joint Surg 1990;72A:272–278.
17. Paya CV, Wilson WR, Fitzgerald RH. Management of infection in total knee replacement. In: Remington JSS, Swartz MN, eds. Current Clininical Topics in Infectious Disease. Vol 9. New York: McGraw Hill, 1988:222–240.
18. Teeny SM, Dorr L, Murata G, Conaty P. Treatment of infected total knee arthroplasty. J Arthroplasty 1990;5:35–39.
19. Ahlberg A, Carlson AS, Lindberg L. Hematogenous infection in total joint replacement. Clin Orthop 1978;137:69–75.
20. Gristina A, Kilkin J. Total joint replacement and sepsis. J Bone Joint Surg. 1983;65A:128–134.
21. Walker RH, Schurman DH. Management of infected total knee arthroplasties. Clin Orthop 1984;186:81–89.
22. Woods GW, Lionberger DR, Tullos HS. Failed total knee arthroplasty. Clin Orthop 1983;173:134–190.
23. Freeman MAR, Sudlow RA, Casewell MW, et al. The management of infected total knee replacements. J Bone Joint Surg. 1985;67-B:764–768.
24. Goksen SB, Freeman MAR. One-stage reimplantation for infected total knee arthroplasty. J Bone Joint Surg 1992;74B:78–134.
25. Insall JN, Thompson FM, Brause BD. Two-stage reimplantation for the salvage of infected total knee arthroplasty. J Bone Joint Surg 1983;65A:1087–1098.
26. Wilson MG, Kelley K, Thornhill TS. Infection as a complication of total knee-replacement arthroplasty. J Bone Joint Surg 1990;72B:878–883.
27. Wilde AH, Ruth JT. Two-stage reimplantation in infected total knee arthroplasty. Clin Orthop 1988;236:23–25.
28. Falahee MH, Matthews LS, Kaufer H. Resection arthroplasty as a salvage procedure for a knee with infection after a total arthroplasty. J Bone Joint Surg 1987;69A:1013–1021.
29. Hagemann WF, Woods GW, Tullos HS. Arthrodesis in failed total knee replacement. J Bone Joint Surg 1978;60A:790–794.
30. Broderson, MP, Fitzgerald RH Jr, Peterson LFA, et al. Arthrodesis of the knee following failed total knee arthroplasty. J Bone Joint Surg 1979;61A:181–185.
31. Knutson KAJ, Jovelius L, Lindstrand A, Lidgren L. Arthrodesis after failed knee arthroplasty. Clin Orthop 1984;191:202–211.
32. Rand JA, Bryan RS, Chao EYS. Failed total knee arthroplasty treated by arthrodesis of the knee using the Ace-Fischer apparatus. J Bone Joint Surg 1987;69A:39–45.
33. Stulberg S. Arthrodesis in failed total knee replacements. Orthop Clin North Am 1982;13:213.
34. Stinchfield FE, Bigliani LU, New HC, et al. Late hematogenous infection of total joint replacement. J Bone and Joint Surg 1980;62A:1345–1350.
35. Bengtson S, Knutson KAJ, Lidgren L. Treatment of infected knee arthroplasty. Clin Orthop 1989;245:173–178.
36. Ivey FM, Hicks CA, Calhoun JH, et al. Treatment options for infected knee arthroplasties. Rev Infect Dis 1990;12:468–477.

88

Revision Technique

Robert E. Booth, Jr.

Preoperative Planning
Preoperative Preparation
Exposure
Component Extraction—Tibial
Component Extraction—Femoral
Component Extraction—Patella
Reconstruction
Defects
Fixation

In the entire spectrum of orthopaedic surgical procedures, there remain few challenges as great as the revision of a failed total knee arthroplasty. The reasons for this parlous state of affairs are many. The etiology of the primary failure may be multifactorial, fully apparent only after inspecting the knee at surgery. Bone and soft tissue defects routinely exceed preoperative expectations. Skin coverage and extensor mechanism management present unique challenges, not found in hip surgery. Occult infections may suddenly become apparent. Instrumentation and revision techniques still lag behind those available for revision hip surgery, often obliging the surgeon to fall back on his cerebral icon of a "generic" total knee for guidance. Although the sequence of steps cannot be planned as predictably as in a primary total knee, some pattern is necessary for a successful result to be achieved.

Preoperative Planning

Although an entire chapter has been devoted to this crucial aspect of revisional knee surgery, certain points are so important that they merit reiteration. First, one must make every possible attempt to identify the precise cause of failure of the index arthroplasty. Exploratory knee surgery has a very low rate of success, which is directly proportional to the surgeon's ability to understand the mode of failure. Secondly, one must have a very high index of suspicion for infection, even in the face of normal preoperative scintigraphic, serologic, and microbiologic tests. The clinical appearance of infection should override these other factors, and the surgeon should err on the side of delayed exchange if the issue is equivocal. Thirdly, the records of prior surgeries must be scrutinized for surgical approach, soft tissue releases, and the make and size of the initial components. Templating for appropriate sizing, using the contralateral limb if necessary, is crucial. Fourthly, one must

have sufficient modular components to accommodate a full range of augmentation and constraint, as additional defects may occur to the joint during the revision operation itself. Lastly, one must remember not to repeat the prior error, perhaps the common failing in revisional knee surgery.

Preoperative Preparation

Every knee arthroplasty undergoing revision should have preoperative aspiration, occasionally multiple times, to obtain adequate culture material for the diagnosis of infection. Particularly if no organism is recovered, one should withhold preoperative antibiotics until fluid and tissue from the joint interfaces can be harvested for further analysis. A tourniquet proportional to the thigh should be placed as far proximally as possible on the limb, since extensile exposure is occasionally required beyond that originally anticipated. Occasionally, it may be necessary to forego tourniquet hemostasis, such as in individuals with vascular bypass grafts or with severely compromised peripheral circulation. The limb should also be examined thoroughly after anesthesia has been induced to confirm motor relaxation and to identify any additional instabilities unmasked by the anesthetic.

Exposure

In the best of circumstances, a longitudinal midline incision will have been used in the index arthroplasty, providing an appropriate approach for the revisional surgery. It is important to avoid the creation of adjacent parallel skin incisions unless absolutely necessary. In this instance, sham incisions to confirm circulatory status may be helpful. One should avoid particularly the creation of large flaps, although this may occasionally be required in those patients who have had eccentric lateral approaches to the primary valgus knee (Fig. 88.1).

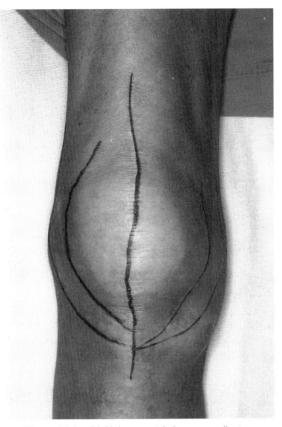

Figure 88.1. Multiple eccentric knee complicate approach.

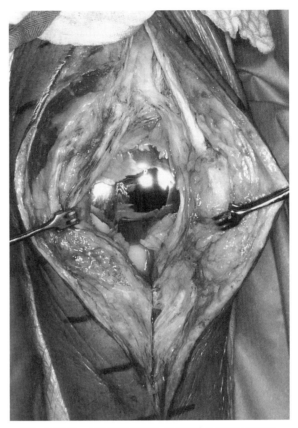

Figure 88.2. Infection merits aggressive synovectomy.

Once the joint has been entered, it is most appropriate and convenient to perform a partial synovectomy and scar excision. Certainly the clearance of a prior scar will facilitate the subsequent exposure and is appropriate at this time. The extent of synovectomy performed depends on the reason for knee failure. If infection is diagnosed, a synovectomy incorporating all nonviable soft tissues should be considered (Fig. 88.2). Viable synovium should be retained, because it is the antibiotic delivery system to the joint that may determine the success of the revision. If particle disease and osteolysis are the cause of failure, a full synovectomy should be performed to clear the joint of particles that might perpetuate osteolytic activity in the revised knee. It is often easiest to begin the synovectomy around the patella, moving from the inferior surface of the patellar tendon proximally across the anterior aspect of the femur and back down along the medial side of the joint (Fig. 88.3). An electrocautery is helpful to define the margins and to remove the material from bone, while providing some hemostasis to these vascular tissues. The margins of the implant should be clearly delineated at this time, because their inspection is necessary later in the case. The posterior synovium usually cannot be reached at this point, but can be debrided later in the case with the limb held in extension by lamina spreaders (Fig. 88.4). A large curette can be used to separate the scar and synovium from posterior capsule. Longitudinal strokes will avoid perforating the capsule and dis-

turbing the neurovascular structures in the popliteal fossa. Posterior synovectomy and scar removal are crucial to rebalancing the knee, just as removal of these tissues anteriorly and laterally is important.

At this juncture, one must make a decision about the management of the eversion of the extensor mechanism. Full eversion is not always necessary, although it is helpful. From preoperative planning, one should know the extent of the prior procedures; in particular, one should know if a lateral retinacular release has been performed. If so, this would be appropriate to recreate at this time, because that aspect of the extensor blood supply has already been compromised. Often debridement of the scar and hypertrophic tissue in the lateral gutter will suffice to free the extensor for full knee flexion and patellar eversion (Fig. 88.5). If a lateral retinacular release is performed for the first time, one must be careful either to preserve or cauterize the lateral geniculate vessels.

A second option includes a turn down of the quadriceps mechanism, either in the form of a V-Y advancement or a transverse "rectus snip." These alternatives should *not* be combined with a lateral retinacular release, since they provide excellent exposure in and of themselves. One would prefer to avoid this approach in a knee that lacked flexion, since early postoperative motion may necessarily be compromised in order to protect the healing extensor.

A third alternative is to perform a very generous tibial tuberosity and anterior tibial crest osteotomy (Fig.

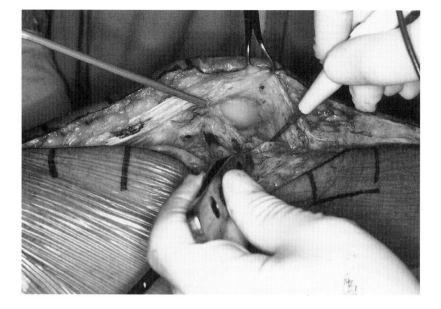

Figure 88.3. Synovectomy should be thorough.

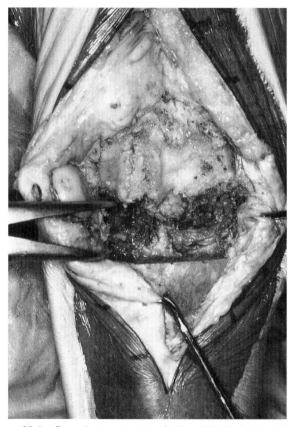

Figure 88.4. Posterior synovectomy facilitated by lamina spreaders.

88.6). This approach also allows superlative exposure and should not be accompanied by a concomitant lateral release, unless absolutely necessary for proper extensor tracking. Another virtue of this particular extensor approach is the ability, at termination of the procedure, to advance and to elevate the osteotomized crest, correcting a patella baja or better accommodating

an artificially elevated joint line. If the lateral soft tissue attachments to the tibial bone are preserved and if the osteotomized fragment is secured with screws or wires, early motion can be accomplished after surgery.

If none of these releases is necessitated, one should still consider protecting the extensor from accidental avulsion as attention is turned to the heavy work of removing the prior components. A towel clip, with one limb through the medial tibial metaphysis and the other limb through the insertion of the patellar tendon, will provide good insurance against the catastrophe of patellar tendon avulsion (Fig. 88.7).

Component Extraction—Tibial

At this point, the standard elevation of the medial tibial sleeve of soft tissue, often incorporating the semimembranosus and posterior capsular tissues can be performed, just as in a standard total knee arthroplasty (Fig. 88.8). This, coupled with the probable severance of any existing fibers of the posterior cruciate ligament, will allow the tibia to be delivered forward from under the femur. Reverse retractors are helpful to perpetuate this position, and the femoral component should be covered with sponges to prevent scratching if there is any thought to its retention. It is helpful at this point to use an electrocautery to define the margins of the tibial component, removing soft tissue and scar so that the interfaces are clearly visible. If the tibial plastic is modular, it should now be removed to create more space and to facilitate the dissection.

It is appropriate to attack the removal of the tibial component first. If the tibial prosthesis is plastic, a reciprocating saw can be used at the prosthesis cement interface to amputate the tray from its stem (Fig. 88.9). The stem and surrounding bone can then be attacked under direct vision. This is a very fortunate circumstance that usually results in almost no loss of tibial bone.

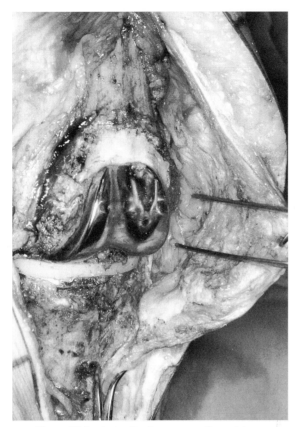

Figure 88.5. Lateral gutter scar merits excision.

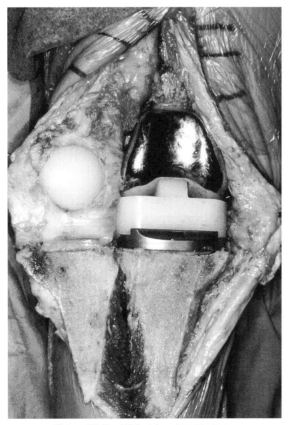

Figure 88.6. Wide tubercle osteotomy.

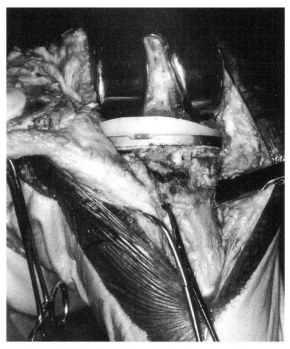

Figure 88.7. Towel clip retards extensor avulsion.

A metal-backed prosthesis may be more difficult to extract. Curved osteotomes should be used, with the attention directed to the prosthesis cement interface at all times, even if the bone cement interface appears loose (Fig. 88.10). Failure to follow this approach will frequently result in the loss of bone from posterior areas still attached to the cement. Once the tibial component has begun to rise from its bed, heavy extraction equipment can be used to pull it free. This should not be attempted, however, until the entire margin of the prosthesis has been separated from the bone beneath.

An uncemented prosthesis may be more difficult to remove, even though it is usually not uniformly attached to bone. One should attempt to identify the areas of spot welds, disrupting them either with an osteotome or a Gigli saw (Fig. 88.11). Screws and other fixation devices that pass through the tray should be removed at the outset. It is crucial in an uncemented component that the periphery be freed before any attempt at extraction. The pattern of bone loss from the removal of porous components is often peripheral—as opposed to the central bone loss typical of cemented components—and may create uncontained defects requiring augmentation or grafting (Fig. 88.12).

Any residual cement or foreign material within the canal can be approached with cement splitting techniques using sharp osteotomes and curved chisels (Fig. 88.13). It is most efficient at this time to complete the preparation of the tibia for the subsequent arthroplasty. External or internal guides can be used now to square the proximal tibial bone, exposing the healthy margins and allowing for proper sizing of a tibial implant. If a stem is to be used, the intramedullary canal of the tibia should be reamed at this point and a trial stem and tray

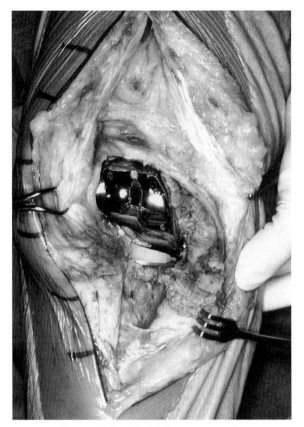

Figure 88.8.   Medial sleeve approach.

implanted to protect the tibial surface from accidental damage during the removal of the femoral and tibial components. No attempt should be made at this time to trim the tibia for bone grafting or augments, because the orientation of these supplements will define the rotation of the tibial component too early in the procedure. This is an option that should be saved for the terminal stages of the operation, when the rotational alignment of the trial components can be assessed collectively.

Component Extraction—Femoral

Secure femoral components can be difficult to remove because of their great conformity to the end of the femur, the often severe osteoporosis or stress shielding of the intercondylar notch, and the difficulty in exposing the posterior condylar regions without compromising the collateral ligaments (Fig. 88.14). The best approach is to use curved or angled osteotomes, beginning at the trochlear flange and progressing distally and then posteriorly to free the prosthesis. Again, one should always attack the prosthesis cement interface, even if the bone cement interface appears loose (Fig. 88.15). It is particularly important to clear the posterior "feet" of the prosthesis, as posterior bone loss is frequently the result of premature extraction. Uncemented components may require a Gigli saw, at least to the level of the femoral lugs, particularly if ingrowth has been extensive. Most stemmed devices are smooth and can be extracted readily. If this is not the case, special techniques such as ultrasonic vibration, proximal femoral fenestration, or prosthesis dismemberment may be necessary. It is helpful at this juncture to use a periosteal elevator to free the posterior capsule from the posterior femoral condyles, an area of frequent scar overgrowth and contracture common to most failed total knees (Fig. 88.16).

Figure 88.9.   Saw excision of all-poly tibial component.

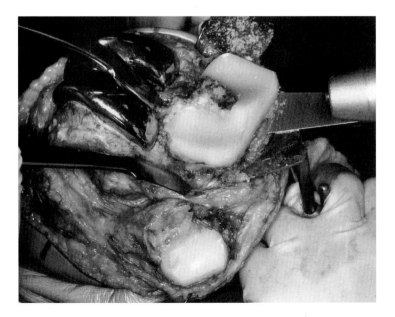

Figure 88.10. Metal-backed prosthesis removal using osteotomes.

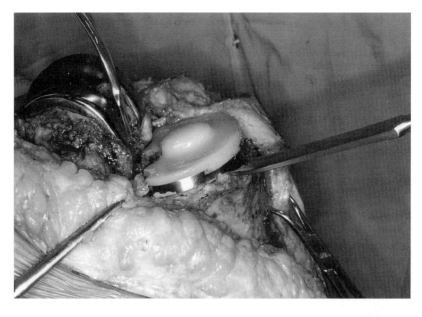

Figure 88.11. Gigli saw in action.

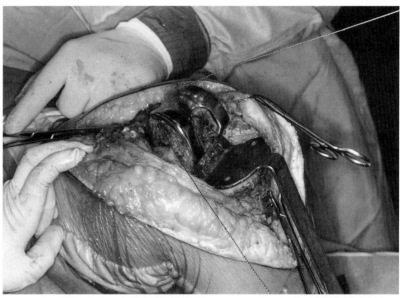

Figure 88.12. Central bone loss.

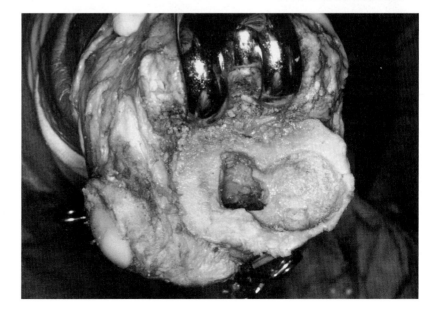

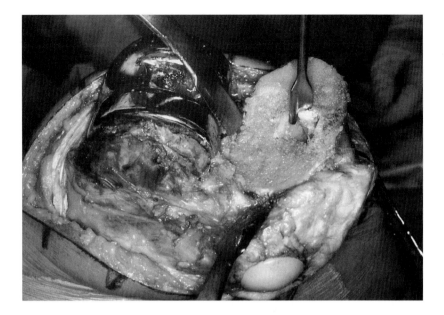

Figure 88.13. Snow removal!

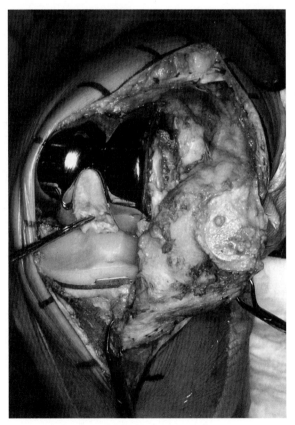

Figure 88.14. PCL too tight.

Component Extraction—Patella

If the patella is to be removed, great care must be taken not to disrupt the residual bone more than necessary. A wet fenestrated towel can be applied about the everted patella, secured by towel clips, to prevent debris from contaminating the joint. All-polyethylene patellae can be sawed flush from their bony bed (Fig. 88.17). The remaining stems and cement can be removed very effec-

tively with a standard burr. Metal-backed patellae are more troublesome, often requiring many small osteotomes or even small diamond tipped circular saws to free their posts when ingrowth has been successful (Fig. 88.18). It is often helpful to use a femoral impactor to provide resistance to osteotomes and other devices, so that the patella is not fractured in the removal process. If the patellar bone is quite thin, as in the case of inset patellae, it may be prudent to retain the prior prosthesis assuming its design is compatible with the trochlear flange of the new femoral device.

Reconstruction

At this juncture, one must now have an organized approach to the reconstruction of the knee arthroplasty. While systems and techniques may differ, several principles currently transcend individual designs and prejudices. The appropriate steps for reconstructing the joint are the following:

1. Reestablish the tibial plateau;
2. Apply the femoral component and balance the knee in flexion;
3. Adjust the femoral component to balance the knee in extension;
4. Reconstruct the patellofemoral articulation.

Since the tibia has already been squared and protected, one need only select the appropriately sized tibial tray to optimize coverage and to support the peripheral tibial cortical bone. Ideally, one would at this point begin recreating the appropriate joint line by restoring—with metal and plastic—appropriate tibial stature (Fig. 88.19). While the competence of the ligaments and the capsule may prejudice our choices, one should attempt to restore the joint line as close as possible to its original anatomic location. This generally lies one fingerbreadth above the tip of the fibular head, one fingerbreadth below the distal pole of the patella, or at the site of the residual meniscal rim scar (Fig. 88.20). A

Figure 88.15. Femoral component excision.

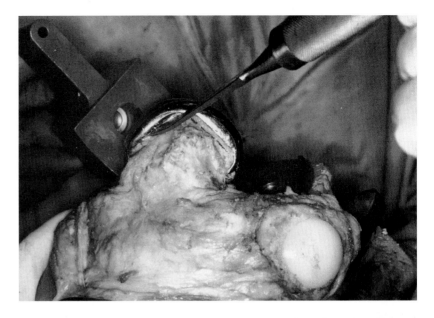

Figure 88.16. Femoral component with large bone loss.

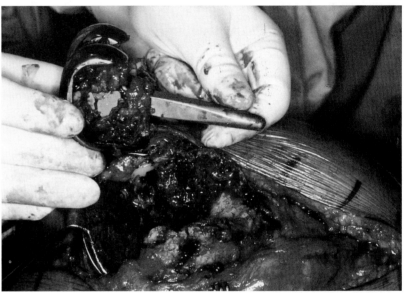

Figure 88.17. All-poly button sawed from bed.

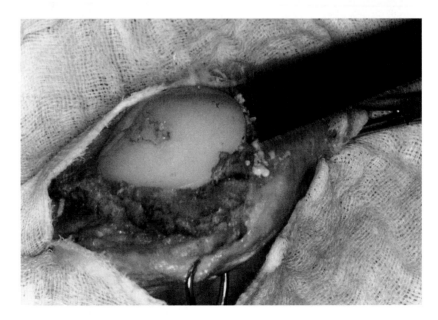

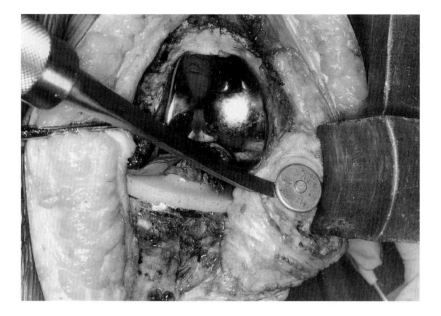

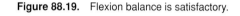

Figure 88.18. Metal-backed patellae hard to remove.

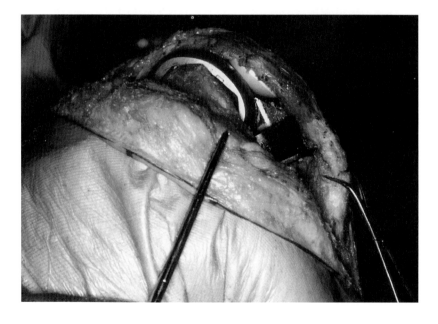

Figure 88.19. Flexion balance is satisfactory.

level and secure tibial platform is the base on which the rest of the arthroplasty will be constructed. If intramedullary rods are to be used, the tibia must be cut perpendicular to its long axis and with little rotational prejudice. Indications for intramedullary rods include the following:

1. The use of organic or prosthetic augmentations;
2. Weakened bone—osteoporotic or fractured;
3. Periprosthetic fractures;
4. Periprosthetic osteotomies.

The next step is to apply the appropriate femoral component and recreate the flexion gap balance. The size of the femoral component should be determined from preoperative templating or premorbid anatomy. In general,

a downsized component may be helpful, particularly in the revision setting, to improve joint motion. The femoral component should be secured in standard fashion at this point, ignoring bony defects of mild to moderate size until later in the reconstruction.

The posterior cruciate ligament, if retained, will reduce the size of the flexion gap but increase the complexity of soft tissue balancing. The vast majority of revision surgeons prefer to substitute for the posterior cruciate ligament in this setting. A tibial plastic is now selected that will confer stability on the knee in flexion. It is crucial that rotational alignment of the femoral component be considered as well, with some element of external rotation relative to the intercondylar line being appropriate to restore flexion balance and to improve patellar tracking. Intramedullary stems may be helpful, even in a tem-

Figure 88.20. Old meniscal scar suggests proper joint line.

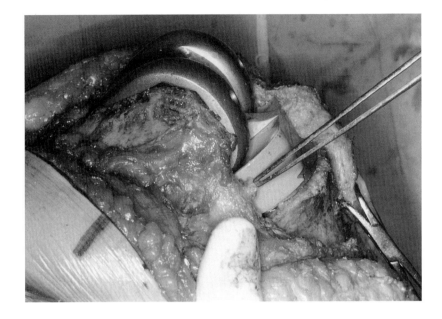

Figure 88.21. Extension gap to be restored.

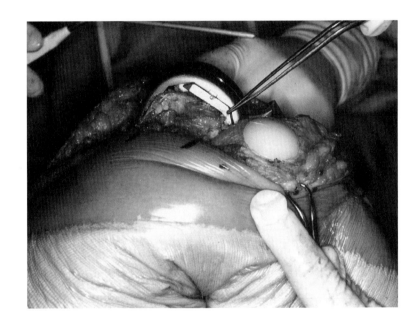

porary fashion, to confirm alignment and to secure the trial prosthesis before terminal implantation.

With the correct size femur in place and the tibial flexion gap already identified, one can now extend the knee and recreate soft tissue balance in extension (Fig. 88.21). Actually, this is quite simple, because one of three conditions will become apparent. If the extension balance fortuitously matches the extension balance, no further adjustment is necessary. If the knee is too loose in extension, distal augments may be added to the femoral component to bring it down on the femur and reestablish appropriate tissue tension (Fig. 88.22). If, as is more common, the knee is too tight in extension, small amounts of distal femoral bone can be removed or further posterior capsular release can be performed to restore full extension. (Fig. 88.23). These adjustments

must be made, however, with due consideration to the modification of the joint line, as determined by the relative position of the extensor mechanism and the old meniscal rim. In general, sacrifice and substitution of the posterior cruciate ligament creates a wider safety range and, thus, a more successful reconstruction.

The finale of the reconstruction is to rebuild the patellofemoral joint. Occasionally, one may prefer to retain the previous patellar prosthesis if it is unworn and secure. If the prior prosthesis has been removed, sufficient bone must remain to stabilize the new patellar button. An unstable or fragile patellar component is worse than none at all, and, occasionally, it may be preferable to tubularize or centralize the extensor tissues without benefit of prosthetic reconstruction. The inferior pole of the patella should never be below the level of the joint

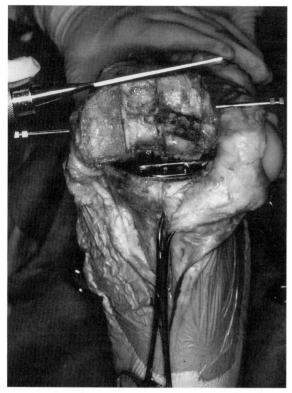

Figure 88.22.   Must establish extension balance.

line, lest excessive forces disrupt the extensor or flexion be incomplete. If this is the case, distal femoral augments can be used to lower the joint line even further. A lateral retinacular release may also be necessary to ensure proper extensor tracking.

Defects

At this juncture, it is appropriate to reconstruct the various bony and soft tissue defects that invariably exist in total knee revisions. While these are also the subject of another chapter, some principles are germane to the general techniques of total knee revision. As a rule, defects 5 mm or less can be filled with cement, 5 mm to 1 cm may require bone grafting or augmentation, and massive defects may require large allografts. At this point in the procedure, it is appropriate to determine the correct rotation of the components, particularly of the tibia, and to add wedges or shims as necessary to fill those gaps. One must remember that the rotation of the tibial and femoral components will be prejudiced by the position of the wedge or augment, and correct extensor tracking must be determined before the bone is trimmed to accept its augments (Fig. 88.24).

Many of the extramedullary devices for cutting tibial wedges are quite bulky and difficult to apply to the anterior bone beneath the patellar tendon. For half wedges, one can merely place the appropriate wedge on the healthy side of the bone, using this slope as a guide to trim the deficient side. At this juncture, one is in reality fitting the patients to the parts, and care must be taken not to resect any more bone than is absolutely necessary. On the femoral side, posterior lateral augments are often helpful to preserve the appropriate external rotation of the component, a common cause for failure of the index arthroplasty. Anterior femoral deficiency is also quite common, but very difficult to resolve (Fig. 88.25). Cement in this area is an unattractive option and often requires a two-stage cementing of the knee. Bone

Figure 88.23.   Release capsule for better extension balance.

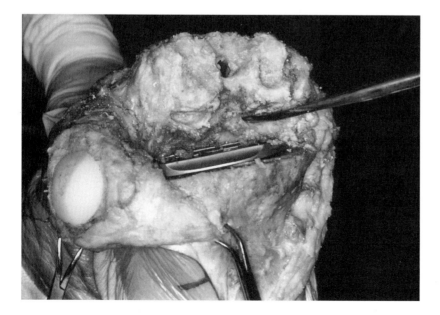

Figure 88.24.   Cutting tibial wedge.

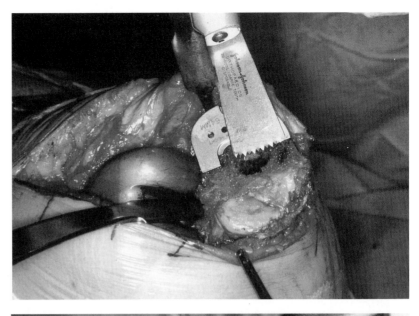

Figure 88.25.   Deficient anterior femur.

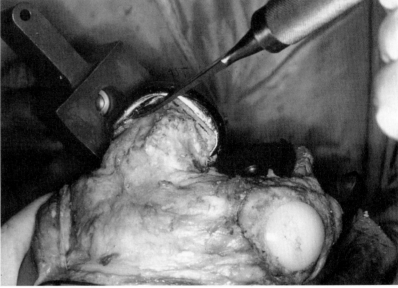

Figure 88.26.   Femoral component in internal rotation with marked epicondyles.

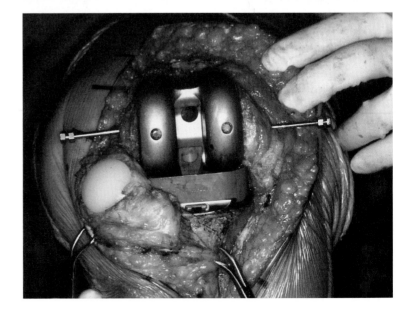

grafts are problematic beneath the trochlear flange, as this is a heavily stressed, shielded area. Currently, there exist no predictable augments for these irregular defects.

The use of intramedullary stems to protect grafts, augments, and weakened bones is very common and quite appropriate. The long-term effects of stress shielding and the multiple junctions of prosthetic devices are causes for future concern. Also, it is generally preferable not to cement stems in either the tibial or femoral canals because of the potential difficulties of subsequent extraction. If cemented stems are used, they would preferably be of a smooth rather than irregular shape to facilitate removal. While this may seem a pessimistic approach, one must always plan for future problems in revisional knee surgery.

Fixation

The vast majority of knee revisions are performed with methylmethacrylate fixation, although some surgeons prefer the uncemented approach. When cement is used, it is crucial that all components be available, assembled, and tested before the cement is mixed. Gelfoam washers are helpful to prevent intrusion of the cement into the femoral or tibial canal. Surface cementing with press-fit stems is the most prevalent approach currently. If allografts or other augmentation devices are used, many prefer to cement the bone or metal parts to the prosthetic component before implantation, in order to reduce the number of variables at the time of terminal assembly. The most skillful of revisional surgeons gen-

erally cement all three components at one time, because this form of assembly allows the knee one last period of autoadjustment in balance and rotation (Fig. 88.26).

While the challenges are often prodigious and the risks quite high, there are few surgical satisfactions that exceed the successful reconstruction of a failed total knee arthroplasty. Hopefully, improved instrumentation and the continued evolution of modular knee systems will further facilitate this demanding procedure.

Suggested Readings

1. Coventry M. Two part total knee arthroplasty: Evolution and present status. Clin Orthop Rel Res 1979;145:29.
2. Dorr LD, Conaty JP, Schreiber R, et al. Technical factors that influence mechanical loosening of total knee arthroplasty. In: Dorr LD, ed. The knee. Papers of the First Scientific Meeting of the Knee Society. Baltimore: University Park Press, 1985: 121–135.
3. Lotke P, Ecker M. Influence of the position of the prosthesis in total knee replacement. J Bone Joint Surg 1977;59A:77.
4. Insall JN, Scott WN, Ranawat CS. The total condylar knee prosthesis–A report of 220 cases. J Bone Joint Surg 1979;61A:173.
5. Ewald FC, Jacobs MA, Miegel PE, et al. Kinematic total knee replacement. J Bone Joint Surg 1984;66A:1032.
6. Gross TP, Lennox DW. Osteolytic cyst-like areas associated with polyethylene and metallic debris after total knee replacement with an uncemented Vitallium prosthesis. J Bone Joint Surg 1992;74A:1096–1101.
7. Tsao A, Mintz L, McRae CR, et al. Failure of the porous-coated anatomic prosthesis in total knee arthroplasty due to severe polyethylene wear. J Bone Joint Surg 1993;75A:19,en>26.
8. Scott RD, Siliski JM. The use of a modified V-Y quadricepsplasty during total knee replacement to gain exposure and improve flexion in the ankylosed knee. Orthopaedics 1985;8:45.
9. Vince KG. Revision knee arthroplasty. In: Chapman M, ed. Operative orthopedics. Philadelphia: JB Lippincott, 1993.
10. Whiteside LA, Ohl MD. Tibial tubercle osteotomy for exposure of the difficult knee arthroplasty. Clin Orthop Rel Res 1990;260:6.

89

Arthrodesis and Resection Arthroplasty

Russell E. Windsor and James V. Bono

Knee Arthrodesis

Knee arthrodesis is an infrequent operation, which is rarely performed primarily for arthritis. It is, however, a salvage procedure for unrevisable failure of total knee arthroplasty. Arthrodesis of the knee in the face of grossly deficient bone stock is difficult to achieve (Fig. 89.1) (3, 17, 19, 51). In limb salvage surgery for malignant and potentially malignant lesions about the knee, resection arthrodesis using an intramedullary rod and local bone grafts has been reported as a successful primary procedure (13). When possible however, every effort is made to maintain knee function with prosthetic distal femoral replacements or special hinged arthroplasties. When performed as a primary procedure after trauma, arthritis, or instability, solid fusion may not always occur. Rates of union by various methods have been reported between 80 and 98%; failure of union results in a fibrous ankylosis, which frequently is painful (7, 8, 17, 28, 48). Knee arthrodesis should be reserved for the carefully selected patient as a salvage procedure for severe infection, bone loss, or instability. Rigid fixation promotes bony union.

Indications

Unilateral Posttraumatic Osteoarthritis in a Young Person (10). In a healthy young male laborer with an isolated, severely damaged knee, an arthrodesis should be recommended. A well-done fusion will be more durable over time than any other reconstructive option. However, arthrodesis is often refused by men and rejected unconditionally by women, which presents a dilemma for the surgeon. In the younger individual, a knee replacement is unlikely to endure a lifetime of hard use and will certainly require future revision. The arthrodesis decision should be made carefully; a knee arthrodesis is final and cannot easily be revised to successful arthroplasty later (22). Fortunately, disabling unilateral, posttraumatic osteoarthritis in a young person is rare, and each case must be judged individually. Occasionally, a joint debridement or a realignment by osteotomy provides temporary relief. Extensive preoperative discussion, including the risks, benefits, expectations, and alternatives to surgery helps the patient decide whether to have surgery, postpone it, or avoid it altogether.

Despite the long-term durability of fusion, the patient may still insist on total knee arthroplasty, hoping for success. In this situation, a preoperative agreement should be made in which the patient accepts arthrodesis if severe early failure of the knee replacement occurs. The patient should understand that the success of arthrodesis following unsuccessful arthroplasty may be less predictable.

Multiply Operated Knee. Occasionally, there are patients who, despite or because of multiple knee operations, complain of a diffusely painful and usually unstable knee; these patients can be depressed, angry, and often hostile. The original insult may have been a ligament injury or patellar dislocation. These patients are challenging to treat. Additional surgery of any kind is unwarranted and inadvisable. Management should consist of simple conservative care, bracing, attendance at a "pain clinic," and perhaps psychiatric consultation. For a select few, arthrodesis may be the correct approach. In this situation, preoperative trial of a cylinder cast is mandatory.

Painful Ankylosis. Ankylosis is defined as motion of no more than 10 or 20 degrees. Patients who develop stiffness from severe rheumatoid arthritis or uncomplicated osteoarthritis may be successfully treated by total knee arthroplasty (40) using quadriceps turn-down techniques, "skeletonization" of the femur, and reestablishment of the medial and lateral gutters by excision of all scarred and contracted tissue. Even in these cases, however, the prospects of gaining normal motion are slim, with the final outcome being less than 90 degrees of motion. In the ankylosed knee following sepsis or an-

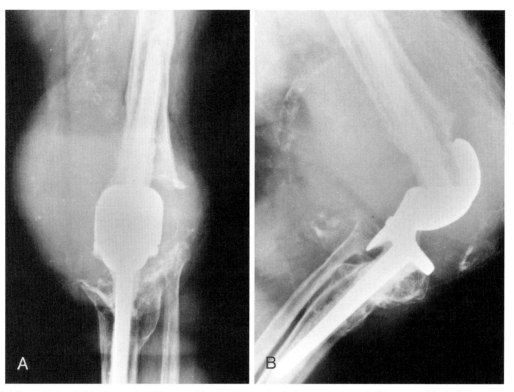

Figure 89.1 AP (**A**) and lateral (**B**) views of a 68-year-old woman following revision total knee arthroplasty with grossly deficient bone stock. The femur and tibia resemble hollow cones with little or no cancellous bone remaining.

cient trauma, an arthroplasty may be either contraindicated or likely to produce a suboptimal result, particularly in terms of motion. A painful ankylosis may benefit from an arthrodesis.

Paralytic Conditions. Poliomyelitis is rare in the United States and western Europe where vaccination is widespread. Muscle weakness can usually be managed successfully by bracing, as the patients often have little pain. However, when associated with genu recurvatum, bracing is difficult and may not be successful. Arthroplasty in this setting is technically demanding (31). In paralytic conditions, arthrodesis adequately addresses the quadriceps weakness and angular deformity.

Neuropathic Joint. Arthrodesis of a neuropathic knee joint has resulted in limited success and frequent nonunion. Thorough debridement of all bone detritus and complete synovectomy increases the rate of bony union (12). Drennan reported 10 cases of arthrodesis of a Charcot knee in nine patients. The best results were obtained after complete removal of the thickened, edematous synovium in these knees. Total knee arthroplasty in Charcot joints has been reported (49). For these cases, bone defects should be treated by implants with metal augments rather than by bone grafting, and constrained-condylar knee replacement designs are recommended. When the Charcot knee is painless, bracing is the treatment of choice. Many Charcot knees are painful, however, and should be carefully selected for knee arthroplasty or arthrodesis.

Malignant and Potentially Malignant Knee Lesions. Certain potentially malignant and low-grade malignant tumors about the knee, such as aggressive giant cell tumor, chondrosarcoma, recurrent chondroblastoma, and carefully selected higher-grade malignant lesions, may be satisfactorily controlled by adequate local resection of the lesion. Reconstruction of the defect created by such resection may be accomplished by (*a*) extremity shortening and arthrodesis, (*b*) arthrodesis with large intercalary bone grafts to preserve length, (*c*) arthroplasty with custom-made prosthetic replacements, and (*d*) allotransplantation of joints (21, 35, 37, 39, 42–45, 52, 53, 57, 58).

Local resection and arthrodesis for tumors about the knee was first described in 1907 by Lexer and others (34, 35, 39, 46, 58). Success in controlling the tumor was frequently complicated by infection, nonunion, and late fatigue fracture. Enneking reported 20 patients with malignant or potentially malignant tumors (osteogenic sarcoma, giant cell tumor, synovial cell sarcoma, chondrosarcoma, and chondroblastoma) in the proximal tibia or distal femur, who were treated by local resection and arthrodesis using an intramedullary rod and autogenous segmental cortical grafts obtained from the same extremity (13). There was only one local recurrence, and rehabilitation lasted about 1 year before the patients resumed a vigorous life-style. A customized bent fluted rod generally provided the most secure fixation (13).

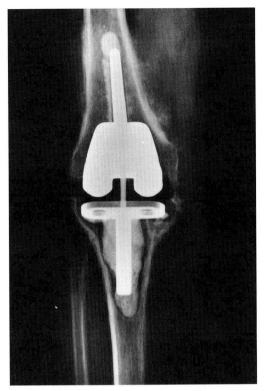

Figure 89.2. Aggressive osteolysis about a stemmed total knee arthroplasty resulting from sepsis.

Failed Total Knee Arthroplasty. Currently the most frequent indication for knee fusion, as well as the most difficult circumstance in which to achieve union, is the failed total knee arthroplasty. Mechanical failure of an arthroplasty can nearly always be better managed by revision. Two-stage reimplantation may be the best choice when the failure is caused by sepsis. Some cases of failed total knee arthroplasty with bone loss and infection can only be managed by removal of the prosthesis and fusion (Fig. 89.2).

Arthrodesis as a salvage procedure for a failed septic knee replacement is indicated in the following circumstances: (*a*) persistent infection recalcitrant to repeated debridements and antibiotic regimes; (*b*) disruption of the extensor mechanism because of infection; (*c*) infection that is sensitive to only severely toxic antibiotic agents, such as *Candida* or other fungi (23, 30, 56); (*d*) a young patient or a disillusioned older one who does not wish to face possible future revision arthroplasties. Occasionally, fusion may be the best choice for a very heavy patient with a septic failure.

Deficiency of the extensor mechanism is a compelling indication for arthrodesis when it occurs in an infected knee arthroplasty (Fig. 89.3). The patient generally displays a profound extensor lag if reimplantation of a new total knee replacement is done. Repair of the extensor mechanism (4) is often impossible because of the destruction of tissue by the infectious organism.

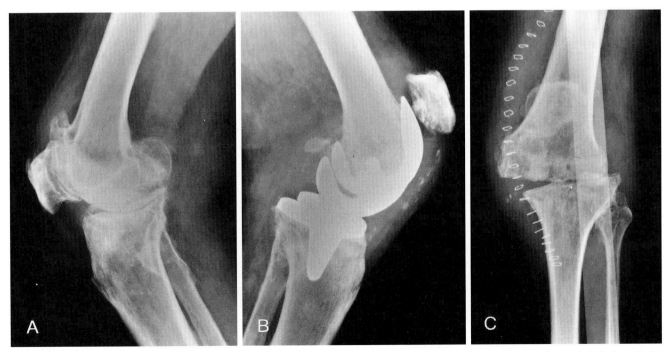

Figure 89.3. A, An 81-year-old woman with severe degenerative arthritis. **B,** Following total knee arthroplasty complicated by sepsis and disruption of the extensor mechanism. **C,** Following removal of components and debridement. A formal arthrodesis is indicated after a 6-week course of antibiotics.

Treatment of fungal infections such as *Candida albicans* requires toxic antibiotics (23, 30). Successful eradication of the infection is difficult, but not impossible, to achieve (33).

Although certain patients insist on reimplantation of a total knee arthroplasty following infection, some do not want to risk recurrent infection and choose arthrodesis to end their treatment.

Arthrodesis may be accomplished by one of four techniques: (*a*) compression arthrodesis with external fixation, (*b*) intramedullary rod fixation, (*c*) compression plating (36, 41), and (*d*) a combination of intramedullary rod fixation and compression plating (50). Intramedullary rod fixation achieves union in a high proportion of patients (11, 15, 16, 18, 20, 25, 29, 38, 47, 55). Knutson obtained fusion in 9 out of 10 knees treated with this method (29). Donley et al. obtained an 85% fusion rate in 20 knees, using intramedullary rod fixation and arthrodesis for the treatment of giant cell tumor, nonunion of a distal femur or proximal tibial fracture, aseptic loosening of a total knee replacement, and treatment of septic total knee replacement (11). Harris (20), Mazet (38), and Griend (18) have reported successful results using this technique. Wilde, however, successfully fused only 6 of 9 (55).

Advantages of the intramedullary rod technique include (*a*) immediate weight bearing and easier rehabilitation, (*b*) the elimination of problems associated with transfixation pins and external frames, (*c*) high fusion rate, (*d*) the potential for dynamization or load sharing, and (*e*) increased stability in bones weakened by atrophy or osteopenia where screws or pins may pull out. The disadvantages include (*a*) the risk of proximal rod migration requiring removal, (*b*) difficulty with alignment, (*c*) dissemination of infection, (*d*) the risk of fat embolism, and (*e*) incompatibility with ipsilateral total hip arthroplasty.

Success has also been achieved with external fixation compression arthrodesis (5–8, 26, 27). Fusion rates of 50% occurred in series that included large numbers of failed hinged prostheses. In this situation, external fixation does not always provide the stability necessary for bone healing. Knutson and colleagues reported 91 attempted fusions for failed knee arthroplasty. Fusions after surface replacement arthroplasties were much more successful than those after hinged prostheses. They believed that both intramedullary rod and external fixation methods were successful and that repeated attempts at fusion were worthwhile (28). External fixator devices must be in place for approximately 3 months; then cast immobilization is necessary until the arthrodesis is healed. One advantage of external fixation for treatment of septic knee replacements is that the device may be removed, leaving no metal in the knee (51).

The advantages of external fixation are (*a*) stable compression across the fusion site (2, 27), especially if half-pins are added anteriorly, (*b*) limb stabilization for management of extensive soft tissue infection, (*c*) technical facility, (*d*) easy removal, and (*e*) "dynamization" and loading across the fusion site. The disadvantages include (*a*) external pin tract problems, (*b*) poor patient

compliance, (*c*) frequent need for premature removal and cast immobilization, and (*d*) nonrigid fixation in cases of severe bone loss.

Technique

Compression Arthrodesis. Compression arthrodesis using a pin and frame technique was popularized by Key (26) and Charnley (5–8). Multiple transfixation pins are now used. Half-pins (6.5-mm Schantz screws) at right angles to the transfixation pins augment stability. Other configurations, such as triangular frames with half-pin fixation, result in high anteroposterior and mediolateral stability (2, 27).

A suitable cancellous surface on both bones optimizes fusion. Bone shortening relaxes the hamstrings and increases flexibility at the hip joint, which is desirable if both knees have to be fused (7). Charnley reported that patients considered limb shortening advantageous for dressing and foot care (7). The desired alignment is 0 to 5 degrees of valgus, with the knee flexed 10 to 15 degrees. More extension can be accepted in the presence of marked bone loss. The patella can be left alone or used to augment the fusion mass.

When arthrodesis is indicated after failed total knee arthroplasty with bone loss, further bone should not be resected; the surfaces must be thoroughly debrided and their irregular surfaces opposed to give the best possible contact. The patella can sometimes be used as a graft to fill large defects. An external fixator device is then applied (e.g., the Hoffman-Vidal apparatus).

Authors' Preferred Technique. Existing midline incisions are used; transverse incisions that divide the quadriceps mechanism may be used in primary cases. Joint surfaces are prepared with a saw. Cutting jigs from a total knee arthroplasty tray are used to make accurate resections and obtain the correct alignment. Three parallel transfixation pins are passed through the distal femur, and three more through the upper tibia. If the knee still demonstrates anteroposterior instability after the frame is applied, additional half-pins, three above and three below the knee, are inserted under radiographic control. The pins are connected to the frame, and compression is applied. Fixation is usually secure enough to allow weight bearing. Currently, the triangular frame configuration is popular, using half-pins 6.5 mm wide at an angle 45 degrees to the anteroposterior and mediolateral planes. This configuration yields rigid stability in both planes and is more tolerable.

Intramedullary Rod Fixation (11, 15, 18, 20, 25, 47, 55). After failure of a hinged arthroplasty, the femur and tibia may resemble hollow cones with little or no remaining cancellous bone (Fig. 89.1); in this setting, external fixation devices cannot provide the stability required for arthrodesis. Cortical bone is often irregular, partially devascularized, or impregnated with metallic debris. Kaufer et al. (25) recommended an initial period of prolonged immobilization; if this results in a stable, painless, fibrous ankylosis, then no further treatment is indicated (14). A period of up to 1 year after removal of the prosthetic components is allowed to pass before performing formal arthrodesis by intramedullary rod fixation.

Intramedullary arthrodesis has gained widespread favor for the salvage of severely infected knee replacements. Most authors recommend doing the procedure in two stages, although Puranen has reported single-stage arthrodesis in a few patients who were infected with organisms exquisitely sensitive to antibiotics (47). However, the best results occurred with a staged arthrodesis having 4 to 6 weeks of intravenous antibiotic therapy administered between the prosthetic removal and the arthrodesis (47). Kaufer recommended a curved Kuntscher rod that was cut down to appropriate length during the procedure (11, 25). Stiehl has reported eight cases of knee arthrodesis using combined intramedullary rodding and plate fixation. By adding a compression plate, intramedullary nail arthrodesis can be extended to situations in which bone loss requires a segmental allograft (50). In severe infections in which a two-stage reimplantation of a new total knee replacement is less likely to succeed, e.g., *Clostridium perfringens* (56) and *Candida albicans* (33), successful arthrodesis has been achieved. New, safer yeast-specific antimicrobial drugs may make salvage of the latter infection possible in the future.

Authors' Preferred Technique. The original longitudinal incision is used whenever possible. The knee joint is exposed in a manner similar to that used in revision arthroplasty, and all scar is removed. Cancellous bone is completely exposed on the distal femur and proximal tibia. An intramedullary ball-tip guide wire is introduced into the tibial shaft to the plafond of the ankle. The canal is sequentially reamed until the cortex is engaged at the tibial isthmus. This canal width determines the size of the rod. The tibial length is measured using the guide rod as a reference.

The ball-tip guide wire is removed from the tibial canal and inserted into the femoral shaft until the tip contacts the piriformis recess. The femoral canal is reamed until it matches the size of the tibial reamer. The femoral length is measured using the guide rod at the piriformis fossa as a reference. Subtracting 1 cm from the combined length of the femur and tibial measurements determines the appropriate rod length. The guide wire is tapped proximally through the piriformis recess with a mallet. The guide wire is advanced until it can be easily palpated under the skin of the thigh, with the leg in an adducted position. An incision is made over the guide wire, and dissection is carried down through the gluteal musculature to the piriformis recess. The recess is reamed progressively to a size 1 mm larger than the tibial and femoral reamer size. After reaming, a 90-cm curved Kuntscher arthrodesis nail (Biomet, Inc.) is cut to the appropriate length using a high-speed cutting tool. An extraction slot is made at the proximal end to allow later removal.

In the treatment of traumatic femoral shaft fractures, an intramedullary nail is inserted with its curve following the anterolateral bow of the femur. However, in intramedullary knee arthrodesis, if the rod follows the anterolateral bow of the femur, it will create varus

alignment with slight hyperextension. For this reason, the rod is inserted with the curve positioned anteromedially down the femoral shaft. The rod will then come through the tibia in valgus and slight flexion at the knee, which is preferred. An axial load is placed on the proximal tibia against the distal end of the femur during rod insertion. Sometimes the rod forces the anterior tibial flare forward, making closure of the arthrotomy difficult. If this occurs, the surgeon may modify the anterior flare with a reciprocating saw. Resected bone should be used as autograft, although some authors consider this unnecessary (11). Wiring of the proximal portion of the rod has been recommended, to prevent proximal migration (11, 25). This may be unnecessary (15, 18, 20, 47).

Complications of Arthrodesis

Regardless of the technique, union may not occur (Fig. 89.4). If the resulting pseudarthrosis is painful, the arthrodesis should be revised. Failed intramedullary fusion with pseudarthrosis may eventually cause breakage of the rod (Fig. 89.5). Fatigue fracture of the rod occurs at or near the pseudarthrosis site. Arthrodesis may be revised using a larger intramedullary nail supplemented by bone grafting (Fig. 89.6). A successful arthrodesis may remain actively infected, particularly if foreign material or necrotic tissue remains. With external fixation, pin tract infections may require premature removal of the apparatus and can seed the intramedullary canal if followed by rod fixation.

The single fused bone that results from successful fusion is vulnerable to increased forces from a larger moment arm; femoral or tibial fractures occur. Back pain has been reported, and patient satisfaction is modest, even with the best arthrodesis. A stiff limb, although painless and functional, can be socially unacceptable. No patient should have an arthrodesis without first having an extended trial in a cylinder cast to appreciate the permanent disadvantages of a stiff limb. Conversion of a sound arthrodesis to an arthroplasty has been reported (22). This procedure is relatively contraindicated for the following reasons: (*a*) collateral ligament integrity is compromised; (*b*) longstanding fusion may result in permanent contracture and scarring of surrounding musculature, limiting knee flexion after conversion; (*c*) muscle atrophy may not be irreversible and leaves a residual extension lag; (*d*) the new arthroplasty is at greater risk of infection or mechanical problems than are routine knee replacements; and (*e*) if subsequent septic or aseptic failure occurs, there is no guarantee of successful fusion.

Resection Arthroplasty

Resection arthroplasty is accomplished by excising the opposing articular surfaces of the distal femur and proximal tibia. Complete removal of scar tissue, synovium, and all foreign material, including metallic hardware, knee replacement components, and acrylic cement, is mandatory (Fig. 90.3) (14, 32). This option is generally reserved for medically fragile patients who

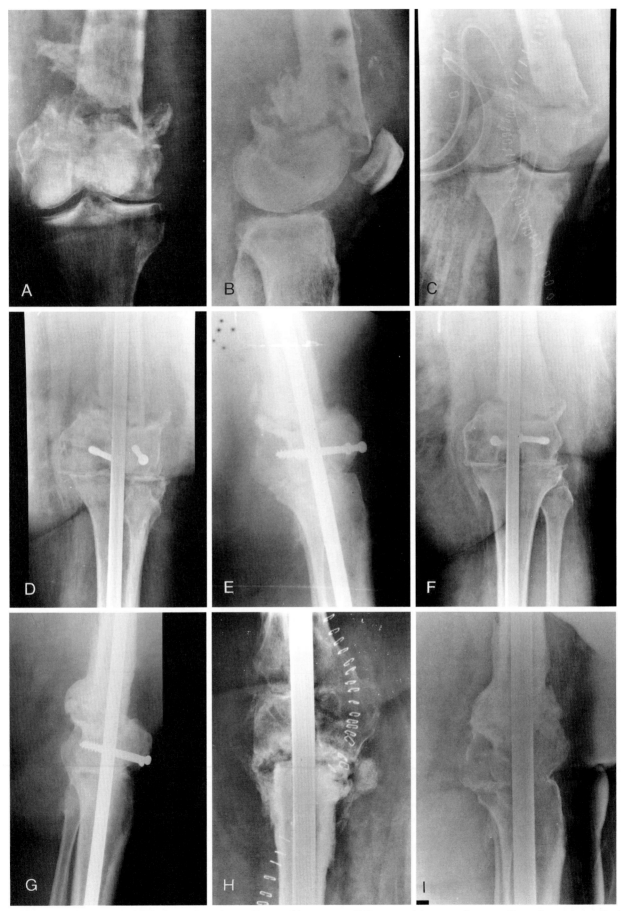

Figure 89.4. AP (**A**) and lateral (**B**) views of an obese 49-year-old woman with an infected supracondylar nonunion following corrective osteotomy. **C,** The wound is debrided, and a 6-week course of antibiotics is administered. **D** and **E,** Following arthrodesis with an intramedullary nail. The patella has been used to augment the fusion mass. **F,** Supracondylar nonunion seen 3 months postoperatively. **G,** Lateral view at 6 months demonstrates persistent supracondylar lucency. **H,** The fusion is revised 7 months after the index fusion. A larger diameter rod is exchanged, and the fusion site is bone grafted. **I,** A solid arthrodesis 11 months after revision of fusion.

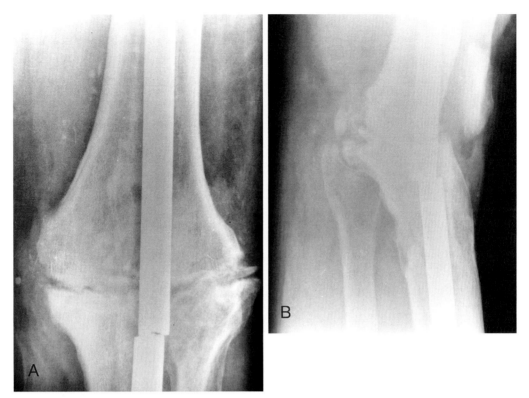

Figure 89.5.   A and **B,** Pseudarthrosis resulting in fatigue fracture of the rod.

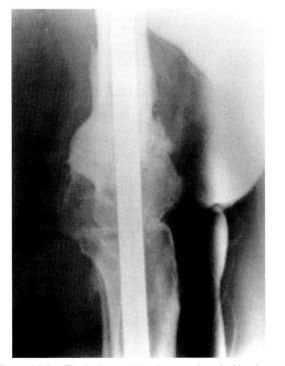

Figure 89.6.   The broken rod has been replaced with a larger diameter rod.

cannot tolerate a two-stage reimplantation protocol. It may also serve as an intermediate step for the patient who has reservations about arthrodesis. Fallahee et al. reported 28 knees that underwent resection arthroplasty for infected total knee arthroplasty (14). Eleven had polyarticular rheumatoid arthritis, 14 had osteoarthritis, and 1 had neuropathic arthropathy in multiple joints. Six patients with prior monarticular o teoarthritis found the resection arthroplasty unacceptable and underwent successful arthrodesis. In three patients, spontaneous bone fusion developed after the resection, with the knee in good position. Patients with more severe disability before the original knee arthroplasty were more likely to be satisfied with the functional results of the resection arthroplasty. Conversely, patients with less disability originally were more likely to find the resection arthroplasty unacceptable. Fifteen patients walked independently. Five of those patients were able to stand and walk without external limb support. The other 10 patients used either a knee-ankle-foot orthosis or a universal knee splint. All 15 patients, however, required either a cane or a walker and remained either moderately or severely restricted in their overall walking capacity.

Resection arthroplasty is useful for the severely disabled sedentary person. The procedure is least suitable for patients with relatively minor disability before their original total joint replacement. The latter group requires arthrodesis or reimplantation of a total knee replacement, if possible, depending on the sensitivity of the organism and adequacy of the antibiotic treatment. The advantage of the resection arthroplasty is that some motion is preserved for sitting and transferring into and out of automobiles and aircraft. The disadvantages are persistent pain and instability with walking.

A modified resection arthroplasty has been presented for problem cases with sepsis or excessive loss of bone stock in which exchange arthroplasty or arthrodesis are inadvisable or impossible (24). The space between the femur and tibia is filled with a bolus of antibiotic-impregnated cement after implant removal. The bolus can improve stability and diminish shortening and maintains a potential space for relatively easier revision arthroplasty in the future (1, 9, 54).

Summary

Arthrodesis as a salvage procedure remains a durable, time-proven technique for treatment of sepsis, tumor, failed arthroplasty, and the flail limb. Fusion should be considered and irreversible. It should be performed selectively, especially in light of modern arthroplasty. Various techniques have been used, each of which has a role in these difficult salvage cases.

References

1. Booth RE Jr, Lotke PA. The results of spacer block technique in revision of infected total knee arthroplasty. Clin Orthop 1989;248:57–60.
2. Briggs B, Chao EYS. The mechanical performance of the standard Hoffmann-Vidal external fixation apparatus. J Bone Joint Surg 1982;64[A]:566–573.
3. Brodersen MP, Fitzgerald RH Jr, Peterson LFA, Coventry MB, Bryan RS. Arthrodesis of the knee following failed total knee arthroplasty. J Bone Joint Surg 1979;61[A]:181–185.
4. Cadambi A, Engh GA. Use of a semitendinosis tendon autogenous graft for rupture of the patellar ligament after total knee arthroplasty. J Bone Joint Surg 1992;74[A]:974–979.
5. Charnley JC. Positive pressure in arthrodesis of the knee joint. J Bone Joint Surg 1948;30[Br]:478–486.
6. Charnley J. Arthrodesis of the knee. Clin Orthop 1960;18:37–42.
7. Charnley J, Baker SL. Compression arthrodesis of the knee. A clinical and histological study. J Bone Joint Surg 1952;34[Br]:187–199.
8. Charnley J, Lowe HG. A study of the end-results of compression arthrodesis of the knee. J Bone Joint Surg 1958;40[Br]:633–635.
9. Cohen JC, Hozack WJ, Cuckler JM, Booth RE. Two-stage reimplantation of septic total knee arthroplasty. J Arthroplasty 1988;3:369–377.
10. Dee R. The case for arthrodesis of the knee. Orthop Clin North Am 1979;10:(1)249–261.
11. Donley BG, Matthews LS, Kaufer H. Arthrodesis of the knee with an intramedullary nail. J Bone Joint Surg 1991;73[A]:907–913.
12. Drennan DB, Fahey JJ, Maylahn DJ. Important factors in achieving arthrodesis of the Charcot knee. J Bone Joint Surg 1971;53[A]:1180–1193.
13. Enneking WF, Shirley PD. Resection-arthrodesis for malignant and potentially malignant lesions about the knee using an intramedullary rod and local bone grafts. J Bone Joint Surg 1977;59[A]:223–236.
14. Falahee MH, Matthews LS, Kaufer H. Resection arthroplasty as a salvage procedure for a knee with infection after total arthroplasty. J Bone Joint Surg 1987;69[A]:1013–1021.
15. Fern ED, Stewart HD, Newton G. Curved Kuntscher nail arthrodesis after failure of knee replacement. J Bone Joint Surg 1989;71[Br]:588–590.
16. Figgie HE III, Brody GA, Inglis AE, Sculco TP, Goldberg VM, Figgie MP. Knee arthrodesis following total knee arthroplasty in rheumatoid arthritis. Clin Orthop 1987;224:237–243.
17. Green DP, Parkes JC II, Stinchfield, FE. Arthrodesis of the knee. A follow-up study. J Bone Joint Surg 1967;49[A]:1065–1078.
18. Griend RV. Arthrodesis of the knee with intramedullary fixation. Clin Orthop 1983;181:146–150.
19. Hagemann WF, Woods GW, Tullos HS. Arthrodesis in failed total knee replacement. J Bone Joint Surg 1978;60[A]:790–794.
20. Harris CM, Froehlich J. Knee fusion with intramedullary rods for failed total knee arthroplasty. Clin Orthop 1985;197:209–216.
21. Higinbotham ML, Coley BL. The treatment of bone tumors by resection and replacement with massive grafts. Instructional Course Lectures, The American Academy of Orthopaedic Surgeons 1950;26–33. Ann Arbor, JW Edwards.
22. Holden DL, Jackson DW. Considerations in total knee arthroplasty following previous knee fusion. Clin Orthop 1988;227:223–228.
23. Iskander MK, Khan MA. *Candida albicans* infection of a prosthetic knee replacement [letter]. J Rheumatol 1988;15(10):1594–1595.
24. Jones WA, Wroblewski BM. Salvage of failed total knee arthroplasty: "beefburger" procedure. J Bone Joint Surg 1989;71[Br]:856–857.
25. Kaufer H, Irvine G, Matthews LS. Intramedullary arthrodesis of the knee. Orthop Trans 1983;7:547–548.
26. Key JA. Positive pressure in arthrodesis for tuberculosis of the knee joint. South Med J 1932;25:909.
27. Knutson K, Bodelind B, Lidgren L. Stability of external fixators used for knee arthrodesis after failed knee arthroplasty. Clin Orthop 1984;186:90–95.
28. Knutson K, Hovelius L, Lindstrand A, Lidgren L. Arthrodesis after failed knee arthroplasty. A nationwide multicenter investigation of 91 cases. Clin Orthop 1984;191:202–211.
29. Knutson K, Lindstrand A, Lidgren L. Arthrodesis for failed knee arthroplasty. J Bone Joint Surg 1985;67[Br]:47–52.
30. Koch AE. *Candida albicans* infection of a prosthetic knee replacement: a report and review of the literature. J Rheumatol 1988;15(2):362–365.
31. Krackow KA, Weiss A-P C. Recurvatum deformity complicating performance of TKA. J Bone Joint Surg 1990;72[A]:268–271.
32. Lettin AW, Neil MJ, Citron ND, August A. Excision arthroplasty for infected constrained total knee replacements. J Bone Joint Surg 1990;72[Br]:220–224.
33. Levine M, Rehm SJ, Wilde AH. Infection with *Candida albicans* of a total knee arthroplasty. Case report and review of the literature. Clin Orthop 1988;226:235–239.
34. Lexer E. Substitution of whole or half joints from freshly amputated extremities by free plastic operation. Surg Gynecol Obstet 1908;6:601–607.
35. Lexer E. Joint transplantations and arthroplasty. Surg Gynecol Obstet 1925;40:782–809.
36. Lucas DB, Murray WR. Arthrodesis of the knee by double plating. J Bone Joint Surg 1961;[43A]:795.
37. Marcove RC, Lyden JP, Huvos AG, Bullough PB. Giant-cell tumors treated by cryosurgery. A report of twenty-five cases. J Bone Joint Surg 1973;55[A]:1633–1644.
38. Mazet R, Urist MR. Arthrodesis of the knee with intramedullary nail fixation. Clin Orthop 1960;18:43–52.
39. Merle D'Aubigne R, Dejouany JP. Diaphyso-epiphyseal resection for bone tumor at the knee. With reports of nine cases. J Bone Joint Surg 1958;40[Br]:385–395.
40. Montgomery WH, Becker MW, Windsor RE, Insall JN. Primary total knee arthroplasty in stiff and ankylosed knees. Orthop Trans 1991;15:54–55.
41. Nichols SJ, Landon GC, Tullos HS. Arthrodesis with dual plates after failed total knee arthroplasty. J Bone Joint Surg 1991;73[A]:1020.
42. Ottolenghi CE. Massive osteoarticular bone grafts. Transplant of the whole femur. J Bone Joint Surg 1966;48[Br]:646–659.
43. Ottolenghi CE. Massive osteo and osteo-articular bone grafts. Technic and results of 62 cases. Clin Orthop 1972;87:156–164.
44. Parrish FF. Treatment of bone tumors by total excision and replacement with massive autologous and homologous grafts. J Bone Joint Surg 1966;48[A]:968–990.
45. Parrish FF. Homografts of bone. Clin Orthop 1972;87:36–42.
46. Phemister DB. Rapid repair of defect of femur by massive bone grafts after resection for tumors. Surg Gynecol Obstet 1945;80:120–127.
47. Puranen J, Kortelainen P, Jalovaara P. Arthrodesis of the knee with intramedullary nail fixation. J Bone Joint Surg 1990;72:433–442.
48. Siller TN, Hadjipavlou A. Arthrodesis of the knee. In: the American Academy of Orthopedic Surgeons, Symposium on reconstructive surgery of the knee. St. Louis: CV Mosby, 1978:161.
49. Soudry M, Binazzi R, Johanson NA, Bullough PG, Insall JN. Total knee arthroplasty in charcot and charcot-like joints. Clin Orthop 1986;208:199–204.
50. Stiehl JB, Hanel DP. Knee arthrodesis using combined intramedullary rod and plate fixation. Clin Orthop 1993;294:238–246.
51. Stulberg SD. Arthrodesis in failed total knee replacements. Orthop Clin North Am 1982;13(1):213–224.

52. Tuli SM. Bridging of bone defects by massive bone grafts in tumorous conditions and in osteomyelitis. Clin Orthop 1972;87:60–73.
53. Volkov M. Allotransplantation of joints. J Bone Joint Surg 1970;52[Br]:49–53.
54. Wilde AH, Ruth JT. Two-stage reimplantation in infected total knee arthroplasty. Clin Orthop 1988;236:23–35.
55. Wilde AH, Stearns KL. Intramedullary fixation for arthrodesis of the knee after infected total knee arthroplasty. Clin Orthop 1989;248:87–92.
56. Wilde AH, Sweeney RS, Borden LS. Hematogenously acquired infec-
tion of a total knee arthroplasty by *Clostridium perfringens*. Clin Orthop 1988;229:228–231.
57. Wilson PD Jr. A clinical study of the biomechanical behavior of massive bone transplants used to reconstruct large bone defects. Clin Orthop 1972;87:81–109.
58. Wilson PD, Lance EM. Surgical reconstruction of the skeleton following segmental resection for bone tumors. J Bone Joint Surg 1965;47[A]:1629–1656.

Index

Page numbers followed by *t* and *f* indicate tables and figures, respectively.

30-degree, 83, 93, 596, 596*f*
70-degree, 83, 93, 596, 596*f*
2.7mm, 596, 596*f*
in osteochondritis dissecans, 387
and portal placement, 553
in treatment of degenerative joint disease, history, 1113
Arthroscopic periosteal elevator, in anterior cruciate ligament reconstruction, two-incision technique, 705, 706*f*
Arthroscopic probe, in anterior cruciate ligament reconstruction, two-incision technique, 710, 711*f*
Arthroscopic rasp, in anterior cruciate ligament reconstruction, 714*f*
Arthroscopic sheath, 545, 545*f*
insertion, 553
Arthroscopic surgery
patient positioning and preparation, 548-551, 549*f*
safety considerations, 551
surgical assistant(s), 550
Arthroscopic Surgery: Principles and Practice, 543
Arthroscopy
advantages and disadvantages, 543-544
anatomy, 77-99
bony, 84
intraarticular, 84-97
with leg holder, 77-78
anesthesia for
general, 563
and postoperative pain, 569-570
local, 561-566
and postoperative pain, 570
peripheral nerve blocks, 561
of anterior cruciate ligament
diagnostic, 601, 601*f*, 692, 700-701, 738, 738*f*
therapeutic, 701-704
endoscopic single-incision technique, 719-726
indications for, 92
instruments for, 548*f*
standard setup for, 547, 548*f*
tunnel placement in, 92-93
two-incision technique, 704-719
applications, 543-544
for arthritis, diagnostic, 1106, 1107*f*
of articular cartilage, 85
degeneration grading, 85, 86*f*
compartment syndrome after, 661, 900
complications, 554-555
general, 900-901
instrument related, 900-901

contraindications to, with knee dislocations, 850
for degenerative joint disease, 1107-1108
complications, 1119
contraindications to, 1107
indications, 1116-1117
patient considerations, in decision making, 1117
studies, 1114
therapeutic, 1113-1120
diagnostic, 543-544, 553-554, 947, 1113-1114
accuracy rate, 543
complication rate, 554
historical review, 1113
indications, 650
intraoperative, importance of, 1119
and magnetic resonance imaging, comparison, 543
and radiography, 1114
in discoid meniscus, 395-399, 396*f*-400*f*
environment for performing, 544-545
extraarticular fluid dissection in tissues during, 900
future, 555
in general hospital, 544
hemarthrosis after, 559
history, 543
image interpretation, 78, 78*f*
inappropriate, 457, 458*t*, 459*f*-460*f*
infection with, risk, 545, 558
instrumentation, 583. *See also specific instrument*
for meniscal repair, 621, 626*f*
for meniscectomy, 595-597, 596*f*-597*f*
for saucerization procedure, 399-400, 400*f*-401*f*
instruments, 543-548, 550
breakage, 900*f*, 900-901
sterilization, 544-545
of intercondylar notch, 78, 79*f*, 80, 82-83, 89
irrigation fluid, 547-548
lasers in, 583, 585-588, 586*f*
for meniscectomy, 597-598
of lateral collateral ligament, 92, 96
of lateral compartment, 96-97
of lateral gutter, 87-88, 87*f*-88*f*
lateral release, with reflex sympathetic dystrophy, 440*t*
ligament reconstruction with, tunnel placement in, 92-95
of ligaments, 89-92
versus magnetic resonance imaging, 328, 328*t*, 329
of medial collateral ligament, 91-92
of medial gutter, 87, 87*f*

meniscectomy
partial, and complete open meniscectomy, comparison, 1114
with reflex sympathetic dystrophy, 440*t*
of menisci, 96, 136, 593, 598-601, 617
after meniscal repair, 623-626
repair procedures. *See* Meniscus/menisci, repair
of meniscotibial ligaments, 95-96
and neoplastic conditions, 457, 460*f*
nerve injury in, 246, 899
and positioning, 558
off axis, 78
operative, complication rate, 554
in osteochondritis dissecans, 386-387, 389*f*
with patellar tracking, 947
of patellofemoral joint, 85-87, 987-989, 1205
diagnostic, 1002
in pediatric patients, 373, 377, 379, 414
of plicae, 88*f*, 88-89
pocket of visualization, 78
of popliteus muscle, 96
portal(s), 79*t*, 79-84, 451, 452*f*, 551-553, 552*f*, 599*f*
accessory, 82*t*, 82-84, 552-553
anterior, 551, 552*f*
anterolateral, 80-81, 551-553
advantages and disadvantages, 79*t*
for meniscectomy, 598, 599*f*
during posterior cruciate ligament reconstruction, 93
anteromedial, 81-82, 551-552
advantages and disadvantages, 79*t*
for meniscectomy, 598, 599*f*
central, for meniscectomy, 599, 599*f*
closure, after meniscectomy, 608
for degenerative joint disease, 1118
far medial and far lateral, 553
incisions for, 551-552
joint line, for meniscectomy, 599*f*, 600
local anesthetic injection, 565-566
medial and medial mid patellar, 553
medial joint line, advantages and disadvantages, 79*t*
for meniscectomy, 598-600, 599*f*
midpatellar, for meniscectomy, 599*f*, 600

placement, 551-553
assessment, 553
improper, 551, 553
posterior compartment, 82-83
advantages and disadvantages, 82*t*
posterolateral, 552, 554
for discoid meniscal evaluation, 396, 397*f*, 399, 400*f*, 401
for meniscectomy, 599*f*, 599-600
posteromedial, 83-84, 552, 554
advantages and disadvantages, 82*t*
for discoid meniscal evaluation, 396
for meniscal repair, 618, 621*f*
for meniscectomy, 599*f*, 599-600
during posterior cruciate ligament reconstruction, 93
proximal superomedial, 553-554
standard, 551-552
superolateral, 79, 80*f*, 552
advantages and disadvantages, 79*t*
for meniscectomy, 599*f*, 600
superomedial, 79-80, 552
advantages and disadvantages, 79*t*
for meniscectomy, 598, 599*f*
transpatellar tendon, 82, 553
advantages and disadvantages, 82*t*
working, 79-82
positioning for, 77, 78*f*, 558
of posterior cruciate ligament, 90-91
30-degree, 93
70-degree, 93
of posteromedial corner, 95-96
postoperative
complications, 453
rehabilitation, 1119-1120
postoperative pain management, 569-571, 577
preoperative
in degenerative joint disease patients, 1117-1118
before realignment osteotomy, 1130
for reflex sympathetic dystrophy, diagnostic, 434-435, 440*t*
regions, 78-79, 79*f*
for relative unicompartmental disease, diagnostic, 1106
for rheumatoid arthritis, 1116
for septic arthritis, 451-452, 452*f*
and arthrotomy, comparison, 451
setup, 543-556

Coagulation factors, changes in, and deep vein thrombosis, 1495
Cobalt-chrome
  biocompatibility, 1361
  markers for, 1352, 1353*f*
  mechanical properties, 1510
Cobalt-chrome-molybdenum alloys, and bone ingrowth, 1371-1372
Cocaine, for local anesthesia, 561
Coccidioides immitis, septic arthritis caused by, 446
Cochlear implants, and magnetic resonance imaging, 327
Co-contraction test, 537, 537*f*
Codivilla technique, for simultaneous repair and lengthening of quadriceps tendon, 914, 914*f*
Codman's triangle, 469
Coherence, of laser light, 584, 584*f*
Cohnheim, J. F., 190
Cold application. *See also* Cryotherapy
  in arthritis, 1080
  to control pain and swelling, 1412
  for reflex sympathetic dystrophy, 1530
Collagen
  absence, in fetal healing, 219
  adipose, 198
  areolar, 198
  in cartilage, 72, 85, 101-103, 103*f*, 105, 106*f*, 115, 199
    early studies, 109-110
  in connective tissue, 191-193, 192*f*
  crimping, 155, 156*f*, 194-195, 195*f*
  fiber-forming, 192
  in fibrocartilage, 199-200
  fibrous, 198
  glutaraldehyde-impregnated bovine implant, 811-812
  implantation, cartilage repair promotion with, 126
  in ligaments, 155, 194
  in menisci, 72, 85, 101-103, 104*f*, 115, 117, 132-133, 133*f*, 200
  and shear modulus, 120-121
  organization, 102, 102*f*, 192, 194-195
    in osteoarthritis, 71
  split-line patterns in, 115, 115*f*, 115*t*
  in soft tissue scars, 205, 212-214, 217*f*, 222
  subtypes, 198
  in synovium, 143, 198
  and tensile strength of wounds, 191
  types, 102, 191-192, 193*t*
  type I, 102-103, 108, 132, 143, 146, 192
    and cartilage repair, 124
    in connective tissue, 192*f*

distribution, 193*t*
  function, 193*t*
  in ligaments, 195
  production, 107
  shear response, 120, 120*f*
type II, 102, 192
  distribution, 193*t*
  function, 193*t*
  production, 107
type III, 143, 146, 192
  distribution, 193*t*
  function, 193*t*
  removal, in scar maturation, 205
type IV, 141, 143, 192
  distribution, 193*t*
  function, 193*t*
type V, 143, 192
  distribution, 193*t*
  function, 193*t*
type VI, 143, 146, 192, 195
  distribution, 193*t*
  function, 193*t*
type VII
  distribution, 193*t*
  function, 193*t*
type VIII, 192
  distribution, 193*t*
  function, 193*t*
type IX, 192, 192*t*, 192
  distribution, 193*t*
  function, 193*t*
type X, 192
  distribution, 193*t*
  function, 193*t*
type XI, 192
  distribution, 193*t*
  function, 193*t*
type XII, 192
  distribution, 193*t*
  function, 193*t*
type XIII, 192
  distribution, 193*t*
  function, 193*t*
Collagenase(s), 193
  and wound healing, 205-206, 1541
Collagenase inhibitors, 206*f*
Collagen fibers
  intermolecular cross-links, 192-193
  in joint capsule, 196
  in skin, 52
Collagen fibrillar compartment, water within, 106
Collagen-glycosaminoglycan matrices, centrifuge formation, 110
Collagen network
  damage, 106
    in osteoarthritis, 123
  mechanical role in shear stiffness and energy storage, 119, 120*f*
  tensile strength, in osteoarthritis, 71
  viscoelasticity, 118
Collagenous materials, tensile properties, 114, 114*f*, 121-122

Collagen-proteoglycan matrix, shear modulus, 119, 120*f*
Collagen/proteoglycan ratio
  of high–weight-bearing regions, 116, 116*f*
  in osteoarthritis, 123
Collateral ligament(s). *See also* Fibular collateral ligament; Lateral collateral ligament; Medial collateral ligament; Tibial collateral ligament
  anatomy, 21-23
  blood supply, 22
  in four-bar linkage mechanism, 17
  functions, 1063
  imbalance, in revision total knee arthroplasty, 1561
  injury(ies), 787-808. *See also* Compartment injury, lateral; Compartment injury, medial; *specific ligament*
    diagnosis, 649-650
    physical examination, 257-258
    with tibia and femur fractures, 660
  innervation, 22
  insertion sites, 371, 371*f*, 373, 375
  magnetic resonance imaging, 332-335, 333*f*-335*f*
  palpation, 255
  sprains, 257
  status, in diagnosis of anterior cruciate ligament tear, 651
  stress testing, 257
  torn fibers, intraoperative placement, in ligament reconstruction, 646
Collimation, of laser light, 584, 584*f*
Communicating veins, 45
Compartment(s), 46-48, 48*f*, 78-79
  anterior, 47, 48*f*
  of calf, 46-47
  definition, 46, 1223
  femur as, 47
  fibula as, 47
  lateral, 47, 48*f*. *See also* Compartment injury, lateral
    arthroscopy, 96-97, 554
    biomechanics, 796-797
    functional anatomy, 795-796
    load distribution in
      as function of anatomic axis, 1156, 1156*f*
      as function of mechanical (load) axis, 1156, 1156*f*
    muscles, 35-36
  leg, 46-48, 48*f*
  medial. *See also* Compartment injury, medial
    arthroscopy, 96-97, 554
    biomechanics, 787-789
    capsular portion, thirds, 787, 788*f*

degeneration, in posterior cruciate ligament-deficient knees, 91
    extracapsular stabilizing structures, 787, 788*f*
    functional anatomy, 787
    load distribution in
      as function of anatomic axis, 1156, 1156*f*
      as function of mechanical (load) axis, 1156, 1156*f*
    osteoarthritis, 864
  patella as, 47
  patellofemoral, evaluation, in surgical decision making, 1104
  posterior
    arthroscopy, 82-83, 93-94, 94*f*
      advantages and disadvantages, 82*t*
      portals, 82*t*, 82-83
    deep, 47-48, 48*f*
    loose bodies in, arthroscopic identification, 83
    superficial, 47, 48*f*
  posterolateral, ligamentous complex, 796, 796*f*
  posteromedial, arthroscopic examination, 554
  soft tissue, 46-47
  of thigh, 47, 47*f*
    anterior, 29*f*, 29-32, 47, 47*f*
    medial, 47, 47*f*
    posterior, 47, 47*f*
  tibia as, 47
  trauma and, 46-47
  tumor spread and, 46-47
Compartment fasciotomies, after revascularization, with knee dislocations, 845, 845*f*
Compartment findings, rating scales for, 287
  IKDC analysis, 295
Compartment injury
  lateral
    acute lateral instability with, repair, 799-801
    classification, 798-799
    combined
      acute, 799
      chronic, 799
    imaging, 798
    incidence, 798
    mechanisms of injury, 797
    physical examination, 797
    repair, surgical technique, 799-807
    treatment, 798-799
  medial
    acute instability with, 790-792
    chronic instability with, 792
    repair, 794-795
    classification, 790-792
    combined injury, 792
    grade I, 790
    grade II, 790
    grade III, 790-791
    grade III rotational instability, 791-792

Dynamic knee simulator, 1449, 1450f
    actuation system, 1449, 1450f
Dynamic posterior shift test, 773, 774f
Dynamic stability, 240
    enhancement, during rehabilitation, 490
        for anterior cruciate ligament injuries, 491
    and neuromuscular control, 241
    patellofemoral joint, 493
Dyprosium-165, radionuclide synovectomy with, 1098

E
ECGF. *See* Endothelial cell growth factor
Edema fluid, spread, and compartments, 46-48
Efficacy, definition, 813
Effusion(s), 934
    and anterior cruciate ligament tear, 684-685
    aspiration, in pediatric patients, 415
    chronic, 940, 996
    effect on quadriceps function, 907
    effects on intraarticular pressure, 147-148, 148f
    after ligament surgery, 907
    magnetic resonance imaging, 345-346
    with meniscal tears, 268
    after meniscal transplantation, 637
    neuromuscular considerations with, 245
    with patellar dislocation, in pediatric patients, 414
    patient history, 253
    in pediatric patients, 372
    physical examination, 255, 255f
    postligament reconstruction, 907
    and proprioception, 245
    radiographic findings in, 319-320, 320f
    rating scales for, 287
    synovial, 147-148, 152
        aspiration, 150
            before instrumented testing, 299
        effects
            on intraarticular pressure, 147-148, 148f
            on joint mechanics, 150
        treatment, 245
EGF. *See* Epidermal growth factor
Ehlers-Danlos syndrome, ligament hypermobility in, 372
Ehrlich, Paul, 191
Eicosanoids, synovial secretion, 147, 149t, 152
Eikenella corrodens, septic arthritis caused by, 446, 447t
Elastic cartilage, 199

Elastic compression stockings, to control swelling, 1412
Elastic fibers, in ligaments, 195, 197f
Elasticity theory, single-phase, 110
Elastic material
    definition, 108
    Hooke's law for, 110
Elastin
    amorphous, 194
    in connective tissue, 192f, 194
    in menisci, 108, 133
Elderly patients. *See also* Age
    falls by, 244
    meniscectomy in, 609-610
    osteosarcomas in, 468
    proprioceptive deficits in, 529
    and treatment of acute anterior cruciate ligament injuries, 692
Electrical muscle stimulation, 577
    rehabilitative, 489
Electrocardiogram, with pulmonary embolism, 1497
Electrocautery, 583
    versus laser surgery, 583
Electrogoniometer, 298
    6-degrees of freedom, 307
        anterior cruciate ligament length measurement with, 180
Electrolyte analysis, during general anesthesia, 560
Electromagnetic digitizer, 6-degrees of freedom, anterior cruciate ligament length measurement with, 180
Electromagnetic tracking devices, kinematic measurement with, 175
Electromyography
    abnormalities, with tourniquet use, 558, 594
    after anterior cruciate ligament injury, 242
    biofeedback, during rehabilitation, 490
Electrotherapy, for postoperative pain, 577
Electrothermal energy. *See* Electrocautery
Elements, trace, and soft tissue healing, 221
Ellison technique, 802
Elmslie-Trillat tibial tubercle osteotomy, 413
ELPS. *See* Excessive lateral pressure syndrome
Elsasser, J. C., 275-276
Embolization, postoperative, 608
    arteriography for, 458
Embryo, wound healing in, 219
Embryology
    of knee, 88
    of lower limb, 37-39, 42
EMG. *See* Electromyography
EMS. *See* Electrical muscle stimulation

Enchondroma, 466
Endoligament, 198, 198f
Endo Model Rotating Hinge System, 1332-1333, 1333t-1335t
Endomysium, 195
Endoneurium, 36
Endoprosthetic implants, after tumor resection, 477
Endorphins, 568
Endoscopic fixation, in chronic anterior cruciate ligament-deficient knee reconstruction, 743-744
Endoscopic reamer, in anterior cruciate ligament reconstruction, single-incision technique, 722, 722f-723f
Endoscopy. *See also* Arthroscopy
    in anterior cruciate ligament reconstruction, 92-93, 719-726, 743-744
        posterior blowout fracture during, 93
Endotenon, 196, 197f, 198, 198f
Endothelial cell(s)
    angiogenic stimulus, after soft tissue injury, 206-207, 207f
    in pathogenesis of deep vein thrombosis, 1494
    of synovial capillaries and venules, 144
Endothelial cell growth factor, 209
Endurance exercise, 490
    in functional rehabilitation, 528
Energy absorption, in brace-knee complex, 509
Energy transmission, in brace-knee complex, 509
Enkephalins, in synovium, 143
Enoxaparin, 1500
Enterobacteriaceae, septic arthritis caused by, therapy for, 448
Enterococci, septic arthritis caused by, treatment, 448t, 450-451
Enterococcus faecalis, septic arthritis caused by, 447-448
    treatment, 448t, 451
Environment
    loading, and soft tissue healing, 222
    mechanical, and soft tissue healing, 222
Environmental temperature, and ligament biomechanical properties, 160-161, 161f
Enzyme(s)
    norepinephrine-producing, in synovium, 143
    proteolytic, in soft tissue healing, 201
    in soft tissue healing, 205
    synovial secretion, 149t
Enzyme solutions, proteoglycan degradation with, to allow clot formation, 125-126

Eosinophil(s), in soft tissue healing, 201
Eosinophilic granuloma, 468
    bone scan in, 458
Epidermal growth factor, 208
Epidural analgesia/anesthesia, 559-560
    advantages and disadvantages, 560
    postoperative, 571-573, 1411
        catheter for, 571
        complications, 572
    complications, 572
    continuous, 1411
    narcotics for, 574
    techniques, 571-572
    in reflex sympathetic dystrophy, 433, 436-438, 438f, 438-439
    versus sympathetic blockade, 436-437
Epidural infusion pump, in reflex sympathetic dystrophy, 438f
Epigastric artery, superficial, 42
Epiligament, 198
Epimorphic regeneration, 218-219
Epinephrine
    in anterior cruciate ligament reconstruction, 703
    in diagnostic arthroscopy, 700, 720
    with local anesthesia, 562-565, 570
    and serum concentrations, 564
    and tourniquet use, 558
Epineurium, 36
Epiphyseal growth plate cartilage, 199
Epiphyseal tumor, magnetic resonance imaging, 459f
Epiphyseal varus angle, measurement, 866, 866f
Epiphyseal varus axis, 866, 866f
Epiphysis
    femoral, 3
    tibial, 5
Epitenon, 198
Ergometry
    cycle, 531, 534f
    upper body, 531
Erosion(s), magnetic resonance imaging, 345
Erythromycin, for septic arthritis, 448t
Escherichia coli, septic arthritis caused by, 445-446, 447t
    treatment, 449-450
Ethyl chloride, coolant sprays containing, 1080
Ethylene oxide
    ligament graft storage in, 167
    sterilization
        of allograft tissue, contraindications to, 646, 673
        of arthroscopic equipment, 545

after ligament
reconstruction/repair,
899
after meniscal transplantation,
637-638
after meniscectomy, 608-609
with open injuries, 659
and patellar tendon rupture,
917
in pediatric patients, 423
prosthetic joint, treatment,
1563-1564
and quadriceps tendon rupture,
912
synovectomy for, 1100
with synthetic grafts, 674
technetium scintigraphy, 354
of total knee arthroplasty, 1563-
1572
after tourniquet use, 558
and wound healing, 1542-1543
Inflammation, 200-201, 489. *See
also* Swelling
absence, in fetal healing, 219
biochemistry, 201-204, 204*f*
rating scales for, 287-288
IKDC analysis, 295
treatment, 970
Inflammatory bowel disease-
associated arthropathy,
disease-modifying
antirheumatic drug therapy
for, 1086-1087
Inflammatory disorders, synovial
biopsy in, 85
Infrapatellar artery, transverse,
12-14
Infrapatellar tendon, anatomy, 910
Inhalation agents, for general
anesthesia, 560
Inhomogeneity
of articular cartilage, 115
definition, 108
of menisci, 117*f*, 117-118
Injury. *See also specific injury*
mechanism, identification, 253
proprioception after,
improvement, 244
reflex prevention, 241
Insall-Burstein Constrained
Condylar system, 1333-
1334, 1337*t*-1339*t*
Insall-Burstein Posterior
Stabilized System, 1321,
1323*f*, 1452, 1455, 1516
I, knee flexion with, 1415-1416
II, 1238, 1238*f*, 1334
contact pressure
distributions in, 1436
results, 1420
Insall-Burstein prosthesis, patellar
strain with, 1484
Insall-Salvati index, 937, 938*f*, 963
Insall-Salvati ratio, 999
In situ lesions, in osteochondritis
dissecans, treatment, 387,
387*f*
Instability, 297
after allograft reconstruction,
478-479

anterior cruciate ligament. *See
Anterior cruciate
ligament, instability*
anterolateral, 796
anterolateral rotary, 797-799
chronic, repair, 801-802, 802*f*-
804*f*
anteromedial, 862
anteromedial rotary, 792, 799
chronic
repair, 794-795
treatment, 792
classification, 265-267
definition, 292, 644
diagnosis, and brace
prescription, 524
drawer, assessment, 506
effect of derotation brace on,
517-518
evolved chronic anterior, 862
functional, definition, 505
grading, 284, 288
as indication for anterior
cruciate ligament
injuries, 684
versus laxity, 254
with ligament injuries, 254, 256-
257
ligamentous, 254, 256-257
and arthritis, treatment, 660
correction, 1185, 1186*f*
high tibial osteotomy with,
1138
after knee dislocation
reduction,
examination for, 844
preoperative, total knee
arthroplasty with,
1339
tibiofemoral joint, bracing
for, 503-526
medial, treatment, 792
medial-lateral, bracing for,
508
and meniscal repair, 626
with meniscal tears, 268
and osteoarthritis
animal experiments, 859
human experience, clinical
history with, 859-860
treatment, 660
patellar. *See Patellar instability*
and patient selection for high
tibial osteotomy, 1122-
1123
posterior, tests, 772-774
posterolateral
chronic, 769
reconstruction, 802-806
tests, 774-775
posterolateral rotary, 797-799
rotational. *See Rotational
instability*
rotatory. *See Rotational
instability*
straight, 265
anterior, 259, 259*f*
classification, 267*t*
diagnosis, 267*t*
testing, 254

valgus, assessment, 506
varus, assessment, 506
Instability brace, for posterior
cruciate ligament injuries,
492
Instrumentation. *See also specific
instrument*
arthroscopic, 583
for meniscal repair, 621, 626*f*
for meniscectomy, 595-597,
596*f*-597*f*
for saucerization procedure,
399-400, 400*f*-401*f*
Instrument breakage
in anterior cruciate ligament
reconstruction,
prevention, 662
in arthroscopic surgery, 554
Instrumented laxity testing, of
acute anterior cruciate
ligament injuries, 687,
687*t*
Instrumented testing, 295, 297-
310
comparison studies, 309
devices
commercially available, 300-
309
experimental, 299-300
history, 297-298
studies, 299
general principles, 298-299
history, 297-298
Instruments, arthroscopic, 545-
548
hand, 546-547
irrigation systems, 547-548
motorized, 1119
motorized shaving systems,
547, 1119
Insufficiency. *See* Deficiency
Insulin, effect on collagen
synthesis, 1542
Insulin growth factor-1, 194
Insulin growth factor-2, 205
Integrins, 146, 194
Intercellular adhesion molecule-1,
146
Intercondylar eminence, 4
Intercondylar notch, 4*f*, 12, 49,
493, 955. *See also*
Notchplasty
anatomy, 646
and anterior cruciate
ligament tears, 680-681
arthroscopic examination, 78,
79*f*, 80, 82-83, 89, 97, 554
arthroscopic view of posterior
triangle through, 599,
599*f*
debridement, for anterior
cruciate ligament
reconstruction, two-
incision technique, 705,
706*f*
developmentally narrow, 89
graft impingement in, 903
after posterior cruciate
ligament reconstruction,
95, 95*f*

preparation, in anterior
cruciate ligament
reconstruction
single-incision technique,
720
two-incision technique, 705,
706*f*
Interference screw
arthroscopic placement, during
anterior cruciate
ligament reconstruction,
93
complications with, 905
Interfibrillar space, water within,
106-107
Interleukin-1, 146-149, 1224
and osseous metabolic activity,
356
in soft tissue healing, 201
Interleukin-2, 150, 1224
Interleukin-6, 148
Interleukin-8, 146
Intermeniscal ligament, 10*f*, 11
Intermittent pneumatic
compression devices
pharmacologic agents
combined with, 1501
prevention of deep vein
thrombosis after knee
surgery, 1500
prevention of thrombus
formation after total
knee arthroplasty, 1503
Internal saphenous vein, 931
International Knee
Documentation
Committee, 275, 289, 292-
293, 297, 643, 652
activity documentation
analysis, 293*f*, 293-294
impairment rating analysis,
294*f*, 294-295
Knee Ligament Standard
Evaluation Form, 289,
290*f*-291*f*
pivot shift test analysis, 293
postoperative scoring scales,
698
symptoms rating analysis, 294*f*,
294-295
Interosseous membranes, 44, 48*f*,
194
Intertrochanteric line, anterior, 30
Intraarticular anatomy,
arthroscopic, 84-97
Intraarticular delivery, of drugs,
and synovium, 150, 151*f*
Intraarticular environment,
synovial regulation, 144-
146, 145*f*, 149, 151
Intraarticular injections, 150
Intraarticular pressure
effects of effusion on, 147-148,
148*f*
and synovial fluid, 151
Intraarticular procedure,
definition, 644
Intracerebral aneurysm clips, and
magnetic resonance
imaging, 327

embryology, 14, 88, 405, 421
force transmission across, menisci in, 11
functions, 503
  neuropathophysiology, 240-241
innervation patterns, 25*f*
instability, 503. *See also* Instability
  types, 505
lateral, layers, 27*f*
lymphatics, 24, 46
mechanical and biologic interactions in, 1063-1065
mechanical axis. *See* Mechanical (load) axis
medial, 26*f*
  layers, 21-22, 22*f*
motion, 503
muscles. *See* Muscle(s); *specific muscle*
nerves. *See* Nerve(s); *specific nerve*
neural anatomy, 237*f*, 237-238
neurophysiology, 238-240
palpation, 255
posterior capsuloligamentous structures, 27*f*
postoperative, evaluation
  with magnetic resonance imaging, 347-350, 350*f*
  with technetium scintigraphy, 360
pressures in, 65-71
  measurement, 65-66
quantitative anatomy, 55-76
sagittal motion, four-bar linkage mechanism in, 17, 20*f*
sensory innervation, 235-237
septic, diagnosis, 443-444
soft tissue restraints, 1063
  active, 503
  passive, 503
stability, 503, 1063, 1067*f*. *See also* Stability
stabilizers
  active, 503
  passive, 503
static, forces acting on, 504
stiffness. *See* Stiffness
terminology, 643, 644*f*
vascular anatomy. *See* I Blood vessels; *specific artery or vein*
Knee abusers, 285-286, 294, 882
Knee-ankle-foot orthosis, after tumor resection, 478
Knee dislocation(s), 837-839. *See also* Dislocation
anterior, 839, 840*f*
  diagnosis, 842, 842*f*
  mechanisms of injuries for, 839, 841*f*
  neurovascular injury with, 838
  reduction, 844
associated with vascular injury, 659

bone-tendon-bone cruciate reconstruction/repair, 853, 855
classification, 839-841
closed
  closed reduction and external immobilization, 847
  early treatment, 847
congenital, 856
  classification, 856*f*
cruciate ligament reconstruction/repair and, 851-852
definition, 643
early reduction, 844
emergency surgery for, 844-846
examination under anesthesia, 850
incidence, 837
initial evaluation, 842-844
initial treatment, 844
injuries associated with, 256-257
irreducible
  open reduction, 844
  repair, 846
lateral, 839, 840*f*, 840-841
  irreducibility, 841
  reduction, 844
lateral collateral structure repairs, 853-854
ligament reconstruction/repair with, 844-845, 847-848
  timing, 849
limb survival after, 845
medial, 839, 840*f*, 840-841
  reduction, 844
nerve injuries with, 838-839
open, 846*f*
  delayed primary closure, 846
  and ligament reconstruction/repair, 846
  repair, 846
posterior, 839, 840*f*
  mechanisms of injury, 839, 841*f*
  neurovascular injury with, 838
  reduction, 844
posterolateral
  irreducible, 841, 844, 846*f*
  mechanism of injury, 841
  radiography, 687
reduction
  examination for ligamentous instability after, 844
  immobilization after, 844
rotational, 839, 840*f*, 841-842
self-reduction, 686
spontaneous reduction, 837, 842
surgery, 849-851
  aftercare, 854-855
  exploration, 851
  general principles, 851
  incisions for, 850
  positioning for, 849-850
  range of motion after, 854

tourniquet use in, 849-850
total, posterior cruciate ligament injury caused by, 91
treatment
  nonoperative, 848-849
  operative, timing, 849
  operative versus nonoperative, 847
  options, 847-848
vascular complications, 842
  with diagnosis, 842-844
vascular injuries with, 837-838, 844-845
vascular reconstruction with, 844-845
  with vascular surgery, 898
Knee extension, 84. *See also* Hyperextension; Total knee arthroplasty, flexion/extension gap
loss
  after anterior cruciate ligament reconstruction/repair, 901
  after injury or surgery, 489
  postoperative, and scarring, 1536-1537
  after total knee arthroplasty, 1416
Knee extensor lag, after anterior cruciate ligament reconstruction, 497
Knee flexion, 84. *See also* Total knee arthroplasty, flexion/extension gap
acquisition, after total knee arthroplasty, 1314-1315
  prerequisites for, 1314-1315
biomechanics and kinematics, 1321-1326
in endoscopic anterior cruciate ligament reconstruction, 93
exercise
  knee extension standing, 1417-1418
  knee extension while walking, 1418
  prone knee extension, 1417
  in standing position, 1417
  supine knee extension stretch, 1417, 1417*f*
  terminal knee extension, 1417, 1417*f*
factors affecting, 1315, 1316*f*
femoral rollback in, 1314, 1314*f*-1315*f*, 1321-1325, 1324*f*-1325*f*
loss, after injury or surgery, 489
over folded pillow, 1416
passive, over side of bed, 1416
patellofemoral joint during, 86, 86*f*
postoperative
  mechanical impediments, 1534-1535
  and scarring, 1536

range, and retinacular balance, 1445
requirements, for activities of daily living, 1314-1315
in sitting position, 1416, 1417*f*
after total knee arthroplasty, 1415-1416
Knee Laxity Tester, 298, 305*f*, 305-306, 698
  compared to other systems, 306
  diagnostic accuracy, 306
  measurements, reproducibility, 306
  studies, 299
Knee Ligament Standard Evaluation Form (IKDC), 289, 290*f*-291*f*
Knee manipulation, under anesthesia
  with osteoarthritis, 869
  for stiff knee arthroplasty, 1532-1533
  after total knee arthroplasty, 1420-1422, 1421*f*
Knee motion
  acquiring, program for, 1416-1418
  axes, 1061
  limits of
    definition, 289
    evaluation, 292-293
  normal, 508
  postoperative, 1415
  preoperative and postoperative, correlation between, 1415-1416
  regaining
    author's preferred program for, 1419-1420
    after total knee arthroplasty, 1414-1418
  requirements, for activities of daily living, 1414-1415
Knee Signature System, 297-298, 306*f*, 306-307
  compared to other systems, 306-307
  diagnostic accuracy, 307
  measurements, reproducibility, 307
  studies, 299
Knee simulator(s)
  apparatus and maneuvers, 1448-1449, 1449*f*-1450*f*
  studies of wear, 1454-1455, 1455*f*
Knee sleeve, 495
Knee Society Clinical Rating System, 1239, 1239*f*
Knee Society Total Knee Arthroplasty Roentgenographic Evaluation and Scoring System, 1240, 1240*f*
Knee testing system
  4-degrees of freedom, 176, 176*f*
  5-degrees of freedom, 177, 177*f*
Knives
  for arthroscopy, 546, 554
    sheathed, 596, 597*f*

Medial collateral ligament—
  continued
  elevation, 1392, 1393*f*
  epiligament, vascularity, 210
  femoral attachment, 16
  functions, 22, 25*f*, 91, 656, 1313
    and bracing, 506
  grade III injuries, 790-791
    rehabilitative knee braces
      for, 515
  healing, 210-211, 788-790
  histology, 18*f*
  injuries, 656-658
    acute instability, 790-792
    with anterior cruciate
      ligament injuries,
      treatment, 693-694
    during arthroscopy, 92
    combined, 792
    mechanism, 656
    mechanisms, 256, 256*f*
    of medial or lateral
      dislocations, 840
    in pediatric patients, 367, 371-
      372
    and prophylactic knee
      braces, 510-511
    radiographic evaluation,
      319
    repair, in anterior cruciate
      ligament-deficient
      knees, 693-694
    rupture of posterior cruciate
      ligament associated
      with, treatment, 655
    stress radiography, 657
    treatment, 656
      goals, 657
      nonoperative, 492
    vascular response to, 210-211
  injury, isolated grades I and II,
    790-791
  instability, 1340
    functional braces for, 520-521
  in knee stability, 1535
  magnetic resonance imaging,
    332-335, 333*f*
  mechanical properties, 168,
    169*f*
  mechanoreceptors in, 488
  open approaches to, nerves at
    risk during, 80
  protection, by functional and
    prophylactic braces, 520
  restraint functions, 256
  rupture
    complete, 656
      treatment, 657-658
    partial, 656
    scar tissue
      biomechanics, 211-216, 222
      vascularity, 211, 211*f*
    sprains, 656
      treatment, 492
    stabilizing role, 178-179
    in anterior cruciate ligament
      deficiency, 681
  stress testing, 257, 258*f*
  stretching, 656
  superficial, 21-22, 22*f*, 92, 95,
    95*f*

elevation of medial
  structures with
  elevator deep to, 1386,
  1386*f*
surgical dissection, 1392, 1393*f*
tears
  magnetic resonance imaging,
    331-333, 333*f*-334*f*
  partial, 657
    treatment, 657
  in pediatric patients, 371
    treatment, 371-372
  tibial attachment, 17, 19*f*
  tightening, 1387
  torn, intraoperative placement,
    in ligament
    reconstruction, 646
  treatment, algorithm for, 657,
    658*f*
Medial collateral structures,
  repair, with knee
  dislocations, 852-853
Medial compartment. *See*
  Compartment(s)
Medial gutter, arthroscopic
  examination, 554
Medial ligamentous complex
  injuries to, gradations, 656-657
  testing, 649
Medial meniscus. *See*
  Meniscus/menisci
Medial patellofemoral ligament,
  anatomy, 930
Medial patellofemoral line, 966
Medial utility incision, 793, 793*f*
Medications. *See* Drug(s); *specific*
  medication
Medicolegal assessments,
  technetium scintigraphy in,
  360
Meissner's corpuscle, 233*f*
Meniscal blade, for saucerization
  procedure, 399-400, 400*f*-
  401*f*
Meniscal femoral ligament(s). *See*
  Meniscofemoral
  ligament(s)
Meniscectomy, 591-613
  in anterior cruciate ligament
    deficiency, 610
  arthroscopic
    versus complete open, 1114
    history, 591-592
    lasers in, 585, 586*f*, 597-598
    radiographic changes after,
      1114-1115
    with reflex sympathetic
      dystrophy, 440*t*
    articular cartilage degeneration
      after, 135, 136*f*
  complete open, versus partial
    arthroscopic, 1114
  complications, 608-609
    with degenerative joint changes
      after anterior cruciate
      ligament injury, 651
  effect on degenerative joint
    disease, 615, 616*f*
  failed, 610
  functional changes after, 136
  guidelines for, 603

historical perspective, 591-592
lateral, as contraindication to
  high tibial osteotomy,
  1122
and load transmission function,
  615
medial
  arthrogenicity, 868
  as contraindication to high
    tibial osteotomy, 1122
  and degenerative joint
    disease development,
    1114
in older patients, 609-610
osteoarthritis after, 860
partial
  arthroscopic
    versus open total, 609
    results, 609
  central. *See* Saucerization
    procedure
  with chronic anterior
    cruciate ligament
    deficiency, 735
  for discoid meniscus, 398
    results, 402
  indications for, 701
  in pediatric patients, 379, 399
  postoperative care, 607-608
  postoperative magnetic
    resonance imaging, 348-
    349, 350*f*
  radiographic changes after, 135,
    135*f*, 320
  regeneration after, 138, 138*f*
  rehabilitation after, 499
  remodeling after, 138*f*, 138-139
  resection techniques, 603-607
  results, 609-610
  surgical techniques, 593-601
  total
    contact area and pressure
      studies with, 70
    and degenerative joint
      disease development,
      1114
  for discoid meniscus, 399, 401
  open
    versus arthroscopic partial,
      609
    results, 609
  tourniquet for, complications,
    661
Meniscofemoral ligament(s), 21,
  21*f*, 91-92, 653, 749
  anterior. *See* Humphry's
    ligament
  magnetic resonance imaging,
    331, 332*f*
  posterior. *See* Wrisberg's
    ligament
Meniscopatellar ligament(s), 24,
  405-406
Meniscosynovial junction,
  arthroscopy, 83, 83*f*, 97
Meniscotibial ligaments, 21, 92.
  See also Coronary
  ligaments
  arthroscopy, 95-96
Meniscus/menisci, 131-140, 199-
  200

abnormalities in, with anterior
  cruciate ligament injury,
  incidence, 651
anatomy, 5-11, 131, 132*f*, 378
  arthroscopic, 96
  arthroscopic repair,
    complications, 555
  arthroscopy, 96, 136, 593, 598-
    601
  in anterior cruciate ligament-
    deficient knee, 601,
    601*f*
  after repair, 623-626
articular surfaces
  canals within, 135, 135*f*
  quantitative anatomic data
    for, 57-58, 58*t*
biochemistry, 131-133
biomechanics, 108-123
  versus articular cartilage,
    108
  history, 109-110
collagen ultrastructural
  organization in, 103,
  104*f*
compressive properties, 112-
  114, 118
constituents, 102-108
creep behavior, compressive,
  112-113, 113*f*
cysts, 602, 603*f*
  aspiration, 607, 607*f*
  incidence, 602
  magnetic resonance imaging,
    346, 347*f*
definition, 5
development, 378, 393-394
discoid. *See* Discoid meniscus
effects of anterior cruciate
  ligament rupture on, 106
extracellular matrix
  composition, 132-133
  synthesis and maintenance,
    131
fibrocartilage, 10
fluid flow through, 110-112
in force transmission across
  knee, 11
functions, 73-74, 96, 101, 135-
  136, 615, 1232
healing response, 615
  after repair
    assessment, 626, 629*f*
    clinical studies, 623-626
  and vascular anatomy, 136,
    138, 615-616, 616*f*
hoop stresses, 70, 96, 103, 118
injuries
  with anterior cruciate
    ligament instability,
    treatment, 693
  degenerative, 592
  diagnosis, 592-593
  epidemiology, 592
  nonmeniscal injuries that
    mimic, 592-593
  in pediatric patients, 378-379
  physical examination for,
    268-269
  traumatic, 592
  treatment, 593

lateral, 4*f*, 5, 6*f*, 8*f*, 10*f*, 11, 18*f*, 23, 27*f*, 34, 44
  anatomy, 131, 132*f*
  anterior horn, 131
  arthroscopic examination, 554
  arthroscopic repair, 97-98, 600-601
  contact pressures on, 70
  detached, repair, 853
  development, 393-394
  discoid. *See* Discoid meniscus
  magnetic resonance imaging, 327
  posterior horn, 12*f*, 28*f*, 131
    arthroscopic view, 83
  repair
    inside-out, 619, 624*f*
    open, 618, 620*f*
  rolled, 397, 398*f*
  tear, physical examination for, 268
  vascular anatomy, 10, 11*f*, 133-134, 134*f*
lesion(s). *See also* Meniscus/menisci, tears
medial
  after anterior ligament rupture, 862
  and anterior tibial translation, 862-863, 867
  osteoarthritis, 865
  in load bearing of tibiofemoral joint, 65
  load distribution by, 101
  loading configurations, 103, 104*f*
  loading direction for, 103, 104*f*
  magnetic resonance imaging, 335-337, 336*f*-339*f*
    pitfalls in, 337-340, 339*f*-340*f*
  mechanical behavior, biphasic theory, 72
  mechanoreceptors in, 135, 488
  medial, 4*f*, 5, 6*f*, 10*f*, 18*f*, 21, 22*f*, 788
    anatomy, 131, 132*f*
    anterior horn, 131
    arthroscopic examination, 554
    arthroscopy, 96
      repair procedures, 97, 600, 600*f*-601*f*
    contact pressures on, 70
    detachment, repair, 853
    development, 393-394
    discoid, 393
    magnetic resonance imaging, 327
    occult derangement, tibial collateral ligament strain with, 10*f*
    posterior horn, 131
    arthroscopy, 83, 83*f*, 97
    function, 95-96
    tears in, arthroscopic repair, 83, 83*f*
  repair
    all-inside, 617, 617*t*, 621-622, 627*f*

inside-out, 618-619, 622*f*-623*f*
  open, 618, 619*f*
surgical dissection, 1392
tears
  arthroscopy, 97
  incidence, 592
  mechanism, 256
  physical examination for, 268
  vascular anatomy, 10, 11*f*, 133-134, 134*f*
mobility, 5
mucoid degeneration, 10-11
neuroanatomy, 135
pain, characteristics, 254
pathology
  at initial anterior cruciate ligament injury, 651-652
  with osteoarthritis, 1114-1115
permeability, 111
positional changes, with flexion and extension, 10*f*
reduction, with knee extension, 397, 398*f*-399*f*
regeneration, 138, 138*f*
remodeling, 138*f*, 138-139
repair, 97-98, 615-622. *See also* Meniscectomy
  with anterior cruciate ligament deficiency, 701, 735
  arthroscopic follow-up, 625-626
  basic science, 136-138, 137*f*
  in competitive athlete, 626-627
  complications, 623
  controversies in, 626-628
  healing response after
    assessment, 626, 629*f*
    clinical studies, 623-626
  historical perspective, 615
  history, 615
  indications for, 616-617
  inside-out technique for, 701
  and patient age, 627
  patient follow-up, 627
  postoperative care, 623, 627, 629*t*
  postoperative magnetic resonance imaging, 350, 350*f*
  rehabilitation after, 499
  reinjury after, 623
  suture orientation, 618, 618*f*, 627
  techniques, 617*t*, 617-622
    all-inside, 617, 617*t*, 621-622, 627*f*
    instrumentation, 621, 626*f*
    choice, 627
    fascial sheath, 622
    fibrin clot, 138, 622, 628*f*
    inside-out, 617*t*, 617-619, 621*f*-624*f*
    and neurovascular anatomy, 623, 629*f*

open, 617*t*, 617-618, 619*f*-620*f*
  outside-in, 617, 617*t*, 619-621, 624*f*-625*f*
  in unstable knee, 626
rolled, 397, 398*f*
sensory innervation, 236-237
shear properties, 118-121, 119*f*-120*f*
shear-weakening effect, 121, 121*f*
stiffness
  compressive, 122
  dynamic, 119-120, 120*f*
stress-relaxation in, 114
stress-strain behavior, 117, 117*t*
structure, 10
tears
  with anterior cruciate ligament injuries, 90, 683-684, 690
  incidence, 651, 731-732, 732*t*
  arthroscopic examination, 554
  arthroscopic management, study, 1114
  bucket-handle (vertical longitudinal), 268, 601, 602*f*, 604*f*
  incomplete, treatment, 605
  magnetic resonance imaging, 337, 338*f*
  in pediatric patients, 378
  simulated, contact area and pressure studies with, 70
  treatment, 604*f*, 604-605
  classification, 137, 601-603, 602*f*, 616, 616*t*
  degenerative (complex), 602, 602*f*, 606*f*
    treatment, 605-606
  diagnosis, 268
    magnetic resonance imaging in, 1105, 1106*f*
  horizontal cleavage, 602, 602*f*, 606*f*
    treatment, 606-607
  incidence, 592, 603, 603*t*, 731
  lateral, and anterior cruciate ligament rupture, 863
  magnetic resonance imaging, 327-329, 331, 337, 337*f*-338*f*, 687, 1187
    false-positive diagnoses, 338, 339*f*
  medial, and anterior cruciate ligament rupture, 862-863
  oblique (flap or parrot beak), 602, 602*f*, 605*f*
    treatment, 605
  patient history in, 253
  in pediatric patients, 378-379
  peripheral
    with anterior cruciate ligament injuries, 617
    stability, 617

radial (transverse), 602, 602*f*
  treatment, 606, 606*f*
red-red, 137, 616*t*, 617
red-white, 137, 137*f*, 616*t*, 617
repair, 137, 603-607. *See also* Meniscus/menisci, repair
repairability, 617
technetium scintigraphy, 357, 359*f*
traumatic, 268
types, 268
white-white, 137, 137*f*, 616*t*
tensile properties, 114*f*, 114-118, 117*f*
tibial attachment, 5
transplantation/replacement, 631-641, 1232
  animal studies, 631-632, 632*f*
  complications, 637-638
  future, 639-640
  history, 631
  immune reaction to, 634
  indications for, 634
  results, 638-639
  sterilization for, 634
  technique, 634-637, 635*f*-636*f*
transplants
  cryopreserved, 632-633
  freeze-dried, 633-634, 638
  fresh, 633
  frozen, 633
  glutaraldehyde-preserved, 634
  preparation, preservation, and storage, 633-634
  shrinking, 638
  treatment, during arthroscopic surgery, 1119
  ultrastructure, 103, 131-133, 132*f*
  vascular anatomy, 10, 11*f*, 133-135, 133*f*-135*f*
  and reparative response, 136, 138, 615-616, 616*f*
viscoelasticity, 118, 121
zones, 616, 616*f*
Meperidine
  for postoperative pain, 566, 574
  epidural, 571
  for reflex sympathetic dystrophy. *See* Demerol, in reflex sympathetic dystrophy
Mepivacaine, for local anesthesia, 561
Merchant classification, of patellofemoral disorders, 405, 406*t*
Merchant's congruence angle. *See* Congruence angle
Merchant view, 84, 317-318, 318*f*
  of patella, 1186-1187, 1188*f*
  patellofemoral joint, 936, 964*f*-965*f*, 965-966, 1000
  of patellofemoral joint, 58, 58*f*
Mercury strain gauges, for ligament testing, 159-160, 181-182

Procaine, for local anesthesia, 561
Profile method, for cross-sectional area measurement, 159
Profunda femoris artery, 3, 31, 42-43, 43f, 47f
    perforating branches, 43, 43f
Proliferation, in soft tissue healing, 200f, 200-201
    biochemistry, 204f, 204-205
Pronation
    hindfoot, 999
    orthotics for, 1003
Prone drawer test, 752
Prone posterior drawer, 773, 774f
Proplast ligament, 810
Propofol
    for general anesthesia, 560
    preoperative, 565
Propranolol, for reflex sympathetic dystrophy, 436
Proprioception
    afferent contribution to, muscle versus joint, 239-240
    and aging, 244-245
    and anesthesia, 245-246
    in anterior cruciate ligament deficiency, 242, 529
    after anterior cruciate ligament reconstruction, 529, 530f
        assessment, 242-243, 242f-243f
        and functional outcome, 243f, 243t, 243-244
    and arthritis, 244-245
    conscious, 529
    deficits, and chronic injuries, 529
    definition, 232, 488, 529
    and effusion, 245
    enhancement, in athletes, 529
    after injury, improvement, 244
    loss, in degenerative joint disease, 244-245, 245f
    mediation, 488
    menisci in, 136
    protective role in acute injury, 529
    range of motion and, 240
    reflex system, 256
    in rehabilitation, 244, 488, 529-530
    sensory pathway for, 233, 233f
    after total knee arthroplasty, 244
    unconscious, 529
Proprioceptive acuity, assessment, 241
Proprioceptive input, of orthoses, 244
Proprioceptive reflex(es), 256, 488, 529
Proprioceptive reflex arcs, 529
    mechanoreceptors in, 90, 488
Proprioceptive testing device, 242, 242f, 529, 529f
Proprioceptive training, 244, 488, 490
    in rehabilitation, 244, 528-530
    after anterior cruciate ligament reconstruction, 497

after posterior cruciate ligament reconstruction, 492, 499
Prostacyclin, in pathogenesis of deep vein thrombosis, 1494
Prostaglandins
    in angiogenic response, 209
    and osseous metabolic activity, 356
    in soft tissue healing, 201
    synthesis, after tissue injury, 568
Prosthesis/prostheses. See also specific prosthesis; Total knee arthroplasty
    constrained, 1237
    definition, 644, 812
    duocondylar design, 1237-1288
    duocondylar/patella-condylar, 1238
    Guepar, 1237
    ICLH, 1238
    as ligament graft, 645
    micromotion, clinical significance, 1358-1360
    nonconstrained, 1237
    polycentric, 1237-1288
    posterior stabilized, 1238, 1243
    rigid-hinge, 1331
    rotating-hinge, 1331
    subsidence (segment motion), 1355
    tibial, 1237
    total condylar, 1238, 1243
    total condylar III, 1238
    UCI, 1238
    unicondylar, 1238
Prosthetic heart valves, and magnetic resonance imaging, 327
Prosthetic joints, for osteoarthritis, 124
Prosthetic replacement, after tumor resection, 470f, 477
    in pediatric patients, 479
Protein(s)
    adhesion, 194, 194t
    chromatographic separation, 191
    in clot formation, 201
    globular, in cartilage, 104
    glycosylation, 193
    link, 105
    and soft tissue healing, 220
    in synovial fluid, 149f, 149-150
Proteinase(s)
    in soft tissue healing, 204-205
    synovial secretion, 147, 150
Proteinase cascade, 206, 206f
Proteinase inhibitors, 206f
Protein C, deficiency, and deep vein thrombosis, 1495
Protein growth factors, in tissue generation/repair, early studies, 191
Protein S, deficiency, and deep vein thrombosis, 1495
Proteoglycan(s)
    aggregates
        formation, 105, 106f

functional properties, 105-106, 106f
    viscoelasticity, 118
    architecture, in osteoarthritis, 71
    in cartilage, 72, 101, 104-106, 108, 199
    and swelling behavior, 121-123
    concentration, and cartilage repair, 124
    in connective tissue, 192f-193f, 193-194
    content, in osteoarthritis, 71
    in fibrocartilage, 199
    function, 194
    inhibition of clot formation by, 125-126
    in ligaments, 195
    matrix, of articular cartilage, 85
    in menisci, 101, 104-106, 108, 133
    molecular weight, 104
    removal, in scar maturation, 205
    shear modulus, 119, 120f
    in soft tissue healing, 205
    structural features, 105
        in osteoarthritis, 123
    structural unit, 104
    in synovium, 143, 146
    that bind to hyaluronic acid, 105
Proteoglycan-collagen matrix, shear modulus, 119, 120f
Proteoglycan/collagen ratio
    of high–weight-bearing regions, 116, 116f
    in osteoarthritis, 123
Proteus mirabilis, septic arthritis caused by, 445-446, 447t
    treatment, 450
Proton density, hydrogen, 325-326
Prototype knee, roentgen stereophotogrammetric analysis studies, 1355-1360, 1356f-1357f
Proximal tibial osteotomy, with reflex sympathetic dystrophy, 440t
Pruritus
    with epidural analgesia, 572
    with patient-controlled analgesia, 573
Pseudallescheria boydii, septic arthritis caused by, 446
Pseudogout
    diagnosis, 453
    and septic arthritis, comparison, 453
    synovectomy in, 1099
Pseudoisometric contraction, 487
Pseudolocking, 959
Pseudomonas aeruginosa
    antibiotic therapy for, 1572
    septic arthritis caused by, 445, 447t
        treatment, 447, 448t, 449-450
Psoas major muscle, 31f
Psoas muscle, 3f, 29f

Psoriatic arthritis
    disease-modifying antirheumatic drug therapy for, 1086-1087
    quadriceps tendon rupture, 912
    total knee arthroplasty for, results, 1245-1246
PTFE. See Polytetrafluroethylene
Pubis, 31f
Pudendal artery(ies)
    deep, 42
    superficial, external, 42
Pudendal nerve, 37f
Pulmonary arteriography, for diagnosing pulmonary embolism, 1497-1498
Pulmonary embolectomy, 1503
Pulmonary embolism, 1496-1497. See also Thromboembolic disease
    arterial blood gases with, 1497
    as arthroscopic complication, 555
    asymptomatic, incidence, 1496, 1498
    after calf thrombosis, 1495
    chest x-ray with, 1497
    diagnosis, 1496-1498
    electrocardiogram with, 1497
    fatal, incidence, 1498-1499
    after high tibial osteotomy, 1161
    incidence, 1493
    after meniscectomy, 608
    pathogenesis, 1497
    prevention, 1493
    risk, 1495
    risk factors for, 1497
    signs and symptoms, 1496-1497
    silent, 1495
    symptomatic, incidence, 1495-1496, 1498
    with total knee arthroplasty, 1279
    treatment, 1503-1504
Pulmonary metastases
    of chondroblastoma, 466
    of osteosarcoma, 470
    radiographic detection, 458
Pulse oximetry, 560
Pulses, distal, evaluation, 842-844
Pusher, Acufex endoscopic spiked, in anterior cruciate ligament reconstruction, 724, 724f
PVNS. See Pigmented villonodular synovitis

Q
Q angle, 14, 17f, 272f, 493-494, 932-933, 933f, 958-959, 1062, 1064f, 1311, 1431, 1451. See also Patellar tracking
    excessive, and patellar instability, 1461, 1464f
    interpretation, 959
    lateral (valgus) force caused by, 1431, 1431f
    measurement, 271-272, 272f, 961, 962f, 996-997

Vancomycin
  indications for, 1572
  prophylactic, 559
  for septic arthritis, 448, 448*t*, 449, 450-451
Varicosities, development, 45
Varus alignment/deformity/ malalignment, 863, 865, 1061, 1064*f*
  and anterior cruciate ligament instability, 744
  assessment, 254
  constitutional arthrogenicity, 865-866
  definition, 865
  exposure, 1385-1386
  of femoral origin, 866
  and frontal imbalance after rupture of anterior cruciate ligament, 867
  high tibial osteotomy for, 1121
    results, 1131
  long bone alignment in, effect on patellofemoral stress distribution, 959, 959*f*
  with oblique joint line, 1070-1071, 1072*f*
  osteoarthritis with, 1067-1072
    general features, 1067-1070
  osteotomy for, 1107-1108, 1108*f*
    technique for, 1126
  overcorrection, 1153-1154
  Q angle with, 1069*f*-1070*f*
  radiographic evaluation, 317
  of tibial origin, 866
  total knee arthroplasty with, 1249-1250
Varus force
  ligament injuries caused by, 256, 257*f*
  rotatory instability caused by, 267
Varus gonarthrosis. *See also* Varus alignment/deformity/ malalignment
Varus instability. *See* Instability, drawer
Varus stress
  during arthroscopy, nerve injuries caused by, 246
  posterior cruciate ligament injury caused by, 91
Varus stress testing, 292
  of instabilities, 266-267, 267*t*
  of lateral collateral ligament, 257
Varus-valgus laxity, in anterior cruciate ligament injury, 686-687, 700
VAS. *See* Visual analog scale
Vascular adequacy, evaluation, in surgical decision making, 1104
Vascular anatomy, 1493-1494
  anterior anastomotic ring, 1539
  of knee, 1539, 1540*f*
Vascular axis, 50
Vascular injuries, with knee dislocations, 837-838

Vascular response, in soft tissue healing, 209-211, 210*f*-211*f*, 223
Vascular surgery
  intraoperative, 898-899
  with knee dislocation, 898
Vasoactive intestinal polypeptide, in synovium, 143
Vasomotor temperament, and reflex sympathetic dystrophy, 432
Vastus intermedius muscle, 29*f*, 29-30, 42
  anatomy, 909
  fibrosis, in pediatric patients, 421
  function, 30
  innervation, 30, 39
Vastus intermedius tendon, anatomy, 956
Vastus lateralis muscle, 3*f*, 29*f*, 29-30, 42, 405, 795-796
  anatomy, 909-910, 910*f*, 956
  blood supply, 42-43
  fibrosis, in pediatric patients, 421
  function, 493
  innervation, 30, 39
Vastus lateralis obliquus muscle, 405
Vastus lateralis tendon, anatomy, 930
Vastus medialis longus muscle, 909
Vastus medialis muscle, 3*f*, 22, 29-30, 29*f*-30*f*, 43, 405
  anatomy, 909-910, 910*f*, 956
  blood supply, 44, 51
  innervation, 30, 39
Vastus medialis obliquus muscle, 30, 405, 787, 909
  advancement, with lateral release
    complications, 1009
    effects, 1005
    results, 1009
  anatomy, 956
  atrophy, 271, 412
  evaluation, 934, 997
  exercises, 493-494
  force vectors, 1004*f*, 1005
  function, 270, 493
  physical evaluation, 271
  training, 969-970
Vastus medialis tendon, anatomy, 930
VDA system. *See* Video dimensional analyzer system
Vein(s)
  oscillating, 26, 50
  superficial, 45, 45*f*-46*f*
Vein thrombosis, as complication of arthroscopic surgery, 1119
Vena cava filters, indications for, 1501-1503
Venography
  for diagnosing deep vein thrombosis, 1495-1496

  intraosseous, of patellofemoral joint, 938
Venous congestion, 50
Venous drainage, of lower extremity, 1493-1494
Venous stasis, 1412
  and deep vein thrombosis, 1494
Venous system
  anatomy, 1493-1494
  physiology, 1494
Venous thrombectomy, 1503
Ventilation-perfusion lung scan, and pulmonary embolism, 1497
  criteria for, 1497, 1498*f*
Vernier calipers, cross-sectional area measurement with, 159
Vessels. *See* Blood vessel(s)
Videocamera, as arthroscopic instrument, 546, 546*f*
Videocamera heads, as arthroscopic instruments, 545*f*
Video dimensional analyzer system
  cross-sectional area measurement with, 159
  ligament strain testing with, 160, 160*f*
Videoprinter, as arthroscopic instrument, 546*f*
Viral transmission. *See also* Human immunodeficiency virus
  with allografts, 907, 1021
  in transfusion, 1281-1282
Virchow, Rudolf, 190
Virchow's triad, 1493-1494
Viscoelasticity, 118
  of articular cartilage and menisci, 118, 121
  of ligaments, 158
  of ligament scar tissue, measurement, 212, 214*f*
Viscoelastic material, definition, 108
Viscoelastic theory, quasilinear, 72
Viscous material, definition, 108
Visual analog scales, 275, 284, 569
Vitamin(s), and soft tissue healing, 220-221
Vitamin A, and soft tissue healing, 220-221
Vitamin C. *See* Ascorbic acid
Vitronectin, 194
VMO. *See* Vastus medialis obliquus muscle
Volkmann, R., 1091
Voloshin, A. S., 591
Vomiting, with postoperative analgesia, 572-574
Von Recklinghausen's disease. *See* Neurofibromatosis
V-Y quadricepsplasty, 984, 984*f*, 1343, 1343*f*, 1343, 1343*f*

W
Walldius prosthesis, 1332
Wall slides, 490

Wang, C. J., 591
Warfarin (Coumadin)
  effect on bone ingrowth, 1371
  mechanism of action, 1499
  prophylaxis after knee surgery, 1499, 1503
  side effects, 1499
  in treatment of deep vein thrombosis, 1501
Watanabe, M., 393-394, 543, 591
Water
  in cartilage, 72, 101, 106-107, 112, 123
    load-equilibrium relationship, 110
    and viscoelasticity, 118
  in connective tissue, 191, 192*f*
  function, 191
  increased, in osteoarthritis, 71
  in ligaments, 163, 191, 192*f*
  in menisci, 101, 106-108, 112
    and viscoelasticity, 118
  in tendons, 163
  transsynovial diffusion, 145, 145*f*
Watson-Jones, R., 393
Wear
  with abrasion, 1255-1256
  adhesive, 1255-1256
  of articulating surfaces, in total knee arthroplasty, 1454-1457
  and contact stress, 1524
  definition, 1255
  design of prosthesis and, 1256-1258
  implant, 1507
  laboratory testing and retrieval analysis, 1258-1264
  mechanisms, 1255-1256
  model of joint dysfunction, 1064-1065, 1068*f*
  normal, 1064
  polyethylene, 1255, 1324, 1467, 1481, 1508, 1509*f*, 1514, 1524-1525, 1525*f*
    design of prosthesis and, 1256-1258
    grade (quality) of polyethylene and, 1266
  posterior, 1324
  of prostheses, recognition, 1256
  third-body, 1255-1256
  and wear rate in knee, 1265
Wear particles
  biological response to, 908, 1363
  cartilaginous, 148
  with synthetic grafts, 674
Wear rate, in knee, 1264-1265
  surface treatments and, 1265-1266
  third-body wear debris and, 1265
Weber technique, for high tibial osteotomy, 1142-1143, 1143*f*
Weight bearing. *See also* High–weight-bearing areas; Low–weight-bearing areas